W9-AWO-556

Fourth Edition

Maternal, Fetal, & Neonatal Physiology

A Clinical Perspective

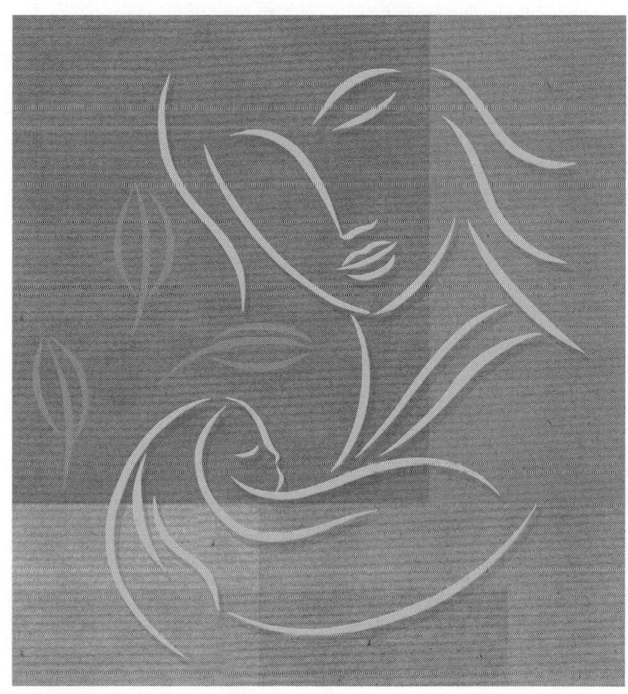

Susan Tucker Blackburn, PhD, RN, FAAN
Professor Emerita
Department of Family and Child Nursing
School of Nursing
University of Washington
Seattle, Washington

ELSEVIER

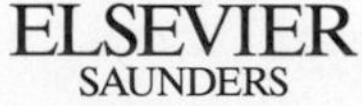

3251 Riverport Lane
Maryland Heights, MO 63043

MATERNAL, FETAL, & NEONATAL PHYSIOLOGY:
A CLINICAL PERSPECTIVE

ISBN: 978-1-4377-1623-8

Notice

Knowledge and best practice in this field are constantly changing. As new research and experience broaden our knowledge, changes in practice, treatment and drug therapy may become necessary or appropriate. Readers are advised to check the most current information provided (i) on procedures featured or (ii) by the manufacturer of each product to be administered, to verify the recommended dose or formula, the method and duration of administration, and contraindications. It is the responsibility of the practitioner, relying on their own experience and knowledge of the patient, to make diagnoses, to determine dosages and the best treatment for each individual patient, and to take all appropriate safety precautions. To the fullest extent of the law, neither the Publisher nor the Author assumes any liability for any injury and/or damage to persons or property arising out of or related to any use of the material contained in this book.

Library of Congress Cataloging-in-Publication Data

Blackburn, Susan Tucker.
Maternal, fetal, & neonatal physiology : a clinical perspective / Susan Tucker Blackburn. -- 4th ed.
p. ; cm.
Maternal, fetal, and neonatal physiology
Includes bibliographical references and index.
ISBN 978-1-4377-1623-8 (hardback)
I. Title. II. Title: Maternal, fetal, and neonatal physiology.
[DNLM: 1. Pregnancy--physiology. 2. Fetus--physiology. 3. Infant, Newborn--physiology. WQ 205]

612.6'3--dc23

2012002845

Executive Content Strategist: Kristin Geen
Content Manager: Laurie K. Gower
Associate Content Development Specialist: Sarah Hembree
Publishing Services Manager: Deborah L. Vogel
Senior Project Manager: Antony Prince
Design Direction: Karen Pauls

Printed in the United States of America

Last digit is the print number: 9 8 7 6 5 4 3 2

Contributors and Reviewers

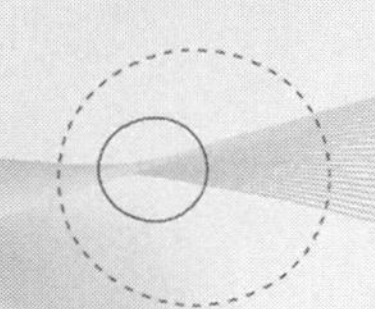

CONTRIBUTORS

Ilana R Azulay Chertok, PhD, MSN, RN, IBCLC
Associate Professor, School of Nursing
West Virginia University
Morgantown, West Virginia
Postpartum Period and Lactation Physiology

Robin Webb Corbett, PhD, RNC-OB
Associate Professor, College of Nursing
East Carolina University
Greenville, North Carolina
Physiologic Basis for Reproduction

Tekoa L. King, CNM, MPH, FACNM
Clinical Professor
Department of Obstetrics, Gynecology, and Reproductive Health
University of California at San Francisco
San Francisco, California
Deputy Editor, Journal of Midwifery & Women's Health
Fetal Assessment

REVIEWERS

Christine Domonoske, BS, PharmD
Neonatal Clinical Pharmacist
Children's Memorial Hermann Hospital
Houston, Texas

Charlotte Stephenson, RN, DSN, CLNC
Clinical Professor, Nelda C. Stark College of Nursing
Texas Woman's University
Houston, Texas

M. Terese Verklan, PhD, CCNS, RNC, FAAN
Professor, Neonatal Clinical Nurse Specialist
University of Texas Medical Branch
Galveston, Texas

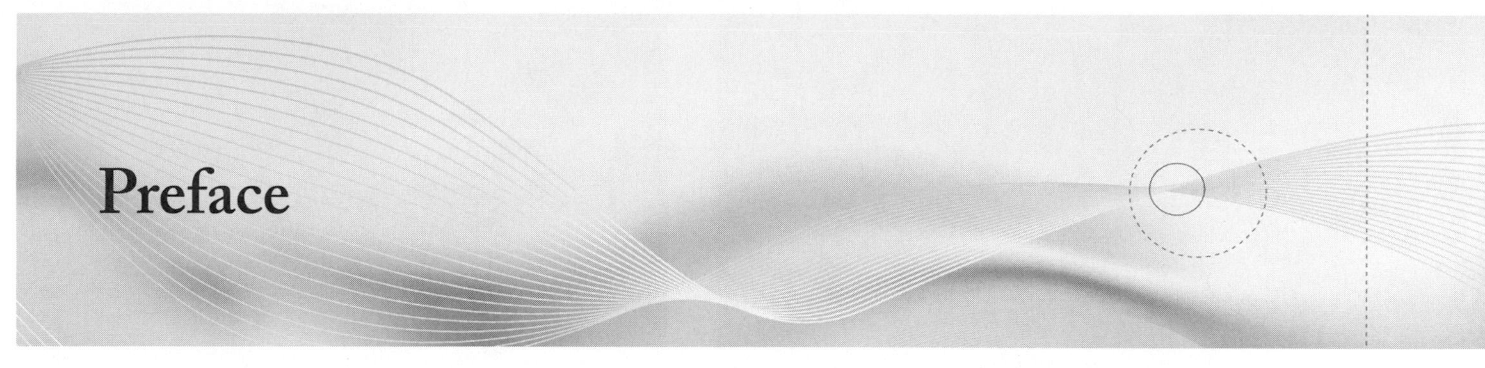

Preface

Accurate assessment and clinical care appropriate to the developmental and maturational stage of the mother, fetus, and neonate depend on a thorough understanding of normal physiologic processes and the ability of the caregiver to understand the effects of these processes on pathologic alterations. Information on normal pregnancy and perinatal physiology and its clinical implications can be found in various sources, including journal articles, general physiology texts, core nursing texts, and medical references. These sources are often either fragmented, too basic in level, too focused on one phase of the perinatal period (and thus lacking integration within the maternal-fetal-neonatal unit), or lacking in the clinical applications relevant to patient care. Thus they do not adequately meet the needs of nurses in specialty and advanced clinical nursing practice.

Therefore the goal of the first and subsequent editions of this book was to create a single text that brought together detailed information on the physiologic changes that occur throughout pregnancy and the perinatal period, with emphasis on the mother, fetus, and neonate and the interrelationships among them. The purpose of this book is not to provide a manual of specific assessment and intervention strategies or to focus on pathophysiology—it is to present current information on the normal physiologic adaptations and developmental physiology that provides the scientific basis and rationale underlying assessment and management of the low-risk and high-risk pregnant woman, fetus, and neonate. Because the focus of this book is on physiologic adaptations, the psychological aspects of perinatal and neonatal nursing are not addressed. These aspects are certainly equally as important but are not within the realm of this text.

This book provides detailed descriptions of the physiologic processes associated with pregnancy and with the fetus and neonate. The major focus is on the normal physiologic adaptations of the pregnant woman during the antepartum, intrapartum, and postpartum periods; anatomic and functional development of the fetus; transition and adaptation of the infant at birth; developmental physiology of the neonate (term and preterm); and a summary of the maturation of each body system during infancy and childhood. Clinical implications of these physiologic adaptations as they relate to the pregnant woman, maternal-fetal unit, and neonate are also examined. Each chapter describes the effects of normal physiologic adaptations on clinical assessment and interventions with low-risk and high-risk women and neonates with selected health problems. Of special interest to those seeking quick access to clinical information are tables with recommendations for clinical practice that are included in each chapter, referencing pages with relevant content that provides the rationale underlying each recommendation.

Advanced practice nursing must be based on a sound physiologic base. Thus I hope that this book will be a useful foundation reference for specialty and advanced practice nurses in both primary and acute care settings, as well as for graduate programs in maternal, perinatal, and neonatal nursing and nurse midwifery. This book may also hold appeal for other health care professionals, including physicians, physical and occupational therapists, respiratory therapists, and nutritionists involved in obstetrics and neonatology.

ACKNOWLEDGMENTS

The help and support of many individuals were critical in making this book a reality. These include former and current students, nursing staff, and colleagues who stimulated me to continue to expand my knowledge of perinatal and neonatal physiology and examine the scientific basis for nursing interventions with pregnant women and neonates. The women, neonates, and their families whom I have cared for and from whom I have learned a great deal also stimulated development of this book. Thank you to Ilana Chertok, Robin Webb Corbett, and Tekoa King for sharing their expertise in the chapters they contributed to this edition. Special thanks to Elizabeth Posey, Susan Skinner and Kristie Marbut for their assistance with manuscript preparation. I am grateful for the efforts of the reviewers, whose constructive comments and suggestions helped in refining the content and in making this book more useful for the intended audience. My appreciation and thanks also goes to the staff at Elsevier, particularly Laurie Gower, Content Manager, Sarah Hembree, Associate Content Development Specialist, and Bridget Healy, Project Manager, for their assistance in the development and production of this book. Finally I would like to thank my family for their support, guidance, and encouragement in all of my endeavors.

Susan Tucker Blackburn

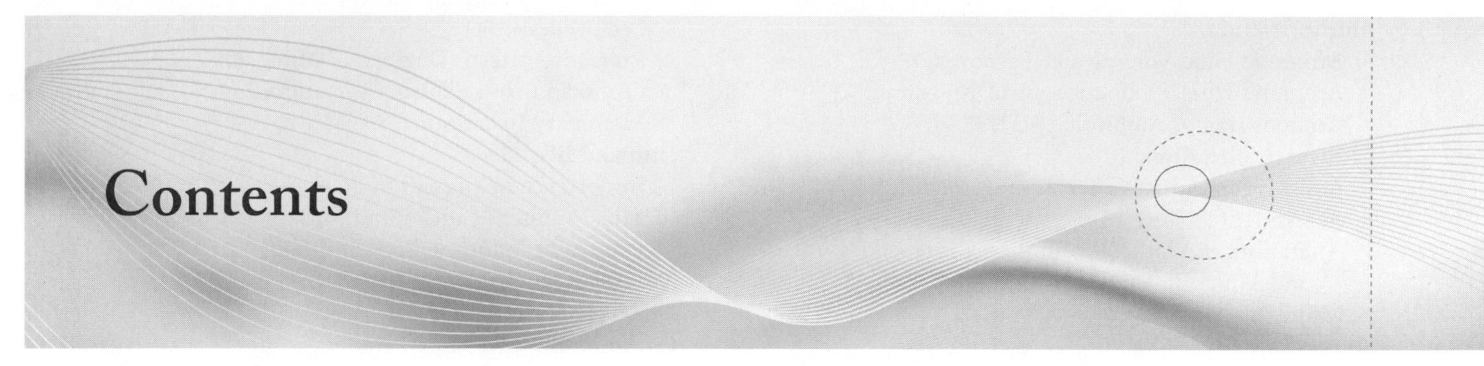

Contents

UNIT III ADAPTATIONS IN METABOLIC PROCESSES IN THE PREGNANT WOMAN, FETUS, AND NEONATE

CHAPTER 1

Biologic Basis for Reproduction

The biologic basis for reproduction includes genetic mechanisms and principles, gametogenesis, and embryonic development of the reproductive system. The process of reproduction is influenced by chromosomal and gene structure and function and many mediating and signaling factors including transcription factors, growth factors, and signaling molecules. Reproduction is also influenced by physiologic processes such as hormonal control mechanisms and the hypothalamic-pituitary-ovarian axis, which are described in Chapter 2.

Our knowledge of genetics continues to expand at a remarkable rate. The Human Genome Project, an international collaborative effort begun in 1990 and completed in 2003, within days of the 50th anniversary of Watson and Crick's description of the deoxyribonucleic acid (DNA) double helix, accomplished its goal of identifying the human DNA sequence, developing an international database, and developing new investigative tools and methods of analysis.[3,34,59] An integral part of the Human Genome Project was the identification and analysis of the ethical, legal, and social issues generated by this new knowledge. One of the outcomes of this project was determining that the human genome (DNA sequences containing all of the individual's genetic information) contains approximately 25,000 genes, far fewer than earlier estimates.[45] The Human Genome Project continues to change our understanding of both human development and the pathogenesis, diagnosis and treatment of diseases.[59] Although the Human Genome Project has significantly altered our knowledge of genetics, there is still much to learn including exact gene numbers, locations and functions, gene regulation, understanding of noncoding DNA sequences, coordination between gene expression, protein synthesis and conservation, and posttranslational events, complex interaction of proteins, gene therapies, developmental genetics, and better understanding of genes involved in complex traits and multigene disorders.[15,34,59]

CHROMOSOMES AND GENES

The human genome is the totality of the DNA sequences, containing all of an individual's genetic information. Each human cell, except for the gametes (ovum and sperm), normally contains 46 chromosomes (diploid number) consisting of 22 pairs of autosomes and 1 pair of sex chromosomes. Autosomal genes are located on the autosomes (chromosomes common to both sexes) and are homologous (a pair of chromosomes with identical gene arrangements). Males have a pair of nonhomologous chromosomes, the X and Y sex chromosomes. In the female, the sex chromosomes (XX) are homologous. One of each chromosome pair comes from the mother and one from the father. The ovum and sperm have only 23 chromosomes (haploid number). This reduction in the number of chromosomes occurs during meiosis. With fertilization and union of the nuclei of the sperm and ovum, the diploid number of 46 chromosomes is restored in the zygote.

Chromosomes

Chromosomes are classified by structure and banding pattern, which varies depending on the stain used or by color if spectral analysis is used. Structural characteristics include the location of the centromere (metacentric, submetacentric, or acrocentric) and the length or size of the chromosomes (Figure 1-1). The upper arm of each chromosome is referred to as the p arm; the lower arm is the q arm. Sections of the p and q arm are numbered according to the banding patterns of mitotic chromosomes so specific loci along each chromosome can be identified. Gismo-trypsin banding (G-banding) has been the most widely used technique, producing up to 300 to 400 metaphase bands. Each band contains many genes. High-resolution banding during late prophase or early metaphase increases the resolution twofold. Newer spectral methods of karyotyping and fluorescent in situ hybridization (FISH) techniques such as chromosome painting, locus-specific mutations FISH, and interphase FISH allow for even greater resolution and specificity of chromosome segments and genes. The karyotype is a pictorial display of chromosomes.

Chromosomes are composed of the DNA double helix and several types of proteins that together are known as *chromatin*. In each chromosome the continuous DNA helix is wound around histone (protein) spools that are coiled around each other to form solenoids. The solenoids are coiled into chromatin threads (Figure 1-2). If unwound, each

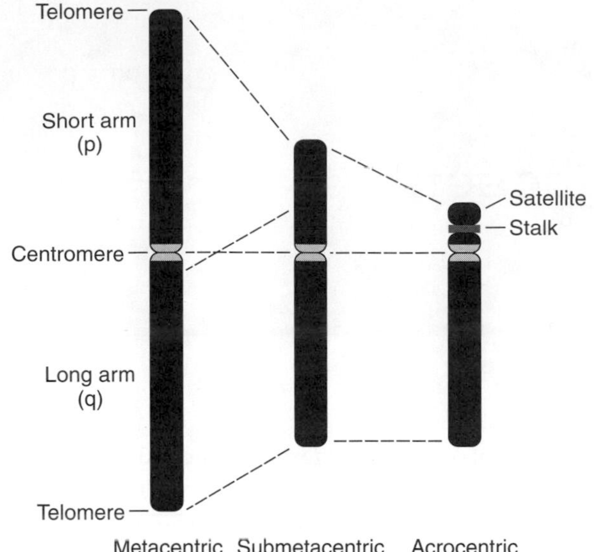

FIGURE 1-1 Schematic diagram of human chromosomes demonstrating metacentric, submetacentric, and acrocentric chromosomes. The location of the centromere, telo-mere, and short (p) and long (q) arms are indicated. (From Morton, C.C. & Miron, P.M. [2004]. Cytogenetics in reproduction. In J.F. Strauss & R. Barbieri [Eds.]. *Yen and Jaffe's reproductive endocrinology: Physiology, pathophysiology, and clinical management* [5th ed.]. Philadelphia: Saunders.)

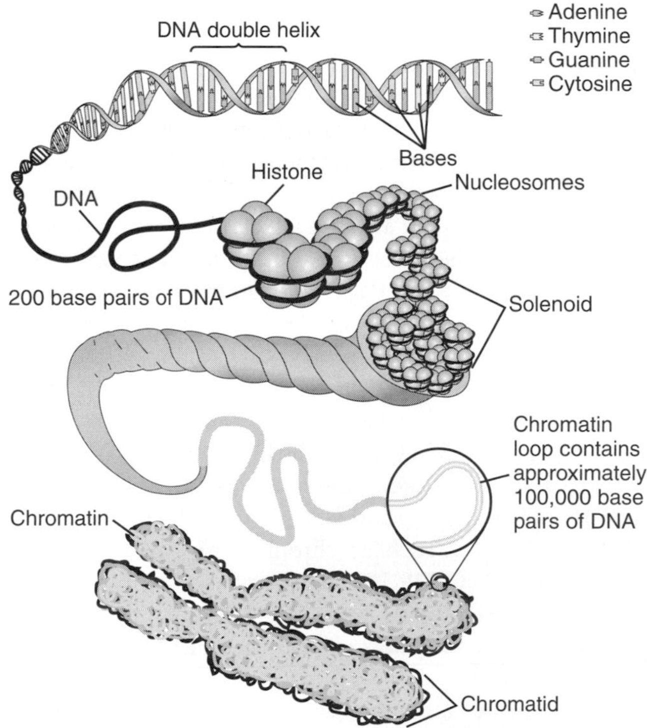

FIGURE 1-2 Structure of DNA and patterns of DNA coiling. DNA is wound around histones to form nucleosomes. These are organized into solenoids that in turn compose chromatin loops. (From Jorde, L.B., et al. [2006]. *Medical genetics* [3rd ed.]. St. Louis: Mosby.)

chromosome would contain approximately 2 m of DNA.[35] The DNA double helix is similar to a flexible ladder, with the sides composed of deoxyribose and phosphate and each rung composed of two nitrogen bases connected by hydrogen bonds (see Figure 1-2). The human genome contains approximately 3 million bases, with 50 to 250 million pairs in each chromosome.[72]

X Chromosomes

Sequencing of the X chromosome identified 1098 genes and 160 million base pairs.[63] In comparison, the Y chromosome contains 78 genes and 23 million base pairs.[63] There is more variation in gene expression in women than in men.[12] More than 300 X-linked disorders have been identified. The X chromosome contains only about 4% of the genes in the human genome, but these genes are responsible for about 10% of all disorders inherited by Mendelian patterns.[63]

In all of a woman's somatic cells (but not in her germ cells), one of the two X chromosomes is inactivated (lyonization) and remains condensed. The inactive X is seen in interphase as the Barr body. The number of Barr bodies is one minus the number of X chromosomes. Therefore a normal male has no Barr bodies and neither does a woman with Turner syndrome (XO); a normal female has 1 Barr body, while a male with Klinefelter syndrome (XXY) has one. In the female, both X chromosomes are reactivated during gametogenesis. Thus the woman produces ova with two active X chromosomes which undergo recombination with each other.[63] In the female zygote, inactivation begins within 7 to 10 days after fertilization.[35] In all cells within the embryo, the inactivated X is random in each cell—it could be the X chromosome the zygote received from its mother or the X chromosome it received from its father—and the same X is inactive in all descendants of that cell. However, in the trophoblast tissue (which is extraembryonic tissue that will become the placenta and chorion) in the preembryonic blastocyst, all the paternally derived X chromosomes are inactivated, whereas all the maternal X chromosomes are active.[35,41,65]

Inactivation is thought to involve methylation of critical segments of DNA and histone deacetylation initiated by the *XIST* gene on the long arm (q13) of X chromosomes.[41,58] The inactive X transcribes RNA from this gene so the X chromosome is coated with *XIST* RNA.[12] Not all genes on the inactive X are inactive; 10% of the genes on the inactive X escape inactivation (thus a woman has a double dose of these genes).[28] The active genes on the inactive X are generally located on the tip of the short arm, which are homologous with some of the genes on the distal end of the Y chromosome.[35]

Genes

Genes are the functional units of heredity consisting of DNA sequences that code for specific amino acids and thus for formation of specific proteins. Currently, each human is thought to have approximately 25,000 genes.[45] Genes make up only about 10% of the human genome.[45] Genes are distributed in clusters along the chromosome, so some areas have many genes, others few.[35] These protein coding sequences of DNA are called *exons* (expression sequences). Exons have a consistent identifying sequence of nucleotides at each end. Interspersed between these are noncoding sequences, called *introns* (intervening sequences), whose exact role is still not completely clear. Much of the DNA consists of series of repeated nucleotides that may be repeated a thousand or more times.[35,45] Some of these sequences are needed for DNA transcription factors, RNA translation, chromosome pairing, and other regulatory functions.[35,45]

Genes are essential in determining and maintaining cell structural integrity and cell function and in regulating biochemical and immunologic processes.[28] Some genes control the function of other genes, others regulate the process of embryonic and fetal development. Genes direct protein synthesis and regulate the rate at which proteins are synthesized. The specific proteins synthesized vary depending on the type of cell. For example, a muscle cell synthesizes myosin for muscle contraction, the pancreatic islet cells synthesize insulin, and the liver cells produce γ-globulin. Although the full complement of genes is present in all cells, genes are selectively switched on and off. Therefore all genes are not active at the same time. This activation process is important during development (see "Developmental Genetics" in Chapter 3) and is influenced by age, cell type, and function. In addition, each gene can produce multiple isotypes, each isotype producing a different product. The different isotypes are produced by the splicing and reorganization of exons within a given gene (Figure 1-3).[44] As a result, a single gene can guide the production of many different forms of messenger ribonucleic acid (mRNA) and thus proteins with individual biologic functions.[10,16]

Genes are arranged in linear order and in pairs on homologous chromosomes, one chromosome and its genes coming from an individual's mother, the other from the father. Each gene has a specific location, called a *locus*, on the chromosome. One copy of a gene normally occupies any given locus. In somatic cells, the chromosomes are paired so that there are two copies of each gene (alleles). The corresponding genes at a given locus on homologous chromosomes govern the same trait, but not necessarily in the same way. If gene pairs are identical, they are homozygous; if they are different, they are heterozygous. In the heterozygous state, one of the alleles may be expressed over the other. This allele is considered dominant, meaning that the trait is expressed if the dominant allele is present on at least one of the pair of chromosomes. Recessive traits can be expressed only when the allele responsible for that trait is present on both chromosomes or when the dominant allele is not present (as with X-linked genes in the XY male, who is hemizygous for that trait). *Genotype* refers to the genetic makeup of an individual or a particular gene pair. The observable expression of a specific trait is referred to as the *phenotype*. A trait may be a

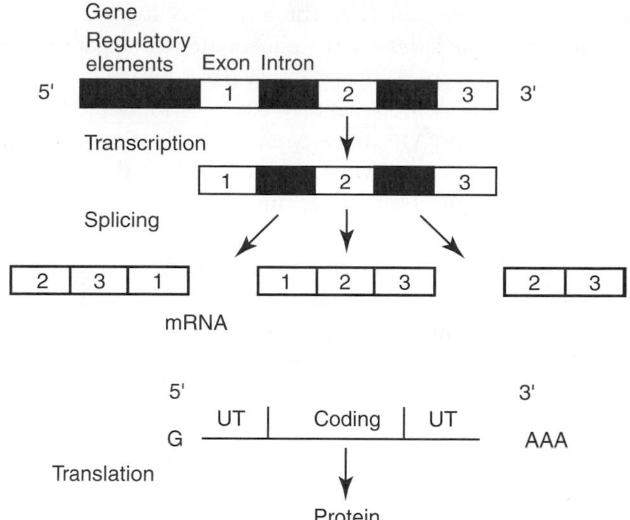

FIGURE 1-3 Scheme for the transcription and translation of a gene within the human genome resulting in multiple gene products using alternative splicing. The gene consists of a 5′ promoter sequence containing multiple regulatory elements (e.g., retinoic acid, vitamin D, or steroid/thyroxine hormone-binding elements), multiple exons (indicated as 1, 2, and 3), which contain the sequence encoding the protein, and intervening noncoding DNA sequences (introns). Following transcription, the messenger ribonucleic acid (mRNA) is processed by splicing out the introns and adding a G residue to the 5′ end and multiple *As* to the 3′ end. Alternate splicing and rearrangement of exons can produce a number of different mRNAs (transcripts) encoding different proteins (i.e., *transcript* 1, exons 2-3-1; *transcript* 2, exons 1-2-3; *transcript* 3, exons 2-3). The designation UT refers to noncoding untranslated regions in the mature mRNA. The mature mRNA is subsequently transported to the cytoplasm and translated into the primary structure of a protein that then is processed and folded to form the biologic substrate. (From Slavkin, H.C. & Warburton, D. [2004]. *Regulation of embryogenesis.* In R.A. Polin, W.W. Fox, & S.H. Abman [Eds.]. *Fetal and neonatal physiology* [3rd ed.]. Philadelphia: Saunders.)

biochemical property, an anatomic structure, a cell or organ function, or a mental characteristic. Thus traits are derived from the action of the gene and not from the gene itself.[28,43,71]

DNA and RNA

The transmission of hereditary information from one cell to another is a function of DNA. DNA also contains the instructions for the synthesis of proteins that determine the structure and function of that cell. The nucleus contains DNA; protein assembly occurs within the cytoplasm in the ribosomes. The transfer of information from the nucleus to the site of synthesis is the role of messenger ribonucleic acid (mRNA), which is synthesized on the surface of DNA.

Both DNA and ribonucleic acid (RNA) are nucleic acids made up of a nitrogenous purine (adenine and guanine) or pyrimidine (cytosine and thymine or uracil) base, a sugar (deoxyribose for DNA and ribose for RNA), and a phosphate group (see Figure 1-2). Together these substrates form a structure that is linked in a linear sequence by phosphodiester bonds. DNA is composed of two antiparallel complementary chains of opposite polarity. These strands form a double helix in which the sides are the phosphate and sugar groups and the crossbars are complementary bases joined by hydrogen bonds. Only complementary bases form stable bonds; therefore adenine (A) always pairs with thymine (T), and guanine (G) always pairs with cytosine (C). Thus the sequence of the bases on one strand determines the sequence of bases on the other.

RNA is a single strand rather than a double helix and contains adenine, cytosine, guanine, and uracil (U), which pairs with adenine, because thymine is not present. There are three major types of RNA: (1) messenger ribonucleic acid (mRNA), (2) ribosomal RNA (rRNA), and (3) transfer RNA (tRNA). Messenger RNA receives information from the DNA and serves as the template for protein synthesis. Transfer RNA brings the amino acids to messenger ribonucleic acid (mRNA) and positions them correctly during protein synthesis. One of the structural components at the protein assemblage site (ribosome) is rRNA. The passage of information from DNA to RNA is called *transcription;* the assemblage of the proper sequence on amino acids is *translation.* Protein synthesis and the sequence of events in transcription and translation are summarized in Box 1-1 below.

The sequence of bases along the DNA makes up the genetic code that specifies the sequence of amino acids in each protein. Each of the 20 amino acids is designated by a specific sequence of three bases (codon). A gene codes for a single protein, which is a series of amino acids. The four bases (A, T or U, C, and G) can be arranged in 64 triplet combinations, of which 61 are used to specify the 20 amino acids. Most amino acids are represented by several codons. For example, AUG codes for methionine, and CAU and CAC both code for histidine. The other three codes are termination codes, which designate the end of a gene (see Box 1-1 below).

GENOMICS

Genetics involves examination of individual genes and their effects. Genomics is "the study of the functions and the interactions of all the genes in the genome."[25] This focus includes gene-environment interactions and will increase our understanding of complex disorders such as diabetes, Alzheimer's disease, hypertension, and cancer.[25] Genomics includes a focus on genetic variations that may alter the risks of disease and on how genes interact with chemical, infectious, environmental, physical, and pharmacologic agents, with an increased emphasis on risk assessment and prevention, development of new diagnostic, treatment, and prognostic techniques and new fields of study such as pharmacogenetics.[39] Genomics will raise additional ethical, legal, and social issues.[14,59]

Genetic polymorphisms are variations in the genome sequence that occur throughout the genome with a frequency of about 1 in 100 basepairs.[68] Polymorphisms may involve the substitution of a single nucleotide base (single nucleotide polymorphisms, or SNPs) or a group of alleles or alternate gene forms that are inherited together (haplotypes). SNPs are the simplest form of DNA variation among individuals.[68] The human genome contains more than 10 million SNPs.[25] Polymorphisms may be nonfunctional and have no effect on the individual or alter expression of a protein that increases the risk of disease, especially with exposure to specific environmental agents or drugs.[38] These variations may be important in altering the effects of exposures to environmental health hazards such as mercury, alcohol, tobacco smoke, air pollutants, and other toxins leading to different levels of risk and susceptibility to disease and to adverse environmental influences within the population.[18,38] Since SNPs can result in individual differences in responses

BOX 1-1 Sequence of Events in Transcription and Translation

TRANSCRIPTION

1. The two strands of the deoxyribonucleic acid (DNA) double helix separate in the region of the gene to be transcribed. One strand acts as a template.
2. Free nucleotide bases pair with the nucleotide bases in DNA.
3. The nucleotide triphosphates paired with one strand of DNA are linked together by DNA-dependent ribonucleic acid (RNA) polymerase to form messenger ribonucleic acid (mRNA) containing a sequence of bases complementary to the DNA base sequence.
4. Once the (mRNA) has formed, the DNA strand rewinds.
5. mRNA is processed before leaving the nucleus. Introns (noncoding areas of DNA) are removed and promoter and terminator structures are added to promote stability and efficiency of translation.

Translation

6. The processed mRNA passes from the nucleus to the cytoplasm, where one end of the mRNA binds to a ribosome.
7. The ribosome is formed from ribosomal RNA (rRNA) and proteins. The mRNA codons are "read" by the ribosome and translated into amino acids.
8. Free amino acids combine with their corresponding transfer RNA (tRNA) in the presence of specific aminoacyl-tRNA synthetase enzymes in the cytoplasm.
9. Amino acid-tRNA complexes bind to sites on the ribosome and the three base anticodons in tRNA pair with the corresponding codons in mRNA.
10. Each amino acid is then transferred from its tRNA to the growing peptide chain, which is attached to the adjacent tRNA.
11. The tRNA freed of its amino acid is released from the ribosome.
12. A new amino acid–tRNA complex is attached to the vacated site on the ribosome.
13. mRNA moves one codon step along the ribosome.
14. Steps 9 to 13 are repeated over and over until all the codons have been read.
15. The completed protein chain is released from the ribosome when the termination codon in mRNA is reached.

Adapted from Vander, A., Sherman, J., & Luciano, D. (2000). *Human physiology: The mechanism of body function* (8th ed.). New York: McGraw-Hill.

to drugs, understanding these variations can individualize pharmacologic management. Research in this area has also identified polymorphic genes and environmental influences that can alter susceptibility to birth defects.[18,79] For example, genetic differences in folate metabolism may increase the risk of neural tube defects and pregnancy loss; a rare transforming growth factor-α polymorphism has been linked with orofacial clefts with exposure to cigarette smoke; differences in enzymes needed for metabolizing anticonvulsant drugs may increase the risk of congenital anomalies in women taking these drugs; polymorphisms in alcohol metabolism may increase the risk of fetal alcohol syndrome; polymorphisms in drug metabolizing enzymes may result in impaired pregnancy maintenance with exposure to cigarette smoke or male infertility with exposure to organophosphate pesticides.[18,79] Study of polymorphisms and gene-environment interactions may lead to better understanding of complex reproductive disorders such as preeclampsia, infertility, and preterm labor as well as disorders such as diabetes, hypertension, infection, coronary artery disease, obesity, and psychiatric disorders.[28,68,79]

CELL DIVISION

Genetic material is passed to daughter cells in two ways: via mitosis in somatic cells and in germ cells via mitosis (during the initial development of germ cells) or meiosis (during gametogenesis). Before onset of either mitosis or meiosis, DNA replication must occur. Before a cell divides, the accurate replication of the genetic material stored within the DNA of the parent cell is essential. During DNA replication, the strands of the double helix uncoil, relax, and separate. The exposed nucleotide bases pair with complementary free nucleotides. DNA polymerase links the nucleotides together, resulting in two identical molecules of DNA to pass on to daughter cells. Enzymes within the cell nucleus "read" the replicated DNA and repair errors. If errors are not repaired, a mutation results. DNA replication is illustrated in Figure 1-4. Mitosis and meiosis are illustrated in Figure 1-5.

Mitosis

Mitosis is the process by which growth of the organism occurs and cells repair and replace themselves. This process maintains the diploid number of 46 chromosomes, forming two daughter cells, each with a single strand of DNA, that are exact replicas of the parent (unless a mutation occurs). The cell cycle consists of four stages: gap 1 (G1), synthesis (S), gap 2 (G2), and mitosis (M). G1, S, and G2 comprise interphase. During G1, the longest stage, proteins needed by the cell are synthesized and substances needed for DNA replication are amassed; DNA replication occurs in the S stage. After completion of DNA replication, each chromosome consists of two identical strands of DNA, called *sister chromatids.* G2 is a resting stage, during which errors in DNA are corrected and the cell prepares for the final M stage, in which the cell

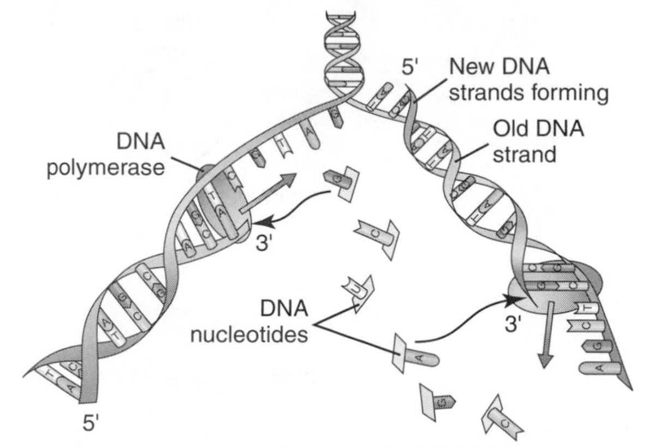

FIGURE 1-4 DNA replication. The hydrogen bonds between the two original strands are broken, allowing the bases in each strand to undergo complementary base pairing with free bases. The process forms two new double strands of DNA. (From Jorde, L.B., et al. [2006]. *Medical genetics* [3rd ed.]. St. Louis: Mosby.)

divides.[45] The length of time for a cell to complete the entire cycle varies with the type of cell and may last hours (epithelial tissues) to weeks (liver cells).[10] The cell cycle is regulated by enzymes such as cyclin-dependent kinases (CDKS), which are control switches for the cycle (i.e., switching from G1 to S or from S to G2); maturation promoting factor, which triggers progression through the cell cycle; protein 63, which blocks the cycle if the DNA is damaged to allow time for DNA repair; and protein 27, which can also block the cycle by binding to cyclins and blocking entry into S.[35] Alterations in these substances can lead to production of mutations and cancerous cells.[10,35]

Thus before initiation of mitosis, DNA replication has occurred (see Figure 1-5). At this point each cell still has 46 chromosomes, but each chromosome has 2 strands of DNA, which is twice the usual amount of DNA. Just before cell division, the duplicated DNA threads (chromatin) change from a loose, relaxed mass and become condensed and tightly coiled, forming the rod-shaped chromosomes. This condensing process facilitates the transfer of DNA to the daughter cells. This change is the first sign of cell division.

As the cell enters prophase, the chromosomes each consist of two DNA threads (sister chromatids). The two chromatids are joined at a single point called the *centromere.* Late in prophase the nuclear membrane begins to disintegrate. The centrioles (two small cylindric bodies) separate and move to opposite sides of the cell. A number of microtubules are observable at this stage. These are spindle fibers that extend from one side of the cell to the other, between the centrioles.

During metaphase the chromatids line up on the metaphase plate in the center of the cell. Other spindle fibers now extend from the centrioles and are attached to the centromere region of the chromosome. In anaphase, the chromosomes divide at the centromere into sister chromatids that are pulled to opposite poles. As the chromosomes reach their respective poles, they begin to uncoil and elongate. A ring of protein appears around the center of the cell and the cell begins to

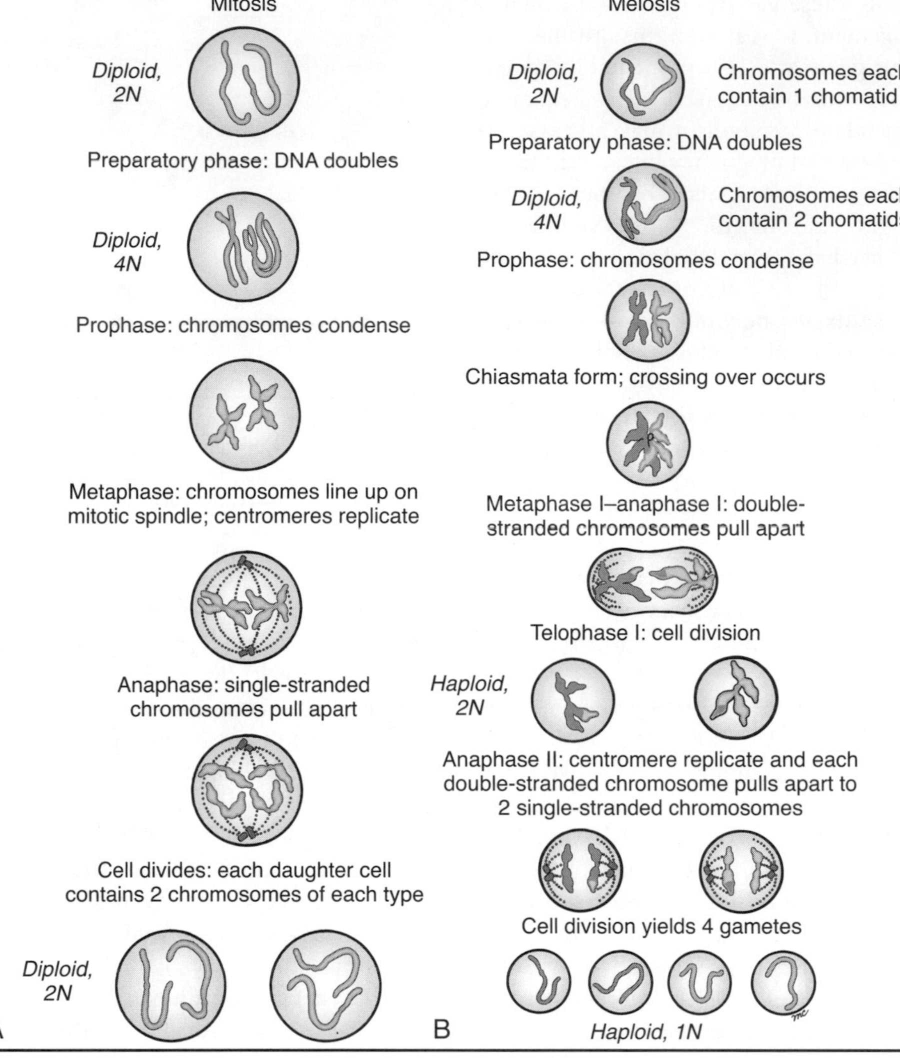

FIGURE 1-5 Summary of stages in mitosis (A) and meiosis (B). (From Schoenwolf, G.C., et al. [2009]. *Larsen's human embryology* [4th ed.]. Philadelphia: Churchill Livingstone Elsevier, p. 22.)

constrict along a plane perpendicular to the spindle apparatus, creating a division in the cell membrane and cytoplasm (cytokinesis). This constriction continues, creating two cells. At the end of this phase (telophase), the nucleus and nuclear membrane re-form and the spindle fibers disappear. Division is complete, and the two daughter cells move into interphase.

Meiosis

Meiosis is the process of germ cell division that is designed to reduce the number of chromosomes from the diploid (46) to haploid (23) number. In this process there are two sequential divisions. The first meiotic division is a reduction division; the second is an equational one (see Figure 1-5). Meiosis results in daughter cells that have 23 chromosomes: one chromosome from each pair of autosomes and one sex chromosome. Each of the 23 chromosomes consists of a single strand of DNA. Fusion of sperm and ovum through fertilization restores the diploid number (46) of chromosomes. Oogonia and spermatogonia arise from the primordial germ cells (see Embryonic and Fetal Development of the Reproductive System). Before initiation of meiosis, the primary oocyte or spermatocyte forms as DNA replicates and each chromosome consists of two chromatids (identical strands of DNA) joined at the centromere.

The first meiotic division consists of four phases (prophase, metaphase, anaphase, and telophase) and results in 4 haploid (23 chromosome) daughter cells, each chromosome having two strands of DNA, or twice the usual amount (see Figure 1-5). Prophase is the longest, accounting for 90% of meiosis I, and most complex phase. Prophase is divided into five stages. In the first stage (leptotene) the chromosomes are threadlike but already duplicated. Although consisting of two chromatids, the chromosome appears as a single strand. The nuclear membrane is intact. The sister chromatids maintain close contact due to formation of a meiosis-specific cohesion complex formed in this stage. Also a synaptonemal complex forms that tethers the homologous chromosomes to each other.[17,46] As the cell moves into the zygotene stage, homologous chromosomes pair up (synapse).

The chromosomes shorten and condense during the pachytene stage. The two chromatids in each chromosome are distinct and can now be seen clearly. Crossover and exchange of segments of genetic material (recombination) occurs at this time between the maternally derived chromatids of one of the chromosome pairs and the paternally derived chromatids of the other homologous chromosome (Figure 1-6). The sites of exchange are called *chiasmata.* Crossing over allows an individual to inherit a mixture of genetic material from maternal and paternal sides, increasing genetic diversity. The pairs of chromatids separate from each other during the diplotene stage. Once this separation is completed, the nuclear membrane dissolves (diakinesis stage). The chromosomes are maximally condensed, chiasmata are terminated, and normal disjunction (separation of chromosomes) occurs.[10,71] The exact mechanism for recombination is not well understood but is regulated by meiotic-specific genes and involves multiple steps.[17] All 23 chromosome pairs are involved in recombination, except that in males the XY pair only does so at the distal ends.[29] Recombination between homologous chromosomes is 1.6- to 1.7-fold greater in females than in males.[46] The reason for this is unknown. Some areas of chromosome pairs have greater frequency of recombination, others less. Decreased recombination has been reported in all trisomies.[46]

Between diakinesis and metaphase I, the nucleus disappears and spindle fibers form. In metaphase the chromosomes line up on the metaphase plate. Homologous chromosomes are paired and attached to spindle fibers at the centromere. The centrioles are at opposite poles. In anaphase I, the centromeres are not divided and the chromatids are not pulled to opposite poles as occurs with mitosis. Instead, each pair of chromosomes separates, with one of each chromosome pair going to each pole (see Figure 1-5). In telophase I, the nuclear membranes re-form and the cell divides to form a secondary oocyte or spermatocyte.[10,71] Each has 23 chromosomes, one member of each original chromosome pair; each chromosome has two chromatids attached at the centromere (i.e., each chromosome has twice the usual amount of DNA). In the female, cell division is unequal, with one daughter cell receiving 23 chromosomes and most of the cytoplasm; the other cell receives 23 chromosomes and minimal cytoplasm (Figure 1-7). This cell is called the first polar body and eventually disintegrates.

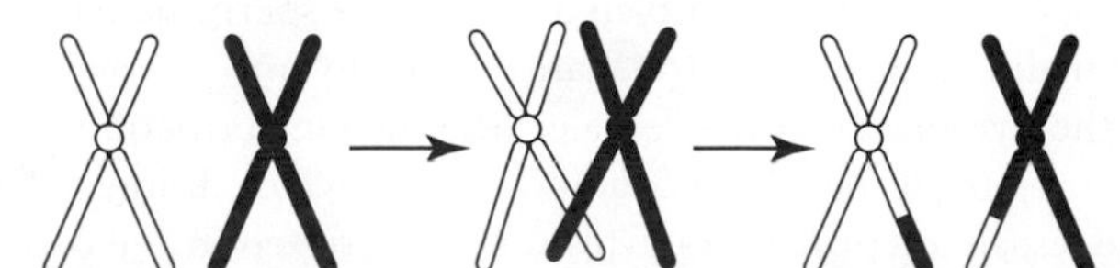

FIGURE 1-6 Illustration of chiasma formation and crossing over during meiosis. Genetic material is exchanged between homologous chromosomes. (From Levine, F. [2012]. Basic genetic principles. In R.A. Polin, W.W. Fox, & S.H. Abman, [Eds.]. *Fetal and neonatal physiology* [4th ed.]. Philadelphia: Saunders.)

In the second meiotic division, no DNA replication occurs. Prophase II is similar to mitosis. During metaphase the chromosomes (only one of each pair is present, each with twice the usual DNA) align along the equator of the cell. Centrioles again appear at the cell poles, and spindle fibers form. As the cell moves from metaphase II to anaphase II, the centromeres divide and the two chromatids from each chromosome separate and move to opposite poles. In telophase II, the nuclear membrane re-forms and cell division occurs, forming the spermatid or ovum.[10,71] The end result is haploid (23 chromosome) cells, with one of each chromosome pair in each cell (see Figure 1-5); each chromosome now has the normal amount of DNA. Again cell division in the females is unequal, resulting in formation of one ovum and the second polar body (see "Oogenesis").

GAMETOGENESIS

Gametogenesis is the process by which the primordial germ cells develop into mature gametes (ova or sperm). These processes are known as *oogenesis* (female) and *spermatogenesis* (male). Oogenesis and spermatogenesis are illustrated in Figure 1-7. Primordial germ cells are discussed further under "Embryonic and Fetal Development of the Reproductive System."

Oogenesis

Oogenesis is the process of ovum development, which, unlike spermatogenesis, begins in fetal life. In the female embryo, germ cell mitosis occurs during migration of the germ cells to the gonadal ridge and continues after the primordial germ cells arrive in the ovary from the yolk sac. During early fetal life (from 2 to 7 months), mitotic proliferation of the oogonia are rapid.[18,28] The oogonia continue to enlarge, their DNA replicates, and they become primary oocytes. The primary oocytes enter meiosis I, then arrest in the diplotene stage of prophase I (see Figure 1-5) and remain dormant until puberty.[56,66,] The nucleus of the arrested primary oocyte swells and becomes the germinal vesicle, which is thought to protect the DNA.[66] Meiosis begins by around 12 weeks' gestation and all oogonia have begun meiosis by the fifth month.[66] All primary oocytes are formed between 2.5 and 7 months' gestation.[18] By birth, a layer of follicular epithelial cells surrounds the primary oocytes, forming the primordial follicles. The follicular cells are important in controlling meiosis, including the meiotic arrest and resumption of meiosis with development of luteinizing hormone (LH) receptors. The meiotic arrest is due to an oocyte maturation inhibiting peptide produced by the surrounding follicular cells.[10,23,67] This peptide is transferred to the oocyte through gap junctions, which are areas of cell-to-cell communication.[10,23] The primary oocytes will remain dormant in this arrested state until sometime after puberty (see Chapters 2 and 3).

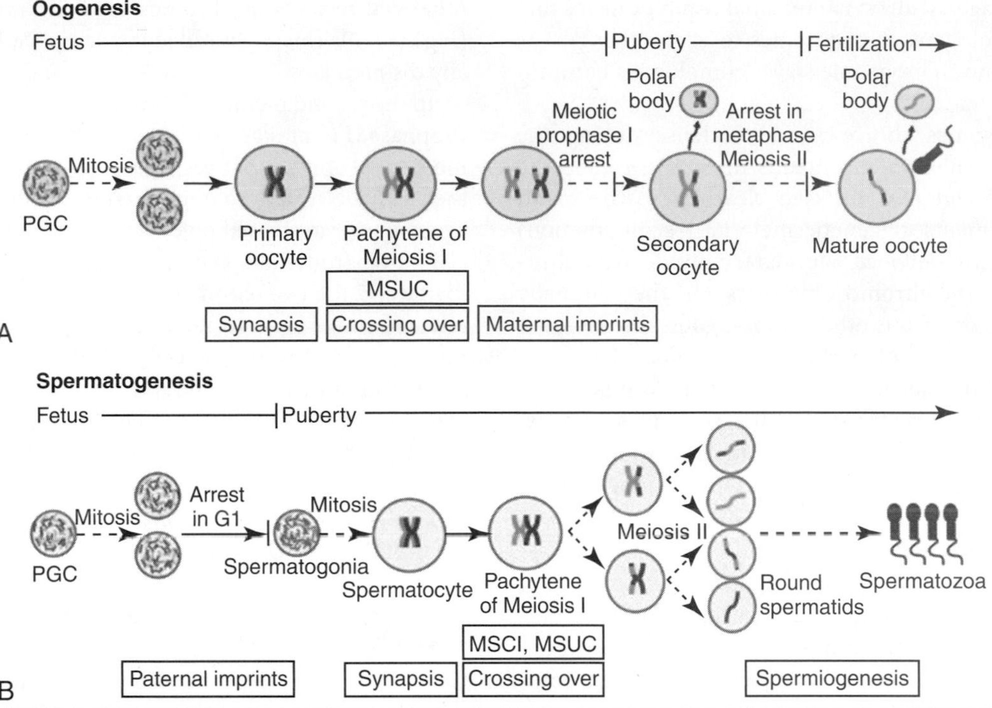

FIGURE 1-7 Developmental transitions in female and male gametogenesis. Primordial germ cells (PGCs) form during embryonic development. **(A)** In the developing ovaries, they undergo mitotic divisions before entering meiosis I after which primary oocytes arrest in prophase I until ovulation. Upon onset of sexual maturation, oocytes complete meiosis I and arrest in metaphase of meiosis II, until fertilization occurs. **(B)** Male PGCs defer meiosis and undergo mitotic proliferation in the developing male gonad until arresting in G1. From sexual maturity onward, spermatogonia resume mitotic proliferation to form spermatocytes, which then activate meiotic differentiation and form four haploid spermatids each, which in turn develop into spermatozoa. For simplicity, meiosis is shown for one pair of homologous chromosomes (in blue and pink). The timing of meiotic recombination, maternal and paternal imprint acquisition, meiotic silencing of unpaired chromatin (MSUC), meiotic sex chromosome inactivation (MSCI), and spermiogenesis are indicated. (From Kota, S.K. & Feil, R. [2010]. Epigenetic transitions in germ cell development and meiosis. *Dev Cell*, 19, p. 676.)

By 20 weeks' gestation, there are 6 to 7 million primary oocytes. This peak is followed by a gradual degeneration of oogonia, which continues to menopause.[18] By birth, 300,000 to 800,000 (average of 200,00 to 400,000) follicles remain; with 40,000 remaining by puberty.[65,66] Of these only about 400 to 500 of these oogonia will become secondary follicles.[10] During oogenesis, arrest, and later oocyte maturation, the oocyte must undergo various changes to become "fertilization competent."[23,30,51] These changes include accumulation of messenger ribonucleic acid (mRNA), proteins, and lipids; development of Golgi, mitochondria, and ribosomal RNA to meet cell needs immediately after fertilization; formation of sperm-specific receptors; and development of mechanisms to block entry of more than one sperm if the cell is fertilized.[10,23,51] These changes are critical since the oocyte supplies the mitochondria and majority of the cytoplasm, including most of the organelles and nonchromosomal molecules to the fertilized ovum.[23]

During each ovarian cycle after puberty, a small number of primary oocytes develop further.[10] Generally only one will mature and be ovulated (see Chapter 2).[30] Follicle-stimulating hormone (FSH) and luteinizing hormone (LH) from the pituitary gland cause an increase in the size of the oocyte as well as formation of the zona pellucida (see Chapter 3) around the oocyte. Before ovulation, the first meiotic division is completed, with an unequal division of the cytoplasm, yielding one secondary oocyte and the first polar body, which degenerates. Although the polar body is nonfunctional, it may divide during the second meiotic division.[10] Once the first meiotic division is completed, the secondary oocyte begins the second meiotic division. Ovulation occurs when the secondary oocyte enters metaphase II, where it again arrests. Meiosis II is completed only if the sperm penetrates the ovum. Meiosis II is also characterized by unequal division of the cytoplasm in the female, resulting in formation of a mature oocyte and the second polar body, which disintegrates. The remaining primary oocytes remain arrested in meiosis I. These processes are controlled by paracrine factors such as KIT ligand (a granulose cell regulator of oocyte development and its receptor, growth differentiating factor-9 and bone morphogenic protein-15), activation of cells receptors and sharing of factors via gap junctions between cells.[40] Reproductive endocrinology and follicle maturation are discussed in Chapter 2. Ovulation is discussed further in Chapters 2 and 3; fertilization is described in Chapter 3.

Spermatogenesis

Sperm development in the seminiferous tubules involves three stages: (1) mitosis (spermatogonial multiplication), (2) meiosis (production of haploid cells), and (3) spermiogenesis (maturation of spermatids to mature spermatozoa). In the male embryo, germ cell mitotic proliferation begins during migration of the germ cells to the gonadal ridge.[41,66] Once these cells reach the ridge, mitosis arrests in the G1 phase of the cell cycle. The Sertoli cells secrete substances to nourish the germ cells (see "Development of the Testes"). After birth mitotic proliferation resumes.[30] Spermatogenesis begins at puberty with the release of androgens. Once begun, the process is continuous for the remainder of the life span.

The androgens and proteins produced locally modulate spermatogenesis within the tubule. Spermatogenesis is regulated by follicle stimulating hormone (FSH) and luteinizing hormone (LH) from the pituitary gland. FSH stimulates development of androgen receptor proteins by the Sertoli cells. Spermatogenesis is regulated by LH which binds to the Leydig cells and stimulates testosterone production which then stimulates the Sertoli cells.[64] Transcription factors act on Sertoli cells to regulate germ cell development during mitosis and meiosis and on spermatids to regulate postmeiotic differentiation into mature sperm.[8,78] Spermatogenesis is also mediated via gap junctions (areas of cell-to-cell communication) between adjacent Leydig cells, adjacent Sertoli cells, and between Sertoli and germ cells, as well as by paracrine and autocrine pathways.[60]

The spermatogonia are located inside the seminiferous tubules. The seminiferous tubule is divided into two zones: the basal compartment, or outer layer (zone 1), of the tubule and the luminal compartment, or inner layer. The basal compartment is composed of type A spermatogonia that are renewed through mitosis. Some of these continue to proliferate and serve as stem cells, whereas others separate from the basal membrane and begin to migrate toward the lumen. These cells are known as *preleptotene spermatocytes* (type B spermatogonia). As migration progresses, the cells undergo further morphologic changes, becoming primary spermatocytes. The first and second meiotic divisions occur with further differentiation in the luminal zone, resulting in formation of secondary spermatocytes and spermatids.

During the first meiotic division, the primary spermatocytes reduce their chromosome count to half (haploid)—each chromosome having two chromatids joined at the centromere and become two secondary spermatocytes; each chromatid has two strands of DNA, or twice the usual amount. The second meiotic division involves separation of the two chromatids of each chromosome (with one going to each daughter cell), forming four spermatids, each with 23 chromosomes and a single strand of DNA (see Figure 1-7). The luminal spermatids undergo spermiogenesis, which is the transformation process from ordinary cell structure to sperm cell with head, acrosome (apical enzyme filled vesicle), midpiece (containing mitochondria to generate energy for movement), and tail with microtubules for propulsion with removal of most of the cytoplasm. The cytoplasm is transferred from the maturing spermatids to the Sertoli cells via tubulobulbar complexes that connect the developing gamete to the Sertoli cells.[66] Changes in chromatin organization within the sperm nucleus occur during postmeiotic spermatogenesis and by imprinting, a process important in differentiation of male versus female germ cells and in the control of fetal growth and development (see Box 1-2 below).[8,13,21,74] From the initial

BOX 1-2 Imprinting

Imprinting involves heritable changes in gene expression that results in a change in gene activity so the imprinted gene remains in a silent state.[9] For most genes, both the maternally inherited and paternally inherited alleles (gene forms) are expressed. With imprinted genes, only one of the two alleles is expressed and that allele is essential for normal development. Genomic imprinting is a "phenomenon that sets a parental signature on a specific deoxyribonucleic acid (DNA) segment during gametogenesis or before fertilization so that it is modified and functions differently depending on the parental origin of the DNA segment."[37]

Imprinted gene expression differs depending on the parent from which the chromosome originated. Genomic imprinting involves four mechanisms: methylation, acetylation, ribonucleic acid (RNA) interference, and chromatin remodeling.[9,75] Methylation is the most studied of these mechanisms. All cells contain two homologous chromosomes: one inherited from one's mother (with female imprints) and another from one's father (with male imprints). During development of germ cells, these imprints are erased in the first meiotic division and new sex-specific imprints established in the gametes. For example, in a male the paternally derived chromosomes have a male imprint and the maternally derived chromosomes have a female imprint. During spermatogenesis the germ cell chromosomes are reprogrammed to have only male imprints. During oogenesis similar types of changes occur during oocyte maturation (see Figure 1-7). As a result the gametes are reprogrammed so that sperm carry only paternal imprints and ova carry only maternal imprints. This reprogramming occurs in two phases.[9,75] Phase 1 occurs in the female during oocyte maturation and in males during spermatogenesis. In this phase the existing imprinting is removed and a new sex-specific imprinting occurs. Phase 2 ". . . occurs after fertilization and involves global demethylation in the embryo prior to implantation. Global remethylation then occurs post-implantation. Most imprinted genes, however, escape the second phase of reprogramming and remain intact throughout embryonic development."[9, p.140] About 100 imprinted genes have been identified and these are found in clusters containing both maternal and paternal genes and a gene that controls the imprinting of the surrounding genes.[9,36,75]

Imprinted genes are inactive in all cells within the body. Loss of imprinting in these genes can lead to disorders such as Prader-Willi and Angelman syndromes (see "Non-Traditional Patterns of Inheritance").

growth phase of the spermatogonia to the final product takes approximately 74 days.[61,65] Once completed, the sperm are set free in the seminiferous tubules and transported via the fluid to the epididymis and ductus deferens, where they are stored until ejaculation (see Chapter 3). At the time of their release from the tubules, the spermatozoa are still morphologically immature and lack motility. While traversing the epididymis, and after ejaculation, they continue to differentiate. The final maturational process in sperm development is capacitation, which involves changes to the acrosome for enzyme release (see Chapter 3).

Abnormal Gamete Development

Abnormal gamete development is the result of either chromosomal or morphologic abnormalities. The impact of maternal or paternal age at the time of conception can be seen in fresh gene mutations. The older the parents are, the greater the likelihood that they will generate germ cells that contain gene mutations that can be passed on to the embryo. DNA damage and replication errors are more likely to occur in males because spermatogenesis involves continual cell division and DNA replication, whereas nondisjunction is more common in females.[57,58] Oocyte fertility begins to decrease after 30 years.[23] The likelihood of chromosomal abnormalities increases after 35 years of age in females, and this may be because of nondisjunction from prolongation of meiosis over many years (see "Alterations in Chromosome Number"). Gametes may also experience alterations in morphology. This is much less common in oocytes than in sperm. Although some oocytes may have two or more nuclei, they probably never mature. In each ejaculate, up to 20% of the sperm are grossly abnormal, having either two heads or two tails. Their ability to fertilize the ovum is probably limited because of decreased or abnormal motility and inability to pass through the cervical mucus, thereby terminating their access to the ovum. An increase in the percentage of abnormal sperm can reduce fertility.[57]

GENETIC AND CHROMOSOMAL DISORDERS

Genetic diseases are the result of detrimental changes in the structure of individual genes (gene disorders) or in the entire chromosome (cytogenetic or chromosomal disorders). These disorders can be inherited (see "Modes of Inheritance") or arise as new mutations or from alterations in chromosomal number or structure during cell division. Mutations are not always deleterious, but rather may introduce genetic variation into the species.[67] Cytogenetic or chromosomal disorders result when a large number of genes are damaged.[45] Individuals born with chromosomal defects often demonstrate both physical and mental alterations.[43] Most gene disorders are mutations in a single or small number of genes, whereas major chromosome errors involve a change in chromosome number or structure. Chromosomal alterations are seen in 60% of spontaneous abortions, 6% to 7% of stillborn infants, and 0.7% of live born infants.[35,58] Chromosomal abnormalities can also be a cause of infertility. Most chromosomal abnormalities arise during gametogenesis, although errors can also occur during fertilization or postfertilization.[58]

Alterations in Chromosome Number

Deviations from euploidy (the correct number of chromosomes) are of two types. *Polyploidy* refers to an exact multiple of the haploid (23) set of chromosomes. For example, *triploidy* refers to a zygote with 69 chromosomes (three of each). Triploidy may arise from fertilization of an ovum (23 chromosomes) with two sperm (each carrying 23 chromosomes) or from fusion of the ovum (23 chromosomes) and polar body (23 chromosomes), which is then fertilized by a sperm (23 chromosomes). Aneuploidy is the term used for cases in which there is not an exact multiple. Monosomy is a subset of the latter, in which one member of a pair of chromosomes is missing. Monosomies are rarely viable. The most common monosomy seen in live born infants is a female with Turner syndrome who has only one X chromosome. Trisomy refers to the presence of an extra chromosome. *Aneuploidy* is seen in 1% to 2% of sperm, about 20% of oocytes and blastocysts, 35% of spontaneous abortions, 4% of stillborn infants, and 0.3% of live born infants.[30] The most common alterations seen in spontaneous abortions are Turner syndrome (XO) and trisomies 16, 21, and 22. The most common trisomies seen in live born infants are trisomies 21 (Down syndrome), 13 (Patau syndrome), and 18 (Edward syndrome). Individuals with Klinefelter syndrome—another example of an alteration in numbers of sex chromosomes—are XXY males. Alterations in chromosome numbers often occur due to nondisjunction during cell division.

Nondisjunction during meiosis is an error in meiotic division. For example, in the case of formation of gametes with a trisomy or monosomy, one gamete will have 24 chromosomes and the other will have only 22 (Figure 1-8). Once fertilization occurs, the gamete with 24 chromosomes forms a zygote with 47 chromosomes (trisomy with an extra copy of one chromosome, such as an extra 21 in trisomy 21). About 95% of Down syndrome cases are due to trisomy 21. In the alternative situation, a 45-chromosome zygote (monosomy for a specific chromosome) is formed from the joining of 22- and 23-chromosome gametes, with one chromosome missing. Most autosomal trisomies and all autosomal monosomies are nonviable.

Nondisjunction is more likely to occur during the recombination that takes place during the first meiotic division. In meiosis I errors, the homologous chromosomes may travel together to the same pole or fail to pair and thus end up at the same pole, or the sister chromatids may separate prematurely. Nondisjunction during the second meiotic division is due to failure of sister chromatids to separate.[30] One model ("limited oocyte pool hypothesis") suggests that a relative scarcity of oocytes at optimal stages of maturation increases the risk of abnormal gametes. Most trisomies that occur in the first meiotic division have a maternal age effect. However, it is unclear

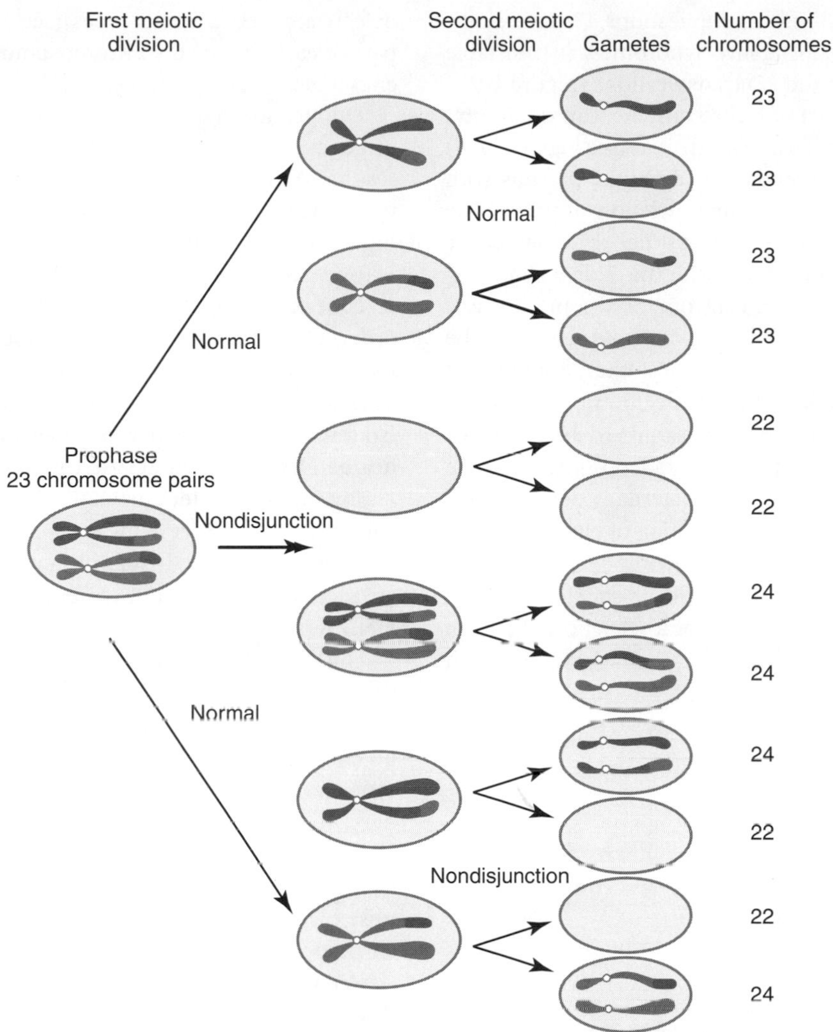

FIGURE 1-8 Possibilities of nondisjunction. *Top arrow,* Normal meiotic division; *middle arrow,* nondisjunction during the first meiotic division; *bottom arrow,* nondisjunction during the second meiotic division. (From Carlson, B.M. [2004]. *Human embryology and developmental biology* [3rd ed.]. St. Louis: Mosby.)

whether the precipitating event occurs prenatally, during oocyte meiotic arrest, or preovulatory when meiosis is resumed, nor is it known what environmental factors may mediate these errors.[30]

Nondisjunction in the autosomes during meiosis, is more frequent in females than in males. Maternal nondisjunction in the first meiotic division accounts for approximately 33% of trisomy 18 and 65% of trisomy 21, whereas maternal nondisjunction in the second meiotic division accounts for approximately 56% of trisomy 18 and 23% of trisomy 21.[30] On the other hand, paternal nondisjunction accounts for 80% of Turner syndrome (XO females) in which the paternal X is lost during meiosis or early after fertilization. Nondisjunction leading to Klinefelter syndrome (XXY male) occurs equally in the mother and father, usually in meiosis I, especially in the father.[30,58] Chromosomal abnormalities are described further in the next section.

Nondisjunction can also occur during mitosis after formation of the zygote. If nondisjunction occurs in the first cell division after fertilization, one daughter cell receives 45 chromosomes and the other 47 chromosomes. The cell with 45 chromosomes usually does not survive; the zygote continues to develop from the 47 chromosome cell and is a trisomy. If mitotic nondisjunction occurs later in development, some cell lines have the normal number of cells and some have an abnormal number. This is called *mosaicism.* Approximately 1% to 2% of individuals with Down syndrome are mosaics; that is, they have some cells with the normal 46 chromosomes and some cells with 47 chromosomes as a result of an extra chromosome 21.

Alterations in Chromosome Structure

Variations in chromosome structure are more common than alterations in chromosomal number. Some have very little effect while others are devastating. Alterations in chromosome structure include (1) deletions, (2) duplications, (3) inversions, (4) isochromosomes, (5) instability syndromes, (6) unstable triplet nucleotide repeats, and (7) translocations (Figure 1-9).

Deletions, the loss of part of a chromosome, can occur anywhere on the chromosome. Terminal deletions (see Figure 1-9, *B*) are those occurring on the ends. For example, persons with cri du chat syndrome have a terminal deletion of part of the short (p) arm of chromosome 5. Interstitial deletions occur along the body of the chromosome, with the ends reattaching. If the broken piece is without a centromere, the piece is lost during cell division. Occasionally, broken fragments may be incorporated into another chromosome. Other examples of deletion syndromes are Wilms tumor (deletion of part of the short arm of chromosome 11), retinoblastoma (deletion of part of the long arm of chromosome 13), Prader-Willi syndrome (deletion of part of the long arm of the paternally derived chromosome 15), Angelman syndrome (deletion of part of the long arm of the maternally derived chromosome 15), Duchenne muscular dystrophy (deletion of part of the short arm of the X chromosome), and DiGeorge syndrome (deletion of part of the long arm of chromosome 22).[28,35] A variation of deletion defects are ring chromosomes (see Figure 1-9, *C*), in which part of each end of the chromosomes are broken off and the ends attach to each other.

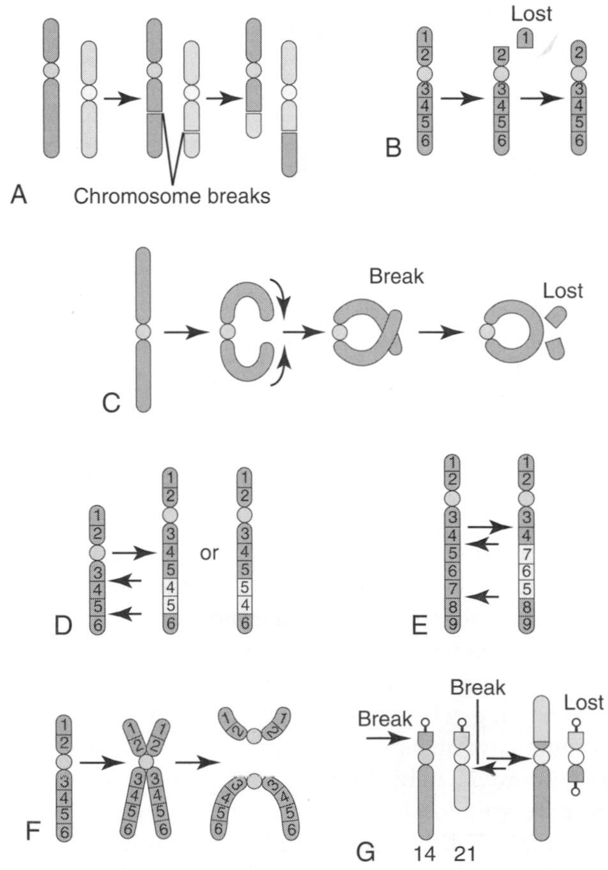

FIGURE 1-9 Diagrams illustrating various structural abnormalities of chromosomes. **A,** Reciprocal translocation. **B,** Terminal deletion. **C,** Ring chromosomes. **D,** Duplication. **E,** Paracentric inversion. **F,** Isochromosome. **G,** Robertsonian translocation. (From Moore, K.L. & Persaud, T.V.N. [2003]. *The developing human: Clinically oriented embryology* [7th ed.]. Philadelphia: Saunders.)

Duplications (see Figure 1-9, *D*) occur when extra copies of genes are created or obtained during crossing-over. The results of this duplication may or may not result in phenotypic changes. Inversions (e.g., a paracentric inversion) (see Figure 1-9, *E*) result from two breaks and the subsequent 180-degree rotation of the broken segment. This results in a sequence change and rearrangement of genes in reverse order. Chromosome pairing cannot occur normally during meiosis, resulting in an increased incidence of spontaneous abortions. This may also explain some cases of infertility. Isochromosomes occur when the chromosome, with its replicated DNA, divides across the centromere (instead of dividing into two sister chromatids), resulting in one chromosome with just upper arms and one with just the lower arms (see Figure 1-9, *F*). Instability syndromes such as Fanconi anemia and xeroderma pigmentosum involve alterations in DNA repair.[35]

Unstable nucleotide repeats are multiple repetitions of a series of three bases at a certain point along the chromosome. These disorders usually demonstrate anticipation, which can be manifest in different ways, in which the disorder becomes more severe with subsequent generations. Examples of disorders in which this defect is seen are myotonic dystrophy, Huntington disease (chromosome 4), and fragile X syndrome (X chromosome). For example, in fragile X syndrome, the unstable CGG nucleotide repeat occurs at the end of the X chromosome. Instead of the usual number of CGG repeats (fewer than 50), there are many more, with severity of the disorder associated with the number of repeats. Expansion of the number of repeats occurs during meiosis in females. Fragile X syndrome is the most common cause of inherited developmental delay and mental retardation and is more common in males than in females. In Huntington disease, the expansion on chromosome 4 occurs primarily in sperm cells; thus the disorder is more likely to occur when passed through males. Age of onset is usually between 40 and 60 years of age. Increased numbers of repeats are associated with a younger age of onset.[35]

Translocations occur following breaks in one or more chromosomes. Genetic material is transferred from one chromosome to another. A balanced translocation occurs when chromosomes exchange pieces and no genetic material is lost. If material is gained or lost, that is considered an unbalanced translocation. Individuals with balanced translocations appear normal; those with unbalanced translocations may have multiple anomalies. Reciprocal translocations (see Figure 1-9, *A*) involve breaks in two chromosomes, with exchange of genetic material. Translocations are also seen with some forms of leukemia and solid tumors.[35]

Robertsonian translocations (see Figure 1-9, *G*) involve chromosomes 13 through 15 and 21 and 22; these occur when the short arms of 2 chromosomes break off and are lost, and the long arms fuse together at the centromere to form a single chromosome. For example, an individual with normal 14 and 21 chromosomes and a 14/21 translocation has an abnormal karyotype and number of chromosomes (i.e., only 45 chromosomes) but a normal phenotype (normal amount of genetic material). However, depending on which combination of 21 and 14 chromosomes are transferred to the gametes, this individual can produce normal, carrier, monosomic (for 21 or 14), or trisomic (for 21 or 14) offspring. Approximately 3% to 4% of Down syndrome is due to translocations, most commonly between chromosomes 14 and 21. These individuals have 46 chromosomes, because the abnormal dose of chromosome 21 is attached to a chromosome 14.

Gene Disorders

Mutations are permanent changes in DNA. Mutations can involve changes in the sequence of bases, involving large amounts of DNA, as occurs with chromosomal abnormalities, or alterations in one or a few bases that result in production of a deficient or defective protein. Mutations can be spontaneous or inherited. If the mutation occurs in a somatic cell, it is transmitted only within that cell line; all other cell lines are free of that mutation. However, if a mutation occurs in a germ cell or gamete, it is transmitted to all somatic and germ cells of the offspring, and thus can be passed to that individual's offspring.

Gene mutations result in inherited biochemical or structural disorders characterized by defective or deficient cellular functioning or altered production of structural components (e.g., skin, muscles, hemoglobin, connective tissue). The consequences of these alterations depend on the type of molecule affected, defect, metabolic reaction, site of action, remaining residual activity, gene interactions, environment, and degree of adaptation.[43] General categories of gene disorders include hemoglobinopathies, disorders of metabolism (carbohydrate, lipid, amino acid, or degradative pathways), deficient or abnormal circulating proteins, alterations in membrane receptors or transport molecules, immunologic disorders, and cancer genetics. There are hundreds of known gene disorders. Table 1-1 lists examples of each major category; several examples are described further in this section.

Hemoglobinopathies may arise from qualitative or quantitative changes in hemoglobin. For example, both sickle cell anemia and β-thalassemia involve mutations in the gene on chromosome 11 for production of β chains. The most common mutation in sickle cell anemia involves a single point mutation (change in just one amino acid, with a valine instead of a glutamic acid inserted into the 146 amino acid sequence that makes up β chains). This mutation results in formation of qualitatively different β globulin chains (HbS). With β-thalassemia, fewer β chains of normal length are produced due to a reduced production rate or absence of synthesis. The α chains have fewer β chains to pair with and accumulate and precipitate. More than 300 different mutations in the β chain gene have been identified in individuals with various forms of β-thalassemia.[35] With α-thalassemia, two pairs of genes (for a total of four genes) control synthesis of α chains for hemoglobin on chromosome 16, with two α globulin genes on each chromosome 16. The clinical status of individuals depends on the number of genes in the two gene pairs that are deleted or abnormal. If just one of the four genes is deleted, the individual is a "silent" carrier. If two genes are absent or inactivated, the individual will have minimal anemia and hemoglobin H disease; three deleted or inactivated genes lead to mild to moderate anemia. Two inactivated genes and one abnormal gene leads to moderate to severe anemia. If all four genes are absent or inactive, these infants develop severe fetal hydrops (edema) and congestive heart failure and are usually stillborn or die soon after birth.[35] However, a few infants have survived with bone marrow transplants.[35]

Metabolic defects result in blocked metabolic pathways, accumulation of toxic precursors, lack of end-product production, and loss of feedback inhibition. For example, phenylalanine is a precursor for tyrosine formation. Tyrosine is then broken down (mediated by tyrosinase), to produce

Table 1-1 Examples of Gene Disorders

TYPE OF DISORDER	EXAMPLES
Hemoglobin disorders	Sickle cell anemia β-Thalassemia α-Thalassemia
Disorders of metabolism: amino acid metabolism	Enzyme defects (phenylketonuria, congenital adrenal hyperplasia) Deficient reabsorption in intestines or kidneys (Hartnup's disease)
Disorders of metabolism: carbohydrate metabolism	Enzyme defects (galactosemia) Excess glycogen accumulation (glycogen storage disorders)
Disorders of metabolism: lipid metabolism	Altered transport (hyperlipidemia) Enzyme defects (medium chain acyl-CoA dehydrogenase deficiency)
Disorders of metabolism: altered degradation pathways	Lysosomal storage disorders Uric acid cycle disorders
Deficient or abnormal circulating proteins	Globulins (immunologic defects) Clotting factors (hemophilia)
Alterations in membrane receptors or regulators	Hypercholesterolemia Cystic fibrosis
Immunologic disorders	Major histocompatibility antigen disease associations (type 1 diabetes, celiac disease, Graves' disease) Immunodeficiency disorders
Cancers	Familial breast and ovarian cancers (BRCA1, BRCA2) Hereditary nonpolyposis colorectal cancer Wilms' tumor Retinoblastoma

Compiled from Jorde, L.B., et al. (2006). *Medical genetics* (3rd ed.). St. Louis: Mosby; Lashley, F.R. (1998). *Clinical genetics in nursing practice* (2nd ed.). New York: Springer.

substances such as melanin and by-products used in synthesis of neurotransmitters. Phenylalanine catabolism is mediated by the enzyme *phenylalanine hydroxylase.* Individuals with phenylketonuria (PKU) have a mutation of the gene required for production of this enzyme. As a result, these individuals have altered enzyme production and have difficulty converting phenylalanine to tyrosine. Phenylalanine and by-products of alternative metabolic pathways accumulate with a deficiency of tyrosine. The accumulated phenylalanine and alternative pathway by-products are excreted in the urine (leading to a musky odor), interfere with tyrosinase function, and are toxic to the central nervous system. The decreased tyrosine results in lack of melanin (leading to the light skin and eye color observed in these cases), altered neurotransmitters, and neurologic abnormalities.

MODES OF INHERITANCE

The way in which a particular trait is transmitted to offspring is referred to as the *mode of inheritance.* The major modes of inheritance are those that follow traditional Mendelian patterns (autosomal and sex-linked inheritance), multifactorial inheritance, and nontraditional patterns. Mendelian patterns follow the principles identified by Mendel (Table 1-2) and influence inheritance of both normal traits and mutated genes. Autosomal dominant traits are the result of a dominant allele at a particular locus on an autosome. When a characteristic is the result of a recessive allele, the mode of inheritance is known as *autosomal recessive.* Genetic diseases resulting from the mutation of a single allele are called *dominant;* those that result from mutation of both alleles are called *recessive.* The traits or disorders expressed by autosomal genes usually occur with the same frequency in males as in females. The latter is not true of sex-linked traits and disorders, which occur with higher frequency in males than in females. This is because the genes located on the X chromosome are present in only one copy in males. Therefore the genes that are on that chromosome are expressed and are considered hemizygous in males.[43] Polygenic traits are governed by the additive effect of two or more alleles at different loci.[43]

Several types of dominance (simple, or complete; partial, or incomplete) and codominance affect the phenotype.[35,43] In simple, or complete, dominance, the heterozygous genotype (dominant allele present on one of the chromosome pair) produces a phenotype similar to that produced by the homozygous genotype (dominant allele present on both of the chromosome pair) for dominant traits. With partial, or incomplete, dominance, the heterozygous genotype (one copy of the recessive gene and one copy of the dominant gene) produces a phenotype that is intermediate between the recessive homozygous (i.e., two copies of a recessive gene) and dominant homozygous (i.e., two copies of a dominant gene) phenotypes. For example, an individual who is a heterozygote (carrier) for familial hypercholesterolemia will have fewer low density lipoprotein receptors and higher blood cholesterol levels than a healthy individual but will have more receptors and lower cholesterol levels than someone with two recessive genes.[35]

Codominance occurs when both alleles are expressed, so that in the heterozygous state, both the dominant and recessive gene products are produced. The gene producing normal β chains for adult hemoglobin (HbA) and the gene producing abnormal β chains (HbS) seen with sickle cell anemia are examples of codominance. If both chromosomes in the pair have the normal β chain gene, HbA is produced; if both chromosomes have the abnormal genes, HbS is produced and the individual has sickle cell anemia. However, if one of the chromosomes has the normal gene and one has the abnormal gene (heterozygote), both HbA and HbS are produced. This individual has the sickle cell trait.

For some traits, such as the ABO blood type, multiple alleles are present. Although any given individual has only two genes for blood type (one on each chromosome in the pair), there are more than two forms of the gene present in the population. For example, although there are genes for types A, B, and O present in humans, any individual has only two alleles. That person may have two identical alleles (AA, BB, or OO), or may have two different alleles (AO, BO, and AB). In the ABO system, A and B are codominant and O is recessive to both A and B. Thus someone who has the AO genotype has the A blood type phenotype. Similarly, a BO individual has the B phenotype. However someone with the AB genotype has AB blood, because A and B are codominant and thus are both expressed.[35,43]

Other factors that influence whether or not an individual with a certain genotype actually manifests the trait are penetrance and variable expression. With differences in penetrance, not everyone with the abnormal gene(s) actually manifests the trait or disorder. This is an "all-or-nothing" type of phenomenon. Reduced penetrance is often seen with autosomal dominant conditions such as retinoblastoma. Variable expression refers to the different manifestations of the phenotype that can be observed in individuals with the same genotype.

Table 1-2 Mendelian Principles of Inheritance

PRINCIPLE	DESCRIPTION
Dominance	In the competition of two genes at the same locus on paired chromosomes, one gene may mask or conceal the other. The individual manifests the dominant gene's characteristic. The concealed trait is termed *recessive.*
Segregation	During meiosis, paired chromosomes are separated to form two gametes. Therefore the genes remain unchanged and are transferred from one generation to the next.
Independent assortment	When displayed traits have alleles at two or more loci, each is distributed within the gametes randomly, independent of each other.

This leads to wide variations in the clinical severity of individuals with some disorders. Examples of disorders with variable expression include neurofibromatosis and osteogenesis imperfecta.[35] Some disorders also exhibit anticipation, which is a tendency for the disorder to become more severe with each subsequent generation. This is frequently seen with disorders characterized by unstable nucleotide repeats such as myotonic dystrophy, Huntington disease, and fragile X syndrome.[35]

Table 1-3 **Major Characteristics of Autosomal Recessive and Dominant Inheritance and Disorders**

AUTOSOMAL RECESSIVE INHERITANCE	AUTOSOMAL DOMINANT INHERITANCE
The mutant gene is located on an autosome.	The mutant gene is located on an autosome.
Two copies of the mutant gene are needed for phenotypic manifestations.	Only one copy of the mutant gene is needed for effects to be evident.
Males and females are affected in equal numbers, on average.	Males and females are affected in equal numbers, on average.
There is usually no sex difference in clinical manifestations.	There is usually no sex difference in clinical manifestations.
Affected individual receives one mutant gene from each parent.	Vertical family history through several generations may be seen.
Family history is usually negative, especially for vertical transmission (in more than one generation).	There is wide variability of expression.
Other affected individuals in family in same generation (horizontal transmission) may be seen.	Penetrance may be incomplete, so the gene may appear to "skip" a generation.
Consanguinity is present more often than in other modes of inheritance.	There is an increased paternal age effect.
Fresh gene mutation is rare.	Fresh gene mutation is frequent.
Age of disease onset is early newborn, infancy, and early childhood.	Later age of onset is frequent.
Often involves enzyme defect or deficiency.	Normal offspring of an affected person have normal children.
Disease course is usually severe.	Structural protein defect is often involved.

Adapted from Lashley, F.R. (1998). *Clinical genetics in nursing practice* (2nd ed.). New York: Springer.

Autosomal Inheritance

The inheritance of these traits is dependent upon the differences between alleles of a particular locus on an autosomal pair. In this type of inheritance, it makes no difference which parent carries the genotype, because the autosomes are the same in both sexes.

Autosomal Recessive Inheritance

A trait governed by a recessive allele is expressed only when the homozygous condition exists.[43] In order for an individual to demonstrate the trait or disorder, both parents must carry the recessive allele. If an affected person reproduces with a homozygous unaffected person, their children will be heterozygous for the trait and will not manifest the disease, but they will be carriers. If two carriers reproduce, then the probability (for each pregnancy) is about 25% that the child will manifest the disease, 50% that the child will be a carrier, and 25% that the child will neither have the disease nor be a carrier. When an affected person reproduces with a carrier, the probability is about 50% that a child will have the disease and 50% that the child will be a carrier. Usually an affected child is the offspring of two heterozygotes who are themselves normal.

Disorders transmitted by recessive inheritance often involve altered enzymes. Normally only 50% of the normal amount of these enzymes is sufficient for normal function.[45] Examples of autosomal recessive disorders include cystic fibrosis, phenylketonuria (PKU), hypothyroidism, Tay-Sachs disease, congenital adrenal hyperplasia, and galactosemia. Hemoglobinopathies such as sickle cell disease are also transmitted by autosomal recessive inheritance. Characteristics of disorders inherited by autosomal recessive inheritance are listed in Table 1-3.

Autosomal Dominant Inheritance

In autosomal dominant inheritance, traits and disorders are expressed in the heterozygote state and the probability of transmission to the offspring is 50% with each pregnancy. Autosomal dominant disorders often involve mutations in genes that regulate complex metabolic pathways or produce structural proteins. Examples of autosomal dominant disorders include Huntington disease (triplet nucleotide repeats), osteogenesis imperfecta (mutations in the collagen gene), and familial hypercholesterolemia (mutations in the receptor for very-low-density lipoproteins).[45] Whenever the gene is present, it is expressed in the phenotype and can be traced through a number of generations. Expression of these genes rarely skips a generation, and a person not affected will not transmit the gene. Therefore the affected individual will have an affected parent, unless the condition is the result of fresh mutation, which is a common finding in most autosomal dominant conditions. An exception to this is Huntington disease, in which new mutations are extremely rare.[35]

Some autosomal dominant disorders (e.g., achondroplasia) are apparent at birth, whereas others (e.g., Huntington disease, adult-onset polycystic kidney disease) have a variable and usually adult onset. Other characteristics of autosomal dominant inheritance include a wide variation in expression in those individuals affected. Penetrance may also not be complete. Penetrance refers to whether or not there is phenotypic recognition of the mutant gene. If a gene is fully penetrant, the trait it controls is always manifested in the individual. If it is not fully penetrant, the disease may appear to skip a generation; that is, a particular genotype produces a particular trait in some individuals but not in others. A parent may be diagnosed with a particular disorder only after having several affected offspring.[45] A paternal age effect is seen with some autosomal dominant disorders.[43] Table 1-3 summarizes characteristics of autosomal dominant inheritance.

Sex-Linked Inheritance

Genes on the X chromosome are identified as X-linked, whereas those on the Y chromosome are Y-linked. There are many X-linked genes; however, there is limited evidence for Y-linked genes except for some associated with the male phenotype. Males can transmit X-linked genes to their daughters but not to their sons, and sons can receive X-linked genes only from their mothers. Female offspring can be either homozygous or heterozygous for X-linked genes because of their dual X chromosomes. Males, on the other hand, are hemizygous for X-linked genes, because they have only one X chromosome.

X-linked inheritance in females is influenced by X-chromosome inactivation (see earlier discussion on X Chromosomes). In all of a woman's somatic cells (but not in her germ cells), one of the two X chromosomes is inactivated, although about 15% of genes on the inactive X remain active.[47,58] The inactive X is reactivated in the oogonium, so that with gametogenesis the woman produces only ova with two active X chromosomes. The inactivated X is random in each cell—it could be the X that the zygote received from the mother or the one it received from the father—and the same X is inactive in all descendants of that cell. Exceptions to the random inactivation are seen in some single gene disorders such as Duchenne muscular dystrophy, in which the normal X tends to be the active one.[47,58] Table 1-4 summarizes characteristics of X-linked inheritance.

X-Linked Recessive Inheritance

In males, an X-linked recessive gene is always expressed, because there is no corresponding gene on the Y chromosome. In females, recessive genes of this nature are usually expressed only when the recessive allele is present in the homozygous form (i.e., on both of the woman's X chromosomes). Occasionally a female may demonstrate the trait secondary to the random inactivation of one of the X chromosomes in each cell. The degree to which this individual expresses the trait depends on the proportion of cells in which the X with the dominant gene has been inactivated. The larger the proportion is, the greater the likelihood that the X-linked trait will be visible. Examples of X-linked recessive inheritance include hemophilia, color blindness, and Duchenne muscular dystrophy.

X-Linked Dominant Inheritance

In this type of inheritance, the trait will be demonstrated in both males and females. Who will be affected and to what degree depend on the genotype of the parents. All the daughters of an affected father will receive the X chromosome with the dominant gene and will express the disease. However, none of the sons of this father will be affected. When the mother is heterozygous and the father is not affected, the probability is 50% that offspring will be affected. If the mother is homozygous, the probability is 100% that children of either gender will be affected. If the father is also affected, the daughters will be homozygous for the disease. X-linked dominant disorders are rare; an example is X-linked hypophosphatemia, or vitamin D–resistant rickets.

Y-Linked Inheritance

Because only males have Y chromosomes and there is no corresponding allele on the X chromosome, these traits occur only in males. If a Y-linked trait is present, it will be expressed. There is no dominance or recessiveness. When a father with a Y-linked chromosome transfers genetic material, all the sons will be affected and none of the daughters will. The Y chromosome also contains at least 12 testes-determining genes that control gonad development and spermatogenesis (see "Development of the Gonads").

Table 1-4 Major Characteristics of X-Linked Recessive and Dominant Inheritance and Disorders

X-LINKED RECESSIVE INHERITANCE	X-LINKED DOMINANT INHERITANCE
The mutant gene is on the X chromosome.	The mutant gene is located on the X chromosome.
One copy of the mutant gene is needed for phenotypic effect in males.	One copy of the mutant gene is needed for phenotypic manifestation.
Two copies of the mutant gene are usually needed for phenotypic effect in females.	X inactivation modifies the gene effect in females.
Males are more frequently affected than females.	Often lethal in males and so may see transmission only in female line.
Unequal X inactivation can lead to manifesting heterozygote female carriers.	Affected families show excess of female offspring.
Transmission is often through heterozygous (carrier) females.	Affected male transmits gene to all his daughters and none of his sons.
All daughters of affected males are carriers.	Affected males have affected mothers (unless it is a new mutation).
All sons of affected males are normal.	There is no male-to-male transmission.
There is no male-to-male transmission.	There is no carrier state.
There may be fresh gene mutations.	Disorders are relatively uncommon.

Adapted from Lashley, F.R. (1998). *Clinical genetics in nursing practice* (2nd ed.). New York: Springer.

Multifactorial Inheritance

Multifactorial inheritance does not follow Mendelian patterns but is due to the interaction of genetic and environmental factors. Multifactorial inheritance includes traits such as height and blood pressure. Multifactorial disorders include birth defects (e.g., neural tube defects, some congenital heart defects, congenital dislocated hips, cleft lip and palate, pyloric stenosis, Hirschsprung's disease) and adult-onset disorders (e.g., some forms of breast and other cancers, bipolar affective disorders, coronary heart disease, types 1 and 2 diabetes). Some disorders can also arise from purely environmental causes as well as via multifactorial inheritance. For example, although some congenital heart defects have a multifactorial inheritance, these defects may also arise as the result of teratogen exposure. Multifactorial disorders are often polygenic and may be additive. The threshold model proposes that a certain threshold or liability must be present for the disorder to occur; the additive polygenic model suggests that multiple genes have an accumulative effect to determine phenotype.[35] Although multifactorial disorders are often polygenic, not all polygenic disorders or traits are multifactorial (i.e., involve an interaction and genetic and environmental factors).[35] The risk of a multifactorial disorder increases with the number of individuals in the family that are affected, closeness of the relationship (highest in first-degree relatives, i.e., parents, siblings, offspring), and severity of the disorder. Thus, the greater the severity of a birth defect, the greater the risk of recurrence in first-degree relatives.[35,43]

Nontraditional Modes of Inheritance

Nontraditional modes of inheritance involve patterns that do not follow traditional Mendelian principles. Examples of these patterns include alterations in genomic imprinting, uniparental disomy, gonadal (germline) mosaicism, and mitochondrial inheritance.

Genomic imprinting (see Box 1-2 on p. 9) is a "phenomenon that sets a parental signature on a specific DNA segment during gametogenesis or before fertilization so that it is modified and functions differently depending on the parental origin of the DNA segment."[37] Thus with genomic imprinting, gene expression differs depending on the parent from which the chromosome originated. Imprinting is a part of normal development, However, disorders can arise from alterations in imprinting. For example, with triploidy (severe growth failure and mental retardation, with most spontaneously aborted), if the extra set of chromosomes comes from the father (i.e., the zygote has 46 paternal chromosomes and 23 maternal), there is marked growth failure in the embryo, with overgrowth of placental tissue. Conversely, if there are two sets of maternal and one set of paternal chromosomes, early embryo growth is normal, with poor placental and chorion development. Complete hydatidiform moles (see Chapter 3) have two sets of paternal chromosomes and none of maternal origin.[58] Loss of imprinting of growth factors may play a role in childhood cancers such as Wilms' tumor.

Another example of genomic imprinting is seen with deletions on the long arm of chromosome 15 (q11-13). If the deletion comes from the father, the offspring has Prader-Willi syndrome; if the deletion is on the maternal chromosome, the offspring has Angelman syndrome. These syndromes have completely different phenotypes. Angelman syndrome is characterized by mental retardation, seizures, absence of speech, frequent smiling, and paroxysmal laughing; Prader-Willi syndrome is characterized by overeating and obesity, behavior problems, and mild to moderate mental retardation. This process is not completely understood but involves epigenetic modifications of the histones by methylation and acetylation that leads to inactivation of certain sites on the chromosome. The initial modifications occur during gametogenesis wherein the previous imprints (i.e., from one's mother or father) are erased and new ones established based on the respective parental pattern.[36] More than 100 imprinted genes, which often occur in clusters, have been identified.[36] The pattern of methylation is unique to the maternal versus paternal genes and the pattern is replicated when the cell divides.[9,75]

Uniparental disomy occurs when the offspring gets both copies of a chromosome from the same parent. For example, Prader-Willi and Angelman syndromes can also arise with uniparental disomy. With Prader-Willi syndrome both number 15 chromosomes come from the mother; with Angelman syndrome, both arise from the father. Other disorders associated with uniparental disomy are Beckwith-Wiedemann syndrome (two paternal number 11 chromosomes), Silver-Russell syndrome (two maternal number 7 chromosomes), and transient neonatal diabetes mellitus (two paternal number 6 chromosomes).[37]

Gonadal (or *germline*) mosaicism refers to mutations that occur in some germ cells. All germ cells (oogonia or spermatogonia) initially undergo mitosis before meiosis and gametogenesis begin. If the mutation occurs at some point during these cell divisions, some cell lines entering meiosis and forming gametes will have the mutation, whereas others will not. This can produce pedigrees that are inconsistent with either dominant or recessive inheritance. For example, a dominant disorder may appear in two offspring of normal parents, or an unaffected parent may have affected children by two different partners. Examples of disorders that have been transmitted by this mechanism are achondroplasia and some forms of osteogenesis imperfecta.[35]

Mitochondrial inheritance is unique in that the mitochondria, which are cytoplasmic organelles involved in cellular respiration and production of energy, have their own unique circular DNA (mtDNA) and genes, which encode proteins needed for oxidative phosphorylation as well as transfer and ribosomal rNA.[35] Mitochondrial genes code for different amino acids than do nuclear DNA. Mitochondria are present in the cytoplasm of the ovum; the sperm does not have any cytoplasm to pass on to the offspring. Thus each person, whether male or female, inherits mitochondrial DNA only from the mother. Mitochondrial disorders are rare and generally involve disorders of the central nervous system, skeletal muscles, eyes, or heart. When they occur, all of the woman's offspring are affected.[35]

EMBRYONIC AND FETAL DEVELOPMENT OF THE REPRODUCTIVE SYSTEM

Embryonic and fetal development of the reproductive system involves the formation of the gonads, genital ducts, and external genitalia from undifferentiated primordial structures (indifferent stage) within the embryo that are adapted to meet the functional needs of the two sexes (Figure 1-10). For the male, the gonads differentiate into the testes, and the duct system becomes the efferent ductules of the testes, the duct of the epididymis, the ductus deferens, the seminal vesicles, and most of the urethra. The external genitalia become specialized to form the penis and scrotum. For the female, the gonads differentiate into the ovaries, and the duct system becomes the uterine (fallopian) tubes, uterus, and vagina. The vulva constitutes the external genitalia.

This developmental process begins at fertilization with the determination of genetic sex, passing through three other stages before birth. These include differentiation of gonadal sex, somatic sex, and neuroendocrine sex. After birth, sexual differentiation continues with the development of social sex, psychologic sex, and secondary sex characteristics. These stages determine the final sexual characteristics and behavior of the individual.

Genetic sex is determined by the genes at the time of fertilization and is defined by the sex chromosome complement. Gonadal sex is defined by the structure and function of the gonads; somatic sex involves all other genital organs; and neuroendocrine sex is established by the cyclic or continuous production of gonadotropin-releasing hormones (GnRHs).

Prenatally the reproductive system develops from analogous undifferentiated structures in both sexes. Table 1-5 illustrates the indifferent structures and their male and female derivatives. The basic pattern is the female phenotype; the male reproductive system develops only when the Y chromosome, testosterone, and other organizing substances are present. Prenatal reproductive system development involves three areas: the gonads, the genital ducts, and the external genitalia. Key genes controlling development of the gonadal ridge into the bipotential gonad are *SF1* and *WTI* in both male and female embryos.[69] In the female embryo the *DAX1* and *Wnt4* genes are also needed for ovarian development;

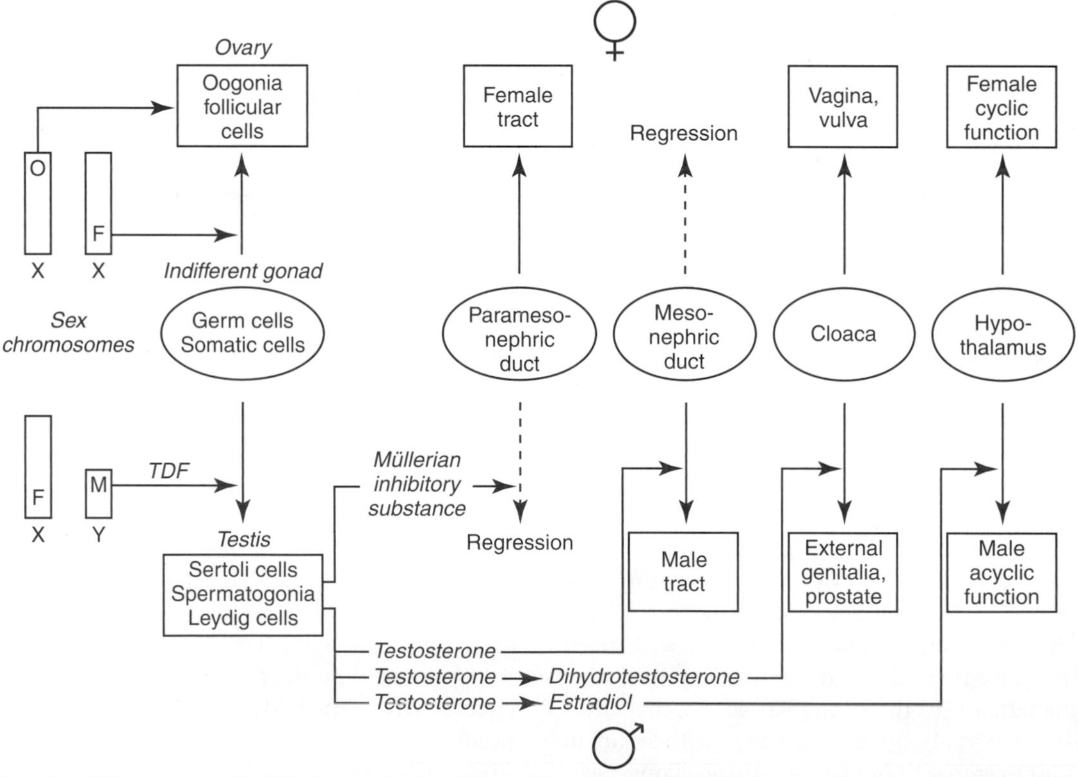

FIGURE 1-10 Proposed regulatory mechanisms in prenatal sexual differentiation. The indifferent stages are in the middle oval blocks. Female structures differentiate upward and male structures downward (solid vertical arrows). Regulatory factors and their source and target are indicated by solid horizontal arrows. Regression is indicated by dashed arrows. *F,* gene for ovarian differentiation; *M,* gene for testicular differentiation; *O,* gene for further ovarian development; *TDF,* testis-determining gene. (From Pelliniemi, L. & Dym, M. [1994]. The fetal gonad and sexual differentiation. In D. Tulchinsky & A.B. Little [Eds.]. *Maternal-fetal endocrinology* [2nd ed.]. Philadelphia: Saunders.)

Table 1-5 Comparison of Male and Female Derivatives of Indifferent Structures in Reproductive System Development

INDIFFERENT STRUCTURE	MALE DERIVATIVE	FEMALE DERIVATIVE
Genital ridge	Testes	Ovary
Primordial germ cells	Spermatozoa	Ova
Sex cords	Seminiferous tubules (Sertoli cells)	Follicular cells
Mesonephric tubules	Efferent ductules	Epoöphoron
	Paradidymis	Paroöphoron
Mesonephric (wolffian) ducts	Appendix of epididymis	Appendix of ovary
	Epididymal duct	Gartner duct
	Ductus deferens	
	Ejaculatory duct	
Paramesonephric (müllerian) ducts	Appendix of testes	Uterine (fallopian) tubes
	Prostate utricle	Uterus
		Upper vagina
Definitive urogenital sinus (lower part)	Penile urethra	Lower vagina
		Vaginal vestibule
Early urogenital sinus (upper part)	Urinary bladder	Urinary bladder
	Prostatic urethra	Urethra
Genital tubercle	Penis	Clitoris
Genital folds	Floor of penile urethra	Labia minora
Genital swellings	Scrotum	Labia majora

From Carlson, B.M. (2004). *Human embryology & developmental biology* (3rd ed.). St. Louis: Mosby.

Wnt4 is also important in development of the müllerian duct into the uterus and fallopian tubes. In males, *SRY*, *SOX9* complemented by *DAX1* are needed for testicular development.[69] Other genes involved in development of the male reproductive system control development and activity of androgen receptors for wolffian duct stabilization and external genitalia development; production of müllerian inhibitory substance and its receptor and genes for formation of testosterone.[69]

Development of the Primordial Germ Cells

The primordial germ cells are first seen at 24 days after fertilization.[10] These cells originate in extraembryonic (yolk sac) mesoderm of the epiblast near the origin of the allantois, following signaling from surrounding tissues.[41] The primordial germ cells proliferate and migrate by amoeboid movements along the dorsal mesentery of the hindgut to the gonadal ridge where they colonize the primitive gonads.[41,57,65,66] The exact mechanism of attraction between the gonadal tissue and the primordial germ cells is unknown, although this migration may be influenced by chemotaxic factors excreted by the primitive gonad.[10] The germ cells express genes that may produce substances to enhance migration. Other genes appear to produce signals to attract the migrating cells to the gonadal ridge and repel them from inappropriate places.[48] If migration is altered and germ cells enter nongonadal tissues, they usually die, but if not, the germ cells might develop into extragonadal teratomas.[10,66] Germ cells induction, proliferation and differentiation is under the control of several sequentially activated genes.[66] Mitotic cell proliferation continues during this migration. The primordial germ cells also undergo changes in chromatin organization during migration. These changes include imprinting with loss of methylation and changes in DNA histone proteins. DNA methylation and imprinting will later be re-established (see Box 1-2 on p. 9). By 42 to 48 days, the germ cells, which have increased from approximately 100 to up to 5000 cells, arrive in the gonadal ridge, where they are incorporated into the mesenchyme.[18,65]

Development of the Gonads

The gonads in the human consist of the ovaries in the female and the testes in the male. These structures are derived from three cellular sources: (1) primordial germ cells, (2) underlying mesenchyme, and (3) coelomic epithelium. Testicular development of the indifferent gonad occurs regardless of whether viable germ cells are present; however, the germ cells must be present for the ovaries to differentiate.[10]

Indifferent Stage

During the fifth week of gestation, a thickening of the coelomic epithelium on the medial side of the mesonephros (see Chapter 11) can be seen; this becomes the genital or gonadal ridge.[57,65] Development of the gonadal ridge is controlled by a group of genes that produce proteins critical for development of this ridge. The surface cells proliferate to form a solid cord of cells that grow downward with fingerlike projections into the mesenchyme, forming the primary sex cords.[57] At the end of 6 weeks, the gonads remain sexually indistinguishable. Two layers can be identified within the gonads: the cortex (coelomic epithelium) and the medulla (mesenchyme). In the XX embryo, the cortex differentiates into the ovary and the medulla essentially regresses. In the XY embryo, the medulla differentiates into the testes and the cortex regresses.

Development of the Testes

Development of the testes begins at 7 to 8 weeks' gestation. The Y chromosome has a strong testis-determining effect on the medulla of the indifferent gonad.[57] The primary sex cords condense and extend into the medulla. Here they branch, canalize, and anastomose to form a network of tubules, the rete testis. These cords are separated from the surface epithelium by a dense layer of connective tissue, the tunica albuginea. Septa grow from the tunica into the medulla to divide the testis into wedge-shaped lobules. Each lobule contains approximately one to three seminiferous tubules, interstitial cells, and supporting cells.

Canalization of the seminiferous cords results in formation of the walls of the tubules by Sertoli (supporting) cells and spermatogenic (germinal) epithelium, which is derived from the primary germ cells.[57,70] The Sertoli cells multiply during growth of the cords until they constitute the majority of the epithelium during fetal life and provide nutrients for the maturing spermatids in adult life.[57,70] The Sertoli cells produce müllerian inhibitory substance (MIS; also called anti-müllerian hormone), which stimulates involution of the müllerian (paramesonephric) ducts. As the Sertoli cells grow, they engulf the germ cells and secrete hormones and factors such as inhibin, activin, cytokines, MIS, and insulin-like growth factor-1 to nourish and sustain the germ cells.[18,48,70] These cells may also secrete a meiosis-inhibiting factor to inhibit spermatogonia meiosis until puberty.[10,48]

The process of cellular reorganization is the first step in male differentiation and is controlled by sex-determining genes on the Y chromosome, including *SRY* and *DAX-1, DAX-2, SOX-9,* and genes needed for steroid production such as *WT-1* and *SF-1*.[18,65,70] These genes produce transcription factors that influence other genes to produce signaling molecules and other proteins that lead to changes characteristic of the male phenotype.[65] Chromosomal translocations, microdeletions and androgen receptor gene mutations are examples of defects that can lead to male infertility. For example, *DAX-1* and *DAX-2* are needed for sperm production and mutations in these genes can result in azoospermia. The *SRY* gene, on the short arm of the Y chromosome, is considered the master gene in testes development, and acts in conjunction with *SOX-9*.[2,10,58,65] *SRY* and *SOX-9* induce the testes to secrete FGF9 which causes tubules from the mesonephric duct to enter the gonadal ridge and increase production of steroidogenesis factor-1 (SF1), which leads to differentiation of Sertoli and Leydig cells. SF1 and *SOX-9* increase production of MIS leading to regression of the paramesonephric duct and SF1 in the Leydig cells up regulates genes for testosterone production.[65]

The mesenchyme contributes masses of interstitial cells (Leydig cells), which proliferate between the tubules. These cells differentiate by 7 to 8 weeks and are functional almost immediately, producing androgens. Testicular testosterone peaks at 12 to 14 weeks, decreases, then peaks again at 28 to 32 weeks' gestation, followed by a decrease to term. Fetal androgens are thought to be important in priming the brain for the male pattern of hormonal release after puberty.[18] The Leydig cells are highly active in the third through fifth gestational months. The rise in testosterone parallels the increase in Leydig cells; after 18 weeks, the number of Leydig cells and testosterone levels decrease. Testosterone and other androgens induce formation of the male genital ducts and masculinization of the external genitalia. In addition, the Leydig cells suppress the development of the müllerian ducts.[57] The testicles start to descend into the inguinal canal during the sixth month, entering the scrotal swellings by 8 to 9 months' gestation. The inguinal canal closes after testes descent.[69]

Development of the Ovaries

In XX embryos, gonadal development begins around 7 weeks' gestation, but occurs more slowly; the ovary is not clearly identifiable until 9 to 10 weeks.[57] The primary sex cords do develop and extend into the medulla of the developing ovary but are not prominent and later degenerate. By the twelfth week, the medulla is mainly connective tissue, with scattered groups of cells that represent the prospective rete ovarii. The rete ovarii appears to be derived from migrating mesonephric cells, which may later give rise to the follicular cells.

During the fourth month, secondary sex cords (cortical cords) are thought to grow into the gonad from the germinal epithelium (surface epithelium).[57] As the cortical cords enlarge, the primordial germ cells are incorporated into them. At around 16 weeks the cords begin to break up into clusters, surrounding the primitive ova (oogonia) with a single layer of flattened supportive follicular cells derived from the cortical cords.[57] After meiotic arrest of the oocyte, the follicular cells become surrounded by a layer of granulosa cells. This complex is the primordial follicle, which will later become the primary follicle (see Chapter 3).[57] Cells of the primordial follicle secrete substances to nurture the oocytes.[48] The surface epithelium becomes separated from the follicles, which lie in the cortex, by a thin fibrous capsule, the tunica albuginea. The ovary, like the testis, separates from the regressing mesonephros, becoming suspended by its own mesentery (mesovarium).[57] The ovary seems to have no significant role in development of the genital ducts and external genitalia.[18]

Female gonadal differentiation occurs in the absence of the testes-organizing genes on the Y chromosome and under the influence of estrogens.[42] *Wnt4, DAX1, FOXL1,* and *RSPO1* are genes that are involved in ovarian development.[42] *Wnt4* up regulates other genes for female genital tract development. For example, *Wnt4* up regulates *DAX1* to inhibit *SOX9* (involved in testicular development).[65] The genes involved in ovarian induction and organization appear to act only if the testes-organizing gene on the Y chromosome is not active. For primary ovarian differentiation, only one X chromosome need be present, so this stage proceeds in 45, X (Turner Syndrome) fetuses. Later development of the female genital system (from about 15 weeks on) requires the presence of 2 X chromosomes, so in most 45, X individuals have abnormal follicular development with oocyte degeneration (gonadal dysgenesis).[53,57] Locally produced estrogen is present by 10 to 14 weeks, peaks at 20 weeks, and may begin to program the hypothalamus for cyclic release of gonadotropins after puberty.[18]

Development of the Genital Ducts

Both male and female embryos have two pairs of genital ducts, the mesonephric (wolffian) duct, which forms at 28 to 39 days, and the paramesonephric (müllerian) duct, which forms at 40 to 42 days.[18] The mesonephric duct originates as part of the urinary system and is incorporated into the developing gonad during the sixth week of gestation. The müllerian ducts initially develop alongside the wolffian ducts in both sexes but reach complete development only in females. The female ducts differentiate autonomously without external regulatory factors, whereas the male system is regulated by testicular androgens and MIS.

Indifferent Stage

The wolffian ducts drain the mesonephric kidneys and develop into the ductus deferens, the epididymis, and the ejaculatory ducts in the male when the mesonephric tubules degenerate. In the female the wolffian ducts almost completely degenerate. The müllerian ducts develop bilaterally alongside the wolffian ducts. The müllerian ducts run caudally parallel to the wolffian ducts, then cross in front of them, fusing to form a Y-shaped canal.[57] The müllerian ducts are retained in the female and regress in the male.

Development of the Male Genital Ducts

MIS stimulates involution of the müllerian ducts in the male during the eighth week. Under the influence of testosterone and other androgens, the wolffian ducts are retained and incorporated into the genital system. The majority of the mesonephric tubules disappear, except those that are in the region of the testes. These 5 to 12 mesonephric tubules lose their glomeruli and join with the rete testis. This creates a communication between the gonads and the wolffian duct. At this point the tubules are called the efferent ductules; these greatly elongate and become convoluted, making up the majority of the caput epididymis. The wolffian duct becomes the ductus epididymis in this region. Below this area, the wolffian duct incorporates muscle tissue and becomes the ductus deferens (vas deferens). The urethra makes up the remainder of the male genital duct system. Development of the male genital ducts is completed by 12 weeks. Local secretion of testosterone from the testes causes differentiation of the ipsilateral wolffian duct; systemic secretion of testosterone influences differentiation of the external genitalia. So a female with excess systemic testosterone (such as occurs with congenital adrenal hyperplasia) will not have development of structures that arise from the wolffian duct (since these structures arise from production of local testosterone from the testes) but will have ambiguous genitalia (influenced by systemic testosterone from adrenals).[69] MIS is produced bilaterally and acts on the side produced. So if only one testes develops, MIS will not be produced and act on that side of the body where the testes is missing so the müllerian duct will not regress on that side.[69]

Development of the Female Genital Ducts

In the female embryo, the wolffian ducts regress at 11 weeks due to lack of testosterone and other androgens, whereas the müllerian ducts are retained due to lack of MIS. Female sexual development, which is under control of the *Wnt* and *HOX* gene families and estrogens, is not dependent upon the presence of ovaries.[52,57] The müllerian ducts become the fallopian tubes, uterus, and proximal vagina in the female. The cranial unfused portions of the müllerian ducts develop into the fallopian tubes; the caudal portion fuses to form the uterovaginal primordium. The latter gives rise to the epithelium and glands of the uterus and to the vaginal wall. The endometrial lining and the myometrium are derived from the surrounding mesenchymal tissue. The vaginal epithelium is derived from the endoderm of the urogenital sinus, and the fibromuscular wall of the vagina develops from the uterovaginal primordium. Initially the vagina is a solid cord (the vaginal plate); the vaginal lumen is formed as the central cells of the plate break down.

The broad ligaments are formed from the peritoneal folds that occur during fusion of the müllerian ducts. The broad, winglike folds extend from the lateral portions of the uterus to the pelvic wall. The folds of the broad ligaments are continuous with the peritoneum and divide the pelvis into anterior and posterior portions. Between the layers of the broad ligament, the mesenchyme proliferates to form loose connective tissue and smooth muscle. This complex of tissue provides support and attachment for the uterus, fallopian tubes, and ovaries.

Development of the External Genitalia

The early development of the external genitalia is similar in male and female embryos. Distinguishing characteristics can be seen during the ninth week of gestation, with definitive characteristics being fully formed by the twelfth week.[57] Development of the external genitalia is summarized in Figure 1-11.

Indifferent Stage

The external genitalia initially appear similar. Early in the fourth week, a swelling can be identified at the cranial end of the cloacal membrane; this is the genital tubercle. Genital (labioscrotal) swellings and genital folds soon develop alongside the cloacal membrane. The genital tubercle elongates at this time and is the same length in both sexes. The urorectal septum fuses with the cloacal membrane, dividing the membrane into a dorsal anal membrane and a ventral urogenital membrane. These membranes rupture around the eighth week, forming the anus and urogenital orifice. The urethral sinus, which is continuous with the urogenital orifice, forms on the ventral surface of the genital tubercle at this time (see Figure 1-11).[57]

Development of the Male External Genitalia

The androgens produced by the fetal testes, especially dihydrotestosterone, induce the masculinization of the external genitalia of the male embryo. The genital tubercle continues to elongate, forming the penis and pulling the genital folds forward. This results in the development of the lateral walls of the urethral groove by the genital folds (see Figure 1-11, *A*). The posterior-to-anterior fusion of the genital folds as they come in contact results in the development of the spongy urethra and the progressive movement of the urethral orifice toward the glans of the penis. The opening, however, remains on the undersurface of the phallus.[57] Backward growth of a plate of ectodermal tissue from the tip of the phallus to the urethra forms the terminal part of the

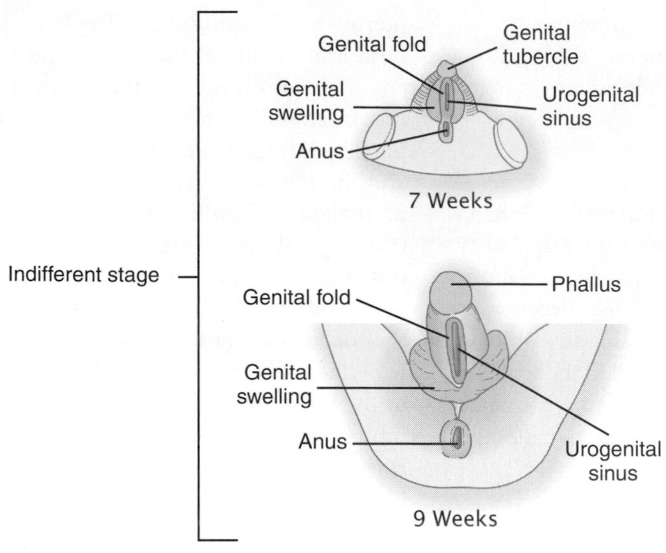

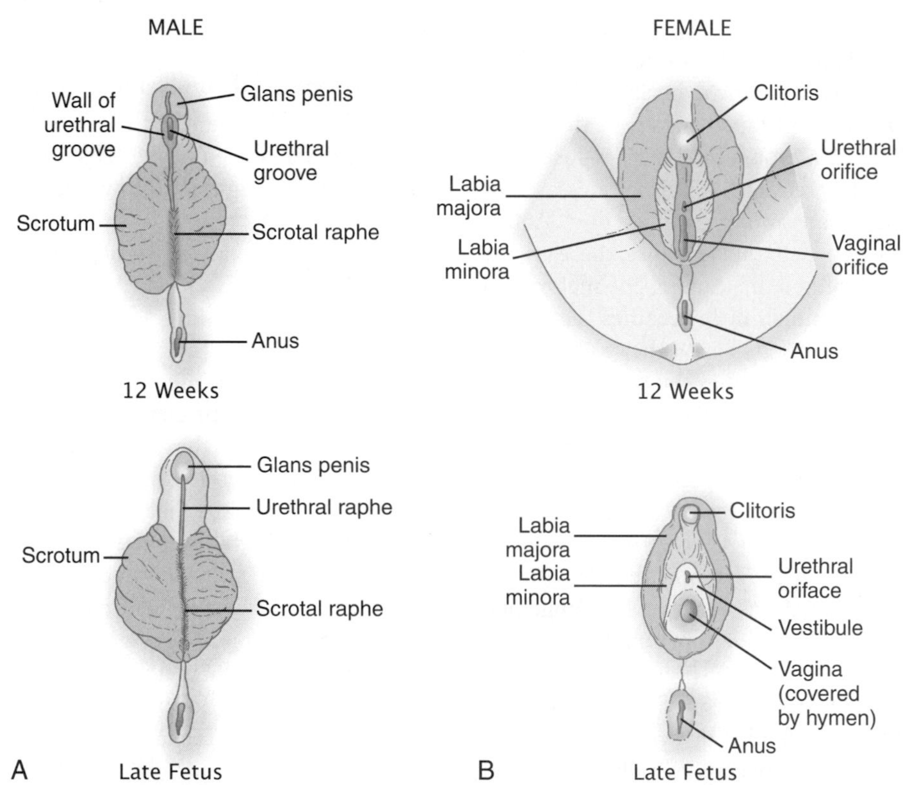

FIGURE 1-11 Differentiation of the external genitalia in males **(A)** and females **(B).** (From Carlson, B.M. [2004]. *Human embryology & developmental biology* [3rd ed.]. St. Louis: Mosby.)

urethra. Once canalized, the urinary and reproductive systems will have achieved an open system. This, along with the descent of the testes into the genital swellings (scrotum), completes the development of the external genitalia (see Figure 1-11, *A*).

After the penile urethra has formed, the connective tissue surrounding the urethra becomes condensed to form the corpus cavernosum urethrae, in which numerous wide and convoluted blood vessels having many arteriovenous anastomoses develop. The genital swellings also grow toward each other and fuse to form the scrotum. External genitalia development in the male is complete by 14 weeks except for continued phallic growth and testicular descent. Tissue swelling occurs in order to dilate the inguinal canal and scrotum in preparation for the descent of the testes, which is usually complete by the eighth month of gestation.

Descent of the testes occurs in two phases: transabdominal descent and inguinoscrotal descent. Descent is moderated by many forces, including the enlargement of the pelvis, trunk growth, and the testes' remaining relatively stationary, as well as the influence of gonadotropins and androgens.[32,57] The teste is released from the urogenital ridge and moves toward the scrotum. At about 32 weeks, the testes actually enter the scrotum. Once passage is complete, the inguinal canal contracts around the spermatic cord. The spermatic cord consists of the vas deferens, blood vessels, and nerves. In 97% of infants, the testes have descended bilaterally before delivery. During the first 3 months following delivery, the majority of undescended testes will descend without intervention.[32,57]

Development of the Female External Genitalia

Without androgens, feminization of the neutral external genitalia occurs and is complete by 11 weeks. Initially, the genital tubercle grows rapidly; however, it gradually slows, becoming the relatively small clitoris. The clitoris develops like the penis, except that the urogenital folds do not fuse. Both the urethra and the vagina open into the common vestibule, which is widely open after the disappearance of the urogenital membrane. The opening is flanked by the urethral folds and the genital swellings, which become the labia minora and majora, respectively (see Figure 1-11, *B*).

Anomalies of the Genital Tract

Anomalies encountered in the reproductive system may be secondary to any of three major factors occurring individually or in combination: (1) genetic makeup, (2) endocrine and hormonal environment, and (3) mechanical events. Each may lead to alterations in development and reproductive ability. Because the embryo is genitally bipotential, when genetic or hormonal factors alter development, the embryo may develop various disorders of sex development.[6,33,42] Mechanical congenital anomalies are related to developmental arrests, interference, or failures that result in changes in normal morphologic patterns.

Disorders of Sex Development

Absence of one or both gonads is a rare disorder. If gonadal agenesis is unilateral, absence of the renal system on the affected side is common. Failure or defective development of nephrogenic mesenchyme is probably the cause, although the etiology of such failure is not known.

Turner syndrome is one of the more common sex chromosome abnormalities. This syndrome is seen in an estimated 0.8% to 1% of spontaneously aborted fetuses and once in every 4000 to 5000 live births. The absence or deletion of an X chromosome usually results in an individual with a 45, XO karyotype, with 80% due to paternal nondisjunction.[2,58] Mosaics (46,XX/45,XO) often have functioning ovaries. In most other cases, however, there is ovarian dysgenesis associated with other somatic abnormalities.[2] Klinefelter syndrome (47,XXY) is seen in 1 out of 1000 live births and is characterized by a small testes and impaired spermatogenesis.

Ovitesticular disorders of sex development are extremely rare.[33,57] Individuals may be 46,XX; 46,XY; or mosaic XX/XY. They have both ovarian and testicular tissue, either as separate organs or as a single ovotestis. Usually the gonadal tissue is not functional, but in some individuals oogenesis and spermiogenesis may occur simultaneously. The external genitalia are ambiguous, but the rest of the physical appearance may be either male or female. This abnormality seems to be the result of an error in sexual determination and lack of dominance of the cortex or medulla of the genital ridge.[57] Possible causes include translocation of testicular differentiation genes to the X chromosome, a mutant gene, or undetected XY cells in the gonad. The presence of uterus and fallopian tubes indicates defective functioning of MIS. In those individuals who are mosaic 46,XX/XY, the etiology involves the union of two zygotes of different genetic sex. The two cell lines develop normally, with limits being set by their topographic distribution during ontogeny.

XY disorders of sex development involve alterations in androgen synthesis or action. Infants have more or less dysgenetic testes with an XY constitution. There is incomplete differentiation of the external genitalia secondary to testicular dysgenesis and insufficient testosterone production.[2] This abnormality may be associated with altered development of the internal genitalia due to inadequate production of MIS and thus the müllerian ducts fail to completely regress.[2] Causes may include a deficiency in the 5α-reductase enzyme necessary to convert testosterone to dihydrotestosterone so that external virilization can occur. In testicular feminization syndrome, there is an inability to bind androgens in target tissues; in other situations, transmission of androgens from the receptor to the nucleus is blocked.[2,57] Externally, the genitalia may be either ambiguous or feminine. Internal structures may also vary. These male infants have varying degrees of phallic and müllerian duct development, even though their karyotype is 46,XY. When differentiation occurs, males with 5α-reductase deficiencies have testosterone and its derivatives in the external genitalia tissue but not in the developing wolffian duct. Testosterone may appear in the wolffian ducts after the period of tissue sensitivity has passed.[7,57] Males with the X-linked gene for testicular feminization (46,XY) have normally differentiated testes; however, these children look like normal females. The vagina ends in a blind pouch, and the uterus and fallopian tubes are nonexistent or rudimentary.[57] The testes are usually intraabdominal or inguinal, or they may descend into the labia majora. There are high levels of circulating testosterone with elevated levels of gonadotropins. Unfortunately, testosterone receptor sites will not bind or incorporate testosterone into the cells in the genital swellings and genital folds.[57] These individuals have female genitalia, and at puberty there is development of female secondary sex characteristics; however, menstruation does not occur. The psychosexual orientation of these children is usually female.[2,57]

XX disorders of sex development involve androgen excess in 46,XX female infants is 46,XX, who have a congenital virilization of the external genitalia. This is usually termed **adrenogenital syndrome** or **congenital adrenal hyperplasia** (CAH), meaning hyperfunction of the adrenal cortices associated with ambiguous genitalia. The most common cause is an excessive production of androgens, which may be due to maternal disease (e.g., adrenal tumor) but is more likely to be of fetal origin. Lack of 21-hydroxylase (an enzyme involved in steroid metabolism) is usually the cause of CAH. Most often these cases involve clitoral hypertrophy, partial fusion of the labia majora, and a persistent urogenital sinus. The infants with this syndrome do have functioning ovaries, fallopian tubes, uterus, and cervix. The wolffian duct does not develop. Often there are other metabolic disorders that require complex care.[2] (CAH is described in more detail in Chapter 19.)

Hypospadias and Epispadias

Hypospadias (urethral orifice on the ventral surface of the penis) may be an isolated abnormality or associated with a disorder of sex development, especially if the penis is very abnormal. The more severe the degree of hypospadias is, the higher the possibility of testicular dysgenesis and of cryptorchidism. This defect occurs in 3 to 5 out of 1000 live births and is probably due to inadequate androgen production, resulting in failure of urogenital fold fusion and incomplete spongy urethra formation.[57,65] The incidence of hypospadius has increased in the past 15 to 20 years for unknown reasons, but possibly due to increased environmental estrogens from industrial chemicals and pesticides.[65] There are four types of hypospadias, with 80% being either glandular or penile. The other 20% are penoscrotal or perineal. Variations in this defect are due to the timing and degree of hormonal failure.[10,57] Epispadias is a relatively rare congenital anomaly, occurring once in every 30,000 live births. The dorsal surface urethral opening is often associated with exstrophy of the bladder. Epispadias may be glandular or penile and is probably due to caudal development of the genital tubercle, resulting in the urogenital sinus being on the dorsal surface once the membrane has ruptured.[10,57]

Uterovaginal Malformation

Fusion defects of the müllerian ducts result in varying degrees of structural duplication. Complete fusion failure leads to the development of two complete genital tracts, in which the vagina is divided in two by a septum, with a separate cervix and uterine body associated with each half (didelphia). If one of the müllerian ducts fails to develop entirely, the result will be uterus unicornis. Various other anomalies may also result, including a single vagina with double cervices, a single vagina and cervix associated with a uterus subdivided into halves, or a single uterus that is incompletely separated by a septum (bicornate, unicornous, vagina simplex). Any of these anomalies may result in infertility.[57]

CLINICAL IMPLICATIONS

Genetic Screening

Carrier screening of adults is done for selected disorders. Usually a population at increased risk for a specific disorder is targeted, for example screening of individuals of Ashkenazi Jewish descent for Tay-Sachs disease. Carrier screening for cystic fibrosis is recommended for couples planning pregnancy or seeking prenatal care.[22] Other disorders may also be screened, depending on risk factors.[62] Issue with genetic screening and diagnosis include interpretation or misinterpretation of data and risks, discrimination (employment, education, insurance), psychologic and social concerns, and issues of the right to know versus the right not to know if one carries a specific gene mutation because genetic disorders are family disorders.

A genetic history should be a routine part of prenatal care to identify women with an increased risk of genetic disorders and birth defects. The family history is a valuable tool in evaluating gene-environment interactions, risk identification, and preventive care.[26] Components of genetic history include family and obstetric history (including a history of pregnancy loss or early infant death, mental retardation or learning disabilities, known genetic disorders, or having infants with anomalies in either of the parents or their families), ethnic background (some recessive disorders occur with markedly increased frequency in specific ethnic groups), maternal and paternal age, and potential teratogen exposures.[67,73] Genetic screening and use of diagnostic techniques such as amniocentesis and chorionic villus sampling (CVS) allow for prenatal identification of increasing numbers of chromosomal, genetic, and other congenital anomalies. Maternal serum screening is used to screen for selected chromosomal anomalies, neural tube defects and other disorders.[4,20] Routine ultrasounds provide an opportunity to observe for major anomalies in the fetus. Ultrasound markers that may allow noninvasive diagnosis have also been identified for infants with Down syndrome and other disorders.[7,27] These techniques and others are described in Chapter 3.

Newborn screening for genetic and other disorders was begun in the 1960s with screening for phenylketonuria (PKU) with additional disorders added in subsequent years. Newborn screening is the only mandated genetic screening. In the United States, each state determines the disorders that will be screened. An expert panel recommended development of a uniform screening panel.[54] Introduction of new techniques such as tandem mass spectrometry (MS/MS) have significantly expanded the numbers of disorders screened. MS/MS can be used to rapidly screen the newborn for up to 55 metabolic disorders in a single analytic run using the dried filter paper blood spot that has been the mainstay of newborn screening since its inception.[5,11,31] The March of Dimes has recently recommended that all infants be screened for 30 disorders, including selected fatty acid, amino acid and organic acid disorders, hemoglobinopathies, congenital hypothyroidism, and other disorders such as congenital adrenal hyperplasia, galactosemia, cystic fibrosis, and biotinidase deficiency.[31,50] Currently all states screen for at least 21 disorders, some screen for up to 54.[31] MS/MS has been determined to be effective in identifying infants with various disorders of fatty acid oxidation, amino acid disorders, and organic acidopathies. MS/MS has also raised questions in that disorders can now be identified for which effective therapies have not yet been developed. More infants are being identified with variations that are not clinically significant variations.[11] In addition, although the number of infants diagnosed with metabolic disorders has increased, it is not clear whether all of these individuals would have eventually become symptomatic or not.[77] Other concerns about newborn screening include the role of written informed parental consent (not currently required in most states) for testing and storage of blood spots for epidemiologic research.[5,11,31] There are also continuing concerns about the effects of false-positive screens on parental stress and parent-infant interaction. Availability of newer techniques such as DNA microarray technology will continue to alter newborn screening.[24,59]

Genetic Disorders and Pregnancy

Genetic disorders can influence the course of pregnancy and have implications for both the mother and the fetus/newborn. In addition, the anatomic and physiologic changes of pregnancy can influence the course of the disorder. Women with severe genetic disorders may have difficulty conceiving. However, with earlier diagnosis after birth and improved therapies, many individuals with genetic disorders are surviving to adulthood and having children. This section will focus on women with two genetic disorders, cystic fibrosis (CF) and phenylketonuria, as examples.

CF is an autosomal recessive multisystem disorder seen most frequently in Caucasian (1 out of 3000 to 3300 live births) and Ashkenazi Jewish (1 out of 3970 live births) populations.[22] CF is due to an abnormal gene on chromosome 7. This gene codes for a protein (CF transmembrane conductance regulator or CFTR) needed for regulating chloride transport across cell membranes. There are more than 1000 CFTR mutations with 70% of CF patients having one of the eight most common mutations. Differences in mutations leads to variations in phenotype and severity. With decreasing mortality, more women with CF are surviving to childbearing age. Although males with CF are often infertile without assisted reproductive technologies, females with CF are able to conceive, although they may have altered fertility, possibly due to impaired ovulation due to the effects of the altered CFTR on the hypothalamus, uterine secretions and cervical mucus and in the endometrium and fallopian tubes.[55] Assuming the partner of a woman with CF is not a carrier, all of their children will be carriers. If the partner is a carrier, there is a 50% risk with each pregnancy of having a child with CF; all nonaffected offspring will be carriers.

CF involves alterations in the exocrine glands and mucus-secreting glands, especially the pancreas and sweat glands, affecting the respiratory, digestive, and reproductive systems. Prepregnancy pulmonary function is a predictor of pregnancy outcome. The normal changes in the respiratory system during pregnancy (see Chapter 10) may stress already compromised pulmonary function resulting in decompensation and increased maternal and fetal mortality and morbidity.[30] Women with mild CF generally do well during pregnancy.[49,55,76] However, women with moderate to severe CF, especially those with hypoxemia, cor pulmonale, and poor nutritional status, often do not do well.[49,76] Particularly ominous is preexisting pulmonary hypertension. In these women, the usual pregnancy increase in cardiac output cannot be accommodated within the pulmonary vasculature. This leads to further desaturation, myocardial hypoxia, decreased cardiac output, and increased hypoxia.[76] Weight loss or poor weight gain during pregnancy is associated with a poor outcome.[49,76] McArdle reviewed as series of 9 studies published since 2000 of pregnancy outcomes in women with CF.[55] Most studies reported an increase prematurity rate with a further increase in preterm births in women with lower pregnancy lung function or diabetes. Forced expiratory volume in 1 sec (FEV_1) <50%-60% was associated with an increased risk of poorer outcomes including increased risk of pregnancy loss, prematurity, and low birthweight and, in some studies, with increased maternal mortality and pregnancy complications. Overall there was no evidence that long term survival was different in women with CF who became pregnant versus those who did not (mean survival in all individuals with CF was 37.4 years in 2008).[19,55]

Phenylketonuria (PKU) is an amino acid disorder due to mutations in a gene on chromosome 12 for production of the enzyme phenylalanine hydroxylase. Severity depends on the mutations, with 400 mutations identified.[1,35] The deficiency of phenylalanine hydroxylase results in elevated levels of phenylalanine that can damage the central nervous system. Outcomes have improved in individuals with PKU due to newborn screening and early initiation of a phenylalanine-restricted diet. Women with PKU have normal fertility. However, their fetuses are at risk if the woman's phenylalanine levels are elevated during pregnancy. Phenylalanine readily crosses the placenta with a 1.5 fetal to maternal plasma ratio.[1] The teratogenic effects of high levels of maternal serum phenylalanine include mental retardation, congenital heart defects, intrauterine growth restriction, spontaneous abortion, altered facies, and microcephaly.[1,35,67] Exposure to high levels of phenylalanine in the first 8 weeks of gestation increases the risk of structural defects; from 8 to 12 weeks, of altered growth of the brain and body; and after 12 weeks, of altered neurologic development.[67] Ninety percent of women with phenylalanine levels greater than 20 mg/dL (1210.8 μmol/L) will have an affected child.[67] Thus dietary control and treatment for 3 months prior to preconception and during pregnancy can reduce sequelae. However, many women of childbearing age with PKU may not adhere to the unpalatable PKU-free diet.[1] Matalon, Acosta and Azen reported that decreasing maternal phenylalanine levels to 600 μmol/L or less was associated with a significant decrease in the incidence of microcephaly.[53]

SUMMARY

The biologic basis for reproduction includes an understanding of basic genetic mechanisms and principles, including cell division, gametogenesis, chromosomal and genetic alterations, and modes of inheritance. Our knowledge in these

BOX 1-3 Selected Genetic Websites

American College of Medical Genetics
www.acmg.net
American Medical Association Family History Tools
www.ama-assn.org/ama/pub/category/2380.html
Gene Tests
www.ncbi.nlm.nih.gov/sites/GeneTests/?db=GeneTests
Genetics and Your Practice
www.marchofdimes.com/gyponline/index.bm2\
Genetics Home Reference
http://ghr.nlm.nih.gov/
Genomics and Its Impact on Science and Society: The Human Genome Project and Beyond
www.ornl.gov/sci/techresources/Human_Genome/publicat/primer2001/index.shtml
Genomics Gallery (Images)
http://genomics.energy.gov/gallery/basic_genomics/gallery-01.html
Human Genome Project
www.ornl.gov/sci/techresources/Human_Genome/home.shtml
International Society of Nurses in Genetics
www.isong.org/
March of Dimes
www.marchofdimes.com
National coalition for Health Professional education in Genetics
www.nchpeg.org/
National Human Genome Research Institute Glossary of Genetic Terms
www.genome.gov/glossary/index.cfm?
National Newborn Screening and Genetics Resource Center
http://genes-r-us.uthscsa.edu
Online Mendelian Inheritance in Man (OMIM)
www.ncbi.nlm.nih.gov/sites/entrez?db=omim
U.S. Surgeon General's Family History Initiative. Family History Tool
www.hhs.gov/familyhistory
Your Genes and Your Health
www.ygyh.org/

Table 1-6 Chromosomes and Reproductive Biology: Clinical Implications for the Care of Mothers and Neonates

Understand the biologic basis for genetic and chromosomal disorders (pp. 1-5, 10-14).
Understand modes of inheritance (pp. 14-18; see also Tables 1-3 and 1-4).
Provide counseling and health teaching to parents regarding genetic disorders and modes of inheritance (pp. 14-18 and Table 1-1).
Perform a genetic and family history as part of routine care (p. 24 and Chapter 3).
Counsel parents about prenatal screening and assist them in interpreting results (p. 24 and Chapter 3).
Teach parents with a familial history of chromosomal or genetic abnormalities about the basis for the disorder (pp. 14-18).
Refer parents with a familial history of chromosomal or genetic abnormalities for genetic counseling (p. 24 and Chapter 3).
Refer neonates born with abnormal genitalia for complete endocrine evaluation, ultrasonography of internal structures, and chromosomal assessment (pp. 23-24).
Teach parents about newborn screening (pp. 24-25).
Understand the effects of genetic disorders on the woman and her fetus during pregnancy (p. 25).
Provide counseling and health teaching to women with genetic disorders before and during pregnancy (p. 25).

areas remains limited but is increasing rapidly. The current revolution in genetic knowledge has markedly altered and challenged our understanding of health and disease and provision of health care, and it will continue to do so. The more nurses and other health care providers understand about the areas and the reproductive processes described in Chapter 2, the more they can work toward ways to improve perinatal outcome. Box 1-3 above lists Internet resources for genetics and genetic disorders. Clinical implications for mothers and neonates can be found in Table 1-6.

References

1. American College of Obstetricians and Gynecologists Committee on genetics. (2009). ACOG Committee Opinion No. 449: maternal phenoketonuria. *Obstet Gynecol, 114*, 1432.
2. Arbolito, V.A. & Vilain, E. (2009). Disorders of sexual development. In J.F. Strauss & R. Barbieri (Eds.). *Yen and Jaffe's reproductive endocrinology: Physiology, pathophysiology, and clinical management* (6th ed.). Philadelphia: Saunders.
3. Austin, C.P. (2004). The impact of the completed human genome sequence on the development of novel therapeutics for human disease. *Ann Rev Med, 55*, 1.
4. Bahado-Singh, R.O. & Argoti, P. (2010). An overview of first-trimester screening for chromosomal abnormalities. *Clin Lab Med, 30*, 545.
5. Banta-Wright, S.A. & Steiner, R.D. (2004). Tandem mass spectrometry in newborn screening: A primer for neonatal and perinatal nurses. *J Perinat Neonatal Nurs, 18*, 41.
6. Barbaro, M., Wedell, A., & Nordenström, A. (2011). Disorders of sex development. *Semin Fetal Neonatal Med, 16*, 119.
7. Benacerraf, B.R. (2010). The history of the second-trimester sonographic markers for detecting fetal Down syndrome, and their current role in obstetric practice. *Prenat Diagn, 30*, 644.
8. Bettegowda, A. & Wilkinson, M.F. (2010). Transcription and post-transcriptional regulation of spermatogenesis. *Philos Trans R Soc Lond B Biol Sci, 365*, 1637.

9. Biliya, S. & Bulla, L.A. Jr. (2010). Genomic imprinting: The influence of differential methylation in the two sexes. *Exp Biol Med (Maywood), 235*, 139.
10. Carlson, B.M. (2008). *Human embryology and developmental biology* (4th ed.). St. Louis: Mosby.
11. Carlson, M.D. (2004). Recent advances in newborn screening for neurometabolic disorders. *Curr Opin Neurol, 17*, 133.
12. Carrel, L. & Willard, H.F. (2005). X-inactivation profile reveals extensive variability in X-linked gene expression in females. *Nature, 434*, 400.
13. Carrell, D.T. & Hammoud, S.S. (2010). The human sperm epigenome and its potential role in embryonic development. *Mol Hum Reprod, 16*, 37.
14. Clayton, E.W. (2003). Ethical, legal, and social implications of genomic medicine. *N Engl J Med 349*, 562.
15. Collins, F.S. & McKusick, V.A. (2001). Implications of the Human Genome Project for medical science. *JAMA, 285*, 540.
16. Collins, P. (2008). Cellular mechanisms in development. In C.R. Rodeck & M.J. Whittle (Eds.). *Fetal medicine: Basic science and clinical practice* (2nd ed). London: Churchill Livingstone.
17. Critchlow, H.M., Payne, A., & Griffin, D.K. (2004). Genes and proteins involved in the control of meiosis. *Cytogenet Genome Res, 105*, 4.
18. Cummings, A.M. & Kavlock, R.J. (2004). Gene-environment interactions: A review of effects on reproduction and development. *Crit Rev Toxicol, 34*, 461.
19. Cystic Fibrosis Foundation. (2009). *Patient registry: Annual data report 2009*. http://www.cff.org; Last accessed April 22, 2011.
20. Dugoff L; Society for Maternal-Fetal Medicine. (2010). First- and second-trimester maternal serum markers for aneuploidy and adverse obstetric outcomes. *Obstet Gynecol, 115*, 1052.
21. Gaucher, J., et al. (2010). From meiosis to postmeiotic events: The secrets of histone disappearance. *FEBSJ, 277*, 599.
22. Goetzinger, K.R. & Cahill, A.G. (2010). An update on cystic fibrosis screening. *Clin LabMed, 30*, 533.
23. Gosden, R. & Lee, B. (2010). Portrait of an oocyte: Our obscure origin. *J Clin Invest, 120*, 973.
24. Green, N.S. & Pass, K.A. (2005). Neonatal screening by DNA microarray: Spots and chips. *Nat Rev Genet, 6*, 147.
25. Guttmacher, A.E. & Collins, F.S. (2002). Genomic medicine: A primer. *N Engl J Med, 347*, 1512.
26. Guttmacher, A.E., Collins, F.S., & Carmona, R.H. (2004). The family history—more important than ever. *N Engl J Med, 351*, 2333.
27. Haak, M.C. & van Vugt, J.M. (2003). Pathophysiology of increased nuchal translucency: A review of the literature. *Hum Reprod Update, 9*, 175.
28. Hamilton, B.A. & Wynshaw-Boris, A. (2009). Basic genetics and patterns of inheritance. In R.K. Creasy, et al. (Eds.). *Creasy & Resnik's Maternal-fetal medicine: Principles and practice* (6th ed.). Philadelphia: Saunders.
29. Handel, M.A. (2004). The XY body: A specialized meiotic chromatin domain. *Exp Cell Res, 296*, 57.
30. Hassold, T. & Hunt, P. (2001). To err (meiotically) is human: The genesis of human aneuploidy. *Nat Rev Genet, 2*, 280.
31. Hiraki, S. & Green, N.S. (2010). Newborn screening for treatable genetic conditions: Past, present and future. *Obstet Gynecol Clin North Am, 37*, 11.
32. Hughes, I.A. & Acerini, C.L. (2008). Factors controlling testis descent. *Eur J Endocrinol, 159*, S75.
33. Hughes, I.A. (2010). The quiet revolution: Disorders of sex development. *Best Pract Res Clin Endocrinol Metab, 24*, 159.
34. Human Genome Project. (2008). http://www.ornl.gov/hgmis/project/about.html; Last accessed April 22, 2011.
35. Jorde, L.B., et al. (2009). *Medical genetics* (4th ed.). St. Louis: Mosby.
36. Kacem, S. & Feil, R. (2009). Chromatin mechanisms in genomic imprinting. *Mamm Genome, 20*, 544.
37. Kalousek, D.K. & Vekemons, M. (2000). Confirmed placental mosaicism and genomic imprinting. *Baillieres Best Pract Res Clin Obstet Gynecol, 14*, 723.
38. Kelada, S.N., et al. (2003). The role of genetic polymorphisms in environmental health. *Environ Health Perspect, 111*, 1055.
39. Khoury, M.J. (2003). Genetics and genomics in practice: The continuum from genetic disease to genetic information in health and disease. *Genet Med, 5*, 261.
40. Kidder, G.M. & Vanderhyden, B.C. (2010). Bidirectional communication between oocytes and follicle cells. Ensuring oocyte developmental competence. *Can J Physiol Pharmacol, 88*, 399.
41. Kota, S.K. & Feil, R. (2010). Epigenetic transitions in germ cell development and meiosis, *Dev Cell, 19*, 675.
42. Kousta, E., Papathanasiou, A., & Skordis, N. (2010). Sex determination and disorders of sex development according to the revised nomenclature and classification in 46, XX individuals. *Hormones (Athens), 9*, 218.
43. Lashley, F.R. (2008). *Essentials of clinical genetics in nursing practice*. New York: Springer.
44. Lee, M.K., et al. (2012). Regulation of embryogenesis. In R.A. Polin, W.W. Fox, & S.H. Abman (Eds.). *Fetal and neonatal physiology* (4th ed.). Philadelphia: Saunders.
45. Levine, F. (2012). Basic genetic principles. In R.A. Polin, W.W. Fox, & S.H. Abman (Eds.). *Fetal and neonatal physiology* (4th ed.). Philadelphia: Saunders.
46. Lynn, A., Ashley, T., & Hassold, T. (2004). Variation in human meiotic recombination. *Annu Rev Genomics Hum Genet, 5*, 317.
47. Lyon, M.K. (1999). X-chromosome inactivation, *Curr Biol, 9*, R235.
48. MacLaughlin, D.T. & Donahoe, P.K. (2004). Sex determination and differentiation. *N Engl J Med, 350*, 367.
49. Mandel, J. & Weinberger, S.E. (2004). Pulmonary diseases. In G.N. Burrow, T.P. Duffy, & J.A. Copel (Eds.). *Medical complications during pregnancy* (6th ed.). Philadelphia: Saunders.
50. March of Dimes. (2010). *Recommended newborn screening tests: 30 disorders*. http://www.marchofdimes.com/baby/bringinghome_recommendedtests.html; Last accessed April 22, 2011.
51. Marteil, G., Richard-Parpaillon, L., & Kubiak, J.Z. (2009). Role of oocyte quality in meiotic maturation and embryonic development. *Reprod Biol, 9*, 203.
52. Massé, J., et al. (2009). The developing female genital tract: From genetics to epigenetics. *Int J Dev Biol, 53*, 411.
53. Matalon, K.M., Acosta, P.B., & Azen, C. (2003). Role of nutrition in pregnancy with phenylketonuria and birth defects. *Pediatrics, 112*, 1534.
54. Maternal and Child Health Bureau. (2005). *Newborn screening: Toward a uniform screening panel and system*. http://mchb.hrsa.gov/screening; Last accessed April 23, 2011.
55. McArdle, J.R. (2011). Pregnancy in cystic fibrosis. *Clin Chest Med, 32*, 111.
56. Miao, Y.L., et al. (2009). Oocyte aging: cellular and molecular changes, developmental potential and reversal possibility. *Hum Reprod Update, 15*, 573.
57. Moore, K.L. & Persaud, T.V.N. (2011). *The developing human: Clinically oriented embryology* (9th ed.). Philadelphia: Saunders.
58. Morton, C.L. & Lee, C. (2009). Cytogenetics in reproduction. In J.F. Strauss & R. Barbieri (Eds.). *Yen and Jaffe's reproductive endocrinology: Physiology, pathophysiology, and clinical management* (6th ed.). Philadelphia: Saunders.
59. Murray, J.C. (2012). Impact of the Human Genome Project on neonatal care. In C.A. Gleason & S. Devaskar (Eds.). *Avery's diseases of the newborn* (9th ed.). Philadelphia: Saunders..
60. Pointis, G., et al. (2010). Physiological and physiopathological aspects of connexins and communicating gap junctions in spermatogenesis. *Philos Trans R Soc Lond B Biol Sci, 365*, 1607.
61. Rajender, S., Rahul, P., & Mahdi, A.A. (2010). Mitochondria, spermatogenesis and male infertility. *Mitochondrion, 10*, 419.
62. Ram, K.T. & Klugman, S.D. (2010). Best practices: Antenatal screening for common genetic conditions other than aneuploidy. *Curr Opin Obstet Gynecol, 22*, 139.
63. Ross, M.T. (2005). The DNA sequence of the human X chromosome. *Nature, 434*, 325.
64. Ruwanpura, S.M., McLachlan, R.I., & Meachem, S.J. (2010). Hormonal regulation of male germ cell development. *J Endocrinol, 205*, 117.

65. Sadler, T.W. (2012). *Langman's medical embryology* (12th ed.) Philadelphia: Lippincott Williams & Wilkins.
66. Schoenwolf, G.C., et al. (2009). *Larsen's human embryology* (4th ed.) Philadelphia: Churchill Livingstone.
67. Seashore, M.R. (2004). Clinical genetics. In G.N. Burrow, T.P. Duffy, & J.A. Copel (Eds.). *Medical complications during pregnancy* (6th ed.). Philadelphia: Saunders.
68. Shastry, B.S. (2009). SNPs: Impact on gene function and phenotype. *Methods Mol Biol, 578*, 3.
69. Shulman, R. M., Palmert, M.R., & Wherrett, D.K. (2011). Disorders of sex development. In R.J. Martin, A.A. Fanaroff, & M.C. Walsh (Eds.). *Fanaroff and Martin's neonatal-perinatal medicine: Diseases of the fetus and infant* (9th ed.). St. Louis: Mosby.
70. Stukenborg, J.B., Colón, E., &, Söder, O. (2010). Ontogenesis of testis development and function in humans. *Sex Dev, 4*, 199.
71. Vander, A., Sherman, J., & Luciano, D. (2004). *Human physiology: The mechanism of body function* (9th ed.). New York: McGraw-Hill.
72. Venter, J.C., et al. (2001). The sequence of the human genome. *Science, 291*, 1304.
73. Wapner, R.J., Jenkins, T.M., & Khalek, N. (2009). Prenatal diagnosis of congenital disorders. In R.K. Creasy, et al. (Eds.). *Creasy & Resnik's Maternal-fetal medicine: Principles and practice* (6th ed.). Philadelphia: Saunders.
74. Ward, W.S. (2010). Function of sperm chromatin structural elements in fertilization and development. *Mol Hum Reprod, 16*, 30.
75. Weaver, J.R., Susiarjo, M., & Bartolomei, M.S. (2009). Imprinting and epigenetic changes in the early embryo. *Mamm Genome, 20*, 532.
76. Whitty, J.E. & Dombrowski, M.P. (2009). Respiratory diseases in pregnancy. In R.K. Creasy, et al. (Eds.). *Creasy & Resnik's Maternal-fetal medicine: Principles and practice* (6th ed.). Philadelphia: Saunders.
77. Wilcken, B., et al. (2003). Screening newborns for inborn errors of metabolism by tandem mass spectrometry. *N Engl J Med, 348*, 2304.
78. Wolgemuth, D.J. & Roberts, S.S. (2010). Regulating mitosis and meiosis in the male germ line: Critical functions for cyclins. *Philos Trans R Soc Lond B Biol Sci, 365*, 1653.
79. Zhu, H., Kartiko, S., & Finnell, R.H. (2009). Importance of gene-environment interactions in the etiology of selected birth defects. *Clin Genet, 75*, 409.

CHAPTER 2

Physiologic Basis for Reproduction

Robin Webb Corbett

Hormones regulate differentiation of the reproductive and central nervous systems in the developing fetus; stimulation of sequential growth and development during childhood and adolescence; and coordination of male and female reproductive systems.

Hormones facilitate sexual reproduction, maintenance of an optimal internal environment, and initiation of corrective and adaptive responses with emergencies. These important physiologic processes are regulated by two major systems: the nervous system and the hormonal system (Figure 2-1). Hormonal regulation of reproductive processes is via the hypothalamic-pituitary-ovarian (HPO) system in the female and the hypothalamic-pituitary-testes (HPT) system in the male.

This chapter will review and discuss the hormonal regulation of the reproductive process for both the male and female. Content addressed includes discussion of reproductive hormones, oogenesis, spermatogenesis, puberty, the ovarian and menstrual cycles, and changes with aging in females and males specific to reproduction.

HYPOTHALAMIC PITUITARY-OVARIAN/ TESTICULAR AXIS

During reproductive life, reproductive function is regulated by cyclic reproductive neuroendocrinology, which is dependent upon the complex interplay of a feedback system involving the ovary or testes, hypothalamus, and anterior pituitary. Expression of hypothalamic-pituitary hormones stimulates ovarian steroid secretion and folliculogenesis (Figure 2-2); the testes produce testosterone which stimulates spermatogenesis. The gonadotropins (follicle-stimulating hormone [FSH] and luteinizing hormone [LH]) and gonadal steroids (estrogen, progesterone, and testosterone) induce follicular maturation, ovulation, and pregnancy in the female and spermatogenesis and steroidogenesis in the male. Thus a woman's and man's reproductive status is entrained to their cyclic neuroendocrine environment.

Hormones

A hormone is a chemical substance secreted into body fluids by a cell or a group of cells that exerts a physiologic effect on other cells of the body, its target cells. Hormones are released into the bloodstream by endocrine glands. The blood carries the hormones to specific cells or organs, hormonal target sites.

Hormone Activators, Receptors, and Messenger Systems

Hormones are chemical messengers that have specific rates and patterns of secretion (e.g., diurnal or other patterns). These patterns, which are pulsatile and have circadian or ultradian rhythmicity, depend on the levels of circulating substrates, calcium, sodium, or the hormone.[12] Various factors affect the circulating level of hormones. Receptor affinity and concentration are regulated by the intracellular and extracellular environment, such as body temperature, calcium and sodium concentrations, and serum pH. Other physiochemical factors affecting hormone release include urea concentration and the lipid matrix of the plasma membrane. Circulating hormone levels are also regulated by growth and development, diet, drugs, sleep-wake cycle, seasonal environmental cues (photoperiod [dark-light cycle]) and exercise.[11,33] Most hormone secretion is episodic (ultradian rhythm) and circadian.[11]

Hormones are constantly excreted by kidneys or deactivated by the liver. Hormones are classified by structure, target gland or origin, effects, or chemical classes. Structural categories of hormones include proteins (prolactin), glycoproteins (FSH and LH), polypeptides (oxytocin), steroids (estrogens, progestins, and testosterone), and fatty acids (prostaglandins and thromboxanes).[11,67] For each hormone, there is a specific cellular receptor, located on the cell surface or within the cell. The majority of hormonal receptors are very large proteins. Hormones bind with appropriate cell receptors, forming a hormone receptor complex, and act on the cell to initiate specific cell functions or activities. Receptor location varies with the type of hormone. For example, protein or peptide hormone receptors are located in or on the cell membrane, whereas steroid hormones such as estrogen diffuse freely across the plasma membrane and have their receptors in the cell cytoplasm. Thyroid hormone receptors are located in the nucleus. Hormone binding with the target cell receptor causes the number of receptors to decrease, a process known as down-regulation (Figure 2-3). In contrast, with up-regulation,

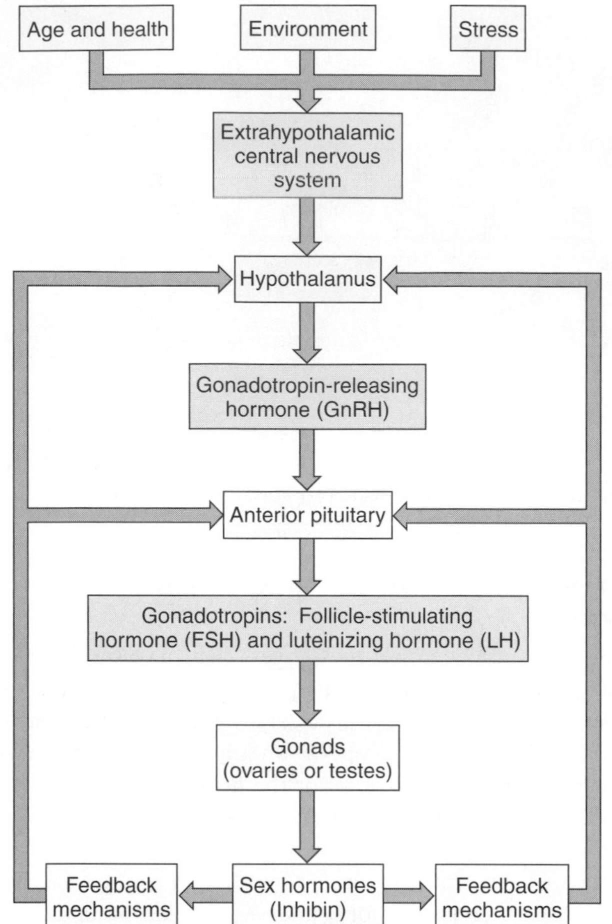

FIGURE 2-1 Hormonal stimulation of the gonads: The hypothalamic-pituitary-gonadal axis. (Adapted from McCance, K.L. & Huether, S.E. [2006]. *Pathophysiology: The biologic basis for disease in adults and children* [5th ed.]. St. Louis: Mosby.)

low concentrations of hormones increase the number of receptors per cell. As receptors decrease with down-regulation, responsiveness of the target tissue decreases. In the unbound state, receptors are inert.

Receptor activation on the target cell may be initiated by a variety of mechanisms such as a first messenger system, a second messenger system, and genetic sequencing. In the first messenger system, the hormone recognizes and binds with its specific receptor. Formation of the hormone receptor complex activates enzymes within the cell with subsequent phosphorylation. The second messenger system may act synergistically or antagonistically to regulate cell activities. Second messengers include cyclic adenosine monophosphate (cAMP), inositol triphosphate, calcium ions, phospholipids, and the calcium-calmodulin complex.

Cellular responses are initiated by transmission of an intracellular signal via a second messenger (Table 2-1) that signals the effect of the hormone on the target cell as membrane transport. Hormone receptor binding increases the intracellular level of second messengers such as cAMP (Table 2-2). The cAMP second messenger system binds with a G protein and converts adenosine triphosphate into cAMP, which then activates a protein kinase A (PKA) pathway, leading to phosphorylation and enzyme activation (Figure 2-4). FSH, LH, and human chorionic gonadotropin (hCG) are hormones that respond to the cAMP second messenger system.[11,77] FSH and LH act on the ovary via the cAMP intracellular signaling pathway.[55,77] Cyclic adenosine monophosphate is a common intracellular messenger during both follicular and luteal phases.[77] GnRH is activated via the phospholipase C second messenger system (Table 2-3).

Hormones bind with the receptor at the cell membrane, catabolizing phosphatidyl-inositol biphosphate into inositol triphosphate and the second messenger diacylglycerol. Similar to cAMP, diacylglycerol activates a protein kinase, phosphorylates, and initiates the cellular response[5] (Figure 2-5). Diacylglycerol activity may result in the synthesis of prostaglandins or combine with calcium, activating cellular metabolic action. Calcium is accessed from the intracellular endoplasmic reticulum and mitochondria by inositol triphosphate, which activates cell functions. Calcium is also mobilized in the calcium-calmodulin second messenger system by binding intracellularly with calmodulin. This binding mediates the use of calcium in the activation, inhibition, or phosphorylation of protein kinases, with subsequent cellular response.[46] After binding with specific receptors, steroid hormones synthesize proteins, which in the nucleus bind with chromosomal deoxyribonucleic acid (DNA) to facilitate the formation of messenger ribonucleic acid (mRNA) and subsequent proteins via genetic instructions.[26]

Hormone Storage

There is no single way in which endocrine glands store and secrete hormones. The amount of hormone stored in the glandular cells is minuscule, but large amounts of precursor molecules, such as cholesterol and its intermediaries, are present within the cell. With specific stimulation, enzymes initiate conversion of these precursors to the final hormone followed by hormone expression. For example, the protein hormone prolactin is initially formed by the endoplasmic reticulum. Known as a preprohormone, this protein is larger than the active hormone and is cleaved while still in the endoplasmic reticulum, yielding a smaller protein molecule—prohormone. The prohormone is transported in vesicles to the Golgi apparatus, where the protein is further processed to form the final active protein hormone. The Golgi apparatus compacts the hormone molecules into small membrane-encapsulated vesicles known as **secretory vesicles.** There the final hormone is stored in the cytoplasmic compartment of the endocrine cell, awaiting its specific signal (nerve, hormonal, or chemical) for hormone secretion.

Hypothalamic and Pituitary Glands

The pituitary gland, also known as the hypophysis, is composed of two segments: the anterior and posterior lobes (Figure 2-6). The hypophysis is pea sized and approximately 15 mm long, sitting in a protected saddle-shaped sphenoid bone cavity

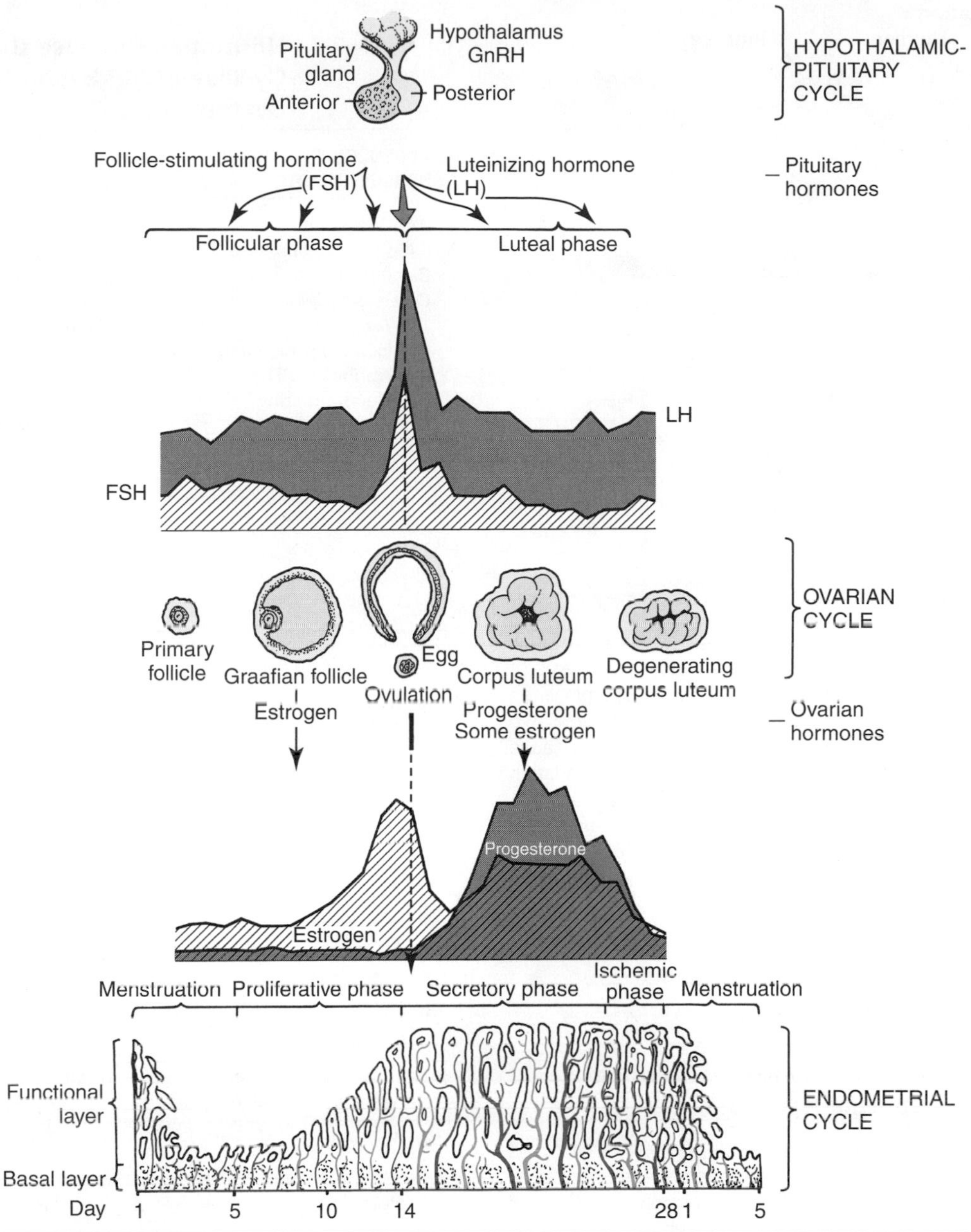

FIGURE 2-2 Menstrual cycle: hypothalamic-pituitary, ovarian, and endometrial. *GnRH,* Gonadotropin-releasing hormone. (From Lowdermilk, D.L. & Perry, S.E. [2007]. *Maternity & women's health care* [9th ed.]. St. Louis: Mosby.)

(the sella turcica) at the base of the brain, directly behind the nasal base. The pituitary gland is slightly heavier in women and may double in size during pregnancy (see Chapter 19). The pars tuberalis, pars distalis, and the intermediate lobe comprise the anterior lobe, the adenohypophysis.[53] The neurohypophysis (i.e., posterior lobe) is composed of the median eminence, infundibular stem, and neural lobe.[46,53] Many hormones are secreted by the anterior pituitary, including growth hormone, adrenocorticotropin, thyroid-stimulating hormone, FSH, LH, and prolactin. Anterior pituitary gland cells known as **gonadotrophs** secrete FSH and LH.[48] About 60% of gonadotrophs (10% to 15% of pituitary cells) are multihormonal, secreting both FSH and LH.[45] Only two hormones are secreted by the posterior pituitary: antidiuretic hormone and oxytocin.

To regulate physiologic processes, communication must occur between the pituitary gland, the hypothalamus, and the target glands and cells. The pituitary gland connects to the hypothalamus directly above the pituitary stalk. The anterior pituitary gland is linked to the hypothalamus via blood vessels known as the hypothalamic-hypophyseal portal system (see Figure 2-6). The pituitary receives blood from the paired superior hypophyseal arteries, which arise from the

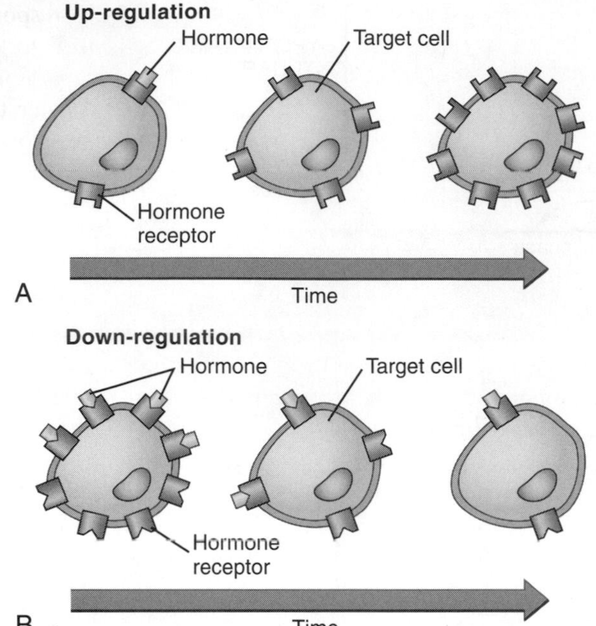

FIGURE 2-3 Regulation of target cell sensitivity. If synthesis of new receptors occurs faster than degradation of old receptors, then the target cell will have more receptors and thus be more sensitive to hormone. This phenomenon **(A)** is called up-regulation because the number of receptors goes up. If the rate of receptor degradation exceeds the rate of receptor synthesis, then the target cell's number of receptors will decrease **(B).** Because the number of receptors and thus the sensitivity of the target cells goes down, this phenomenon is called down-regulation. Shading represents hormone concentration. (From Thibodeau, G.A. & Patton, K.T. [2007]. *Anatomy and physiology* [6th ed.]. St. Louis: Mosby.)

Table 2-1 Second Messengers Identified for Specific Hormones

SECOND MESSENGER	ASSOCIATED HORMONES
Cyclic AMP	Adrenocorticotropic hormone (ACTH)
	Luteinizing hormone (LH)
	Human chorionic gonadotropin (hCG)
	Follicle-stimulating hormone (FSH)
	Thyroid-stimulating hormone (TSH)
	Antidiuretic hormone (ADH)
	Thyrotropin-releasing hormone (TRH)
	Parathyroid hormone (PTH)
	Glucagon
Cyclic GMP	Atrial natriuretic hormone
Calcium	Angiotensin II
	Gonadotropin-releasing hormone (GnRH)
	Antidiuretic hormone (ADH)
IP_3 and DAG	Angiotensin II
	Luteinizing hormone-releasing hormone (LHRH)

From McCance, K.L. & Huether, S.E. (2006). *Pathophysiology: The biologic basis for disease in adults and children* (5th ed.). St. Louis: Mosby. *AMP,* Adenosine monophosphate; *DAG,* diacylglycerol; *GMP,* guanosine monophosphate; *IP_3,* inositol triphosphate.

Table 2-2 Hormones That Use the Adenyl Cyclase-cAMP Second Messenger System

ADRENOCORTICOTROPIC HORMONE (ACTH)	GLUCAGON
Angiotensin II (epithelial cells)	Human chorionic gonadotropin (hCG)
Calcitonin	Luteinizing hormone (LH)
Catecholamines (β-receptors)	Parathyroid hormone (PTH)
Corticotropin-releasing hormones (CRH)	Secretin
Follicle-stimulating hormone (FSH)	Thyroid-stimulating hormone (TSH)
	Vasopressin (V_2 receptor, epithelial cells)

From Guyton, A.C. & Hall, J.E. (2006). *Textbook of medical physiology* (11th ed.). Philadelphia: Saunders.

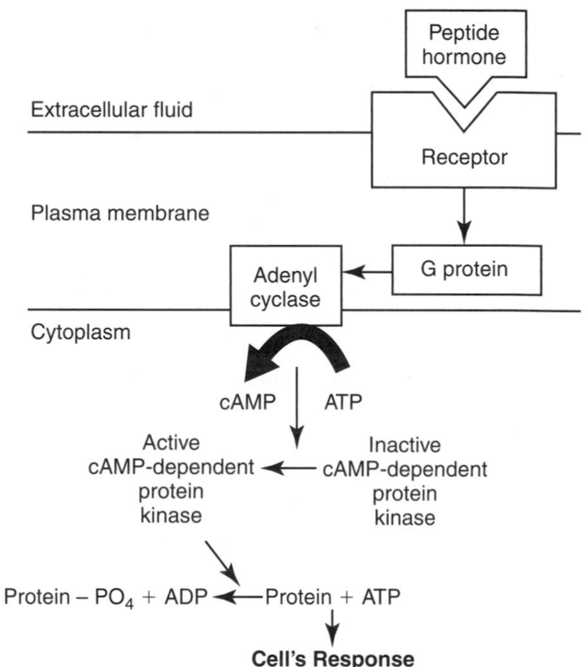

FIGURE 2-4 Cyclic adenosine monophosphate (cAMP) mechanism, by which many hormones exert their control of cell function. *ADP,* Adenosine diphosphate; *ATP,* adenosine triphosphate. (From Guyton, A.C. & Hall, J.E. [2006]. *Textbook of medical physiology* [11th ed.]. Philadelphia: Saunders.)

internal hypophyseal artery, which is a branch of the internal carotid arteries, and merge at the upper pituitary stalk.[11,46] The inferior hypophyseal and trabecular arteries supply the neural lobe. The anterior pituitary sinusoids receive blood from the hypophyseal portal vessels, long and short portal veins that arise in the median hypothalamic eminence.[11]

Hypothalamic hormones, which are either releasing hormones (RHs) or inhibiting hormones (IHs), control

Table 2-3 Hormones That Use the Phospholipase C Second Messenger System

ANGIOTENSIN II (VASCULAR SMOOTH MUSCLE)	OXYTOCIN
Catecholamines (α-receptors)	Thyroid-releasing hormone (TRH)
Gonadotropin-releasing hormone (GnRH)	Vasopressin (V_1 receptor, vascular smooth muscle)
Growth hormone–releasing factor (GHRF)	

From Guyton, A.C. & Hall, J.E. (2006). *Textbook of medical physiology* (11th ed.). Philadelphia: Saunders.

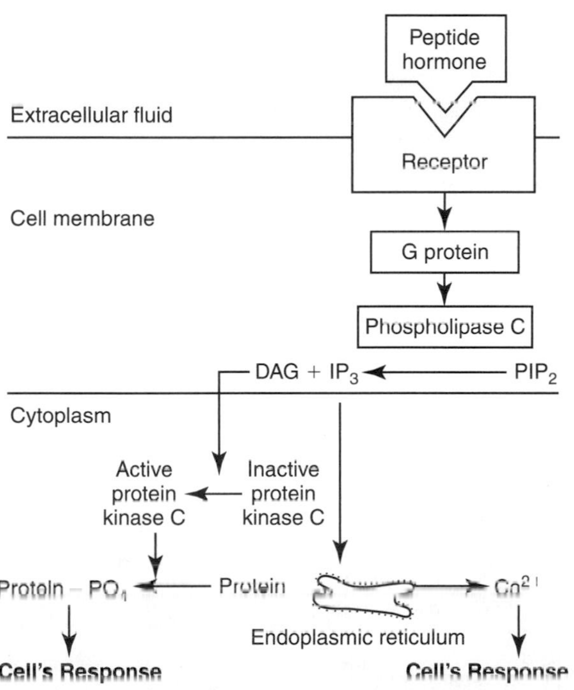

FIGURE 2-5 The cell membrane phospholipid second messenger system, by which some hormones exert their control of cell function. *DAG,* Diacylglycerol; *IP*$_3$, inositol triphosphate; *PIP*$_2$, phosphatidyl-inositol biphosphate. (From Guyton, A.C. & Hall, J.E. [2006]. *Textbook of medical physiology* [17th ed.]. Philadelphia: Saunders.)

expression of the anterior pituitary hormones. RHs and IHs are discharged into the blood vessels of the hypothalamic-hypophyseal portal system. The vascular system permits transport of gonadotropin-releasing hormones (GnRHs) from the hypothalamus down the pituitary stalk to the anterior pituitary lobe, where they trigger the release of anterior pituitary gonadotropins (FSH and LH). Blood vessels end in capillaries at both ends, allowing movement of RHs that moderate pituitary secretion from the hypothalamus (see Figure 2-6). When hypothalamic neurons (neurosecretory neurons) are stimulated, these neurosecretory cells respond by releasing RHs, into the portal circulation and then to the anterior pituitary.[75] Hypothalamic RHs travel via nerve fibers to the infundibulum of the neurohypophysis and enter the peripheral circulation by the perigomitolar capillary network.[23] Long and short portal vessels travel parallel to the pituitary stalk and terminate in the anterior pituitary capillaries.[23]

The posterior pituitary lobe receives nerve fibers from the supraoptic and paraventricular nuclei of the anterior hypothalamus through the pituitary stalk, known as the neurohypophysis. The posterior pituitary, an extension of the hypothalamus, is composed of glial-like cells (i.e., pituicytes), the supporting structure for terminal nerve fibers and terminal nerve endings. Axon terminals comprise the major part of the neural lobe. Axon terminals are derived from the magnocellular secretory neurons (one type of hypothalamic neurosecretory cell) of the paraventricular and supraoptic nuclei of the hypothalamus (see Figure 2-6). A cell body located in the supraoptic or paraventricular hypothalamic nucleus projects its neuronal process into the neural lobe and the neurohormone (posterior pituitary hormones) is released from the nerve endings. The axon terminals traverse the internal zone median eminence and in association with the capillary plexus secrete posterior pituitary hormones into the hypophyseal veins and subsequently the general circulation.[47] Posterior pituitary hormones travel from the hypothalamus to the neurohypophysis via neurosecretory neurons.[11] Neurohypophyseal hormones travel to the neurohypophyseal tract through the pituitary stalk for storage in the posterior pituitary capillary nerve endings via neurophysins (protein binders).[26] Nerve endings, which are shaped like bulbous knobs, lie on the surfaces of the capillaries, onto which are secreted vasopressin and oxytocin.

REPRODUCTIVE HORMONES IN FEMALES AND MALES

The hypothalamic-pituitary-ovarian/testicular axis is regulated by hormones synthesized and expressed by the hypothalamus, pituitary, ovaries, testicles, and adrenals (Figure 2-7). Some of these hormones and their physiology are well known, including LH, FSH, activin, inhibin, follistatin, estrogens, progesterone, dehydroepiandrosterone sulfate (DHEAS), dehydroepiandrosterone (DHEA), 5x–dihydrotestosterone (DHT), androsterone, and testosterone (Table 2-4). Other hormones are less well known. These include oocyte maturation inhibitor, luteinization inhibitor, and gonadotropin surge–inhibiting factor. Hormonal innervation is independent but also interdependent with other hormones, specifically dose response and receptor proliferation and sensitivity.

Hormones synthesized by the hypothalamus include GnRHs, which mediate anterior pituitary hormone secretion. In response to stimulation by GnRH, the anterior pituitary expresses the hormones known collectively as gonadotropins (i.e., FSH, LH) that enhance follicular proliferation and maturation and subsequent ovulation in females. The ovaries

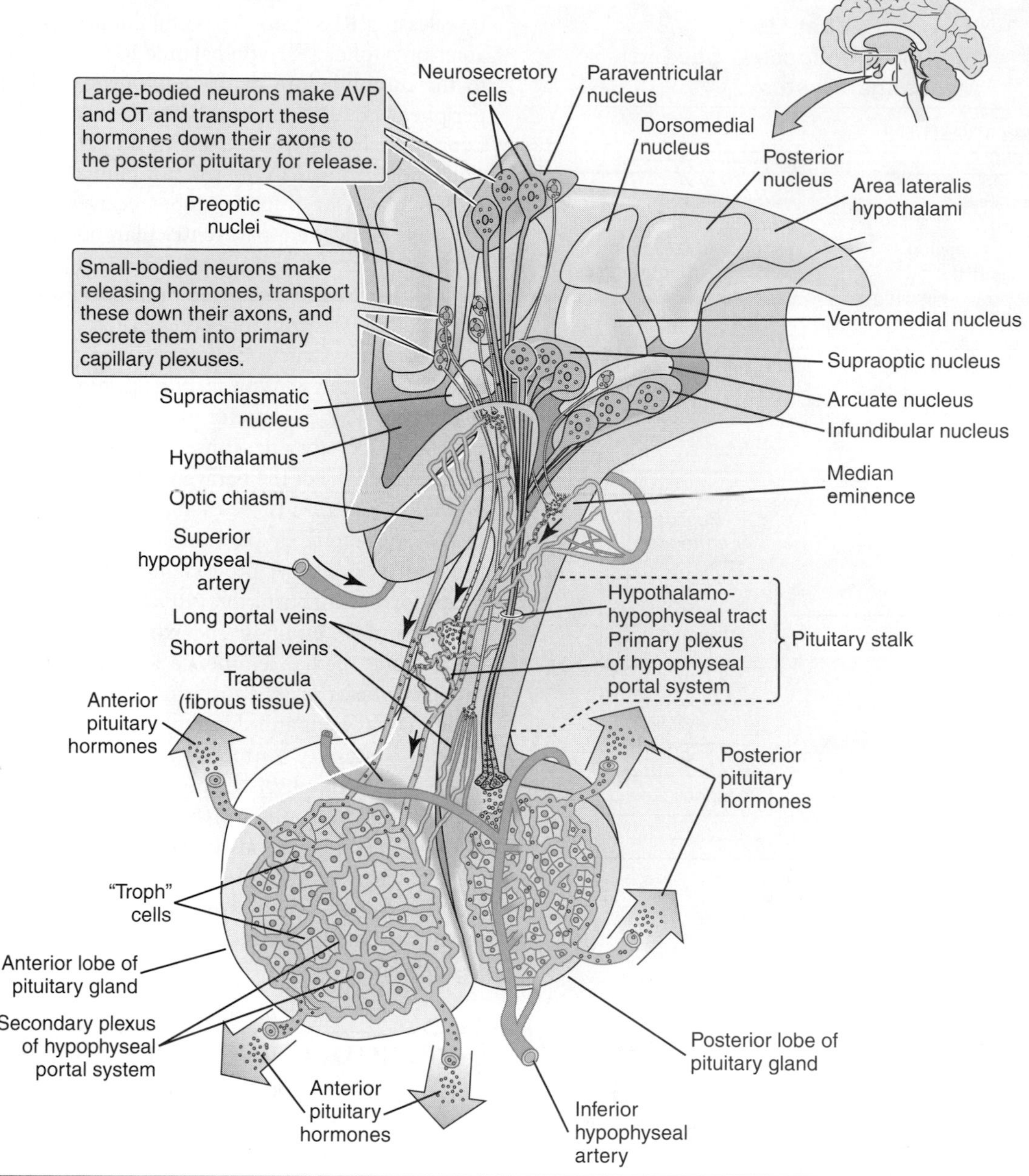

FIGURE 2-6 The hypothalamic-pituitary portal system. (From Boron, W.F. & Boulpaep, E.L. [2005]. *Medical physiology*. Philadelphia: Saunders.)

and adrenal cortices synthesize DHEA, the precursor hormone for the steroidal hormones estrogen, progesterone, and testosterone. Steroidal hormones (i.e., estrogen, progesterone) and gonadotropins enhance follicular proliferation and maturation of the dominant follicle in preparation for the mid-cycle LH surge and ovulation.

In males, the gonadotropins regulate steroidogenesis and gametogenesis in the testes. The FSH/LH ratio is lower in males than females. Leydig cells, in response to LH synthesize and secrete testosterone. FSH acts on the seminiferous tubules, where stimulation by FSH enhances germ cell maturation. Receptors for testosterone and FSH are located on the Sertoli cell's germinal epithelium. Sertoli cells are responsible for sperm production, with approximately 1.54 sperm per sertoli cell.[51]

Luteinizing Hormone

LH is a glycoprotein that is secreted by the anterior pituitary. LH is the primary hormone involved in ovulation. This hormone promotes theca interstitial cell androgen biosynthesis with the eventual conversion to estradiol in the presence of FSH.[11,23] Small but sustained increments of LH enhance the development and growth of small antral follicles to preovulatory stage. Receptors for LH are located in the ovarian thecal and luteal cells and testicular Leydig cells.[11]

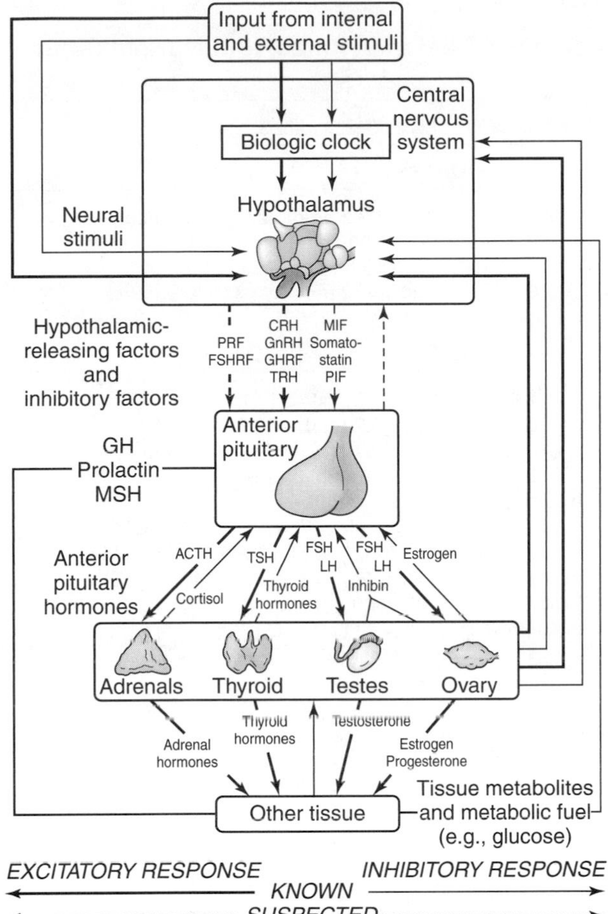

FIGURE 2-7 Schematic drawing of the relationships and feedback mechanisms of the hypothalamus and pituitary glands. Hypothalamic releasing and inhibitory factors include the following: corticotropin-releasing hormone (CRH), gonadotropin-releasing hormone (GnRH), growth hormone–releasing factor (GHRF), thyrotropin-releasing hormone (TRH), dopamine, somatostatin, prolactin-inhibiting factor (PIF), and prolactin-releasing factor (PRF). Anterior pituitary hormones include the following: growth hormone (GH), prolactin, adreno-corticotropic (ACTH); thyrotropin, or thyroid-stimulating hormone (TSH), follicle-stimulating hormone (FSH), and luteinizing hormone (LH). Posterior pituitary hormones include arginine vasopressin and oxytocin. *FSHRF*, Follicle-stimulating hormone–releasing factor; *MIF*, melanocyte-stimulating hormone–inhibiting factor; *MSH*, melanocyte-stimulating hormone. (From Frohman, L.A. [1980]. In D.T. Krieger & J.C. Hughes [Eds.]. *Neuroendocrinology: A hospital practice book*. Sunderland, MA: Sinauer Associates. Illustration by Nancy Lou Gahan and Albert Miller. Copyright by The McGraw-Hill Companies, Inc.)

Under the influence of FSH and LH, ovarian granulosa cells acquire LH receptors in mid to late follicular phase. These gonadotropins synergistically promote follicular development, increase ovarian granulosa cells, and produce inhibin.[41] In the preovulatory phase, LH levels rise dramatically, a process known as the LH surge. Within 10 to 12 hours of LH peak levels (or 28 to 32 hours of the onset of the LH surge), ovulation occurs.

Nicotine (tobacco use) inhibits pulsatile LH secretion in males but not in females.[18] LH stimulates the synthesis and secretion of testosterone by Leydig cells in the testis.[51]

Follicle-Stimulating Hormone

FSH is a glycoprotein gonadotropin secreted by the anterior pituitary. FSH promotes follicular growth and differentiation, FSH and LH receptors, inhibin and activin activities, and estrogen synthesis. Receptors for FSH are located on the ovarian granulosa and testicular Sertoli cells.[11] FSH is instrumental in estrogen formation, pubertal development, and follicular maturation.[36] FSH is also instrumental in the induction of aromatase in ovarian granulosa cells for estrogen production.[66] Although not mandatory for early follicular development, FSH is necessary for follicular development beyond the small antral follicle size.[36] Antral formation is enhanced in response to FSH expression.[53] In concert with estradiol, FSH increases FSH receptors and LH receptors located on the granulosa cells.[66] Testosterone suppresses the secretion of GnRH and FSH and LH; inhibin and follistatin inhibit FSH secretion. In contrast, activin stimulates the secretion of FSH.[51] FSH receptors are located on the germinal epithelium of the Sertoli cells with FSH acts specifically on the seminiferous tubules. Proliferation of the Sertoli cell is correlated with FSH and LH exposure.

Activin

Activin is a glycoprotein that activates the release of FSH.[27,42] Composed of dimers of the β-inhibin subunits, activin A is synthesized in gonadal tissue but may also be synthesized in nongonadal organs, such as bone marrow.[8] During pregnancy, activin A has been isolated in the placenta and fetal membranes.[30] Higher activin concentrations overcome the effect of inhibin, with a resulting increase in FSH expression. Activin levels are independent of FSH stimulation.[8] Activin levels are highest midcycle and in the late luteal–early follicular phase. Levels are even higher during pregnancy, peaking at term.[30,66] Jenkin and colleagues[30] suggest that elevated activin A concentrations are associated with fetal distress. Activin from ovarian granulosa cells promote FSH-induced growth of LH receptors on granulosa cells and inhibits synthesis of thecal cell LH, progesterone, and estrogen. In addition, activin may promote maturation of oocytes.[66] Activin levels do not vary according to age or gender.[23] However, activin A concentrations during the menstrual cycle range from 100 to 200 pg/mL, whereas postmenopausal levels may be five times higher than these levels.

Inhibin

Inhibin, another glycoprotein, suppresses FSH secretion from the hypophysis.[27,42] Inhibin is synthesized primarily by the ovarian granulosa cells and is secreted into the follicular fluid.[21] Synthesis of inhibin is regulated in response to gonadotropins or factors that increase intracellular cAMP. There are two different forms of inhibin: inhibin A and inhibin B. Inhibin A and B have similar biologic characteristics; the primary difference is that hormonal synthesis is regulated differently during the follicular and luteal phases (Figure 2-8). FSH regulates inhibin production by the ovarian granulosa cells. LH augments inhibin production in the granulosa cells with the acquisition of

Table 2-4 **Blood Production Rates, Secretion Rates, Metabolic Clearance Rates, and Normal Serum Concentration of Sex Steroid Hormones**

STEROID HORMONE	REPRODUCTIVE PHASE	MCR (L/DAY)	PR (MG/DAY)	SR (MG/DAY)	REFERENCE VALUES
MEN					**TESTES**
Androstenedione		2200	2.8	1.6	80.2-209.7 ng/dL (2.8-7.3 nmol/L)
Testosterone		950	6.5	6.2	198.8-1000 ng/dL (6.9-34.7 nmol/L)
Estrone		2050	0.15	0.11	10-67.56 ng/dL (37-250 pmol/L)
Estradiol		1600	0.06	0.05	<10.1-57.2 pg/mL (<37-210 pmol/L)
Estrone sulfat		167	0.08	Insignificant	600-2500 pmol/L
WOMEN					**OVARY**
Androstenedione		2000	3.2	2.8	88.8-349.6 ng/dL (3.1-12.2 nmol/L)
Testosterone		500	0.19	0.06	20.2-80.7 ng/dL (0.7-2.8 nmol/L)
Estrone	Follicular	2200	0.11	0.08	2.9-10.8 ng/dL (110-400 pmol/L)
	Luteal	2200	0.26	0.15	310-660 pmol/L
	Postmenopausal	1610	0.04	Insignificant	22-230 pmol/L
Estradiol	Follicular	1200	0.09	0.08	<10.1-98.1 pg/mL (<37-360 pmol/L)
	Luteal	1200	0.25	0.24	190.1-340.5 pg/mL (699-1250 pmol/L)
	Postmenopausal	910	0.006	Insignificant	<10.1-38.1 pg/mL (<37-140 pmol/L)
Estrone sulfate	Follicular	146	0.10	Insignificant	700-3600 pmol/L
	Luteal	146	0.18	Insignificant	1100-7300 pmol/L
Progesterone	Follicular	2100	2.0	1.7	0.3-3.0 nmol/L
	Luteal	2100	25.0	24.0	19.0-45.0 nmol/L

From Strauss, J.F. (2004). The synthesis and metabolism of steroid hormones. In Strauss, J.F. & Barbieri, R.L. (Eds.). *Yen and Jaffe's reproductive endocrinology* (5th ed.). Philadelphia: Saunders. *MCR,* Metabolic clearance rate; *PR,* production rate; *SR,* secretion rate.

its LH receptors. In addition, ovarian insulin growth factor 1 (IGF-1) and vasoactive intestinal peptide stimulate inhibin synthesis. Levels of inhibin vary in the menstrual cycle from 100 IU/L to 1500 IU/L. In the follicular phase, inhibin concentrations are low, with increased levels in the luteal phase. In response to rising FSH levels in the luteal-follicular phase, inhibin levels drop dramatically. With menopause, inhibin concentrations are reduced, with decreases in inhibin B noted initially.[27]

Inhibin A is produced by the luteinized ovarian granulosa cells and expressed by the dominant follicle or corpus luteum.[27] Inhibin A slowly increases during the late follicular phase, stimulated by incremental LH expression, and is present in high levels during early and midfollicular phase, peaking in the midluteal phase. This is followed by a decreasing inhibin A in the late follicular phase.[27] The initial late follicular reduction in inhibin A is followed by a decreased but consistent level thereafter. During the second half of the menstrual cycle, concentrations of inhibin A increase markedly parallel to increasing concentrations of estradiol. FSH and LH stimulate expression of inhibin A by the dominant follicle.[27] Levels of inhibin A are positively correlated with follicular size.[66] Levels increase in midpuberty.[23]

Inhibin B is produced by the ovarian granulosa cells and Sertoli cells of the testis.[27] Inhibin B decreases FSH synthesis and obscures the effects of low activin levels.[42,51] In the early follicular phase, there are increased levels of FSH and estradiol. These hormones stimulate inhibin B expression from the luteinized granulosa cells. Thus inhibin B levels increase during the early follicular phase and reach their highest point at the early to midfollicular phase of menstrual cycle.[27] Levels are highest in the granulosa cells of small luteal antral follicles. Then inhibin B levels continuously decrease, becoming undetectable following the LH surge.[66] No association has been noted with inhibin B levels and follicular size.[66] Levels of inhibin B increase during childhood, peaking in midpuberty and decreasing thereafter.[23]

Follistatin

Follistatin is derived from the ovarian granulosa cells of small antral and preovulatory follicles. This polypeptide, like inhibin, suppresses FSH expression and may modulate the effects of activin on FSH.[23,27,66] However, follistatin is only about one third as active as inhibin.[29] Other physiologic roles of follistatin include the protein binding of activin (which restricts the bioavailability of activin) and the synthesis of progesterone.[64,66] Concentrations of follistatin remain relatively constant throughout the menstrual cycle.[29,66] Levels of follastatin do not vary during puberty although increases occur with normal menses.[23] Follistatin levels increase in pregnancy with peak levels at term.[30]

Steroid Hormones

The steroidal hormones—androgens, estrogens, and progestogens—are primarily produced by the gonads and adrenals (see Table 2-4). Steroid hormones are not stored but are produced as needed.[67] Cholesterol is the precursor for steroid hormones (Figure 2-9). Steroidogenic cells express

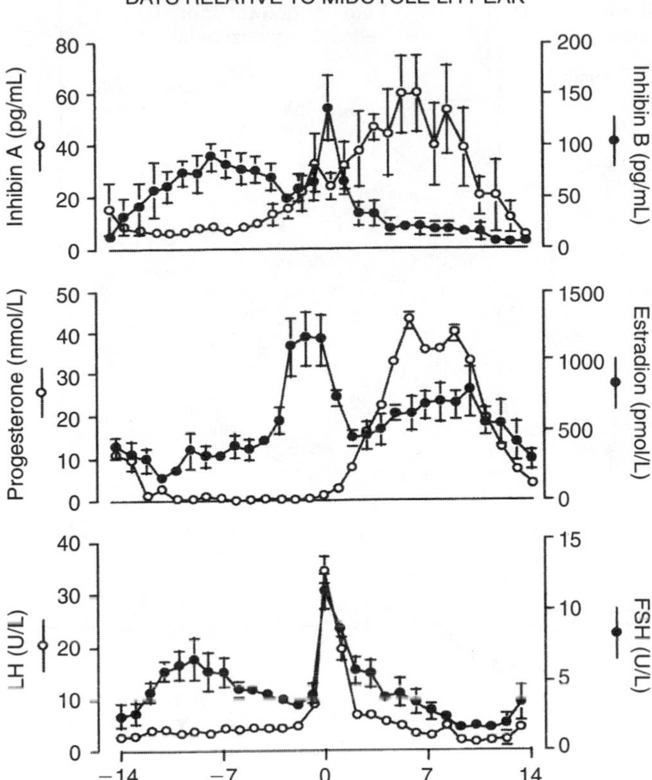

FIGURE 2-8 Plasma concentrations of inhibins A and B (*top*), progesterone and estradiol (*middle*), and luteinizing hormone (LH) and follicle-stimulating hormone (FSH) (*bottom*) during ovulatory cycles in women. Data are aligned to the day of the midcycle LH peak (day 0). Mean ± SE is shown. (From Groome, N.P., Illingworth, P.J., O'Brien, M., et al. [1969]. Measurement of dimeric inhibin B throughout the human menstrual cycle. *J Clin Endocrinol Metab, 81,* 1401. Note this figure is pulled from Jameson, L. & DeGroot, L. [2010]. *Endocrinology: Adult and pediatric Vol II* [6th ed.]. Philadelphia: Saunders Elsevier [Figure 128-2, p. 2328].)

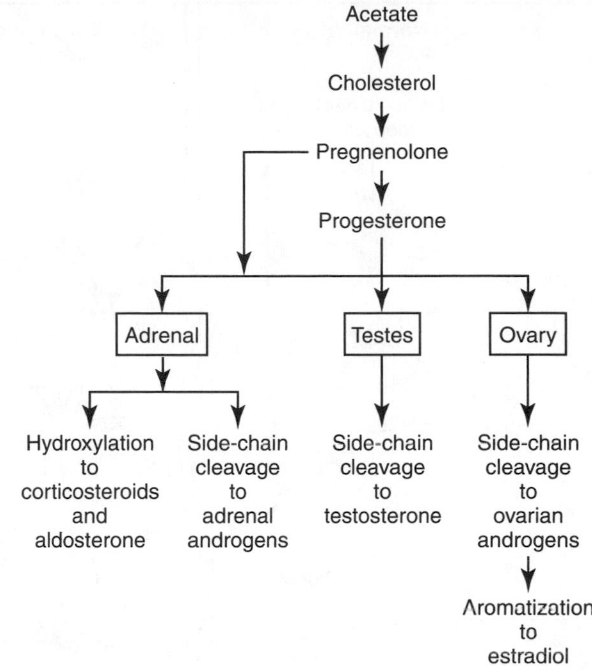

FIGURE 2-9 The unified concept of steroid hormone synthesis. Characteristic steroid secretory functions of the ovary, testes, and adrenal gland are shown. The pathway from acetate to progesterone is common to all. (From Ryan, K.J. [1972]. Steroid hormones and prostaglandins. In D.E. Reid, K.J. Ryan, & K. Benirschke [Eds.]. *Principles and management of human reproduction.* Philadelphia: Saunders.)

low-density lipoprotein (LDL) receptors, in particular, and high-density lipoprotein (HDL) receptors to uptake cholesterol. Steroidogenesis commences with LH stimulating the conversion of cholesterol to pregnenolone within the mitochondria of the cells of the theca interna cells (Figure 2-10, *A*). Transfer of the cholesterol within the mitochondria is enhanced by a steroidogenic acute regulatory protein (StAR).[67] Steroid synthesis employs a number of enzymes including hydroxylases, dehydrogenases, reductase, transferases, steroid sulfatase, sulfotransferases, and an aromatase (Table 2-5).[67] The hydroxylases and aromatase arise from the P450 family and act as a catalyst to steroidogenesis.[67] Aromatase transcription for hormonal synthesis is evoked with follicular development at the 7-mm stage.[60]

The gonads (i.e., ovaries, testes) produce the majority of the steroidal hormones; the adrenal cortex produces minimal amounts of estrogens and dihydrotestosterone. Progesterone and pregnenolone are also synthesized by the placenta from cholesterol precursors. Synthesis of steroidal hormones may follow one of two pathways: the pregnenolone pathway or the progesterone pathway (Figure 2-11). From the pregnenolone pathway the hormones dehydroepiandrosterone and androstenediol are produced. Dehydroepiandrosterone and androstenediol, hormones derived from the pregnenolone pathway, may enter the progesterone pathway in the synthesis of the hormones androstenedione and testosterone, respectively. The progesterone pathway synthesizes the prohormones androstenedione and testosterone, with final conversion to the hormone dihydrotestosterone. Also from this pathway, androstenedione is converted to estrone (E_1) and testosterone is converted to estradiol. In women, approximately 60% of circulating testosterone is derived from the peripheral conversion of androstenedione. Steroidal hormonal levels vary in the reproductive cycle and in the reproductive life of the woman and man (Table 2-6).[68]

Dehydroepiandrosterone Sulfate, Dehydroepiandrosterone, 5X-Dihydrostestosterone, and Androstenedione

Major androgen precursors are DHEAS, DHT, DHEA, and androstenedione. These androgen precursors precede steroidal synthesis. Secreted by the ovaries and adrenals, the androgen precursors begin to increase in early adolescence and decline in the fifth and sixth decades. DHEA increases during adrenarche around 7 to 9 years of age, peaking in the early twenties and then declines.[63] Thereafter, follicular maturation, increased estradiol levels, and

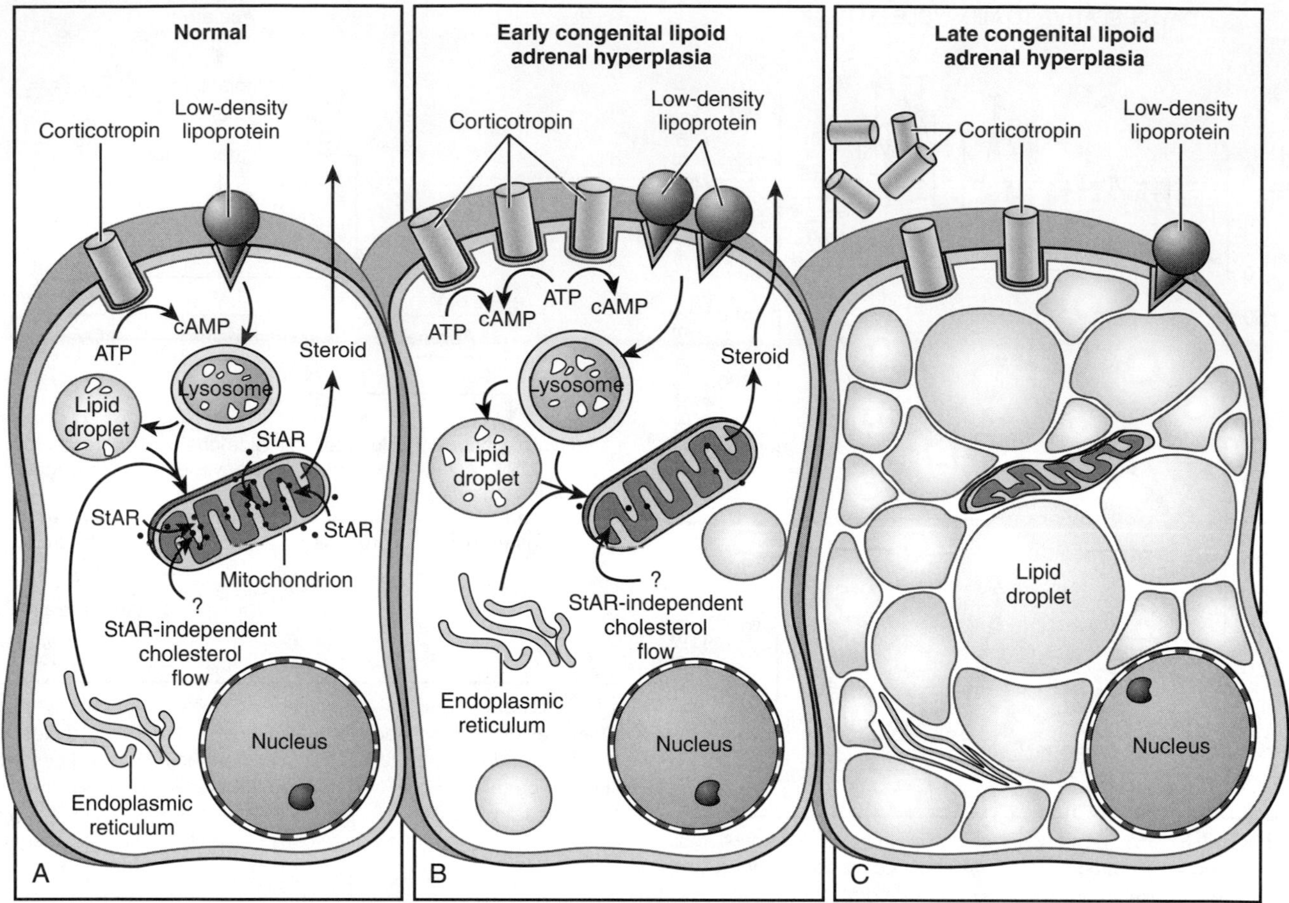

FIGURE 2-10 Steroidogenic acute regulatory protein (StAR). In the healthy steroidogenic cell, binding of adrenocorticotropic hormone (ACTH) stimulates transport of low-density lipoprotein (LDL) cholesterol into the cell by endocytosis. LDL is processed by lysosomes and either stored in lipid droplets or transferred to the mitochondria. Meanwhile, cholesterol is also synthesized independently by the endoplasmic reticulum mechanisms that may be STAR dependent or independent. (From Bose, H.S., et al. [1996]. The pathophysiology and genetics of congenital lipoid adrenal hyperplasia. *N Engl J Med, 335,* 1870. Jameson, L. & DeGroot, L. [2010]. *Endocrinology: Adult and pediatric Vol II* [6th ed.]. Philadelphia: Saunders Elsevier [Figure 118-7, p. 2175].)

Table 2-5 Enzymes Used in Steroidogenesis

ENZYME	DESIGNATION
Cholesterol side chain cleavage	CYP11A
17α-Hydroxylase	CYP17
17,21-Lyase	CYP17
21-Hydroxylase	CYP21
11β-Hydroxylase	CYP11B1
Aldosterone synthetase	CYP11B2
Aromatase	CYP19
3β-Hydroxysteroid dehydrogenase	3βHSD
17β-Hydroxysteroid dehydrogenase	17βHSD
5β-Reductase	5βRed

From O'Malley, B.W. & Strott, C.A. (1999). Steroid hormones: Metabolism and mechanism of action. In S.C. Yen, R.B. Jaffe, & R.L. Barbieri (Eds.). *Reproductive endocrinology: Physiology, pathophysiology, and clinical management* (4th ed.). Philadelphia: Saunders.

LH stimulation are necessary for ovarian androgen synthesis. Androgens are the precursors of estrogen and progesterone synthesis.

During the menstrual cycle, particularly the follicular phase, two thirds of testosterone is derived from peripheral conversion of androstenedione. During pregnancy, the fetal adrenal produces DHEA, the precursor of placental estrogen synthesis. DHEA is a hormone produced primarily by the adrenals and less so by the ovaries. The physiologic role of dehydroepiandrosterone is unknown.[14] Age is the most important determinant in DHEA hormonal variance, although the cause of the decreased levels with aging is unknown.[70] Hormonal concentrations of DHEA decline with age more so than do estrogen, progesterone, or testosterone.[70]

Testosterone synthesis into DHT in males takes place principally in the target glands. Testosterone is primarily secreted in the blood, with only a small amount stored in the testis. The testis produces approximately 6 to 7 mg testosterone per day.[51] Androgen receptors in the testis are expressed in the Sertoli cells, peritubular cells and the Leydig cells (Figure 2-12). These

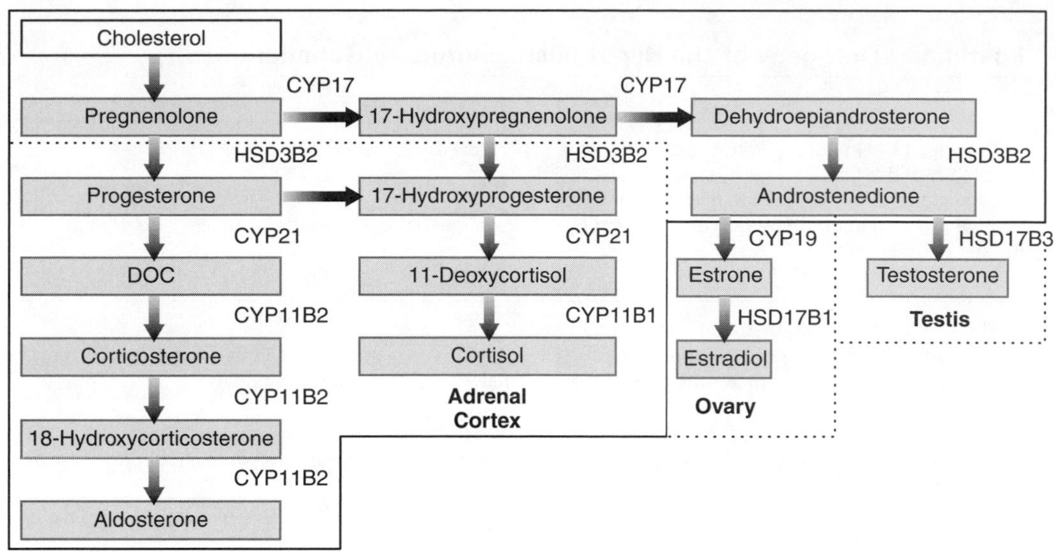

FIGURE 2-11 Steroidogenesis. This figure shows pathways of adrenal, ovarian, and testicular steroidogenesis. Dark solid lines indicate predominant pathways for adrenal steroidogenesis. Dashed lines indicate predominant pathways for gonadal steroidogenesis. (From Witchel, S.F. & Lee, P.A. [2002]. Ambiguous genitalia. In M.A. Sperling [Ed.]. *Pediatric endocrinology* [2nd ed.]. Philadelphia: Saunders.)

receptors are essential for spermatogenesis, spermatocyte and spermatid development, and testosterone production. The spermatic vein is the primary route of transport to the general circulation. DHT from testosterone acts on the epididymis, vas deferens, seminal vesicles, and prostate. Aspermia may result from a lack of testosterone. Estradiol, testosterone, and DHT are necessary for these effects. Wolffian duct expression with subsequent masculinization of fetal sexual differentiation is primarily related to testosterone (see Chapter 1). Changes in the external genitalia, prostate, and urethra are due to DHT. Both DHT and testosterone are necessary for growth of the penis. Testosterone production is greatest during the time of differentiation of the external genitalia, between 9 and 14 weeks' gestation and subsequently decreases.[51]

Estrogens

Estrogens include estrone (E_1), estradiol, and estriol (E_3) (Figure 2-13). In nonpregnant women, the ovaries are the primary source of estrogens; the adrenal cortices also produce small amounts. Before ovulation, the follicles secrete estradiol, which is dependent upon thecal cell androgen production. During pregnancy, the placenta produces significant quantities of estrogens. The principal estrogen of the reproductive years is estradiol produced by the ovaries. Estriol, a weak estrogen, is derived from the conversion of either estradiol or estrone. Estrone is derived from androgens of the adrenals and ovaries. Estradiol has 12 times the estrogenic potency of estrone and 80 times that of estriol.[26] During the reproductive years, estrone concentrations are greater than those of estradiol, with levels ranging from 1000 pg/mL (3699 pmol/L) in the follicular phase to luteal levels of 1800 pg/mL (6658.2 pmol/L). The greater biologic potency of estradiol establishes it as the dominant estrogen at this time. Conversely, estradiol levels dramatically decrease with menopause and there is a higher estrone-estradiol ratio, with estrone becoming the dominant estrogen of the menopausal period. The "two-cell, two-gonadotropin" theory proposes that two cells (i.e., thecal, granulosa cells) and the two gonadotropins (i.e., FSH, LH) stimulate estrogen synthesis (Figure 2-14).[24,47,66]

Androgen formation from cholesterol occurs in the theca interna with LH stimulation. Androgen is then converted to estrogens. In addition, antral follicles produce estradiol and these follicles ovulate in response to gonadotropin stimulation (Figure 2-15).[15,57] Stress can negatively affect hormonal stimulation. Estradiol blood levels are significantly lower in women diagnosed with depression.[11]

Estradiol stimulates follicular maturation. Increased levels of estrogen by day 5 in the ovarian cycle act to inhibit FSH and LH release. Estrogen priming facilitates FSH development of granulosa LH receptors. Increasing estrogen levels stimulate LH secretion. During the follicular phase, estrogen facilitates endometrial changes of the proliferative phase. Endometrial tissue depth increases from 1 to 2 mm to 3.5 to 5 mm, with tortuous gland development, increased mitotic activity, and expansion of the spiral arteries. In response to estrogen, the cervical mucus becomes more watery and clear, with increased stretch ability prior to ovulation (spinnbarkeit). During the follicular phase, the cervical os opens, closing during the luteal phase. Uterine and fallopian tube changes in response to rising estrogen levels include rhythmic contractions to facilitate sperm motility and ovum retention, respectively.

Increased breast sensitivity during the luteal phase is thought to be related to estrogen levels. Following ovulation, the corpus luteum produces estrogen and progesterone. Increased levels of estrogen, in concert with progesterone, inhibit

Table 2-6 **Postulated Ontogeny of the Hypothalamic Pituitary Gonadal Circuit**

FETUS
Medial basal hypothalamic LHRH neurosecretory neurons (pulse generator) operative by 80 days' gestation
Pulsatile secretion of FSH and LH by 80 days' gestation
Initially unrestrained secretion of LHRH (100 to 150 days of gestation)
Maturation of negative gonadal steroid feedback mechanism by 150 days' gestation—sex difference
Low level of LHRH secretion at term
EARLY INFANCY
Hypothalamic LHRH pulse generator highly functional after 12 days of age
Prominent FSH and LH episodic discharges until approximately 6 months of age in males and 12 months of age in females, with transient increase in plasma levels of testosterone and estradiol in males and females, respectively
LATE INFANCY AND CHILDHOOD
Intrinsic CNS inhibition of hypothalamic LHRH pulse generator operative; predominant mechanism in childhood; maximal sensitivity by approximately 4 years of age
Negative feedback control of FSH and LH secretion highly sensitive to gonadal steroids (low set point)
LHRH pulse generator inhibited; low amplitude and frequency of LHRH discharges
Low secretion of FSH, LH, and gonadal steroids
LATE PREPUBERTAL PERIOD
Decreasing effectiveness of intrinsic CNS inhibitory influences and decreasing sensitivity of hypothalamic-pituitary unit to gonadal steroids (increased set point)
Increased amplitude and frequency of LHRH pulses, initially most prominent with sleep (nocturnal)
Increased sensitivity of gonadotrophs to LHRH
Increased secretion of FSH and LH
Increased responsiveness of gonad to FSH and LH
Increased secretion of gonadal hormones
PUBERTY
Further decrease in CNS restraint of hypothalamic LHRH pulse generator and of the sensitivity of negative feedback mechanism to gonadal steroids
Prominent sleep-associated increase in episodic secretion of LHRH gradually changes to adult pattern of pulses about every 90 minutes
Pulsatile secretion of LH follows pattern of LHRH pulses
Progressive development of secondary sexual characteristics
Spermatogenesis in males
Middle to late puberty—operative positive feedback mechanism and capacity to exhibit an estrogen-induced LH surge
Ovulation in females

Adapted from Grumbach, M.M., et al. (1974). Hypothalamic-pituitary regulation of puberty in man: Evidence and concepts derived from clinical research. In M.M. Grumbach, G.D. Grave, & F.E. Mayer (Eds.). *Control of the onset of puberty.* New York: John Wiley & Sons (p. 115); P.R. Larsen, et al. (Eds.). (2003). *Williams textbook of endocrinology* (10th ed.). Philadelphia: Saunders.

CNS, Central nervous system; *FSH,* follicle stimulating hormone; *LH,* luteinizing hormone; *LHRH,* LH-releasing hormone.

FSH and LH secretion. As the corpus luteum degenerates, estrogen levels decrease. GnRH levels rise in response, with a subsequent increase in FSH and LH to initiate folliculogenesis.

In males, testosterone is converted to DHT by testicular 5X-reductase and then to estradiol by testicular aromatase. Estrogen receptor-B and aromatase activity are located in the germ cells and Sertoli cells. Estrogens in concert with androgens are necessary for the changes in prostate development and proliferation.[51] The role of estrogens in regard to testicular function is not clear.[51]

Progestogens

Progesterone is the only naturally occurring steroidal progestogen. The ovaries produce progesterone primarily early in the follicular phase, but large amounts of progesterone are converted by the granulosa cells to estrogens. With the LH surge, there is a subsequent increase in progesterone. In concert with estrogen, progesterone stimulates significant FSH secretion and a subsequent increase in granulosa LH receptors (see Figure 2-8). Follicular wall elasticity is secondary to increased progesterone levels.

Progesterone production in the follicular phase is 2.5 mg/day, whereas luteal phase production is 25 mg/day.[42] For the first 6 to 10 weeks following conception, the primary site of progesterone production is the corpus luteum.[45] Progesterone levels rise significantly, peaking at approximately day 8 of the luteal phase. Increased levels of progesterone—along with estrogen via negative feedback—limit the expression of FSH and LH. With involution of the corpus luteum, progesterone levels drop dramatically. In contrast with

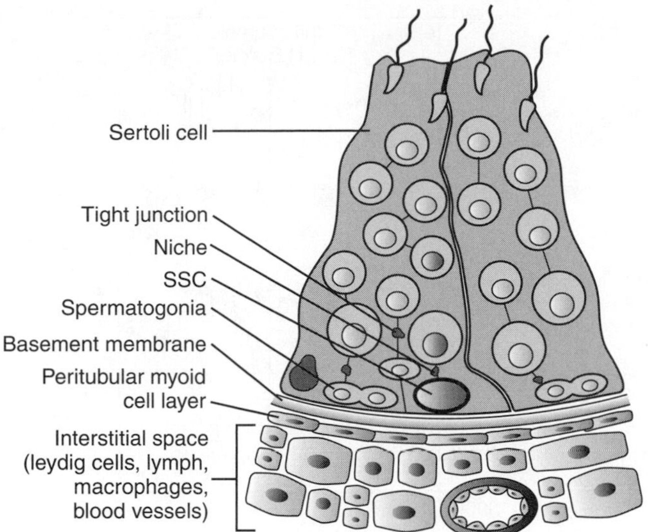

FIGURE 2-12 The site of the spermatogonial stem-cell (SSC) niche in the seminiferous epithelium. SSCs are in contact with the basal lamina and are found in the basal compartment of the seminiferous epithelium, below the Sertoli cell tight junctions and surrounded by Sertoli cell cytoplasm. In addition to factors produced by Sertoli cells that regulate SSCs, the nearby peritubular cells and Leydig cells are possible additional sources of molecules that influence SSC functions. (From Johnston, D.S., Wright, W.W., DiCandeloro, P., et al. [2008]. Stage-specific gene expression is fundamental characteristic of rat spermatogenic cells and Sertoli cells. *Proc Natl Acad Soc USA, 105, 8315.* In L. Jameson & L. DeGroot (Eds.). *Endocrinology: Adult and pediatric Vol II* [6th ed.]. Philadelphia: Saunders [Figure 136-6, p. 2444].)

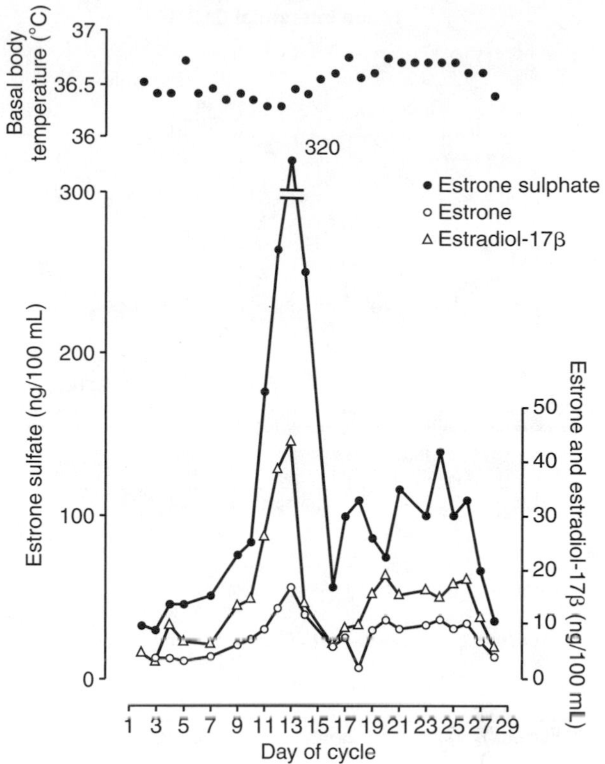

FIGURE 2-13 Circulating levels of estrone, estradiol-17β, and estrone sulfate during the menstrual cycle. (From Fraser, I.S., et al. [1998]. *Estrogens and progestogens in clinical practice.* Philadelphia: Churchill Livingstone.)

fertilization of the oocyte, the placenta becomes the primary producer of progesterone after approximately 10 gestational weeks.[42] Progesterone modulates the effects on the reproductive organs, including the "quieting" of the fallopian tubes during the luteal phase to assist the fertilized ovum in its transport to the uterus. This quieting also extends to the uterus to facilitate trophoblast implantation (see Chapter 3).[42] In addition, progesterone suppresses T cell processes, inhibiting fetal tissue rejection (see Chapter 13).[42] Progesterone levels are negatively correlated with body mass index.[70] Ethnicity also contributes significantly to variances in progesterone levels.[70]

The role of progesterone in the testis is not clear, though progrestone receptors have been identified on spermatozoa and in peritubular cells.[51]

Testosterone

Testosterone is an androgen derived from the androgenal precursors DHEA and DHEAS.[56] In females, from 30% to 50% of androgens originate in the adrenals and ovaries, with the remainder deriving from peripheral tissue conversion as liver and adipose tissue.[56]

At birth, male newborns have testosterone levels comparable to normal adults; levels decrease by the seventh day, increase again in the second month, and then fall significantly during the sixth month after birth and remain low until puberty. At approximately 7 years, androgens are produced in response to dehydroepiandrosterone by the adrenal gland. Gonadotropin secretion, beginning around 10 years, leads to nocturnal pulsatile LH secretion with increased testosterone levels. With maturity, testosterone has a circadian pattern with 25% lower levels at night in comparison with the early morning levels. With aging, as with females, testosterone concentrations decrease.[51]

Secretion of androgens in females commences at approximately 6 to 8 years of age and is influenced primarily by elevated DHEAS and less so by androstenedione levels.[56] Levels begin to reach adult levels during adolescence and begin to decline in the fifties. Premenopausally, mean testosterone production rates decrease from 200 mcg/day to 150 mcg/day perimenopausally. Synthesis of testosterone occurs early in the follicular cycle by the ovaries. The majority of testosterone is converted into estrogens by the granulosa cells. Testosterone levels decline with age. Body mass index is the most important predictor of testosterone levels.[70]

In males, the maximal levels of DHEA and DHEAS are from the ages of 20 to 25 years with a decrease in subsequent years. At 60 years of age, DHEA(S) levels are only a third of DHEA(S) of previous levels.[51] Testosterone and DHT decrease the pulsatile GnRH frequency at the hypothalamus.[51]

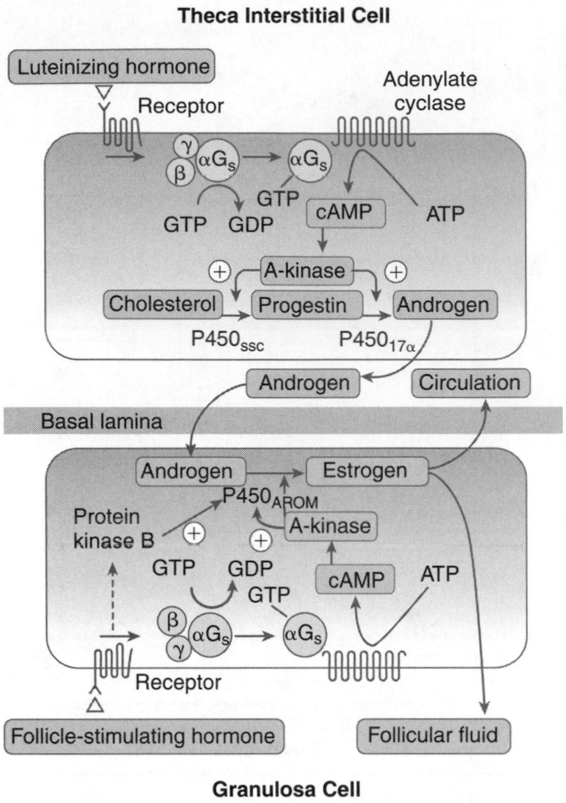

Theca Interstitial Cell
Luteinizing hormone
Receptor
Adenylate cyclase
γ β αG_s αG_s
GTP GDP GTP
cAMP
ATP
A-kinase
Cholesterol Progestin Androgen
$P450_{SSC}$ $P450_{17\alpha}$
Androgen
Circulation
Basal lamina
Androgen Estrogen
$P450_{AROM}$
Protein kinase B
A-kinase
GTP GDP GTP
cAMP
ATP
β γ αG_s αG_s
Receptor
Follicle-stimulating hormone
Follicular fluid
Granulosa Cell

FIGURE 2-14 The two cell, two-gonadotropin system for estradiol synthesis in the follicle. LH and FSH are shown to stimulate adenylate cyclase via G-protein–coupled receptors. The cAMP generated from ATP activates protein kinase A to stimulate expression of the respective steroido-genic enzymes in theca and granulose cells. In addition, in granulose cells, FSH binding to the FSH receptor leads to activation of protein kinase B, probably via a phosphatidyl inositol second message, which augments aromatase expression. *ATP,* adenosine triphosphate; *cAMP,* cyclic adenosine monophosphate; *FSH,* follicle stimulating hormone; *LH,* Luteinizing hormone. (Adapted from Erickson, G.F. & Shimasaki, S. [2001]. The physiology of folliculogenesis: the role of novel growth factors. *Fertil Steril, 76,* 943.)

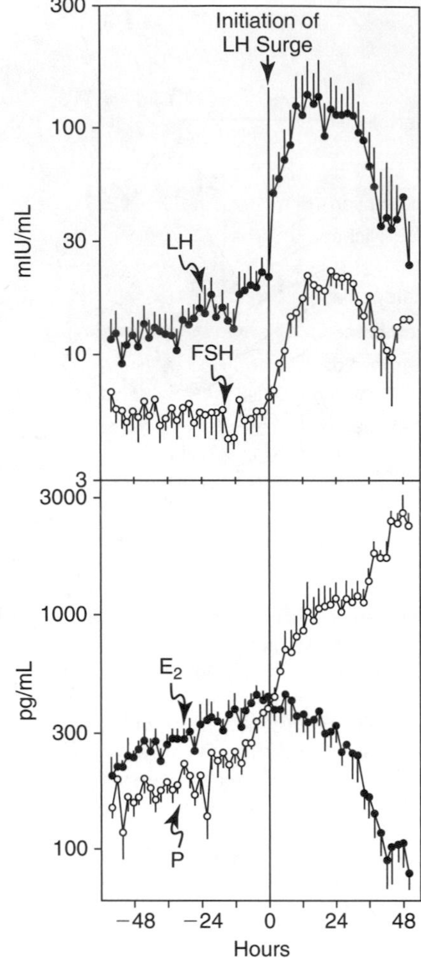

FIGURE 2-15 Mean (±SE) luteinizing hormone (LH), follicle-stimulating hormone (FSH), estradiol (E_2), and progesterone (P) levels measured every 2 hours for 5 days at midcycle in seven studies. Data were centered at the initiation of the gonadotropin surge. Note that the data were plotted on a logarithmic scale. (From Hoff, J.D., Quigley, M.E., & Yen, S.S.C. [1983]. Hormonal dynamics at midcycle: A reevaluation. *Endocrinol Metab,* 57, 792.) Note this figure is in Jameson, L. & DeGroot, L. (2010). *Endocrincology: Adult and pediatric Vol II* (6th ed). Philadelphia: Saunders Elsevier (Figure 128-4, p. 2330).

Oocyte Maturation Inhibitor

The factor leading to oocyte meiotic arrest in the prophase stage is thought to be oocyte maturation inhibitor.[26,47] Meiosis is postulated to resume with the complex interplay of oocyte maturation inhibitor and ovarian granulosa cumulus cells (see Chapter 3).

Luteinization Inhibitor

The existence of another chemical factor, luteinization inhibitor, is suggested by the ability of granulosa cells from large preovulatory follicles to initiate spontaneous luteinization.[66]

Gonadotropin Surge–Inhibiting Factor

Gonadotropin surge–inhibiting factor is thought to be a nonsteroidal substance that inhibits the LH surge and FSH expression as normally occurs by either estradiol or GnRH. In contrast to inhibin, which inhibits only FSH expression, gonadotropin surge–inhibiting factor suppresses both FSH and LH. The ovaries are the source of this short-acting factor.[66]

Relaxin

Relaxin is produced by the luteal cells of the corpus luteum and thought to facilitate decidualization of the endometrium and suppress contractions of the uterine myometrium. Relaxin is associated with collagen remodeling and cervical softening.[42] Levels are highest in the first trimester, peaking at 1.2 ng/mL between 8 and 12 weeks' gestation and decreasing approximately 20% for the remainder of the pregnancy.[66]

Feedback Systems

Hormone secretion is regulated by feedback systems, which can be negative or positive (Figure 2-16). The negative feedback

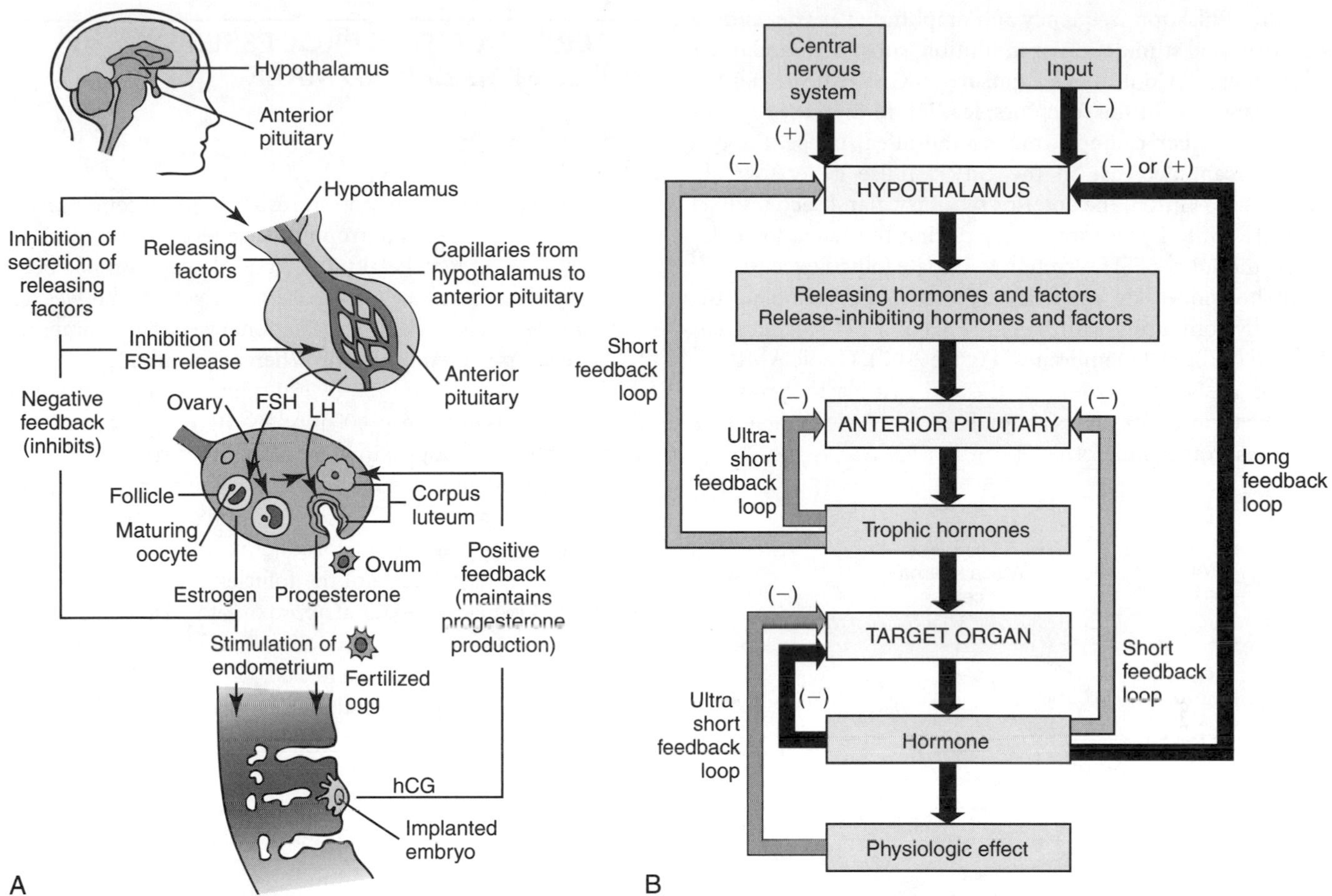

FIGURE 2-16 Feedback loops. **A,** Endocrine feedback loops involving the hypothalamus-pituitary gland and end organs (endocrine regulation). **B,** General model for control and negative feedback regulation is possible at three levels: target organ (ultrashort feedback), anterior pituitary (short feedback), and hypothalamus (long feedback). (From McCance, K.L. & Huether, S.E. [2006]. *Pathophysiology: The biologic basis for disease in adults and children* [5th ed.]. St. Louis: Mosby.)

system is the most common. As the level of a hormone rises, it inhibits the initiation of further release of that hormone. Secretion of a pituitary hormone to a level above the set point causes a decrease in secretion of that same pituitary hormone into the blood. For example, the administration of moderate amounts of estrogen will lower the secretion of FSH and LH into the blood. In the normal menstrual cycle, high levels of progesterone and moderate levels of estrogen during the luteal phase will lower gonadotropin secretion by a long-loop negative feedback. With positive feedback, a rising hormone level will increase secretion of the same hormone. High levels of estrogen in blood increase the secretion of LH and FSH from the adenohypophysis, resulting in a surge of gonadotropins (FSH and LH).[17,27]

Physiologic effects are produced by peripheral target tissues (gonads) and travel via the bloodstream to the brain and pituitary gland. In addition to the negative and positive feedback loops, there are long, short, and ultrashort loops. In the long-loop feedback, the gonadotropins (FSH and LH) increase the gonadal secretion of steroidal hormones. These steroidal hormones (i.e., estrogen, progesterone) influence the secretion of LH and FSH by their feedback effects on the systems controlling gonadotropin secretion. In the short-loop feedback system, LH or FSH circulates in the vascular system, returns to the median eminence of the hypothalamus, and subsequently decreases the secretion of GnRH from the neurosecretory axons.[6,17,26] This is a more direct negative feedback system that does not involve gonadal steroid hormones. In the ultrashort-loop feedback, the GnRH may directly stop GnRH secretion from the neurosecretory axons in the median eminence. At present, only the short and ultrashort feedback loops have been demonstrated to be negative. On the other hand, the long-loop feedback system may be either positive or negative. High serum levels of estrogen increase the secretion of LH and FSH from the adenohypophysis, resulting in an LH surge with ovarian release of the ovum.

Gonadotropin-Releasing Hormone

Gonadotropin-releasing neurons are located in the arcuate nucleus of the medial basal hypothalamus and in the preoptic area of the anterior hypothalamus.[6,23] The GnRH pulse generator exhibits pulsatile secretion at 60- to 90-minute intervals from the medial basal hypothalamus with ultradian rhythm. Pulsation frequency and amplitude vary depending on hormonal stimulation or inhibition, substrates, and other hormones.[6,23] Continuous exposure to GnRH decreases the responsiveness of the receptors, leading to increased down-regulation.[2] For example, during the luteal phase, there is a significant decrease in the GnRH pulse generator.[24] In response to GnRH, the anterior pituitary gland secretes FSH and LH. GnRH pulse frequency during the luteal follicular phase modulates FSH secretion to initiate folliculogenesis.[17,73] Both hormones are small glycoproteins that stimulate the ovary by combining with specific FSH and LH receptor cells located in the cell membranes (Figure 2-17). Cyclic AMP, the second messenger system in the cell cytoplasm, promotes mobilization and expression of FSH and LH from storage granules in the gonadotropes.[24]

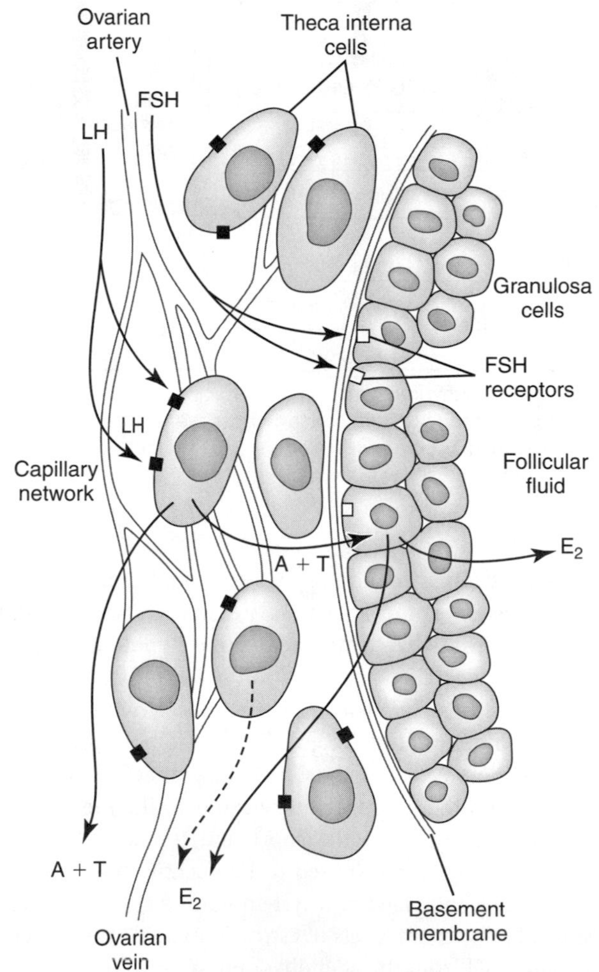

FIGURE 2-17 Diagram of action of gonadotropins on the follicle and the synthesis of estrogens. Luteinizing hormone (LH) interacts with receptors on the theca cells to stimulate production of androgens and small amounts of estradiol (E_2). Follicle-stimulating hormone (FSH) activates the aromatase enzyme system in the granulosa cells by interacting with receptors. *A*, Androstenedione; *T*, testosterone. (From Band, D.T. [1984]. The ovary. In C.R. Austin & R.V. Short [Eds.]. *Hormonal control of reproduction [vol. 3]*. Cambridge: Cambridge University Press.)

REPRODUCTIVE PROCESSES IN THE FEMALE AND MALE

Gametogenesis

Oogenesis

In utero, the ovaries function in response to placental secretion of chorionic gonadotropin. Oogenesis commences as early as week 3.[21,47,66] Fetal pituitary FSH secretion has been detected in the fetus as early as 12 to 14 gestational weeks.[2] Serum FSH levels at 20 to 28 gestational weeks are comparable to levels postmenopausally. Whereas the adult pulse generator frequency is from 60 to 120 minutes, the fetal GnRH frequency pulsates every 60 minutes. By 6 to 7 gestational weeks, there are approximately 10,000 germ cells. At approximately 20 gestational weeks, the maximal number (6 to 7 million) of primordial follicles are present; this number decreases throughout the reproductive life of the woman, the climacteric.[6,66] Atresia of the follicles begins at 24 weeks' gestation. Oogenesis ceases at approximately 28 weeks' gestation, with no further ova production.[66] At birth, the newborn ovaries contain approximately 200,000 to 400,000 follicles arrested in the prophase stage of meiosis.[47,66] (Oogenesis is described further in Chapter 1.)

Spermatogenesis

Sperm production takes place within a complex endocrine environment. The development of mature germ cells in the seminiferous tubules involves three stages: (1) mitosis, spermatogonial multiplication; (2) meiosis, production of haploid cells; and (3) spermiogenesis, maturation of spermatids to mature spermatozoa. The androgens and proteins produced locally modulate spermatogenesis seen within the seminiferous tubule (see Chapter 1).

The seminiferous tubule is divided into basal and luminal compartments. The basal compartment is the outer layer (zone 1) of the tubule, whereas the luminal compartment is the inner layer. The basal compartment is composed of stem cells (type A spermatogonia) that are renewed through mitosis. Some of these continue to proliferate and serve as stem cells, whereas others (preleptotene spermatocytes or type B spermatogonia) separate from the basal membrane and begin to migrate toward the lumen. As migration progresses, the cells undergo further morphologic changes, becoming primary spermatocytes. The first and second meiotic divisions occur with further differentiation in the adluminal zone, resulting in the formation of secondary spermatocytes and spermatids. The luminal spermatids undergo a complex sequence of changes within the cell organelles (spermiogenesis). (Spermatogenesis and spermiogenesis are discussed further in Chapter 1.)

Spermatogenesis is the differentiation and proliferation of diploid germ cells, via a six-stage system.[51] There are two types of spermatogonia, type A and type B. Type A can be classified as Ap and Ad with Ap differentiating to type B, the spermatogonium. The spermatocytes, via first meiotic division, become secondary spermatocytes over 1 to 3 weeks. With the second meitotic division, lasting only 1 to 2 days, there is a reduction in the chromosome number with development of the spermatids. Spermiogenesis is the process by which the spermatids undergo shaping of the cell nucleus and formation of the flagellum. During spermiogenesis there are four phases: Golgi, cap, acrosomal, and maturation phases. In the Gogi phase, craniocaudal symmetry occurs. During the cap phase, the spermatids and acrosome develop and the spermatids become elongated. During the acrosomal phase, the cell nucleus chromatin becomes greatly condensed and the spermatids become more enlongated. The expulsion of the remaining cytoplasm, known as the residual body, occurs during the maturation phase. Sperm are then released into the tubular lumen, passing into the epididymis. Sperm development from an Ap spermtogonium into a mature sperm requires minimally four spermatogenic cycles, with each cycle lasting approximately 16 days. As sperm are present in the epididymis at varied stages, a spermatogenesis cycle ranges from 64 to 74 days.[51]

The sperm move down the tubules by contraction and fluid secretion by the Sertoli cells. The evolution process takes approximately 74 days. Of these 74 days, about 50 days are spent in the seminiferous tubule. Each stage of spermatogenesis has a specific time frame, 16 to 18 days for spermatogonia, 23 days for primary spermatocytes, 1 day for secondary spermatocytes, and about 23 days for spermatids.[31] At the time of their release into the seminiferous tubules, the spermatozoa are still morphologically immature and lack motility. While traversing the epididymis (which takes 14 to 21 days), they continue to differentiate. Forward motility is achieved in the proximal epididymis. (Ejaculation, sperm transport, and fertilization are described in Chapter 3.)

Puberty

Although not completely understood, puberty is thought to be controlled via the central nervous system. Gonadotropin-releasing hormone (GnRH) is released from the hypothalamic GnRH neurons. Neurotransmitters, such as catecholamines, prostaglandins, and serotonin, act to either inhibit or stimulate the process. Other contributing factors include body mass index, nutritional status, steroid hormones, and ethnicity.[40]

During pregnancy, at approximately midgestation, increased levels of LH and FSH are secreted with levels increasing throughout the remaining pregnancy. Following birth, there is an initial increase in LH and FSH, decreasing over subsequent days. In the first 6 to 12 weeks following birth, these levels peak as a result of increased hypothalamic-pituitary-gonadal (HPG) axis activity. Levels then decrease over the subsequent months,[40] with serum FSH levels higher in female infants than male infants.[35] During childhood, hypothalamic activity is suppressed by the central nervous system. Although quiescent during this juvenile pause, by the age of 5 to 7 years there is increased LH and FSH secretion, even before the physiologic changes accompanying puberty.[40]

The GnRH neurons, located in the arcuate nucleus of the hypothalamus, release episodic pulses of GnRH into the hypothalamic hypophyseal portal plexus. Receptors in the anterior pituitary gland, gonadotropes release FSH and specifically LH in the portal system with subsequent stimulation of the gonads.[40] Increased serum LH levels are sleep dependent and are accompanied during puberty with a rise in amplitude of nocturnal gonadotropin pulses.[35] Ovarian response requires episodic secretion of GnRH at 70- to 90-minute intervals. Ovarian granulosa cells in response to FSH secrete androstenedione, a primary component for estradiol production. In contrast in the male, the Leydig cells produce testosterone in response to LH stimulation and with spermatogenesis production by FSH stimulation.[40]

GnRH episodic pulses increase in frequency at about 10 years of age (Figure 2-18) increasing at night during sleep.[35,40,73] With puberty, estradiol stimulus via positive feedback initiates the hypothalamic pulse generator (Figure 2-19). This hormonal stimulus is dependent upon an adequate LH pool for the LH surge, ovarian follicles responsive to FSH, and a pituitary gland responsive to GnRH. LH pulses have been detected as early as mid-childhood. With the onset of puberty, there is a greater increase in LH pulse amplitude in comparison to pulse frequency.[35] There is a progressive increase in FSH and LH daytime pulsatility, with a subsequent decrease in sleep-entrained pulse amplification (Figure 2-20).[35] Prepubertal girls have high FSH concentrations. FSH is necessary for pubertal development, and rising FSH levels accompany follicular development.[37] Ovary activation occurs in response to increasing LH pulses.[65]

There is increased gonadotropin sensitivity to GnRH with the cessation of the gonadostat.[20] Control of GnRH release is mediated via a neuroendocrine cascade composed of neuropeptides, neurotransmitters, and neuro-steroids. These neuropeptides include opioids, neuropeptide Y, galanin, and

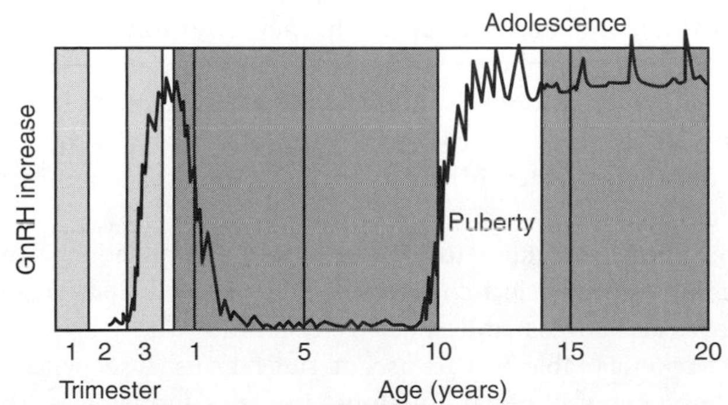

FIGURE 2-18 Diagrammatic representation of the ontogeny of gonadotropin-releasing hormone (GnRH) secretion from fetal life to adolescence. Note the prepubertal nadir and upswing of GnRH secretory activity at the onset of puberty. This is followed by irregular luteinizing hormone surges during adolescence. (From Yen, S.S.C. [1987]. Reproductive strategy in women: Neuroendocrine basis of endogenous contraception. In R. Rolland [Ed.]. *Neuroendocrinology of reproduction*. Amsterdam: Excerpta Medica.)

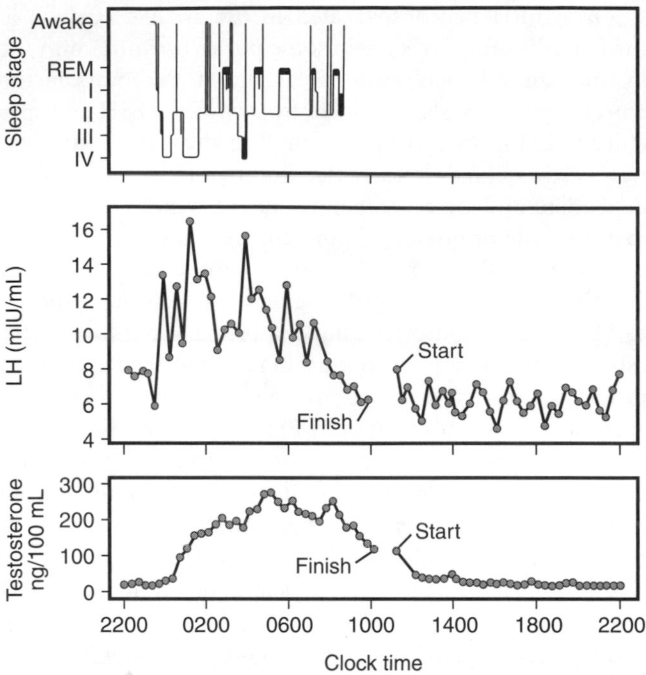

FIGURE 2-19 Plasma luteinizing hormone (LH) and testosterone sampled every 20 minutes in a 14-year-old boy in pubertal stage 2. The histogram displaying sleep stage sequence is depicted above the period of nocturnal sleep. Sleep stages are rapid eye movement (REM) with stages I to IV shown by depth of line graph. Plasma LH is expressed as mIU/mL. Plasma testosterone is expressed as nanograms per 100 mL. To convert LH values to international units per liter, multiply by 1.0 to convert testosterone values to nanomoles per liter, multiply by 0.03467. (From Boyar, R.M., Rosenfeld, R.S., & Kapen, S., et al. [1974]. Human puberty: Simultaneous augmented secretion of luteinizing hormone and testosterone during sleep. *J Clin Invest* 54, 609. Copyright of the American Society for Clinical Investigation. Kronenberg, H., Melmed, S., Polonsky, K., & Larsen, R. (2008). *Williams textbook of endocrinology* (11th ed.), Philadelphia.)

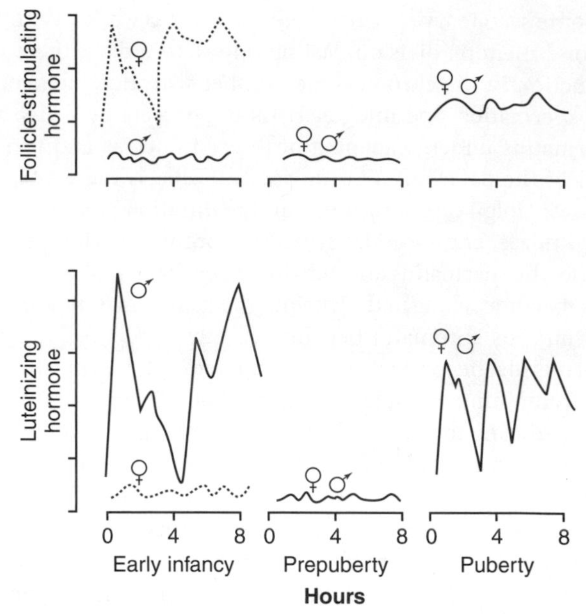

FIGURE 2-20 Changes in the patterns of follicle-stimulating hormone and luteinizing hormone secretion at puberty. (From Klein, K., et al. [1996]. In S.G. Hillier, H.C. Kitchener, & J.P. Neilson [Eds.]. *Scientific essentials of reproductive medicine.* Philadelphia: Saunders.)

corticotropin-releasing factor (CRF). Neurotransmitters include dopamine, melatonin, serotonin, γ-aminobutyric acid (GABA), and noradrenaline. The neurotransmitters dopamine, norepinephrine, and epinephrine stimulate GnRH secretion. Serotonin is norepinephrine mediated. DHEA (an antagonistic neurosteroid) and allopregnanolone (an agonistic neurosteroid) are also important factors in initiating puberty.[20]

Puberty, secondary to gonadal hormone stimulation, is the initiation of physical changes in both the male and female. Physical changes manifest between 8 and 13 years of age. Tanner criteria (Table 2-7) are used to stage the usual sequence of attainment of pubertal milestones in males and females. The staging criteria evaluate breast, pubic hair, and male genital development, with stage 1 as prepubertal and stage 5 as adult.

Male Puberty

Adrenarche, the increased production of adrenal sex steroids (DHEA, DHEAS, and androstenedione) occurs before production of gonadal steroids.[74] Following adrenarche, the gonadal sex steroids testosterone and estradiol are secreted. Testosterone secretion marks the gonadarche, occurring before physiologic changes of puberty. Secreted diurnally, levels of testosterone are higher earlier in the day. Estradiol levels vary considerably, increasing later at night than testosterone and peaking by mid-morning.[35] In puberty, gonadal steroids rise gradually, increasing with successive Tanner stages.[40] Other sex steroids of adrenal and gonadal origin—DHEA, estrone, androstenedione, and 17-hydroxyprogesterone—are also secreted. In response, sex steroid binding protein levels increase.[40]

Reproductive capability in men begins with spermarche. Unlike menarche, which occurs toward the end of puberty, spermarche begins early in puberty, preceding the peak growth spurt and beginning at an average of 13.5 years of age. Puberty generally takes about 4 years to complete, beginning somewhere between 11 and 16 years of age. During this time there is growth and development of the reproductive organs, rapid physical growth, and development of secondary sex characteristics.

The specific stimulus or mechanism for initiating puberty is unclear. An increase in the release of pituitary gonadotropins stimulates the production of androgens, particularly testosterone. Testosterone levels increase following nocturnal pulsatile LH secretion, peaking in the early morning.[35] Spontaneous morning erections are secondary to these increased testosterone levels. Synthesis of testosterone and other androgens results in the changes in the reproductive system and somatic tissue.

The major changes include the enlargement of the testes and penis; development of pubic, axillary, facial, and body

Table 2-7 Stages of Pubertal Development (Tanner)

STAGE	BREAST	PUBIC HAIR	
GIRLS			
1	Prepubertal	No pigmented hair	
2	Budding with larger areolae	Small amount of coarse, pigmented hair mostly along labia majora	
3	Enlargement of breast and areolae	Spread of coarse, pigmented hair over mons pubis	
4	Secondary mound of areolae	Almost adult pattern	
5	Mature contour	Adult pattern	
STAGE	**GENITALIA**	**PUBIC HAIR**	**TESTICULAR VOLUME**
BOYS			
1	Prepubertal	No pigmented hair	<3 mL
2	Thinning and darkening of scrotum, increased size of penis	Small amount of coarse, pigmented hair at base of penis	3-8 mL
3	Increased diameter of penis	Coarse, pigmented hair extends above penis	10-15 mL
4	Increased diameter and length of penis	Almost adult pattern	15-20 mL
5	Adult size and shape	Adult pattern	≥25 mL

From Witchel, S.F. & Plant, T.M. (2004). Puberty: Gonadarche and adrenarche. In Strauss, J. & Barbieri, R. (Eds.). *Yen and Jaffe's reproductive endocrinology* (5th ed.). Philadelphia: Saunders.

hair; rapid skeletal growth; hypertrophy of the larynx, with subsequent deepening of the voice; increased activity of the sweat and sebaceous glands; and muscular hypertrophy. Along with these changes, the seminiferous tubules begin sperm production. Before this point, a meiosis-inhibiting factor may be secreted by the Sertoli cells to inhibit spermatogonia meiosis. For males, testicular enlargement from the growth of the seminiferous tubules is the best indicator of pubertal activation of the HPT axis and occurs before other physical changes. Increased testicular volume usually occurs between 9 and 14 years.[74] Pubertal development before 9.5 years of age in males is considered precocious puberty.[40,74] At midpuberty in males, gynecomastia, sperm production with ejaculation, and increasing height and weight occur. Sperm production with ejaculation may occur at midpuberty but mature sperm is not present until about a year after the growth of the penis.

Other physiologic changes accompanying later adolescence include development of facial and chest hair and extension of pubic hair.[40] The mean age of Tanner stage 2 (see Table 2-7) pubic hair development is 12 years and in African-American males at an earlier age of 11.2 years.[40] Tanner stage 5 pubic hair development also varies by ethnicity with median ages of 16, 15, and 15.8 years for whites, African-Americans, and Mexican-Americans, respectively.[40] In contrast to females, in males, pubertal linear growth begins in Tanner stage 3 and may continue after stage 5. Therefore males are taller at the time of peak height velocity.[40]

Female Puberty

In females, the mean age of menarche, defined as the initial menses, is 12 years of age and has been for the previous 30 years. Although the age of menarche has decreased by 2 to 3 months per decade since the mid-1800s, present research does not document its continuation. Earlier menarche is posited to be the result of better nutrition, increased body mass, increased light exposure, and decreased disease. Median pubertal stages among females vary by ethnicity.

Breast development, termed *thearche,* is the best indicator of pubertal activation of the hypothalamic-pituitary-ovarian (HPO) axis.[40] The NHANES III survey found the onset of breast development is 10.4 years for white girls, 9.5 years for African-American girls and 9.8 years for Mexican-American girls.[40] Even though the onset of development may vary, the survey found the median age for complete adult breast development is 14 years for the population as a whole.[40] Breast development before 8 years of age is considered precocious puberty.[17,74] Pubertal growth is the result of increasing estradiol levels, beginning before stage 2 breast development. Peak height growth occurs before menarche, during breast stage 3.[40] Following menarche, female pubertal growth decelerates. Therefore, even though girls have an earlier onset of puberty within the normal range, both girls and boys complete puberty at approximately the same age. Attainment of physical parameters is not earlier for girls despite a longer "growing season."[43]

Following birth, the ovaries are dormant until puberty, although some primordial follicles partially respond to the FSH of childhood.[4] At puberty, 300,000 to 600,000 follicles await activation; however, only approximately 400 to 500 oogonia mature as secondary follicles for ovulation.[4,9,50,66] Oocytes are arrested in the prophase stage of the first meiotic division, converting oogonia to primary oocytes until ovulation. With ovulation, meiosis commences and the first polar body is formed.[6,66] Atresia of the remaining ovarian follicles occurs in response to apoptosis. Apoptosis is the programmed cell self-destruction without an accompanying inflammatory response. (Meiosis is discussed further in Chapter 1.)

After puberty, with increased FSH and LH expression, the ovaries and follicles are stimulated. Oocytes are surrounded by a single layer of granulosa cells that are believed to nourish the ovum and secrete oocyte maturation inhibiting factor. Oocyte maturation inhibiting hormone maintains the ova as primordial follicles in the first stage of meiotic division as in fetal development.[47,66]

Ovarian Cycle

The ovarian cycle consists of the follicular phase and the luteal phase (Figure 2-21). During the follicular phase there is ovarian follicular maturation and ovulation. The luteal phase includes the development of the corpus luteum from luteinization of the granulosa and theca interna cells. With involution of the corpus luteum, a new ovarian cycle begins.

The follicular phase commences with follicular growth in response to gonadotropin stimulation. A primordial follicle contains an oocyte with a single layer of granulosa cells. Developing into preantral follicles or primary follicles, the oocyte is covered with multiple layers of granulosa cells. FSH expression by the granulosa cells parallels formation of the antral cavity. Follicles mature from primordial to preantral follicles even without LH and FSH stimulation, but subsequent maturation does not occur without FSH stimulation.[37]

Follicular maturation to the antral stage is thought to require a 3-month trajectory (85 days).[6,24,47] The "trajectory of follicle growth"—from follicle recruitment to follicle selection to dominant follicle—is interdependent with gonadotropins (Figure 2-22).[6,22,24] Gonadal steroids act to "guide" the process from primordial follicle to the secondary follicular stage.[22,24]

The GnRH pulse generator has a frequency of approximately one discharge per hour (60 to 90 minutes), resulting in a GnRH pituitary portal circulation bolus. Research suggests that there is a corresponding LH pulse for each GnRH pulsation.[24] Hormone priming (i.e., small doses over a period of time) induces an increased LH pulse amplitude, which over 4 hours enhances GnRH receptors. Activation of the system initiates a sequence of reproductive endocrinology events (Figure 2-23). Specialized neurons in the hypothalamus synthesize and secrete GnRH in response to hormonal and neural stimuli. The GnRH pulse generator varies, dependent upon cycle timing. In the early follicular phase, the LH generator pulses approximately every 94 minutes (compared to late follicular phase pulsations every 60 to 70 minutes, 100 minutes during the early luteal, and every 200 minutes during the late luteal phase.[6] More rapid pulses are associated with increased LH secretion and slower pulses associated with FSH secretion.[6] Both ovaries have an equal opportunity for stimulation and alternate ovulation.

The neurosecretory cells integrate neuronal input from the feedback signals of the developing ovarian follicle. GnRH is secreted into the capillary venous network, bathing the anterior pituitary gland through the portal circulation. GnRH binds to membrane receptors located in the pituitary gonadotropes via cAMP and calcium mobilization, stimulating gonadotropin release.[76] Then pituitary gonadotropes secrete LH and FSH in pulses into the peripheral circulation. During the follicular phase of the ovarian cycle, the GnRH pulse generator operates at the same frequency as in its unmodulated state (i.e., independent of hypothalamic-pituitary-ovarian stimulation), releasing GnRH from secretory packets.

Differentiation of follicles is believed to be multifactorial. Endocrine, paracrine, and autocrine factors modulate the effect of FSH on the growing follicles.[59] Rising FSH

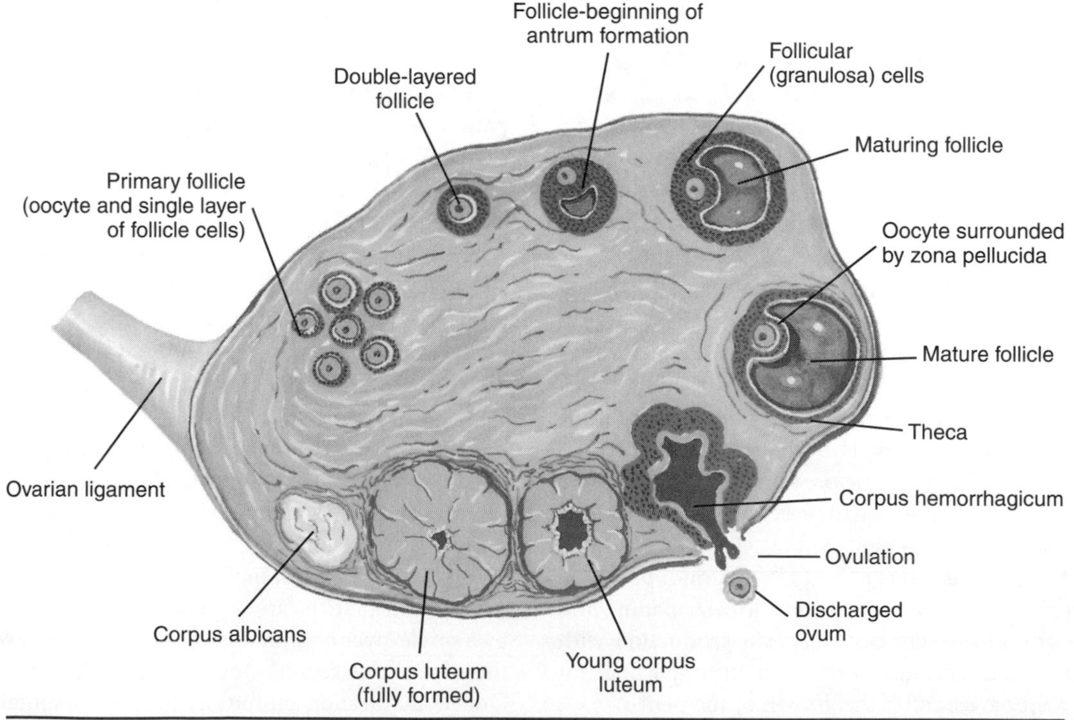

FIGURE 2-21 Cross-section of the ovary during reproductive years. (From Thibodeau, G.A. & Patton, K.T. [2007]. *Anatomy and physiology* [6th ed.]. St. Louis: Mosby.)

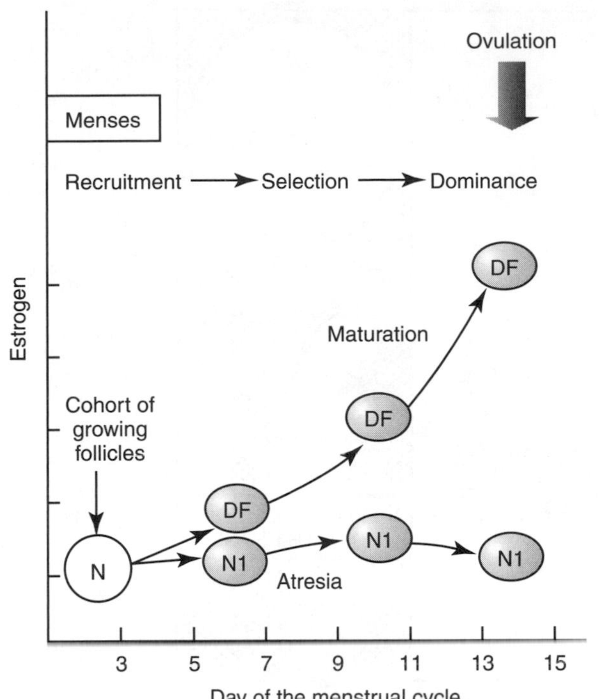

FIGURE 2-22 Time course for recruitment, selection, and ovulation of the dominant ovarian follicle (DF) with onset of atresia among other follicles (N_1) of the cohort. (From Hidgen, G.D. [1986]. Physiology of follicular maturation. In H.W. Jones, Jr., et al. [Eds.]. *In vitro fertilization.* Baltimore: Williams & Wilkins.)

levels are noted in the early follicular phase, stimulating increased inhibin B secretion (Figure 2-24).[72,73] FSH and LH secretion increases significantly. The increase in FSH precedes that of LH by several days. With FSH stimulation, follicular development progresses. Follicular recruitment consists of follicular maturation from a primordial follicle to a secondary follicle. A primordial follicle (30 to 60 μm in diameter) is a primary oocyte in the late diplotene phase that is surrounded by a single layer of approximately 15 pregranulosa cells.[66] Primordial follicles have been detected as early as 16 weeks' gestation, with formation ceasing by 6 months postpartum. Follicular growth is accelerated when the germinal vesicle reaches approximately 20 μm in diameter.

Primary follicles (greater than 60 μm in diameter) are primary oocytes surrounded by a single layer of granulosa cells.[66] Spindle cells of the ovarian stroma develop into granulosa cells, which rapidly proliferate. Granulosa cells give rise to the theca follicular cells, which are composed of two sublayers: the theca interna and theca externa. The theca interna (the inner sublayer) develops the follicular blood supply and secretes steroidal hormones, androgens which aromatize to estradiol.[4] The theca externa (the external layer) becomes the capsule of the maturing follicle as it comes in contact with the surrounding stroma. The theca externa is thought to produce an angiogenic factor. Differentiation of the thecal cells concludes the primary follicle stage. Development of the zona pellucida is characteristic of a preantral primary follicle.[66] Mucopolysaccharides secreted by the granulosa cells comprise the zona pellucida.[10]

Secondary follicles (less than 120 μm) are primary oocytes surrounded by approximately 600 granulosa cells, arranged in several layers.[66] Follicular enlargement is secondary to oocyte growth, proliferation of granulosa cells, and thecal cell differentiation. Accompanying the proliferation of granulosa cells and secondary follicles is the development of FSH, estrogen, and androgen receptors that become coupled as gap junctions.[66]

Ovarian activin promotes FSH expression. Rising FSH levels in turn promote accelerated growth of 6 to 12 primordial follicles each cycle.[26] Follicular recruitment of secondary follicles follows FSH and LH expression and occurs in the first 4 to 5 days of the cycle, leading to a selected follicle cohort from days 5 to 7. Until day 7 of the early follicular phase, all maturing follicles possess gametogenic potential for follicular selection.[24]

As follicles develop (ranging from 200 to 400 μm in diameter) in response to increase FSH, antral formation follows.[66] Follicular fluid that is high in estrogen is expressed by the granulosa cells (see Figure 2-21). Antral development heralds follicle maturation as a vesicular follicle and graafian follicle. With antral formation, the follicle is called a vesicular follicle; rapid proliferation of the granulosa and theca cells continues with estradiol expression.[7,62] Continued follicular maturation as a vesicular follicle is dependent upon activation of the granulosa and thecal cells by increased FSH and follicular estrogen. In response to the rising follicular estrogen levels, the granulosa cells develop increased FSH receptors and sensitivity.[24] Receptors for FSH and LH are present on the follicular granulosa cells and thecal cells (antral follicles), respectively.[2] Vesicular follicular enlargement results.

The follicle dominance attained during the midfollicular and late follicular phases is determined by rising serum FSH levels and by specific follicular sensitivity to FSH.[59,66] Initially, there is an intercycle rise in FSH that promotes follicular development. Dominant follicles have a greater sensitivity to FSH than the remaining growing follicles. Granulosa cells secrete inhibin and follistatin, both peptides that suppress FSH secretion during the midfollicular phase. Also, with increasing ovarian levels of follistatin and inhibin B in the middle to late follicular phase (the time of follicle selection), there is a corresponding decrease in FSH secretion. During the mid and late follicular phases, the number of developing dominant follicles decreases in response to lower serum FSH levels and sensitivity.[59] With follicle selection, secondary to gonadotropic stimulus, one single follicle matures and is dominant (days 8 to 12). Follicle dominance is determined by the late follicular phase (approximately 7 days before ovulation) and is established when the follicle is 3 to 8 mm.[60,66] When follicular cells are 10 mm, LH receptors are located on the granulosa cells.[4] In contrast to follicular recruitment that transcends ovarian cycles, the follicular selection and dominant phase is completed within one cycle.

Factors contributing to follicle dominance include the ability of the follicle to aromatize androgens from the midfollicular

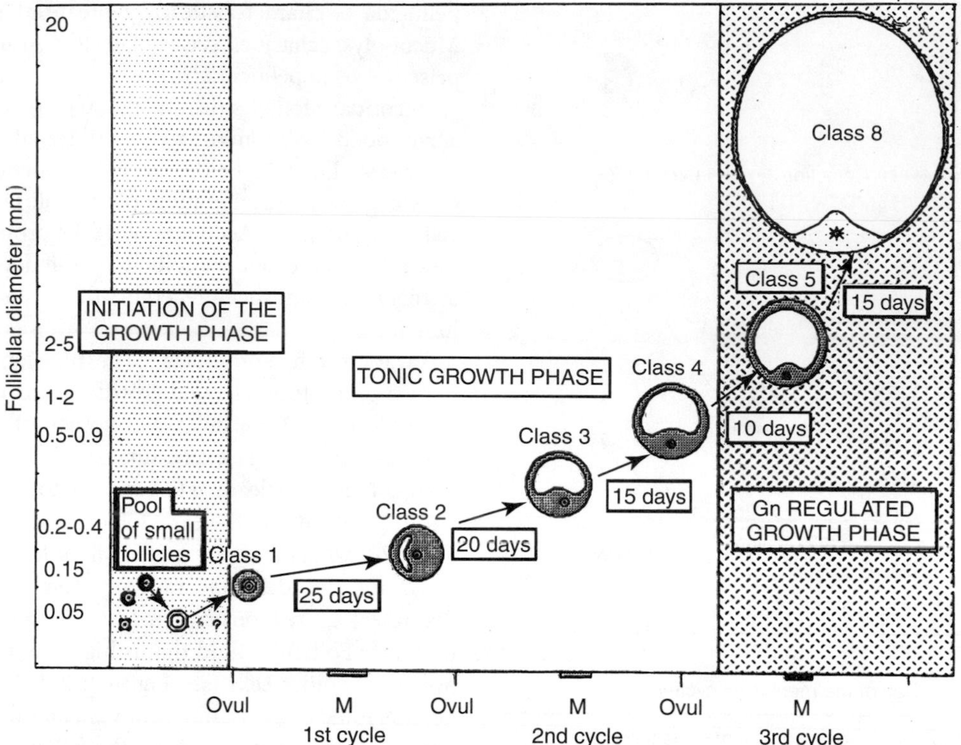

FIGURE 2-23 Complete follicular growth trajectory. Class 1 follicle is a secondary follicle with theca cells and is presumed to become responsive to gonadotropins. Although the tonic (early) stage of follicle development (class 1 to 4) is likely to be gonadotropin dependent (albeit to a lesser extent), the final stages of follicular development (class 5 to 8) are the ones heavily dependent on gonadotropins. According to this view, late luteal phase, class 5 follicles constitute the cohort from which the follicle destined to ovulate in the following cycle is recruited. The exponential gonadotropin dependent growth phase (class 5 to 8) takes place during the follicular phase of the cycle following the third menses from initiation of the growth phase. During this time, follicular selection and dominance are accomplished. The total duration of the process wherein a class 1 follicle is converted into preovulatory class 8 follicle is estimated to be 85 days and spans three ovulatory cycles. *M*, Menses; *Ovul*, ovulation; *Gn*, gonadotropin. (From Larsen, P.R., et al. [2003]. *Williams textbook of endocrinology* [10th ed.]. Philadelphia: Saunders.)

phase on, specifically estradiol and a high granulosa cell mitotic index.[24,53,66] As the dominant follicle matures, it expresses increased estradiol, with a subsequent rise in serum estradiol levels.[65] About 90% of circulating estradiol is secreted by the dominant follicle.[2,24] In addition, the dominant follicle contains FSH and estrogen intrafollicularly. Late follicular phase estradiol levels are at their highest levels within the follicle and blood. During follicular maturation when plasma estradiol levels exceed a threshold level of approximately 250 pg/mL (917.8 pmol/L) for 36 hours, the negative feedback system is overridden by a positive feedback result. Estrogen's positive system feedback relationship with the hypothalamus stimulates increased secretion of GnRH and follows the "priming" of the adenohypophysis by high-frequency GnRH.[2] Estrogen modulates the release of FSH and LH by the gonadotropin pulse generator when "read" by the pituitary gland. Hormonal patterns are illustrated in Figure 2-25.

Higher levels of interleukin-8 (IL-8) and interleukin-11 (IL-11), both chemotaxic cytokines, are found in more dominant follicles.[58] IL-8 activates neutrophils and promotes cell proliferation and angiogenesis.[58] In addition, genes are involved in ovarian development and function. Many of these genes are yet to be identified but include transcription factors, extracellular growth factors, and RNA binding proteins.[66]

Follicular growth may also be categorized by class or phase (see Figure 2-23).[66] The tonic growth phase involves the conversion of a preantral follicle (class 1) to an antral follicle up to 2 mm in diameter (class 4). Follicular development during the tonic growth phase is gonadotropin dependent. With development of the theca interna, class 1 follicles are activated by gonadotropin stimulation. Tonic follicular growth occurs over three menstrual cycles. During the first menstrual cycle, secondary follicles mature as class 1 follicles in the early luteal phase (days 15 to 19). In the following menstrual cycle, which is designated the second cycle, class 1 follicles are converted into class 2 follicles (days 11 to 15 of the second cycle). Early antral development is noted in class 2 follicles. Also during the second cycle, approximately 20 days later, class 2 follicles mature to class 3 follicles (end of luteal phase). In the late follicular phase of the third menstrual cycle, class 3 follicles become class 4 follicles.

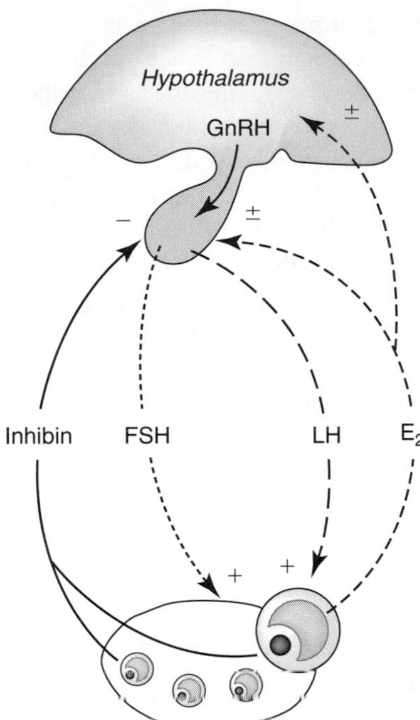

FIGURE 2-24 Diagrammatic representation of the hypothalamic-pituitary-ovarian axis in women during the follicular phase. Estradiol (E_2) feeds back at both the hypothalamus and anterior pituitary to inhibit the secretion of follicle-stimulating hormone (FSH) and luteinizing hormone (LH) (negative feedback). Under certain conditions, it can provoke the discharge of LH (positive feedback). Inhibin arising from both dominant and small antral follicles suppresses the synthesis and release of FSH by the anterior pituitary. *GnRH,* Gonadotropin-releasing hormone. (From Hillier, S.G. [1998]. Biosynthesis and secretion of ovarian and adrenal steroids. In I.S. Fraser, et al. [Eds.]. *Estrogens and progestogens in clinical practice.* Philadelphia: Churchill Livingstone.)

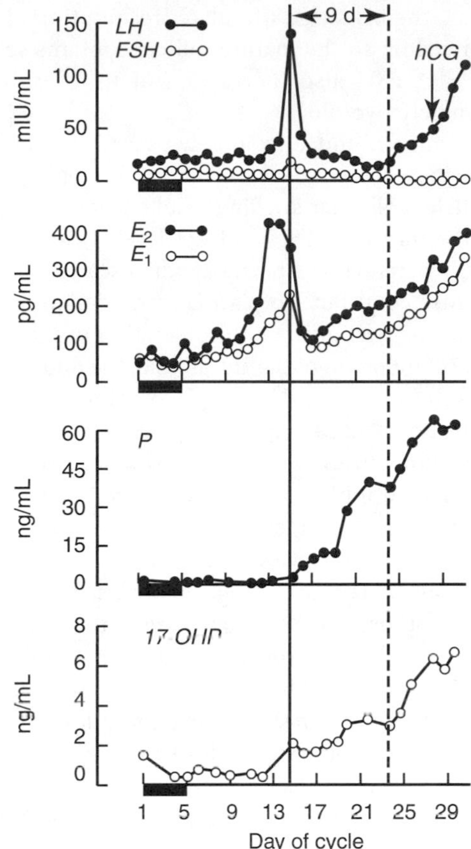

FIGURE 2-25 Hormonal patterns of human chorionic gonadotropin (hCG), luteinizing hormone (LH), follicle-stimulating hormone (FSH), estradiol (E_2), estrone (E_1), progesterone (P), and 17α-hydroxyprogesterone (17-OHP) during a menstrual cycle. Note the rise in hCG, which is detectable on cycle days 26 and 27. (From Creasy, R.K., Resnik, R., & Iams, J.D. [Eds.]. [2004]. *Maternal-fetal medicine: Principles and practice* [5th ed.]. Philadelphia: Saunders.)

Conversion of class 4 follicles to class 5 is gonadotropin dependent and occurs in the late luteal phase of cycle 3. All follicular maturation beyond class 4 is strongly dependent upon FSH and LH.[66] Follicular recruitment during the late luteal phase for the succeeding cycle will occur from class 5 follicles. During this phase, which is even more gonadotropin dependent, follicles mature from class 5 to class 8 before ovulation, averaging 5 days per class. Follicular selection and dominance occurs during this gonadotropin growth phase. Maturation of the follicle is accompanied by follicular growth, with an increase from 5 to 20 mm in diameter.

The hypothalamus responds via negative feedback to the moderately increased estrogen levels by inhibiting the secretion of gonadotropins. Decreasing FSH concentration and FSH sensitivity initiate follicle atresia of the nondominant follicles.[24] Higher follicular fluid levels of IL-11 have been noted in atretic follicles.

Over 2 to 3 days, the rising ovarian estradiol levels sensitize the LH pulse generator in the anterior pituitary gland to secrete LH but suppress FSH expression. In the mid to late follicular phase, rising estrogen and inhibin B levels result in reduced FSH but increased LH secretion.[66,72] The pituitary gland gonadotropes respond with a preovulatory surge of gonadotropins (specifically LH) into the peripheral circulation.[24] Thus estrogen levels signal the hypothalamus, which regulates the pulsatile expression of gonadotropin.[21] Follicles greater than 18 mm in diameter are the source of the increased estradiol secretion, which subsequently signals the LH surge.[2,8] The LH surge prior to ovulation is accompanied by decreases in intrafollicular estradiol and androstenedione. In contrast, increases in progesterone and 17α-hydroxyprogesterone are noted intrafollicularly. Inhibin A levels increase concurrently with rising estradiol levels and follicular maturation. Thecal vascularity of the dominant follicle is more than twice that of the nondominant follicles by day 9. This increased vascularity contributes to the elevated LH secretion on day 12 in the ovarian cycle, approximately 2 days before ovulation.[66]

Ovulation

LH secretion increases significantly (i.e., sixfold to tenfold), peaking approximately 12 to 24 hours before ovulation.[50] Known as the LH surge, this dramatic increase in LH precedes ovulation by up to 36 hours (see Figure 2-2).[66]

In addition, the LH surge stimulates resumption of the first meiotic division, so the mature follicle contains secondary oocytes.[21,24,66] FSH also increases, but to a lesser degree (approximately twofold).

The ovum surrounded by loosely packed follicular cells is known as the *cumulus oophorus* and is located to one side of the follicle. Follicular swelling results from the synergistic effect of the increased FSH and LH levels before ovulation. Follicular hyperemia and prostaglandins secreted in the follicular tissues contribute to plasma transudation and subsequent follicular swelling. With proliferation of the granulosa cells and accumulation of the antral fluid, the follicle enlarges, moving to the surface of the ovary approximately 5 to 6 days before ovulation.[66] LH action on the granulosa cells 2 to 3 days before ovulation causes decreased estrogen secretion but, conversely, increased inhibin and progesterone levels.[4] Therefore one day before ovulation, estrogen levels are decreasing with increasing incremental levels of progesterone.

The LH surge lasts, on average, 48 hours, with a rapid ascension for approximately 14 hours before the peak and with a descending limb of approximately 20 hours. In response to the ovulation-inducing LH surge, the dominant follicle ruptures (days 13 to 15), with subsequent formation of the corpus luteum. While accompanied by drastic decreases in estradiol and inhibin B, there are rising levels of inhibin A and the second increase in progesterone at approximately 36 hours after initiation of the LH surge. Ovulation occurs approximately 35 to 44 hours after the LH surge.

As the follicle enlarges, a small cystlike protrusion (i.e., the stigma) develops in the outer follicular wall. Proteolytic enzyme digestion of the mature follicle capsule wall, prostaglandin contraction of the thecal externa smooth muscle, and possibly plasminogen activators and matrix metalloproteinase together promote stigma rupture. Initially, fluid oozes from the follicle. The oocyte, surrounded by the zona pellucida, extrudes and is carried out by the viscous follicular fluid.

Luteal Phase

Progesterone dominates during the luteal phase of the ovarian cycle. The remaining granulosa cells of the ruptured follicle are changed into lutein cells via stimulation by LH remaining from the LH surge.[24] With luteinization, granulosa cells fill with lipids and become yellowish.[66] Thecal cells of the corpus luteum produce androgens. Androgens are progressively converted to androgenic steroids and then to estrogens and progesterone.[66] The luteinization process is enhanced by rising LH levels accompanying the LH surge and is dependent on the degree of exposure. The process continues with only the initial LH surge, although with decreased secretion of androgens and a shortened corpus luteum life span. The corpus luteum, along with lutein cells, secretes increasing amounts of estrogen and progesterone, particularly progesterone, producing approximately 25 to 50 mg per day (see Figure 2-6).[66] The corpus luteum is dependent on trophoblastic hCG for progesterone secretion, glandular growth, and prevention of involution.[66]

During the luteal phase of the ovarian cycle, FSH and LH levels drop drastically in response to high levels of estrogen and, to a lesser extent, progesterone as secreted by the corpus luteum. Gonadotropin concentrations, especially that of FSH, further decrease secondary to the increased hormone concentration of inhibin A secreted by the luteal cells as signaled by the anterior pituitary gland.[2] Secretion of the hypothalamic pulsatile GnRHs declines, leading in turn to decreased LH pulses in response to increased progesterone levels and hypothalamic signaling.[2] In contrast to the early follicular phase, secretion of the LH pulse generator declines from pulses every 60 to 90 minutes to one pulse every 7 to 8 hours with an increase in the pulse amplitude.

Luteal cells of the corpus luteum constitute the principal source of progesterone (the hormone of pregnancy) and, to a lesser degree, estrogen during the first 10 weeks of gestation (Figure 2-26). Progesterone levels during the luteal phase suppress FSH levels. Decreased FSH levels (lowest of the cycle) prevent folliculogenesis. LH levels after ovulation differ little from those of the follicular phase secondary to the increased amplitude of the LH pulse generator.[24] LH is necessary to maintain the corpus luteum.

Midluteally, peak levels of progesterone and estrogen are noted. These peak ovarian steroid levels are coupled with an endometrium favorable to trophoblastic implantation. During the luteal phase, uterine contractility decreases, becoming nearly quiescent at the time of blastocyst implantation.[15]

The placental hormone hCG (see Chapter 3) "rescues" or enhances corpus luteum development and continuation during its first 3 to 4 months.[24,42,66] Luteinization-inhibiting hormone prevents corpus luteum formation and the subsequent luteinization process until ovulation has occurred.

Corpus Luteum Demise

The corpus luteum involutes in approximately 9 to 11 days unless the oocyte is fertilized.[12] Decreased LH levels signal the corpus luteum (approximately 1.5 cm) to begin the involution process at day 21. By day 26, the corpus luteum has progressively involuted to become the corpus albicans, which

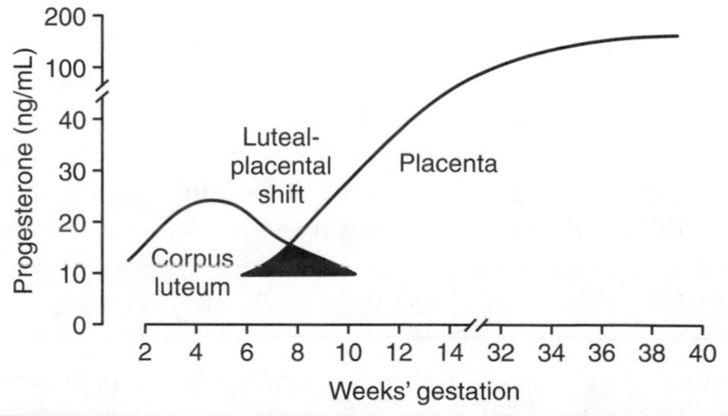

FIGURE 2-26 Diagrammatic representation of the shift in progesterone production from the corpus luteum to the placenta between the seventh and ninth week of gestation. (From Creasy, R.K., Resnik, R., & Iams, J.D. [Eds.]. [2004]. *Maternal-fetal medicine: Principles and practice* [5th ed.]. Philadelphia: Saunders.)

over the following weeks is replaced by connective tissue. As the corpus luteum involutes, estrogen, progesterone, and inhibin levels fall, removing the feedback inhibition of the anterior pituitary gland. As a result, the anterior pituitary begins to secrete progressively more FSH and, in a few days, LH.

With involution, progesterone continues to decrease to a level similar to that of the follicular phase. The declining inhibin A levels 48 hours before menstruation (in concert with rising FSH levels) contribute to follicular recruitment. One day before menstruation, the LH pulse generator frequency increases and amplitude decreases, with a subsequent increase in inhibin B and follicular development. Increased GnRHs are secreted in response to the lower progesterone and estrogen levels, initiating a new ovarian cycle. Menstruation begins. The new ovarian cycle commences with follicular recruitment, selection, and dominance.

Menstruation

Menarche is the first menstrual cycle; the mean age of menarche ranges from 12 to 12.7 years of age in the United States.[40,49,74] As noted earlier, the decline in the age of menarche has been associated with improved nutrition, increased body mass, increased light exposure, and decreased disease. According to Tanner's staging, menarche commonly occurs at stage 4.[40] Menarche commonly occurs 2 to 3 years following the initiation of breast development.[74]

With early menstrual cycles, the developing follicles secrete only estrogens. Estrogen secretion is variable and is unopposed by progesterone.[65] As a result, early cycles are anovulatory and irregular for 1 to 2 years, with variable menstrual flow.[65,74] Generally within 1 to 2 years, menstrual frequency stabilizes at 28 days, ranging from 26 to 34 days, with pattern variations noted at the extremes of reproductive ages.[24] The interval between menstrual cycles averages 28.1 days for women reporting cycle lengths ranging from 15 to 45 days.[12] Cycle length variations primarily occur in the follicular-proliferative phase.[24] Lasting 4 days (give or take a day), most menstrual discharge occurs within the first 24 hours, with the maximal flow occurring on day 2.[3,24] The duration of the menses ranges from 4 to 6 days, is very individualistic but is normally consistent each cycle. Menses of less than 2 days and greater than 7 days are considered abnormal.[65]

Over 3 to 8 days, uterine blood loss averages approximately 35 mL (ranging from 25 to 60 mL), with an equal amount of serous fluid loss per menstrual cycle.[3,12,15] Intersubject menstrual blood loss variations are also noted.[3,28] Iron loss accompanying menstruation is believed to be approximately 0.4 to 1 mg/day of the cycle up to 12 mg/cycle.[3,12,61] Menstrual blood loss of greater than 60 mL per menses is positively correlated with iron deficiency anemia.[65] Menstrual discharge has a distinctive fleshy, musky odor secondary to tissue necrosis and endometrial ischemia and anoxia.

Endometrial Cycle

The endometrial cycle of the uterus is composed of proliferative and secretory phases and menstruation. During the proliferative phase there is development of vascular, endothelial and stromal cells with thickening of the endometrium while during the secretory phase there is ongoing growth and changes in the spiral arteries and endometrial cells to facilitate implantation. With menstruation, there is regression of the endometrium and spiral artery coiling with subsequent endometrial hypoxia, ischemia and endometrial degeneration.[12]

Whereas the ovary is sensitive to FSH and LH, the uterus is more sensitive to estrogen and progesterone (Figure 2-27).

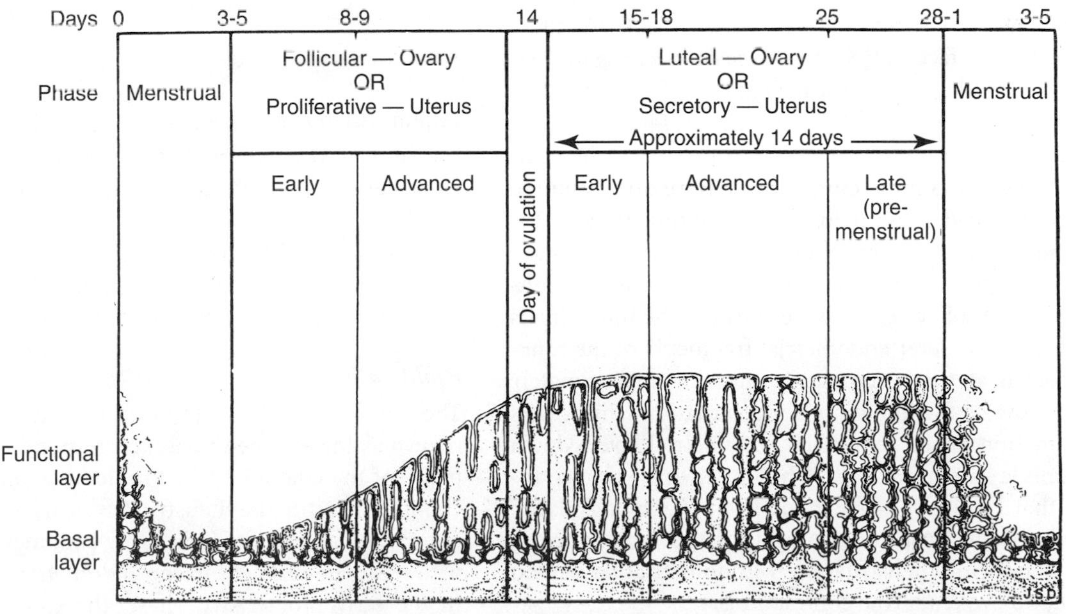

FIGURE 2-27 Cyclic changes in thickness and morphology of endometrium and the relation of these changes to those of the ovarian cycle. (From Cunningham, F.G., et al. [1993]. The endometrium and deciduas: Menstruation and pregnancy. In *Williams' obstetrics* [19th ed.]. Stamford: Appleton & Lange, p. 81.)

The uterine endometrium is comprised of three layers: the functionalis, containing the stroma (mesenchymal connective tissue); the spongy zone; and the germinal basalis layer, which is adjacent to the myometrium (Figure 2-28).[19,24,65] Whereas the functionalis layer is denuded each menstrual cycle, the germinal basalis remains constant throughout.[24,65] During the proliferative phase there is re-ephithelization of the functionalis endometrium and angiogenesis in the basilis layer. Also, in the basilis layer, the stroma become more dense and there is glandular hyperplasia, while in the functionalis the stroma is looser and the glands more separated.[12]

With fertilization, the endometrial tissue changes from secretory tissue to decidual tissue in preparation for implantation.[12] Under the influence of progesterone, the endometrial stroma is transformed to decidual cells.[12] The decidual tissue contains bone marrow cells and immunologic substances such as cytokines, relaxin, inhibin, growth factors, and prorenin to facilitate "acceptance" of the implanting trophoblast.[12] A number of leukocytes and lymphocytes are found in the reproductive tract, specifically in the endometrium. In varying levels, these leukocytes facilitate implantation and protect the fetus and the woman from ascending organisms during pregnancy and menstruation, This natural immunity includes an increase in neutrophils during the perimenstrual phase, with macrophages increasing from the proliferative to the menstrual phases and CD8 cells increasing in the proliferative phase. Natural killer (NK) cells, present in the perimenstrual endometrium, increasing in the secretory phase and with pregnancy, are found in the decidua during the first trimester.[65]

Uterine blood is supplied by the uterine and ovarian arteries, which branch to form the arcuate arteries. These arcuate arteries further branch to form the spiral (coiled) arteries and the basal (straight) arteries (see Figure 2-28). Spiral arteries supply primarily the endometrial basal layer and are responsive to vasoconstrictive factors; basal vessels are not responsive to vasoconstrictive factors.[12] Spiral arteries underlying the placenta undergo marked changes with pregnancy (see Chapter 3).

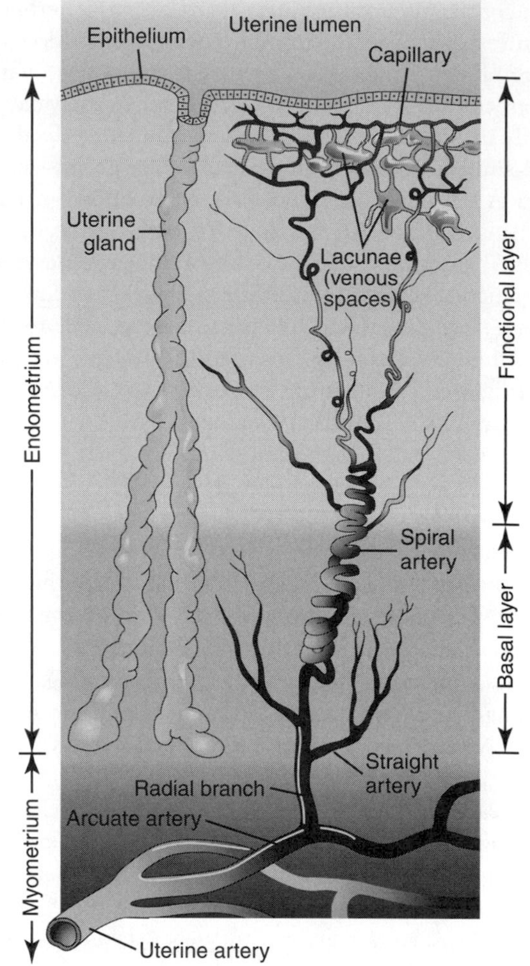

FIGURE 2-28 Diagram of the glands and vasculature of the endometrium. (From Moore, K.L. & Persaud, T.V.N. [2003]. *The developing human: Clinically oriented embryology* [7th ed.]. Philadelphia: Saunders.)

Menstrual Phase

Menstrual bleeding is initiated with arterial vasoconstriction, subsequent hematoma formation, and relaxation of the endometrial arteries, followed by bleeding, with resultant anoxia.[12] Apoptotic changes occur in the endometrial tissue throughout the endometrial cycle.[62] Fissures form in the functionalis layer, and necrotic outer endometrial fragments of the functionalis detach at the hemorrhagic sites for approximately 48 hours following the initiation of menstruation. This results in desquamation of the superficial endometrial layers down to the basalis layer within 48 to 72 hours, leaving a thin endometrium that cyclically regenerates from the spongy layer. Two thirds of the functionalis layer of the endometrium may be shed during menstruation.[12] Endometrial tissue and seeping blood evoke uterine contractions.

Menstrual blood clotting and fibrinolysis are orchestrated by hormonal endometrial stimulation.[12] Progesterone facilitates production of tissue factor and plasminogen activator inhibitor–1 for blood coagulation. In contrast, plasminogen activator is released with the necrotic endometrium and enhances the nonclotting properties of the menstrual fluid.[12] In addition, leukocytes and prostaglandins are released with the desquamated tissue and blood.[12] Uterine leukocytes are thought to protect the uterus from infection, although the endometrium is completely desquamated.

Proliferative Phase

The proliferative phase (the first 11 days of the cycle) is also known as the estrogen phase, corresponding to the follicular phase of the ovarian cycle. Proliferative phase variations account for most of the menstrual cycle irregularities.[24] Following menstruation, a thin layer of endometrial stroma is left, with few epithelial cells in the endometrial glands and crypts. In the early proliferative phase, the endometrial glands are simple and straight.[24] With increasing ovarian estrogen, the endometrium spongy layer, stromal and epithelial cells, and glandular and stromal mitoses proliferate.[12,57] Neutrophils adherent to the endometrium may be the source of vascular endothelial growth factor, promoting endometrial angiogenesis.[19] During the late proliferative phase there is continued growth of the stroma and glands, with corkscrew convolutions, edema, lymphocytes, and macrophages. Cervical mucus significantly increases. From days 12 to 14 of the cycle, there is maximized endometrial growth and proliferation. Growth of the endometrial tissue ranges from 0.5 mm to 5 mm (Figure 2-29).[12,24]

Secretory Phase

The secretory phase, or the following 12 days, corresponds to the luteal phase of the ovarian cycle, with increased secretion of estrogen and progesterone. At ovulation, the endometrium is 3 to 4 mm thick and the endometrial glands secrete a thin, stringy mucus. These mucus strings line the cervical canal, providing channels to guide the sperm. There are increased endometrial lipid and glycogen deposits, along with stromal cytoplasm and tortuosity of blood vessels.[24] In response to progesterone, vacuoles are formed approximately 36 to 48 hours after ovulation.[12] Stromal edema contributes to enlargement of the endometrium. Increased endoplasmic reticulum and mitochondria are noted in the endometrial epithelial cells.

Midsecretory and Late Secretory Phases

Spotting or breakthrough bleeding may result from decreased estradiol levels at ovulation. Midcycle pain, also referred to as **mittelschmerz,** occurs on the side of the dominant follicle.[50] Accompanying the LH surge is a basal temperature nadir.[25] The basal temperature increases 0.5° F to 1° F (0.3° C to 0.6° C) on day 16 of the cycle (following the LH surge) and remains elevated for approximately 11 to 14 days (Figure 2-30).[25] The endometrium responds to the increased progesterone with edema and further secretory development. Endometrial venules and sinusoidal

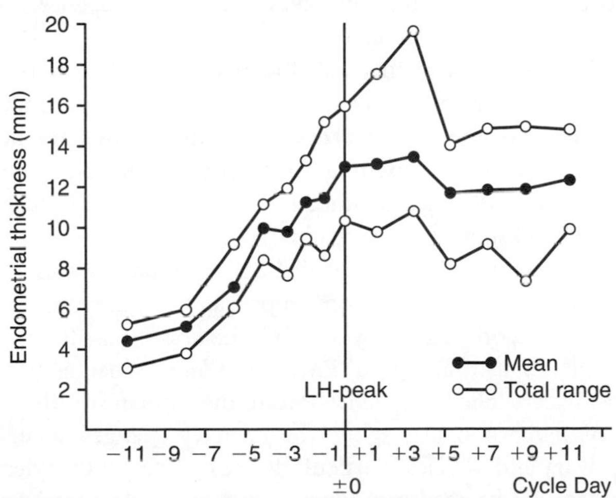

FIGURE 2-29 The endometrial thickness (in mm) measured by transvaginal ultrasound, presented as mean and total range, in 16 women during an ovulatory cycle. Each point on the curve represents a minimum of six observations. (From Bakos, O., Lundkvist, O., & Bergh, T. [1993]. Transvaginal sonographic evaluation of endometrial growth and texture in spontaneous ovulatory cycles. A descriptive study. *Hum Reprod,* 8, 799.)

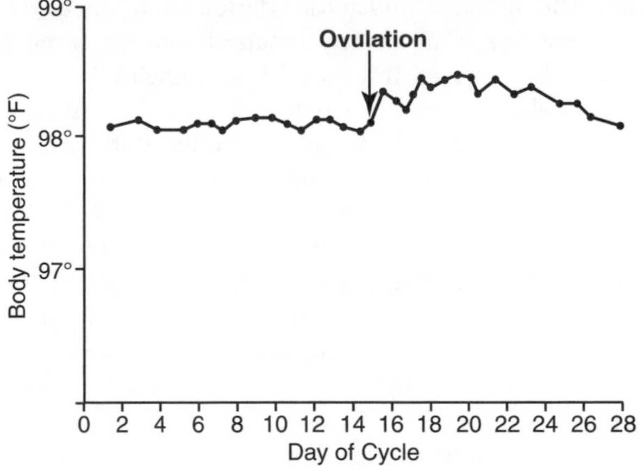

FIGURE 2-30 Elevation of body temperature shortly after ovulation. (From Guyton, A.C. & Hall, J.E. [2006]. *Textbook of medical physiology* [11th ed.]. Philadelphia: Saunders.)

spaces fill with blood and stromal cells accumulate cytoplasm, forming the predecidual endometrial layer. Decidualization is facilitated by transforming growth factor–β and progesterone.[12]

Endometrial spiral arteries coil and lengthen, and the endometrial glands become increasingly tortuous. Endometrial secretory activity is greatest 6 days after ovulation.[24] Increased estradiol and progesterone contribute to maximal stroma edema on day 22.[24] The highly vascularized endometrium is then 5 to 6 mm thick and secreting tissue factors, coagulation factor, plasminogen activator inhibitor–1, and other factors.[12] Coiled arteries lengthen rapidly in the thickening endometrium. Endometrial secretions increase, preparing for implantation of the fertilized ovum.

If fertilization of the oocyte does not occur, the corpus luteum degenerates secondary to decreased estrogen and progesterone levels. Blood vessels of the secretory endometrium undergo vasoconstriction, arterial relaxation, bleeding, ischemia, and endometrial tissue necrosis. Menstruation occurs.

With fertilization, the secretory endometrium is further transformed to decidual tissue (see Chapter 3). In response to increased estrogen and progesterone, the endometrial stromal cells become decidual cells surrounded by a membrane.[12] Growth of the decidua ranges from 5 to 10 mm in depth in preparation for implantation.[12] Embryonic expression of the heparin-binding epidermal growth factor promotes implantation and trophoblast invasion through paracrine and autocrine signaling.[38] This process helps cells penetrate the stroma and displace the arteriole endothelium. The hCG produced by the syncytiotrophoblast (outer layer of the trophoblast) rescues the corpus luteum, thereby increasing estrogen and progesterone levels. The blastocyst implants and pregnancy occurs. (Implantation is discussed further in Chapter 3.)

Premenstrual/Ischemic Phase

The uterus responds to the declining gonadal steroids by stimulating the uterine endometrial cells followed by involution on days 26 to 28. Without support from the corpus luteum, vasospasm occurs in the arterioles and coiled arteries and blood vessels in the endometrial mucosa from 4 to 24 hours before menstruation.[12,26] Endothelin 1 from the endometrial epithelium or stroma promotes vasospasm and vasoconstriction of the endometrial arteries. With vasospasm and decreased estrogen and progesterone, necrosis of the basal layer of the endometrium and stratum vascular blood vessels results and blood pools beneath the endometrium.[24] About 1 to 2 days before menstruation, stroma and epithelial cells of the endometrium produce IL-8 and monocyte chemotactic protein–1, which are chemotactic factors for neutrophils and monocytes.[12] As the corpus luteum ceases to function, there is resorption of the endometrial edema, with subsequent endometrial shrinking.

Gestational Follicular Development

During pregnancy, limited follicular maturation continues in response to gonadotropin stimulation. Although follicular growth may continue until delivery, atresia soon follows. Atresia of the follicles occurs before the follicles can grow to ovulatory size.

Male Reproductive Endocrinology

The earlier section on reproductive hormones discussed male endocrinology. This section provides a summary of these processes. The hormones of the male reproductive system are released by the hypothalamus, anterior pituitary, and testes. Release is both systemic and local, being continuous or acyclic after puberty. Slight diurnal changes in plasma testosterone levels occur. The release of male reproductive hormones is controlled by a negative feedback loop along the hypothalamic-pituitary-testicular axis (see Figure 2-7).

Testosterone is an androgen produced by the Leydig cells of the testes. Initial production of testosterone early in embryonic development is responsible for development of the male reproductive organs and external genitalia. Production becomes active again at puberty. Testosterone is necessary for spermatogenesis, development of male secondary sex characteristics, bone growth, growth and development of male reproductive organs, sexual drive, and potency. The testes also produce small amounts of other androgens.

The hypothalamus regulates the testicular environment by secreting GnRH, which is moderated further by norepinephrine, serotonin, endorphin, melatonin, and dopamine. GnRH secretion occurs once every 60 to 90 minutes.[67] The pulsatile pattern is required for the production and release of LH and FSH by the anterior pituitary.

Both LH and FSH act directly on the testes, stimulating spermatogenesis and testosterone production. Both hormones have a high affinity for their respective receptors. Once bound, they activate the protein kinase cascade via cAMP. LH stimulates the Leydig cells to initiate steroidogenesis by synthesizing androgens from cholesterol precursors. Along with androgen production, LH is responsible for triggering spermatogenesis.

The effects of FSH complement those of LH. FSH binds to receptor sites in the Sertoli cells, stimulating the production of proteins that in turn affect spermatogenesis. FSH is also responsible for facilitating mitosis in the spermatogonia and initiating meiosis in the spermatocyte. Lastly, FSH seems to be necessary for the maturation of the spermatid. Normal levels of FSH are necessary to maintain normal sperm quality.

Testicular testosterone is thought to act directly on the germ cells and Sertoli cells. Through diffusion and active transport, testosterone supports the germinal epithelium and regulates spermatogenesis.

Climacteric

Menopause and the **climacteric** are both terms referring to a woman's transition from a reproductive to a nonfertile state. This transition encompasses a myriad of physiologic and psychosocial changes. Although they are sometimes used interchangeably, the terms climacteric and menopause have different meanings. The climacteric is the transitional period encompassing the perimenopausal, menopausal, and postmenopausal years. From 37.5 years of age onward, there is increased follicular atresia and the ovaries are less responsive, resulting in decreased female fertility.[9,13] Decreased female fertility precedes menopause. The climacteric continues for approximately 2 to 5 years after menopause and includes the physiologic and psychosocial changes accompanying estrogen deprivation.

The term *menopause* (from the Greek word for "to stop") means cessation of menses and is confirmed by amenorrhea for 12 months. The mean age of menopause is 51.4 years of age, with a range of 42 to 58 years.[9,13] By their early 50s, the majority of women (90%) experience menopause.[10] Premature menopause (menopause at age younger than 40 years of age) occurs in approximately 1% of women.[9] Other factors may also contribute to menopausal changes. For example, tobacco use may accelerate ovarian aging. Women who smoke may experience menopause as much as 2 years earlier than nonsmokers.[66] In addition, a strong association has been noted between maternal and daughters' ages at menopause, suggesting a genetic component.[9]

The 2 years preceding and following menopause are referred to as perimenopause.[14] Women who are perimenopausal experience menstrual cycles that are irregular and have greater variation in length and intensity.[1] Figure 2-31 shows reproductive staging as defined by the Stages of Reproductive Aging Workshop.[10] The reproductive interval is stages −5 to −3, with stages −2 to −1 called the menopausal transition and stages +1 to +2 as postmenopausal.[10] Postmenopausal is further categorized as *early,* which is the first 5 years following the final menstrual period (FMP), and *late* defined as beginning 5 years following the FMP until the woman's death.[9]

With reproductive aging, the primary changes occur in the ovary and follicles (particularly the oocytes).[10] Oocytes in women of advanced reproductive age (40 to 45 years) have been found to have abnormal chromosomal alignment at metaphase and increased meiotic nondisjunction.[66] Although ovarian follicles may form more rapidly, they are the same size as in earlier years. At menopause, the ovaries are atrophic and weigh less than 10 g. The ovarian medulla is large and

Final menstrual period (FMP)

Stages:	−5	−4	−3	−2	−1	0	+1	+2
Terminology:	Reproductive			Menopausal Transition			Postmenopause	
	Early	Peak	Late	Early	Late*		Early*	Late
				Perimenopause				
Duration of stage:	Variable			Variable		ⓐ 1 yr	ⓑ 4 yrs	Until demise
Menstrual cycles:	Variable to regular	Regular		Variable cycle length (>*7 days different from normal)*	≥2 skipped cycles and an interval of amenorrhea *(≥60 days)*	*Amen × 12 mos*	None	
Endocrine:	Normal FSH		↑FSH	↑FSH			↑FSH	

*Stages most likely to be characterized by vasomotor symptoms ↑ = elevated

FIGURE 2-31 The Stages of Reproductive Aging Workshop (STRAW) staging system. *Amen*, Amenorrhea. (From Soules, M.R., et al. [2001]. Executive summary: Stages of Reproductive Aging Workshop (STRAW). *Fertil Steril*, 76, 874.)

contains sclerosed blood vessels. With aging, there is a decrease in the total follicular population and in each type of follicle, although no difference has been noted in the total number of follicles of the right and left ovaries. The ovaries secrete primarily androstenedione at levels four times the premenopausal levels, contributing to increased ovarian vein testosterone levels (15 times higher).

During perimenopause, minimal follicles are present at various stages (i.e., primordial to atretic) of development. It is thought that in the decade before menopause there is a significant increase in follicular atresia, which accounts for the minimal ovarian follicles. For 1 to 5 years perimenopausally, menstrual cycles lengthen, and ovulation frequency and reproductive hormone levels vary (see Figure 2-31).[52] In a woman's mid-30s and 40s, the hormone inhibin B begins to progressively decline.[17] Subsequently, FSH levels increase as a compensatory mechanism.[9,16,71] Initially, LH levels stabilize at approximately premenopausal levels, although they begin to rise following amenorrhea of 12 months and then plateau.[34] Changes in inhibin and FSH concentration may precede decreased levels of estrogen and progesterone.

During menopause, estrone becomes the major estrogen; it is derived primarily from peripheral aromatization of adrenal androstenedione, mainly in adipose tissue.[9] Thus the daily production of estrone is significantly related to the woman's body mass index.

With ovarian aging, there is a decrease in estradiol synthesis. Only about 10% of the ovaries secrete estradiol.[13] With aging, androstenedione decreases, with a subsequent decrease in estradiol production. After menopause, androstenedione expression decreases by approximately 50%. Postmenopausally, estradiol production declines to about 12 mcg/day compared to up to 500 mcg/day during the reproductive years. In contrast, estrone levels increase to 80 mcg/day during menopause compared to premenopausal levels of 40 mcg/day.[9] The hypothalamic-pituitary-estrogen positive-feedback mechanism no longer initiates LH secretion.[71] As ovulation frequency decreases, anovulatory cycles increase, with a subsequent decrease in progesterone.

Reproductive hormone levels change with menopause (see Table 2-4). Hormonal confirmation of menopause includes a 10% to 20% increase in FSH levels and LH levels three to five times greater than those in earlier menstrual cycles. FSH levels increase gradually but do so significantly. LH levels greater than 40 IU/L and early follicular FSH levels greater than 30 IU/L are frequently clinical markers for ovarian reserve.[47] FSH levels maximize approximately 1 to 3 years after menopause. Postmenopausally, testosterone levels decrease from 200 mcg/day to 150 mcg/day. Therefore an androgen excess state exists.[13]

Menopausal declines in estradiol particularly and the other sex steroids have numerous physiologic and psychologic effects (Figure 2-32), including vasomotor instability, breast tissue reduction, sleep difficulties, depression, atrophy of urogenital epithelium, atrophy of vaginal tissue and dermis, osteoporosis, coronary heart disease, lethargy, headaches, and concentration difficulties.[13] Vasomotor symptoms (hot flashes or night sweats) are reported by 65% to 76% of perimenopausal women. The prevalence of vasomotor symptoms is positively correlated with serum FSH levels.[9,55]

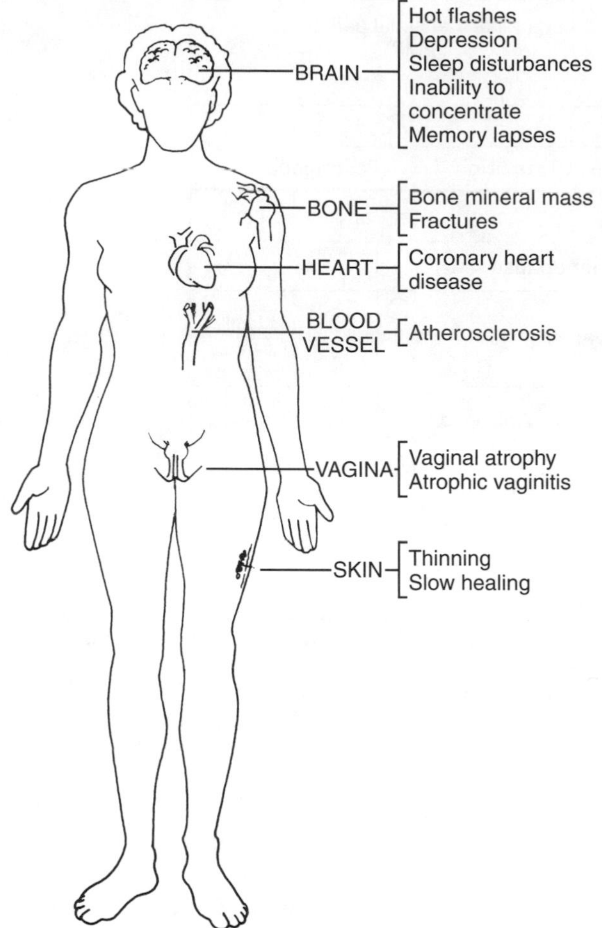

FIGURE 2-32 Effect of estrogen deprivation or reduced estrogen on different organ and tissue systems at or after menopause. (From Dawood, M.Y. [2000]. Menopause. In L.J. Copeland [Ed.]. *Textbook of gynecology* [2nd ed.]. Philadelphia: Saunders.)

Aging Male

Males do not experience a cessation in reproductive ability in the same manner that females experience menopause. There is a gradual decline in testosterone production and in spermatogenesis with aging, but this finding varies.[51] Reproductive ability is usually not compromised, however. The production rate of sperm for a 20-year-old male is approximately 6.5 million sperm per gram per day. By the age of 50 to 90 years of age, a decline is noted and averages 3.8 million sperm per gram per day.[31] With advancing age, it is purported there is incompetence in the hypothalamic-pituitary-testicular feedback system with resulting inadequate LH levels.[51] In addition, there is a decrease in normal morphologic and motile sperm. In later life, atrophy of the external genitalia may occur.[51] Concomitantly involution of the testes and degenerative changes in the Leydig cells, diminishes production of testosterone. With declining health or exacerbation of chronic diseases, there is a decrease in sperm production and ejaculate volume.[51] The age at which these events occur is variable among individual men, and some do not experience them at all.

SUMMARY

Reproductive endocrinology is an orchestrated cascade of events initiated in utero and mediated by hormonal control. Episodic pulses of gonadotropin-releasing factors and hormones modulate the secretion of gonadal steroids, estrogen, progesterone, and testosterone. Cyclical follicular development and maturation, in concert with endometrial changes, prepare for the fertilized oocyte. Hormonal regulation of testicular function and spermatogenesis are necessary for fertilization of the oocyte. Knowledge of the hypothalamic-pituitary-ovarian/testicular axis undergirds reproductive health and obstetric, infertility, gynecologic, and andrologic nursing. Recommendations for clinical practice related to the physiologic basis for reproduction are summarized in Table 2-8.

Table 2-8 Summary of Recommendations for Clinical Practice Related to the Physiologic Basis for Reproduction

Understand the basic processes involved in the hypothalamic-pituitary-ovarian-testicular axis (pp. 29-44, 58; Figures 2-5, 2-7, 2-16, and 2-26).
Understand the basic processes involved in steroidogenesis (pp. 36-41; Figures 2-10, 2-11, and 2-14).
Counsel women and men regarding physical and physiologic changes during puberty, reproduction, premenopause, menopause, postmenopause, and reproductive functions in the aging male (pp. 45-58; Figures 2-19 and 2-32; Tables 2-4, 2-6, and 2-7).
Provide teaching to families regarding physical and physiologic changes during puberty, reproduction, the climacteric for females and reproductive functions for the older male (pp. 45-58; Figures 2-18, 2-19, Figure 2-21, and 2-32; Tables 2-4, 2-6, and 2-7).
Counsel families regarding follicular growth and development (pp. 48-53, 56; Figure 2-24).
Understand the usual patterns of reproductive hormone production and counsel men, women, and families regarding the changes during the woman's life span (pp. 33-42, 45-47, 53, 57-58; Figures 2-25 and 2-32; Tables 2-2 and 2-4).
Provide health teaching regarding the ovarian cycle and changes during the woman's life span (pp. 45-47, 48-53, 56-58; Figures 2-23, 2-24, and 2-27).
Provide health teaching regarding the endometrial cycles and changes during the woman's life span (pp. 45-47, 53-58; Figures 2-24, 2-27, 2-28, 2-29, 2-30, and 2-31).
Provide health teaching regarding spermatogenesis and changes during the men's life span (pp. 44-47, 56, 58).
Educate and provide support to families undergoing reproductive alterations (pp. 45-47, 53, 56-58).
Teach families who have experienced reproductive problems the basic principles of neuroendocrinology (pp. 29-44, 58; Figure 2-7).

References

1. Astrup, K. (2004). Menstrual bleeding patterns in pre- and perimenopausal women. A population-based prospective diary study. *Acta Obstet Gynecol Scand, 83*, 197.
2. Baird, D.T. (1998). Feedback mechanisms. In I.S. Fraser (Ed.). *Estrogens and progestogens in clinical practice*. Philadelphia: Churchill Livingstone.
3. Baldwin, R.M., Whalley, P.J., & Pritchard, J.A. (1961). Measurements of menstrual blood loss. *Am J Obstet Gynecol, 81*, 739.
4. Beckman, C., et al. (2006). *Obstetrics and gynecology* (5th ed.). Philadelphia: Lippincott Williams & Wilkins.
5. Bulun, S. (2005). Hormone action. In B. Carr, R. Blackwell, & R. Azziz (Eds.). *Azziz's essential reproductive medicine*. New York: McGraw-Hill.
6. Bulun, S.E. & Adashi, E.Y. (2008). The physiology and pathology of the female reproductive axis. In H.K. Kronenberg, et al. (Eds.). *Williams textbook of endocrinology* (11th ed.). Philadelphia: Saunders.
7. Carr, B. (2005). The ovary and the normal menstrual cycle. In B. Carr, R. Blackwell, & R. Azziz (Eds.). *Essential reproductive medicine*. New York: McGraw-Hill.
8. Casper, F.W., et al. (2001). Concentrations of inhibins and activin in women undergoing stimulation with recombinant follicle-stimulating hormone for in vitro fertilization treatment. *Fertil Steril, 75*, 32.
9. Cedars, M. & Evans, M. (2008). Menopause. In R. S. Gibbs, et al. (Eds.). *Danforth's obstetrics and gynecology* (10th ed.). Philadelphia: Lippincott Williams & Wilkins.
10. Chiquoine, A.D. (1960). The development of the zona pellucida of the mammalian ovum. *Am J Anat, 106*, 149.
11. Clifton, D. & Steiner, R. (2010). Neuroendocrinology of reproduction. In J.F. Strauss & R.L. Barbieri (Eds.). *Yen and Jaffe's reproductive endocrinology: Physiology, pathophysiology, and clinical management* (6th ed.). Philadelphia: Saunders.
12. Cunningham, F.G., et al. (2010). *Williams' obstetrics* (23rd ed.). New York: McGraw-Hill.
13. Dawood, M.Y. (2000). Menopause. In L.J. Copeland (Ed.). *Textbook of gynecology* (2nd ed.). Philadelphia: Saunders.
14. Ebeling, P. & Koivisto, V.A. (1994). Physiological importance of dehydroepiandrosterone. *Lancet, 343*, 1479.
15. Fanchin, R., et al. (2001). Uterine contractility decreases at the time of blastocyst transfers. *Hum Reprod, 16*, 1115.
16. Freeman, E.W., et al. (2001). Hot flashes in the late reproductive years: Risk factors for African-American and Caucasian women. *J Women's Health Gender-Based Med, 10*, 67.
17. Fritz, M. & Speroff, L. (2011). *Clinical gynecologic endocrinology and infertility*. (8th ed.). Philadelphia: Lippincott Williams & Wilkins.
18. Funabashi, T., et al. (2005). Nicotine inhibits pulsatile luteinizing hormone secretion in human males but not in human females, and tolerance to this nicotine effect is lost within one week of quitting smoking. *J Clin Endocrinol Metab, 90*, 3908.
19. Gargett, C.E., et al. (2001). Focal vascular endothelial growth factor correlates with angiogenesis in human endometrium. Role of intravascular neutrophils. *Hum Reprod, 16*, 1065.
20. Genazzani, A.R., et al. (2000). Neuropeptides, neurotransmitters, neurosteroids, and the onset of puberty. *Ann N Y Acad Sci, 900*, 1.
21. Gill, S. & Hall, J. (2005). Neuroendocrinology. In B. Carr, R. Blackwell, & R. Azziz (Eds.). *Essential reproductive medicine*. New York: McGraw-Hill.
22. Goodman, A.L. & Hodgen, G.D. (1983). The ovarian triad of the primate menstrual cycle. *Recent Prog Horm Res, 39*, 1.
23. Gordon, C. & Laufer, M. (2005). The physiology of puberty. In S.J. Emans, M.R. Laufer, & D.P. Goldstein (Eds.). *Pediatric & adolescent gynecology* (5th ed.). Philadelphia: Lippincott Williams & Wilkins.
24. Gordon, K. & Oehninger, S. (2000). Reproductive physiology. In L.J. Copeland (Ed.). *Textbook of gynecology* (2nd ed.). Philadelphia: Saunders.
25. Greene, C.A. & O' Keane, J.A. (2000). Investigation of the infertile couple. In L.J. Copeland (Ed.). *Textbook of gynecology* (2nd ed.). Philadelphia: Saunders.
26. Guyton, A.C. & Hall, J.E. (2011). *Textbook of medical physiology* (12th ed.). Philadelphia: Saunders.
27. Hall, J.E. (2009). Neuroendocrine control of the menstrual cycle. In J.F. Strauss & R.L. Barbieri (Eds.). *Yen and Jaffe's reproductive endocrinology: Physiology, pathophysiology, and clinical management* (6th ed.). Philadelphia: Saunders.
28. Hallberg, L., et al. (1966). Menstrual blood loss—a population study. Variation at different ages and attempts to define normality. *Acta Obstet Gynecol Scand, 45*, 320.
29. Halvorson, L.M. & Chin, W.W. (1999). Gonadotropic hormones: Biosynthesis, secretion, receptors, and action. In S.C. Yen, R.B. Jaffe, & R.L. Barbieri (Eds.). *Reproductive endocrinology: Physiology, pathophysiology, and clinical management* (4th ed.). Philadelphia: Saunders.
30. Jenkin, G., et al. (2001). Physiological and regulatory roles of activin A in late pregnancy. *Mol Cell Endocrinol, 180*, 131.
31. Jones, E. & DeCherney, A. (2003). The male reproductive system. In W. Boron & E. Boulpaep (Eds.). *Medical physiology*. Philadelphia: Saunders.
32. Knobil, E. (1989). The electrophysiology of the GnRH pulse generator in the rhesus monkey. *J Steroid Biochem, 33*, 669.
33. Kronenberg, H.M., et al. (2008). Principles of endocrinology. In H.K. Kronenberg, et al. (Eds.). *Williams textbook of endocrinology* (11th ed.). Philadelphia: Saunders.
34. Kwekkeboom, D.J., et al. (1990). Serum gonadotropins and a subunit decline in aging normal postmenopausal women. *J Clin Endocrinol Metab, 70*, 944.
35. La Rosa, C., Traggiai, C., & Stanhope, R. (2004). Normal childhood, puberty and adolescence. In S. Creighton, et al. (Eds.). *Paediatric and adolescent gynaecology: A multidisciplinary approach*. New York: Cambridge University Press.
36. Lazar, M.A. (2008). Mechanism of action of hormones that act on nuclear receptors. In H.K. Kronenberg, et al. (Eds.). *Williams textbook of endocrinology* (11th ed.). Philadelphia: Saunders.
37. Layman, L.C. & McDonough, P.G. (2000). Mutations of follicle stimulating hormone-β and its receptor in human and mouse: Genotype/phenotype. *Mol Cell Endocrinol, 161*, 9.
38. Leach, R.E., et al. (1999). Multiple roles for heparin-binding epidermal growth factor-like growth factor are suggested by its cell-specific expression during the human endometrial cycle and early placentation. *J Clin Endocrinol Metab, 84*, 3355.
39. Lee, P. & Kulin, H. (2005). Normal pubertal development. In T. Moshang (Ed.). *Pediatric endocrinology: The requisites in pediatrics*. St. Louis: Mosby.
40. Lee, P. (2005). Early pubertal development. In T. Moshang (Ed.). *Pediatric endocrinology: The requisites in pediatrics*. St. Louis: Mosby.
41. Levy, D.P., et al. (2000). The role of LH in ovarian stimulation-exogenous LH: Let's design the future. *Hum Reprod, 15*, 2258.
42. Liu, J.H. (2004). Endocrinology of pregnancy. In R.K. Creasy, R. Resnik, & J.D. Iams (Eds.). *Maternal-fetal medicine: Principles and practice* (5th ed.). Philadelphia: Saunders.
43. Llop-Vinolas, D., et al. (2004). Onset of puberty at eight years of age in girls determines a specific tempo of puberty but does not affect adult height. *Acta Paediatr, 93*, 874.
44. Lobo, R.A. (2009). Menopause and aging. In J.F. Strauss & R.L. Barbieri (Eds.). *Yen and Jaffe's reproductive endocrinology: Physiology, pathophysiology, and clinical management* (6th ed.). Philadelphia: Saunders.
45. Longcope, C. (1998). Metabolism of estrogens and progestogens. In I.S. Fraser, et al. (Eds.). *Estrogens and progestogens in clinical practice*. Philadelphia: Churchill Livingstone.
46. Low, M. (2008). Neuroendocrinology. In H.K. Kronenberg, et al. (Eds.). *Williams textbook of endocrinology* (11th ed.). Philadelphia: Saunders.
47. Macklon, N.S. & Fauser, B.C.J.M. (1999). Aspects of ovarian follicle development throughout life. *Horm Res, 52*, 161.
48. Melmed, S. & Kleinberg, D. (2008). Anterior pituitary. In H.K. Kronenberg, et al. (Eds.). *Williams textbook of endocrinology* (11th ed.). Philadelphia: Saunders.
49. Mitan, L.A.P. & Slap, G.B. (2000). Adolescent menstrual disorders. *Adolesc Med, 84*, 851.

50. Moore, K.L. & Persaud, T.V.N. (2008). *Before we are born: Essentials of embryology and birth defects* (8th ed.). Philadelphia: Saunders.
51. Nieschlag, E., Behre, H., & Nieschlag, S. (Eds.) (2010). *Male reproductive health and dysfunction* (3rd ed.). New York: Springer.
52. O'Connor, K.A., Holman, D.J., Wood, J.W. (2001). Menstrual cycle variability and the perimenopause. *Am J Hum Biol, 13*, 465.
53. Palter, S.F., et al. (2001). Are estrogens of import to primate/human ovarian folliculogenesis? *Endocr Rev, 22*, 389.
54. Piano, M. & Huether, S. (2002). Mechanisms of hormonal regulation. In K.L. McCance & S.E. Huether (Eds.). *Pathophysiology: The biologic basis for disease in adults and children.* (4th ed.). St. Louis: Mosby.
55. Randolph, J., et al. (2005). The relationship of longitudinal change in reproductive hormones and vasomotor symptoms during the menopausal transition. *J Clin Endocrinol Metab, 90*, 6106.
56. Rittmaster, R.S. (2000). Hyperandrogenism. In L.J. Copeland (Ed.). *Textbook of gynecology* (2nd ed.). Philadelphia: Saunders.
57. Rogers, R.J., et al. (2001). Dynamics of the membrana granulosa during expansion of the ovarian follicular antrum. *Mol Cell Endocrinol, 171*, 41.
58. Runesson, E., et al. (2000). Gonadotropin- and cytokine-regulated expression of the chemokine interleukin 8 in the human preovulatory follicle of the menstrual cycle. *J Clin Endocrinol Metab, 85*, 4387.
59. Scheele, F. & Schoemaker, J. (1996). The role of follicle-stimulating hormone in the selection of follicles in human ovaries: A survey of the literature and a proposed model. *Gynecol Endocrinol, 10*, 55.
60. Schneyer, A.L., et al. (2000). Dynamic changes in the intrafollicular inhibin/activin/follistatin axis during human follicular development: Relationship to circulating hormone concentrations. *J Clin Endocrinol Metab, 85*, 3319.
61. Scott, D.E. & Pritchard, J.A. (1967). Iron deficiency in healthy young college women. *JAMA, 199*, 147.
62. Shikone, T., et al. (1997). Apoptosis of human ovary and uterine endometrium during the menstrual cycle. *Horm Res, 48*, 27.
63. Siiteri, P. (2005). The continuing saga of dehydroepiandro-sterone (DHEA). *J Clin Endocrinol Metab 90*, 3795.
64. Sidis, Y., et al. (2001). Follistatin: Essential role for the N-terminal domain in activin binding and neutralization. *J Biol Chem, 276*, 17718.
65. Strauss, J.F. & Lessey, B.A. (2009). The structure, function, and evaluation of the female reproductive tract. In J.F. Strauss & R.L. Barbieri (Eds.). *Yen and Jaffe's reproductive endocrinology: Physiology, pathophysiology, and clinical management* (6th ed.). Philadelphia: Saunders.
66. Strauss, J.F. & Williams, C.J. (2009). The ovarian life cycle. In J.F. Strauss & R.L.Barbieri (Eds.). *Yen and Jaffe's reproductive endocrinology: Physiology, pathophysiology, and clinical management* (6th ed.). Philadelphia: Saunders.
67. Strauss, J.F. (2009). The synthesis and metabolism of steroid hormones. In J.F. Strauss & R.L. Barbieri (Eds.). *Yen and Jaffe's reproductive endocrinology: Physiology, pathophysiology, and clinical management* (6th ed.). Philadelphia: Saunders.
68. Styne, D.M & Grumbach, M.M. (2008). Puberty: Ontogeny, neuroendocrinology, physiology, and disorders. In H.K. Kronenberg, et al. (Eds.). *Williams textbook of endocrinology* (11th ed.). Philadelphia: Saunders.
69. Tena-Sempere, M., Levallet, J., & Huhtaniemi, I. (2004). Gonadotrophin receptors. In S. Creighton, et al. (Eds.). *Paediatric and adolescent gynaecology: A multidisciplinary approach.* New York: Cambridge University Press.
70. Ukkola, O., et al. (2001). Age, body mass index, race and other determinants of steroid hormone variability: The HERITAGE Family Study. *Eur J Endocrinol, 145*, 1.
71. Weiss, G. (2001). Menstrual irregularities and the perimenopause, *J Soc Gynecol Invest, 8*, S65.
72. Welt, C.K., et al. (2001). Differential regulation of inhibin A and inhibin B by luteinizing hormone, follicle-stimulating hormone, and stage of follicle development. *J Clin Endocrinol Metab, 86*, 2531.
73. Welt, C.K., et al. (1997). Frequency modulation of follicle-stimulating hormone (FSH) during the luteal-follicular transition: Evidence for FSH control of inhibin B in normal women. *J Clin Endocrinol Metab, 82*, 2645.
74. Witchel, S.F. & Plant, T.M. (2009). Puberty: Gonadarche and adrenarche. In J.F. Strauss & R.L. Barbieri (Eds.). *Yen and Jaffe's reproductive endocrinology: Physiology, pathophysiology, and clinical management* (6th ed.). Philadelphia: Saunders.
75. Woodruff, T.K. & Mather, J.P. (1995). Inhibin, activin and the female reproductive axis. *Annu Rev Physiol, 57*, 219.
76. Young, E.A., et al. (2000). Alteration in the hypothalamic-pituitary-ovarian axis in depressed women. *Arch Gen Psychiatry, 57*, 1157.
77. Zeleznik, A.J. (2001). Modifications in gonadotropin signaling: A key to understanding cyclic ovarian function, *J Soc Gynecol Invest, 8*, S24.

The Prenatal Period and Placental Physiology

CHAPTER 3

The prenatal period encompasses the period from conception to birth. During this period the pregnant woman experiences major physiologic and psychologic changes that support maternal adaptations, support fetal growth and development, and prepare the mother for the birth process and transition to parenthood. Simultaneously the embryo and fetus are developing from a single cell to a complex organism. Supporting this development are the placenta, fetal membranes (amnion and chorion), and amniotic fluid. These structures protect and nourish the embryo and fetus and are essential for the infant's survival, growth, and development.

Alterations in maternal physiology, endocrine function, embryonic and fetal development, or placental function and structure can lead to maternal disorders and fetal death, malformations, poor growth, or preterm birth. Prenatal screening and diagnosis can be used to evaluate fetal status. Assessment of placental size and function and amniotic fluid volume and composition is useful in evaluating fetal growth and health status during gestation. This chapter describes events that result in conception and provides an overview of pregnancy; related endocrinology; and development of the embryo, fetus, and placenta. Specific clinical implications related to normal and abnormal development are discussed.

OVERVIEW OF PREGNANCY

The duration of pregnancy averages 266 days (38 weeks) after ovulation, or 280 days (40 weeks) after the first day of the last menstrual period (Figure 3-1). This equals 10 lunar months, or just over 9 calendar months. During these months, the almost solid uterus, with a cavity of 10 mL or less, develops into a large, thin-walled organ. The total volume of the contents of the uterus is 5 L or more at term, 500 to 1000 times the original capacity.[33]

Most of the changes encountered during pregnancy are progressive and can be attributed to either hormonal responses or physical alterations secondary to fetal size. The preimplantation endocrine system controls the reproductive cycle. In the woman, this involves the cyclic release of pituitary gonadotropins and secretion of estrogen and progesterone by the ovary (see Chapter 2).

The postimplantation endocrine systems of the mother, placenta and fetus control the integrity and duration of gestation. These processes include (1) maintenance of the corpus luteum by human chorionic gonadotropin (hCG); (2) production of estrogen, progesterone, human placental lactogen (hPL), and other hormones and growth factors by the placenta; and (3) release of oxytocin (by the posterior pituitary), prolactin (by the anterior pituitary), and relaxin (by the ovary, uterus, and placenta).

Changes in specific organ systems and metabolic processes during pregnancy and clinical implications are described in detail in Units II and III. This section presents an overview of physiologic changes during each trimester of pregnancy based on the time from the start of the last menstrual period. Concomitant with these adaptations and equally significant are psychologic adaptations; these adaptations are not discussed because the focus of this text is on physiologic changes.

First Trimester

During the first trimester, the woman experiences the first signs and symptoms of pregnancy. The first sign of pregnancy is usually cessation of menses. The average cycle length is 28 days, with a range of 15 to 45 days. The first missed period is suggestive of pregnancy; by the time the second period is missed, pregnancy becomes probable. Brief or scant bleeding may occur during pregnancy, most commonly in the first trimester around the time of implantation.

Breast tenderness and tingling, especially around the nipple area, often occurs beginning at 4 to 6 weeks. Increased breast size and vascularity are usually evident by the end of the second month and are due to growth of the secretory duct system. Colostrum leakage may occur by 3 months. Enlargement of the sebaceous glands around the nipple (Montgomery's glands) may also be apparent.

Nausea with or without vomiting may occur any time of the day or night. This symptom usually begins about 6 weeks after the onset of the last menstrual period and continues for 6 to 12 weeks or longer in some women. An increase in frequency of urination is seen during the first trimester. Excessive fatigue is often experienced and may last throughout the first 12 weeks. The cause of this fatigue is unknown,

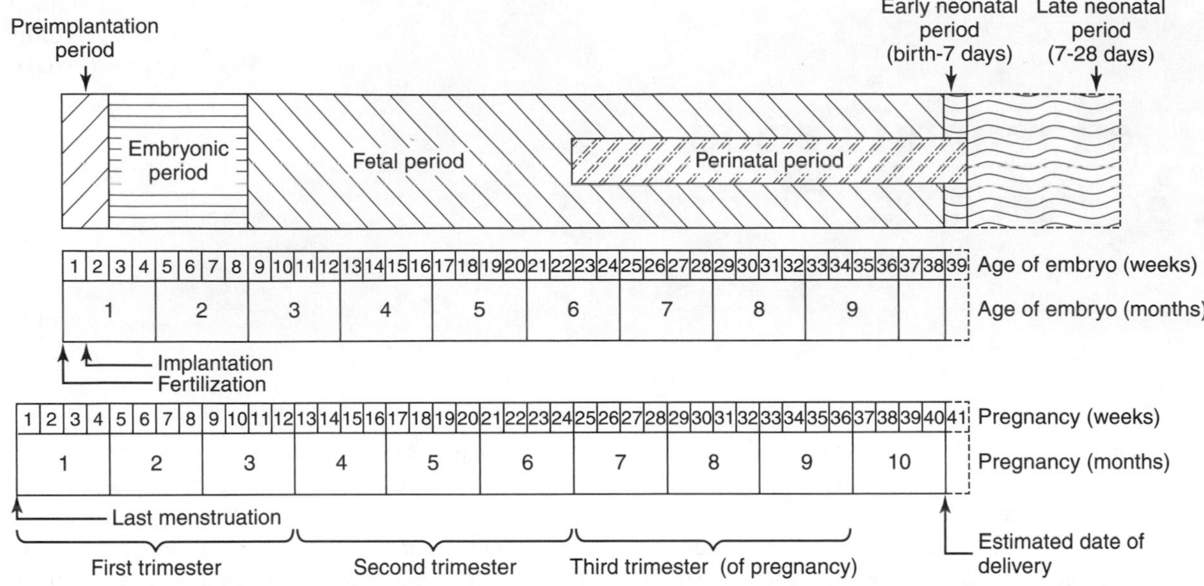

FIGURE 3-1 The two time scales used to depict human development. Embryonic development, in the upper scale, is counted from fertilization (or from ovulation [i.e., postovulatory days]). The clinical estimation of pregnancy is counted from the last menstrual period and is shown on the lower scale. Note that there is a 2-week discrepancy between these scales. The perinatal period is very long because it includes all of the preterm deliveries. (From Standring, S. [2005]. *Gray's anatomy: The anatomical basis of clinical practice* [39th ed.]. Edinburgh: Churchill Livingstone.)

but it may be a response to hormonal shifts. Hormonal changes are also thought to be responsible for the dyspnea experienced during this period.

Physical signs associated with pregnancy include Goodell's sign (softening of the cervix and vagina with increased leukorrheal discharge), Hegar's sign (softening and increased compressibility of the lower uterine segment), and Chadwick's sign (bluish purple discoloration of the vaginal mucosa, cervix, and vulva) by 8 weeks. Although a presumptive sign of pregnancy, Chadwick's sign is only useful in primiparous women. By 8 to 10 weeks, fetal heart tones can be auscultated by Doppler ultrasonography. Real-time ultrasound can pick up fetal heart movements earlier. Maternal cardiovascular changes are also occurring, with stroke volume and cardiac output increasing and systemic vascular resistance decreasing. These changes contribute to increased renal plasma flow and glomerular filtration.[33] Weight gain during the first trimester is usually small.

Second Trimester

This trimester is characterized by marked maternal changes as the fetus's presence becomes more evident. The uterus, which starts as a pear-shaped organ, becomes ovoid, as length increases over width. With this growth, the uterus moves into the abdominal cavity and begins to displace the intestines. The tension and stretching of the broad ligament may lead to painful sensations. Normally contractions during the second trimester are irregular and usually painless.

The increasing vascularity of the vagina and pelvic viscera may result in increased sensitivity and heightened arousal and sexual interest. Mucorrhea is not uncommon as a result of the hyperactivity of the vaginal glandular tissues. This change may increase the pleasure experienced during sexual intercourse. Spontaneous orgasm and multiple orgasms may occur as a result of the increased congestion. Leukorrhea often occurs, with thick, white, acidotic (pH of 3.5 to 6.0) discharge that may contribute to inhibition of pathogenic colonization of the vagina.[33] Perineal structures also enlarge as a result of the vasocongestion, increased vascularity, hypertrophy of the perineal body, and fat deposition that began during the first trimester.

The breasts become increasingly more nodular. Colostrum can be easily expressed at this stage. The nipples become larger and more deeply pigmented. The areolae have also broadened. Increased skin pigmentation occurs elsewhere as well. The line from the umbilicus to the symphysis pubis (linea alba) may darken very distinctly and is referred to as the *linea nigra*. Darkening of the skin over the forehead and cheeks (melasma or chloasma gravidarum) can also result from hormonal changes. Most pigmentation changes fade by a year following delivery, but some may persist.

Other cutaneous changes include the appearance of spider nevi and capillary hemangiomas. The former usually resolve; the latter may shrink but often do not completely disappear after delivery. The breakdown of underlying connective tissue may result in reddish, irregular stretch marks on the abdomen, buttocks, thighs, or breasts. Little can be done to prevent the formation of stretch marks, which may fade with time.

Increased estrogen levels may result in hyperemic, soft, swollen gums that bleed easily. Increased salivation also may occur. Good oral and dental care is important. Elevated progesterone levels decrease the motility of the gastrointestinal tract. By the end of the second trimester, esophageal regurgitation may lead to heartburn. Fluid retention and constipation also may occur as pregnancy progresses.

Maternal blood volume rises significantly during these months, and hematocrit and hemoglobin levels begin to fall due to hemodilution. Blood pressure decreases slightly, whereas the heart rate increases by 10 to 20 beats per minute. Hemodynamic changes continue. Most women develop a systolic murmur during the second or third trimesters. Glomerular filtration rate increases. Bladder and ureter tone is decreased, and the ureters become more tortuous, increasing the risk of urinary tract infection.

Protein and carbohydrate needs increase markedly, contributing to the weight gain during this phase. The mother first perceives fetal movement (quickening) at 16 to 20 weeks' gestation (earlier in successive pregnancies). These movements become perceptible to a hand on the mother's abdomen toward the end of this period. By 20 weeks, the uterus will be at the level of the umbilicus.

Third Trimester

In the third trimester fatigue, dyspnea, and increased urinary frequency are experienced. Fatigue and dyspnea are related to the increased weight and pressure exerted by the greatly enlarged uterus. Thoracic breathing predominates. Increased urinary frequency is due to pressure of the presenting part against the bladder.

The uterine wall thins to 5 to 10 mm by term. The fetus can be easily palpated through the uterine wall, and fetal movements are quite visible. The uterus reaches almost to the liver, and broad ligament pain may become more intense as tension is increased. Uterine contractions become more regular and uncomfortable and are easily detected and palpable near term.

The heart is displaced slightly to the left as a result of the increased pressure from the enlarged uterus. Blood pressure rises slightly, and cardiac output remains unchanged. Blood volume peaks at 28 to 34 weeks' gestation. Dependent edema frequently occurs as blood return from the lower extremities is reduced. Increasing pelvic congestion, relaxation of the smooth muscle in the veins, and the increased pressure of the growing fetus may result in varicosities of the perineum and rectum. Constipation and obesity may lead to development of engorged blood vessels.[33]

The growing uterus displaces the intestines and stomach. A hiatal hernia may develop along with increasing heartburn and a decreased stomach capacity. The bladder is pulled up and out of the true pelvis by the growing uterus. This stretches the urethra and increases the susceptibility to urinary tract infection.

The increased elasticity of connective and collagen tissue leads to relaxation and hypermobility of the pelvic joints. Separation of the symphysis pubis results in instability of the sacroiliac joint. The center of gravity shifts lower with development of a progressive lordosis to compensate for the anterior shift of the uterus. Balance is maintained by an enhanced cervicodorsal curvature, leading to difficulty in walking and the characteristic waddling gait. Stress on the ligaments and muscles of the middle and lower back and spine may lead to discomfort and back pain.[33]

Most women tolerate these changes without difficulty; however, many become tired of pregnancy late in gestation. The process of conception and the changes related to pregnancy are truly remarkable events. The coming together of all factors brings about the appropriate and necessary environment for the nurturance and development of the next generation.

CONCEPTION

For conception to occur, a precise set of sequential events must take place. The probability of a viable conception per menstrual cycle is less than 40% to 50%.[25,103] The process of conception and fetal survival is selective, as evidenced by implantation failures and the approximately 50% anomaly rate encountered in spontaneously aborted fetuses.[103,130] Gametogenesis is described in Chapter 1. The ovarian and endometrial cycles necessary for conception and early support of the fertilized ovum, as well as follicle maturation, are described in Chapter 2. This section will examine ovulation, sperm transport, fertilization, cleavage, and zygote transport.

Ovulation

The ovary is responsible for two important functions: gametogenesis and steroid hormone synthesis. Integration of ovarian steroid synthesis, follicle maturation, ovulation, and corpus luteum function is essential for fertilization and implantation. Estrogen and progesterone have significant effects on tubal and uterine motility, endometrial proliferation, and the properties of the cervical mucus.[33] In order for fertilization to take place, the oocyte must become "fertilization competent" (see Chapter 1). The close proximity of the oocytes and follicular cells in the ovary allows the follicle and oocyte to communicate bidirectionally via gap junctions (intracellular membrane channels) in order to work together to control meiotic arrest and resumption, follicle maturation; ovulation; and corpus luteum formation, function, and regression.[26] The hypothalamus and anterior pituitary regulate these latter morphologic changes through secretion of gonadotropin-releasing hormone (GnRH) and gonadotropins. Follicle-stimulating hormone (FSH) and luteinizing hormone (LH) act synergistically (see Chapter 2). Endocrine interactions in follicle maturation are illustrated in Figure 3-2.

Usually only one follicle matures and is ovulated, although the exact mechanism for this is unknown. At the beginning of the menstrual cycle, up to 15 to 20 primary (pre-antral) follicles are stimulated by FSH, but only 6 to 12 enlarge. Of these growing follicles, several develop into antral follicles. Eventually one follicle becomes dominant and begins to function independent of FSH. This follicle secretes inhibin,

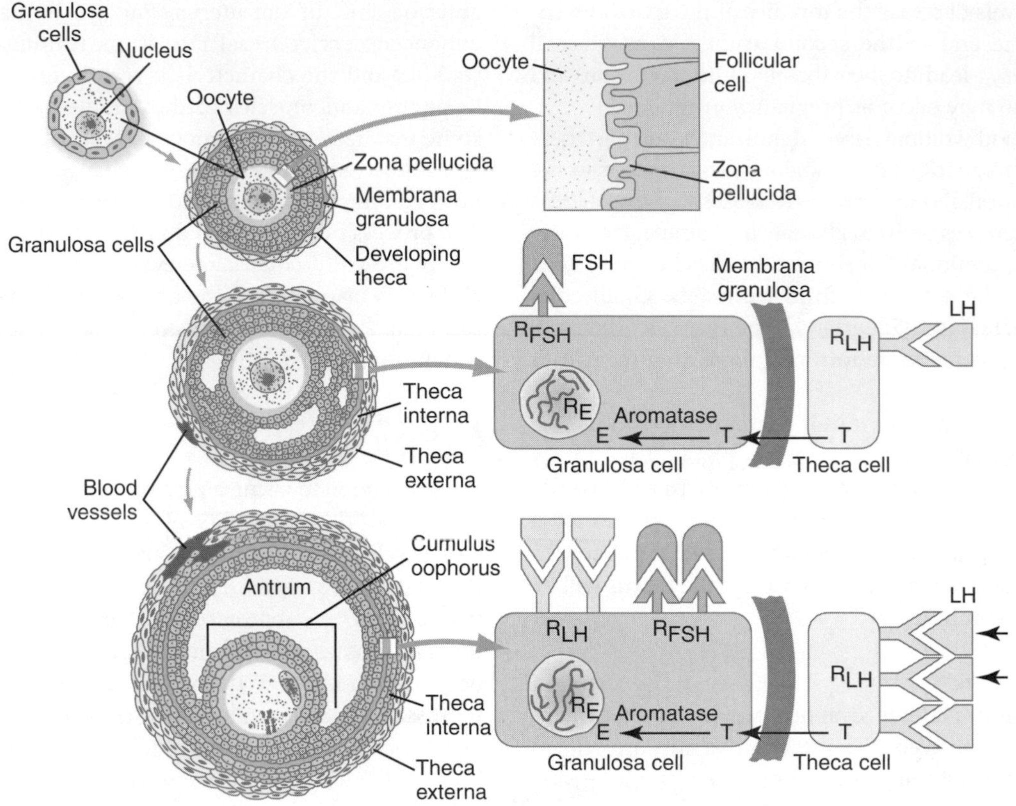

FIGURE 3-2 Growth and maturation of a follicle along with major endocrine interactions in the theca and granulosa cells. *E,* Estrogen; *FSH,* follicle stimulating hormone; *LH,* luteinizing hormone; *R,* receptor; *T,* testosterone. (From Carlson, B.M. [2004]. *Human embryology and developmental biology* [3rd ed.]. St. Louis: Mosby.)

which inhibits pituitary FSH. Because the other maturing follicles are still dependent on FSH, which is now decreased, they begin to regress and degenerate.[25] The process of follicular development and maturation is described in the section on the Ovarian Cycle in Chapter 2. The ovary during reproduction is illustrated in Figure 2-21.

In the fully developed follicle (Graafian or tertiary follicle), multiple layers of granulosa cells line the antral side of the basement membrane (membrane granulosa), and a cumulus of granulosa cells surrounds the oocyte. Proliferation of these cells is stimulated by growth differentiation factor 9 (GDF9), which is a member of the transforming growth factor β family.[130] GDF9 is also important for oocyte maturation and differentiation. Oxygen and nutrients diffuse across the granulosa cells to the oocyte. Antral fluid contains proteins, enzymes, proteoglycans, and hormones such as FSH and steroids.[25] The oocyte is surrounded by the zona pellucida, which contains sperm receptors. The external theca layers around the follicle consist of the outer theca externa (capsular like covering) and vascularized, glandular inner theca interna. Under the stimulation of FSH, the theca and granulosa cells produce large amounts of estrogen (primarily estradiol), which peak about 24 hours before ovulation. Production of estrogen stimulates proliferation of the endometrium, thinning of cervical mucus, and LH secretion.[130]

LH levels rise, which increases production of progesterone and inhibin A by the dominant follicle through interaction of LH with LH receptors on granulosa cells. The rise in progesterone occurs 12 to 24 hours before ovulation and elicits a rapid and marked surge in LH secretion, paralleling the mid-cycle FSH peak (see Chapter 2). The LH peak is essential for ovulation, which occurs 28 to 36 hours later.[25,33] The mid-cycle surge of LH initiates ovulation by stimulating prostaglandin (PGE and PGF) synthesis, leading to formation of collagenase and other proteolytic enzymes with disruption of the gap junctions between the oocyte and follicular cells.[25] The LH surge also increases concentration of maturation promoting factors, which disrupts meiotic inhibition and initiates completion of the first meiotic division.[130] The oocyte completes its first meiotic division 10 to 12 hours before ovulation, forming the secondary oocyte (23 chromosomes plus most of the cell cytoplasm) and first polar body (23 chromosomes and minimal cytoplasm). The small polar body is nonfunctional and degenerates (see Chapter 1). The LH surge also causes a decrease in estradiol production.

Ovulation begins with a protrusion or bulge on the ovarian wall. A small avascular spot (stigma) develops, forms a vesicle, and ruptures, extruding the secondary oocyte, follicular fluid, and surrounding cells. Rupture is thought to be caused by enzymatic digestion of the follicular wall via the action of proteases (e.g., collagenase, plasmin, and hyaluronic acid), which dissolve connective tissues.[58,103] The oocyte is surrounded by the zona pellucida and corona radiata (radially arranged granulosa cells). The second meiotic division begins with ovulation, then arrests in metaphase.[130] The second meiotic division is not completed until fertilization. The oocyte is swept by the fimbriae into the fallopian tube. Muscular contraction of the tube and, primarily, beating of the cilia move the ovum along the tube to the ampulla (the usual site of fertilization). If unfertilized, the ovum usually dies within 24 hours.[103]

Corpus Luteum

After ovulation, the follicular walls and theca collapse inward and become vascularized (Figure 3-3). The granulosa cells undergo a luteinizing process to form the corpus luteum. The corpus luteum secretes progesterone, beginning within 30 to 40 hours of the LH surge. A small amount of estrogen is secreted by the theca cells.[25] If fertilization has taken place, implantation occurs during the latter part of this week. Around the time of implantation, the trophoblast tissue secretes human chorionic gonadotropin (hCG), a luteotropin that stimulates the corpus luteum to continue to function. hCG may alter the metabolism of the uterus to prevent the release of substances that result in luteal regression. The corpus luteum can only produce progesterone for about 10 days without hCG stimulation.[25] If implantation does not occur, hCG is not produced, the corpus luteum begins to regress, undergoing apoptosis (mediated by uterine leutolytic factors such as prostaglandins), and involution begins.[25] The decline in steroid hormones results in menstruation.

The corpus luteum is essential for continuation of the pregnancy until the placenta has developed the capacity to secrete estrogens and progesterone. Removal of the corpus luteum prior to this time usually leads to a miscarriage.[130] From 6 to 10 weeks, there is a transition period in which both the placenta and corpus luteum are producing hormones; by 7 weeks the placenta is capable of producing sufficient progesterone to maintain pregnancy if needed. At 6 to 8 weeks, there is a dip in progesterone levels, indicating a decline in corpus luteum functioning. This is followed by a secondary rise in progesterone (presumably as a result of placental takeover) without a rise in the metabolite 17α-hydroxyprogesterone (secreted by the corpus luteum). Around 32 weeks there is a more gradual rise in this metabolite, indicating increased placental utilization of fetal precursors.

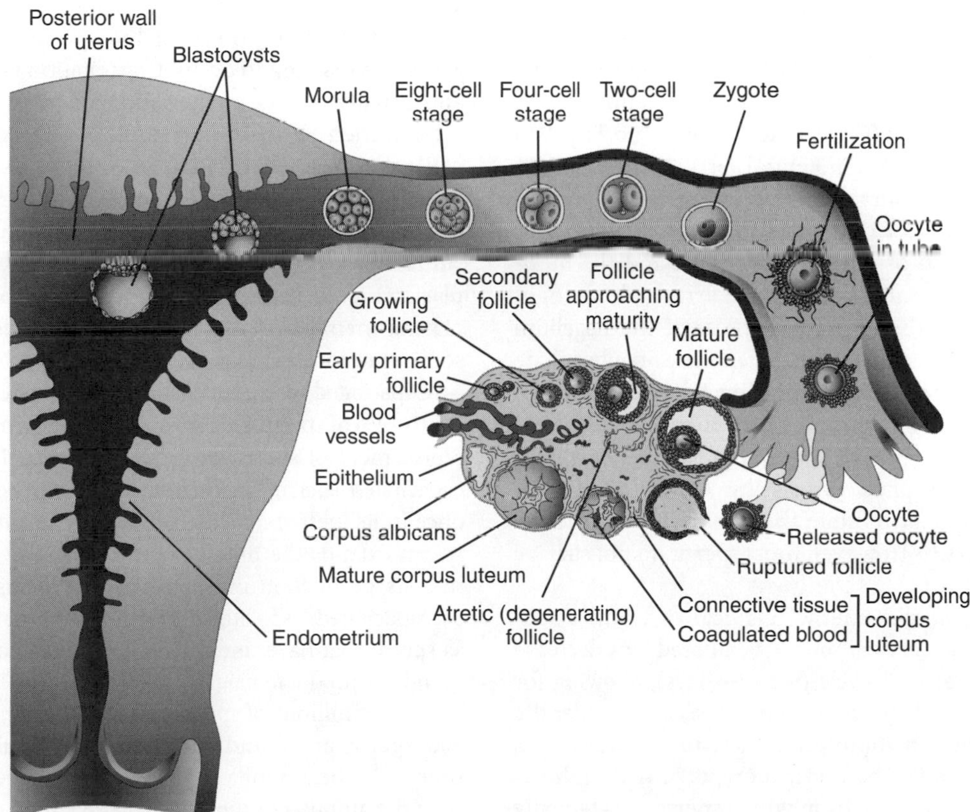

FIGURE 3-3 Diagrammatic summary of the ovarian cycle, fertilization, and human development during the first week. (From Moore, K.L. & Persaud, T.V.N. [2003]. *The developing human: Clinically oriented embryology* [7th ed.]. Philadelphia: Saunders.)

Sperm Transport

Spermatozoa have not completely differentiated when they are released into the lumen of the seminiferous tubules (see Chapter 1). They are nonmotile and incapable of fertilization. Mature sperm have a condensed and genetically inactive nucleus. Reactivation of the nucleus occurs once the sperm enters the cytoplasm of the ovum.[161] Sperm are moved down the seminiferous tubules and through the epididymis and vas deferens by (1) the pressure of additional sperm forming behind them, (2) seminal fluid, and (3) peristaltic action. Biochemical and morphologic maturation of the sperm occurs during their 14 to 21 day passage through the epididymis. Further modifications occur after ejaculation so that the sperm can bind to the zona pellucida of the ovum. Sperm are stored in the vas deferens and epididymis before ejaculation. Ejaculation occurs through the urethra with contraction of the ampulla and the ejaculatory duct upon orgasm.

The volume of ejaculate ranges from 2 to 6 (mean 3.5) mL and usually contains 100 million sperm per mL.[103] Men with less than 10 million sperm per mL are likely to be sterile.[103] Some spermatozoa are immature, senescent, or abnormal, and generally only the normal and strongest sperm are able to complete the journey within the female reproductive tract to the upper end of the fallopian tube. As sperm move along the epididymis, they begin to gain motility. Sperm become fully motile in the semen after entering the female reproductive tract.[161] Semen provides fructose for energy and an alkaline pH for protection against the acid environment of the vagina; it also dilutes the sperm to improve motility. Sperm move at 2 to 3 mm per minute. Motility is slower in the acidic vaginal environment and faster in the alkaline uterine environment.[103] Failure of sperm to achieve motility is a cause of male infertility; for potential fertility, at least 40% should be motile by 2 hours after ejaculation.[103]

The neck and midpiece of the spermatozoa contain a pair of centrioles, the base of the tail apparatus, and the mitochondrial sheath. The mitochondria are arranged in a tight helical spiral around the anterior portion of the flagellum (tail). Mitochondria supply the adenosine triphosphate (ATP) required for independent motility. Sperm must reach the ovum within an allotted time or they exhaust their energy supply and die. Sperm survival in the uterus is relatively short because phagocytosis by leukocytes begins within a few hours. Sperm retain their ability to fertilize the ovum for 1 to 3 days.[132] However, most sperm do not survive for more than 48 hours.[25,103]

Once deposited at the external cervical os, some ejaculated sperm cross the cervical mucus facilitated by a decrease in mucus viscosity at mid-cycle (9 to 16 days), allowing for more rapid migration. Within minutes, these sperm enter the uterine cavity, although some get caught in cervical crypts and endometrial glands. The cervical crypts provide a short-term reservoir or storage site from which sperm are gradually released; this may increase the chance of fertilization.[103] Uterine motility, stimulated by prostaglandins in seminal fluid that cause smooth muscle contraction, facilitates initial sperm transport.[68] Other sperm move more slowly (2 to 3 mm/hr) or are stored in cervical crypts and slowly released.[25]

Sperm chemotaxis (organized movement of the sperm toward the ovum) is stimulated by chemoattractants in follicular fluid, and possibly the cumulus oorphus and ovum. Other components of follicular fluid that may also act as chemoattractants include heparin, progesterone, atrial natriuretic peptide, epinephrine, oxytocin, calcitonin, and acetylcholine.[44] Capacitated sperm appear to be responsive to a sperm chemotrophic factor and other chemicals released by the follicle ovum and use these substances to "find" the ovum.[132]

Fertilization

The process of fertilization has been defined in three different ways: (1) the instant of sperm and ovum fusion, (2) time from sperm-ovum fusion to development of the male and female pronuclei, and (3) time from sperm-ovum fusion to the first mitotic division (about 24 hours). Fertilization begins with contact between the sperm and secondary oocyte, arrested in the metaphase of the second meiotic division (see Chapter 1). Fertilization usually occurs in the upper third of the fallopian tube, usually in the ampulla. Before fertilization, the sperm must undergo two final maturational changes: capacitation and the acrosome reaction.

Capacitation involves removal of the glycoprotein coat and seminal plasma proteins from the plasma membrane over the acrosome (head of the sperm), which allows the acrosome reaction to occur. Capacitation takes about 7 hours and usually occurs in the fallopian tubes while the sperm are attached to the tubal epithelial lining, but may begin while the sperm is still in the uterus.[25] This process is stimulated by substances in the female genital tract and follicular fluid.[58,103] For example, albumin in genital tract secretions stimulates loss of fatty acids and cholesterol from the sperm plasma membrane. This increases permeability of the sperm plasma membrane and initiates capacitation and the acrosome reaction.

Capacitated sperm are chemotaxically active.[44] Approximately 2% to 14% of sperm are capacitated at any time, with continued replacement of sperm that lose their capacitation with newly capacitated sperm. Each sperm can only become capacitated once in its lifespan.[44] This constant replacement of capacitated sperm extends the time when fertilization is possible by continuous production of "ripe" sperm.[44] Thus after ejaculation precapacitated, capacitated, and postcapacitated sperm, as well as sperm that have undergone the acrosomal reaction, can be found within the female genital tract.

Of the millions of sperm in the ejaculate, only up to 300 to 500 sperm are found in the fallopian tubes at any given time.[25,130] The ampulla of the ovulatory tube has more sperm than the ampulla of the nonovulatory tube. Although it takes only one sperm to penetrate the ovum, it appears that several hundred are necessary to effect passage of the spermatozoa through the corona radiata to the ovum. The number of spermatozoa that are ejaculated does not appear to influence the number of sperm that enter the fallopian tubes unless very low counts occur.

The acrosome reaction with release of enzymes through small holes in the acrosomal membrane must occur for successful penetration of the corona radiata and zona pellucida by the sperm. The acrosome is a saclike structure on the head of the sperm containing many enzymes, including acid glycohydrases, proteases, phosphatases, esterases, and hyaluronidase.[103] Acrosin, a serine protease, may be most important.[25] The capacitated sperm binds to the zona pellucid of the ovum, initiating the acrosome reaction (sperm activation).[155] The sperm penetrates the zona pellucida and binds to the outer membrane of the oocyte (Figure 3-4).

The zona pellucida is an ovum-specific extracellular membrane composed of three glycoproteins (ZP1, ZP2, ZP3) that act as ligands (molecules that bind to receptors) for sperm receptors. ZP3 mediates sperm binding and the acrosomal reaction.[130] Roles of the zona pellucida include sperm activation (acrosome reaction), preventing fertilization by more than one sperm, protecting the ovum before fertilization and protecting the fertilized ovum until shortly before implantation.[155] Binding of the sperm to ZP3 is mediated by a sperm surface protein (SED1).[132] Once a sperm has bound to ZP3, a zonal reaction occurs with release of lysosomal enzymes. This reaction causes physicochemical alterations in the zona pellucida that make it impenetrable to other sperm.

The sperm head traverses the perivillous space between the plasma membranes and zona pellucida and attaches to the surface of the oocyte, and their plasma membranes fuse. This process is mediated by integrins (adhesion molecules) on the ovum surface along with FERTILINβ (also known as ADAM2), IZUMO and other substances produced by the sperm.[132] The head and tail of the sperm enter the oocyte, leaving the outer plasma membrane of the sperm attached to the outer membrane of the oocyte. The ovum has a layer of cortical secretory granules along the inside of its plasma membrane. After sperm entry, the sperm-ovum interaction releases a wave of calcium along the zona pellucida resulting in fusion of the cortical granules with the plasma membrane of the ovum and release of hydrolytic enzymes, proteases, and polysaccharides into the perivillous space.[25] This modifies the zona pellucida glycoproteins, preventing activation and entry of other sperm.[154]

After entering the cytoplasm of the oocyte, the sperm undergoes rapid morphologic changes. The tail of the sperm degenerates and the head enlarges to form the male pronucleus. Each pronucleus has 23 chromosomes (22 autosomes

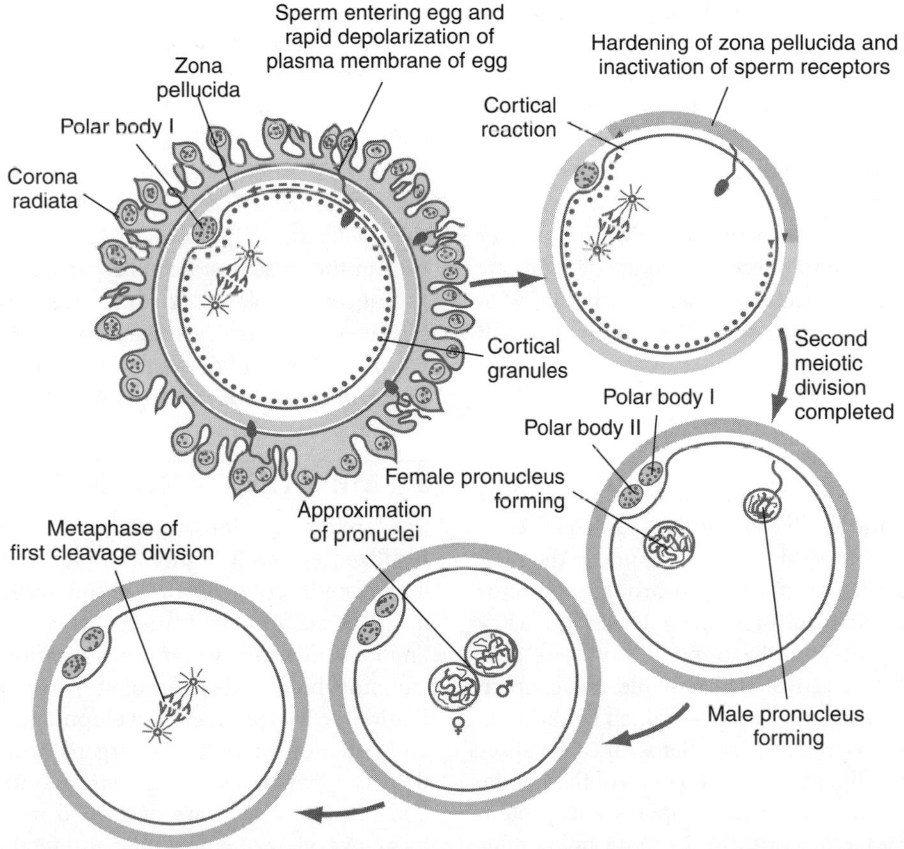

FIGURE 3-4 Summary of the main events involved in fertilization. (From Carlson, B.M. [2004]. *Human embryology and developmental biology* [3rd ed.]. St. Louis: Mosby.)

and 1 sex chromosome). Sex of the offspring is determined by the male and depends on whether the sperm that enters the ovum contains an X or Y chromosome. The sperm nucleus becomes reactivated so that it can again synthesize DNA and RNA.[161] This processing involves removal of the nuclear membrane with exposure of the sperm chromatin to the cytoplasm of the ovum. The nuclear protein is remodeled and the nucleus decondenses, becoming larger and more spherical. A new nuclear envelope develops, forming the male pronucleus and activating DNA transcription and replication. This is thought to be mediated by factors in the cytoplasm of the ovum. This process takes about 3 to 4 hours, during which the developing male pronucleus gradually approaches the female pronucleus.[161]

The ovum must be metabolically activated. Entry of the sperm into the ovum triggers two events: (1) the cortical and zonal reactions described earlier, which blocks entry of other sperm; and (2) a transient increase in intracellular calcium accompanied by an increase in oxidative metabolism.[25] The increased calcium stimulates the oocyte to complete its second meiotic division with extrusion of the second polar body into the perivitelline space. The nucleus enlarges and is called the female pronucleus. The oocyte is now mature and metabolically active.[154] Failure of calcium signaling can lead to complete failure (triploidy) or partial failure (abnormalities of chromosomal number of the second meiotic division, cleavage arrest, and alterations in development of the inner cell mass and trophectoderm [trophoblast]). These alterations can result in implantation failure and miscarriage.[143]

The female and male pronuclei approach each other, their membranes disintegrate, and the nuclei fuse (see Figure 3-4). Chromatin strands intermingle, and the diploid number (46) of chromosomes is restored. The *zygote* (from the Greek, meaning "yoked together") is formed, and mitotic division (cleavage) begins. The zygote measures 0.2 mm in diameter and carries the genetic material necessary to create a unique human being. Fertilization results in species variation, with half of the chromosomes coming from the mother and half from the father, mixing the genes each parent originally received from their parents.[103]

Cleavage and Zygote Transport

Cleavage involves a series of rapid mitotic cell divisions that begins with the first mitotic division of the zygote and ends with formation of the blastocyst. Cleavage is under the control of mitosis-promoting or maturation-promoting factor (MPF).[25] The zygote divides into two daughter cells (blastomeres) about 30 hours after fertilization; each of these cells divides into two smaller cells, which also divide, and so forth (see Figure 3-3). The dividing cells are contained by the zona pellucida and become progressively smaller with each subsequent division, with no change in the total mass of the zygote. The trophoblast secretes an immunosuppressant protein called early pregnancy factor (EPF) by 24 to 48 hours after fertilization. Pregnancy tests within the first 10 days after fertilization use EPF in maternal serum.[103]

Cell division occurs every 12 to 24 hours. By 3 to 4 days, the zygote has divided into 8 to 16 blastomeres. Around the eight- to nine-cell stage, the blastomeres realign and form a tight ball of cells mediated by cell surface adhesion glycoproteins. This process, called compaction, allows increased interaction between cells needed for formation of the inner cell mass. This occurs via gap and tight junctions.[25]

The zygote remains in the ampulla for the first 24 hours, then is propelled down the fallopian tube by ciliary action over the next few days. At the 12- to 16-cell stage (about 3 days after fertilization), the zygote becomes a solid cluster of cells called the *morula* (from the Latin word for "mulberry," which it resembles).[25] The zygote reaches the uterine cavity 3 to 4 days after fertilization (about 90 hours or 5 days after follicle rupture). Development is now under control of the embryonic genome. Fluid (which provides nutrients) from the uterine cavity enters the morula as the blastocyst is formed.

The blastocyst consists of four distinct components: (1) zona pellucida, a thick glycoprotein membrane that is beginning to stretch and thin; (2) trophectoderm (trophoblast), a one-cell-thick outer layer of flattened cells that will form the placenta and chorion; (3) inner cell mass (embryoblast), a one- or two-cell-thick, crescent-shaped cluster of cells that will form the embryo; and (4) fluid-filled blastocyst cavity.[103] The zona pellucida protects the zygote from adhering to the mucosa of the fallopian tube and from rejection by the maternal immune system (see Chapter 13). Position of individual cells and gene transcription factors influence which cells become trophoblast and which become inner cell mass. For example, *Oct4* and *Nanog* are transcription factors found in all blastomeres in the morula. In the cells that become the inner cell mass, these transcription factors continue to be expressed, but are turned off in the cells of the future trophoblast.[132] If these gene transcription factors are deficient, all or most of the cells in the blastocyst become part of the trophectoderm, resulting in a molar pregnancy (see Gestational Trophoblast Disease). The blastocyst floats free in the uterine cavity from 90 to 150 hours after ovulation, then begins to implant 6 to 7 days after fertilization (Figure 3-5).

EMBRYONIC AND FETAL DEVELOPMENT

The infant develops progressively from the single-cell fertilized egg to a highly complex multicellular organism. The genetic constitution of the individual is established at the time of fertilization. During development of the embryo and fetus, genetic information is unfolded to control morphologic development. Alterations in genetic information or morphologic development can modify structure and function of cells and organs and result in congenital defects. Principles of genetic control of development and morphogenesis are described in this section, followed by an overview of embryonic and fetal development. Development of specific body systems is described in Units II and III.

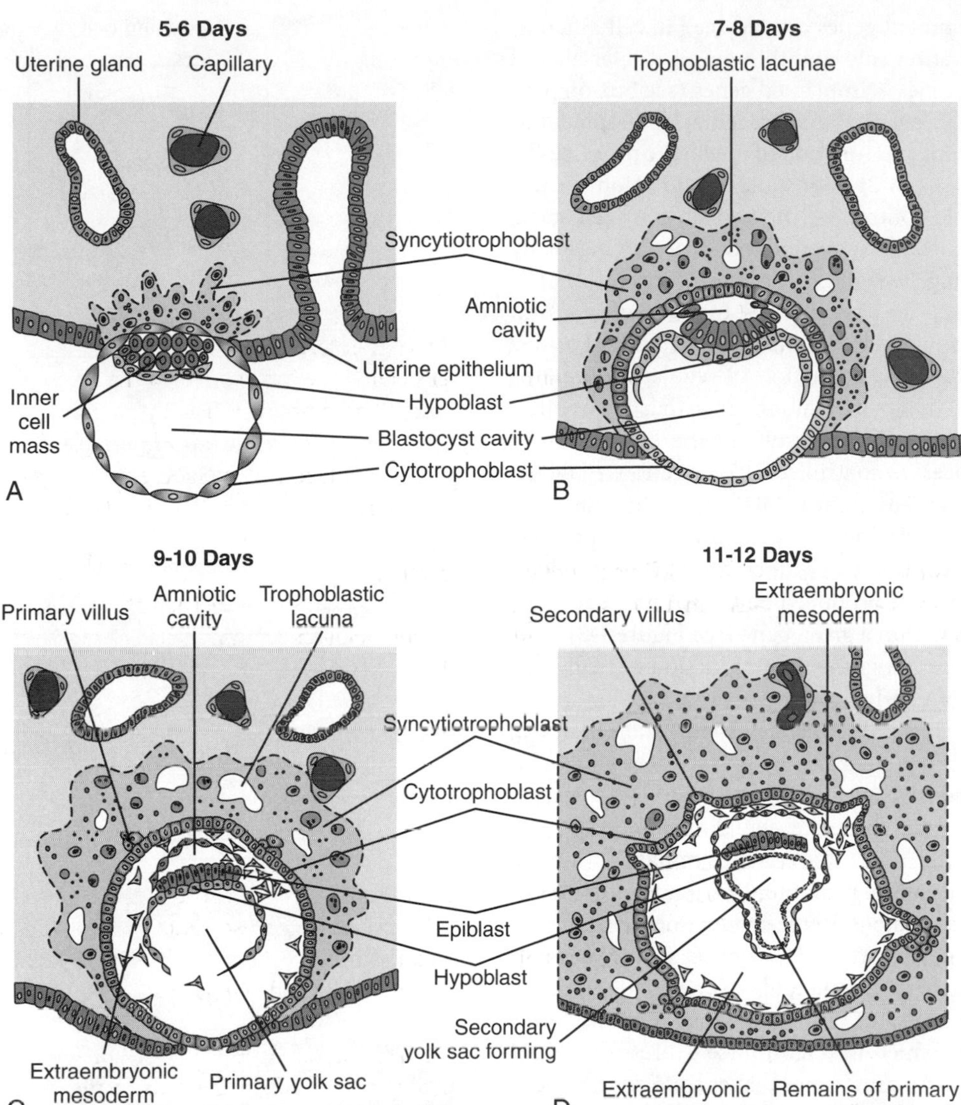

FIGURE 3-5 Implantation and early development of the embryo. **A,** Syncytiotrophoblast invades endometrium. **B,** Most of the embryo is embedded in the endometrium with early formation of trophoblastic lacunae. The amniotic cavity and primary yolk sac are beginning to form. **C,** Implantation is almost complete; primary villi are forming and the embryonic mesoderm is appearing. **D,** Implantation is complete; secondary villi and the secondary yolk sac are forming. (From Carlson, B.M. [2004]. *Human embryology and developmental biology* [3rd ed.]. St. Louis: Mosby.)

GENETIC CONTROL OF DEVELOPMENT

Embryonic development combines growth, differentiation, and organization of cellular components at all levels. As development progresses, differential synthesis is established, resulting in cellular differentiation. Growth is the process of creating more of a substance that is already present through increase in cell size and number. In contrast, differentiation is the creation of new types of substances, cells, tissues, and organs that were not previously present. Organization is the process by which these elements are coordinated into functional integrated units. Morphogenesis is the production of a special form, shape, or structure of a cell or group of cells and occurs by the precise organization of cell populations into distinct organs.[71]

The mechanisms controlling morphogenesis are complex and incompletely understood.[25] Development is controlled by developmental gene families within the embryo.[21,25,31,52,85] Much of the knowledge of developmental genes to date comes from animal models. Often the names of these genes or their products reflect characteristics of the animals or situations in which they were first identified. Developmental genes control the definition of body axes (ventral/dorsal, anterior/posterior, left/right, medial/dorsal)—and the arrangement of different cells to form tissues and organogenesis.[151] These processes involve the coordination of signaling molecules and other proteins, DNA transcription factors, extracellular matrix components, enzymes, and transport systems.[40,73] Development genes are involved in cell differentiation and proliferation into adulthood and if later altered can lead to malignancies.[56] Imprinted genes (see box on p. 9) are also important in prenatal and placental development as well as in development and function of metabolic processes.[121]

Although the first cell divisions after fertilization are under maternal genetic control, by the two- to four-cell stage, the embryonic genome is activated and is producing many intercellular signaling proteins and transcription factors.[40,61] Transcription factors are proteins that turn other genes on and off, thus controlling expression of these genes. Positive feedback induces further production of regulatory proteins and gene transcription factors that influence that cell or other target cells. Negative feedback results in the production of inhibitors. This process is controlled by interactions of developmental genes with environmental factors that turn the gene on and off at precise intervals. Each gene can produce multiple isotypes, each isotype producing a different product. The different isotypes are produced by the splicing and reorganization of exons within a given gene (see Figure 1-3).[85] As a result, a single gene can guide the production of many different forms of mRNA and formation of proteins with unique biologic functions. Thus individual developmental genes may have different functions at different stages of development and with development of specific organs.[21,25,31,52]

Developmental genes produce signaling molecules and transcription factors. Transcription factors remain within the cell and bind to DNA at the promoter or enhancer regions of specific genes or regulate mRNA production.[25,56] Often a cascade is set up, wherein the transcription factor turns on various genes which in turn can regulate other genes. Initially these regulatory genes send out signals that induce expression of other genes, which in turn induce expression of still other genes and so forth until genes that encode development of specific structures or functions of cells or tissues within the embryo are expressed.[132] The proteins produced regulate cell activities, such as causing a cell to differentiate in a specific way, and are modulated by positive and negative feedback loops.[52] Examples of developmental gene families include the *homeobox (HOX)* and *PAX* gene families. For example, the *HOX* genes are involved with craniocaudal organization; the *PAX* gene family is involved with development of the urogenital system, central nervous system (CNS), thyroid gland, and eye, among other sites.[25]

Intercellular signaling molecules (first messengers), many of which are growth factors, influence other cells by binding to receptor molecules (Figure 3-6). Signaling molecules act in a paracrine fashion, that is, they are secreted into the spaces surrounding the cell where the molecules are produced and diffuse between cells in that area.[73,130] These molecules act to bind (as ligands) to receptor molecules on cell membranes. After a series of protein interactions, a transcription factor is activated and a signal is sent to the cell nucleus and a gene is expressed resulting in production of specific proteins needed to guide development.[25,130] Receptor molecules can be intracellular or on the cell surface. Extracellular receptors are binding sites for ligands (hormones, growth factor, or cytokine). Binding to the receptor alters the receptor and stimulates an intercellular response (signal transduction) either directly via a protein kinase or indirectly via a second messenger such as cyclic adenosine monophosphate (cAMP). Signaling molecules may also act by inhibiting other signaling molecules.[25] Justacine signaling also occurs via three mechanisms: (1) interaction of a protein on one cell membrane with a receptor on the surface of another cell; (2) via gap junctions (see Chapter 4 for a discussion of gap junctions), or

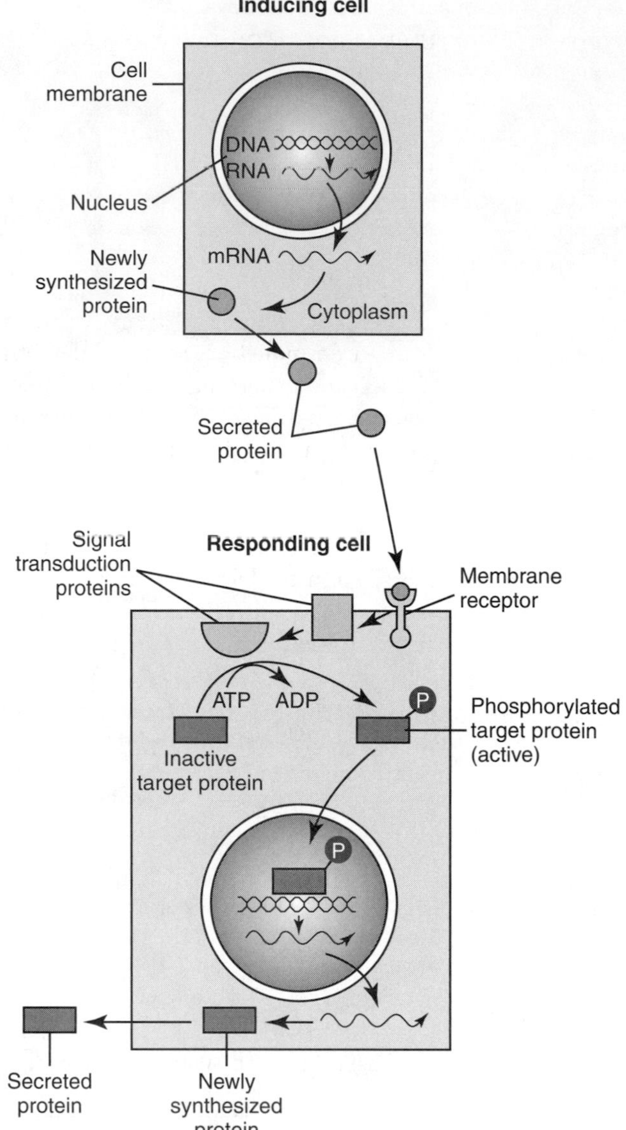

FIGURE 3-6. Example of signal transduction. Inducing cells influence their neighbors by secreting small proteins (growth factors) that diffuse to adjacent cells (responding cells) and bind to their membrane receptors. This initiates an intracellular signaling cascade through a series of signal transduction proteins and phosphorylation events. Phosphorylated proteins enter the nucleus, where they alter gene expression, leading to the synthesis of new proteins. (From Schoenwolf, G.C., et al. (2009). *Larsen's human embryology* (4th ed.). Philadelphia: Churchill Livingstone Elsevier.)

(3) interaction of extracellular matrix ligands (collagen, proteoglycans, fibronectin, and laminin) with receptors on neighboring cells.[130]

Major signaling pathways are *Wnt, Hedgehog, transforming growth factor β (TGF-β) family, tyrosine kinase, Notch, Integrin,* and retinoic acid signaling.[73,130,132] The *Wnt* family is involved in the dorsal/ventral axis and formation of the midbrain, muscles, gonads, and kidneys. Alterations are associated with tumors and possibly congenital anomalies.[73] The hedgehog family, such as the sonic hedgehog *(Shh)* gene, is involved in patterning of many tissues and organs, including axis formation, motor neuron induction, somite differentiation, neural tube induction and patterning, and limb patterning.[25,56,130,132] Mutations are associated with central nervous system (e.g., holoprosencephaly), axial skeletal, and limb abnormalities as well as with some basal cell carcinomas.[25,73] The TGF-β family includes TGF-β, which is important in mesoderm induction and myoblast proliferation, activin (granulose cell proliferation, mesoderm induction), inhibin (inhibition of gonadotropin secretion by the pituitary), müllerian inhibitory substance (regression of the paramesonephric duct (see Chapter 1), bone morphogenetic proteins, and decapentaplegic (limb development).[21,25,31,52,130,132] The TGF-β family is also involved in angiogenesis, axon growth, mesoderm differentiation and epithelial branching in the lung and kidneys.[130] Defects in TGFβ signaling can lead to vascular and skeletal disorders as well as pulmonary hypertension and cancer.[132]

Tyrosine kinase signaling involves growth factors (GFs) such as fibroblast growth factor (FGF), epidermal GF (EGF), insulin-like GFs, platelet derived GFs, and vascular endothelial GF.[130,132] FGFs are found in bone, so mutations in FGF receptor genes can lead to skeletal dysplasia and disorders such as achondroplasia, Crouzon syndrome, Apert syndrome, and some forms of craniosyntosis.[73] Defects in Notch signaling can lead to skeletal disorders such as Alagille syndrome and spondylocostal dysostosis as well as cancers such as T-cell acute lymphoblastic leukemia.[132] Integrins are receptors that are involved in linking the extracellular matrix and cell cytoskeleton and in signal transduction that can lead to changes in cell size, shape, and position.[132] Defective integrin signaling can lead to alterations in skin and connective tissue such as epidermolysis bullosa and cancers of the breast, intestine, and reproductive organs.[132] Retinoic acid (derived from vitamin A) acts as a morphogen, which is "a diffusible substance that determines cell fate during development in a concentration-dependent manner."[132, p. 161]

Alterations in developmental genes and their products can result in congenital anomalies through various mechanisms.[41] Mechanical failures involve defects in structural genes such as collagen resulting in qualitative or quantitative differences. For example, collagen mutations are seen in osteogenesis imperfecta, Apert syndrome, and epidermolysis bullosa; a fibrillin defect is seen in Marfan syndrome. Alterations in cell numbers due to regulatory failures can lead to overgrowth, such as occurs in Beckwith-Wiedemann syndrome, or undergrowth, such as occurs with some forms of microcephaly. Failure of cell migration during development leads to anomalies such as lissencephaly (failure of neuronal migration) or Hirschsprung's disease (failure of neural crest cells to migrate and form ganglia). Failure of the developmental switch, turning genes on and off, can upset the development timetable and also lead to defects.[41]

Mechanisms of Morphogenesis

The human embryo's progression through stages of development is shared by many other creatures (phylogenetic recapitulation). As a result, animal models can be useful in understanding developmental processes and deviations in humans. Development and maturation generally proceed in a cephalocaudal direction. Morphogenesis is accomplished by a variety of genetically controlled mechanisms. Various tissues and organs are at different stages of maturity throughout development. For example, the gut and bladder are essentially structurally complete at birth, whereas the long bones and lung alveoli do not reach maturity for years after birth. Therefore various organs are more or less vulnerable to insults and toxic agents at different stages of development. Thus morphogenic mechanisms are induced by the signaling pathway and transcription factors describe in the previous section.

Cell Differentiation

Initially all cells are similar and unspecialized, but each must eventually become 1 of 350 different cell types found in the human body.[139] Cells pass through two phases in order to become specialized. In the first phase (determination), the cell becomes restricted in its developmental capabilities and loses the ability to develop in alternative ways. Cell determination occurs for the first time in the blastocyst, with formation of the inner cell mass (which forms the embryo) and trophoblast (which becomes the placenta). In the second phase (differentiation), cells develop distinctive morphologic and functional characteristics. Initially, cell position determines the fate of the cell. Specific differentiation is regulated by interactions between cell populations and is controlled by *HOX* and other gene families that are switched on to produce specific signaling molecules in a sequential manner.[139] Cell differentiation often involves induction (see below) in which one tissue signals (induces) a second tissue (responder) to differentiate into a specific structure. Signals are sent between cells in both directions (cross-talk) to complete the differentiation.[130]

Induction

Induction is the process by which cells in one part of the embryo influence cells around them to develop in a specific way. Induction requires inductors, or cells that stimulate reactions in surrounding cells via signal transduction and induced tissue, which is made up of cells that have the capacity or competence to respond to these protein signals via cell membrane receptor molecules (see Figure 3-6). At some point, inductors and inducers lose their ability to perform these actions.[31]

Secondary induction is a cascade of developmental events and is a common way many parts of the embryo are formed. For example, in the nervous system, the notochord is a primary inductor or organizer for brain development. The forebrain reacts to secondary inductors in the mesoderm to form the optic cup, which then induces adjacent ectoderm to form the eye lens. The eye lens then induces epidermis around it to form the corneal epithelium. Other examples of induction are in the formation of the gastrointestinal system, where the gut endoderm induces the surrounding mesenchyme to differentiate into organs such as the liver or pancreas (see Chapter 12) or in the renal system where the utereic bud causes the surrounding mesenchyme to become nephrons (see Chapter 11).[130]

If any of these steps is interfered with, the next stage in development may not occur, or it may occur abnormally. If these alterations occur early in the developmental sequence, complete organ agenesis may result.[103] An example of chemical pathway activity during secondary induction is the interaction of activin and TGF-β, which influences branching of epithelial tubes in the kidney, pancreas, and salivary glands.[85,130]

Differential Cell Proliferation

Differential cell proliferation results from localized differences in rates of cell division. Proliferation is controlled by cell signaling mechanisms and growth factors. These differences may lead to a buildup of cells in certain areas or may result in a phenomenon called *invagination,* in which cells growing more slowly than surrounding cells appear to be "sinking" into tissues. In fact, one set of cells is overtaking the other cells in growth. This phenomenon can be seen during the development of the neural groove, the oral cavity, and the nostrils. The rate of cell proliferation is modulated by interactions of receptor molecules on the surface of the cells with systemic and local growth factors that stimulate proliferation during organogenesis. A period of rapid cell proliferation often precedes differentiation. Proliferation inhibition by teratogenic agents may cause defects. Growth inhibition can also be caused by lack of space (when space runs out, tissues stop proliferating). For example, with a diaphragmatic hernia, the intestinal contents are in the thoracic cavity and may inhibit lung development.

Programmed Cell Death

Programmed cell death or apoptosis is a precisely timed event—under genetic control and cell feedback mechanisms—that occurs in many of the embryonic tissues as part of normal development. The process involves the release of lysosomal hydrolytic enzymes that dissolve cells, thereby altering the tissues. This mechanism is responsible for lumen formation in solid tubes (trachea and parts of the gut) and the disappearance of the webbing between the fingers and toes. If enzyme release is inhibited, syndactyly, some forms of bowel atresia, or imperforate anus may result. If enzyme activity is increased, micromelia (shortened limbs) may result.[139]

Cell Size and Shape Changes

Cell size and shape changes occur with elongation or narrowing and swelling or shrinkage. Elongation or narrowing is accomplished by the coordinated activities of cell microfilaments and microtubules. Microtubules are long cylinders containing tubulin, a substance that alters its length when polymerized (i.e., joined together to form a molecule of higher molecular weight [MW]). Certain chemicals (including some found in microorganisms) inhibit tubulin polymerization and normal microfilament action. Changes in osmotic balance or interference in transport of elements across the membranes results in swelling or shrinkage of cells.

Cell Migration

During development some cells move around in a fashion similar to that of an amoeba. This process is dependent on microtubular and microfilament elongation and contraction. Migration involves the elongation of the leading edge of the cell, followed by adhesion of the cell to a new contact point. Contraction of the cell toward the new adhesion site results in movement of the cell. Alterations or interference may limit cell migration and result in a defect. Hirschsprung's disease (absence of intestinal ganglion cells) results from failure of neural crest cells to migrate. From 3 to 6 months' gestation, millions of neurons and glial cells within the central nervous system migrate from their point of origin in the periventricular area to their eventual loci in the cerebrum and cerebellum. Alterations in this migration can result in alterations in CNS organization and function (see Chapter 15).[103,139]

Cell Recognition and Adhesion

This mechanism involves the adhesion of certain cells, such as the neural folds, which meet and fuse to form the neural tube. The recognition and adhesion process involves interaction of specific substrates (e.g., integrins, glycoproteins, cell surface enzymes) on one cell with complementary substrates, enzymes, or adhesion molecules on the membrane of another cell. A similar mechanism is seen with adhesion during cell migration. Interference with cellular membrane substrates may prevent adhesion. Alterations in this mechanism may be responsible for cleft palate or neural tube defects.

Folding of the Embryo

The embryo begins as a relatively straight line of cells. As new cells form, the embryo is forced to conform to available space. To adapt to the confined space, the embryo folds (curves) in both transverse and longitudinal planes. Folding in the transverse plane causes the embryo to become cylindrical in shape; longitudinal folding results in the head and tail folds. Structures within the embryo (e.g., heart, intestines) also undergo folding to conform to the space available to them. Folding is mediated by signaling and other proteins.

Overview of Embryonic Development

Preembryonic development occurs from the time of conception and zygote formation until 2 weeks' gestation. By the time of implantation, the inner cell mass consists of 12 to 15 cells. At about 7 days, the first of three germ cell layers that give rise to the embryo—the hypoblast, or primitive endoderm—appears.[25] During the second week the bilaminar embryo develops as the inner cell mass differentiates to form the epiblast along the inner part of the amniotic cavity.

The developing organism appears as a flat disk with a connecting stalk that will become part of the umbilical cord. Cytotrophoblast cells around the inner wall of the blastocyst cavity form the primitive yolk sac (see Figure 3-5, *C*) and extraembryonic coelom, which serves as transfer interface and nutrient reservoir.[69] Connective tissue (extraembryonic mesoderm) fills in the space between the cytotrophoblast cells and the extraembryonic coelomic membrane. Near the end of the second week, cavities appear in the extraembryonic mesoderm and fuse to form the extraembryonic coelom. A secondary yolk sac (see Figure 3-5, *D*) develops from the primary sac (which gradually disintegrates) and provides for early nutrition of the embryo. Part of it is eventually incorporated into the primitive gut. The fluid in this cavity is an ultrafiltrate of maternal serum with placental and secondary yolk sac products.[69] An endodermal cell thickening (prochordal plate) appears at one end of the disk and is the future site of the mouth and cranial region.

The embryonic period lasts from 2 weeks after fertilization until the end of the eighth week. This period is the time of organogenesis. Figure 3-7 summarizes the major stages in development of specific organ systems. Development of specific organ systems is described in detail in Chapters 8 to 20. This section provides an overview of major events during embryogenesis.

The third week of development coincides with the first missed menstrual period (see Figure 3-1). During the third week, growth becomes more rapid, with development of the mesoderm and establishment of the trilaminar embryo; formation of the neural tube (CNS), somites (bones and other supporting structures), and coelom (body cavities); and development of a primitive cardiovascular system.

The primitive streak (thick band of epiblast cells) appears at 15 days in the midline of the dorsal aspect of the embryonic disk.[103] Cells in the primitive streak migrate between the endoderm and ectoderm to form the mesoderm; the epiblast layer becomes the ectoderm, establishing the trilaminar embryo. Cells from the mesoderm later migrate out into the embryonic body to become mesenchyme and form supporting tissues.

The ectoderm layer eventually forms the central and peripheral nervous systems, epidermis, hair, nails, inner ear, epithelium of the sensory organs, nasal cavity and mouth, salivary glands, and mucous membranes. The middle mesoderm layer develops into the dermis; muscle; connective tissue; skeleton (tendon, bones, cartilage); circulatory and lymphatic systems; kidneys; gonads; and the lining of the pericardial, pleural, and peritoneal cavities. The endoderm forms the epithelium of the digestive, respiratory, and urinary tracts as well as the thyroid and parathyroid glands.[25,103]

Development is in a cranial-to-caudal direction, with the embryo initially being a pear-shaped disk with a broad cephalic end and a narrow caudal end. The primitive streak elongates cranially to form a midline rod of cells, or notochord. The notochord extends to the prochordal plate, where the endoderm and ectoderm fuse into the oropharyngeal membrane. Other cells from the primitive streak migrate around the notochord and prochordal plate to form a cardiogenic area where the heart will develop. At the caudal end the endoderm and ectoderm fuse into the cloacal membrane.[25,103]

The ectoderm over the notochord thickens to form the neural plate, which will eventually form the neural tube, which gives rise to the brain and spinal cord. The mesoderm on either side of the notochord thickens to form two long columns that divide into paired cuboidal bodies (somites). Somites give rise to the skeleton and its associated musculature and much of the dermis. Somite development can be used to distinguish the stage of embryonic development. The foregut and body cavities begin to develop. Mesoderm cells aggregate in the cardiogenic area at 18 to 19 days to form two endocardial tubes, which fuse by 19 to 20 days.[25,103] Primitive blood cells and vessels develop in the yolk sac, chorion, and embryo, and by 21 days' gestation they link with heart tubes to form a primitive cardiovascular system.

The fourth week is a time of body building. The embryo becomes cylindrical and begins to assume a C-shape as a result of transverse and longitudinal folding. The neural tube fuses during days 21 to 28. The cranial area enlarges and develops cephalic and cervical flexure, with the head oriented in the characteristic flexed position. The heart is prominent and begins beating at 20 to 22 days. Small swellings become visible on the lateral body walls at 26 (arm buds) and 28 (leg buds) days. The branchial arches (from which the face, mandible, and pharynx will develop) become visible; however, facial structures are not distinct and human likeness is not clear yet. The embryo is 2 to 5 cm long.[25,103]

As the embryo enters the fifth week, the form develops a humanlike appearance.[103] Head growth is rapid as a result of brain development. The embryo further flexes into the characteristic C-shape and the facial area comes into close approximation with the heart prominence. The forelimbs begin to develop, and paddle-shaped hand plates with digital ridges are visible. The heart chambers are forming, and five distinct areas in the brain are visible. The cranial nerves are present. Retinal pigment and the external ear begin to appear.

Limb differentiation continues in the sixth week, short webbed fingers develop, and toe rays form. The face is much more distinct, the jaws are visible, and the nares and upper lip are present. Heart development is almost complete, and circulation is well established. The liver is prominent and producing blood cells. The intestines enter the proximal portion of the umbilical cord.

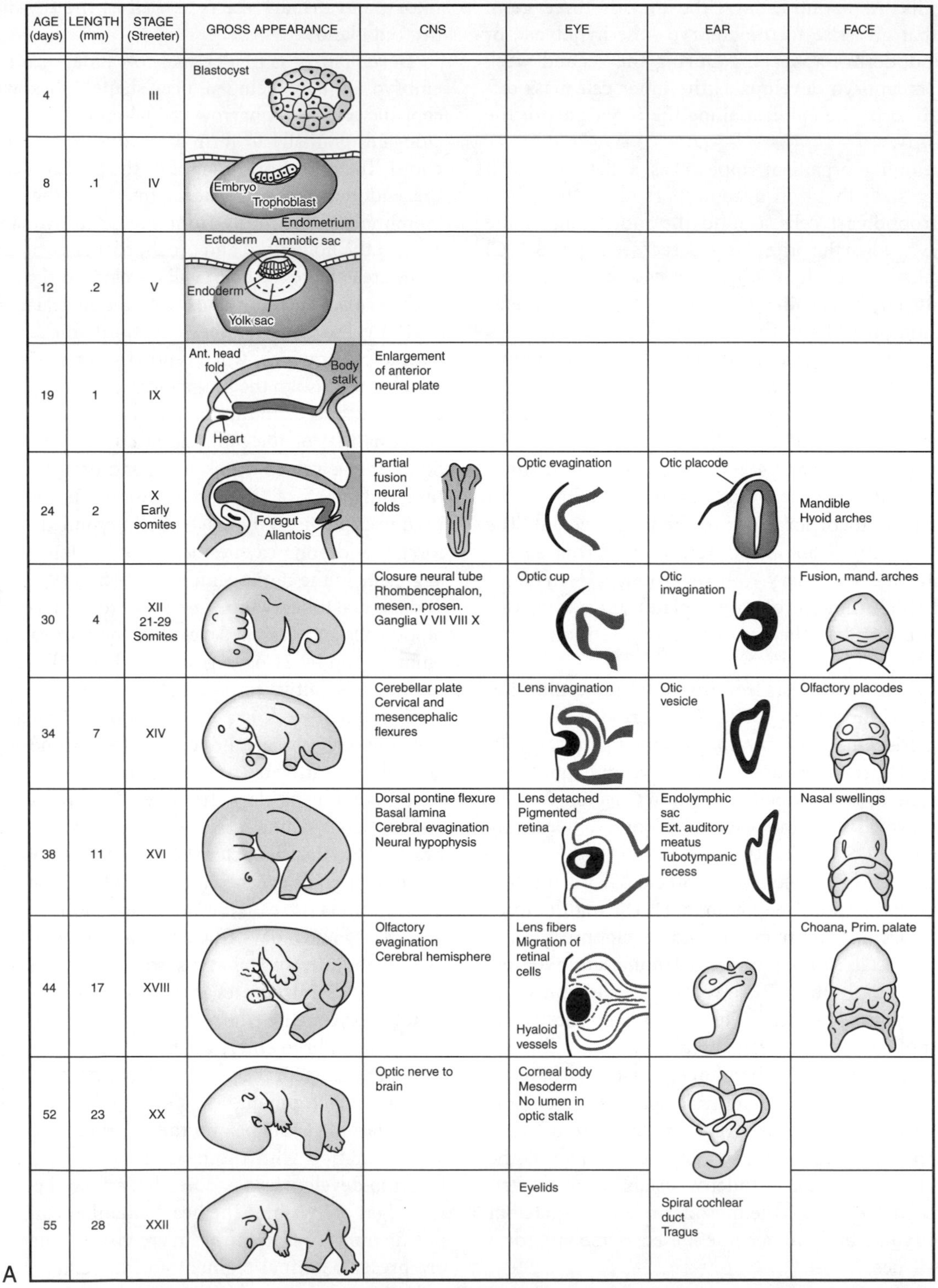

EMBRYONIC DEVELOPMENT

AGE (days)	LENGTH (mm)	STAGE (Streeter)	GROSS APPEARANCE	CNS	EYE	EAR	FACE
4		III	Blastocyst				
8	.1	IV	Embryo Trophoblast Endometrium				
12	.2	V	Ectoderm Amniotic sac Endoderm Yolk sac				
19	1	IX	Ant. head fold Body stalk Heart	Enlargement of anterior neural plate			
24	2	X Early somites	Foregut Allantois	Partial fusion neural folds	Optic evagination	Otic placode	Mandible Hyoid arches
30	4	XII 21-29 Somites		Closure neural tube Rhombencephalon, mesen., prosen. Ganglia V VII VIII X	Optic cup	Otic invagination	Fusion, mand. arches
34	7	XIV		Cerebellar plate Cervical and mesencephalic flexures	Lens invagination	Otic vesicle	Olfactory placodes
38	11	XVI		Dorsal pontine flexure Basal lamina Cerebral evagination Neural hypophysis	Lens detached Pigmented retina	Endolymphic sac Ext. auditory meatus Tubotympanic recess	Nasal swellings
44	17	XVIII		Olfactory evagination Cerebral hemisphere	Lens fibers Migration of retinal cells Hyaloid vessels		Choana, Prim. palate
52	23	XX		Optic nerve to brain	Corneal body Mesoderm No lumen in optic stalk		
55	28	XXII			Eyelids	Spiral cochlear duct Tragus	

A

FIGURE 3-7 Timetable of human embryonic and fetal development. (From Jones, K.L. [1996]. *Smith's recognizable patterns of human malformation* [5th ed.]. Philadelphia: Saunders.)

The embryonic ages for Streeter's stages XII-XXII have been altered in accordance with the human data from Iffy, L., et al.: Acta Anat., 66:178, 1967.

EXTREMITIES	HEART	GUT, ABDOMEN	LUNG	UROGENITAL	OTHER
					Early blastocyst with inner cell mass and cavitation (58 cells) lying free within the uterine cavity
					Implantation Trophoblast invasion Embryonic disk with endoblast and ectoblast
		Yolk sac			Early amnion sac Extraembryonic mesoblast, angioblast Chorionic gonadotropin
	Merging mesoblast anterior to prechordal plate	Stomodeum Cloaca		Allantois	Primitive streak Hensen's node Notochord Prechordal plate Blood cells in yolk sac
	Single heart tube Propulsion 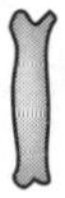	Foregut		Mesonephric ridge	Yolk sac larger than amnion sac
Arm bud 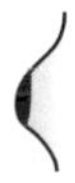	Ventric. outpouching Gelatinous reticulum 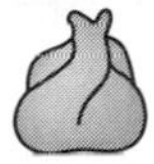	Rupture stomatodeum Evagination of thyroid, liver, and dorsal pancreas	Lung bud 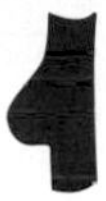	Mesonephric duct enters cloaca	Rathke's pouch Migration of myotomes from somites
Leg bud 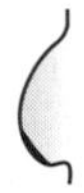	Auric. outpouching Septum primum 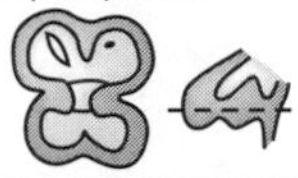	Pharyngeal pouches yield parathyroids, lat. thyroid, thymus Stomach broadens	Bronchi 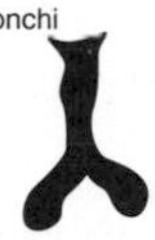	Ureteral evag. Urorect. sept. Germ cells Gonadal ridge Coelom, Epithelium 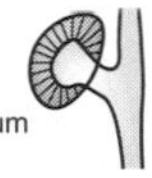	
Hand plate, Mesench. condens. Innervation 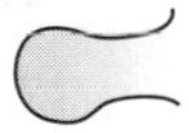	Fusion mid. A-V canal Muscular vent. sept. 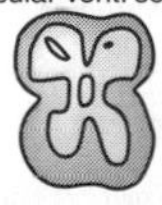	Intestinal loop into yolk stalk Cecum Gallbladder Hepatic ducts Spleen	Main lobes 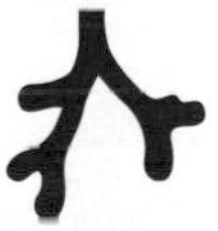	Paramesonephric duct Gonad ingrowth of coelomic epith 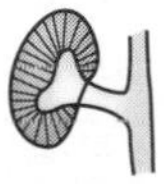	Adrenal cortex (from coelomic epithelium) invaded by sympathetic cells = medulla Jugular lymph sacs
Finger rays, Elbow 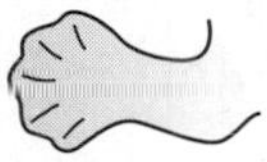	Aorta Pulmonary artery Valves Membrane ventricular septum	Duodenal lumen obliterated Cecum rotates right Appendix	Tracheal cartil. 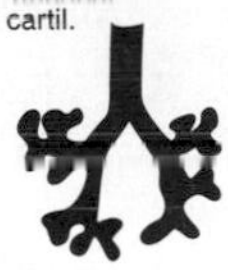	Fusion urorect. sept. Open urogen. memb., anus Epith. cords in testicle 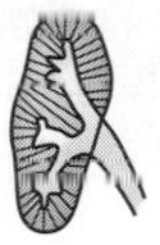	Early muscle
Clearing, central cartil. 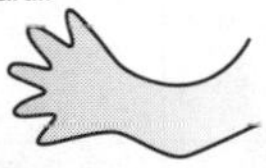	Septum secundum 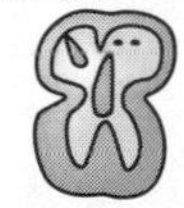			S-shaped vesicles in nephron blastema connect with collecting tubules from calyces	Superficial vascular plexus low on cranium
Shell, Tubular bone 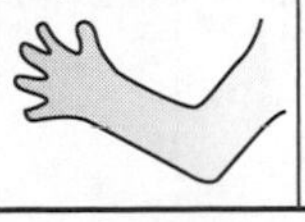				A few large glomeruli Short secretory tubules Tunica albuginea Testicle, interstitial cells	Superficial vascular plexus at vertex

B

FIGURE 3-7, cont'd Timetable of human embryonic and fetal development. (From Jones, K.L. [1996]. *Smith's recognizable patterns of human malformation* [5th ed.]. Philadelphia: Saunders.)

(Continued)

FETAL DEVELOPMENT

AGE (weeks)	LENGTH (cm) C-R	LENGTH (cm) Tot.	WT (g)	GROSS APPEARANCE	CNS	EYE, EAR	FACE, MOUTH	CARDIO-VASCULAR	LUNG
7½	2.8			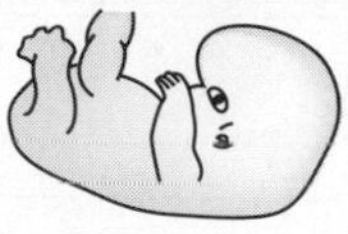	Cerebral hemisphere 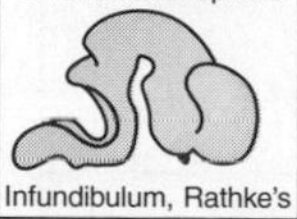 Infundibulum, Rathke's	Lens nearing final shape	Palatal swellings 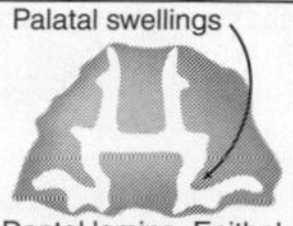 Dental lamina, Epithel.	Pulmonary vein into left atrium	
8	3.7			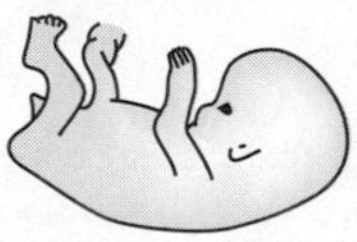	Primitive cereb. cortex 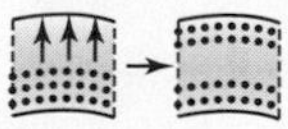 Olfactory lobes Dura and pia mater	Eyelid Ear canals	Nares plugged Rathke's pouch detach. 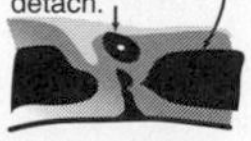 Sublingual gland	A-V bundle Sinus venosus absorbed into right auricle	Pleuroperitoneal canals close 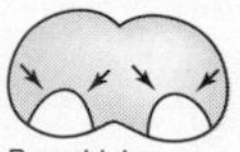 Bronchioles
10	6.0				Spinal cord histology 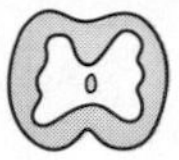 Cerebellum	Iris Ciliary body Eyelids fuse Lacrimal glands Spiral gland different	Lips, Nasal cartilage Palate 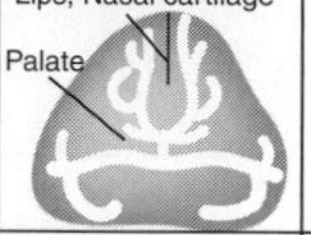		Laryngeal cavity reopened
12	8.8			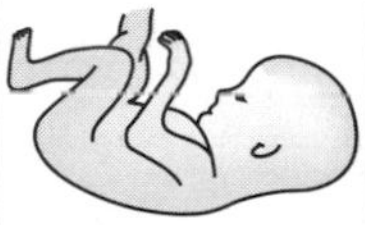	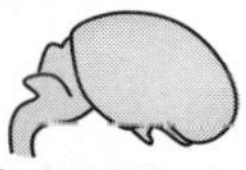 Cord-cervical and lumbar enlarged, Cauda equina	Retina layered Eye axis forward Scala tympani	Tonsillar crypts Cheeks 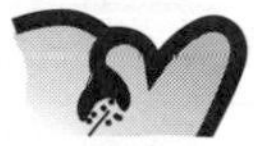 Dental papilla	Accessory coats, blood vessels	Elastic fibers
16	14				Corpora quadrigemina Cerebellum prominent Myelination begins	Scala vestibuli 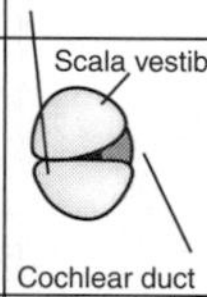 Cochlear duct	Palate complete Enamel and dentine	Cardiac muscle condensed	Segmentation of bronchi complete
20				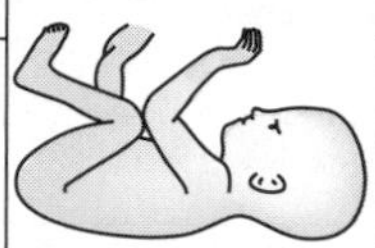		Inner ear ossified	Ossification of nose		Decrease in mesenchyme Capillaries penetrate linings of tubules
24		32	800		Typical layers in cerebral cortex Cauda equina at first sacral level		Nares reopen Calcification of tooth primordia		Change from cuboidal to flattened epithelium Alveoli
28		38.5	1100	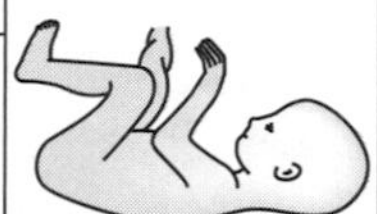	Cerebral fissures and convolutions	Eyelids reopen Retinal layers complete Perceive light			Vascular components adequate for respiration
32		43.5	1600	Accumulation of fat		Auricular cartilage	Taste sense		Number of alveoli still incomplete
36		47.5	2600						
38		50	3200		Cauda equina, at L-3 Myelination within brain	Lacrimal duct canalized	Rudimentary frontal maxillary sinuses	Closure of: foramen ovale, ductus arteriosus, umbilical vessels, ductus venosus	
First postnatal year +				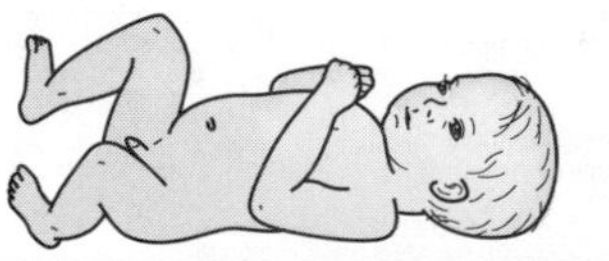	Continuing organization of axonal networks Cerebrocortical function, motor coordination Myelination continues until 2-3 years	Iris pigmented, 5 months Mastoid air cells Coordinate vision, 3-5 months Maximal vision by 5 years	Salivary gland ducts become canalized Teeth begin to erupt 5-7 months Relatively rapid growth of mandible and nose	Relative hypertrophy left ventricle	Continue adding new alveoli

C

FIGURE 3-7, cont'd Timetable of human embryonic and fetal development. (From Jones, K.L. [1996]. *Smith's recognizable patterns of human malformation* [5th ed.]. Philadelphia: Saunders.)

GUT	UROGENITAL	SKELETAL MUSCLE	SKELETON	SKIN	BLOOD, THYMUS LYMPH	ENDOCRINE
Pancreas, dorsal and ventral fusion	Renal vesicles	Differentiation toward final shape	Cartilaginous models of bones Chondrocranium Tail regression	Mammary gland		Parathyroid associated with thyroid Sympathetic neuroblasts invade adrenal
Liver relatively large Intestinal villi	Müllerian ducts fusing Ovary distinguishable	Muscles well represented Movement	Ossification center Sternum	Basal layer	Bone marrow Thymus halves unite Lymphoblasts around the lymph sacs	Thyroid follicles
Gut withdrawal from cord Pancreatic alveoli Anal canal	Testosterone Renal excretion Bladder sac Müllerian tube into urogenital sinus Vaginal sacs, prostate	Perineal muscles	Joints	Hair follicles Melanocytes	Enucleated RBCs Thymus yields reticulum and corpuscles Thoracic duct Lymph nodes; axillary iliac	Adrenalin Noradrenalin
Gut muscle layers Pancreatic islets Bile	♀ ♂ Seminal vesicle Regression, genital ducts		Tail degenerated Notochord degenerated	Corium, 3 layers Scalp, body hair Sebaceous glands Nails beginning	Blood principally from bone marrow Thymus—medullary and lymphoid	Testicle—Leydig cells Thyroid— colloid in follicle Anterior pituitary acidophilic granules Ovary—prim. follicles
Omentum fusing with transverse colon Mesoduodenum, asc. and desc. colon attach to body wall Meconium Gastric, intest. glands	Typical kidney Mesonephros involuting Uterus and vagina Primary follicles	In-utero movement can be detected	Distinct bones	Dermal ridges hands Sweat glands Keratinization		Anterior pituitary—basophilic granules
	No further collecting tubules			Vernix caseosa Nail plates Mammary budding	Blood formation decreasing in liver	
						Testes—decrease in Leydig cells
						Testes descend
	Urine osmolarity continues to be relatively low			Eccrine sweat Lanugo hair prominent Nails to fingertips		
			Only a few secondary epiphyseal centers ossified in knee		Hemoglobin 17-18 g Leukocytosis	
			Ossification of 2nd epiph. centers—hamate, capitate, proximal humerus, femur. New ossif. 2nd epiph. centers till 10-12 yrs. Ossif. of epiphyses till 16-18 yrs.	New hair, gradual loss of lanugo hair	Transient (6 wk) erythroid hypoplasia Hemoglobin 11-12 g 7S gamma globulin produced by 6 wks. Lymph nodes develop cortex, medulla	Transient estrinization Adrenal—regression of fetal zone. Gonodotropin with feminization of ♀ 9-12 yr. (onset); masc. of ♂ 10-14 yr. (onset)

D

FIGURE 3-7, cont'd Timetable of human embryonic and fetal development. (From Jones, K.L. [1996]. *Smith's recognizable patterns of human malformation* [5th ed.]. Philadelphia: Saunders.)

The last 2 weeks of the embryonic period are a time of facial, organ system, and neuromuscular development. The head is rounded and more erect although still disproportionately large. The eyes are open, and the eyelids are developing. The eyelids fuse by the end of the eighth week and do not open again until about the twenty-fifth week. The mouth, tongue, and palate are complete. The external ear is distinct, although it is still low on the head. The regions of the limbs are distinct, and elbow and wrist flexion are possible. Fingers are longer and the toes are differentiated. The feet have moved to the midline. The forearms gradually rise above the shoulder level, and the hands often cover the lower face. The abdomen is less protuberant, and the body is covered by thin skin.[25,103]

Neuromuscular development leads to movement, which can be seen on ultrasound although not felt. The gastrointestinal and genitourinary systems have separated, and the kidneys have achieved their basic structure, although nephron development will continue until 34 to 36 weeks' gestation. Although the internal genitalia have differentiated, the external genitalia have not. The rectal passage is complete, and the anal membrane is perforated, resulting in an open digestive system.[25,103]

Overview of Fetal Development

The fetal period extends from the end of the eighth week of gestation until term. All major systems and external features are established or have begun to develop by the beginning of this period. During the early fetal period (9 to 20 weeks), there is further differentiation of body structures, with a gradual increase in functional ability. By 6 months, the fetus has achieved 60% of its eventual length and 20% of its weight.[103] During the late fetal period (20 weeks to term), further maturation of organ and body systems occurs, along with a marked increase in weight. Organization is a prominent feature of this period.

During weeks 9 through 12, the embryo is 5 to 8 cm long and weighs 8 to 14 g. The head is half the body length. The body length doubles during these weeks. Head growth slows down, the neck lengthens, and the chin is lifted off the chest. The face is broad with widely set eyes, fused lids, and low-set ears. Teeth begin forming under the gums, and the palate fuses. Fingernails become apparent, and the arms reach their final relative length.[25,103]

Micturition and swallowing of amniotic fluid begin. The esophageal lumen forms, and the intestines reenter the abdominal cavity and assume their fixed positions. The bone marrow begins blood formation. The external genitalia differentiate, and by 12 weeks' gestation sexual determination is possible visually.

From 13 to 16 weeks, rapid growth continues. The length of the embryo almost doubles during these weeks. The embryo weighs 20 g by the end of the sixteenth week.[103] The eyes and ears have achieved more normal positions, giving the face a distinctively human look. Fetal skin is extremely thin, and lanugo is present. There is increased muscle and bone development, which along with establishment of initial neuromuscular connections results in increased fetal movements. Skeletal ossification continues during this period. Brown fat deposition and meconium formation begin.[25,103]

Growth slows slightly during the next month (17 to 20 weeks), and the legs reach their final relative positions. During this period, fetal movement is felt by the first-time mother (earlier with successive pregnancies). Fetal heart tones are now audible with a stethoscope. Myelinization of the spinal cord begins. Head hair, eyelashes, and eyebrows can be seen. The sebaceous glands are active, resulting in vernix caseosa deposition. Lung development continues as bronchial branching is completed and terminal air sacs begin to develop. The pulmonary capillary bed is forming in preparation for gas exchange. By 20 weeks' gestation, the fetus weighs about 300 g and is 25 cm long.[103]

After 20 weeks, weight increases substantially. By 24 to 25 weeks, the fetus weighs 650 to 780 g and is 30 cm long.[103] The body is better proportioned. The skin is translucent, and subcutaneous fat has yet to be laid down. Fingerprint and footprint ridges are formed, and the eye is structurally complete.

During weeks 25 to 28, the gas exchange ability of the lungs improves so that extrauterine life can be sustained. Subcutaneous fat begins to form, and head hair and lanugo are well developed. The eyes open as the lids unfuse. CNS development allows initiation of rhythmic breathing movements and partial temperature control. The testes begin to descend into the scrotum.

From 29 weeks to term, fat and muscle tissue are laid down and skin thickness increases. Although the bones are fully formed, ossification is not complete. Vernix caseosa and lanugo begin to disappear as term gestation is approached and growth slows. The testes descend into the scrotum. The infant fills the uterine cavity, and the extremities are flexed against the body. Myelinization and skeletal ossification progresses, and sleep-wake cycles are established. By 38 to 40 weeks, fetal size averages 3000 to 3800 g and 45 to 50 cm.[103]

Intrauterine Environment

The uterine environment normally provides the ideal stimulation for the development and refining of organ systems for transition to and interaction with the extrauterine environment. The amniotic fluid provides the space for the developing fetus to grow and protection from the external environment. Amniotic fluid cushions against external pressure, allowing pressure to the uterus to be transmitted from one side to the other with minimal exertion on the fetus. The weightless space allows for the symmetric development of the face and body. Adequate volume facilitates normal lung development and, until late gestation, exercise and neuromuscular development. The amniotic sac and uterine wall give the fetus something to push against during "practice" activities.

The maternal body provides the fetus with a darkened environment, which may become grayer as the uterus grows and stretches. Auditory stimuli are rich and include the sound of blood flow through the umbilical cord. Most of these sounds are patterned and rhythmic. Extrauterine sounds, such as voices and music, are transmitted in a muted form to the fetus. The maternal system maintains a warm thermal environment. Kinesthetic and vestibular stimulation are provided by maternal movement and changes in position. Other stimuli that influence the activity and responses of the fetus and neonate include maternal biorhythms and diurnal, circadian, and sleep-wake cycles. Exposure of the fetus to these stimuli and events provides appropriate experiences that enhance neurologic organization and establishment of synaptic connections (see Chapter 15). These activities are critical for successful transition to extrauterine life and for establishing physiologic and social relationships necessary to ensure survival.

THE PLACENTA AND PLACENTAL PHYSIOLOGY

The human placenta is a hemochorial villous organ that is essential for transfer of nutrients and gases from the mother to the fetus and for removal of fetal waste products. Alterations in placental development and function markedly influence fetal growth and development and the ability of the infant to survive in intrauterine and extrauterine environments.

Placental Development

Implantation

Implantation is mediated by a coordinated sequence of interactions between maternal and embryonic cells.[42] Implantation involves three distinct processes: (1) loss of the zona pellucida ("hatching" of the blastocyst) 5 days after fertilization, followed by rapid proliferation of the trophectoderm to form the trophoblast cell mass; (2) adherence of the blastocyst to the endometrial surface, which leads to the decidual reaction; and (3) erosion of the epithelium of the endometrial surface, with burrowing of the blastocyst beneath the surface.[46,84,132] With hatching, the blastocyst acquires the ability to attach to the uterus.[67] This involves expression of Perlecon (a heparin sulfate proteoglycans), which binds specifically to extracellular matrix proteins.[132] Both implantation and placentation require ongoing communication (cross-talk) between the developing blastocyst and maternal endometrium via hormones, cytokines, growth factors, and other immunoregulatory substances.[42]

The endometrium must undergo physiologic changes in order for implantation to occur, with a narrow period of maximal uterine receptivity ("window of implantation") for implantation.[42] The ideal window for synchronization between the uterus and blastocyst and thus normal implantation is thought to occur around 8 days after ovulation.[87,112,130] Specific receptors (particularly $\alpha v\beta 3$) appear opening the implantation window; this window is closed several days later.[42,68,87,130] Implantation can also occur in other tissues, resulting in ectopic pregnancy, without this restricted time interval. The endometrium prepares for implantation by the cyclic secretion of 17β-estradiol and progesterone. These hormones regulate the expression of growth factors and cytokines in the uterus, which in turn alter the endometrial surface.[42]

Uterine receptivity is characterized by increased vascularity and edema of the endometrium, increased secretory activity of the endometrial glands, decrease in the polysaccharide matrix surface coating of the epithelial cells, and development of pinopods (microprotrusions) on the epithelial surface.[111,132] The pinopods interact with microvilli on the trophoblast during initial attachment of the blastocyst. Markers of endometrial receptivity are the appearance of pinopods (that last only 1 to 2 days), cell adhesion molecules such as intregrins, cytokines (especially the interleukin family), homeobox genes and their transcription factors (see "Genetic Control of Development"), growth factors (especially the transforming growth factor-β family), proteases and their inhibitors, and endocrine mediators including estrogens, progesterone, calcitonin, human chorionic gonadotropin (hCG), prolactin, and corticotropin-releasing hormone (CRH).[80,112] Adhesion molecules (integrins) form cell surface receptors that develop from days 20 to 24 of the menstrual cycle.

Uterine receptivity must be synchronized with preimplantation, implantation, and placentation signaling by the zygote and blastocyst. Substances involved in this signaling include (1) early pregnancy factor (EPF); (2) preimplantation factor (PIF); (3) growth factors such as epidermal growth factor, transforming growth factor–α, platelet-derived growth factor, insulin-like growth factors (IGFs), tumor necrosis factor–α (TNF-α), and colony stimulating factor–1; (4) immunoregulatory cytokines such as interleukin-1 (IL-1), interleukin-6 (IL-6), and TGF-β; (5) cyclooxygenase-2 and prostaglandins; (6) platelet activity factor (PAF); (7) vascular endothelial growth factor; and (8) hCG.[42,67,81,112] Growth factors such as TNF-α are found by the two- to eight-cell stage; others appear several days later.[47] The zygote develops receptors for cytokines and growth factors by the two cell stage; by the blastocyst stage, these receptors are seen only on trophectoderm tissue.[42] Before implantation the trophoblast is activated. This process occurs 5 to 6 days after fertilization and lasts about 24 hours.[77] The initial signaling between the trophoblast and luminal epithelium is closely linked with immunologic mechanisms (see Chapter 13).[55,67,81,112]

By 5 to 6 days after fertilization (7 to 9 days after ovulation), the blastocyst rests on and adheres to the endometrium.[67] Metabolism increases, with localized changes seen at the eventual site of the implantation beginning up to 24 hours before adherence of the blastocyst to the endometrium.[84] The place of attachment is usually on the upper posterior wall of the uterus, near the side where the ovary with the corpus luteum is located, but it can occur at various other intrauterine and extrauterine sites.[87]

Ligands (molecules that bind to receptors) such as cytokines, growth factors, and hormones on the trophectoderm of the hatched blastocyst bind to cell surface adhesion molecules on the surface of the luminal endometrium.[77] Initial attachment may be mediated by L-selectin (a carbohydrate binding protein) on the trophoblast and carbohydrate receptors on the uterine epithelium. Further attachment and invasion is mediated by integrins (transmembrane glycoproteins with α and β subunits that can be up-regulated via interaction with other substances), IL-10, metalloproteinases, vascular endothelial GF and L-selectin.[68,123] Integrins serve as cell surface receptors for fibrinogen, fibronectin, collagen, and laminin.[87] Laminin promotes attachment; fibronectin promotes invasion of the blastocyst into the uterine epithelium.[130] In addition, near the time of implantation expression of heparin-binding epidermal growth factor-like GF is up regulated near implantation sites.[132] Adhesion (apposition) is initially unstable, relying on interaction between uterine epithelial pinopods and trophoblast microvilli, then stabilizes and is followed by trophoblast invasion of the endometrium.[112] The blastocyst orients itself so that the embryonic pole containing the embryo-forming inner cell mass contacts the endometrial surface first.

The trophectoderm (trophoblast) attaches to endometrial extracellular matrix proteins and secretes proteases to degrade these proteins and begins to invade the endometrium. Fingerlike projections of trophoblast cells protrude between the cells of the endometrial epithelium into the endometrial stroma.[50] The trophoblast cells then migrate between the cells of the endometrial extracellular matrix until they reach maternal blood vessels. Regulatory substances found on both trophoblast and endometrial tissue enhance interaction, invasion, and trophoblast proliferation. These substances include (1) metalloproteinases (e.g., collagenases, gelatinases, stomelysins); (2) plasminogen activation; (3) plasmin-regulating factors; (4) cytokines such as IL-1β (stimulates trophoblast invasion); and (5) growth factors such as epidermal GF and TGFβ (limits invasion and induces syncytium formation).[5,6,42,62,87] Other factors limit trophoblast invasion and develop as part of the decidual reaction. For example, the decidua (i.e., the altered endometrium during pregnancy) secretes protease inhibitors such as TGF-β and tissue inhibitor of metalloproteinase (TIMP). The trophoblast may also autoregulate its invasion via secretion of TGF-β, TIMP, and hCG.[42] If trophoblast invasion is too extensive, placenta accreta can result; if invasion is too little, the risk of miscarriage or placental abruption is increased.

By the seventh day after fertilization, the trophoblast begins to differentiate into two layers: the inner cytotrophoblast and the outer syncytiotrophoblast layer.[50] The mononuclear cytotrophoblast is a mitotically active layer that forms new syncytial cells, the chorionic villi, and the amnion. The cytotrophoblast serves as a stem cell population to generate new trophoblast cells.[55] The syncytiotrophoblast is a thick multinuclear mass, without distinct cell boundaries, that puts out fingerlike projections that invade the endometrial epithelium, engulfing uterine cells (see Figure 3-5). Slight bleeding may occur during this process, which may be mistaken for a scanty, short menstrual period. The trophoblast, primarily the syncytiotrophoblast, produces hCG (which maintains the corpus luteum during early pregnancy) as well as estrogens, progesterone, hPL, and other substances (see "Placental Endocrinology"). The functions of the trophoblast are summarized in Table 3-1.

Several forms of extravillous trophoblast are derived from the cytotrophoblast. Interstitial trophoblast migrates into the uterine tissue and attaches the anchoring villi of the placenta to the decidua. HLA-G is expressed on the anchoring trophoblast and helps protect fetal tissue from the maternal immune system (see Chapter 13).[55] Other extravillous trophoblast migrates out from the placenta into the endometrium and spiral arteries. This type of trophoblast has two roles: (1) conversion of the maternal spiral arteries into low-resistance, high-capacity vessels and (2) formation of plugs at the top of the spiral arteries to limit maternal blood flow into the placenta during the first trimester (see Placental Circulation).[55,68,79,87] Implantation is complete by 10 days after fertilization.[50] At this point, the blastocyst lies beneath the endometrial surface and is covered by a blood clot and cellular debris. By 10 to 12 days, the endometrial epithelium has regenerated in this area.[112]

Many ova that are fertilized never implant. One third to one half of all zygotes never become blastocysts; 70% to 75% of blastocysts implant and 51% of these survive to the second week.[103] Implantation can be selectively inhibited by administration of low-dose estrogen for several days following sexual intercourse ("morning-after" pill). Estrogen preparations

Table 3-1 **Functions of the Trophoblast**

FUNCTION	EFFECTORS
Erosion of maternal tissue to make space for implantation and growth	Proteases (e.g., plasminogen system, matrix metalloproteinases)
Hormone secretion	hCG, hPL, estrogen, progesterone and others
Transport nutrients and waste products	Substrate specific transporters, trophoblast, endothelial plasma membranes
Placental attachment	Adhesion molecules in the extracellular matrix and at the cell surface
Migration and arterial transformation	Adhesion molecules, proteases, extracellular matrix components

Adapted from Aplin, J. (2000). Maternal influences on placental development. *Semin Cell Dev Biol, 17,* 116. *hCG,* Human chorionic gonadotropin; *hPL,* human placental lactogen.

such as diethylstilbestrol act by altering the normal balance of estrogen and progesterone during the secretory phase of the endometrial cycle, making the endometrial lining unsuitable for implantation. Estrogen may also accelerate passage of the zygote along the fallopian tube so that it arrives in the uterus before the secretory phase of the endometrial cycle is established.[103]

Ectopic Pregnancy. Extrauterine implantation results in an ectopic pregnancy in 1 in every 80 to 250 pregnancies.[103] The incidence of ectopic pregnancy has increased fourfold since 1972 and accounts for 10% to 11% of maternal mortality in the United States.[33] Ectopic pregnancy is the most common cause of maternal death in the first 20 weeks of pregnancy. Much of the increased incidence in recent years is thought to be a result of the prevalence of sexually transmitted diseases (STDs) and pelvic inflammatory disease (PID). The most common site for an ectopic pregnancy is the isthmus and ampulla of the fallopian tubes.[103] This probably results from delay in transport of the zygote from the site of fertilization to the uterine cavity. If transport is delayed, the blastocyst emerges from the zona pellucida while in the fallopian tube and adheres to and implants in tubal mucosa. The delay may be due to tubal adhesions or mucosal damage from PID.[103] PID and salpingitis disrupt and damage the tubal mucosa, decreasing the number of cilia, which are essential for timely movement of the zygote along the tube. Alterations in the concentrations of progesterone, estrogen, and prostaglandins may also delay ovum transport.

Endometrium and Decidua

The uterine endometrial lining consists of an epithelial layer that contains ciliated and mucus-secreting cells. These cells penetrate into the endometrial stroma and may enter the underlying myometrium. The endometrium is divided into two functional zones (see Figure 2-28). The deepest basalis layer lies adjacent to the myometrium. This layer responds to progesterone stimulus with secretory activity and provides the base for endometrial regeneration after menstrual sloughing.[98] The superficial (functionalis) layer of endometrium includes the outer compacta and the middle spongiosa, which contains glands and blood vessels. During the secretory phase of the menstrual cycle, the endometrium undergoes physical changes in preparation for implantation (see Chapter 2).

With conception these changes become more extensive. Under stimulation of progesterone and estrogen, the epithelium and stromal cells become progressively hypertrophic and develop subnuclear vacuoles rich in glycogen and lipids.[84,122,146] Early nutrition of the blastocyst is from digestion of substances in endometrial tissue and surrounding capillaries. The endometrial changes during pregnancy are known as the decidual reaction, and the altered endometrial lining is known as the decidua. The decidual reaction involves remodeling of the extracellular matrix with changes in collagen, proteoglycans, and glycoproteins. Estrogen and progesterone pathways that control epithelial and stromal function during implantation and decidualization include (1) CCATT/enhancer binding protein-β (transcription factor); (2) homeobox-10 (transcription factor); (3) bone morphogenetic protein-2 (morphogen); (4) Wnt4 (morphogen); (5) Indian hedgehog (morphogen); and (6) gap junctions.[122] A poor decidual reaction is associated with placenta accreta and ectopic pregnancy.[42] In addition these pathways are altered in endometriosis leading to impaired implantation.[122] Decidualization also involves alterations in local immune cells and processes and changes in maternal spiral arteries (see "Placental Circulation").[19] As decidualization increases, the window of receptivity for implantation is closed.[79]

In addition to its role in early nutrition of the embryo, the decidua may protect the endometrium and myometrium from uncontrolled invasion by the trophoblast cell mass.[84] The decidua also acts as a physical barrier and—via production of cytokines that promote trophoblast attachment, not invasion—to protect the endometrium during the period when trophoblast cells migrate out of the placenta to the maternal spiral arteries (see "Maternal Uteroplacental Circulation").[79] A somewhat hypoxic environment appears to be needed in early pregnancy for trophoblast invasion and differentiation; high oxygen levels may alter morphogenesis.[68,79,157]

The decidua is divided into three sections (Figure 3-8). The *decidua capsularis,* just above the area of trophoblast proliferation, initially covers the growing embryo. With development of the chorion, the decidua capsularis gradually regresses. The portion of the decidua on which the blastocyst rests forms a soft, spongy vascular bed known as the *decidua basalis,* site of the future placenta.[4] Large numbers of maternal macrophages, especially maternal natural killer cells, migrate into the decidua basalis (see Chapter 13).[108,146] Decidual macrophages are important in maternal tolerance of the implanting blastocyst and cooperate with fetal trophoblast cells in remodeling maternal spiral arteries during pregnancy (see "Placental Circulation").[108] At the interface between the trophoblast and decidua basalis is a specialized extracellular matrix rich in fibrin and fibronectin that supports trophoblast adhesion and migration.[4] The remaining portion is known as the *decidua parietalis* (or decidua vera).

The decidua basalis forms the maternal portion of the placenta and the stratum in which separation of the placenta will occur at delivery.[33,103] With embryonic growth, the decidua basalis is progressively compressed. The glands and blood vessels become distorted and assume oblique and horizontal courses. As the embryo fills the lumen of the uterus, the decidua capsularis disappears. By 18 to 20 weeks after conception, the chorion laeve and decidua parietalis meet and fuse, obliterating the uterine cavity (see Figure 3-8).[51,84,124]

Development of the Amniotic Cavity

The amniotic cavity appears during the second week following fertilization as the blastocyst is burrowing into the endometrium. Small spaces appear between the inner cell mass

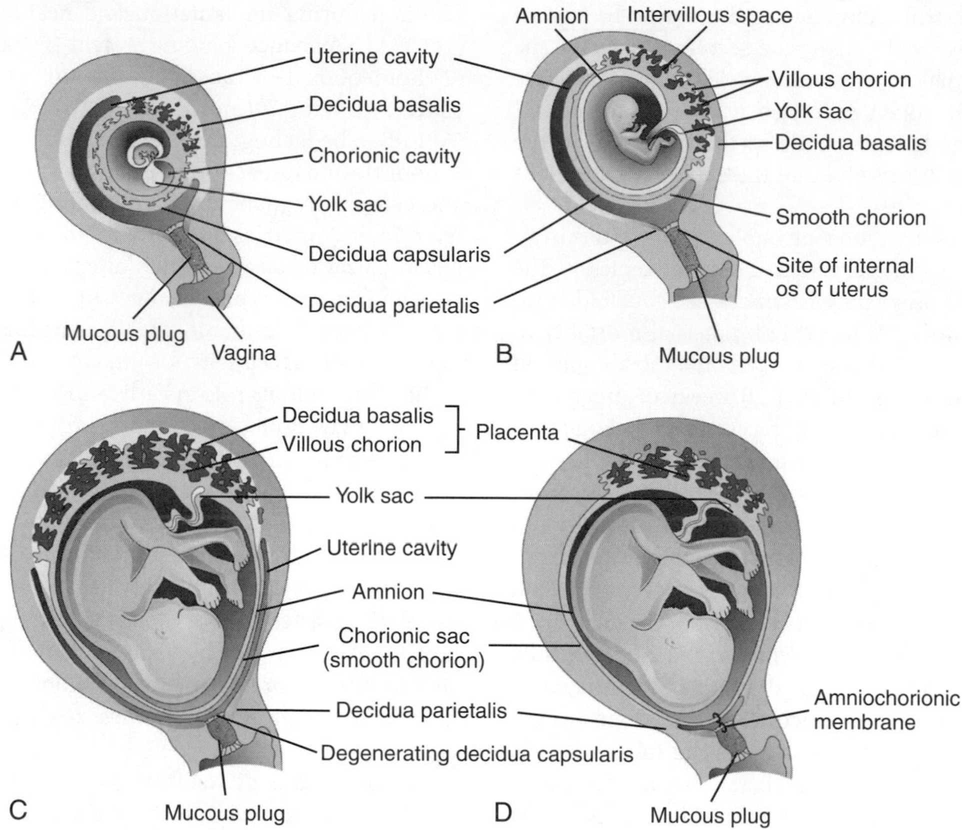

FIGURE 3-8 Changes in the decidual layers with growth of the embryo and fetus. **A** to **D**, Drawing of sagittal sections of the gravid uterus from the fifth to twenty-second weeks, showing the changing relations of the fetal membranes to the decidua. In **D**, the amnion and chorion are fused with each other and the decidua parietalis, thereby obliterating the uterine cavity. Note also in **D** that the chorionic villi persist only where the chorion is associated with the decidua basalis; here they form the villous chorion (fetal portion of the placenta). (From Moore, K.L., Persaud, T.V.N., & Torchia, M.G. [2013]. The developing human: Clinically oriented embryology [9th ed.]. Philadelphia: Saunders [Figure 7-1, C-F].)

and cytotrophoblast. These spaces coalesce to form a narrow amniotic cavity that gradually enlarges to completely surround the fetus (Figure 3-9).

The amniotic cavity develops a thin epithelial roof or lining. This lining is the amnion, which arises from amnioblasts (amniogenic cells) from the cytotrophoblast. The floor of the amniotic cavity is formed from the embryonic epiblast germ layer. Initially a small amount of fluid may be secreted by the amniotic epithelial cells, but the major early source of amniotic fluid is probably maternal serum. With advancing gestation, the epithelial cells of the amnion become more cuboidal or columnar and are covered with microvilli.[103]

Placentation

As the syncytiotrophoblast proliferates and invades the endometrial stroma, the blastocyst slowly sinks into the endometrium. By 7 to 8 days after fertilization, intersyncytial spaces or lacunae are seen in the syncytiotrophoblast (see Figure 3-5).[51] Capillaries in the endometrium grow and surround the syncytiotrophoblast forming a capillary plexus connected to the early lacunae.[164] The lacunae fill with a nutritive substance or filtrate containing primarily glandular fluid derived from maternal blood that diffuses through the trophoblast to the embryo. Individual lacunae fuse into lacunar networks that will later develop into the intervillous spaces (IVS) and become filled with maternal blood. Endometrial capillaries around the implanted embryo become congested and dilated, forming sinusoids.

Blood flow into the IVS is limited in the first trimester and the IVS is probably filled primarily with this filtrate of maternal serum and secretions from the endometrial glands.[22,23,68,70,116] The highly oxygenated maternal blood does not fill the IVS until fetal vessels are established in the villi and mechanisms to protect the fetus against oxidative stress are established.[22,68,70,79] This begins at 8 to 9 weeks and increases after 10 to 12 weeks.[22] Before that time, trophoblast plugs fill the tops of the spiral arteries, controlling arterial pressure and limiting blood flow into the IVS.[76,124] Oxygen concentration in the IVS at 8 weeks is ≤20 mmHg (3% to 5% O_2) versus 60 mmHg (8% to 10% O_2) in the surrounding decidua.[116] Thus initial placental and embryonic development occurs in a relatively hypoxic environment. This environment may stimulate production of vascular endothelial growth factor and stimulate chorionic

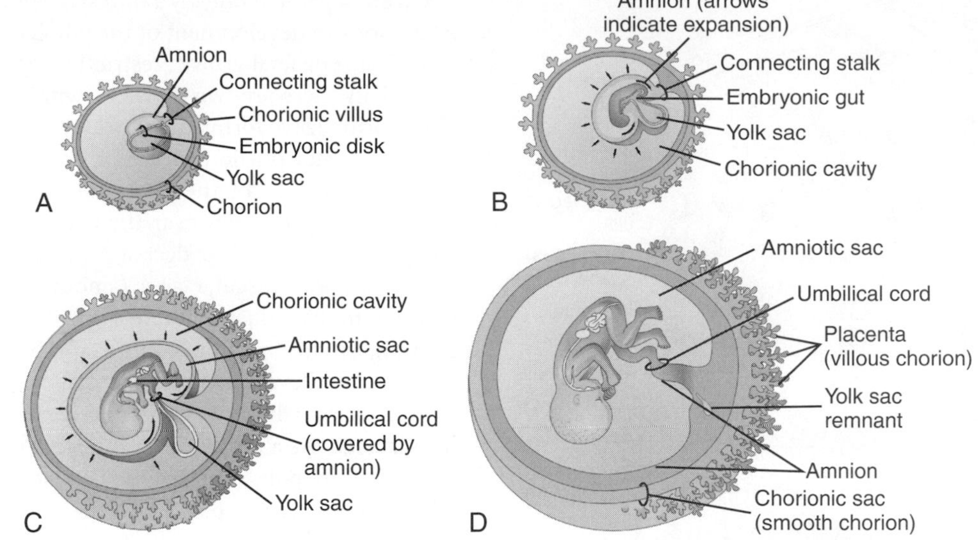

FIGURE 3-9 Development of the amniotic cavity, amnion, and chorion. **A,** 3 Weeks. **B,** 4 Weeks. **C,** 10 Weeks. **D,** 20 Weeks. (From Moore, K.L. & Persaud, T.V.N. [2003]. *The developing human: Clinically oriented embryology* [7th ed.]. Philadelphia: Saunders.)

vascularization.[22,68,70] Low O_2 levels may be essential for control of early cardiovascular development by hypoxia inducible factors (HIF).[157]

HIFs act as mediators to allow cells to adjust to low O_2 conditions and facilitate placental vascularization and signaling for trophoblast differentiation.[116] HIFs are activated by both hypoxia and nonhypoxic factors such as the renin-angiotensin system, GFs, and cytokines.[116,119] For example, HIF-1 regulation via angiotensin II increases extravillous trophoblast growth, cellular proliferation, and soluble fms-like receptor-1. Alterations are seen in the pathophysiology of preeclampsia (see Chapter 9). HIF-1 and TGFβ inhibit trophoblast invasion, while HIF-1 and insulin-like growth factor 2 increase trophoblast growth.[116,119]

Early flow of maternal blood into the IVS has been reported to be primarily in the periphery of the developing placenta.[70] Jauniaux and colleagues postulate that higher oxygen flow in the periphery may induce regression of villi and formation of the chorion laeve (chorion).[22,70] Increased flow in the central area of the developing placenta may increase the risk of early pregnancy loss due to oxidative damage to the trophoblast.[70] By 11 to 12 weeks the spiral arteries become patent and maternal blood flow into the IVS and fetal oxygen levels increase. Vascular changes in the uteroplacental vessels are described further in "Placental Circulation."

Development of the Villi. The placenta consists of the outer epithelial layer, derived from trophoblast cells, and an inner vascular network and connective tissue stroma, derived from embryonic mesoderm. Initially the lacunae are separated by trabecular columns of syncytiotrophoblast (primary villous stems), which provide the framework for development of the placental chorionic villi. The cytotrophoblast differentiates into vascular cytotrophoblast, which fuses to form chorionic villi and the extravascular invasive trophoblast, which is involved in remodeling of the spiral arteries (see "Placental Circulation").[78] Chorionic villi begin to appear toward the end of the second week of gestation as proliferation of the cytotrophoblast layer produces columns of cells or fingerlike processes known as *primary chorionic villi*.[78] A mesenchymal core grows within these primary villi, forming secondary villi. Blood vessels within the villi arise from this mesenchymal core within a few days, forming tertiary villi.[78,84]

As the columns of cytotrophoblast cells proliferate, they extend through the syncytiotrophoblast, expanding laterally to meet and fuse with adjoining cytotrophoblast columns. This forms the cytotrophoblastic shell and divides the syncytiotrophoblast into an inner layer and a peripheral layer. The peripheral layer degenerates and is replaced by fibrinoid material.[50,84] Villous development is stimulated by growth factors such as vascular endothelium growth factor (VEGF) and placental-like growth factor and by the relatively hypoxic environment. VEGF is found in maternal plasma by 6 weeks' gestation and peaks at the end of the first trimester, similar to the pattern seen with hCG. During the third trimester, placental growth factors enhances formation of terminal villi.[78] The low-oxygen environment stimulates angiogenesis, trophoblast formation, and increased numbers of highly vascularized terminal villi.[78]

The cytotrophoblastic shell is the point of contact between the fetal tissue and maternal tissue; it attaches the chorionic sac to the basal plate. The basal plate is formed by the compact and spongy zones of the maternal decidua basalis, remnants of the trophoblast, and fibrinoid material. By the end of the fourth month, the shell has regressed, with replacement of the cytotrophoblast cell columns by fibrinoid material (Rohr layer) and formation of clumps (islands) of cytotrophoblast cells.[50] A layer of fibrinoid material

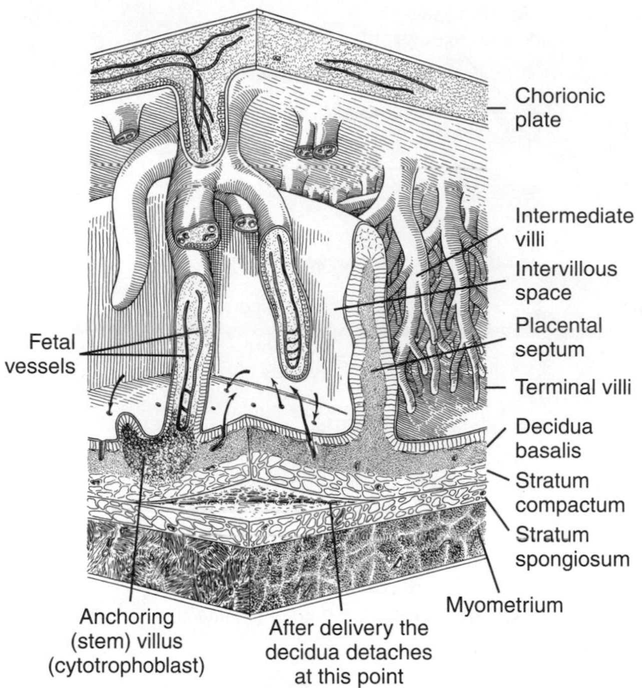

FIGURE 3-10 Diagrammatic composition of placental tissues near term. *Arrows* indicate the blood flow from uteroplacental arteries to the intervillous space and back to the uteroplacental veins. (From Duplessis, G.D.T. & Haegel, P. [1971]. *Embryologie.* New York: Masson. English edition by Springer-Verlag; Chapman and Hall; and Masson, [1972].)

(Nitabuch layer) also develops within the spongy zone of the decidua basalis. This is the level of placental separation at delivery (Figure 3-10).

Villi containing blood vessels (tertiary villi) arise around 20 days postconception.[51,164] By 21 to 22 days, a primitive fetoplacental circulation is established between blood in the vessels of the villi, vessels forming in the embryo, primitive heart, and blood islands in the yolk sac (see Chapters 8 and 9). The villi that arise from the chorionic plate and attach to the maternal decidua basalis are known as anchoring (or stem) villi. Initially embryonic and fetal blood vessels develop within stem villi by branching angiogenesis.[76,78] Stem villi, which contain arteries and veins as well as some arterioles and venules, make up about one third of the villi in the mature placenta.[51] Mature intermediate villi grow from the sides of stem villi and project into the IVS (see Figure 3-10). These intermediate villi, which constitute approximately 25% of the villi in the mature placenta, contain primarily fetal capillaries with a few small arterioles and venules.[50,51] Intermediate villi and their branches (terminal villi), constitute the major area of exchange between maternal and fetal circulations. After fetal viability, terminal villi are formed by nonbranching angiogenesis in mature intermediate villi.[76] Terminal villi contain multiple dilated capillaries or sinusoids and account for 30% to 40% of the mature villous tree.[51] Terminal villi bulge into the villous cytotrophoblast so that maternal and fetal blood are separated only by a thin syncytiotrophoblast layer.[78] Alterations in development of the villous system may lead to miscarriage or fetal growth restriction.[164]

Initially there are two divisions within the chorionic villi. The chorion laeve forms the chorion; the chorion frondosum forms the fetal portion of the placenta. At first, villi cover the entire surface of the chorionic sac. Beginning around 8 weeks' gestation, villi near the decidua capsularis become compressed, blood flow decreases, and the villi degenerate, leaving a bare avascular area (smooth chorion, or chorion laeve). Simultaneously, villi near the decidua basalis (villous chorion, or chorion frondosum) rapidly enlarge, increase in number, and develop a mesenchymal core and blood vessels.

Anchoring villi grow more slowly than other portions of the placenta. As a result, during the third month, folds of the basal plate are pulled up into the IVS (see Figure 3-10). These folds (known as the placental septa) do not extend to the chorionic plate and have no known morphologic or physiologic function.[50,84]

By 40 to 50 days after ovulation, the trophoblast has invaded far enough into the endometrium to reach and begin to erode maternal spiral arterioles. Trophoblast plugs fill the tops of the spiral arteries until around 10 to 12 weeks' gestation, when the arteries open up and begin to supply blood to the IVS.[4] This is the time when the mature placenta is established. The chorion laeve fuses onto the decidua vera, forming the chorion or outer fetal membrane. The inner membrane, the amnion, is derived from the amniogenic cells (amnioblasts) of the cytotrophoblast (see "Development of the Amniotic Cavity").

Placental Growth

By 4 months, the placenta has achieved its full thickness, with no new lobules or stem villi added after 10 to 12 weeks. Circumferential placental growth continues with further ramification of stem villi (via growth and extension of new trophoblast sprouts, followed by growth of the mesenchymal core and development of blood vessels), lengthening of existing villi, and increases in the size and number of placental capillaries.[33,103] Much of the expansion of villi after 20 weeks is in the terminal villi. Mature intermediate villi elongate in the third trimester, which assists in generation of new terminal villi branches.[99] As a result of the proliferation of terminal villi, the surface area for placental exchange continues to increase until late in gestation. In addition, the thickness of the tissue layers separating maternal and fetal blood thins, thus enhancing diffusion. Trophoblast sprouts not used to form new villi break off, enter the maternal circulation, lodge in the mother's lung capillaries, and are cleared by proteolysis.

After 30 weeks' gestation, syncytial knots develop, pulling the syncytium and its nuclei into "piles" several layers thick and leaving a thin, attenuated, anuclear membrane in the intervening areas.[103] These areas (known as the *vasculosyncytial membrane*) appear to, but do not actually, fuse with dilated fetal capillaries and are thought to be specialized regions that facilitate placental gas exchange.[50,84]

The placenta eventually occupies one third of the inner uterine surface. Until 15 to 16 weeks, the placenta is larger than the fetus; the fetus then becomes larger than the placenta, so that by term the fetus is five to six times heavier than the placenta. The early growth of the placenta establishes a wide area of maternal blood flow (so the placenta is not dependent on relatively few blood vessels for perfusion) and adequate trophoblast tissue for production of sufficient hCG to maintain the corpus luteum and thus the pregnancy.

Increases in villous surface area and thinning of placental tissue layers increase the functional efficiency of the placenta during pregnancy. During the first 2 months, the relatively few villi are greater than 170 μm in diameter, are vascularized by a small central fetal vessel, and are covered by two layers of trophoblast (syncytiotrophoblast outer layer and inner layer of cytotrophoblast) of uniform thickness. At this stage, the villous stroma consists of a loose network of primitive mesenchymal tissue and many Hofbauer cells (tissue macrophages).[50] From 8 to 30 weeks, the number of villi increase and the average diameter decreases to about 70 μm. The stroma becomes thinner and more compact and contains fibroblasts and collagen fibers with fewer Hofbauer cells.[50] By term the placental villi are approximately 35 to 40 μm in diameter. The trophoblast layer and stroma have thinned considerably, and few cytotrophoblast cells are seen.[51]

The area-to-volume ratio of the placenta progressively increases. Surface area increases from 3.4 m^2 (28 weeks) to 12.6 m^2 (term), and the syncytium decreases in thickness from 10 mm^2 to 1.7 mm^2 late in gestation. The actual surface area is closer to 90 m^2 because of the presence of extensive microvilli on the surface of the syncytiotrophoblast covering the villi.[33,46] Transfer efficiency of placental tissue increases sixfold. The trophoblast layer and connective tissue thin so that the capillaries lie closer to the syncytial trophoblast, decreasing the distance that nutrients and waste products have to travel.

By term the placenta weighs approximately 480 g (±135 g) with a diameter of 18 to 22 cm and thickness of 2 to 2.5 cm, although considerable variation is seen.[134] Although villous growth continues to near term, the placenta begins to undergo degenerative changes. These changes include increased syncytial knots, intervillous thrombi, fibrin deposits, infarcts, and calcifications.

Abnormal growth of the placenta may also occur. Hypoplasia of the syncytiotrophoblast can alter implantation and result in abortion, abruptio placentae, or poor development of terminal villi and increase the risk of stillbirth or preterm delivery. Hyperplasia and reactivation of the syncytial growth layer, possibly due to suboptimal oxygenation, have been observed in women with hypertension and prolonged pregnancy. Although the amount of cytotrophoblast decreases with gestation, the remaining tissue retains its proliferative capacity so the cytotrophoblast can be reactivated to replace damaged or destroyed syncytiotrophoblast.[50] However, this hyperplasia may be followed by degenerative changes.[33]

Placental Structure

Although the mature placenta contains maternal and fetal components, it is primarily a fetal structure composed of extensively branching, closely packed fetal villi containing fetal blood vessels (see Figure 3-10). Three main types of chorionic villi can be identified: (1) stem (or anchoring) villi, which consist of multiple branches and function to stabilize the villous tree; (2) mature intermediate villi, located between the stem and terminal villi; and (3) terminal villi, which are the major areas of maternal-fetal exchange.[84] On the fetal side, the placenta is covered by the chorionic plate, a thin membranous structure continuous with the fetal membranes. On the maternal side, the outer layer of trophoblast cells fuse to the decidua basalis.

The fetal portion of the placenta is divided into 50 to 60 lobes, each arising as a primary stem villus supplied by primary branches of the umbilical vessels from the chorionic plate. Each lobe is divided into one to five subunits or lobules. Lobules are globular structures with a central cylindrical space that is relatively empty.[50] This space may arise because of preferential growth of villi in relation to entry of maternal arteries into the IVS. Beneath the chorionic plate the primary stem villi divide into secondary stem villi. These villi run parallel to the chorionic plate, dividing into tertiary stem villi, which project downward through the parenchyma of the placenta around the central space and anchor onto the basal plate (see Figure 3-10).[50] Each primary stem villus may give rise to varying numbers of secondary stem villi and lobules.[50] The terminal villi branch off of the tertiary stem villi.

The placental septa divide the maternal surface of the placenta into 10 to 40 (average 15 to 20) lobes, each containing at least one and usually more main stem villi and their branches.[33,51] The term *cotyledon* is sometimes used to describe these lobes. Fox suggests that, because the maternal lobes are just areas between placental septa with no physiologic or morphologic significance, *cotyledon* should really be used to describe portions of the villus tree that arise from a single primary stem villus.[50]

Maternal and fetal circulations are separated by several layers of tissue. These tissues are called the *placental membrane* or *placental barrier*. A substance, such as glucose, moving from the maternal to the fetal circulation must initially pass from maternal blood through five layers to reach the fetal blood: (1) the microvillous membrane of the syncytiotrophoblast, (2) the syncytiotrophoblast cells, (3) the basal membrane of the syncytiotrophoblast, (4) the connective tissue mesenchyme of the villus, and (5) the epithelium of the fetal blood vessel (Figure 3-11). The cytotrophoblast ceases to form a continuous layer after about 12 weeks and is replaced by a fibrinoid layer.[103] As gestation continues, the connective tissue thins, and the fetal capillaries increase in number and size.

UMBILICAL CORD

The umbilical cord can be seen on ultrasound by 42 days and is well established by 8 to 9 weeks.[97] It normally contains two arteries and one vein surrounded by Wharton jelly, a substance containing collagen, muscle, and mucopolysaccharide. The cord epithelium is formed by amnion. No other blood

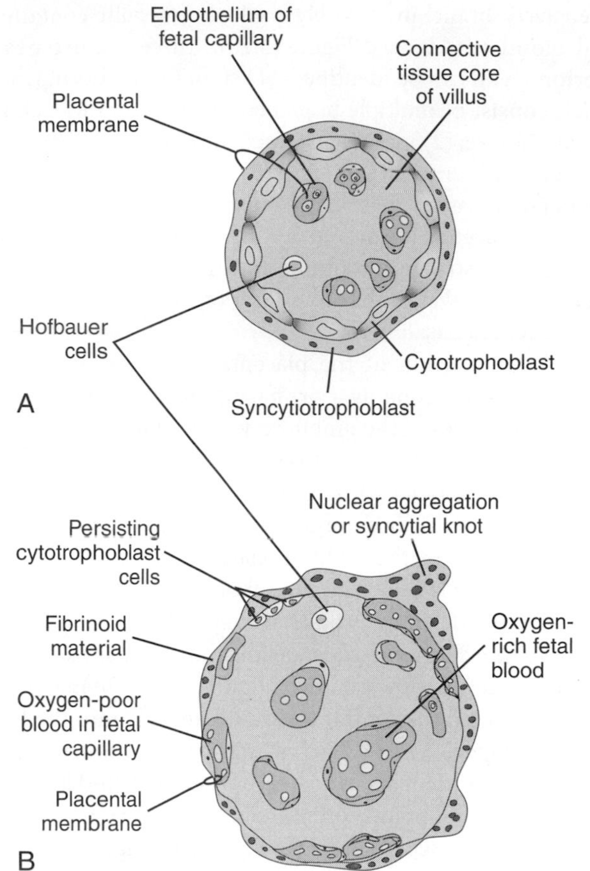

FIGURE 3-11 The placental membrane or barrier. **A,** and **B,** Drawings of sections through a chorionic villus at 10 weeks and at full term, respectively. (From Moore, K.L. & Persaud, T.V.N. [2003]. *The developing human: Clinically oriented embryology* [7th ed.]. Philadelphia: Saunders.)

vessels are found in the cord; neural tissue is also absent. Vasoresponsiveness of the cord to stimuli or drugs is thought to be myogenic.[84]

The umbilical vessels are longer than the cord and tend to twist and spiral within the cord. The umbilical arteries contain four muscle layers: an inner circular layer, a longitudinal layer, and two helical layers. The helical layers function independently to coil both the arteries and the umbilical cord. The twist or spiral of the cord is established by 9 weeks' gestation. A left (counterclockwise) twist is more common than a right (clockwise) twist; however, bidirectional twisting is sometimes seen. The direction of the twist is not significant.[134] Coiling is thought to protect the cord against tension, compression, and entanglement. Up to 30% of cords may be uncoiled at 20 weeks, but less than 5% by term.[97] Lack of coiling has been associated with fetal growth restriction, oligohydramnios, fetal anomalies, and preterm delivery.[97]

The cord is usually inserted near the center of the placenta but may be attached at any point. Centric and eccentric insertion of the cord have no significance and reflect differences in the plane of implantation and placental growth. However, velamentous and marginal insertion of the cord are abnormal.

The cord arises from fusion of the connecting stalk with the yolk sac stalk and allantois at the end of the fourth week of gestation.[103] The umbilical vessels arise from the allantois and initially consist of four vessels. One of the two original umbilical veins invariably atrophies by 6 weeks after fertilization, followed by dilation of the remaining (left) vessel. Occasionally one umbilical artery, usually the left, also regresses sometimes or does not form, resulting in a two-vessel cord, which may sometimes be associated with other anomalies (see "Abnormalities of the Cord and Placenta").[97]

The cord reaches its maximal length by 30 weeks and averages 55 to 60 cm (range, 30 to 90 cm) with a width of 1 to 2 cm (thicker in large for gestational age infants).[47,97,134] Cord length is determined both genetically and by intrauterine space and fetal activity, which places tension on the cord.[47,97] The minimum cord length for vaginal delivery is thought to be 32 cm.[134] Occasionally the arteries may fuse near the placenta, so observation of the number of placental vessels should occur at least 3 cm from the placenta.[134]

The umbilical vessels constrict soon after delivery. Constriction of the umbilical arteries begins within 5 seconds of birth and is complete by 45 seconds; the umbilical vein begins to constrict within 15 seconds of delivery and is functionally closed by 3 to 4 minutes.[84] Placental transfusion and issues regarding timing of cord clamping are discussed in Chapter 8.

AMNION AND CHORION

The amnion and chorion begin to develop soon after fertilization and continue to grow until about 28 weeks' gestation. After this point, further mitotic activity is rare, and enlargement takes place by stretching of the existing membranes.[84] The layers of the fetal membranes at term are: the innermost amniotic epithelium (involved in amniotic fluid exchange and pH regulation), lamina propria, chorionic connective tissue, cytotrophoblastic layer (which along with the chorionic connective tissue becomes the chorionic basal plate at the placental margin), and decidual layer.[51] By 7 to 10 weeks, the amnion and chorion are in contact with each other, and their mesenchymal layers may fuse in places.[51]

The chorion, or outer membrane, contains blood vessels that atrophy as pregnancy advances, but no nerves. The blood vessels carry nutrients for the chorion that cross via diffusion to supply the amnion. The chorion is composed of 2 to 10 layers of polygonal cells and is up to 0.4 mm thick. The amnion is a thick (0.08 to 0.12 mm), avascular, and nerveless membrane with cuboidal and columnar cells. Its surface is strengthened by surface desmosomes and microvillar interdigitations that lie over a basement membrane with a collagenous extracellular matrix.

The amnion and chorion are connected by an extracellular matrix (fibrous proteins embedded in polysaccharide gelatinous matter). The chorion adheres to the decidua. The chorion is relatively fixed. The amnion is passively pushed against and moves over the chorion aided by mucus from the spongy layer. As a result, the amnion can rupture, forming shreds of tissue (amniotic bands), while the chorion remains intact. The amniotic bands may wrap around, constrict, or amputate fetal parts. The reason for rupture of the amnion is unknown but may be related to trauma.[84]

The fetal membranes are metabolically active and are involved in amniotic fluid turnover (see "Amniotic Fluid Volume and Turnover") and initiation of labor (see Chapter 4). The fetal membranes are a major site of prostaglandin (PG) synthesis and metabolism. During most of pregnancy many PGs are converted to inactive metabolites due to a balance between prostaglandin synthetase (need for PG synthesis) and 15-hydroxyprostaglandin dehydrogenase (PGDH; needed for PG inactivation). However near term, PG synthesis increases and PGDH decreases in preparation for labor onset.[107] The amnion is a reservoir for storage of arachidonic acid, an essential prostaglandin precursor, and the chorion is a reservoir for progesterone.[84] The membranes and decidua are rich sources of enzymes (e.g., phospholipase A2) needed for formation of prostaglandins. Cells of the amnion are involved in protein synthesis; protein and lipid secretion; and exchange of water, electrolytes, and other solutes. The amnion has a metabolic rate similar to that of the liver. The chorion synthesizes substances such as renin and prostaglandins. 11-β-hydroxysteroid dehydrogenase type 1 (11β-HSD1) is also found in fetal membranes. 11β-HSD1 converts inactive cortisone to active cortisol. Fetal membrane 11β-HSD1 contributes to the increase in glucocorticoid concentrations in the third trimester needed for fetal organ maturation and initiation of labor (see Chapter 4).[107]

The ability of the membranes to stretch and resist rupture from increasing fetal size and amniotic fluid volume until the end of pregnancy is thought to be related to the collagen-rich tissue of the amnion, which has great tensile strength that is maintained throughout gestation. With delivery, the decidua and chorion must separate to allow expulsion of the membranes. This process involves fetal fibronectin, an extracellular matrix protein found at the decidual-chorionic interface.[107] Rupture of the membranes is discussed in Chapter 4. Premature rupture of the membranes (PROM), or rupture before onset of uterine contractions, may be due to factors such as mechanical stress (polyhydramnios, multiple gestation), alterations in membranous collagen, or chorioamnionitis. In chorioamnionitis a variety of vaginal and cervical microorganisms have been demonstrated to produce proteases that alter membrane integrity and reduce the pressure needed for rupture. PROM may be mediated by collagenetic enzymes from the placenta and amniotic fluid that increase in activity with increasing gestational age.

Placental Circulation

Adequate blood flow to and through the placenta from both fetal and maternal circulations is essential for sufficient exchange of nutrients, gases, and waste products. However, nearly half of the combined maternal-fetal blood flow to the placenta is not involved in maternal-fetal transfer due to maternal and fetal shunts within the uteroplacental circulation.[46] The fetal shunt is the portion of umbilical blood flow that does not supply the area of exchange between maternal and fetal blood. Approximately 17% to 25% of the total umbilical blood flow is used to supply the fetal membranes and placental tissue. Maternal shunt is the portion of uterine blood flow that does not supply the IVS. Approximately 20% to 27% of uterine arterial blood supplies the myometrium and cervix. At term the uterus extracts 30 to 35 mL of oxygen per minute from maternal blood.[50]

Fetal-Placental Circulation

Deoxygenated blood from the fetus passes via the two umbilical arteries, which spiral around the umbilical vein, to the placenta. Each artery supplies half of the placenta. Before entering the placenta, the two umbilical arteries are connected by several anastomosed vessels. These arteries tend to fuse close to the surface of the placenta. As the cord enters the placenta, the arteries divide and branch radially onto the chorionic plate before entering the villi. The chorionic vessels branch into 20 to 40 villous trunks or lobular arteries, which branch further into multiple smaller villous vessels, forming an extensive arteriovenous system within each villus. The veins converge back into the umbilical vein at the umbilical cord.

The rate of fetal blood flow in the placenta is about 500 mL/min.[50] Blood flow is dependent on fetal heart activity and regulated by the interaction of blood pressure, fetal right-to-left shunts, and systemic and pulmonary vascular resistance.[46] Contraction of smooth muscle fibers in stem villi may help pump blood from the placenta back to the fetus. The placenta is a low-resistance circuit in the fetal circulatory system (see Chapter 9) as a result of minimal umbilical innervation.

Maternal Uteroplacental Circulation

Blood flows to the uterus via the uterine arteries, which are branches of the internal iliac and ovarian arteries from the abdominal aorta, and then into the uterine spiral arteries (see Figure 2-28). The proportion of the maternal cardiac output supplying the uterus and IVS increases during pregnancy, peaking at 10% to 20%.[102] The increased blood flow is mediated by the low-resistance uteroplacental circuit, alterations in maternal cardiac output and systemic and peripheral vascular resistance, and hormonal and chemical influences (see Chapter 9). Blood reaches the placenta via the altered spiral arteries of the uterus. The spiral arteries are also altered during the menstrual cycle, elongating in the proliferative phase and becoming coiled (spiraled) during the secretory phase.[76] However, more extensive changes occur during pregnancy along with destruction of muscular and elastic elements of the walls of these arteries.

Maternal blood enters the IVS via uteroplacental arteries (altered spiral arteries) in the endometrium. By term, blood in these spaces is supplied by 100 to 200 (decreasing to 50 to 100 by term) maternal uteroplacental arteries and removed by 50 to 200 veins.[51] Blood flow enters the IVS through arterial inlets near the center of a lobule as a funnel-shaped stream flowing toward the chorionic plate or "roof" of the placenta (see Figure 3-10).[103] The blood then flows radially around the villi, allowing exchange of materials between maternal and fetal circulation. Blood leaves the IVS via wide venous outlets at the periphery of villous trees and flows into the uteroplacental veins and subchorial, interlobular, and marginal venous lakes.[51]

Overall the pressures within this system are low due to anatomic changes in maternal uterine blood vessels. As a result, the maternal arterial blood pressure is not transmitted to the IVS, and pressure gradients from the arterial to venous sides are relatively small (i.e., pressure averages 25 mmHg [3.25 kPa] in the uteroplacental arteries, 15 to 20 mmHg [1.99 to 2.66 kPa] in the IVS, and 5 to 10 mmHg [0.66 to 1.33 kPa] in the uterine veins).[50,84]

The IVS in the mature placenta contains about 150 mL of blood, which is completely replenished three to four times a minute. The rate of blood flow within the maternal side of the placenta increases during pregnancy from 50 mL/min at 10 weeks to 500 to 600 mL/min by term.[33,46] Uterine contractions limit the entry of blood into the IVS but do not squeeze out a significant amount of blood. Thus oxygen transfer to the fetus may be decreased during a normal contraction but does not cease, because transfer continues from blood remaining in the IVS.

The arteries of the endometrium (decidua) and myometrium undergo marked physiologic changes during pregnancy that convert the uterine spiral arteries into uteroplacental arteries. These changes are mediated by extravillous invasive trophoblast that invades the spiral arteries in the decidua and upper third of the myometrium. Interstitial extravillous trophoblast migrates into the decidua and surrounds the spiral arteries, destroying their muscular walls and elastic elements, causing them to swell. A subtype of extravillous trophoblast, endovascular trophoblast, migrates into the luminal walls replacing the spiral artery endothelium (Figure 3-12).[23,42,50,63,146] Trophoblast invasion involves

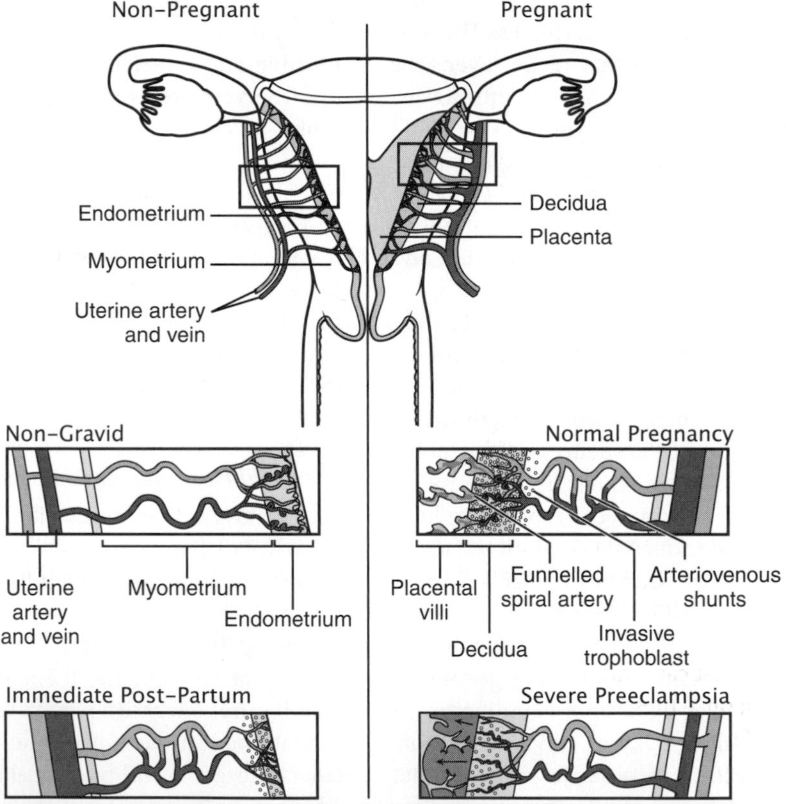

FIGURE 3-12 Diagrammatic representation of uterine and placental vasculature (dark gray shading = arterial; light gray shading = venous) in the non-pregnant, pregnant, and immediate post-partum state. Normal pregnancy is characterized by the formation of large arteriovenous shunts that persist in the immediate post-partum period. By contrast, pregnancies complicated by severe preeclampsia are characterized by minimal arteriovenous shunts, and thus narrower uterine arteries. Extravillous cytotrophoblast invasion in normal pregnancy (diamonds) extends beyond the decidua into the inner myometrium resulting in the formation of funnels at the discharging tips of the spiral arteries. Contrast with severe preeclampsia. (Prepared by Ms. Leslie Proctor, MSc.) (From Burton, G.J., et al. (2009). Rheological and physiological consequences of conversion of the maternal spiral arteries for uteroplacental blood flow during human pregnancy. *Placenta, 30,* 473.)

a combination of migratory and proteolytic activities mediated by matrix metalloproteinases, serine proteases, tissue plasminogen activator, and urokinase.[51,63] Much of the arterial wall is replaced by a fibrinoid extracellular matrix that arises from maternal fibrin and from proteins secreted by the trophoblast so that the smooth muscle of the wall and elastic lamina are lost.[19,23,76,113]

These alterations change the vessels from narrow to large caliber, widely dilated vessels, enhancing the capacity of the uteroplacental vessels to accommodate the increased blood volume needed to supply the placenta.[76] The vessels become funnel shaped with a four-fold increase in diameter.[23] The terminal coils of the arteries may reach 2 to 3 mm in diameter.[23] These vessels are also functionally denervated due to decreased neurotransmitter sites. As a result, the spiral arteries (now called *uteroplacental arteries*) underlying the placenta are almost completely dilated and become distended, flaccid, saclike structures with low resistance, able to accommodate the blood needed to supply and provide a reservoir for the IVS.[146] These arteries are no longer responsive to systemic circulatory pressor agents or influences of the autonomic nervous system.[47] Control of the uteroplacental circulation is at the level of the radial arteries and is mediated primarily by local (uteroplacental) influences, including placental production of prostacyclin (PGI_2). PGI_2, the most potent vasodilator produced by the placenta, is thought to maintain vasodilation of these vessels, prevent platelet aggregation, and enhance cell disengagement (needed for disruption of elastic and muscular elements).

As the trophoblast migrates into the decidua, it acquires an endothelial cell adhesion molecule phenotype, switching from a proliferative function to an invasive function. This switch is controlled by down- and up-regulation of specific genes and gene products, including integrins, and mediated by trophoblast and decidual factors, such as growth factors, enzymes, and binding proteins.[63,65] Proinvasive factors include trophoblast proteases and decidual activators and attractants; antinvasive factors include decidual barrier properties and local inhibitors. If the balance between proinvasive and inhibiting factors is altered, abnormally decreased or increased invasion occurs.[79] The depth of the invasion is limited because extravillous trophoblast can only proliferate while in contact with anchoring villi; once these cells migrate out they can only invade for the lifespan of the migrating cell.[51] In addition, the extravillous trophoblast is thought to be under the influence of a paracrine signal, probably IGF-1, secreted by the villous mesenchyme. As the extravillous trophoblast migrates farther away, the paracrine signal and thus trophoblast invasiveness diminishes.[83] Altered invasion is associated with miscarriage, fetal or intrauterine growth restriction (IUGR), preeclampsia (see Figure 3-12), preterm labor with intact membranes, preterm rupture of membranes, spontaneous abortion, and placental abruption.[18,23,63,127,155] Excessive blood flow to the IVS in the first trimester may result in an oxidative insult to the developing embryo and decreased angiogenesis in the placenta.[70]

The invasive trophoblast not only remodels the spiral arteries but also temporarily occludes the tips of the spiral arteries, limiting maternal blood from entering the IVS in significant amounts until 10 to 12 weeks' gestation (see Placentation).[22,23,68,70,79,124] The trophoblast plugs, seen particularly in the central areas, probably allow seepage of plasma through intracellular clefts.[22] These changes reduce placental oxygen concentration until about 10 weeks, when concentrations increase rapidly. At the same time, as maternal blood begins to flow more readily into the IVS, fetal antioxidant systems increase.[70] Thus first trimester placental circulation is very different from that in the second and third trimesters.[68] The low oxygen environment in the first trimester may protect the developing embryo, who has not yet developed protective mechanisms against oxidative stress.[68,70] Failure of conversion of the spiral arteries results in maternal blood entering the IVS at a greater velocity. This can lead to morphologic changes in the placenta including reduction in anchoring villi, impaired maternal-fetal oxygen exchange, and increased intermittent perfusion of the IVS leading to placental oxidative stress.[23]

The extravillous invasive trophoblast migrates into the maternal tissue in two phases. During the initial phase from about 6 to 10 or 12 weeks, spiral arteries in the decidua are altered; during the second phase, beginning at 14 to 16 weeks and lasting for 4 to 6 weeks (generally completed by 20 to 22 weeks), spiral arteries in the inner one third of the myometrium are altered.[19,50,65,76,84,146] Only spiral arteries underlying the placental bed are modified. This process is controlled by the interaction of ovarian and placental hormones, local cytokines, immune cells, and vascular growth factors.[76]

The importance of these changes for fetal survival and growth can be appreciated by examining situations such as spontaneous abortion, preeclampsia, and IUGR in which invasion of the spiral arteries by invasive cytotrophoblast does not occur or is abnormal.[18,23,63,65,68] Early pregnancy loss is often associated with defective placentation (thin, fragmented trophoblast shell and decreased cytotrophoblast invasion at the ends of the spiral arteries). Failure of plugging of these arteries exposes the placenta and embryo to intermittent oxidative stress that may increase the risk of pregnancy complications.[22,23,106] Recurrent spontaneous abortion in some women may be due to absent or inadequate conversion of spiral arteries to uteroplacental arteries.[22] Absence of changes in the decidual portion of the spiral arteries has been associated with late first trimester loss; absence of changes in the myometrial portion has been associated with second trimester loss.[118] Failure of the normal cytotrophoblastic invasion of the decidua and myometrium and subsequent arterial changes occurs in some types of fetal growth restriction. Underperfusion of the IVS may lead to occlusion of small arterioles within the villi. These changes can markedly alter fetal growth and health status and are similar to changes reported with some growth-restricted fetuses.

Preeclampsia is associated with alterations in the normal invasion of the spiral arteries by the invasive trophoblast (see Figure 3-12).[76,79,105] This defect, which may have a genetic basis, is postulated to be an initial event in the development of preeclampsia. Generally the first invasive trophoblast phase proceeds normally, but there is failure of the second phase.[50,84] Thus decidual spiral arteries undergo the usual physiologic changes, but the myometrial arteries do not. The uninvaded arterial segments may also develop atherosclerosis with necrosis and invasion of the damaged wall by fibrin and other substances. Alterations in the normal changes within the uterine arteries in women with preeclampsia lead to (1) decreased perfusion of the IVS due to the retained muscular coat and inability of the vessels to dilate sufficiently to accommodate the increased blood flow, and (2) hypertension in the uteroplacental arteries due to continued sensitivity of these vessels to circulatory pressor agents and the influences of the autonomic nervous system.[84,118]

The basis for this defect in preeclampsia is unclear. It may be a primary defect in invasive trophoblast, alterations in endometrial metabolism, altered endometrial immunologic reactions, or due to an altered environment.[79] Preeclampsia has been associated with abnormal expression of integrin molecules limiting trophoblast invasion into the decidua, resulting in decreased uteroplacental blood flow.[65] If the spiral arteries are not converted into low-resistance circuits, the placenta secretes vasoactive substances that increase maternal blood pressure.[79] Alterations in production of placental PGI_2 and thromboxane (TXA_2) occur with preeclampsia. Prostacyclin (PGI_2) is produced in many tissues and is a potent vasodilator and inhibitor of platelet aggregation and uterine contractility, which acts to promote increased uteroplacental blood flow during pregnancy. Conversely, TXA_2 is a potent vasoconstrictor that opposes the action of prostacyclin. An imbalance in levels of these mediators produced by the placenta, with a relative elevated TXA_2 and decreased prostacyclin, may alter the usual changes in the uterine blood vessels.

Placental Function

The placenta has four major activities: metabolic, endocrine, immunologic, and transport. The placenta also serves as a "radiator," with 85% of fetal heat production transmitted to the mother via the placenta.[133]

Placental Metabolism

Placental metabolism contributes to the quality and quantity of the fetal nutrient supply. Placental metabolic functions are particularly important early in pregnancy in providing nutrition and energy for the developing fetus and for the placenta itself. The placenta has a high metabolic rate. Rates of oxygen consumption and glucose utilization by the placenta approximate those of the brain.[78] Glucose use by the placenta equals 50% to 70% of the uterine glucose uptake.

The placenta is an active synthesizer of glycogen, fatty acids, cholesterol, and enzymes. The placenta produces protective and enhancement enzymes such as sulfatase, which enhances the excretion of fetal estrogen precursors, and insulinase, which increases the barrier to the transfer of insulin.[46] Relatively large amounts of ammonia and lactate are produced by the placenta and may be important in stimulating metabolic activity of the fetal liver. The impact of alterations in these metabolic processes on placental function and transport during pathologic states is not clear, but they decrease the capacity of the fetus to tolerate labor and transition to extrauterine life. Placental metabolic functions are described further in Chapter 16.

Placental Endocrinology

Placental endocrine activities are important in maintaining pregnancy and inducing metabolic adaptations in the mother and fetus. The placenta synthesizes polypeptide hormones (such as hCG and human placental lactogen [hPL]) and steroid hormones (estrogens and progesterone) as well as mediators such as pregnancy-associated plasma proteins (PAPP), neurohormones and neuropolypeptides, binding proteins, cytokines, and growth factors (Table 3-2). Growth factor receptors appear on the trophoblast early in gestation. Growth factors are short polypeptides that are produced in many different types of tissues. Growth factors act in paracrine and autocrine manner on specific localized target tissues by interacting with receptors on the target cell's membrane. This stimulates, via second messengers, signal transduction within the cell, initiating specific changes within the cell such as glucose uptake, RNA and protein synthesis, amino acid transport, and DNA synthesis and cell replication.[87]

Four major hormones synthesized by the placenta are hCG, hPL, progesterone, and estrogens. The placenta also produces pituitary-like and gonad-like peptide hormones (i.e., placental corticotropin, human chorionic thyrotropin, melanocyte stimulating hormone, β-endorphin, β-lipoprotein), hypothalamus-like releasing hormones (i.e., human chorionic somatostatin, CRH), and gut hormones (i.e., gastrin, vasoactive intestinal peptide). The placenta, membranes, and fetus also synthesize a variety of peptide growth factors including EGF, nerve growth factor (NGF), platelet-derived growth factor (PDGF), skeletal growth factor, and IGF-1 and IGF-2 (see Table 3-2).[45,87]

Placental growth factors regulate cell growth and differentiation, hormone release at the local level, and uterine contractility.[87] For example, IGF-1 and IGF-2 regulate cell proliferation and differentiation to maintain normal fetal growth. IGF works by enhancing amino acid and glucose uptake and preventing protein breakdown. Transforming growth factor–α (TGF-α) and EGF have primary roles in regulating cell differentiation.[87] TGF-β has both proliferative and antiproliferative actions to stimulate and inhibit cell differentiation. This factor is also involved in embryogenesis and neural migration and differentiation. Activin stimulates and inhibin decreases placental hCG and progesterone. Follistatin inhibits follicle-stimulating hormone (FSH) release.[87] Human placental growth hormone (GH-V) regulates IGF-1.

Until 15 to 20 weeks, maternal pituitary GH (GH-N) is the major maternal growth hormone; after that time, levels of GH-V increase and maternal GH-N is supressed.[45,87] GH-V

Table 3-2 Examples of Growth Factors, Neuropeptides, and Proteins Identified in Placental Tissues

PROTEIN/PEPTIDE HORMONE	NEUROHORMONE/ NEUROPEPTIDE	GROWTH FACTOR	BINDING PROTEIN	CYTOKINE
Human chorionic gonadotropin Human placental lactogen Growth hormone variant Adrenocorticotropic hormone	Gonadotropin-releasing hormone Thyrotropin-releasing hormone Growth hormone-releasing hormone Somatostatin Corticotropin-releasing hormone Oxytocin Neuropeptide Y β-Endorphin Met-enkephalin Dynorphia	Activin Follistatin Inhibin Transforming growth factor (α and β) Epidermal growth factor Insulin-like growth factor 1 (IGF-1) IGF-2 Fibroblastic growth factor Platelet-derived growth factor	Corticotropin-releasing-hormone-binding protein (CRH-BP) Insulin-like growth factor-binding protein-1 (IGFBP-1) IGFBP-2 IGFBP-3 IGFBP-4 IGFBP-5 IGFBP-6	Interleukin-1 (IL-1) IL-2 IL-6 IL-8 Interferon-α Interferon- β Interferon-γ Tumor necrosis factor-α

From: Liu, J.H. (2009). Endocrinology of pregnancy. In R.K. Creasy, et al. (Eds.). *Creasy & Resnik's Maternal-fetal medicine: Principles and practice* (6th ed.). Philadelphia: Saunders Elsevier, p.117.

may alter maternal metabolism by stimulating gluconeogenesis and lipolysis in the second half of pregnancy to increase nutrient availability for the fetus (see Chapter 16).[45,87] Parathyroid hormone–related protein (PTHrP) mediates placental calcium transport (see Chapter 17). PTHrP also has a role in development of the bone and epithelial organs and in the interaction of epithelial and mesenchymal cells.[141] Leptin is involved in regulating energy homeostasis, weight, and reproductive processes in pregnancy and may play a role in regulating fetal growth and development and possibly in placental development, angiogenesis, and hematopoiesis.[45,96] In addition to the hypothalamus, corticotropin-releasing hormone (CRH) is synthesized by the placenta (the major source of CRH during pregnancy), amnion, chorion, and decidua and stimulates release of prostaglandins. CRH has a major role in initiation of myometrial contractility and labor onset (see Chapter 4).

The placenta also produces cytokines that help regulate placental function (see Table 3-2). Cytokines are regulatory peptides or glycoproteins produced by most nucleated cells that regulate cell function via paracrine (intercellular) or autocrine (intracellular) signals. For example, interleukins induce syncytiotrophoblast release of hCG that in turn stimulates release of progesterone from the corpus luteum. Other cytokines and peptides produced by the placenta are involved in immunoregulation (see Chapter 13).

Human Chorionic Gonadotropin. Human chorionic gonadotropin (hCG) is a heterodimer glycoprotein with α and β subunits that is biologically similar to LH, FSH, and thyroid stimulating hormone. In early pregnancy there are more β subunits found, and then similar numbers of each type are seen; after 22 weeks there are more α than β subunits.[30] Measurement of free β subunits is used in first and second trimester maternal serum screening (see "Assessment of the Embryo and Fetus"). The major function of hCG is to maintain the corpus luteum during early pregnancy in order to ensure secretion of progesterone and other substances until placental production is adequate.[87] In addition, hCG may stimulate the fetal testes and adrenal gland to enhance testosterone and corticosteroid secretion, stimulate production of placental progesterone, promote angiogenesis, uterine growth and quiescence, enhance fetal growth and development, and suppress maternal lymphocyte responses to prevent rejection of the placenta by the mother.[30,114] hCG may also have a role in preventing cervical ripening during pregnancy.[75] Release of hCG is enhanced by gonadotropin-releasing hormone (GnRH), IL-1, IL-2, IGF, EGF, and activin and inhibited by inhibin, opioids, and TGF-β.[117] hCG is produced primarily by syncytiotrophoblast cells in the placenta, although small amounts may be produced by other types of trophoblast tissue.[50] Several variants of hCG are produced, including hyperglycosalated hCG (hCG-H). hCG-h is produced by the extravillous trophoblast and promotes implantation and cytotrophoblast growth.[30]

hCG can be detected in maternal serum and urine 7 to 8 days after ovulation, or around the time of implantation and has been found in the preimplantation blastocyst.[75,87] hCG is used as the basis of pregnancy tests using maternal urine. Generally, enough hCG has been produced to give a positive indication of pregnancy by 3 weeks after conception (7 to 8 days before the expected menses).[87] Concentrations of hCG in maternal serum double every 2 to 3 days until peak values (100,000 mU/mL) are reached 60 to 90 days after conception (Figure 3-13).[75,87] Concentrations of hCG decrease after 10 to 11 weeks and reach a plateau at low levels at 18 to 20 weeks.[43] By 2 weeks after delivery, hCG disappears. Persistently low levels may indicate an abnormal placenta or ectopic pregnancy; levels remain elevated in women with hydatidiform moles.[33] Higher levels are also seen with multiple gestations.[131]

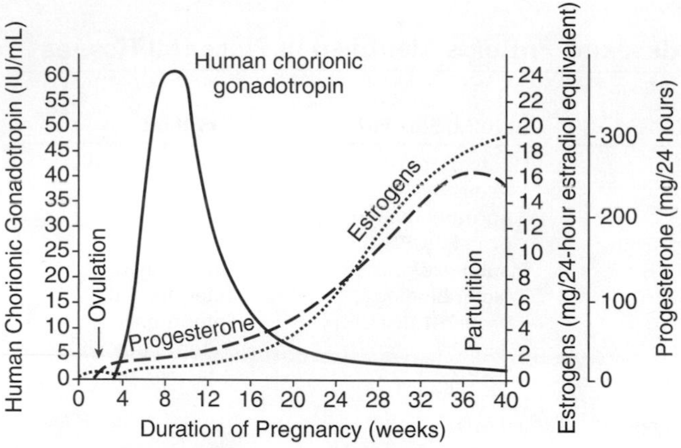

FIGURE 3-13 Patterns of excretion of human chorionic gonadotropin, progesterone, and estrogen during pregnancy. (From Guyton, A.C. [1987]. *Human physiology and mechanisms of disease* [4th ed.]. Philadelphia: Saunders.)

Human Placental Lactogen. hPL, also called *human chorionic somatomammotropin (hCS) or chorionic growth hormone,* consists of a single polypeptide chain similar in structure to human growth hormone and prolactin. hPL promotes fetal growth by altering maternal protein, carbohydrate, and fat metabolism (see Chapter 16). The primary role of hPL is regulating glucose availability for the fetus. hPL is an insulin antagonist that increases maternal metabolism and use of fat as an energy substrate and reduces glucose uptake and use by maternal cells. As a result, more glucose is available for transport to the fetus.[50] Thus hPL acts as a growth-promoting hormone, promoting fetal growth by altering maternal metabolism. The functions and regulation of hPL are not completely understood.[87]

Production of hPL by the syncytiotrophoblast begins 12 to 18 days after conception (5 to 10 days after implantation), rises during pregnancy, and peaks near term. hPL is the most abundant placental secretory product.[87,131] Secretion of hPL is regulated by glucose; decreased serum glucose leads to increased hPL secretion and increased maternal lipolysis. As early as 4 weeks after conception, hPL can be detected in maternal serum; little is found in maternal urine. hPL has a short half-life, so maternal serum levels reflect the rate of production.

Steroidogenesis. Progesterone and the estrogens are steroid hormones whose placental synthesis increases during pregnancy (see Figure 3-13). Early in gestation, the corpus luteum is the main synthesis site, but by 6 to 8 weeks the placental syncytiotrophoblast has taken over as the major producer.[74] Steroidogenesis during pregnancy is based on a complex set of interactions by systems in the mother, fetus, and placenta. Each system lacks essential enzymes necessary for creation of the final hormone. Placental production of progesterone and estrogens is an example of a function that requires cooperative efforts of the mother, placenta, and fetus. The main source of cholesterol for steroidogenesis is maternal low-density lipoproteins.[74] The placenta lacks certain enzymes needed for production of estriol; these enzymes are present in the fetal adrenal gland. The fetus is the major source of specific precursors for the estrogens, and the mother is the major source of precursors for the progesterone (Figure 3-14). Placental progesterone also serves as a precursor for fetal synthesis of corticosteroids, testosterone, and androgens.[33,71,74]

Progesterone. Progesterone is produced by the corpus luteum (under the influence of hCG) during the first 6 to 10 weeks after fertilization.[87] After that period, progesterone is synthesized primarily by the placenta using maternal cholesterol and low-density lipoproteins as precursors. A fetus is not essential for placental progesterone production, which continues even after fetal death. Progesterone production in late pregnancy is about 250 mg/day; 90% is secreted into maternal circulation.[50,74] Active progesterone metabolites such as deoxycorticosterone (DOC) contribute to the altered response to the pressor action of angiotensin II during pregnancy (see Chapter 11).

During pregnancy, progesterone acts to decrease myometrial activity and irritability; constrict myometrial vessels; decrease sensitivity of the maternal respiratory center to carbon dioxide; inhibit prolactin secretion; help suppress maternal immunologic responses to fetal antigens, thereby preventing rejection of the fetus; relax smooth muscle in the gastrointestinal and urinary systems; increase basal body temperature; and increase sodium and chloride excretion.[33]

An important role of progesterone in the fetus is to serve as the substrate pool for fetal adrenal gland production of glucocorticoids and mineralocorticoids. The fetal adrenal gland lacks enzymes in the 3β-hydroxysteroid dehydrogenase, δ4-5 isomerase system necessary for synthesis of some important corticosteroids. Therefore the fetus must utilize progesterone substrate from the placenta to accomplish this.

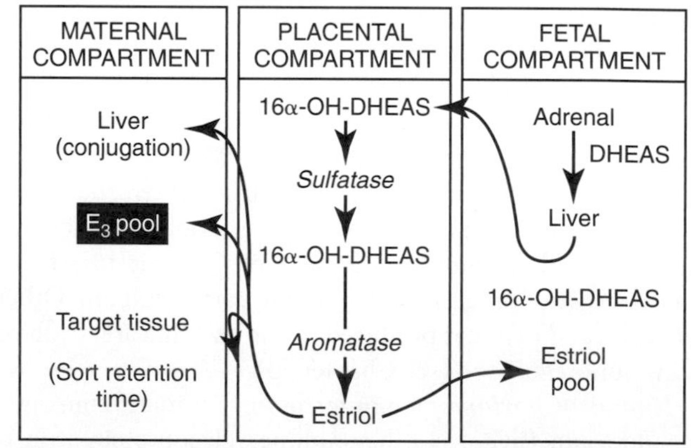

FIGURE 3-14 Roles of the maternal-fetal-placental compartments in the formation of estriol. The roles of each compartment in the formation of estriol (E_3) from the fetal precursor 16α-hydroxydehydroepiandrosterone (16α-OH-DHEAS). *DHEA,* Dehydroepiandrosterone. (From Liu, J.H. [2009]. Endocrinology of pregnancy. In R.K. Creasy, et al. (Eds.). *Creasy & Resnik's Maternal-fetal medicine: Principles and practice* (6th ed.). Philadelphia: Saunders Elsevier, p. 116.)

Estrogens. The three major estrogens are estrone, estradiol, and estriol. During pregnancy, production of estrogens, particularly estriol, increases markedly. Estrone and estradiol production increases about 100 times; estriol production increases about 1000 times. At term, estriol production by the placenta is 35 to 45 mg/day.[74] During pregnancy, estrogens act to enhance myometrial activity, promote myometrial vasodilation, increase sensitivity of the maternal respiratory center to carbon dioxide, soften fibers in the cervical collagen tissue, increase pituitary secretion of prolactin, increase serum binding proteins and fibrinogen, decrease plasma proteins, and increase the sensitivity of the uterus to progesterone in late pregnancy.[33]

Early in pregnancy, estriol is derived from estrone and estradiol. Production of estrogens, and particularly estriol, is dependent on interaction of the maternal-fetal-placental unit. Approximately 90% of the precursors for estriol are derived from the fetus; 40% of the precursors for estrone and estradiol come from the mother and 60% from the fetus.[33,87] The primary source of estriol precursors (dehydroepiandrosterone sulfate [DHEAS]) is the fetal adrenal gland under stimulation by fetal adrenocorticotropic hormone (ACTH). DHEAS is hydroxylated in the fetal liver and further metabolized by the placenta to form estriol. By term the fetal adrenal is producing 100 to 200 mg/day of DHEAS.[74] Estriol is secreted by the placenta into maternal circulation and eventually excreted in maternal urine. Maternal serum and urinary estriol levels rise rapidly during early pregnancy, more slowly between 24 and 32 weeks, and then increase rapidly again in the last 6 weeks. Although not currently used, estriol assays were one of the earlier methods of assessing fetal well-being and placental function for management of complicated pregnancies.[33,93]

Placental Immunologic Function

The immunologic functions of the placenta include protection of the fetus from pathogens and prevention from rejection by the mother. Many bacteria are too large to cross the placenta, although most viruses and some bacteria are able to cross. The placenta also allows passage of maternal antibodies of the immunoglobulin G (IgG) class primarily via pinocytosis, although some may cross by diffusion. This may also be a disadvantage, because both protective and potentially deleterious antibodies cross the placenta. The fetus differs in genetic makeup from the mother, yet it is not rejected. Possible explanations for this phenomenon and placental immunologic functions are discussed in Chapter 13.

Placental Transport

Placental transfer or transport involves bidirectional movement of gases, nutrients, waste materials, drugs, and other substances across the placenta from maternal-to-fetal circulation or from fetal to maternal circulation (Figure 3-15). Transport across the placenta increases during the course of gestation due to changes in placental structure (decreasing distance between maternal and fetal blood), increased fetal and maternal blood flow, and greater fetal demands. Relative concentrations of substance in maternal versus fetal circulation may be higher in the fetus, higher in the mother or similar in mother and fetus. For example, amino acids, calcium, and phosphorus are higher in fetal than maternal plasma; total proteins, globulins, fibrinogen, phospholipids, glucose, and fatty acids are higher in maternal than fetal plasma, while concentrations of sodium, chloride, and urea are similar.[72]

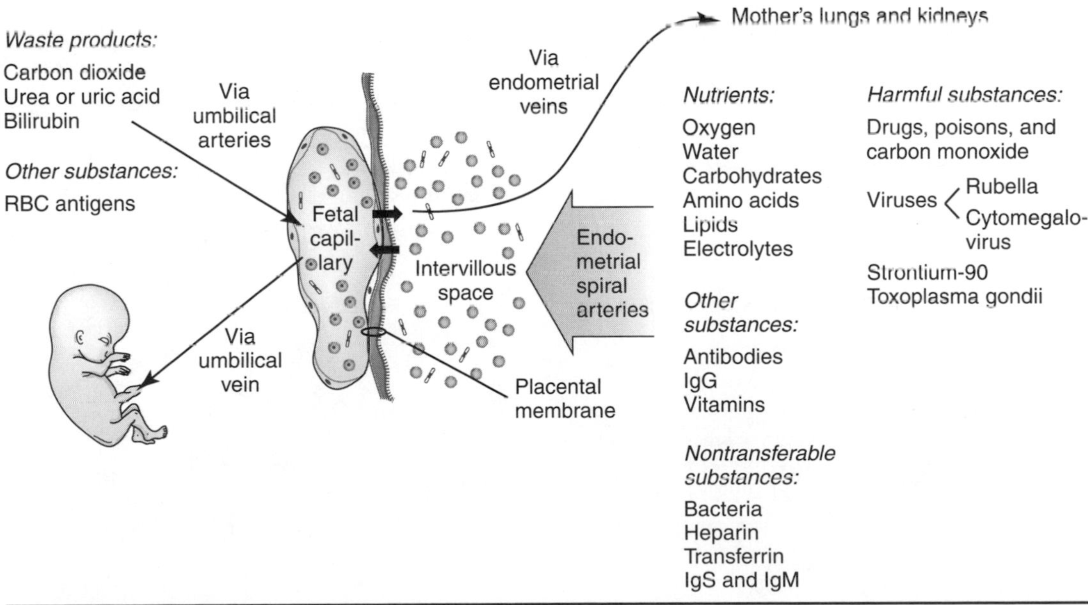

FIGURE 3-15 Summary of transfer of substances across the placenta between the mother and the fetus. (From Moore, K.L. & Persaud, T.V.N. [2008]. *The developing human: Clinically oriented embryology* (8th ed.). Philadelphia: Saunders, p. 119.)

The syncytiotrophoblast is the site of transport with substances moving from the apical membrane (facing maternal blood in the IVS), across the cell wall and villous stoma to the basal membrane (facing the fetal capillary epithelium).[92] The mechanisms by which substances are transferred across the placenta include simple (passive) diffusion, facilitated diffusion, active transport, pinocytosis, endocytosis, bulk flow, solvent drag, accidental capillary breaks, and independent movement. Facilitated diffusion and active transport are mediated by protein carriers and other transporters. Transporters are located on both the maternal-facing brush border syncytiotrophoblast (facing the IVS) and the fetal-facing basal membrane (facing the fetal villous stroma).[54] Transporters include both nutrient (see Chapter 16) and drug (see Chapter 7) transporters.[32,66,148,158] Transfer can be modified by maternal nutritional status; exercise; and disease, such as diabetes mellitus (glucose transport increases due to maternal hyperglycemia), hypertension (decreased nutrient transfer as a result of reduced uteroplacental blood flow), and alcoholism (ethanol impairs placental uptake of amino acids and glucose).

Simple (Passive) Diffusion. Diffusion is movement of a substance from higher to lower concentration or electrochemical gradients (Figure 3-16, *A*). The quantity of a substance transferred is illustrated by the Fick diffusion equation:

$$Q/t = \frac{KA(C1 - C2)}{L}$$

Q/t is the quantity transferred/unit of time, K is the diffusion constant, A is the fetal surface area available for exchange, C1 − C2 is the concentration gradient across the placenta, and L is the thickness of the membrane across which the substance is to move.

Diffusion is the major mechanism of placental transfer. Simple diffusion is generally limited to smaller molecules that can pass through pores in the cell wall. Because the cell walls have a high lipid content, some lipid-soluble substances may cross directly through these lipid regions.[33] Water-soluble substances cross easily if less than 100 molecular weight (MW); lipid-soluble molecules less than 600 MW cross unimpeded. The cell walls can act as a barrier to some large non–lipid-soluble substances such as muscle relaxants used with anesthesia. Substances that cross the placenta via simple diffusion include water, electrolytes, oxygen, carbon dioxide, urea, simple amines, creatinine, fatty acids, steroids, fat-soluble vitamins, narcotics, antibiotics, barbiturates, and anesthetics.[46] Fat-soluble vitamins and cholesterol diffuse as lipoprotein complexes. Compounds such as histamine, serotonin, angiotensin, and epinephrine diffuse readily, but significant concentrations may never reach the fetus due to enzymatic deamination within the placenta.[33] Free water crosses at a rate of 180 mL/second, faster than any other known substance.[46]

Carbon dioxide is highly soluble in the placental membrane and diffuses readily. Oxygen diffuses with greater difficulty and therefore requires a considerable gradient of oxygen pressure on either side of the membrane. The average gradient is about 20 mmHg (2.66 kPa) for oxygen and 5 mmHg (0.66 kPa) for carbon dioxide. The oxygen gradient is higher because the placenta and myometrium also extract oxygen.[46] The rate of gas exchange across the placenta is limited by maternal blood flow supplying oxygen to the placenta. The placenta consumes about 10% to 30% of the oxygen delivered to it.[84]

Although the placenta is similar to the lungs in relation to the efficiency of gas exchange, the PO_2 levels of maternal and fetal blood leaving the placenta differ. These differences are

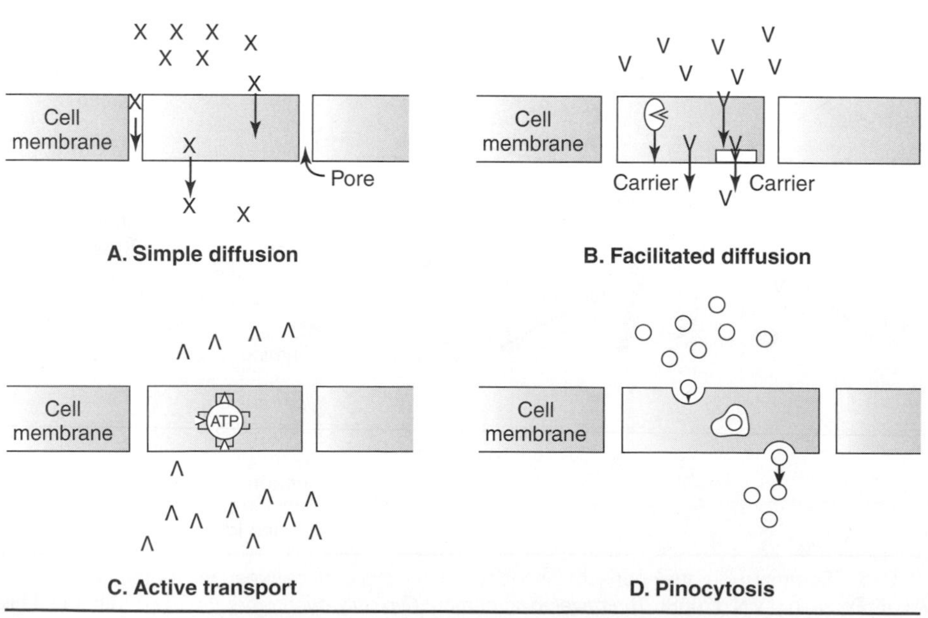

FIGURE 3-16 Mechanisms of placental transfer.

due to the previously described vascular shunts in maternal and fetal circulations, nonuniform distribution of maternal and fetal blood flow, and differences in the positions of the maternal and fetal oxygen hemoglobin dissociation curves (see Chapters 6 and 10). When maternal blood flow exceeds fetal flow, the exchange of oxygen with fetal blood results in only minimal changes in maternal PO_2. Blood from these compartments contributes heavily to the PO_2 of mixed venous blood leaving the uterus. Conversely, oxygen exchange in areas in which fetal blood flow exceeds maternal flow depletes maternal reserves and equilibrates at a level similar to the fetal PO_2.[103] Placental gas exchange is discussed further in Chapter 6.

Facilitated Diffusion. Facilitated diffusion (or transplacental protein mediated diffusion) involves transport via protein transporters to move substances across the placental membrane (see Figure 3-16, *B*). Movement is from higher to lower concentration or electrochemical gradients. Glucose (fetal levels are 70% to 80% of maternal values) and possibly some oxygen are transported from maternal-to-fetal circulation via facilitated diffusion. Placental glucose metabolism may partially account for differences in maternal and fetal glucose concentrations. Glucose transport occurs via glucose transport proteins or GLUT (see Chapter 16).[72,123] Waste products such as lactate are transported from fetus to mother via facilitated diffusion.

Active Transport. Active transport utilizes energy-dependent carrier systems and other protein transporters to move substances against concentration or electrochemical gradients (see Figure 3-16, *C*). Amino acids, potassium, water-soluble vitamins, calcium, phosphate, iron, and iodine cross the placenta via active transport.[46,72,117] Active transport systems become saturated at high concentrations. Similar molecules may compete, reducing the movement of some substances across the placenta.

Amino acids such as alanine, glutamine, threonine, and serine that are transported by multiple carrier systems are found in high concentrations in placental tissue. Thirteen amino acid monomeric or heterodimeric transporter protein systems have been described.[72] Umbilical vein concentrations of most amino acids are higher than maternal plasma concentrations from midgestation to term.[72] The net movement of many amino acids is greater than that estimated for fetal growth needs, suggesting that the fetus also uses these substances for energy or the synthesis of other amino acids.[72] The amount of amino acids transported across the placenta increases markedly late in pregnancy due to increased numbers of carriers. Most polypeptides and larger proteins that cross the placenta do so via endocytosis/pinocytosis or accidental capillary breaks.

Endocytosis and Exocytosis. Endocytosis is an invagination in the surface of a cell that forms intracellular membrane–bound vesicles; exocytosis occurs on the opposite side of the cell with fusion of the vesicle to the membrane and release of the vesicles' contents.[72] Endocytosis involves the engulfing of microdroplets of maternal plasma or small solutes (pinocytosis) (see Figure 3-16, *D*) or large particles (phagocytosis) by trophoblast cells. Substances in maternal plasma such as globulins (IgG), phospholipids, lipoproteins, and antibodies are transferred to the fetus or metabolized by the placenta. These mechanisms are necessary to transfer molecules too large for diffusion or for which no carrier transport exists and allow some molecules of up to 150,000 MW (i.e., IgG) to cross the placenta.

Maternal antibodies of the IgG class readily cross the placenta during the third trimester. This is a facilitated process that becomes more efficient in late gestation.[29] Transfer may be mediated by fetal Fc receptors.[29] IgG antibodies from the mother can be protective (e.g., antibodies against diphtheria, measles, mumps, herpes simplex virus) or potentially damaging (as occurs in Rh incompatibility or with maternal Graves' disease or myasthenia gravis) to the fetus (see Chapter 13). Maternal immunoglobulin A (IgA) antibodies do not cross in significant amounts; immunoglobulin M (IgM) antibodies are not transferred.

Bulk Flow, Solvent Drag, and Water Channels. Water crosses the placenta rapidly. Bulk flow may occur with changes in hydrostatic or osmotic forces. Ions cross either by simple diffusion or by solvent drag as dissolved electrolytes are pulled across the placenta by the movement of water. This mechanism is useful in maintaining water and osmotic balances between maternal and fetal circulations.[46] This mechanism may involve aqueous pores and is most effective for molecules with low MW. Water movement varies within the placenta depending on the concentrations of various osmotically active substances and the hydrostatic pressure.[72] At least five different aquaporin (AQP) water channels are expressed on the placenta and fetal membranes.[34] These channels play a role in the transfer of water across the fetal membranes into fetal circulation via osmotic gradients.[34,135]

Accidental Capillary Breaks. Accidental capillary breaks and breaks in the villous covering permit passage of intact blood cells between maternal and fetal circulations. Small amounts (0.1 to 0.2 mL) of fetal cells can be found in maternal circulation intermittently during pregnancy. More extensive (≥1 to 2 mL) fetomaternal hemorrhage may occur with placental separation and increase the risk of isoimmunization (see Chapter 13).[46]

Independent Movement. Maternal leukocytes or organisms such as *Treponema pallidum* may cross the placenta under their own power. Although many viruses can infect the fetus, the specific mechanisms through which they cross the placenta are unclear. Some viruses may be carried across via pinocytosis.[67]

Transfer of Substances Across the Placenta

Dancis noted that in thinking about placental transfer: "Ask not whether a maternal nutrient [or other substance] crosses the placenta. Ask rather, how, how much, and how fast. Ask also as to fetal need."[35] There are few compounds—endogenous or exogenous—that are unable to cross the placenta in detectable amounts given sufficient time and sensitivity of detection.[35] Placental transfer is influenced by the area of the placenta, physicochemical characteristics of the diffusing substance, concentration gradients, electrical potential differences, diffusing distance, degree of binding of a substance to hemoglobin or other blood proteins, permeability of the placental barrier, and the rates of maternal and fetal blood flow through the intervillous space and villi.[46]

Diffusion of a substance across the placenta can be expressed as follows:

$$\text{Diffusion} = \frac{\text{Substance characteristics} \times \text{surface area} \times \text{concentration gradient}}{\text{Distance}}$$

Increased surface area for exchange (as occurs with growth of the placenta), increased concentration gradients, and decreased diffusing distance enhance transfer across the placenta. As the placenta matures, the distance between maternal and fetal blood decreases due to thinning of the syncytiotrophoblast and mesenchyme as well as increases in the size and number of capillaries in the villi. Transfer may be reduced with decreased surface area (e.g., small placenta, placental infarcts) or increased diffusing distance (e.g., placental edema, infection).

Physicochemical characteristics that influence movement across the placenta include lipid solubility, MW, degree of ionization, and protein binding. These characteristics can increase, decrease, or prohibit movement of potentially harmful drugs and other substances from maternal-to-fetal circulation (see Chapter 7).[33,46] Placental transfer may be increased or enhanced if a substance is lipid soluble (e.g., lipoproteins) or nonionized (e.g., phenobarbital), has an MW less than 600 (e.g., propylthiouracil), or lacks significant binding to albumin (e.g., ampicillin). Increased maternal-to-fetal concentration or electrochemical gradients also increase transfer. A substance may be prevented from crossing the placenta because it has a certain charge or molecular configuration (e.g., heparin) or certain size (e.g., bacteria, IgM), is altered or bound by enzymes within the placenta (e.g., amines, insulin), or is firmly bound to the maternal red blood cell or plasma protein (e.g., carbon monoxide).[46,50]

The rate of maternal blood flow to and through the IVS and fetal blood flow to and through the villi influence placental transfer. Blood flow is the limiting factor in gas exchange across the placenta and also affects transfer of nutrients and waste products. During uterine contractions, the entry of blood into the IVS is limited. Transfer of oxygen and other nutrients to the fetus may decrease but does not cease during contractions.[46,50] The decrease in afferent blood flow during a contraction may be due to: (1) compression and obliteration of the uteroplacental veins with increased IVS pressure, (2) occlusion of the uteroplacental arteries, or (3) increased intraluminal pressure within the uterus with alteration in the arteriovenous pressure gradients within the IVS.

The fetus may become hypoxic and acidotic if contractions are hypertonic or if resting time between contractions is insufficient. If placental transfer is compromised by small placental size, infarcts, or edema, fetal distress may arise at lower levels of uterine activity. Because the quantity of oxygen reaching the fetus is primarily flow limited, reduction of uteroplacental blood flow increases the risk of fetal hypoxia.

In addition to uterine contractions, factors that may alter uteroplacental blood flow include maternal position; anesthesia; nicotine and other drugs; emotional or physical stress; and degenerative changes within the placenta that are seen with hypertension, prolonged pregnancy, diabetes, or renal disease. Maternal blood flow to and through the IVS can be altered by (1) changes in the systemic circulation (cardiac disease, small uterine artery); (2) changes in the number or size of the uteroplacental blood vessels (infection, degeneration); (3) compression of the uteroplacental blood vessels (tetanic or other abnormal contractions, polyhydramnios, multiple gestation); and (4) degenerative changes in the IVS associated with high-risk conditions such as maternal hypertension.[46]

Separation of the Placenta

Placental separation and expulsion occur during the third stage of labor. The "afterbirth" consists of maternal and fetal tissues (see Figure 3-10). Maternal tissues include the decidua basalis (maternal portion of the placenta), decidua parietalis, and any remaining decidua capsularis. Fetal tissues include the chorion frondosum (fetal portion of the placenta), chorion laeve (chorion), amnion, and umbilical cord. Retained fragments of the placenta and membranes can lead to uterine atony, hemorrhage, or infection.

The sudden emptying of the uterus with delivery of the fetus rapidly reduces the surface area of the placental site to an area approximately 10 cm in diameter. This reduction in the base of support for the placenta leads to compression and shearing of the placenta from the uterine wall.[84] The usual site of placental separation is within the spongy layer of the decidua basalis (see Figure 3-10). This layer has been described as "like the lines of perforation found between postal stamps."[84] The placenta may separate from the central area to the margins with inversion so that the fetal surface presents first (Schultze mechanism), or from the margins toward the center with initial presentation of the maternal surface (Duncan mechanism). Placentas implanted in the fundus of the uterus are more likely to separate via Schultze mechanism; those implanted lower on the uterine wall usually separate by Duncan mechanism (although these placentas may invert before expulsion).

AMNIOTIC FLUID

Amniotic fluid provides space for symmetric fetal growth, maintains constant temperature and pressure, protects and cushions the fetus, allows free movement of the fetus, and distributes pressure from uterine contractions evenly over the fetus.[33] Amniotic fluid antibacterial factors, such as transferrin (which binds iron needed by some bacteria and fungi for growth), fatty acids (which have a detergent effect on bacterial membrane), immunoglobulins (e.g., IgG, IgA), and lysozyme (which is bactericidal for gram-positive bacteria), help protect the fetus from infection (see Chapter 13).[11]

Amniotic Fluid Volume and Turnover

The exact mechanisms for regulation of amniotic fluid volume are unclear, although the primary components of flow (fetal swallowing, urination, and lung fluid) are highly regulated.[11] Fetal swallowing, lung fluid, and fetal urine are regulated to meet fetal needs of those organs and not to produce or remove amniotic fluid. Any amniotic fluid volume regulation appears to be via changes in intramembranous exchange and may be mediated by endothelial growth factor.[128] Maternal fluid status and hydration can alter amniotic fluid volume. For example, especially in early pregnancy, subnormal maternal plasma volume expansion reduces amniotic fluid volume.[128] Maternal hydration can significantly increase amniotic fluid volume.[64]

Amniotic fluid first appears as a droplet dorsal to the embryonic pole at about 3 weeks.[103] There are approximately 7 mL of amniotic fluid by 8 weeks, 30 mL by 10 weeks, and 190 mL by 16 weeks, and an average of 700 to 800 mL by term (with wide variations) decreasing to about 400 mL by 42 weeks.[11,104,160] Amounts of amniotic fluid vary widely in the third trimester. The net volume turnover of amniotic fluid is about 1000 mL/day.[11] Turnover rate is independent of volume.

Amniotic Fluid Production and Disposition

The cells of the amnion are separated by intracellular channels leading directly into the amniotic cavity that allow bulk flow of water and solutes. Transfer of water and most solutes across the amnion and chorion is governed by hydraulic, osmotic, and electrochemical forces. Water movement occurs as a result of a net imbalance between intramembrane hydrostatic pressure and effective osmotic pressure.[103] Some of the free water in amniotic fluid is thought to come from this intramembrane pathway. In the last half of pregnancy, fetal urine output is the major source of amniotic fluid followed by lung fluid; the primary removal pathways are fetal swallowing and intramembranous movement. Major sources for amniotic fluid production and exchange include the following:

1. *Fetal renal/urinary tract.* Hypotonic urine is present in the amniotic space by 9 to 11 weeks. The fetus produces an average of 700 to 800 mL/day in the third trimester.[11,160] After 40 weeks, fetal urine production declines.
2. *Fetal respiratory tract.* The fetal lungs secrete an average of 150 to 200 mL of lung fluid/day.[102] Lung fluid contains phospholipids such as lecithin, sphingomyelin, and phosphatidylglycerol that are used to assess fetal lung maturity (see Chapter 10). About half of this is swallowed; the remainder contributes to amniotic fluid. Oral and nasal secretions may have a minor contribution to amniotic fluid volume.[11]
3. *Fetal gastrointestinal tract.* Fetal swallowing is a major route for disposal of amniotic fluid. Fetal swallowing begins at 8 to 11 weeks. The fetus swallows an average of approximately 500 to 700 mL/day late in pregnancy.[11,104,160]
4. *Placenta, fetal membranes (intramembranous pathway).* The fetal membranes are thought to be the second most important route of amniotic fluid clearance (after fetal swallowing) during the second half of gestation and account for an estimated 200 to 500 mL/day of amniotic fluid removal.[11] Water crosses the membranes by either nondiffusional fast bulk flow or slower diffusional flow, facilitated by AQP water channels in the amnion and placenta.[34,135,160] The net transfer of water is probably small except at the site of the placenta, where the chorioamniotic membrane is relatively close to maternal blood. The umbilical cord arises from the same cell type as the amnion and is also involved in fluid exchange after 4 weeks, with development of intracellular channels in cord membranes. Vascular endothelial GF is thought to be involved in intramembranous absorption.[160]
5. *Uterine wall via sinusoidal vessels of the decidua (transmembranous pathway).* This is a minor pathway, with only small amounts (≈10 mL/day) of fluid removed via this pathway near term.[11]
6. *Fetal skin.* Before complete keratinization of the fetal skin at 22 to 25 weeks (see Chapter 14), the skin is a site for transfer of water and solutes.

These pathways with maximum volumes for each route are summarized in Figure 3-17. Amniotic fluid volume may also be influenced by other factors, including changes in tonicity of maternal serum and amniotic fluid prolactin, which seems to influence permeability of the amnion and chorion membranes.[160]

Composition of Amniotic Fluid

Amniotic fluid is 98% to 99% water, with the remainder consisting of electrolytes, creatinine, urea, bile pigments, renin, glucose, hormones, fetal cells (including stem cells), lanugo,

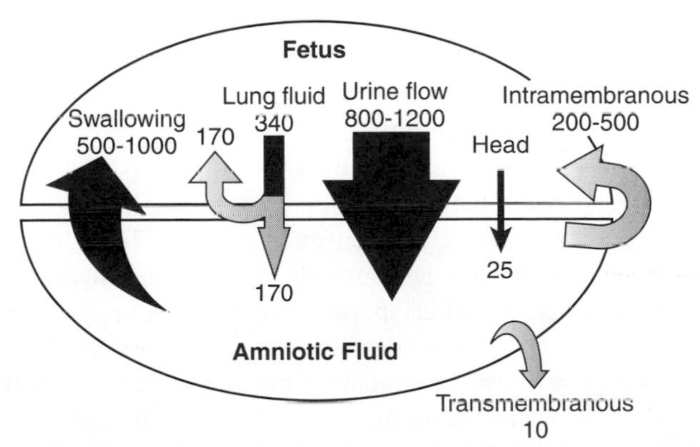

FIGURE 3-17 Summary of volume flows in and out of the amniotic space in late gestation. Arrow size is proportional to flow rate. (From Brace, R.A. [1997]. Physiology of amniotic fluid volume regulation. *Clin Obstet Gynecol, 40,* 286. Modified from original from Gilbert, W.M. & Brace, R.A. [1993]. Amniotic fluid volume and normal flows to and from the amniotic cavity. *Semin Perinatol, 17,* 150.)

and vernix caseosa. The composition of amniotic fluid changes with gestation. In early pregnancy, amniotic fluid is similar to maternal and fetal serum with little particulate matter. Amniotic fluid osmolality decreases from 290 mOsm/kg in the first trimester to 255 mOsm/kg near term and is similar to dilute fetal urine with added phospholipids and other substances from the fetal lungs.[11,160] Urea, creatinine, and uric acid concentrations increase as pregnancy progresses; whereas sodium and chloride levels decrease as fetal renal function matures.

CLINICAL IMPLICATIONS

Assisted Reproductive Technology

Issues surrounding conception relate to the ability of couples to conceive and maintain pregnancies until the fetus can survive outside the uterus. Infertility is the principal symptom of conception failure. Failure to conceive can result from disorders of ovulation, spermatogenesis, and gamete transport. Recent years have brought increased knowledge of these factors, with development of assisted reproductive technologies (ART) such as in vitro fertilization (IVF), gamete intrafallopian transfer (GIFT), zygote intrafallopian transfer (ZIFT), and associated interventions such as artificial insemination, therapeutic donor insemination, ovulation induction, microsurgery, laser surgery, intracytoplasmic sperm injection (ICSI), cryopreservation, frozen embryo transfer (FET), donation of eggs or preembryo, and surrogate mothering for couples having difficulty achieving conception.[145] Emotional, physical, and financial stress is high for these families.

The most common ART procedure used in the United States is IVF with GIFT and ZIFT used in less than 1% of cycles. During 2009, most cycles (70.1%) used fresh nondonor eggs.[27] The rate of clinical pregnancies using fresh nondonor eggs or embryos was 36.9%, with no pregnancy in 62.5%; the success rate for frozen embryos was lower.[27] Of those cycles that resulted in pregnancy, approximately 81% led to a live born infant.[27] Of these, 69.5% were singletons and 28.9% multiples. Major reasons for ART in 2009 were multiple male and female factors (17.8%), male factor infertility (18.8%), multiple female factors (10.6%), tubal factors (7.7%), ovulatory dysfunction (6.8%), and endometriosis (4.2%).[27] Preimplantation genetic diagnosis was usually done.

Artificial insemination with donor sperm has been used to treat infertility since the nineteenth century. This therapy may be employed when azoospermia, oligospermia, decreased sperm motility, or other sperm abnormalities are present. When vasectomy is nonreversible or the risk of genetic disorders is high artificial insemination may be an option. Single women who desire a child may also opt to use this method in order to conceive. Candidates for insemination must ovulate regularly or respond to ovulation-inducing drug therapy. The techniques used include deposition of sperm into the upper vagina at the cervical os, or inside the cervical canal, or directly into the uterus. Reported success rates are 5% to 20% per month with 70% to 90% of women conceiving within 6 months. Fresh semen is rarely used, because of concern over sexually transmitted diseases and infection with human immunodeficiency virus.

In vitro fertilization means fertilization that takes place outside the body. The first infant conceived in this manner was born in 1978. Since that time, thousands of infants have been born utilizing this technique. Originally, IVF was developed for women with blocked or absent fallopian tubes. This continues to be one of the main reason for use of IVF, but other indications include endometriosis unresponsive to conventional therapy, low sperm counts, immunologic disorders unresponsive to therapy, hostile cervical mucus or sperm antibodies, control of sex-linked disorders, and idiopathic infertility.

The procedure is done in four stages: ovulation induction and monitoring, follicular aspiration, fertilization, and embryo transfer. The goal of ovulation induction is recruitment of a large number of follicles to increase the number of embryos that can be transferred or frozen for use in subsequent cycles and thus the percentage of successful pregnancies. Drugs given on day 2 or 3 of the menstrual cycle induce maturation of more than one follicle. The maturing ova are monitored and, once adequate follicular size is achieved or preovulatory estradiol levels are appropriate, follicular aspiration can occur.[17,25,103]

The woman is given human chorionic gonadotropin (hCG) to enhance the final stages of follicular maturation and to control timing of ovulation. After follicle aspiration and processing of the semen sample from the father, the ova are identified, placed in a special nutrient culture medium and incubated at body temperature. Capacitated sperm are then mixed with the ova, and the mixture is incubated again for 48 to 72 hours to allow for fertilization and adequate early cell division. Generally around 100,000 sperm are needed, and at least 100,000 sperm per oocyte are preferred.[17]

Embryo transfer generally occurs when the zygote has reached a six- to eight-cell stage on day 3 to 5 after fertilization; timing varies between different centers.[17,87] Transfer at 3 days (at least 6 to 8 cell stage) is associated with a 12% to 25% change of implantation; transfer at 5 days after fertilization (morula or blastocyst stage) is associated with a 30% to 50% implantation rate (not all of these will survive).[87] If two or three embryos are transferred, there is a 35% to 45% chance of a clinical pregnancy.[87] The zygotes are injected via a catheter into the cervix. More than one zygote may be transferred to increase the likelihood of pregnancy this increases the risk of multiple pregnancy. Progesterone by injection is begun on the day of transfer to support the corpus luteum. A serum β-hCG assay is done at 2 weeks to determine if implantation has occurred. Progesterone supplements are continued for up to 10 weeks if implantation has taken place. Unused zygotes may be frozen and stored.

GIFT is the process of transferring eggs and sperm directly into the fallopian tube via a fine catheter. This therapy was developed for use in infertile couples when there was doubt that the gametes would be able to reach the fallopian tubes or when male factor or idiopathic infertility existed; it is rarely used currently.[103] Women must have at least one healthy patent fallopian tube in order to qualify for this treatment modality. The three stages of GIFT are induction, oocyte retrieval, and gamete transfer to fallopian tubes. Ovarian induction is the same as in IVF. Oocyte retrieval is by laparotomy or transvaginal using ultrasonographic techniques. The ova are mixed with capacitated sperm, and the mixture is transferred to the fallopian tubes. Fertilization takes place within the natural environment and successive events progress normally.

The process for ZIFT is similar to IVF, but after fertilization the zygote is returned to the fallopian tube without further incubation. Currently, ZIFT is rarely used. As with GIFT, women must have one patent fallopian tube.

Procedures used in conjunction with IVF and other ART's include use of donor oocytes, assisted hatching (creation of an opening in the zona pellucida to assist with implantation), and ICSI.[145] ICSI is used with an increasing number of IVF and involves injecting the sperm into the ova.[27] ICSI can be used for males who have had vasectomies, who have severe sperm abnormalities, or who are unable to ejaculate and has improved pregnancy rates in couples with male factor infertility.[17]

Multiple gestations, particularly dizygotic twins and other dizygotic multiples, are increased due to transfer of multiple embryos. Monozygotic twinning is also increased and may be due to blastocyst or zona pellucida damage with embryo splitting.[70,90] There may be an increased risk of chromosomal abnormalities with ICSI.[109] It is unclear whether there are increased risks of congenital anomalies from the procedure or if the increase reported in some studies is due to the reason for the infertility (usually male factor infertility) or the increase in multiples, who have higher rates.[49,109] An association between IVF and a minor increase in the incidence of birth defects has also been reported in some studies.[49] The rate of ectopic pregnancy is higher with ART.[17]

Assessment of the Embryo and Fetus

Prenatal Screening

Prenatal screening begins in the preconception period with evaluation of risks and discussion of potential risks and approaches to decrease risk. These approaches include folic acid supplementation in all women of childbearing age (see Chapter 15), identification of women at risk for preterm birth, and genetic screening (see Chapter 1) or strategies to decrease risk in women with chronic disorders such as diabetes mellitus, cardiovascular problems, or genetic disorders.

Techniques available for prenatal screening include history, risk assessment, carrier testing, first trimester genetic screening, second trimester genetic screening, and ultrasound (which is done as part of both first and second trimester screening). A genetic history should be a routine part of preconceptional and prenatal care to identify women with an increased risk of genetic disorders and birth defects. Components of genetic history include family and obstetric history (including a history of pregnancy loss or early infant death, mental retardation or learning disabilities, known genetic disorders, or previous anomalies in either the parents or their families), ethnic background (some recessive disorders occur with markedly increased frequency in specific ethnic groups), maternal and paternal age, and potential teratogen exposures.[153] Based on family and ethnic background, carrier screening may be offered for specific autosomal recessive disorders such as Tay-Sachs disease (in Ashkenazi Jewish heritage), sickle cell disease (African and Mediterranean background), or thalassemias (Mediterranean and Asian background).[20] The American College of Obstetricians and Gynecologists (ACOG) and American College of Medical Genetics recommend cystic fibrosis screening in the preconception or prenatal periods, particularly for couples of northern European Caucasian and Ashkenazi Jewish background (1 carrier per 3300 tests).[2,20] Recently ACOG recommended screening of all patients regardless of ethnicity.[3] Cystic fibrosis screening does not test for all of the hundreds of mutations that have been identified in the cystic fibrosis gene, but only for those with a frequency in the U.S. population of greater than or equal to 0.1%.[125]

Fetal aneuploidy risk can be evaluated prenatally "on the basis of a combination of maternal age, prior family history, maternal serum biochemical tests and fetal ultrasound markers."[14] Ultrasound markers for both first and second trimester screening have been identified for infants with Down syndrome.[94,111,153] The genetic sonogram involves examination for markers found on second trimester ultrasounds that are observed more frequently in infants with chromosomal abnormalities.[140] These findings include shortened femur or humerus, increased nuchal fold, intracardiac echogenic foci, echogenic bowel, renal pyelectasis.[20,138] Doppler flow studies are used to assess fetal status (see first and second trimester screening) and risk of maternal complications. Abnormal ductus venosus (DV) wave forms at 11 to 13 weeks are associated with an increased risk of aneuploidy, congenital heart defects, and twin to twin transfusion syndrome (TTTS) in monochorionic twins.[94] DV wave forms can be used for fetal surveillance later in pregnancy with fetal growth restriction, monochorionic twins with TTTS, fetal hydrops, and fetal supraventricular tachycardia.[10] Alterations in cardiac preload or afterload can produce changes in pressure gradients and DV wave forms.[10,94] Uterine artery Doppler has been used in the first trimester for screening for early onset preeclampsia and fetal growth restriction in at-risk women.[7] Biomarkers of these disorders to be used in conjunction with Doppler flow, including placental GF, inhibin-A, pregnancy-associated plasma protein-A (PAPP-A) and PP-13 are also being investigated.[1,7,110]

First Trimester Screening. First trimester screening methods include maternal serum screening and ultrasound and Doppler flow studies for increased nuchal translucency (NT), abnormal ductus venosus (DV) blood flow, tricuspid valve regurgitation and increased hepatic artery flow.[94,111,153] NT is due to the subcutaneous accumulation of fluid behind fetal neck, possibly due to delayed development of the lymphatic system to drain fluid that flows into the nuchal area. Infants with trisomies tend to have more collagen and elastic connective tissue, allowing for accumulation. NT is associated with an increased risk of spontaneous abortion, other aneuploidies, and fetal anomalies. NT may also be useful in early diagnosis of some congenital heart defects (due to excess extravascular fluid).[38] The optimal time to assess NT and DV and tricuspid flow alterations is at 11 to 13 weeks.[10]

Maternal serum is screened for the free β subunit of hCG and PAPP-A from 10 through 13 weeks. Free β subunit of hCG (see Placental Endocrinology), which is detectable 10 days after ovulation, initially doubles every 1.5 to 2 days, peaking at 8 to 10 weeks.[75] PAPP-A is a large molecular weight glycoprotein synthesized by the placental syncytiotrophoblast and released directly into maternal serum. PAPP-A is detectable at approximately 6 weeks of pregnancy and doubles every 6 days, plateauing at 14 weeks. Maternal smoking decreases PAPP-A; multiple gestation increases both hCG and PAPP-A.[111]

Increased levels of the free β subunit of hCG are seen in infants with trisomy 21 and decreased in infants with trisomy 13 and 18.[111] Decreased levels of PAPP-A are seen with trisomy 21, 13, and 18, impending death, and impaired fetal well-being. Reported detection rates (and false positive rates) for trisomy 21 using maternal age (MA) and first trimester screening parameters are 75% to 89% (5%) for MA and fetal NT; 60% to 70% (5%) for MA, serum free β–hCG and PAPP-A; 85% to 95% (5%) for MA, serum free β–hCG, PAPP-A and NT; and 93% to 96% (2.5%) for all of the above plus nasal bone or DV or tricuspid flow.[111] First trimester screening does not screen for neural tube defects, although these and other defects may be detected on first trimester ultrasound.[7]

Second Trimester Screening. Second trimester screening has become a standard of prenatal care. Second trimester screening is called maternal serum multiple marker screening (MMS), enhanced or expanded maternal serum α-fetoprotein (AFP) screening, triple screen, or quad screen (depending on the components used). Screening is done on maternal serum at 15 to 20 weeks (optimum is 16 to 18½ weeks). Different combinations of components are used. The screen initially involved three components: AFP, unconjugated estriol (uE3), and the free β subunit of hCG with the more recent addition of inhibin A (for the quad screen).

AFP is an oncofetal glycoprotein that moves from fetal to maternal blood via diffusion across the fetal membranes. AFP is initially synthesized in the yolk sac and from the third month in the fetal gastrointestinal system and liver.[43,153] AFP normally increases until 10 to 14 weeks, then decreases.[59,153] AFP levels are elevated in infants with neural tube defects and low with fetal loss, some trisomies, and growth restriction.[100] AFP may also be elevated in infants with ventral wall defects such as omphalocele and gastroschisis, esophageal atresia, some skin defects (such as epidermolysis bullosa and aplasia cutis), and renal nephrosis.[153] An elevated AFP has also been associated with placenta previa, abnormal placental adherence (placenta acreta), gestational hypertension, preeclampsia, fetal growth restriction and abruption; low AFP has been associated with preterm birth and macrosomia.[43]

Unconjugated estriol (uE3) is a reflection of fetal functional maturity since precursors for placental production must be produced by the fetus. Levels are decreased in infants with trisomies, Turner syndrome, anencephaly, congenital adrenal hyperplasia, fetal growth restriction, and fetal loss.[43] Inhibin A is a glycoprotein from the placenta and provides negative feedback to the pituitary to prevent FSH release, and has a role in cell differentiation and immune function.[43] Inhibin A normally increases to 10 weeks, then plateaus to 25 weeks, followed by a rise to term. Levels are decreased in infants with trisomy 21.[20] Increased levels of AFP and hCG in women with normal fetuses have been associated with an increased risk of stillbirth, abruption, preterm labor, pregnancy-induced hypertension, miscarriage, and low birth weight. Similarly, decreased uE3 has been associated with increased risk of preeclampsia, fetal growth restriction, miscarriage, and intrauterine fetal death. Increased second trimester free β-hCG is associated with placental dysfunction with preeclampsia, fetal loss, preterm birth, and fetal growth restriction.[43]

Maternal serum second trimester screening is used to screen for Down syndrome, trisomy 18, and neural tube defects (spina bifida and anencephaly). Some infants with Turner syndrome may also be identified. AFP and hCG are most useful in screening for Down syndrome, whereas AFP is most useful for screening for neural tube defects (see Chapter 15). Each laboratory has its own cut-off for positive screen, so results are usually reported in multiples of the median (MoM). Abnormal values for AFP are generally less than 0.5 and greater than 2.5 MoM.[152] About 100 in 1000 women will have a positive screen; of these women, only 2 or 3 will have a fetus with a defect.[59] Factors that can influence screen results include maternal age, race and weight, gestational age, and maternal diabetes.

If a woman has a positive screen, follow-up ultrasound and/or amniocentesis are indicated. Second trimester ultrasound markers for trisomy 21 include nucal fold ≥5 mm, hypoplastic or absent nasal bone, shortened humerus and femur, echogenic intracranial foci, hyperechogenic bowel (also seen with cystic fibrosis, cytomegalovirus and severe fetal growth restriction).[153] Reported detection rates (and false positive rates) for trisomy 21 using MA and second trimester screening parameters are 60% to 65% (5%) for MA, serum AFP and free β-hCG; 65% to 70% (5%) for MA, serum AFP, free β-hCG and uE3 (triple screen); and 65% to 70% (5%) for MA, serum AFP, free β-hCG, uE3 and inhibin A (quadruple screen).[111] Stepwise screening, combining first and second trimester screening results, i.e., MA, NT, PAPP-A (11-13 weeks) and quadruple screen has a detection rate of 90% to 94% with a 5% false positive rate.[111]

Prenatal Diagnosis

Assessment of fetal status and placental function and analysis of the constituents of amniotic fluid are useful in evaluating the growth and health of the fetus, the ability of the fetus to withstand the stresses of labor and delivery and timing of delivery.[57] Newer techniques have improved monitoring of fetal and placental status with high-risk pregnancies. Techniques for evaluation of placental function consist of biochemical monitoring of the fetoplacental unit, antepartum fetal heart rate surveillance, fetal blood gas monitoring, and the biophysical profile. These are discussed in Chapter 6. Chorionic villus sampling (CVS) and amniocentesis allow for prenatal diagnosis of increasing numbers of chromosomal, genetic, and other congenital anomalies. Percutaneous umbilical blood sampling can be used for both prenatal diagnosis and therapy. Routine ultrasound studies provide an opportunity to observe for major and minor anomalies in the fetus. Ultrasound can also be used to monitor fetal growth and well-being. Causes of congenital anomalies are found in Table 3-3.

Table 3-3 Causes of Congenital Anomalies

CAUSE	PERCENTAGE
Chromosomal abnormalities	6-7
Gene abnormalities	7-8
Environmental agents	7-10
Multifactorial inheritance	20-25
Unknown etiology	50-60

Data from Moore, K.L. & Persaud, T.V.N. (2003). *The developing human: Clinically oriented embryology* (7th ed.). Philadelphia: Saunders.

Genetic screening and use of diagnostic techniques such as CVS, amniocentesis, and the genetic ultrasound allow for prenatal identification of increasing numbers of chromosomal, genetic, and other congenital anomalies. Timing of these techniques is illustrated in Figure 3-18. All of these techniques are associated with increased parental anxiety and concern.[47] The goal of prenatal diagnosis is to provide parents with the assurance that they will have a child who is unaffected by the specific disorders being evaluated. Most women participate in prenatal testing for reassurance; 90% to 95% will have a normal fetus. If an abnormality is identified, prenatal diagnosis provides parents with an opportunity to prepare for the birth of an affected infant; plan for delivery, care, and management of the infant; or elect to terminate the pregnancy. In some cases, early diagnosis provides options for fetal therapy, such as intervention for urinary tract obstructions to reduce prenatal renal damage (see Chapter 11), some forms of neural tube defects (see Chapter 15), some forms of congenital heart defects (see Chapter 9), transfusions for hematologic conditions (see Chapter 8), or pharmacologic interventions (see Chapter 7).[37] Indications for prenatal diagnosis include maternal age greater than 35; paternal age greater than 50 or 55; history of two or more miscarriages; previous pregnancy

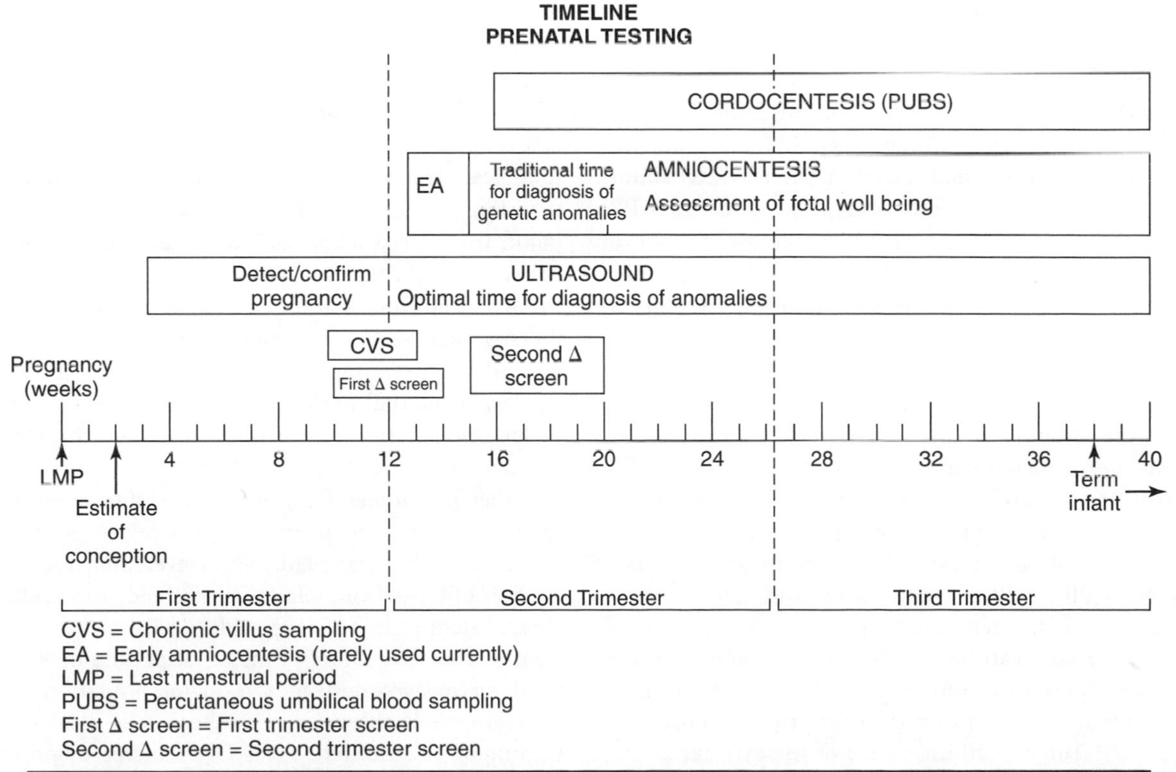

FIGURE 3-18 Usual timeline for prenatal testing. (Modified from a figure originally developed by Brock, K.A. [1990]. Seattle: University of Washington.)

or family history of genetic or chromosomal disorder; parents who are known or suspected carriers of a specific genetic disorder; previous child with or family history of a neural tube or other birth defect, especially defects known to have a multifactorial inheritance pattern; exposure to known teratogens; and women with positive first or second trimester screening results.[153]

Preimplantation Genetic Diagnosis. Genetic analysis of the oocyte or polar body is sometimes done as part of IVF, usually because of a family history of a specific genetic disorder or to detect aneuploidy. Preimplantation genetic diagnosis, also with IVF, is done at the eight-cell stage, usually around 3 days after fertilization removing one or two blastomeres at 3 days or 5 to 12 cells from trophectoderm in the 5 to 7 day blastocyst.[153] The cells are evaluated using fluorescent in situ hybridization (FISH) or polymerase chain reaction techniques.[11]

Chorionic Villus Sampling. CVS is an alternative to genetic amniocentesis. CVS is generally performed 10 to 13 weeks after the last menstrual period (see Figure 3-18). Earlier, chorionic villi may not be sufficiently developed for adequate tissue sampling and risk of limb anomalies is increased; later, the chorion laeve is disappearing and the chorion frondosum is forming the definitive placenta. Both transabdominal and transcervical (because the uterus is still in the pelvis) approaches can be used after the gestational sac and implantation site are located by ultrasound. However, transabdominal approaches are preferred because of a lower miscarriage rate.[115]

Trophoblast tissue is aspirated from several sites on the chorion. This tissue can be analyzed for chromosome anomalies or with enzyme assay (for inborn errors of metabolism) or DNA analysis (hemoglobinopathies and other disorders).[153]Advantages of CVS include early diagnosis before the pregnancy is obvious to others and, for some assays, a decreased waiting period for results. Disadvantages include a risk of spontaneous abortion, infection, bleeding, and amniotic fluid leakage; uncertainty about long-term effects on the infant; and inability to do AFP assays for diagnosis of neural tube defects at this stage of gestation.[153,159] CVS before 10 weeks' gestation has been associated with an increased risk of limb defects and is not recommended.[159] CVS between 10 and 13 weeks is a safer alternative for first trimester prenatal diagnosis than early amniocentesis.[159] Transabdominal CVS can also be done in the second and third trimesters.[115,153]

Amniocentesis. Genetic amniocentesis has traditionally been performed in most centers at 15 to 16 weeks (range, 15 to 20 weeks) (see Figure 3-18), because at this time amniotic fluid volume has reached 150 to 250 mL (so approximately 20 to 30 mL can easily and safely be removed), the uterus has reached the pelvic brim (so a transabdominal approach can be used), adequate fetal cells are available, and diagnostic studies can be completed in time for a second trimester abortion (if this option is chosen by the parents).[159] The overall incidence of miscarriage is 1% to 1.7%; the risk is higher with advanced maternal age.[115,153] The incidence of other maternal and fetal complications (spotting, fluid leak, bleeding, infection) is low.[159] Early amniocentesis before 14 to 15 weeks has also been used in some centers, although it is currently uncommon. An increased risk of fetal loss, amniotic fluid leakage, and 10-fold increase in talipes equinovarus has been reported with early amniocentesis.[115,153,159]

Cellular and biochemical components of amniotic fluid change with gestational age and are useful indicators of fetal maturity and well-being. Amniotic fluid contains cells from the amnion, fetal skin, buccal and bladder mucosa, and tracheal lining. Amniotic fluid cells can be examined to determine fetal sex (important with sex-linked disorders) and to diagnose genetic and chromosomal disorders using DNA and enzymatic analysis. Polymerase chain reaction techniques can be used to identify in utero infection such as cytomegalovirus, toxoplasmosis, or parvovirus B19.[115] Rapid detection of trisomies 21, 13, and 18, and alterations in sex chromosome numbers can be obtained within 24 hours using FISH techniques with uncultured cells.[159] Amniotic fluid can be cultured for karyotype (to identify other chromosomal abnormalities) or for biochemical assay (to identify specific inherited metabolic disorders), analyzed using DNA hybridization and restriction enzyme techniques (for detecting gene deletions that occur with disorders such as hemoglobinopathies), and analyzed for quantification of AFP (screening for neural tube defects and other anomalies). Newer microarray technology (also called molecular karyotyping) has been used when multiple congenital anomalies are seen on ultrasound and conventional karyotyping is normal to detect microdeletions, duplications, and other alterations.[163] Cellular and biochemical components of amniotic fluid can be used to evaluate fetal health and maturity, including fetal lung maturity (see Chapter 10).

Umbilical Blood Sampling. Cordocentesis, or percutaneous umbilical blood sampling (PUBS), involves use of the umbilical cord to obtain fetal blood samples. Umbilical blood sampling has been used in the prenatal diagnosis of inherited blood disorders (hemoglobinopathies and coagulopathies), in detection of congenital infection, to assess fetal anemia (in Rh isoimmunization and in thrombocytopenia), and in fetal therapy such as blood transfusions. This technique is performed using real-time ultrasound as early as 16 weeks after the last menstrual period (see Figure 3-18). Complications include infection, preterm labor, bleeding, thrombosis, and transient fetal arrhythmia.

Other Techniques. Celocentesis, aspiration of extra-amniotic fluid, has been used from 6 to 10 weeks; long-term effects still need to be evaluated.[115,147] Developing technology for analysis of DNA from fetal nucleated red blood cells, mesenchymal stem cells, and trophoblast cells in maternal circulation, or free fetal DNA in maternal plasma may reduce the need for invasive testing.[82] A major limitation in analysis of fetal cells is the paucity of these cells; thus enrichment techniques are needed. Fetal DNA increases progressively, accounting for 3% to 6% of the DNA in maternal plasma; levels increase with fetal aneuploidy.[82] In addition, newer imaging techniques, such as fetal magnetic resonance imaging and three-dimensional ultrasonography, enhance diagnosis of fetal anomalies.[82,140]

Alterations in Placenta, Umbilical Cord, and Amniotic Fluid

An intact and adequately functioning placenta and amniotic fluid are critical for fetal survival and well-being. Without the placenta the fetus could not survive, because it would have no alternatives for essential processes such as respiratory gas exchange and nutrition. This section discusses alterations in the placenta and amniotic fluid in low- and high-risk pregnancies, the implications for the fetus and neonate from placental dysfunction and alterations in amniotic fluid volume, and the basis for common cord and placental abnormalities. Alterations in placental structure and function may lead to alterations in fetal programming (see Chapters 12, 16, and 19) and increase the risk of later disease.[88,144] Longtine & Nelson note that "placental structure and function are affected by developmental plasticity, epigenetic effects, as well as by exogenous or endogenous stressors, nutrient limitation, or metabolic imbalances. The resulting placental dysfunction can affect fetal development in utero and predispose the adult to a variety of diseases."[88]

Alterations in the Appearance of the Placenta and Membranes

The appearance of the placenta (color, size, consistency) often provides clues to maternal or placental dysfunction or pathologic processes in the fetus. The color of the placenta is determined by fetal hemoglobin. Pale placentas suggest fetal anemia. The placenta is paler in immature infants and congested in infants of diabetic mothers. Edematous, pale, and bulky placentas are seen with immune and nonimmune hydrops fetalis, twin-to-twin transfusion syndrome (in the donor twin), fetal congestive heart failure, and infection.[123,124] These placentas may also contain more Hofbauer cells, an immature trophoblast layer, and other changes similar to those seen with hypoxia. Placentas less than 2 to 2.5 cm thick are often seen with IUGR; those more than 4 cm thick may be seen with diabetes mellitus and fetal hydrops.

The placenta responds to hypoxia and ischemia with formation of excessive syncytial knots, proliferation of villous cytotrophoblast (Langhans) cells, nucleated erythrocytes, fibrinoid necrosis of the villi, increased perivillous fibrin, and thickening of the trophoblast basement membrane.[50,123] The placentas from women with preeclampsia often have infarcts, hematomas, and characteristic histologic changes such as excessive proliferation of cytotrophoblast tissue within the villi and fibrin deposits.[84,99] Infarctions are also seen in placentas of infants with IUGR whose placentas are also small and in placentas from women with elevated hemoglobin levels (more than 13 g/dL [130 g/L]) in the second half of pregnancy. In this latter group, the infarctions may be due to increased blood viscosity and thrombosis. Placentas of women who smoke may demonstrate increased thickness of the villous membrane that may reduce efficiency of diffusion.[99] Pathologic changes in placentas of infants with fetal growth restriction are linked to reductions in placental blood flow and include thickening of villous trophoblastic basal membrane, villous infarction, thrombi, hematomas, villitis, and decreased mean placental weight and fetal-placental weight ratios.[150]

Thrombi in the veins along the chorionic plate appear as yellow streaks on the surface of the placenta. These thrombi are associated with velamentous insertion of the cord and may embolize. Infarctions are often seen near the margins of the placenta; central infarctions are less common and more serious, in that they may disrupt IVS circulation. Infarctions are areas of ischemic necrosis of primary villi resulting from obstruction of IVS blood flow due to thrombi or marked impairment of blood flow in the spiral arteries.[33,50] Initially these infarcted areas are red, later turning brown, gray, and then white with fibrin deposition; they may be covered with necrotic decidua. Hematomas and thrombi may be seen in the intervillous spaces (IVS). Infarctions may be a way the fetus responds to villi that have inadequate maternal perfusion; that is, the flow of blood to the affected villus is reduced so blood normally flowing to that villus can be redistributed to areas where maternal circulation is adequate.

Multiple plaques or nodules on the fetal surface of the placenta are found with amnion nodosum (associated with oligohydramnios and renal agenesis), squamous metaplasia (benign disorder), and infection.[4,33] With chorioamnionitis, the placenta often has an opaque surface and may be foul smelling or edematous.[124] Infection with *Candida albicans* is associated with white or yellow nodules on the placental surface.[33]

Meconium staining of the membranes may also occur. Because meconium is not discharged until after fetal gastrointestinal peptides (e.g., motilin) have reached critical levels, meconium passage is infrequent in preterm infants and more common in post term infants. Green membranes are not necessarily due to meconium, in that accumulations of hemosiderin (as may occur with hemolysis and circumvallation) also stain the membranes green.[123] Green pigment can be found in amniotic macrophages an hour after meconium is discharged and in chorionic macrophages by 2 to 3 hours. With extended exposure to meconium, extraplacental membranes become edematous and the membranes and placenta become tan-green or brown.

Alterations in Amniotic Fluid Volume

An understanding of the processes involved in the production of amniotic fluid and the pattern of fluid accumulation during pregnancy is necessary for assessing uterine growth and identifying women who need further evaluation (see "Amniotic Fluid"). Alterations in production and removal of amniotic fluid can lead to polyhydramnios (hydramnios) or oligohydramnios.

Polyhydramnios. Polyhydramnios (also called *hydramnios*), has traditionally been defined as accumulation of more than 2.1 L of fluid in a single amniotic sac at term.[160] More recently the amniotic fluid index (AFI) based on the largest amniotic fluid pocket seen on ultrasound has been used (≥25 cm at any gestational age or a maximum vertical pocket [MVP] of ≥8 cm in depth).[160] Polyhydramnios has an overall incidence of 1% to 3%. It can occur gradually during pregnancy or rapidly over a few days or weeks. Polyhydramnios is idiopathic in 60% of women but is also associated with maternal disease; multiple gestation; immune and nonimmune hydrops fetalis; Down syndrome and other chromosomal anomalies; and fetal gastrointestinal, cardiac, and neural tube anomalies. However, women with any of these complications can also have normal amniotic fluid volume.[129] Idiopathic or essential polyhydramnios (i.e., due to no known cause) is thought to arise from an unexplained imbalance in water exchange between the fetus, mother, and amniotic fluid. Increased aquaporin (AQP) water channel expression has been described in pregnancies complicated by idiopathic polyhydramnios.[34,95,162] Second trimester polyhydramnios resolves spontaneously in 40% to 50% with good fetal outcomes.

Although multiple gestation frequently results in increased accumulation of amniotic fluid, in most cases this is not true polyhydramnios, because the fluid is distributed among several sacs, each sac containing usual amounts of fluid. An increased incidence of polyhydramnios has been reported in monozygotic (MZ) monochorionic twins with arteriovenous anastomoses within their shared placenta and twin-to-twin transfusion syndrome (see "Placental Abnormalities in Multiple Gestation"). Development of polyhydramnios in these pregnancies may be the result of excessive urination, polycythemia, and transudation of fluids. The elevated venous pressure and altered fluid dynamics seen with hydrops fetalis and some cardiovascular disorders may lead to excessive accumulation of amniotic fluid. Polyhydramnios is more frequent in diabetic women, perhaps because of fetal polyuria caused by fetal hyperglycemia or because of alterations in osmotic gradients as a result of increased amniotic fluid glucose.

Congenital anomalies are reported in 12% to 19% of pregnancies complicated by polyhydramnios.[129] Neural tube defects, particularly anencephaly, may result in polyhydramnios as a result of decreased fetal swallowing or transudation of fluid from the exposed meninges. Polyhydramnios associated with chromosomal anomalies may be related to reduced fetal swallowing and, in some infants with Down syndrome, duodenal atresia. Although polyhydramnios is seen in many infants with esophageal or duodenal atresia (presumably due to decreased fetal swallowing and decreased gut absorption), these pregnancies may also have normal amniotic fluid volume.[129] The basis for this finding is unclear but suggests that amniotic fluid homeostasis is a very complex mechanism involving the interaction of many variables.

Treatment options include fetal therapy (e.g., if the cause is due to fetal hydrops or arrhythmias); serial amniocenteses; and administration of prostaglandin synthetase inhibitors such as indomethacin. Indomethacin is thought to work by increasing fluid reabsorption by the fetal lungs, decreasing fetal urine production, and increasing fluid movement across the membranes to the mother. Indomethacin has potential maternal and fetal side effects.

Oligohydramnios. Oligohydramnios is ≤5 cm or MVP ≤1 cm on AFI evaluation.[160] Oligohydramios can occur at any time during gestation and is seen in 1% to 2% of pregnancies.[160] Oligohydramnios is rarer than polyhydramnios and is associated with amnion abnormalities, placental insufficiency, and fetal urinary anomalies.[139] Any alterations in formation or excretion of urine by the fetus in the second half of gestation can result in oligohydramnios. Oligohydramnios may lead to umbilical cord compression in labor and fetal distress.

Inadequate amniotic fluid during labor can be due to premature rupture of the membranes, oligohydramnios, or early amniotomy. A lack of adequate fluid removes the natural protective cushioning effect of this fluid and increases the risk of cord compression and fetal heart rate decelerations during contractions. Interventions for alterations in fetal heart rate patterns are discussed in Chapter 6.

Severe fetal renal anomalies (agenesis, dysplasia, or obstructive disorders) may lead to oligohydramnios because of decreased or no urine output. Bilateral renal agenesis in conjunction with pulmonary hyperplasia, musculoskeletal abnormalities, and a characteristic facies is known as Potter syndrome and is associated with oligohydramnios. Several of the findings in Potter syndrome may be deformation defects arising from lack of amniotic fluid.[71]

Movement produced by fetal muscular activity is an integral component of normal morphologic development. Mechanical forces can lead to defects either from intrinsic forces (e.g., fetal myoneuropathy, development of an organ in an abnormal and excessively small site, or alterations in the normal flow or volume of body fluids) or from external forces (e.g., a bicornate uterus, fibromas, or oligohydramnios) that interfere with fetal mobility.[101]

The constraints on fetal movement imposed by oligohydramnios can result in a cascade of developmental events resulting in fetal anomalies. These anomalies include congenital contractures (due to relative or complete immobilization of the joints in a confined space); lung hyperplasia (lack of room for development of the thorax and for the subsequent stretch or distention of lung tissue required for normal lung growth); shortened umbilical cord (length is related to stretching from fetal activity); dysmorphic facies including micrognathia, low-set ears, small alae nasi, and hypertelorism (molding of the face by compressive forces); growth restriction (fetal motor activity seems important for normal development of muscle mass and weight gain); perhaps microgastria (lack of stretching and distention because the volume of amniotic fluid available for swallowing is reduced); and "loose" skin (stretched by the attempts of the constrained fetus to move).[101] This sequence has been termed the fetal akinesia/hypokinesia deformation sequence.[101]

Oligohydramnios is also associated with amnion nodosum. In this disorder, yellow-gray nodules or plaques consisting of desquamated fetal epidermal cells, hair, and vernix are found in and on the amnion and on the placental surface (fetal side). This debris is probably pressed into the amnion by close approximation of the fetal skin and amnion in the presence of oligohydramnios. Oligohydramnios may also occur with IUGR (as a result of decreased urine flow rates) or with prolonged pregnancy.

Abnormalities of the Cord and Placenta

Abnormalities of the cord and placenta arise from alterations in implantation and placentation or from disorders of the trophoblast. Occasionally these abnormalities may have minimal effect on the fetus and the outcome of the pregnancy; more often, serious and sometimes fatal conditions develop so that the pregnancy cannot be maintained or fetal development and survival are threatened. At times, maternal survival and reproductive function may also be compromised.

Abnormalities of Implantation and Separation. The major abnormalities of implantation and separation of the placenta are placenta previa, abruptio placentae, and placenta accreta. Placenta previa is implantation of the placenta over or near the internal cervical os so that it encroaches on a portion of the dilated cervix. Placenta previa may be classified as total, partial, or marginal; low-lying placentas are sometimes included in this classification. Various theories have been proposed to explain the pathogenesis of placenta previa, including defective vascularization of the endometrium, alteration of the normal ovum transport mechanism, and development of the placenta in the decidua capsularis.[33,50]

If the blastocyst implants in endometrium that is poorly vascularized due to atrophic or inflammatory changes, the placenta may develop a larger decidual surface area to compensate for an inadequate blood supply and grow downward into the lower uterine segment.[33] If vascularization of the endometrium in the upper uterine segment is poor, the blastocyst may continue to descend, implanting by chance in healthier endometrium in the lower uterine segment. Altered transport of the blastocyst due to abnormal uterine motility, deviations in the size or shape of the uterine cavity, scars or fluid in the cavity can also result in displacement of the blastocyst to the lower uterus.[33]

Normally the chorionic villi initially surround the entire embryo but later degenerate beneath the decidua capsularis, forming the chorion laeve. By 4 months, the growing fetus fills the uterine cavity and the decidua capsularis fuses with the decidua vera (see Figure 3-8). If chorionic villi near the lower uterus fail to degenerate as the decidua capsularis fuses with the decidua vera, these villi can become incorporated into the placenta and impinge on the lower uterine segment.[33,50] The incidence of a low lying placenta is higher in early gestation than at term due to growth of the lower uterine segment.[97]

A placental abruption is separation of a normally implanted placenta before the delivery of the fetus. Abruptio placentae is initiated by hemorrhage into the decidua basalis with formation of a hematoma that leads to separation and compression of the adjacent portion of the placenta. Hemorrhage may develop secondary to degenerative changes in the arteries supplying the intervillous space and with thrombosis, degeneration of the decidua, and vessel rupture with formation of a retroplacental hemorrhage.[50] Possible causes include maternal hypertension (secondary to essential hypertension, preeclampsia, chronic renal disease, or cocaine use or alterations in the transformation of the spiral arteries), compression or occlusion of the inferior vena cava, circumvallate placenta, or trauma.[33,50,97,127] The incidence of abruptio placentae is markedly increased with maternal cocaine use. These drugs induce vasoconstriction of placental blood vessels and a sudden elevation in maternal blood pressure.

Placenta accreta is a general term used to describe any placental implantation in which there is abnormally firm adherence of all or part of the placenta to the myometrium. As a result, there is partial or total absence of the decidua basalis and attachment of the chorionic villi to the fibrinoid (Nitabuch) layer or myometrium. Occasionally the villi invade the myometrium (placenta increta) or penetrate through the myometrial wall (placenta percreta). Placenta accreta usually occurs when decidual formation is defective, such as with implantation over uterine scars or in the lower uterine segment. Placenta acreta occurs in 3 out of 1000 deliveries and its prevalence has increased in the past decade.[120] Placenta accreta is associated with placenta previa, particularly in the presence of a uterine scar, and with significant morbidity including severe hemorrhage, uterine perforation, infection, and hysterectomy.[33,50,120]

Abnormalities of Placentation. The size and configuration of the placenta are influenced by the degree of vascularization of the decidua and the number and arrangement of the primitive villi that later comprise the fetal portion of the placenta.[33] The major clinically significant abnormalities of placental configuration result in circumvallate, marginate, or succenturiate placentas.

With circumvallate placenta, the area of the chorionic plate is reduced. As chorionic villi invade the decidua, the fetal membranes fold back upon themselves, creating a dense, grayish-white raised ring encircling the central portion of the fetal surface (Figure 3-19). The fetal vessels forming the cord stop at this ring rather than covering the entire fetal surface of the placenta. The risk of abruptio placenta is increased with circumvallate placentas. Marginate (or circumarginate) placentas (see Figure 3-19) also arises from a chorionic plate that is smaller than the basal plate. In these placentas the white ring composed of the fetal membranes coincides with the margin of the placenta, without the folding back of the membranes seen in circumvallate placentas.[50]

The etiology of circumvallate and marginate placentas is uncertain, although partial or complete forms are seen in up to 25% of gestations.[134] Possible causes include subchorial infarcts, formation of insufficient chorion frondosum, and an abnormally deep implantation of the blastocyst causing part of the fetal surface to be covered by the decidua vera. These placentas are often asymptomatic, but circumvallate

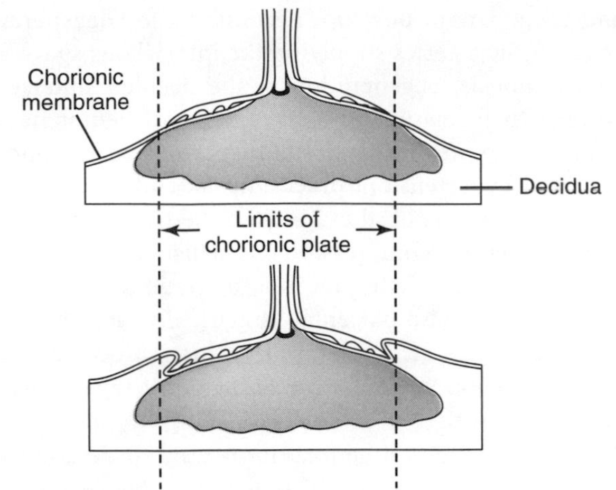

FIGURE 3-19 Diagrammatic representation of a marginate placenta *(top)* and a circumvallate placenta *(bottom)*. (From Fox, H. [1997]. *Pathology of the placenta* [2nd ed.]. Philadelphia: Saunders.)

placentas have been linked to threatened abortion, preterm labor, painless vaginal bleeding after 20 weeks, placental insufficiency, and intrapartum and postpartum hemorrhage.[33,50]

Succenturiate placenta involves development of one or more smaller accessory lobes in the membranes that are attached to the main placenta by fetal vessels. This abnormality arises when a group of villi distant to the main placenta fail to degenerate, implantation is superficial, or implantation occurs in a confined site (e.g., a bicornate uterus) so that attachment of the trophoblast also occurs on the opposing wall.[33,50] The accessory lobes may be retained, leading to postpartum hemorrhage or infection. These placentas are often associated with malrotation of the implanting blastocyst with velamentous insertion of the cord.[33]

Abnormalities of the Umbilical Cord. The umbilical cord may develop knots, loops, torsion, or strictures. These alterations are associated with increased fetal mortality and morbidity.[50,84] Excessively long cords (greater than 75 to 100 cm) are more likely to develop knots, torsion, or prolapse. Excessively long cords are associated with increased fetal activity. Abnormally short cords (less than 30 to 32 cm) are associated with asphyxia at birth as a result of traction on the cord with fetal descent.[33,134] Abnormally short cords are also associated with decreased fetal activity because tension on the cord normally promotes growth. Decreased fetal activity is seen with Down syndrome, neuromuscular disorders, and fetal malformations may result in short cords.

A single umbilical artery occurs in about 1% of newborns and probably arises from agenesis or degeneration of the missing vessel early in gestation.[126] This anomaly is associated with an increased incidence of fetal cardiovascular and urinary tract anomalies.[126] In infants with an isolated single umbilical artery, the incidence of renal anomalies is approximately 7%.[97]

Battledore placenta, or insertion of the cord at or within 1.5 cm of the margin of the placenta (seen in 5% to 7% of placentas), may be clinically benign but has been linked to preterm labor, fetal distress, and bleeding in labor due to cord compression or vessel rupture.[97,134] With velamentous insertion (1% to 2% of placentas), the cord inserts into the membranes so that the vessels run between the amnion and chorion before entering into the placenta.[97] These variations in insertion of the cord probably arise at the time of implantation. Velamentous insertion is more common in multiple births.

Normally the blastocyst implants with the inner cell mass adjacent to the endometrium and the trophoblast that will form the placenta. The body stalk, which will become the cord, aligns with the center of the placenta. Rotation of the inner cell mass (and body stalk) gives rise to eccentric insertions of the cord. The degree of rotation will influence how far the umbilical cord will be from the center of the placenta (i.e., eccentric, marginal, velamentous). Velamentous insertion may lead to rupture and fetal hemorrhage associated with a high fetal mortality, particularly with vasa praevia (when the fetal vessels are located along the lower uterine segment, crossing the internal cervical os, and presenting ahead of the fetus).[33,53,97]

Gestational Trophoblast Disease

Gestational trophoblast disease includes hydatidiform mole and gestational trophoblast tumors (derived from neoplastic hyperplastic changes). Both forms of trophoblast disease are associated with markedly elevated levels of hCG.[33] Hydatidiform moles result from deterioration of the chorionic villi into a mass of clear vesicles. Histologically, hydatidiform mole is characterized by hyperplasia of the syncytiotrophoblast and the cytotrophoblast, edema of the avascular villous stroma, and cystic cavitations within the villous stroma. The villi become converted into molar cysts connected to each other by fibrous strands.[28] There may be no fetus (complete mole) or the remains of a degenerating fetus or amniotic sac (partial or incomplete mole). Rarely the fetus in an incomplete molar pregnancy survives to delivery.[33]

The karyotype of a complete mole is usually 46,XX (90%) and is derived from duplication of a haploid X-carrying (23,X) sperm. The remainder are 46 XY and arise from fertilization of the ovum by two sperm with failure of the maternal genome to participate in development.[15] Thus the mole is usually androgenic in origin; that is, the ovum develops under the influence of a spermatozoon nucleus. The nucleus of the ovum is inactivated or lost before fertilization. A complete mole is associated with increased risk of later choriocarcinoma.

In an incomplete or partial mole, the hydatidiform changes are focal; that is, there is slowly progressive swelling of some villi (which are usually avascular), whereas other vascular villi develop with a functioning fetoplacental circulation.[33] The karyotype of this type of mole is usually triploid (69,XXX; 69,XXY; or 69,XYY). An incomplete mole results from fertilization of a normal haploid ovum (23,X) by two haploid sperm (dispermy) or a single diploid sperm.[15,50] A third type involves heterozygous diploid fertilization of an empty ovum with two haploid sperm (46,XX or 46,XY). This form of mole is associated with an increased risk of gestational trophoblast tumors.

Multiple Gestation

The incidence of twins in the United States is 33 per 1000 live births and has doubled in the last 20 years.[156] This increase is attributed to delayed childbearing and increased use of ART.[13] The arrangement of membranes and placentas in twin gestations is determined by the type of twin and the stage of gestation at which twinning occurs. The incidence of twin conceptions is greater than that of twin births. Ultrasound studies indicate that up to 12% of pregnancies begin as twins, but are converted to singleton pregnancies by the asymptomatic loss of one embryo.[50] Spontaneous reduction in the number of embryos is seen in 36% of pregnancies that begin as twins, 53% of triplet pregnancies, and 63% of quadruplet pregnancies.[39]

The basic types of twins are monozygotic (MZ) (arising from division of a single ovum after fertilization) and dizygotic (DZ) (simultaneous fertilization of two ova enclosed within a single follicle or theca, or ovulation of two ova from one or both ovaries that are then fertilized independently). Most (70%) twins are DZ. A third type of twinning has been proposed to occur due to simultaneous fertilization of an ovum and the first polar body by two sperm, although supporting evidence is scanty.[13] This section focuses on twins, because higher-order multiples (e.g., triplets, quadruplets) can be MZ, DZ, or multizygotic, with attributes that are variations of findings characteristic of twins.

Twin zygosity cannot be determined solely by the number of placentas. Two types of placentas are seen: monochorionic, which occurs with MZ twins, and dichorionic, which may occur with either MZ or DZ twins. Dichorionic placentas may be separate or fused (with a ridge in the central fusion plane). Examinations to determine zygosity often require morphologic examination of the chorion, amnion, and yolk sac as well as DNA analysis, which can be done quickly and reliably by restriction fragment length polymorphism (RFLP) analysis.[13] Placentas and membranes of twins and other multiple births should always be saved and sent for pathologic examination for morphologic and DNA analysis.

MZ twins may have one or two placentas (which may be separate or fused). The placentas and membranes of MZ twins may be monochorionic-monoamniotic, monochorionic-diamniotic, or dichorionic-diamniotic (fused or separate). About 70% of MZ twins are monochorionic and 30% are dichorionic.[13,36] With higher-order multiple births, placentas and membranes may be monochorionic-monoamniotic, monochorionic-multiamniotic, or multichorionic-multiamniotic (Figure 3-20). Although DZ twins always have two dichorionic-diamniotic placentas, the placentas may be fused and appear

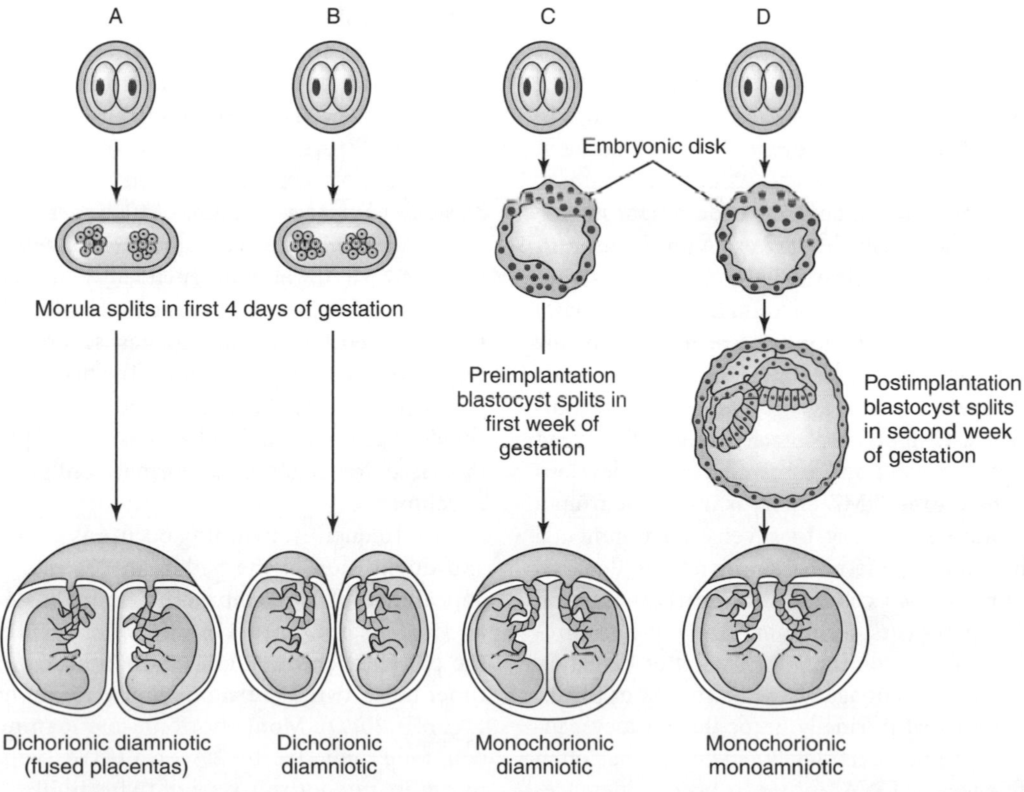

FIGURE 3-20 Diagrammatic representation of the development and placentation of monozygotic twins. (From Fox, H. [1997]. *Pathology of the placenta* [2nd ed.]. Philadelphia: Saunders.)

to be single. Fused placentas increase the risk of growth restriction in one or both infants as a result of competition for space and abnormal cord insertions. About 80% of twins can be differentiated according to zygosity (i.e., as MZ or DZ) at or shortly after birth as follows (percentages are approximate): (1) 23% are monochorionic and therefore the infants are MZ; (2) 30% are dichorionic with a male and female twin and are almost always DZ; and (3) 27% are same-sex twins but with different blood types and thus usually DZ. The remaining 20% are same-sex twins with similar blood types who are either MZ twins with dichorionic placentas (either separate or fused) or DZ twins of the same sex (with separate or fused placentas).[13,36] Monochorionic twins of opposite sexes occur occasionally, possibly due to reciprocal chimerism or embryo fusion followed by later separation.[16] Determination of the zygosity of these twins requires more intensive investigation and DNA analysis.

Perinatal mortality is 3 to 11 times higher in twins than in singletons.[13] This risk is affected by zygosity and placental and membrane characteristics. For example, mortality is two to three times higher in monochorionic twins than in dichorionic (either DZ or MZ) twins. Monochorionic twins tend to weigh less and are more frequently growth restricted in utero than are dichorionic twins. The incidence of congenital anomalies is higher in MZ twins than in DZ twins.[36,142] Structural defects in MZ twins may arise from deformations due to limited intrauterine space, disruption of blood flow due to placental vascular anastomoses, or localized defects in early morphogenesis.

Monozygotic Twins

Spontaneous MZ twins occur in 3.5 to 4 in 1000 births.[13] The rate of MZ twinning is relatively constant worldwide and in most cases is probably a random event that is an accident in embryonic development. However, while not common, familial MZ twinning with an autosomal dominant inheritance pattern has been described.[90] The exact mechanism for monozygotic twinning is unclear but there are two main theories: splitting theory (splitting of a single inner cell mass) and co-dominance theory (development of more than one organizing axis).[156] MZ twinning may involve a teratogenic exposure.[13] Evidence for a teratogenic basis include an increased frequency with increased maternal age, discordant malformations in twin pairs and susceptibility for development of co-dominant axes.[90] MZ embryos may arise from a delay in implantation secondary to adverse environmental conditions such as inadequate nutrition or oxygen deprivation or to formation of two cell lines from early mosaicism (see Chapter 1) that triggers separation. The increased frequency of MZ twins reported in ART and after ovulation induction may be due to damage to the blastocyst or breaks in the zona pellucida that normally keeps the blastocyst intact.[60,90] MZ twins are not completely "identical" but often have subtle differences in DNA, minor to major differences in birth weight, or the presence of congenital defects in one twin due to unequal allocation of blastomeres. Postzygotic genetic events that can lead to MZ pair differences include postzygotic crossing-over or nondisjunction, imprinting differences, discordant cytoplasmic segregation, chromosomal mosaicism, altered patterns of X-chromosome inactivation in female MZ twins, or late gene mutations (see Chapter 1).[90,156] Separation may interrupt left-right axial orientation resulting in "mirror-image" twins. This is seen in 10% to 15% of MZ twins and involves mirror imaging of physical characteristics, but not situs inversus.[60] MZ twinning can occur at three different stages of development: (1) during the early blastomere stage, (2) during formation of the inner cell mass, and (3) with development of the embryonic disk (Figure 3-20). The stage of development determines the number of placentas and arrangement of membranes (Figure 3-21).

Separation of the ovum during the early blastomere stage, accounting for 25% to 30% of MZ twins, usually occurs about 2 days after fertilization while the blastomere is in the two- to four-cell stage (see Figure 3-20, *A* and *B*).[60] Because this is before differentiation of any cells, the two blastomeres will develop independently into morulae, blastocysts, and embryos, each with separate placentas, chorions, and amnions (dichorionic-diamniotic). These blastocysts will implant at separate sites. If these sites are close together, the placentas may fuse (see Figure 3-20, *A*). Membranes separating the embryos will contain the amnion-chorion of infant 1 and the chorion-amnion of infant 2 separated by their fused placentas. This arrangement of infants, placentas, and membranes, which is identical to that of same-sex DZ twins, requires blood typing, DNA analysis, and other analyses to determine zygosity.

Separation and duplication of the inner cell mass during development of the blastocyst 4 to 7 days after fertilization give rise to the most common (70% to 75%) form of MZ twins (see Figure 3-20, *C*).[60] The trophoblast layer that will become the placenta and chorion has already formed in the blastocyst before separation of the inner cell mass. The amnion and amniotic cavity, however, have not yet begun to form and will develop independently in each embryo. Thus this form of twinning is monochorionic-diamniotic with a single placenta. The membranes separating the embryos consist of two layers of amnion. The placenta of these infants is larger than the placenta found with a single infant but smaller than two single placentas. These placentas have an increased frequency of abnormal configurations and cord attachments.[13]

Less frequently, twinning occurs as a result of separation and duplication of the rudimentary embryonic disk, with appearance of two embryonic nodes instead of one at 7 to 15 (possibly up to 17) days after fertilization. Because the placenta, chorion, and amnion have all formed at this time, these twins are monochorionic-monoamniotic (see Figure 3-20, *D*). Monochorionic-monoamniotic infants account for only 1% to 2% of all MZ twins.[12,60] Perinatal mortality rate for this type of twins is 50% to 60% because of twisting, knotting, and entanglement of the two umbilical cords within the single amniotic sac.[13,50] Mortality

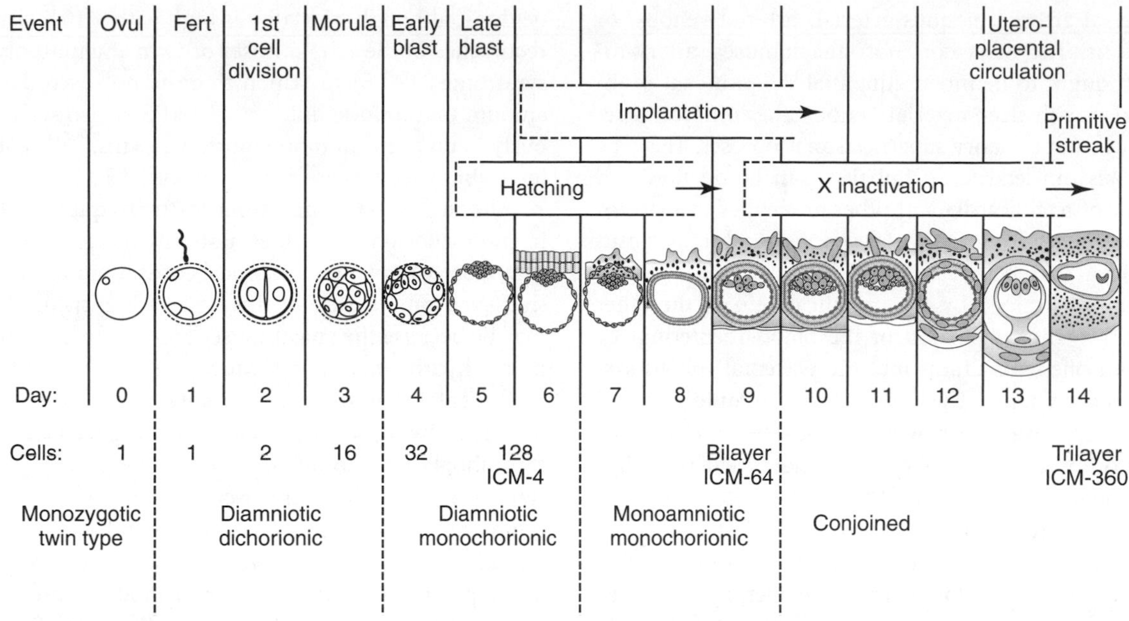

FIGURE 3-21 Schematic drawing of normal human embryonic development with timing of monozygotic twinning superimposed. *ICM,* Inner cell mass. (From Hall, J.G.. [2001]. Twins and twinning. In D.L. Rimoin, J.M. Connor, & R.E. Pyeritz, [Eds.]. *Emery and Rimoins's principles and practice of medical genetics* (vol 1, 4th ed.). New York: Churchill Livingstone.)

usually occur before 32 weeks.[13] If this form of twinning occurs prior to 13 to 14 days, two separate embryos are formed (see Figure 3-20).

Separation at 15 to 17 days, or after formation of the primitive streak, is usually incomplete; that is, the embryonic disk divides but remains united at one or more points (fission theory), resulting in the formation of conjoined twins. Development of conjoined twins has also been explained as arising after normal division of the embryonic disk into two cell masses that subsequently abut and join together (collision or fusion theory).[90] Conjoined twins occur in 1 in 50,000 live births.[90] The most common areas of fusion (either singularly or in combination) are the thorax, abdomen, and umbilical cord. Late separation can also lead to acardiac or amorphous fetuses.

Dizygotic Twins

The incidence of spontaneous DZ twins varies markedly among different racial groups, ranging from 1 in 20 to 25 births in certain Nigerian tribal groups to 1 in 80 in U.S. Caucasians, 1 in 70 in African-American populations, and 1 in 150 in Japanese women.[142] The incidence of DZ twinning is related to the frequency of double ovulation which is influenced by a variety of endocrine, endogenous, genetic exogenous, and iatrogenic (administration of gonadotropins for treatment of infertility) factors.[13] DZ twinning has a strong maternal familial tendency. For example, the incidence of twins in female relatives of mothers of twins is 19% versus 10.7% among female relatives of fathers of twins. A gene on chromosome 3 has been linked to DZ twinning.[24] Approximately 7% to 15% of the population are estimated to carry this gene.[60] Endocrine factors suggested in the etiology of DZ twins usually relate to increased levels of follicle-stimulating hormone (FSH) with overstimulation of the ovaries, leading to release of more than one ovum.[13] Endogenous factors associated with an increased incidence of DZ twinning include increased parity, maternal age (peaking at 35 years), maternal height and weight (perhaps related to nutrition), and increased frequency of intercourse.[13] Because DZ twins arise from separate ova, they have separate placentas, chorions, and amnions (dichorionic-diamniotic), although their placentas may fuse if implanted close to each other.

Placental Abnormalities in Multiple Gestations

Bardawil and colleagues categorized pathologic placental lesions associated with multiple gestation into four groups: (1) specific pathology directly due to the twinning process (conjoined twins, acardiac or amorphous fetuses, and vascular anastomoses); (2) pathologic lesions or conditions that arise as a consequence of group 1 lesions (entanglement of umbilical cords in monoamniotic twins, twin-to-twin transfusion, polyhydramnios, amnion nodosum, chimera in DZ twins); (3) lesions related to physical problems of accommodation due to decreased intrauterine space (circumvallate changes, velamentous or marginal cord insertion, vasa praevia); and (4) incidental lesions that can occur in any placenta and are not related to twinning specifically.[8]

Vascular connections or anastomoses occur in nearly all common monochorionic placentas shared by MZ twins.[13] Thus twin-to-twin transfusion is a normal event in monochorionic pregnancies but is not usually significant because blood flow is balanced.[12] Placental vascular anastomoses can be arterial-arterial, venous-arterial, arterial-venous, or venous-venous. The most common anastomoses, artery-to-artery, are thought to be inconsequential.[13] Significant problems can arise with deep arterial-venous anastomoses, especially without compensatory superficial anastomoses. This type of anastomosis can lead to an imbalance in blood flow and development of fetal acardia and other anomalies or twin-to-twin transfusion syndrome. Arterial-venous anastomoses usually occur in a shared lobe supplied by an umbilical artery of one twin and drained by the umbilical vein of the other (Figure 3-22).[13] Thus a portion of the blood reentering the placenta from one fetus drains into the placental venous system of the second fetus. The vascular flow is unidirectional and, unless compensated for by anastomoses in the opposite direction or other artery-to-artery anastomoses, will result in a hydrodynamic imbalance.[13]

Twin-to-twin transfusion syndrome (TTTS) is seen in about 9% of MZ twins.[86,137] TTTS usually results from arterial-venous anastomoses. The donor twin is smaller, hypovolemic, and anemic and may develop congestive heart failure. In the donor twin the reduced circulating volume stimulates the renin-angiotensin system with increased production of angiotensin II. This stimulates vasoconstriction to increase vascular volume, but can lead to hypertension (which can further decrease renal and placental perfusion and lead to fetal growth restriction).[9,12] This infant has decreased urine volume, and oligohydramnios may be present. The larger, recipient twin is hypervolemic and hypertensive with excessive urination often leading to polyhydramnios. This infant responds to the increased blood volume by increasing atrial natriuretic peptide, which leads to increased glomerular filtration, decreased tubular reabsorption and suppression of arginine vasopressin and polyuria.[9,12] This infant may develop hydrops and cardiomegaly.[13] The volume overload can lead to ventricular hypertrophy and increased aortic and pulmonary outflow.[94] TTTS may occur with significant differences in volume without significant differences in hemoglobin levels (twin oligo-polyhydramnios sequence or TOPS).[136,137] Most cases of TTTS develop at 15 to 25 weeks; the earlier the discordant growth in TTTS, the greater the mortality.[149] Fetoscopic laser coagulation of the placental anastomoses can be done, although mortality is high with a 10% risk of either recurrence of the anastomoses or twin anemia-polycythemia syndrome (TAPS) in which there is no discordance in the amount of amniotic fluid.[48,86,89] TAPS is also seen spontaneously in up to 5% of monochorionic twins.[136,137] Later neurologic abnormalities are increased with TTTS.[9]

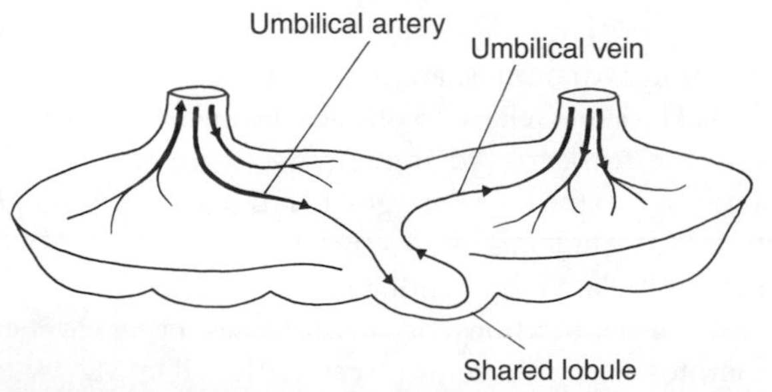

FIGURE 3-22 Vascular anastomoses in shared placental lobules with twin-to-twin transfusion. (From Wigglesworth, J.S. [1996]. *Perinatal pathology* [2nd ed.]. Philadelphia: Saunders.)

Although vascular anastomoses are frequent and extensive in monochorionic-monoamniotic twins, especially in those with closely implanted umbilical cords, twin-to-twin transfusion syndrome is rare in this type of MZ twin. This finding may be because the anastomoses are so extensive that there is no net hydrodynamic imbalance.

Placental vascular anastomoses can also be present between a living and a dead twin, with subsequent passage of thromboplastic substances to the living twin. These substances can initiate intravascular coagulation, thrombosis, infarction, necrosis, alterations in organ function, and death. Vascular abnormalities have been suggested as a cause for development of acardia or amorphous fetuses (shapeless mass of necrotic tissue and fibrin).[36,91,142,156] This anomaly, called *twin reversed arterial perfusion syndrome* (TRAP), occurs in 1% of MZ twins.[90] TRAP likely arises in association with large artery-to-artery and vein-to-vein anastomoses. If pressure in the umbilical artery of the normal twin exceeds that in the artery of the other twin, circulation in the recipient twin may be reversed (i.e., blood flows to the twin via the umbilical arteries and returns to a large placental vein-to-vein anastomosis via the umbilical vein). The resultant low perfusion pressure, poor oxygenation, and circulatory reversal lead to development of multiple severe structural defects. The abnormal twin continues to develop only if there is perfusion by the normal twin, who may subsequently develop cardiac hypertrophy, congestive heart failure, and hydrops fetalis.[91]

Anastomoses in dichorionic fused placentas are rare (1 in 1000) but may account for chimerism in DZ twins. Chimerism may complicate the determination of zygosity.[16] The chimerous twin carries within its system genetically dissimilar blood or tissue from its fraternal twin. Movement of material from one twin to the other is thought to involve transfer of precursor blood cells or other immature cells through vascular communication during early stages of gestation when the fetal immune system is poorly developed. In chimerism, the recipient twin becomes tolerant of the foreign blood cells or tissue from its twin.[84]

SUMMARY

The prenatal period involves major progressive changes in the pregnant woman that support and occur simultaneously with the growth and development of the embryo, fetus, and placenta. The respiratory, nutritive, immunologic, and endocrinologic functions of the placenta are critical for fetal growth and development and pregnancy outcome. A major component of nursing care for women with normal, at risk, and complicated pregnancies is providing appropriate counseling and health teaching to promote optimal fetal development

Table 3-4 Summary of Recommendations for Clinical Practice Related to the Prenatal Period and Placental Physiology

Counsel women regarding physical and physiologic changes during pregnancy and postpartum (pp. 61-63 and Chapters 7 to 20).
Understand the basic processes involved in embryonic and fetal development (pp. 68, 72 and Figure 3-7).
Provide teaching to families regarding embryonic and fetal development at each stage of gestation (pp. 73-78).
Provide appropriate counseling and health teaching to promote optimal fetal development and health (pp. 73-79).
Counsel women regarding the use of drugs or exposure to other environmental agents during pregnancy (pp. 78-79 and Chapter 7).
Recognize and monitor women at risk for ectopic pregnancy (p. 81).
Understand the usual patterns of human chorionic gonadotropin production and counsel women regarding pregnancy testing (pp. 68, 91).
Provide health teaching regarding placental development and growth during gestation (pp. 79-85).
Recognize and monitor for factors that can alter placental growth and development or lead to pregnancy loss (pp. 79-85).
Understand the dynamics of placental function throughout gestation and the factors influencing transfer (pp. 90-96).
Recognize and monitor for factors that can alter maternal-fetal-placental circulation (pp. 87-90).
Recognize the potential effects of maternal disorders on placental function and fetal development (pp. 87-90, 103).
Monitor fetal growth and development (pp. 78-79 and Chapter 12).
Identify fetal risk situations during the antepartum and intrapartum periods related to alterations in placental function (pp. 87-90 and Chapter 6).
Understand endocrine functions of the placenta and interaction of the maternal-fetal-placental unit (pp. 90-93 and Figure 3-14).
Counsel women regarding the effects of estrogen and progesterone on body function and structure during pregnancy (pp. 92-93).
Perform a risk assessment and genetic history as part of routine care (p. 99 and Chapter 1).
Counsel parents about prenatal screening and assist them in interpreting results (pp. 99-100).
Understand the bases and risks of prenatal diagnostic tests (pp. 101-103).
Educate and provide support to families undergoing prenatal diagnosis (pp. 99-103).
Recognize factors that may alter the composition, production, and removal of amniotic fluid (pp. 96-98, 103-105).
Monitor infants with a history of maternal polyhydramnios for congenital defects (pp. 103-104).
Monitor infants with a history of maternal oligohydramnios for congenital anomalies and fetal growth restriction (pp. 104-105).
Inspect the placenta, membranes, and umbilical cord after delivery (pp. 103, 105-106).
Know the implications of placental, umbilical cord, and trophoblastic disorders, and monitor at-risk women and their infants (pp. 103, 106-107).
Teach women who have experienced a multiple birth the basis for development of monozygotic and dizygotic twins (or triplets, quadruplets, and other multiples) and implications of the arrangements of placentas and membranes (pp. 107-109).
Recognize and monitor for fetal and neonatal effects of placental abnormalities with multiple gestation (pp. 109-110).

and health and to prevent exposure of the fetus to adverse environmental influences. To accomplish this goal and to assess maternal and fetal responses to compromised placental function and identify fetal risk situations during the antepartum and intrapartum periods, the nurse must understand the factors influencing transfer of substances across the placenta. An understanding of endocrine functions and interactions of the maternal-fetal-placental unit provides a basis for assessing, monitoring, and teaching pregnant women undergoing various tests for clinical assessment of placental function and fetal well-being. Recommendations for clinical practice are summarized in Table 3-4.

References

1. Akolekar, R., et al. (2009). Maternal plasma inhibin A at 11-13 weeks of gestation in hypertensive disorders of pregnancy. *Prenat Diagn, 29*, 753.
2. American College of Obstetricians and Gynecologists and the American College of Medical Genetics. (2001). *Preconception and prenatal carrier screening for cystic fibrosis: Clinical and laboratory guidelines.* Washington, DC: ACOG.
3. American College of Obstetricians and Gynecologists Committee on Genetics. (2011). ACOG Committee Opinion No. 486: Update on carrier screening for cystic fibrosis. *Obstet Gynecol, 117*, 1028.
4. Aplin, J. (1999). Maternal influences on placental development. *Semin Cell Dev Biol, 11*, 115.
5. Aplin, J.D. & Kimber, S.J. (2004). Trophoblast-uterine interactions at implantation. *Reprod Biol Endocrinol, 2*, 48.
6. Aplin, J.D., Jones, C.J., & Harris, L.K. (2009). Adhesion molecules in human trophoblast—a review. I. Villous trophoblast. *Placenta, 30*, 293.
7. Bahado-Singh, R.O. & Jodicke, C. (2010). Uterine artery Doppler in first-trimester pregnancy screening. *Clin Obstet Gynecol, 53*, 879.
8. Bardawil, W.A., Reddy, R.L., & Bardawil, L.W. (1988). Placental considerations in multiple pregnancy. *Clin Perinatol, 15*, 130.
9. Baschat, A., et al. (2011). Twin-to-twin transfusion syndrome (TTTS). WAPM Consensus Group on Twin-to-Twin Transfusion. *J Perinat Med, 39*, 107.
10. Baschat, A.A. (2010). Ductus venosus Doppler for fetal surveillance in high-risk pregnancies. *Clin Obstet Gynecol, 53*, 858.
11. Beall, M.H. & Ross, M.G. (2009). Amniotic fluid dynamics. In R.K. Creasy, et al. (Eds.). *Creasy & Resnik's Maternal-fetal medicine: Principles and practice* (6th ed.). Philadelphia: Saunders Elsevier.
12. Bebbington, M. (2010). Twin-to-twin transfusion syndrome: Current understanding of pathophysiology, in-utero therapy and impact for future development. *Semin Fetal Neonatal Med, 15*, 15.
13. Benirschke, K. (2009). Multiple gestation: The biology of twinning. In R.K. Creasy, et al. (Eds.). *Creasy & Resnik's Maternal-fetal medicine: Principles and practice*

(6th ed.). Philadelphia: Saunders Elsevier.
14. Benn, P., et al. (2011). Aneuploidy screening: A position statement from a committee on behalf of the Board of the International Society for Prenatal Diagnosis. *Prenat Diagn, 31*, 519.
15. Berkowitz, R.S. & Goldstein, D.P. (2009). Current management of gestational trophoblastic diseases. *Gynecol Oncol, 112*, 654.
16. Boklage, C.E. (2006). Embryogenesis of chimeras, twins and anterior midline asymmetries. *Human Reproduction, 21*, 579.
17. Boyle, K.E., Vlahos, N., & Jarow, J.P. (2004). Assisted reproductive technology in the new millennium: Part II. *Urology, 63*, 217.
18. Brosens, I., et al. (2011). The "Great Obstetrical Syndromes" are associated with disorders of deep placentation. *Am J Obstet Gynecol, 204*, 193.
19. Brosens, J.J., Pijnenborg, R., & Brosens, I.A. (2002). The myometrial junctional zone spiral arteries in normal and abnormal pregnancies: A review of the literature. *Am J Obstet Gynecol, 187*, 1416.
20. Bubb, J.A. & Matthews, A.L. (2004). What's new in prenatal screening and diagnosis? *Prim Care, 31*, 561.
21. Burdine, R.D. & Schier, A.F. (2000). Conserved and divergent mechanisms in left-right axis formation. *Genes Dev, 14*, 763.
22. Burton, G.J. & Jauniaux, E. (2004). Placental oxidative stress: From miscarriage to preeclampsia. *J Soc Gynecol Invest, 11*, 342.
23. Burton, G.J., et al. (2009). Rheological and physiological consequences of conversion of the maternal spiral arteries for uteroplacental blood flow during human pregnancy. *Placenta, 30*, 473.
24. Busjahn, A., et al. (2000). A region on chromosome 3 is linked to dizygotic twinning. *Nat Genet, 4*, 398.
25. Carlson, B.M. (2008). *Human embryology and developmental biology* (4th ed.). St. Louis: Mosby Elsevier.
26. Cecconi, S., et al. (2004). Granulosa cell-oocyte interactions. *Eur J Obstet Gynecol Reprod Biol, 115*, S19.
27. Centers for Disease Control Reproductive Health Information Source. (2009). Assisted reproductive technology success rates: National summary and fertility clinic reports. Available online at *http://www.cdc.gov/art/ART2009_Full_.pdf.*
28. Cheung, A.N. (2003). Pathology of gestational trophoblastic diseases. *Best Pract Res Clin Obstet Gynaecol, 17*, 849.
29. Chucri, T.M., et al. (2010). A review of immune transfer by the placenta. *J Reprod Immunol, 87*, 14.
30. Cole, L.A. (2010). Hyperglycosylated hCG, a review. *Placenta, 31*, 653.
31. Collins, P. (1999). Cellular mechanisms in development. In C.R. Rodeck & M.J. Whittle (Eds.). *Fetal medicine: Basic science and clinical practice*. London: Churchill Livingstone.
32. Cross, J.C. (2006). Nutritional influences on implantation and placental development. *Nutrition Rev, 64*, 512.
33. Cunningham, G., et al. (2009). *Williams obstetrics* (23rd ed.). New York: McGraw-Hill.
34. Damiano, A.E. (2011). Review: Water channel proteins in the human placenta and fetal membranes. *Placenta, 32*, S207.
35. Dancis, J. (1981). Placental transport of amino acids, fats and minerals. In *Placental transport*. Mead Johnson Symposium on Perinatal and Developmental Medicine (No. 18). Evansville, IN: Mead Johnson.
36. Denbow, M.L. & Fisk, N.M. (1998). The consequences of monochorionic placentation. *Baillieres Clin Haematol, 12*, 37.
37. Deprest, J.A., Gratacos, E., & Lewi, L. (2009). Invasive fetal therapy. In R.K. Creasy, et al. (Eds.). *Creasy & Resnik's Maternal-fetal medicine: Principles and practice* (6th ed.). Philadelphia: Saunders Elsevier.
38. Devine, P.C. & Simpson, L.L. (2000). Nuchal translucency and its relation to congenital heart disease. *Semin Perinatol, 24*, 343.
39. Dickey, R., et al. (2002). Spontaneous reduction of multiple pregnancy: Incidence and effect on outcome. *Am J Obstet Gynecol, 186*, 77.
40. Dobson, A.T., et al. (2004). The unique transcriptome through day 3 of human preimplantation development. *Hum Mol Genet, 13*, 1461.
41. Donnai, D. & Read, A.P. (2003). How clinicians add to knowledge of development. *Lancet, 362*, 477.
42. Duc-Goiran, P., et al. (1999). Embryo-maternal interactions at the implantation site: A delicate equilibrium. *Eur J Obstet Gynecol Reprod Biol, 83*, 85.
43. Dugoff, L. & Society for Maternal-Fetal Medicine. (2010). First- and second-trimester maternal serum markers for aneuploidy and adverse obstetric outcomes. *Obstet Gynecol, 115*, 1052.
44. Eisenbach, M. & Tur-Kaspa, I. (1999). Do human eggs attract spermatozoa? *Bioessays, 21*, 203.
45. Evain-Brion, D. (1999). Maternal endocrine adaptation to placental hormones in humans. *Acta Paediatr Suppl, 428*, 12.
46. Faber, J.J. & Thornburg, K.L. (1983). *Placental physiology*. New York: Raven Press.
47. Filly, R.A. (2000). Obstetrical sonography: The best way to terrify a pregnant woman. *J Ultrasound Med, 19*, 1.
48. Fisk, N.M., Duncombe, G.J. & Sullivan, M.H. (2009). The basic and clinical science of twin-twin transfusion syndrome. *Placenta, 30*, 379.
49. Fortunato, A. & Tosti, E. (2011). The impact of in vitro fertilization on health of the children: An update. *Eur J Obstet Gynecol Reprod Biol, 154*, 125.
50. Fox, H. (2007). *Pathology of the placenta* (3rd ed.). Philadelphia: Saunders.
51. Frank, H-G. (2012). Placental development. In R.A. Polin, W.W. Fox & S.H. Abman (Eds.). *Fetal and neonatal physiology* (4th ed.). Philadelphia: Saunders.
52. Freeman, M. (2000). Feedback control of intercellular signaling in development. *Nature, 408*, 313.
53. Gagnon, R., et al. (2009). Guidelines for the management of vasa previa. *J Obstet Gynaecol Can, 31*, 748.
54. Ganapathy, V. (2000). Placental transporters relevant to drug distribution across the maternal-fetal interface. *J Pharmacol Exp Ther, 294*, 413.
55. Goldman-Wohl, D. & Yagel, S. (2002). Regulation of trophoblast invasion: From normal implantation to pre-eclampsia. *Mol Cell Endocrinol, 187*, 233.
56. Goodman, F.R. (2003). Congenital abnormalities of body patterning: Embryology revisited. *Lancet, 362*, 651.
57. Gribbin, C. & James, D. (2004). Assessing fetal health. *Best Pract Res Clin Obstet Gynaecol, 18*, 411.
58. Guyton, A.C. & Hall, J.E. (2010). *Textbook of medical physiology* (12th ed.). Philadelphia: Saunders Elsevier.
59. Haddow, J.E. & Palomaki, G.E. (1999). Biochemical screening for neural tube defects and Down syndrome. In C.H. Rodeck & M.J. Whittle (Eds.). *Fetal medicine: Basic science and clinical practice*. London: Churchill Livingstone.
60. Hall, J.G. (2003). Twinning. *Lancet, 362*, 735.
61. Harper, J.C., Pergament, E., & Delhanty J.D. (2004). Genetics of gametes and embryos. *Eur J Obstet Gynecol Reprod Biol, 115*, S80.
62. Harris, L.K., Jones, C.J. & Aplin, J.D. (2009). Adhesion molecules in human trophoblast—a review. II. Extravillous trophoblast. *Placenta, 30*, 299.
63. Harris, L.K. (2010). Review: Trophoblast-vascular cell interactions in early pregnancy: How to remodel a vessel. *Placenta, 31*, S93.
64. Hofmeyr, G.J. & Gulmezoglu, A.M. (2002). Maternal hydration for increasing amniotic fluid volume in oligohydramnios and normal amniotic fluid volume. *Cochrane Database Syst Rev, 1*, CD000134.
65. Hubel, C.A. (1999). Oxidative stress in the pathogenesis of preeclampsia. *Proc Soc Exp Biol Med, 222*, 222.
66. Hutson, J.R., Koren, G., & Matthews, S.G. (2010). Placental P-glycoprotein and breast cancer resistance protein: Influence of polymorphisms on fetal drug exposure and physiology. *Placenta, 31*, 351.
67. Imakawa, K., Chang, K.T., & Christenson, R.K. (2004). Pre-implantation conceptus and maternal uterine communications:

molecular events leading to successful implantation. *J Reprod Dev, 50*, 155.

68. Jaffe, R. (1998). First trimester utero-placental circulation: Maternal-fetal interaction. *J Perinat Med, 26*, 168.
69. Jauniaux, E. & Gulbis, B. (2000). Fluid compartments of the embryonic environment. *Human Reprod Update, 6*, 268.
70. Jauniaux, E., et al. (2003). Trophoblastic oxidative stress in relation to temporal and regional differences in maternal placental blood flow in normal and abnormal early pregnancies. *Am J Pathol, 162*, 115.
71. Jones, KL. (2005). *Smith's recognizable patterns of human malformation* (6th ed.). Philadelphia: Saunders.
72. Jones, R.L., et al., (2012). Mechanisms of transfer across the human placenta. In R.A. Polin, W.W. Fox, & S.H. Abman (Eds.). *Fetal and neonatal physiology* (4th ed.). Philadelphia: Saunders.
73. Jorde, L.B., et al. (2009). *Medical genetics* (4th ed.). St. Louis: Mosby Elsevier.
74. Kallen, C.B. (2004). Steroid hormone synthesis in pregnancy. *Obstet Gynecol Clin North Am, 31*, 795.
75. Keay, S.D., et al. (2004). The role of hCG in reproductive medicine. *BJOG, 111*, 1218.
76. Khong, T.Y. (2004). Placental vascular development and neonatal outcome. *Semin Neonatol, 9*, 255.
77. Kimber, S.J. & Spanwick, C. (2000). Blastocyst implantation: The adhesion cascade. *Semin Cell Dev Biol, 11*, 77.
78. Kingdom, J. (2000). Development of the placental villous tree and its consequences for fetal growth. *Eur J Obstet Gynecol Reprod Biol, 92*, 35.
79. Kliman, H.J. (2000). Uteroplacental blood flow: The story of decidualization, menstruation, and trophoblast invasion. *Am J Pathol, 157*, 1759.
80. Kodaman, P.H. & Taylor, H.S. (2004). Hormonal regulation of implantation. *Obstet Gynecol Clin North Am, 31*, 745.
81. Krussel, J.S., et al. (2003). Regulations of embryonic implantation. *Eur J Obstet Gynecol Reprod Biol, 110*, S2.
82. Kumar, S. & O'Brien, A. (2005). Recent developments in fetal medicine. *BMJ, 328*, 1002.
83. Lacey, H., et al. (2002). Mesenchymally-derived insulin-like growth factor 1 provides a paracrine stimulus for trophoblast migration. *BMC Dev Biol, 2*, 5.
84. Lavery, J.P. (1987). *The human placenta: Clinical perspectives.* Rockville, MD: Aspen.
85. Lee, M.K., et al., (2012).. Regulation of embryogenesis. In R.A. Polin, W.W. Fox, & S.H. Abman (Eds.). *Fetal and neonatal physiology* (4th ed.). Philadelphia: Saunders.
86. Lewi, L. & Verh, K. (2010). Monochorionic diamniotic twin pregnancies pregnancy outcome, risk stratification and lessons learnt from placental examination. *Acad Geneeskd Belg, 72*, 5.
87. Liu, J.H. (2009). Endocrinology of pregnancy. In R.K. Creasy, et al. (Eds.). *Creasy & Resnik's Maternal-fetal medicine: Principles and practice* (6th ed.). Philadelphia: Saunders Elsevier.
88. Longtine, M.S. & Nelson, D.M. (2011). Placental dysfunction and fetal programming: The importance of placental size, shape, histopathology, and molecular composition. *Semin Reprod Med, 29*, 187.
89. Lopriore, E., et al. (2009). Risk factors for neurodevelopment impairment in twin-twin transfusion syndrome treated with fetoscopic laser surgery. *Obstet Gynecol, 113*, 361.
90. Machin, G. (2009). Non-identical monozygotic twins, intermediate twin types, zygosity testing, and the non-random nature of monozygotic twinning: A review. *Am J Med Genet Part C Semin Med Genet, 151C*, 110.
91. Machin, G.A. (2004). Why is it important to diagnose chorionicity and how do we do it? *Best Pract Res Clin Obstet Gynecol, 18*, 515.
92. Macias, R.I., Marin, J.J., & Serrano, M.A. (2009). Excretion of biliary compounds during intrauterine life. *World J Gastroenterol, 15*, 817.
93. Magriples, U. & Copel, J.A. (2004). Obstetric management of the high-risk patient. In G.N. Burrow, T.P. Dully, & J.A. Copel (Eds.). *Medical complications during pregnancy* (6th ed.). Philadelphia: Saunders.
94. Maiz, N. & Nicolaides, K.H. (2010). Ductus venosus in the first trimester: Contribution to screening of chromosomal, cardiac defects and monochorionic twin complications. *Fetal Diagn Ther, 28*, 65.
95. Mann, S.E., et al. (2006). Steady-state levels of aquaporin 1 mRNA expression are increased in idiopathic polyhydramnios. *Am J Obstet Gynecol, 194*, 884.
96. Mantzoros, C.S. (2000). Role of leptin in reproduction. *Ann N Y Acad Sci, 900*, 174.
97. Marino, T. (2004). Ultrasound abnormalities of the amniotic fluid, membranes, umbilical cord, and placenta. *Obstet Gynecol Clin North Am, 31*, 177.
98. Maruyama, T., et al. (2010). Human uterine stem/progenitor cells: Their possible role in uterine physiology and pathology. *Reproduction, 140*, 11.
99. Mayhew, T.M. & Burton, G.J. (1997). Stereology and its impact on our understanding of human placental functional morphology. *Microsc Res Tech, 38*, 195.
100. Mizejewski, G.J. (2003). Levels of alpha-fetoprotein during pregnancy and early infancy in normal and disease states. *Obstet Gynecol Surv, 58*, 804.
101. Moessinger, A.C. (1989). Morphological consequences of depressed or impaired fetal activity. In W.P. Smotherman & S.R. Robinson (Eds.). *Behavior of the fetus.* Caldwell, NJ: Telford Press.
102. Monga, M. (2009). Maternal cardiovascular, respiratory and renal adaptation to pregnancy. In R.K. Creasy, et al. (Eds.). *Creasy & Resnik's Maternal-fetal medicine: Principles and practice* (6th ed.). Philadelphia: Saunders Elsevier.
103. Moore, K.L., Persaud, T.V.N & Torchia, M.G. (2008). *The developing human: Clinically oriented embryology* (9th ed.). Philadelphia: Saunders.
104. Moore, T.R. (2011). The role of amniotic fluid assessment in evaluating fetal well-being. *Clin Perinatol, 38*, 33.
105. Myatt, L. & Webster, R.P. (2009). Vascular biology of preeclampsia. *J Thromb Haemost, 7*, 375.
106. Myatt, L. (2010). Review: Reactive oxygen and nitrogen species and functional adaptation of the placenta. *Placenta, 31*, S66.
107. Myatt, L. & Sun, K. (2010). Role of fetal membranes in signaling of fetal maturation and parturition. *Int J Dev Biol, 54*, 545.
108. Nagamatsu, T. & Schust, D.J. (2010). The immunomodulatory roles of macrophages at the maternal-fetal interface. *Reprod Sci, 17*, 209.
109. Neri, Q.V., Takeuchi, T., & Palermo, G.D. (2008). An update of assisted reproductive technologies results in the United States. *Ann N Y Acad Sci, 1127*, 41.
110. Nicolaides, K.H., et al. (2006). A novel approach to first-trimester screening for early pre-eclampsia combining serum PP-13 and Doppler ultrasound. *Ultrasound Obstet Gynecol, 27*, 13.
111. Nicolaides, K.H. (2011). Screening for fetal aneuploides at 11 to 13 weeks. *Prenat Diagn, 31*, 7.
112. Norwitz, E.R., Schust, D.J., & Fisher, S.J. (2001). Implantation and the survival of early pregnancy. *N Engl J Med, 345*, 1400.
113. Osol, G. & Mandala, M. (2009). Maternal uterine vascular remodeling during pregnancy. *Physiology (Bethesda), 24*, 58.
114. Panesar, N.S. (1999). Human chorionic gonadotropin: A secretory hormone. *Med Hypotheses, 53*, 136.
115. Papp, C. & Papp, Z. (2003). Chorionic villus sampling and amniocentesis: What are the risks in current practice? *Curr Opin Obstet Gynecol, 15*, 159.
116. Patel, J., et al. (2010). Regulation of hypoxia inducible factors (HIF) in hypoxia and normoxia during placental development. *Placenta, 31*, 951.
117. Petraglia, F., et al. (1998). Paracrine regulation of human placenta: Control of hormonogenesis. *J Reprod Immunol, 39*, 221.
118. Pinjnenborg, R. (1998). The human decidua as a passageway for trophoblast invasion. *Trophoblast Res, 11*, 229.
119. Pringle, K.G., et al. (2010). Beyond oxygen: Complex regulation and activity of hypoxia inducible factors in pregnancy. *Hum Reprod Update, 16*, 415.
120. Publications Committee, Society for Maternal-Fetal Medicine, & Belfort, M.A. (2010). Placenta accreta. *Am J Obstet Gynecol, 203*, 430.
121. Radford, E.J., et al. (2011). Genomic imprinting as an adaptative model of developmental plasticity. *FEBS Lett, 585*, 2059.

122. Ramathal, C.Y., et al. (2010). Endometrial decidualization: Of mice and men. *Semin Reprod Med, 28,* 17.
123. Redline, R. (2011). Placental pathology. In R.J. Martin, A.A. Fanaroff, & M.C. Walsh (Eds.). *Fanaroff and Martin's neonatal-perinatal medicine: Diseases of the fetus and infant* (9th ed.). Philadelphia: Mosby Elsevier.
124. Redline, R.W. (2004). Placental inflammation. *Semin Neonatol, 9,* 265.
125. Richards, C.S. & Haddow, J.E. (2003). Prenatal screening for cystic fibrosis. *Clin Lab Med, 23,* 503.
126. Rittler, M., et al. (2010). Single umbilical artery and associated malformations in over 5500 autopsies: Relevance for perinatal management. *Pediatr Dev Pathol, 13,* 465.
127. Romero, R., et al. (2011). Placental bed disorders in preterm labor, preterm PROM, spontaneous abortion and abruptio placentae. *Best Pract Res Clin Obstet Gynaecol, 25,* 313.
128. Ross, M.G. & Brace, R.A. (2001). National Institutes of Child Health and Human Development conference summary: Amniotic fluid biology—basic and clinical aspects. *J Matern Fetal Med, 10,* 2.
129. Ross, M.G. & Nijland, M.J. (1997). Fetal swallowing: Relation to amniotic fluid regulation. *Clin Obstet Gynecol, 40,* 352.
130. Sadler, T.W. (2012). *Langman's medical embryology* (12th ed.) Philadelphia: Lippincott, Williams & Wilkins.
131. Schindler, A.E. (2004). First trimester endocrinology: Consequences for diagnosis and treatment of pregnancy failure. *Gynecol Endocrinol, 18,* 51.
132. Schoenwolf, G.C., et al. (2009). *Larsen's human embryology* (4th ed.). Philadelphia: Churchill Livingstone Elsevier.
133. Schroder, H.J. & Power, G.G. (1997). Engine and radiator: Fetal and placental interactions for heat dissipation. *Exp Physiol, 82,* 403.
134. Schuler-Maloney, D. (2000). Placental triage of the singleton placenta. *J Midwifery Womens Health, 45,* 104.
135. Sha, X.Y., et al. (2011). Maternal-fetal fluid balance and aquaporins: From molecule to physiology. *Acta Pharmacol Sin, 32,* 716.
136. Slaghekke, F., et al. (2009). TAPS and TOPS: Two distinct forms of fetal-fetal transfusion in monochorionic twins. *Z Geburtshilfe Neonatol, 213,* 248.
137. Slaghekke, F., et al. (2010). Twin anemia-polycythemia sequence: Diagnostic criteria, classification, perinatal management and outcome. *Fetal Diagn Ther, 27,* 181.
138. Sonek, J. & Nicolaides, K. (2010). Additional first-trimester ultrasound markers. *Clin Lab Med, 30,* 573.
139. Staples, D. & Rankin, J. (2010). *Physiology in childbearing with anatomy and related biosciences* (3rd ed.). Edinburgh: Bailliere Tindall.
140. Stewart, T.L. (2004). Screening for aneuploidy: The genetic sonogram. *Obstet Gynecol Clin North Am, 31,* 21.
141. Strewler, G.J. (2000). The physiology of parathyroid hormone-related protein. *N Engl J Med, 20,* 177.
142. Taylor, M.J. & Fisk, N.M. (2000). Prenatal diagnosis in multiple pregnancy. *Baillieres Best Pract Res Clin Obstet Gynaecol, 14,* 663.
143. Tesarik, J. (1999). Calcium: Signaling in human preimplantation development: A review. *J Assist Reprod Genet, 16,* 216.
144. Thompson, J.A. & Regnault, T.R. (2011). In utero origins of adult insulin resistance and vascular dysfunction. *Semin Reprod Med, 29,* 21.
145. Thornton, K.L. (2000). Advances in assisted reproductive technologies. *Obstet Gynecol Clin North Am, 27,* 517.
146. Trundley, A. & Moffett, A. (2004). Human uterine leukocytes and pregnancy. *Tissue Antigens, 63,* 1.
147. Tsui, D.W., Chiu, R.W., & Lo, Y.D. (2010). Epigenetic approaches for the detection of fetal DNA in maternal plasma. *Chimerism, 1,* 30.
148. Vähäkangas, K. & Myllynen, P. (2009). Drug transporters in the human blood-placental barrier. *Br J Pharmacol, 158,* 665.
149. Valsky, D.V., et al. (2010). Selective intrauterine growth restriction in monochorionic twins: Pathophysiology, diagnostic approach and management dilemmas. *Semin Fetal Neonatal Med, 15,* 342.
150. Vedmedovska, N., et al. (2011). Placental pathology in fetal growth restriction. *Eur J Obstet Gynecol Reprod Biol, 155,* 36.
151. Veraksa, A., Del Campo, M., & McGinnis, W. (2000). Developmental patterning genes and their conserved functions: From model organisms to humans. *Mol Genet Metab, 69,* 85.
152. Wald, N.J., et al. (2000). Assay precision of serum alpha fetoprotein in antenatal screening for neural tube defects and Down's syndrome. *J Med Screen, 7,* 74.
153. Wapner, R.J., Jenkins, T.M., & Khalek, N. (2009). Prenatal diagnosis of congenital disorders. In R.K. Creasy, et al. (Eds.). *Creasy & Resnik's Maternal-fetal medicine: Principles and practice* (6th ed.). Philadelphia: Saunders Elsevier.
154. Wassarman, P.M. & Litscher, E.S. (2001). Towards the molecular basis of sperm and egg interaction during mammalian fertilization. *Cells Tissues Organs, 168,* 36.
155. Wassarman P.M., et al. (2004). Egg-sperm interactions at fertilization in mammals. *Eur J Obstet Gynecol Reprod Biol, 115,* S57.
156. Weber, M.A. & Sebire, N.J. (2010). Genetics and developmental pathology of twinning. *Semin Fetal Neonatal Med, 15,* 313.
157. Webster, W.S. & Abela, D. (2007). The effect of hypoxia in development. *Birth Defects Res C Embryo Today, 81,* 215.
158. Weier, N., et al. (2008). Placental drug disposition and its clinical implications. *Curr Drug Metab, 9,* 106.
159. Wilson, R.D. (2000). Amniocentesis and chorionic villus sampling. *Curr Opin Obstet Gynecol, 12,* 81.
160. Wolf, R.B. & Moore, T.R. (2011). Amniotic fluid and nonimmune hydrops fetalis. In R.J. Martin, A.A. Fanaroff, & M.C. Walsh (Eds.). *Fanaroff and Martin's Neonatal-perinatal medicine: Diseases of the fetus and infant* (9th ed.). Philadelphia: Mosby Elsevier.
161. Wright, S.J. (1999). Sperm nuclear activation during fertilization. *Curr Top Dev Biol, 46,* 133.
162. Zhu, X., et al. (2010). The expression of aquaporin 8 and aquaporin 9 in fetal membranes and placenta in term pregnancies complicated by idiopathic polyhydramnios. *Early Hum Dev, 86,* 657.
163. Zuffardi, O., et al. (2011). Array technology in prenatal diagnosis. *Semin Fetal Neonatal Med, 16,* 94.
164. Zygmunt, M., et al. (2003). Angiogenesis and vasculogenesis in pregnancy. *Eur J Obstet Gynecol Reprod Biol, 110,* S10.

CHAPTER 4

Parturition and Uterine Physiology

During parturition the actions of the myometrium, decidua, fetus, placenta, and membranes must be integrated to achieve birth of the fetus without compromising fetal or placental perfusion. This process requires synchronization between myometrial activity and changes in cervical structure and is mediated by a cascade of events and signals that convert the uterus from the quiescent phase seen throughout much of pregnancy to the activated structure needed for birth. Although our understanding of these factors has increased markedly in recent years, many aspects remain unknown.

This chapter reviews the structure of the uterus and individual myometrial cells; changes during pregnancy; physiology of parturition, with respect to cervical dilation, initiation of labor, and myometrial contractions; and clinical implications related to preterm and post term labor onset, labor induction, and dystocia. Maternal pain during labor is discussed in Chapter 15.

UTERUS

The uterus is a major site of physiologic activity during the childbearing years. Alterations in the endometrium occur with the monthly menstrual cycle (see Chapter 2) and during pregnancy (see Chapter 3). Myometrial activity is associated with menstruation, sperm transport, zygote transport, implantation, pregnancy, and parturition.[2] During pregnancy the uterus supports growth and development of the embryo and fetus. At the end of pregnancy, the uterine myometrium must move from a relatively inactive state to produce the strong, synchronous, coordinated contractile forces needed to expel the fetus and placenta. Knowledge of the physiologic changes that bring about this transition in uterine function is incomplete at present but is the focus of much interest and research.

Uterine Structure

The uterine wall consists of three layers: (1) internal endometrium, (2) myometrium, and (3) external serous epithelial layer, with an area known as the junctional zone between the first two layers.[33,88] The thin serosa protects the uterus and provides a relatively inelastic base upon which the myometrium develops tension to increase intrauterine pressure. During early pregnancy the endometrial cells enlarge and a hypersecretory state develops with changes in cellular composition as the endometrium is remodeled into the decidua to support implantation, placental development, and fetal nutrition (see Chapter 3).[96]

The myometrium consists of four muscle layers separated by a vascular zone. The muscle layers form a web that supports and protects the developing fetus. The inner layer, below the decidua, is circular and perpendicular to the long axis of the uterus. This layer runs clockwise and counterclockwise in a spiral. The middle layer consists of interlacing fibers in a figure-eight shape interspersed with blood vessels. The outer two layers run parallel to the longitudinal axis of the uterus.[96,145] These muscle layers are composed of smooth muscle cells arranged in interconnected bundles of 10 to 50 partially overlapping cells set in a matrix of collagenous connective tissue and ground substance.[18,47] The ground substance transmits the contractile forces from individual myometrial cells along the muscle bundle.[18] Around the bundles of smooth muscle cells are fibroblasts, blood and lymphatic vessels, and nerve cells. The subendothelial myometrium forms the junctional zone where myometrial contractions arise in the nonpregnant uterus.[88,96] Myocytes in the junctional zone have a greater nuclear area, decreased extracellular matrix, less water content, and greater blood perfusion than those in the outer myometrium.[88] Because the uterine muscle layers have different embryonic origins, they have distinct hormonal responses and thus may respond differentially to uterotonic agonists and antagonists.[88]

The uterus is innervated primarily by the sympathetic nervous system along with some fibers from the cerebrospinal tract and the parasympathetic nervous system.[33] These include adrenergic neurons (postganglionic sympathetic fibers from lumbar and mesenteric ganglia), cholinergic neurons (sparse, primarily innervating the cervix), and peptidergic neurons.[96] Adrenergic fibers are most dense in the fallopian tubes, cervix, and vagina and are relatively sparse in the uterine corpus and fundus. In comparison to other smooth muscle cells, which tend to be richly innervated, the uterus has a relatively low density of nerves to smooth muscles cells.[47] The myometrium normally contracts spontaneously unless this ability is altered by endocrine, paracrine, or apocrine factors.

This intrinsic ability is suppressed during pregnancy, then enhanced during labor.[2]

The role of the nervous system in myometrial activity is poorly understood. The adrenergic and peptidergic nerves may play a role in suppressing myometrial contractility during pregnancy.[18,47] Adrenergic fibers in the uterine wall disappear near term, leaving only those in the cervix and uterine horns. Peptidergic and sympathetic nerves also decrease markedly during pregnancy.[182] Thus control of contractility during pregnancy changes to local control, particularly prostaglandins (PGs) in the decidua and chorion and oxytocin in the myometrium. Communication between myometrial cells during labor occurs primarily via gap junctions (see "Gap Junction Formation").

Uterine Growth

The nonpregnant uterus weighs 40 g to 50 g, increasing to 1100 g to 1200 g by term; uterine volume increases from 10 mL to 5 L.[131] The elastic properties of the uterus support its growth during pregnancy. The uterus increases in weight, length, width, depth, volume, and overall capacity during pregnancy. Uterine growth begins after implantation. Initially, growth primarily involves hyperplasia and is influenced by estrogen and growth factors (e.g., insulin-like growth factor 1 [IGF-1], epidermal growth factor, transforming growth factors, fibroblast growth factor-β), and is independent of the effects of stretching from the growing embryo.[19,96,116,176] This early uterine growth occurs regardless of whether the embryo is implanted in the uterus or at an extrauterine site.[136,145]

Later uterine growth involves primarily hypertrophy of the myocytes, stimulated by estrogens, and remodeling of the extracellular matrix, mediated by distention of the uterus by the enlarging fetus.[96,116,131] As the uterus grows, the ratio of ribonucleic acid (RNA) to deoxyribonucleic acid (DNA) increases due to increased RNA synthesis and total protein. By 3 to 4 months, the uterine wall has thickened from 10 to 25 mm. With further distention the wall thins to 5 to 10 mm at term. Myometrial smooth muscle fibers increase in length from 50 to 500 μm and width from 5 to 15 μm due to a progressive increase in actin and myosin content.[116,136,145] The isthmus becomes thinner and more distensible forming the lower uterine segment.[131] Smooth muscle cell creatinine phosphatase, adenosine triphosphate (ATP), and adenosine diphosphate (ADP) also increase to term.[136] The isthmus does not undergo hypertrophy and becomes thin and distensible in order to allow passage of the fetus.[116]

The height of the uterine fundus reaches the maternal umbilicus by about 20 weeks' gestation and the xiphoid process of the sternum by 8 months. As the fetal head descends into the pelvis ("lightening") late in gestation, the fundal height becomes slightly lower.

After 12 to 16 weeks' gestation, as the fundus changes from a spherical shape to become more dome shaped, distention occurs primarily in a cephalic direction.[116] The shape of the fundus influences intrauterine pressure. In a sphere, tension is a geometric function of the radius of curvature; in a cylinder, tension is a linear function (and thus is lower).[136] In the absence of contractions, intrauterine pressure peaks at midpregnancy, then decreases as the shape of the fundus changes. The pressure remains low until term in spite of the increasing intrauterine volume.

Uterine smooth muscle undergoes phasic contractile activity. At mid-gestation, contractions of the circular muscles of the uterus are weaker than those of the longitudinal muscles. Contractile strength increases in the circular muscles so that by term these muscles are similar to longitudinal muscles in their contractile ability. The basis for this change is thought to be differences in membranous electrical events, cell-to-cell coupling via gap junctions, and intracellular calcium release.[47]

MYOMETRIUM

The myometrium has two basic properties: contractility and elasticity. Contractility is the ability to lengthen and shorten. Elasticity is the ability to grow and stretch to accommodate the enlarging uterine contents, maintain uterine tonus, and permit involution following delivery.

Myometrial Cell Structure

The contractile units of the uterus are the smooth muscle cells in a connective tissue matrix. Movement of contractile forces along the uterus occurs from transmission of tension generated by individual smooth muscle cells to other smooth muscle cells and the connective tissue matrix.[47] Uterine smooth muscles are unique in that active, synchronous contraction of these muscles occurs only during the birth process.

Myometrial cells contain three types of protein myofilaments (actin, myosin, and intermediate), microtubules, and protein structures called dense bodies. Myosin is a hexamer approximately 160 nm long. Myosin is the principal contractile protein. Myosin is laid down in thick (15 to 18 nm) myofilaments that optimize interaction with actin and generation of force.[18,96] Myosin filaments consist of two heavy chains, with a molecular weight of 200 kilodaltons (kDa), arranged in a head-and-tail structure and two light chains. The helical heavy chains unite at one end of the filament to form two globular heads that protrude from the myosin at regular intervals (Figure 4-1).[1,116] The two light chains (molecular weights of 20 and 17 kDa) are bound to the head in the neck region (see Figure 4-1). The longer light chain (molecular weight 20 kDa) has a regulator role in muscle contraction and can bind to calcium and magnesium and become phosphorylated.[1,18,96,116] In addition to the two light chains, the myosin head also contains sites for magnesium adenosine triphosphatase (Mg-ATPase) (an enzyme necessary for the interaction of actin and myosin and subsequent generation of force) and an actin binding site where the actin and myosin interact.[18,96] The helical tail, formed by the heavy chains, transmits the force (tension) generated by the interaction of myosin and actin. Myosin filaments are unidirectional and

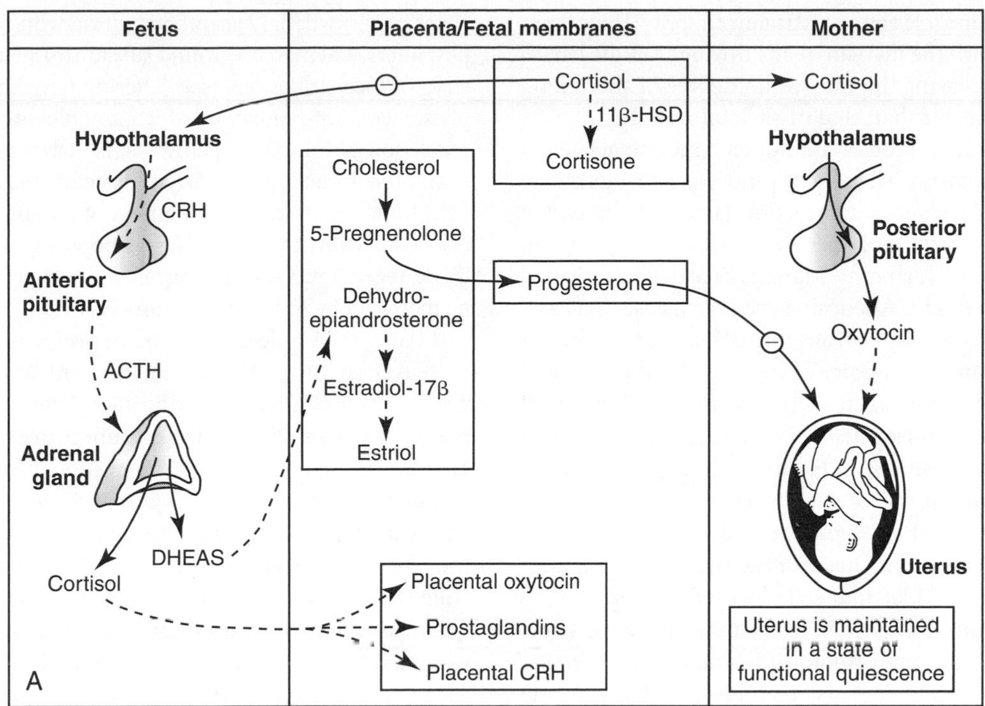

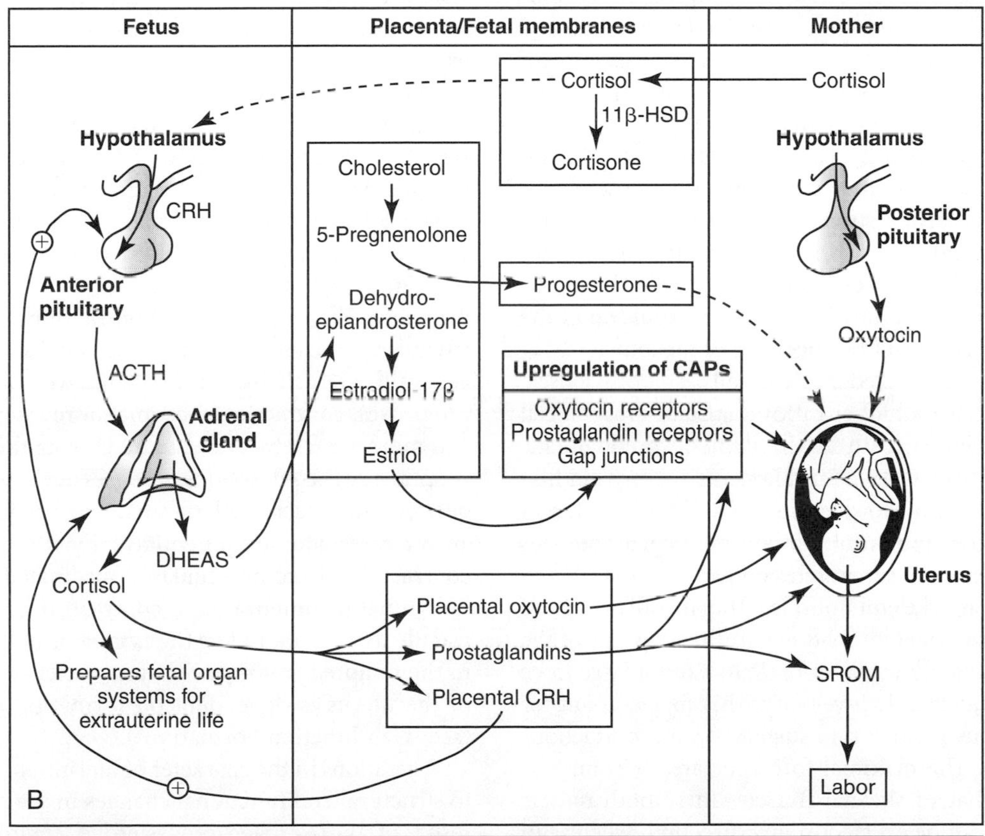

FIGURE 4-1 Proposed parturition cascade for labor induction at term. The spontaneous induction of labor at term in the human is regulated by a series of paracrine and autocrine hormones acting in an integrated parturition cascade. **A,** The factors responsible for maintaining uterine quiescence throughout pregnancy are shown. **B,** The factors responsible for the onset of spontaneous labor are shown. They include the withdrawal of the inhibitory effects of progesterone on uterine contractility and the recruitment of cascades that promote estrogen (estriol) production and lead to up regulation of the contraction-associated protein in the uterus. *ACTH,* Adrenocorticotropic hormone (corticotropin); *CAPs,* contraction-associated proteins; *CRH,* corticotropin-releasing hormone; *DHEAS,* dehydroepiandrostenedione; *11β-HSD,* 11β-hydroxysteroid dehydrogenase; *SROM,* spontaneous rupture of membranes. (From Norwitz, E.R. & Lye, S.J. [2009]. Biology of parturition. In R.K. Creasy, et al. [Eds.]. *Creasy & Resnik's Maternal-fetal medicine: Principles and practice* (6th ed.). Philadelphia: Saunders Elsevier, p. 71.)

longer in smooth muscle than in striated muscle. This allows actin to interact with the myosin heads throughout the length of the myosin, increasing the maximum degree of shortening to 5 to 10 times greater than that of skeletal muscle.[18,96]

Actin is a globular protein monomer (molecular weight 45 kDa) with six isoforms. The α-actin and γ-actin isoforms are the ones primarily involved in contraction; β-actin forms part of the cytoskeleton.[1] Actin polymerizes into long, thin (6 to 9 nm) filaments. These filaments originate in and are distributed between dense bodies.[116] Adenosine triphosphatase (ATPase) activity on the myosin head initiates formation of cross-links or bonds between actin and myosin. The myosin head rotates and as a result pulls on the actin filament, creating tension (force) and a relative spatial displacement (shortening).[96] Interaction of myosin and actin is illustrated in Figure 4-1.

The intermediate fibers form a structural network. These fibers may be involved in signal transduction, contractile activity, and secretion of collagen and extracellular matrix components.[1,19] Interstitial-like cells located on the borders of myometrial smooth muscle bundles may also have a role in cell signaling.[68] The microtubules, formed by tubulin, are involved in myometrial hyperplasia and hypertrophy during pregnancy. Tubulin is a substrate for G-protein receptor kinase, a substance involved in myosin phosphorylation and down-regulation of β_2-adrenoreceptors.[19] The dense protein bodies are scattered throughout the cytoplasm and on the inner surface of the cell membrane and are attached to the poles of the smooth muscle cell by intermediate (10-nm thick) filaments and actin thin filaments. The dense bodies and their filaments form a supportive structure for the contractile filaments and a network of actin attachment sites (adhesion plaques).[18,19,96] These structures enable the uterus to enlarge and generate forces sufficient for expulsion of the fetus regardless of the weight or position of the fetus.

In comparison to striated muscle cells, smooth muscle cells are smaller, have a higher ratio of surface area–to–cell volume, and have less myosin. Actin filaments predominate, with approximately 11 to 15 actin filaments per myosin filament versus a 6:1 ratio in skeletal muscle.[18,96] Filaments in smooth muscle occur in random rather than regular bundles throughout the cell, so these muscles do not have the striated appearance seen in skeletal muscle. The myofilaments in smooth muscle are oriented obliquely to the long axis of the muscle fibers, which allows the muscle to exert a large force along a short distance at low velocity. This may account for the ability of the myometrium to sustain strong contractions over many hours. The maximal force per area is similar to or greater than that of skeletal muscle. In smooth muscle the pulling force can be exerted in any direction, whereas in skeletal muscle the force generated and the resultant contraction are aligned with the axis of the muscle fibers.[18]

Changes During Pregnancy

During pregnancy the myometrium is thought to undergo changes in cellular phenotype. These proposed phases include (1) early proliferative phase with myocyte hyperplasia (see "Uterine Growth"); (2) synthetic phase with myocyte hypertrophy, interstitial matrix (ground substance) synthesis and remodeling of local adhesions (see "Uterine Growth"); (3) contractile phase with up-regulation of contractile proteins and down-regulation of inhibitory pathways; (4) labor phase with expression of contraction-associated proteins (CAPs), synthesis of uterotonic agents and development of intense contractions; and (5) postpartum involution with apoptosis, wound repair, and tissue regenerations (see Chapter 5).[163] Postpartum repair may be mediated by myometrial stem cells.[101,163]

Myometrial quiescence during pregnancy is mediated by increases in progesterone, relaxin, nitric oxide (NO), and prostacyclin (PGI_2).[96] Uterine blood flow increases during pregnancy from 2% of cardiac output prior to pregnancy to 10% to 20% by term.[131] Uterine blood flow is redistributed from similar amounts flowing to endometrium and myometrium in the nonpregnant uterus to 80% to 90% flowing to the placenta during pregnancy, with the remainder divided equally between the endometrium and myometrium.[131] Changes in uterine blood flow are due to decrease placental vascular resistance as a result of remodeling of the spiral arteries, which results in increased vessel diameter and decreased resistance (these changes are described in Chapter 3), estrogens, vascular endothelial growth factor, angiotensin II, nitric oxide, and prostacyclin.[131]

The uterus is never completely quiescent; low-frequency, low-amplitude activity occurs even in the nonpregnant state.[1,18,96,115] The frequency of contractions increases during pregnancy with an increase of approximately 5% per week.[118] Diurnal periodicity has been reported with increased frequency at night (five to six per hour) and lowered frequency in the early afternoon (two to three per hour) near term.[118] Initially these contractions tend to be mild, irregular, nonsynchronized, and focal in origin and are generally not felt by the pregnant woman. As pregnancy progresses, contractions become more intense and frequent and more are felt by the woman. During the third trimester, spontaneous contractions progressively increase in frequency with decreased negative membrane potential and an increase in action potentials.[139] With the onset of labor, contractions become regular, coordinated, and intense as individual myometrial cells contract in harmony. The contractile force is about five times greater in the pregnant than in the nonpregnant myometrium. Synchronous contraction of the uterus is dependent on formation of gap junctions (see "Gap Junction Formation").[47,115,116]

Alterations in the character of uterine contractions are due to structural and functional changes in the myometrium as a result of the estrogen-progesterone environment of pregnancy. These changes include the following:

1. Change in the velocity and timing of action potentials. In the nonpregnant uterus, action potentials occur at the peak of a contraction at a velocity of about 6 cm/sec. In pregnancy the action potential occurs much closer to the beginning of the contraction wave and at 1 to 2 cm/sec.

2. Hypertrophy and hyperplasia of the myometrial cells, with increased contractile proteins, under the influence of estrogen.
3. Increased sensitivity of the myometrium to the effects of myosin light chain kinase phosphorylation.
4. Alteration in the arrangement of muscle bundles. In pregnancy these bundles are arranged in closer contact enhancing gap junction formation.
5. Development of the sarcoplasmic reticulum. This enhances calcium movement.
6. Increased number of mitochondria and cellular adenosine triphosphate (ATP). This enhances energy production by the myometrial cell.[1,47,103,115,116,131]

Near labor onset the myometrial contractile capacity increases as the myometrium undergoes activation (see "Parturition"). There is enhanced communication among the cells of the uterus at term, so that the action potential covers the entire uterus in 2 to 3 seconds, resulting in nearly simultaneous contraction of the myometrium. This phenomenon may result from the increased velocity of the action potentials, the closer arrangement of muscle bundles with gap junction formation, and the increased number of muscle cells.[47,118]

CERVIX

During pregnancy the cervix increases in mass, water content, and vascularization. The connective tissue of the uterus (particularly the cervix) undergoes changes in its viscoelastic plasticity so that, by term, "it combines the properties of a rubber band with those of saltwater taffy."[136] In order for the fetus to be expelled, the cervix must first change from a relatively rigid to a soft, distensible structure. Myometrial contractions exert a slow, steady pull on the cervix, resulting in cervical stretching but with little rebound between contractions. This leads to progressive cervical dilation.

Structure of the Cervix

The cervix is composed of an extracellular connective tissue matrix (composed primarily of collagen, elastin, and proteoglycans) covered by a thin cellular layer of smooth muscle and fibroblasts that penetrate into the connective tissue matrix.[95,116] Approximately 85% to 90% of the cervix is connective tissue matrix and 10% to 15% is smooth muscle.[78,160] The amount of smooth muscle varies between the upper (25%), middle (16%), and lower (6%) portions of the cervix. The extracellular matrix is made from substances secreted by the fibroblasts.[8] This matrix consists of a dense network of interlacing collagen and elastin fibers embedded in a gel-like ground substance (proteoglycans).

The collagen fibers form a relatively rigid rod-shaped structure (important during pregnancy to retain the fetus) and impart tensile strength to the cervix.[18] Collagen in the cervix is primarily types I and III (found mainly in the connective tissue stroma) and type IV (associated with smooth muscle and vascular components).[78] About 80% of the collagen in the stroma is type I and 20% is type III.[160] The collagen fibers are arranged in cross-linked triple helices. The cross-linking protects the collagen fibers from being broken down by collagenase and proteases.[95] Elastin is haphazardly arranged parallel to and between collagen fibers, imparting elasticity to the cervical tissue and contributing to the integrity of the tissue.[47,95] The elastin-to-collagen ratio is greatest at the internal os. Elastin can stretch in any direction to twice its length and thus may be important in the ability of the cervix to distend in labor and then return to its normal shape after parturition.[95,115]

The ground substance (proteoglycans) is composed of glycosaminoglycans attached to a glycoprotein core. The major glycosaminoglycans in the cervix are dermatan sulfate (70%), heparan sulfate (15%), and hyaluronan (15%).[18] These substances are large charged molecules that bind together, attract water, and coil around and lock the collagen fibrils in place.[18]

Changes During Pregnancy

Cervical remodeling is noted throughout pregnancy and includes softening, ripening dilation, and subsequent repair.[150,181] Softening begins in the first trimester and is a slow process mediated by progesterone. Changes in collagen structure with decreased cross linking and increased solubility, decreased tensile strength and increased epithelial repair, and protective factors are all characteristics of cervical softening.[181]

In the nonpregnant cervix, collagen fibers are in bundles forming cable-like structures. As pregnancy progresses the bundles become less dense with thinner and more loosely packed fibers.[95] Hyaluronan (which has a high affinity for water) and cervical water content increase.[95] The total collagen increases and is remodeled to maintain cervical integrity. However, the relative amount of collagen decreases 30% to 50% as a result of increases in other proteins and in the water content of the extracellular matrix.[188] Decorin, a dermatan sulfate proteoglycan that coats the collagen fibers, increases during later pregnancy and labor.[95,116] Decorin and hyaluronan separate the collagen fibrils, increasing fibril dispersion and disorganization.[188] Smooth muscle cells in the cervix enlarge, then later undergo programmed cell death at term.[95]

Fibroblasts, leukocytes, macrophages, and eosinophils proliferate in the cervix during pregnancy. These changes may be important in altering vasopermeability to increase cervical water content and in secretion of proteases for cervical ripening. The fibroblasts are also involved in the metabolism of collagen and glycosaminoglycans. Fibronectin is also found in the cervix and decreases at labor onset.[95] Fibronectin may act as a "biologic glue." Collagenase activity increases threefold, beginning as early as 10 weeks; elastase activity increases toward the end of pregnancy and after parturition.

Cervical Ripening and Dilation

The rigid cervix of pregnancy must become distensible in order to expel the fetus.[18] Cervical ripening and distention begins several weeks before delivery and involves biochemical changes in the cervix that are mediated by both hormonal factors (estrogens, progesterone) and mechanical factors (cervical stretch and the pressure from the descending fetal head).[131] This process is accompanied by localized decreases in progesterone and increases in estrogen levels, increased tissue water content, increased high molecular weight hyaluronan, increased tissue monocytes and vascularization, and a marked decrease in tensile strength.[181] After delivery, postpartum repair is mediated by synthesis of extracellular matrix molecules, metabolism of high molecular weight hyaluronan to the low molecular weight form, proinflammatory gene expression, increased neutrophils, and macrophage activation.[181]

Ripening and dilation are inflammatory processes that involve changes in collagen, proteoglycans, and smooth muscle with enzymatic degradation of collagen.[136,150,175] Factors responsible for the maintenance of cervical integrity during pregnancy and cervical ripening at the end of pregnancy include remodeling of the extracellular matrix and apoptosis mediated by increases in degradative enzymes such as matrix metalloproteinases (MMPs), synthesis of extracellular matrix proteins, increased collagen turnover, disruption of collagen fibrils, increase in the decorin-to-collagen ratio, increased hyaluronan and thus cervical water content, and infiltration of the cervix by neutrophils and macrophages.[26,131,144,150,188] These processes are mediated by cytokines such as interleukin-1 (IL-1), interleukin-6 (IL-6), interleukin-8 (IL-8), and tumor necrosis factor–α (TNF-α). IL-1 and TNF-α alter the adhesiveness of vascular epithelium. IL-6 increases prostaglandin (PG) and leukotriene (LT) production. This dilates cervical blood vessels and enhances movement of neutrophils into the cervix. IL-8 is a proinflammatory chemokine (chemokines are a type of cytokine that mediates chemoattraction) that stimulates MMP-8 and increases neutrophil chemotaxis.[78,175,188] IL-8 and similar substances attract inflammatory cells that release proinflammatory cytokines such as IL-1β and THF-α. These cytokines activate the nuclear factor-kappa B (NF-κB) signaling pathway, which can block progesterone receptor mediated actions.[150]

Collagen is degraded by MMPs such as collagenase, elastase, and other nonspecific proteolytic enzymes, resulting in a loss of collagen fibrils. The MMP system is a series of proteins that, with zinc as a cofactor, act in a cascade to degrade collagen. Both MMPs and MMP inhibitors increase during pregnancy. During most of pregnancy these are in balance, but in late pregnancy there is a net increase in MMPs, leading to collagen degradation and disorganization. Hyaluronan (which loosely binds collagen fibrils) stimulates MMP production in the cervix and neutrophil chemotaxis.[95] Neutrophils and macrophages also secrete MMP and are a major source of MMP-8 (neutrophil collagenase).[78] MMP activity is enhanced by IL-1 and IL-8. Hyaluronan increases by 50% with labor onset, then decreases rapidly after delivery, accompanied by a decrease in dermatan sulfates, especially decorin (which tightly binds collagen fibrils thus resulting in loosening and dispersal of collagen bundles), and an increase in the water content of the cervix.[40,95,116] This weakens the structure of the cervix by decreasing the cross-bridges between collagen fibers and decreases the collagen content by 50%.[40]

A proposed mechanism for the process of cervical ripening and dilation is illustrated in Figure 4-2. In summary, cervical ripening involves an inflammatory cascade with

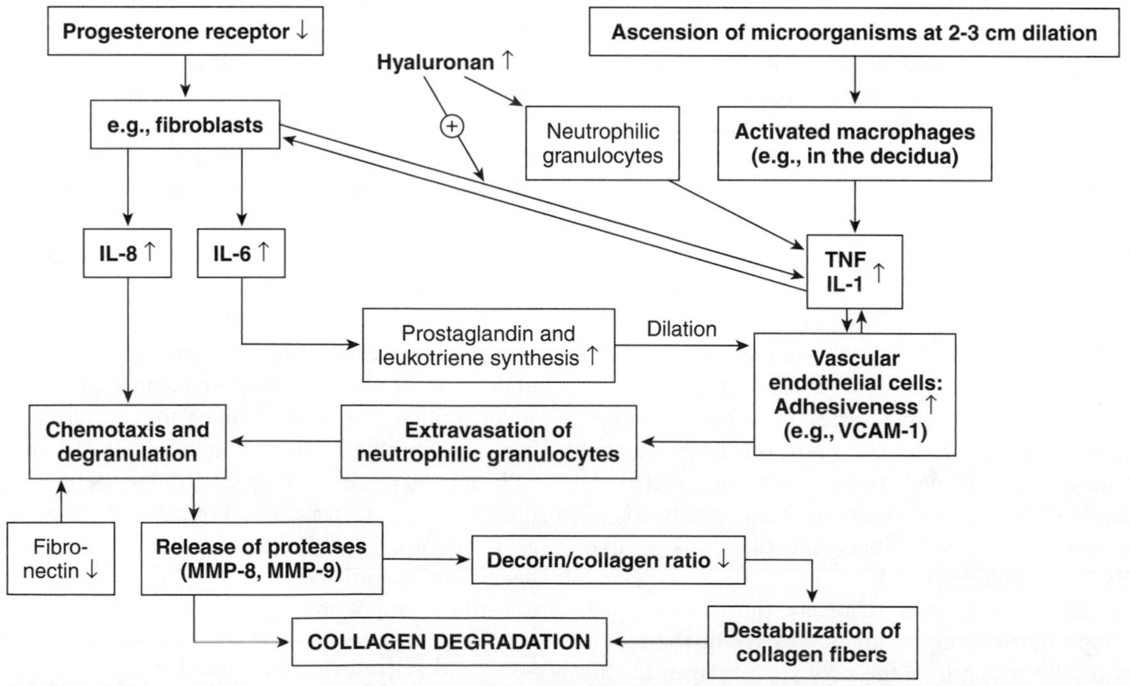

FIGURE 4-2 Hypothetical model for the biochemical changes during cervical dilation at term. *IL*, Interleukin; *MMP*, matrix metalloproteinase; *TNF*, tumor necrosis factor *VCAM*, vascular cell adhesion molecule. (From Winkler, M. & Rath, W. [1999]. Changes in the cervical extracellular matrix during pregnancy and parturition. *J Perinatol Med, 27*, 58.)

release of proinflammatory cytokines (e.g., IL-1, IL-6, especially IL-8, TNF-α), leading to infiltration of the cervix by leukocytes and macrophages, which in turn release and activate MMPs. MMPs alter the synthesis of extracellular matrix proteins, and increase collagen turnover and retention of water.[27] As a result, collagen is degraded and collagen fibers are disrupted and dispersed.

Hormonal control of cervical ripening is a complex process that involves a cascade of changes in estradiol, progesterone, and relaxin mediated by PGI_2, PGE_2, $PGF_{2\alpha}$, nitric oxide (NO), and cytokines.[18,26,27,114,122] Progesterone inhibits collagen breakdown. Alterations in the estrogen-to-progesterone ratio correlate with increased procollagenase activity, collagen degradation, and apoptosis (programmed cell death). Increased cervical relaxin may activate collagen peptidase and mediate changes in water and mucopolysaccharide content of the cervix.[18] Uterine activity is enhanced by mechanical stretching of the cervix (Ferguson reflex). This response may be due to the effects of $PGF_{2\alpha}$ and oxytocin release stimulated by cervical stretching.

PGE_2 and $PGF_{2\alpha}$ have a localized influence on cervical softening. PGE_2 action on the cervix is independent of uterine contractile activity and is used to improve cervical inductability (i.e., responsiveness of the cervical tissue) before induction of labor (e.g., when delivery is indicated because of risk factors). PGE_2 also dilates small blood vessels in the cervix—increasing leukocyte extravasation—and stimulates neutrophil chemotaxis.[96] Prostaglandins also enhance collagenase activity, increase production of proteoglycans that bind water, and decrease decorin, which is needed for collagen stability.

NO in the cervix increases near term and may act with PGE_2 to induce cervical vasodilatation and neutrophil infiltration, and may regulate MMP activation.[26,27,122] Inductable nitric oxide synthetase (iNOS) is present in macrophages and regulates NO in response to inflammatory stimuli. NO stimulates release of PGE_2 and regulates cyclooxygenase-2 (COX-2, an enzyme needed to convert arachidonic acid to PGs) to locally increase PGE_2.[175,186]

RUPTURE OF FETAL MEMBRANES

The fetal membranes are a major site of prostaglandin synthesis and metabolism. The fetal membranes also contain abundant 11-beta hydroxysteroid dehydrogenase-1 (11β-HSD1), which converts inactive cortisone to active cortisol, and thus plays a role in regulating metabolism and transport of cortisol between fetal and maternal circulations (see Chapter 19).[121] A possible feedback loop within the fetal membranes has been postulated involving glucocorticoids, proinflammatory cytokines, surfactant protein-A, 11β-HSD1, prostaglandins, and cortisol to enhance fetal organ maturation and labor onset (see "Initiation of Labor").[121]

The amnion and chorion are connected by an extracellular matrix (fibrous proteins embedded in polysaccharide gelatinous matter). The chorion adheres to the decidua. With delivery, the decidua and chorion must separate to allow expulsion of the membranes. This process involves fetal fibronectin, an extracellular matrix protein found at the decidual-chorionic interface.[121,150]

The exact mechanism for rupture of the membranes is unknown, but is thought to be due to "a programmed biochemical set of events leading to collagen remodeling and superimposed physical stretch forces leading directly to tissue damage" and thus rupture.[84] The fetal membranes are distended 40% at 25 to 27 weeks' gestation, 60% at 30 to 34 weeks and 70% at term.[150] Membrane rupture is associated with disruption of the extracellular matrix and basement membrane by matrix metalloproteinases (MMPs) that alter collagen (a major component of the amnion and chorion) and degrade components of these structures.[43,53,185]

The tensile strength of the membranes, which is greater in the amnion, is imparted by type I, III, and IV collagenous fibers that maintain the noncollagenous components (elastin, proteoglycans, microfibrils, decorin, plasminogen, and integrins) of the extracellular matrix.[111,135] The extracellular matrix and the membranes themselves undergo continual remodeling by MMPs during pregnancy to adapt to changes in uterine pressure and volume.[111] This process is regulated by a balance between MMPs and tissue inhibitors of MMPs (TIMPs) mediated by prostaglandins (PGs), cytokines, and chemokines.[53,111] Labor is associated with an increase in MMPs and a decrease in TIMPs. Increases in neutrophils, macrophages, and monocytes and in the decidual-chorionic interface right before labor onset, coinciding with increases in proinflammatory cytokines and chemokines enhances this process.[43,53,122,123,185] IL-1 and TNF-α, which increase during labor, may in turn mediate up-regulation of MMPs, induce apoptosis, and increase PGE_2.[84] Regional induction of MMPs in the membranes over the internal cervical os before labor may target this area for later rupture.[101,112] This area is reported to have increased MMP-9, decreased TIMP, and increased apoptosis with labor.[41,53,117,135,150]

Hyperdistention with pressure of the presenting part along with increased hydrophobicity results in loss of phospholipids that normally lubricate the chorion-amnion interface, leading to increased shear force with cellular fracturing and rupture. Stripping of the membranes results in mechanical disruption as well as increasing phospholipase A_2 release, both of which increase $PGF_{2\alpha}$.[179]

Premature rupture of the membranes (PROM), or rupture before onset of uterine contractions, may be due to factors such as mechanical stress (polyhydramnios, multiple gestation), alterations in membranous collagen, or chorioamnionitis.[111] These events may result in increases in extracellular matrix degrading enzymes and inappropriate MMP activation.[111] Women with PROM have alterations in membranes such as decreased collagen fibers, disruption of collagen fiber patterns and deposition of amorphous material between the fibers.[150] With chorioamnionitis a variety of vaginal and cervical microorganisms have been demonstrated to produce proteases that alter membrane integrity and reduce the pressure needed for rupture. PROM may be mediated by collagenalytic enzymes from the placenta and amniotic fluid that increase in activity with increasing gestational age. Deficiency of protease inhibitors and abnormal expression of certain MMPs have been reported in PROM.[183,185]

PARTURITION

"Parturition is a multifactorial physiologic process that involves multiple interconnected positive feed forward and negative feedback loops. Each of these loops is connected to others in a carefully time-regulated fashion. When parturition occurs normally, both maternal and fetal processes are involved."[126] Parturition is an inflammatory event modulated by environmental, endocrine, and physical factors. At term this inflammatory process is a response to hormonal signals from the fetus and mechanical stretch; in preterm labor it may be due to infection or other processes that alter tissue integrity.[109] Initiation of labor is associated with migration of leukocytes and macrophages into the myometrium, cervix and fetal membranes, release of chemotaxic factors leading to increased expression of proinflammatory cytokines and increased NF-κB (transcription factor that regulates gene expression).[52,109,150] Mendelson proposed that this inflammatory response and NF-κB activation "promote uterine contractility via (1) direct activation of contractile genes (e.g., COX-2[cyclooxygenase-2], oxytocin receptor, and connexin 43) and (2) impairment of the capacity of PR [progesterone receptor] to mediate uterine quiescence."[109] Parturition involves anatomic, biochemical, immunologic, endocrinologic, and clinical events.[150] The major events in parturition are fetal membrane rupture, cervical dilation, myometrial contractility, placental separation, and uterine involution.

Initiation of Labor

Initiation of labor involves a complex interplay of maternal and fetal factors and endocrine signaling whose specific interrelationships and significance are still not completely understood.[22,74,152] Labor initiation is regulated by the fetal genome via two integrated pathways: endocrine (fetal hypothalamic-pituitary-placental axis) and mechanical (fetal growth places tension of the uterine wall), which leads to myometrial biochemical and molecular changes that increase contraction-associated proteins (CAPs) involved in myometrial excitability.[163] Prostaglandins are the final common pathway ion mechanisms of labor onset. Challis and colleagues proposed that parturition is divided into four phases: (1) phase 0, quiescence; (2) phase 1, activation; (3) phase 2, stimulation; and (4) phase 3, involution.[19] Phase 0 occurs for 95% of pregnancy. During this phase, progesterone and other uterotonic inhibitors—including PGI_2, relaxin, NO, and parathyroid hormone–related peptide (PTHrP)—maintain myometrial quiescence.[109]

Phase 1, activation, accounts for about 5% of the duration of pregnancy. During this phase, levels of uterotonic inhibitors decrease, whereas estrogen increases, mediated by transcription factors that up regulate expression of contraction-associated proteins (CAPs).[52,163] CAPs include gap junction proteins (particularly connexin 43 [Cx43]), myometrial oxytocin receptors, PGE_2 receptors (EP_1 to EP_4), $PGF_{2\alpha}$ receptors (FP), and calcium channels.[19,96] Activation involves an increase in expression of genes that encode CAPs. A major transcription factor that regulates CAP expression is NF-κB and its mediators, TNFα, IL-1β, IL-8, and COX-2.[32,109] NF-κB activity is decreased during pregnancy due to progesterone/progesterone receptor blocking and upregulation of NF-κB inhibitors. At term signals from the fetus increases with macrophage activation and migration, release of cytokines and chemokines, and NF-κB activation.[109] Signals from the fetus include secretion of surfactant lipids and surfactant-protein-A (SP-A), augmented placental corticotropin-releasing hormone (CRH) production, and increased uterine stretch by the growing fetus.[109] SP-A synthesis begins only after 80% of gestation has been completed.[109] Surfactant phospholipids and SP-A contains arachidonic acids that serves as a precursor for prostaglandin (PG) production (see Box 4-1 below) by the amnion. With maturation of the fetal hypothalamic-pituitary-adrenal system (see Chapter 19), fetal and placental CRH are increased, stimulating production of estrogens, locally altering the estrogen to progesterone ratio with functional withdrawal of progesterone (see "Progesterone"), altering the hormonal milieu.[19,97,102,131] These changes increase myometrial excitability, responsiveness to uterotonics (e.g., PGs, oxytocin), and electrical coupling.[18,19,26,27,102]

Stretching of the uterus may regulate myometrial contractility by increasing CAP gene expression and myometrial activation.[19,63] During much of gestation this expression is blocked by progesterone. The functional progesterone withdrawal at term results in activation and CAP expression. In multiple gestations, one of the reasons that the risk of preterm labor is increased is that stretch-attenuating pathways are overwhelmed by the greatly increased myometrial tensile stress, shifting the balance regulating myometrial contractility toward activation.[19,94]

Myometrial activation is part of a conditioning or preparatory stage during which there is activation of uterine contractility, cervical ripening, and activation of fetal membranes (Figure 4-3).[27] The activation stage involves interaction of the uterus, cervix, and fetal membranes and involves endocrine, immune, and neural control mechanisms.[26,27] Once myometrial activation has occurred, current tocolytics may be less effective in suppressing contractions.[96] During phase 1, myometrial contractions become more regular, with higher frequency and amplitude.[19] Transition from phase 0 to phase 1 is a normally gradual process over the last few weeks of pregnancy.[19]

Phase 2, which accounts for about 0.2% of pregnancy duration, involves stimulation of the myometrium by uterotonics, primarily PGs and oxytocin, and initiation of coordinated forceful contractions.[19] Once labor is initiated, myometrial contraction and relaxation proceed via the enzymatic phosphorylation and dephosphorylation of myosin and subsequent promotion and inhibition of myosin-actin interaction. Phase 3, involution (see Chapter 5), is primarily mediated by oxytocin.[19,96]

BOX 4-1 Prostaglandins

Prostaglandins (PGs) are "bioactive lipids and members of the eicosanoids family derived from arachidonic acid, which act in a paracrine or autocrine manner and function via binding to specific G-protein-coupled receptors, activating intracellular signaling and gene transcription".[79] PGs act as intermediaries, exerting their major effect at the subcellular level at or near the site of production. PGs are usually metabolized locally but may enter the blood to be rapidly inactivated by pulmonary and hepatic enzymes. PGs are classified into subgroups based on the configuration of their 5-carbon ring. PGE_2, $PGF_{2\alpha}$, and prostacyclin (PGI_2) are the most important in reproductive processes. During pregnancy, PGs are needed for maternal cardiovascular changes, including preventing hypertension and increasing uteroplacental blood flow, and in cervical ripening and the initiation of labor. Surfactant secreted into the amniotic fluid by the fetal lung also provides another source of arachidonic acid for PG synthesis by the amnion.[109,163] SP-A from the fetal lung and the decidua may play a role in regulating PG production during pregnancy.[109,163,171] PGs are synthesized rapidly, are relatively unstable, and have a short half-life. PGs are formed by enzymatic oxidation of arachidonic acid, a polyunsaturated fatty acid precursor found in an esterified form (glycophospholipid). Formation of PG requires that arachidonic acid be changed to a nonesterified form either directly by cellular phospholipase A_2 or indirectly by phospholipase C. Nonesterified arachidonic acid can be further metabolized by specific microsomal or cytosolic enzymes via several pathways (including cyclooxygenases and lipoxygenases). There are two forms of cyclooxygenase: COX-1 and COX-2. COX-1 is normally produced to maintain physiologic homeostasis; COX-2 is inductable by exogenous signals such as myometrial activation or infection. PGs and thromboxane A_2 (TXA_2) are formed via the cyclooxygenase pathway under the influence of prostaglandin synthetase and thromboxane synthetase. TXA_2 is a platelet aggregation factor and vasoconstrictor whose actions are balanced by the opposing actions of PGI_2. Nonsteroidal anti-inflammatory agents such as aspirin and indomethacin inhibit formation of PGs and TXA_2, by blocking cyclooxygenase activity. Since PGs mediate the action of the hypothalamus in responding to pyrogens released during an infection, aspirin effectively reduces fever. Arachidonic acid metabolism via the lipoxygenase pathway leads to the production of various acids followed by the formation of leukotrienes (LTs). Leukotrienes are chemotaxic and chemokinetic for leukocytes. PGs act on G-protein coupled receptors tied to different effector systems. There are eight subtypes of PG receptors found in different tissues: TXA_2, PGI_2, PGF, PGD, and four types of PGE receptors. Eicosanoids are signaling molecules synthesized primarily from arachidonic acid. The four major groups are prostaglandins, prostacyclins, thromboxanes, and leukotrienes.[8] Thromboxanes are platelet aggregation factors and potent vasoconstrictors that oppose the action of PGI_2.

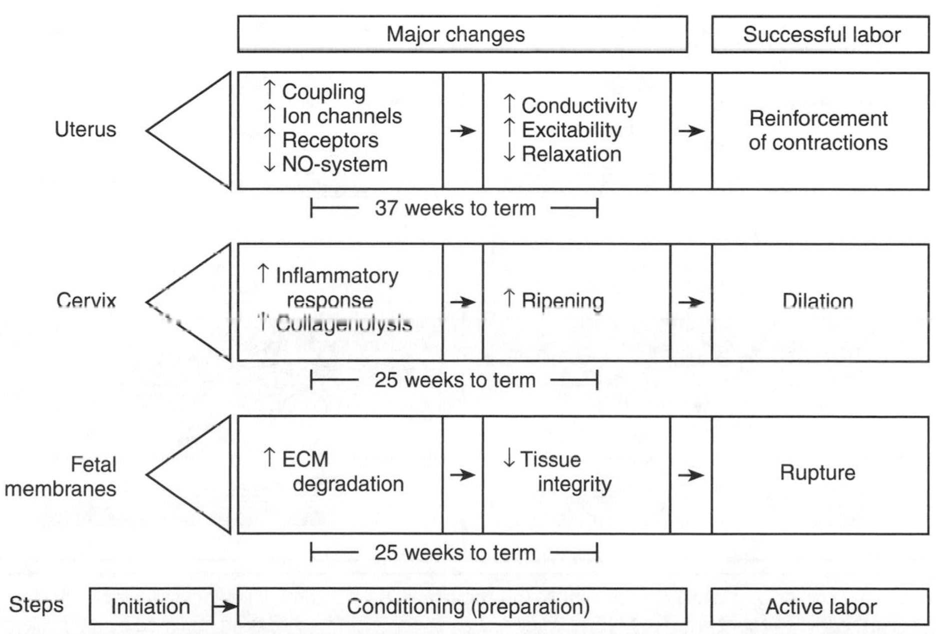

FIGURE 4-3 Model of changes in the uterus, cervix, and fetal membranes for initiation of labor. (From Maul, H., et al. [2003]. The physiology of uterine contractions. *Clin Perinatol, 30*, 669.)

Labor is a phenomenon that depends on complicated interactions and genetic influences between the fetus and mother.[21,131] Labor onset is thought to be controlled by the fetal genome via several interrelated pathways involving endocrine and mechanical signaling.[22,131] Gestational age upregulation of genes within the fetal HPA axis is critical for timing and control of labor. Timing of the maturation of the fetal HPA axis is probably set soon after implantation, however stress or other factors may alter the clock.[131]

The endocrine pathway operates primarily between the fetus and placenta. Increased expression of fetal genes and increased placental CRH leads to increased fetal cortisol and dehydroepiandrosterone sulphate (DHEAS). Cortisol stimulates further placental CRH; DHEAS increases placental estrogen production. Thus the concomitant functional withdrawal of progesterone results from local alterations in the estrogen-to-progesterone ratio. Estrogen acts on PG synthesis to promote further placental CRH secretion, up-regulates CAPs to enhance gap junction (Cx43) formation, increase activity of $PGF_{2\alpha}$ and possibly oxytocin receptors, and enhance expression of myosin light chain kinase and calmodulin needed for myometrial smooth muscle contraction.[131] The increase in cortisol also up-regulates prostaglandin H_2 synthetase enzymes, which increase synthesis and release of PGE_2 and $PGF_{2\alpha}$ from the cells of the amnion, chorion, and decidua.[22] PGs promote further CRH secretion by the placenta. The mechanical pathway is stimulated by uterine growth. Uterine stretch stimulates expression of CAP genes and CAP activation, which increase the contractility of the myometrium and its responsiveness to prostaglandins.[22]

A proposed mechanism for the initiation of labor at term is illustrated in Figure 4-4. This interaction can be altered by stress, infection, hemorrhage, excess stretch, and other factors leading to preterm labor.[22] Endocrine, paracrine, and other factors believed to influence uterine quiescence, activation, contractility, and the onset of labor are described in this section.

Corticotropin-Releasing Hormone

CRH is a neuropeptide produced primarily in the hypothalamus and, during pregnancy, by the placenta and myometrium. Placental CRH is the major source of CRH during pregnancy, with increased levels found in maternal and fetal circulations before labor onset.[11] Placental CRH concentrations increase up to 50- to 100-fold in the last 6 to 8 weeks of gestation, paralleling the increase in fetal cortisol.[91,102] CRH is also produced by the decidua, chorion, and amnion. CRH receptors found in the myometrium, placenta, decidua, fetal membranes, adrenal gland and other organs are up-regulated near term.[11,20,63,188] CRH actions are mediated by a network of G-protein coupled membrane bound receptors.[54]

During pregnancy, CRH affects the myometrium by inhibiting PGE_2, increasing cyclic adenosine monophosphate (cAMP),

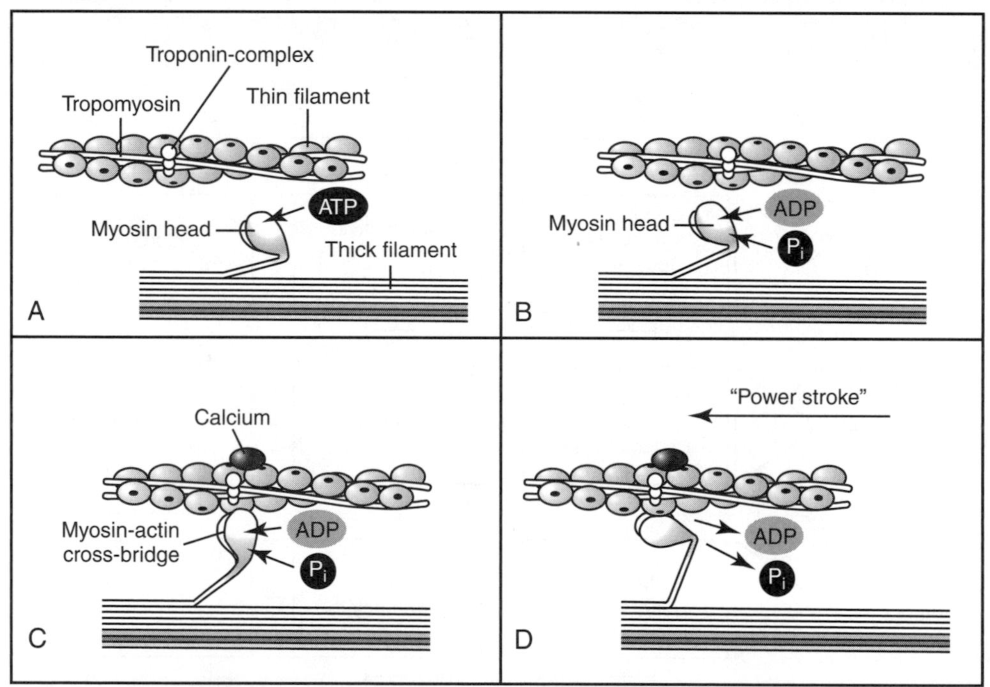

FIGURE 4-4 Mechanics of muscle contraction. **A,** The appearance of the contractile unit is illustrated. The thick filament refers to myosin; the thin filament is actin. Myosin binding sites on the actin filaments are covered by a thin filament known as tropomyosin that obscures the myosin-binding sites, therefore preventing the myosin heads from attaching to actin and forming cross-bridges. Adenosine triphosphate (ATP) binds to the myosin head. The troponin complex is attached to the tropomyosin filament. **B,** The hydrolysis of ATP into adenosine diphosphate (ADP) and inorganic phosphate (Pi) allows the myosin head to assume its resting position. **C,** The binding of calcium to the troponin complex results in a conformational change that allows binding site between actin and myosin to be exposed with the formation of actin-myosin cross-bridges. **D,** The formation of actin-myosin cross-bridges results in release of ADP and Pi, causing the myosin heads to bed and slide past the myosin fibers. This "power stroke" results in a shortening of the contractile unit and the generation of force within the muscle. At the end of the power stroke, the myosin head releases the actin-binding site, is cocked back to its furthest position, and binds to a new molecule of ATP in preparation for another contraction. The binding of myosin heads occurs asynchronously (i.e., some myosin heads are binding actin filaments while other heads are releasing them), which allows the muscle to generate a continuous smooth force. Cross-bridge formations must therefore form repeatedly during a single muscle contraction. (From Norwitz, E.R. & Lye, S.J. [2009]. Biology of parturition. In R.K. Creasy, et al. [Eds.]. *Creasy & Resnik's Maternal-fetal medicine: Principles and practice* [6th ed.]. Philadelphia: Saunders Elsevier, p. 78.)

and up-regulating nitric oxide (NO) synthetase.[63,131,140] CRH has a role in trophoblast growth, tissue remodeling via matrix metalloproteinases (MMPs), immune function, and control of placental vasomotor tone.[140] Placental CRH influences the onset of labor by inducing fetal cortisol production via positive feedback to the placenta to further increase CRH, which increases myoactivity.[11] Increased cortisol stimulates production of PG by the fetal membranes and increases DHEAS and thus estrogen production. Estrogens induce CAP formation and release of oxytocin and MMP-9 needed for membrane rupture and placental separation.[11] Thus CRH has "a protective role for the myometrium by preventing uterine contractions [during pregnancy], whereas at term CRH enhances the myometrial contractile response to $PGF_{2\alpha}$, PGE_2 and oxytocin."[19]

In the mother, serum CRH (primarily from the placenta) increases steadily to 35 weeks, then increases markedly with the onset of labor.[140,167] Before 35 weeks, most of the CRH is neutralized by binding to CRH-binding protein (CRH-BP) produced in the maternal liver, placenta, decidua, amnion, and chorion.[11,63,188] Levels of this binding protein decrease 50% in the last 6 weeks of gestation.[188] Several weeks before labor onset, CRH concentrations exceed concentrations of CRH-BP with an increase in circulating free (physiologically active) CRH to term.[52,91,102,140,188] The increased CRH stimulates an increase in myometrial PG receptors, PG release, and fetal cortisol.[11,22,91,140] Increased fetal cortisol stimulates PG synthesis by increasing prostaglandin-H synthetase-2 (PGHS-2) and decreasing PG catabolism by decreasing 15-hydroxyprostaglandin dehydrogenase (PGDH) expression.[22,91,140] PGDH activity in pregnancy may be maintained by activation of glucocorticoid receptors (GRs), which respond to both progesterone and cortisol. Near labor onset, the increased cortisol displaces progesterone from the GRs. This inhibits PGDH activity and production.

CRH levels are maximal at the end of labor, decreasing rapidly immediately after birth and reaching prepregnancy levels by 24 hours postpartum.[52,167] Elevated levels of CRH in the second trimester have been associated with an increased risk of spontaneous preterm delivery.[52,140,188] CRH levels are lower with a slower rise with post term labor.[188]

As noted above, CRH is involved in increasing placental estriol and fetal glucocorticoid production.[11,91,170] Placental CRH is thought to stimulate fetal ACTH, which in turn stimulates the fetal adrenal cortex to produce glucocorticoids such as cortisol and DHEAS.[91,170] DHEAS is needed by the placenta to produce estrogens, particularly estriol. Cortisol stimulates fetal lung maturation (see Chapter 10) and further placental CRH production. This is in contrast to the effect of increased cortisol on the hypothalamus, where it has an inhibitory effect. In the placenta, glucocorticoids stimulate CRH receptors and increase CRH production.[91,140,170]

Urocortins are CRH-related peptides that act as ligands (ions or molecules that bind to other molecules to create a complex). Urocortins are found in many tissues including fetal membranes and the placenta. Their role is not yet well understood. Urocortins influence estrogen biosynthesis in the placenta, acts as a uteroplacental vascular relaxant, via activation of the nitric oxide (NO) cyclic guanosine 3′-5′ monophosphate (cGMP) system, and may have a role in regulating placental vascular resistance and modulating myometrial contractility.[54,109,140,201]

Progesterone

Progesterone, acting via progesterone receptors (PR), has a major role in controlling uterine and cervical function and suppressing uterine excitement throughout gestation. Progesterone interacts with cell membrane receptors to stimulate cAMP, which, along with cGMP, sequesters intracellular calcium in the sarcoplasmic reticulum (SR), thus decreasing contractility. Progesterone also enhances uterine quiescence by down-regulating genes needed to produce the CAPs needed for labor, limiting production of stimulatory PGs, suppressing release of proinflammatory cytokines that increase PG formation, suppressing NF-κB activity, and up-regulating the NO system and other relaxants.[19,52,103,109,170] Progesterone metabolites may inhibit oxytocin binding and signaling as well as proinflammatory cytokines to help keep the uterus in a relatively quiescent state during pregnancy.[131] Studies have shown that progesterone supplementation decreases the incidence of preterm birth in some high risk women ("Preterm Labor").[34,44,72,106]

Systemic progesterone levels do not fall in humans and regional differences in progesterone levels are seen. A functional withdrawal of progesterone action is seen in the myometrium in late pregnancy that is mediated by transcription factors. Near labor onset, NF-κB is activated and induces a proinflammatory cascade.[109] This is associated with increased expression of oxytocin receptors, contractile genes and PGHS-2, which along with activation of NF-κB, impairs PR function by down regulating PR activation, increasing metabolism of progesterone and upregulating inhibitory PR isoforms such as progesterone receptor-A (PR-A) and progesterone receptor-C (PR-C).[19,52,109,120,131]

Progesterone interacts with both nuclear (transcriptional) and extramembrane PRs in myometrial cells. The nuclear PRs modulate gene expression and protein activation; the membrane PRs act via direct coupling that induces intracellular signaling cascades.[114] Both of these effects influence myometrial contractility. The functional progesterone withdrawal also involves changes in the expression of progesterone receptor isoforms PR-A and PR-B.[52,114,133,188] PR-A inhibits PR-B mediated by NF-κB. PR-B activates progesterone responsiveness in tissues.[20,32,52,113,114,169,174,188] The PR-A/PR-B ratio increases in late pregnancy, thus the inhibitory effect of PR-A becomes more dominant, reducing the progesterone responsiveness of PR-B.[20,113,133,169,174,188] As a result, PR-B activation is decreased leading to a functional progesterone withdrawal; decreasing progesterone enhances further activation of NF-κB.[52] PR-C may inhibit up-regulation of progesterone-PR signaling in the myometrium.[114,131,188]

The local functional withdrawal of progesterone removes the progesterone-induced suppression of estrogen receptors, thus increasing myometrial contractility. In addition, the cortisol dominant estrogen effects from the fetal-placental unit near term may override the effects of progesterone.[131] Progesterone and cortisol have antagonistic effects, so the functional decrease in progesterone in late pregnancy when cortisol levels are increased enhances contractility.[170] Cortisol may also compete with progesterone for progesterone receptor binding.

Estrogen

Estrogen levels rise beginning at 34 to 35 weeks. Estrogens promote formation of gap junctions; upregulates oxytocin receptors in the myometrium; enhance lipase activity and release of arachidonic acid, thus stimulating PG production; increase binding of intracellular calcium; and increase myosin phosphorylation.[18,47,52,91] Estrogen (particularly estriol) production by the placenta (see Chapter 3) is dependent on fetal adrenal precursors. The placenta produces more than 90% of the estriol in pregnancy. DHEAS from the fetal adrenal is hydroxylated to 25-OH-DHEAS in the fetal liver. 25-OH-DHEAS is used by the placenta to produce estriol. Increased CRH stimulates ACTH to increase DHEAS output by the fetal adrenal, which leads to increased estrogen in late gestation. Concentrations of estradiol and estrone in amniotic fluid increase 15 to 20 days before onset of either term or preterm labor. Estrone produced locally in the chorion and decidua may influence the intrauterine progesterone-to-estrogen ratio, promote production of stimulatory PGs ($PGF_{2\alpha}$, PGE_2), and decrease production of inhibitory PGs (PGI_2). Increased stimulatory PGs and estrogens increase expression of oxytocin and PG receptors, L-type calcium channels, myosin light chain kinase, calmodulin, PGHS, and gap junctions (Cx43).[170]

Prostaglandins

Prostaglandins (PGs) (see Box 4-1 on page 123) are produced in the decidua and fetal membranes and have a central role in the initiation of labor. PGs bind to the cell membrane, increase the frequency of action potentials, and stimulate actual muscle contraction. Prostaglandins are the final common pathway in mechanisms of labor onset.[79,150] $PGF_{2\alpha}$, thromboxane, PGE_1 and PGE_2 promote myometrial contractility by increasing gap junction formation and calcium influx into the myometrium; PGE_2, PGD_2, and PGI_2 inhibit contractions.[131]

During most of pregnancy, PG synthesis is low and PG receptors in the myometrium are down-regulated.[91,131] PGDH expression, which is stimulated by progesterone, is high in the chorion, reducing transfer of PGs from the fetal-placental unit to the decidua and myometrium during much of pregnancy.[131] Up-regulation and increased PG production near the end of pregnancy are stimulated by CRH, cortisol, and uterine stretch and mediated by increased PGHS and decreased PGDH.[150,188] Levels of PGE_2 and $PGF_{2\alpha}$ increase before and during labor in maternal plasma and amniotic fluid.[91,150] PGs mediate labor onset and enhance contractility through increasing expression of gap junction proteins (connexin 43), oxytocin receptors and PG receptors, inducing MMP synthesis in the fetal membranes and cervix to enhance membrane rupture and cervical ripening, increasing expression of PR-A and PR-B, and increasing sarcoplasmic calcium levels in the cytoplasm and extracellular calcium entry into myometrial smooth muscle cells.[91,116,150] PGs are needed for changes in the extracellular matrix during cervical ripening and for decidual and fetal membrane changes leading to membrane rupture and placental delivery at birth.[150,175,186]

The amnion is a major site of PG synthesis with high levels of PGHS and minimal PGDH activity at the time of labor onset.[120] In the amnion, the major PG is PGE_2, The decidua also has high levels of PGHS and minimal PGDH. PGDH predominates in the chorion, located between the amnion and decidua.[19,144] The decidua produces large amounts of PGI_2 and to a lesser extent $PGF_{2\alpha}$ and PGE_2. PGHS is found in two forms. One form (PGHS-1) is always present for normal homeostasis; the other form (PGHS-2 or COX 2) is up-regulated by cytokines, growth factors, and glucocorticoids.[19] Expression of COX-2, produced in the fetal membranes and myometrium, is regulated by NF-κ and induced by proinflammatory cytokines.[32,131] COX-2 activity increases to term with further marked increase in labor. COX-2 activity in the amnion is the rate limiting step in production of PGs. Increased COX 2 activation is associated with a decrease in PGDH in the chorion, which allows PGs produced in the amnion to cross the chorion and enter the myometrium to stimulate contractions.[150] Increases in cortisol increase COX 2 expression in the fetal membranes and down regulates PGDH in the chorion. This promotes cervical ripening and myometrial contractions.[131]

PGs act by interacting with specific PG cell membrane receptors that are coupled with G-proteins and tied to different effector substances.[8,62] Activation of PGF, thromboxane A_2 (TXA_2), EP_1 receptors (increases intracellular calcium), and EP_3 receptors (inhibits adenyl cyclase) stimulates contractions. Activation of PGD_2, EP_2 receptors (stimulates adenyl cyclase), and PGI_2 receptors inhibits contractions.[8] Uterine quiescence may be enhanced by this coupling and by increases in relaxant PGs, such as PGI_2.[120] Coupling near term increases with up-regulation of PGE_2 contractile receptors (EP_1 and EP_3) and the $PGF_{2\alpha}$ receptor (FP) and loss of relaxatory PGE_2 receptors (EP_2 and EP_4).[62,120] Contractile receptors are most abundant in the fundus, whose forces are needed for propulsion of the fetus, whereas relaxatory receptors are more abundant in the lower uterine segment and may enhance passage of the fetal head and shoulders.

The placenta produces PGE_2, PGD_2, PGI_2, and TXA_2. Following delivery, placental TXA_2 may be important in enhancing hemostasis after placental separation. PGI2 is produced by the pregnant and the nonpregnant myometrium as well as by the placental vasculature; it helps maintain uterine quiescence.[96] PGI_2 increases in late pregnancy and with uterine distention by the fetus.[96] PGI_2 is a potent vasodilator that inhibits platelet aggregation and protects the vascular epithelium. PGI_2 is important in maintaining blood flow to the placenta and in ensuring adequate uterine blood flow during labor.[18] Suppression of PGI_2 formation leads to vasoconstriction and is thought to have a role in preeclampsia (see Chapter 9).

Oxytocin

Oxytocin is synthesized in the hypothalamus and released from the posterior lobe of maternal and fetal pituitary glands. Oxytocin is also produced in the myometrium, decidua, placenta, and fetal membranes. Concentration in the maternal circulation are stable during pregnancy, but increase during the second stage of labor.[131] The rate of fetal oxytocin secretion increases after spontaneous initiation of labor.[131] Under the influence of estrogen, the sensitivity of the myometrium to the effects of oxytocin changes markedly during pregnancy. Alterations in myometrial sensitivity to oxytocin are mediated by changes in the density and affinity of oxytocin receptors.[116,180] Up-regulation of oxytocin receptors before labor may also be regulated by mechanical stretch.[180]

Oxytocin receptors (OTR) in the myometrium increase 50- to 100-fold in early pregnancy and up to 200-300-fold by term.[116,131,140] The greatest concentration of OTR is found in the fundus with few in the lower uterine segment and cervix.[131] OTRs are G-protein–coupled receptors whose effects are mediated by phospholipase C, which mediates production of nonesterified arachidonic acid and thus PGs. This increases inositol 1,4,5-triphosphate (InsP3), which increases intracellular calcium and thus myometrial contractility.[8] Binding of oxytocin to OTRs on the cell membrane increases the frequency of pacemaker potentials and lowers the threshold for initiation of action potentials. Failed induction and postdate pregnancies are associated with a decreased concentration of oxytocin receptors. Oxytocin is a stimulant that is used to induce or augment labor. Oxytocin does not work as well as a labor stimulant for induction of labor before term, possibly due to the lack of adequate oxytocin receptors.

Relaxin

Relaxin is an insulin-like ovarian hormone produced initially by the corpus luteum and then by the myometrium and placenta. Relaxin levels are greatest during the first trimester but remain detectable in maternal circulation throughout gestation, falling rapidly after delivery.[18,140] Relaxin is involved in decidualization and implantation (see Chapter 3), modulation of MMP activity and myometrial quiescence.[51] Relaxin also induces vasodilatation and plays a role in maternal hemodynamic, musculoskeletal and renal changes during pregnancy (see Chapters 9, 11 and 15).[31,105] Relaxin increases cAMP, inhibits calcium increases in the myocyte, decreases affinity of myosin light chain kinase for calmodulin and myosin, and activates potassium channels.[116] Activation of these channels hyperpolarizes the membrane with uterine relaxation.[96] Relaxin acts synergistically with progesterone in blocking uterine activity and maintaining myometrial quiescence during pregnancy and may suppress oxytocin release.[162] Relaxin enhances cervical ripening and may help regulate gap junction permeability.

Nitric Oxide

Nitric oxide (NO) is produced by the decidua, fetal membranes, placental syncytiotrophoblast, and fetal and placental vascular epithelium. NO regulates vascular tone via release of PGI_2 from endothelial cells. NO and its substrate, L-arginine, are thought to be important in maintaining myometrial quiescence, cervical rigidity, and maternal systemic vasodilatation during pregnancy and in regulating fetal and uteroplacental blood flow.[15,116] NO and progesterone are thought to work together as gene regulators to down-regulate the genes needed for CAP production for parturition.[26] Levels of NO are elevated in the myometrium but not in the cervix during pregnancy. NO relaxes the myometrium and maintains cervical rigidity.[27] Near term, levels of NO decrease in the uterus and increase in the cervix. In the myometrium, NO activates the guanylate cyclase pathway, increasing cGMP, which leads to decreased intracellular calcium concentrations and interferes with myosin light chain kinase activity.[93,131] Thus a fall in NO is involved in initiation of labor, whereas an increase in NO is thought to help cervical ripening.[27]

NO synthesis is mediated by nitric oxide synthetase (NOS). NOS isoforms found in the fetal membranes and decidua may have different roles during pregnancy: nNOS (NOS-1) enhances uterine quiescence, eNOS (NOS-III) is important in uteroplacental and fetal circulation, and Inductable nitric oxide synthetase (iNOS) (NOS-II) from macrophages plays a role in cervical ripening.[173] Levels of NOS in the uterus decrease near term and disappear during labor. Alterations in NOS production have been reported with placental insufficiency.[83]

Cytokines and Other Factors

Inflammatory processes and mediators are a major component in enhancing uterine contractility and cervical ripening.[52,193] Cytokines such as IL-1, IL-6, IL-8 (especially), TNF-α, interferon, and transforming growth factor-β (TGF-β) play important roles in mediating the events of parturition.[45,52,109,134] IL-1 stimulates PG production by the amnion, decidua, and myometrium; IL-6 stimulates PGHS for PG production by the amnion, chorion, and decidua; and IL-8, produced by the chorion, decidua, placenta, myometrium, and endometrium, induces neutrophil chemotaxis and activation, production of MMPs, cervical ripening, and may play a role in formation of the lower uterine segment.[22] TNF-α also stimulates PG production by the amnion and decidua. TGF-β is involved in regulating the effects of progesterone on PTHrP, Cx43, and gap junction formation. Epidermal growth factor promotes uterine contractions by increasing intracellular calcium and increasing PG synthesis in the decidua and fetal membranes.[131] Parathyroid hormone related peptide (PTHrP) has a relaxant effect on myometrium that is removed near labor onset with a decrease in amniotic fluid PTHrP near term labor onset.[131] PTHrP is a vasorelaxant and also has a role in placental calcium transport (see Chapter 17).[140] Magnesium competes with calcium for calmodulin binding, reducing myosin light chain kinase prompting uterine relaxation.[140] Endothelin levels and receptors also increase during pregnancy. Endothelin is a peptide that modulates fetoplacental circulation and enhances myometrial contractility by increasing intracellular calcium and myosin light chain phosphorylation.[116,131]

Myometrial Contraction

Myometrial contraction is mediated via interaction of actin and myosin. In smooth muscle such as myometrium, contraction and relaxation are regulated primarily via enzymatic phosphorylation and dephosphorylation of myosin. The key enzyme is myosin light chain kinase (MLCK), the principal control mechanism for smooth muscle contractility.[94] Activity of MLCK is regulated by calcium, calmodulin, and cAMP-mediated phosphorylation, which are in turn influenced by hormones and pharmacologic agents. The mechanisms for myometrial smooth muscle contraction are described here and summarized in Figure 4-5.

Initiation of action potentials in uterine smooth muscle is primarily dependent on the influx of Ca^{2+} across the cell membrane, although ions such as Na^{+} and K channels are also involved. Intracellular calcium is essential for activation of MLCK, and calcium levels increase significantly with contractions. MLCK is associated with the long light chain of myosin and is activated by changes in intracellular calcium. Excitation of the myometrial cell increases concentrations of free calcium in the cytoplasm.[18,47] The calcium may be released from intracellular stores in the sarcoplasmic reticulum mediated by InsP3. Because calcium stores in the sarcoplasmic reticulum are relatively sparse, calcium from other sources (i.e., intracellular membrane-bound calcium vesicles, mitochondrial stores, or extracellular calcium) is also required.[47,96]

The main mechanisms for transport of extracellular calcium across the cell membrane into myometrial cells are as follows: L-type voltage-dependent Ca^{2+} channels activated by the action potential, adenosine triphosphate (ATP)-dependent pumps (via Ca,Mg-ATPase), and Ca^{2+}-activated K^{+}channels (which set the threshold for activation of the cell membrane).[1,94,154] Magnesium may trigger further intracellular calcium release. Voltage-dependent channels are the major channels and allow passage of calcium when the potential across the cell membrane falls to a critical level. In smooth muscles, the action potential is carried by calcium rather than by sodium as in nerve cells. Repolarization involves movement of K^{+} into the myocyte and inactivation of the calcium channels.[1,154] These channels are G-protein–coupled. Movement of calcium across these channels can be blocked by calcium antagonists or slow channel blockers such as nifedipine.

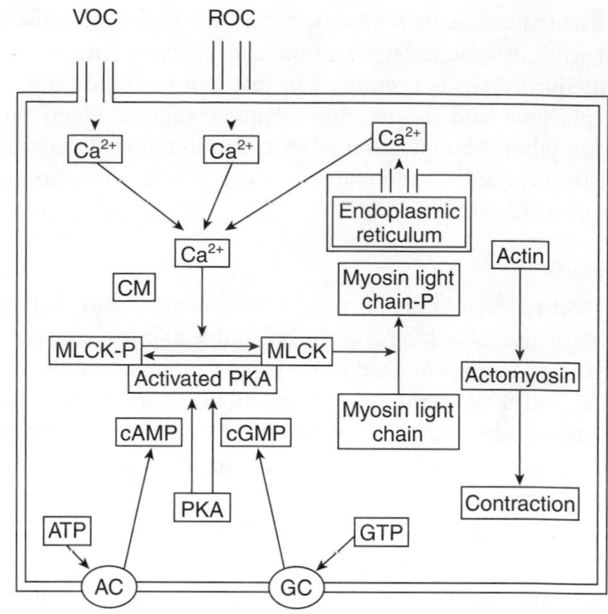

FIGURE 4-5 Biochemistry of myometrial contraction and relaxation. Myosin light chain kinase (MLCK) is the central molecule regulating uterine contractility. It is activated by calcium (Ca^{2+}) bound to calmodulin (CM). Cytoplasmic calcium concentration is the result of calcium released from deposits in the endoplasmic reticulum plus the influx of extracellular calcium through channels that are voltage operated or receptor operated. MLCK is deactivated by protein kinase A (PKA), which in turn is activated by cAMP and cGMP. β-agonists inhibit uterine contractions by activating adenyl cyclase (AC) with formation of cAMP, whereas nitric oxide has the same effect by activating guanylate cyclase (GC) and increasing production of cGMP. Calcium channel blockers relax muscle by inhibiting calcium influx through voltage-operated channels (VOCs). *P*, Phosphorus; *ROC*, receptor-operated channel. (From Arias, F. [2000]. Pharmacology of oxytocin and prostaglandins. *Clin Obstet Gynecol, 43*, 457.)

Intracellular free calcium levels must be 10^{-6} to 10^{-7} M for MLCK activation.[96] Although the amount of free calcium is critical in determining whether or not the muscle contracts or relaxes, calcium does not act independently. Calcium must first bind with calmodulin, forming a calcium-calmodulin complex, which in turn activates MLCK.[1,18] Calmodulin is a cytoplasmic regulatory calcium-binding protein that is activated by increases in unbound intracellular calcium.[1,18] Calcium binding to calmodulin changes its configuration so calmodulin can modulate the activities of enzymes and protein such as MLCK. Activated MLCK catalyzes phosphorylation (addition of a phosphate group) of the myosin light chain. Phosphorylation activates the ATPase on the myosin head with the release of chemical energy needed for the subsequent binding of myosin and actin (actomyosin). The result is release of adenosine diphosphate (ADP) and a phosphorus molecule, which changes the configuration of the myosin with flexion of the head on the tail. This flexion pulls on the actin filament and the muscle contracts (see Figure 4-1).[18,94,96] Other proteins involved in regulation of actin-myosin interaction include tropomyosin, caldesmon, and calponin.[116]

Myometrial relaxation occurs when calcium is removed. As soon as intracellular Ca^{2+} levels increase, mechanisms to remove calcium are stimulated. These mechanisms include uptake by the SR, extrusion across the cell membrane mediated by Ca^{2+} extruding proteins and decreased MLCK sensitivity to calcium.[125] Relaxation involves the action of the enzyme–myosin light chain phosphatase. With removal of the phosphate group from the myosin head, the actin no longer recognizes the myosin. Actin-myosin interaction is inhibited and the muscle cell relaxes. Reduction in MLCK activity due to decreased calcium-calmodulin levels also leads to muscle relaxation, as does inhibition of phosphorylation by increased levels of cAMP and cGMP.[1,18] cAMP and cGMP are second messengers (i.e., they carry the message of a hormone to the site where the hormonal effect is realized) that lower the affinity of myosin for calcium-calmodulin or reduce intracellular calcium by stimulating calcium return to intracellular stores or extrusion across the cell membrane.[47]

The relative activity of adenyl cyclase (mediates cAMP synthesis) and phosphodiesterase (mediates cAMP breakdown) influences myometrial contractility by altering cAMP levels within the cell. Adenyl cyclase increases intracellular cAMP, which reduces calcium-calmodulin complexes and intracellular calcium levels and thus MLCK (see Figure 4-5). Hormones and pharmacologic agents influence activity of MLCK and cAMP. For example, adenyl cyclase is activated by β-adrenergic agonists, resulting in increased cAMP and reduced contractility. Substances such as α-adrenergic agonists that inhibit phosphodiesterase, which normally mediates cAMP breakdown, also result in elevated levels of intracellular cAMP.[19,94]

Oxytocin and $PGF_{2\alpha}$ enhance contractility by increasing intracellular calcium levels and the rate of MLCK phosphorylation. Oxytocin also releases calcium from intracellular stores and inhibits calcium uptake by the sarcoplasmic reticulum, extending actin-myosin interaction and thus muscle contraction. Relaxin increases cAMP, which inhibits MLCK phosphorylation and induces muscle relaxation.

The myosin head contains magnesium adenosine triphosphatase (Mg-ATPase) sites where ATP is hydrolyzed, converting chemical energy to mechanical force. Energy (released from ATP by myosin ATPase) is critical for myometrial contraction. ATP is used for both actin-myosin interaction and ion transport. If adequate oxygen and glucose are not available for ATP formation, as may occur with prolonged labor, the contractile process will be inhibited.

PGs and oxytocin promote release of calcium from intracellular pools or prevent uptake of calcium into these pools. This promotes contractility. On the other hand, agents that inhibit myometrial activity (e.g., progesterone, relaxin, PGI_2, and β-agonists) promote calcium sequestration or extrusion (via cAMP-dependent enzymes) and thus myometrial relaxation.[18,19,94]

In summary, control of myometrial activity is dependent on enzymatic phosphorylation of myosin by MLCK to allow interaction of actin and myosin. Hormonal, biochemical, and physical factors mediate MLCK activity, uterine activity, and myometrial structural and functional alterations. Before onset of labor, the myometrium undergoes activation, with decreases in substances that maintain uterine quiescence and increases in CAPs (see Figure 4-3) that enhance uterine contractility.

Coordination of Uterine Contractions

Electrical and contractile activity in smooth muscle cells is controlled by myogenic, neurogenic, and hormonal control systems.[18,46] Myogenic activity, the spontaneous activity of the myometrium that occurs in the absence of any neural or hormonal input, includes the intrinsic excitability of the muscle cell, the ability of the muscle to contract spontaneously, and the mechanisms that produce rhythmic contractions. Neurogenic and hormonal control systems are superimposed on the muscle's inherent myogenic properties to initiate, augment, and suppress myometrial activity.[18,46] Myogenic control is dominated by hormonal influences, especially those of estrogen and progesterone, which influence myogenic characteristics through their generally opposing actions, as well as the mechanical forces from uterine stretching.[63,103] Estrogen increases and progesterone decreases the potential for contraction. Neurogenic control is not critical, since labor can occur in women with spinal injury (see Chapter 15), although the length of labor may be altered.

Coordination of contractions occurs by coupling of myometrial cells via electrical (e.g., gap junctions) and chemical (e.g., PGs, oxytocin) mechanisms. Polarization and depolarization of the cell membranes moves the electrical signals across the myometrium.[2] These electrical signals are generated by movement of calcium through ion channels into the myometrial cell. Action potentials propagate rapidly throughout the uterus, initiating movement of calcium into the cells via voltage-dependent channels, which activate myofilaments, resulting in a contraction.

Spontaneous cycles of activity in myometrial cells are characterized by (1) slow, rhythmic fluctuations in the magnitude of electrical potential across the cell membrane and (2) spikes of electrical activity that occur in bursts at the crests of slow waves (action potentials) and become synchronous at parturition (a single spike can initiate a contraction; multiple spikes are needed to maintain forceful contractions).[116] Action potentials occur in bursts; with progression of labor, electrical activity becomes more organized with and increase in amplitude and duration.[131] The more frequent the action potential, the more frequent the contraction; the duration of the action potential is the duration of the contraction; and the number of spikes is reflected in the force of the contraction.[116,131]

Any myometrial cell is thought to have pacemaker potential and be able to generate spontaneous activity (the exact mechanism is unknown), which depolarizes the cell membrane to a critical threshold. The location of the pacemakers may change with each contraction.[188] Cells that act as pacemakers within the uterus have higher resting transmembrane potential and spontaneously initiate action potentials.[131] Cell depolarization triggers a change in the Na^+, Ca^{2+}, and K^+conductance (action potential). The action potential increases membrane permeability to calcium and release of intracellular calcium stores.[47] As long as extracellular K^+ concentrations are high, action potentials increase in frequency. When maximum ion concentrations are reached within the cell, ionic stability is restored by active outward transport of Na^+ and Ca^{2+}, intracellular uptake of calcium, and by recapturing of intracellular K^+. The muscle cell returns to a resting state.

As action potentials are conducted to neighboring myometrial cells, groups of cells contract, leading to what is perceived by the woman as a uterine contraction. Coordination of uterine contractions occurs when all myometrial cells contract nearly simultaneously. Coordination and synchronization of contractions is mediated by the low-resistance gap junctions between myometrial cells. These junctions allow propagation of the action potential between cells and thus throughout the uterus and are critical for the effectiveness of myometrial contractility during labor.[150]

Gap Junction Formation

Smooth muscle bundles normally separated from each other within connective tissue may come into closer approximation to form intercellular gap junctions (low-resistance bridges or intercellular communication channels). Gap junctions allow transfer of current-carrying ions and exchange of second messengers between the cytoplasm of adjacent cells.[96] Thus gap junctions are the site where the action potential is propagated from cell to cell. Increased gap junction interaction is associated with improved propagation of electrical impulses, increased conduction velocity, and coordinated contractility of the myometrium.[46,47]

Gap junction proteins are called connexins (Cx). The major connexin in uterine gap junctions is Cx43.[116] Cx43 increases to term and is maximal during labor. Increased Cx43 is associated with decreased electrical resistance and thus myometrial contractility.[96] Connexins within the cell membranes of adjacent smooth muscle cells align to create symmetric openings (gap junctions) between their cytoplasm. Each opening or pore contains multiple channels; each channel consists of six connexins aligned symmetrically in a hexametric structure with six connexins in the adjacent cell.[96,116] These pores are separated by a narrow gap and provide a pathway for transport of ions, metabolites, and second messengers.[18] Gap junctions can be open or closed, thus controlling intercellular communication. Increased permeability across the junctions increases synchrony of electrical conduction and muscular contraction and subsequently more effective labor.[150]

The number and size of gap junctions increase markedly during gestation, reaching approximately 1000 per cell in late pregnancy or during labor.[47,116] Gap junctions are absent or infrequent in nonpregnant myometrium and decline markedly within 24 hours of delivery.[18,47] An increase in gap junctions is seen in women in preterm labor; delay in the formation of gap junctions is associated with prolonged pregnancy.[18,47,100] Myometrial stretch may also increase gap junctions.[63]

Estrogen stimulates gap junction formation by stimulating synthesis of connexins. One way progesterone may function to inhibit labor and maintain the pregnancy is by inhibition of estrogen-enhanced connexin synthesis.[47] Some PGs stimulate whereas others inhibit gap junction formation, either directly or indirectly via estrogen and progesterone activities.[47] Gap junction formation is also inhibited or decreased by indomethacin, relaxin, isoxsuprine, and isoproterenol; oxytocin has little effect. Lack of adequate concentrations of gap junctions decreases the effectiveness of oxytocin; as a result, oxytocin may not be effective with women experiencing preterm or post term labor. Increased intracellular calcium reduces coupling, and increased cAMP in the uterus decreases gap junction permeability.[46,47] One mechanism by which relaxin, PGI_2, and β-agonists are thought to inhibit myometrial contractility is by increasing intracellular cAMP, which uncouples gap junctions, thus preventing synchronous uterine activity.[46,116]

Physiologic Events During a Uterine Contraction

A normal uterine contraction spreads downward from the cornus within about 15 seconds. Although the actual contractile phase begins slightly later in the lower portion of the uterus, functional coordination of the uterus is such that the contraction peak is attained simultaneously in all portions. The intensity of the contraction decreases from the cornus downward and is essentially absent in the cervix.

Resting baseline tonus in labor is at an intrauterine pressure of approximately 10 to 12 mmHg (1.33 to 1.59 kPa), which may increase to 30 mmHg (3.99 kPa) with hypertonia.[136] Uterine contractions can be palpated abdominally with intrauterine pressure greater than 10 to 20 mmHg (1.33 to 2.66 kPa) and perceived by the woman at 15 to 20 mmHg (1.99 to 2.66 kPa) (Figure 4-6).[115] During early first stage, intrauterine pressure increases 20 to 30 mmHg (2.66 to 3.99 kPa) above resting values, increasing to greater than 50 mmHg (6.65 kPa) in the active phase and to 100 to 150 mmHg (13.3 to 19.95 kPa) during a Valsalva maneuver with maximal expulsive efforts.[115] A laboring woman generally perceives pain at pressures greater than 25 mmHg (3.32 kPa) or more, although this varies with individual thresholds. Thus the duration of a contraction assessed from palpation or patient perception will be shorter than the actual contraction, and the duration between contractions will seem longer.[115] Women exhibit marked individual variation in the intensity, frequency, and duration of contractions. Position and the use of oxytocin, analgesics, and anesthesia also influence contractions.

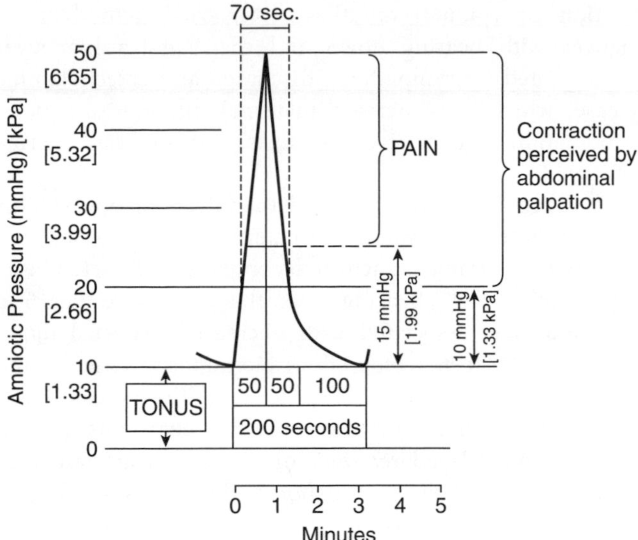

FIGURE 4-6 Correlation between abdominal palpation and intrauterine pressure tracing. (Data from Caldeyro-Barcia, R. *Second World Congress F.I.G.O.* Montreal. Libraire Beauchemin, Ltd.)

CLINICAL IMPLICATIONS FOR THE PREGNANT WOMAN AND HER FETUS

Labor and delivery place additional stressors on the maternal-fetal unit, which may be further increased in high-risk situations. Alterations in the physiologic processes of parturition can have a significant impact on the well-being of the mother, fetus, and neonate. Knowledge of these processes is critical in understanding the basis for nursing care and therapies to initiate or inhibit labor and the etiologic factors in dystocia and preterm or post term labor onset.

Maternal Position During Labor

Position during labor is influenced by cultural factors, obstetric practices, place of delivery, technology, and the preferences of the mother and health care providers.[90,110] Maternal position during labor influences the characteristics and effectiveness of uterine contractions, fetal well-being, maternal comfort, and course of labor.[37,56,110,148,149]

Historically a variety of positions have been used for labor and delivery. Delivery positions currently used in many U.S. institutions include lithotomy, lateral (Sims), semisitting, dorsal (or modified lithotomy), squatting, and occasionally kneeling.[149] Although lithotomy has often been used routinely, primarily for the comfort and convenience of the person delivering the infant, this position has no physiologic advantages and may interfere with expulsive efforts. Therefore alternative positions are currently being used in many settings.

Several positions have advantages or disadvantages from an anatomic and physiologic standpoint. During the first stage of labor, upright positions, such as sitting, standing, squatting, and kneeling, allow the abdominal wall to relax, and the influence of gravity causes the uterine fundus to fall forward. This directs the fetal head into the pelvic inlet in an anterior position and applies direct pressure to the cervix, which helps stimulate and stretch the cervix. An upright position during the second stage has been associated with a decrease in cesarean birth and instrumental delivery and a reduction in labor duration.[147] Feedback from the cervix to the myometrium may stimulate more intense contractions and shorten labor.[90] The lateral recumbent position reduces pressure on maternal blood vessels and promotes venous return and cardiac output, thus increasing uterine perfusion and fetal oxygenation.[110] Side-lying may be effective during labor with a posterior fetus, by allowing the weight of the uterus and fetus to tip away from the back and permitting application of counter pressure over the lumbosacral area.

Position at delivery should optimize alignment for fetal descent and maximize the capacity of the pelvis and efficiency of maternal expulsive efforts.[149] Squatting enhances engagement and descent of the fetal head and increases maternal pelvic diameters. In this position the upper portion of the symphysis pubis is compressed and the bottom part separated slightly. This results in an outward movement and separation of the innominate bones and backward movement of the lower sacrum. The pelvic outlet increases 28% with increased transverse (1 cm) and anteroposterior (0.5 to 2 cm) diameters. Thigh pressure against the abdomen during squatting may also promote fetal descent and correction of unfavorable fetal positions. Sitting or semisitting (30-degree angle) may have similar advantages.[42,90,168]

Dorsal and supine positions have been associated with adverse effects on maternal hemodynamics and fetal status and with the supine hypotension syndrome.[42,149,168] A supine position is a disadvantage during engagement and descent of the fetal head because this position does not optimize fetal alignment, maximize pelvic diameter, or maximize efficiency of maternal expulsive efforts.[90] Supine positions have also been associated with an increase in instrumental deliveries and episiotomies and with a statistically, but not clinically significant decrease in estimated blood loss at delivery.[37]

Most studies of maternal position during labor have compared the effects of two positions, so findings vary with the positions used. A **Cochrane Review** of 19 studies (n = 5794) of maternal positioning during second-stage labor concluded that any upright or lateral position as compared to a supine or lithotomy position decreased the length of the second stage, need for forceps, episiotomy, severe pain, and abnormal fetal heart rate patterns; increased the risk of blood loss (particularly with use of birthing chairs or stools); and slightly increased the risk of perineal tears.[56] In the supine position, contractions were more frequent but less intense than in the side-lying position. The use of the supine position during the first stage of labor compromised effective uterine activity, prolonged labor, and increased use of drugs to augment labor.[148] Placing a woman in the side-lying position increased the intensity and decreased the frequency of contractions and promoted greater uterine efficiency.[18,19,38,168] Frequency and intensity of contractions and uterine activity increased with sitting or standing. Upright positions (e.g., standing, sitting, squatting, kneeling), as opposed to supine positions, were associated with more regular and intense contractions, less likelihood of an epidural and shorter duration of first and second stages and total labor.[87,90,202] The lateral recumbent position (as opposed to sitting) led to more intense, less frequent contractions and greater uterine efficiency during the first stage.[37,148] Squatting has been reported to be the most effective position for pushing.[50,195]

Positional effects appear as soon as the maternal position is changed and last as long as the position is maintained.[148] Changes are more marked with spontaneous than with induced labor and do not seem to be affected by parity or fetal position. Alternating positions after the woman has maintained one position for a period of time can enhance the effectiveness of contractions. If the woman prefers a supine position, alternating this position with standing or side-lying can increase the efficiency of contractions.[148]

Although many studies have not found specific alterations in fetal status associated with maternal position, positions that increase the efficiency of contractions and decrease the duration of labor may reduce fetal stress.[56,148] For example, semisitting positions during delivery may shorten the length of the second stage and reduce fetal acidosis.[149]

Use of hands and knees positioning has been suggested as an intervention to promote rotation of an occipitoposterior fetal head to occipitoanterior during labor via the effects of gravity and buoyancy.[65,67,149,177] However a Cochrane review of the use of a hands-and-knees position found only three studies that met review criteria and did not recommend use of this position for correction of an occipitoposterior fetal postion.[65,67,149,177] However this position was found useful for persistent back pain during the first stage.[67]

Maternal comfort is also an important consideration. Many women prefer lateral or standing positions over supine.[110] Position preferences may change during labor. A woman may prefer sitting or walking during early labor and later may prefer semirecumbent or side-lying with pillow support as labor progresses. Roberts summarizes factors to consider in selecting a position conducive to labor progress and maternal comfort: "potential mechanical advantage of the position; the associated hemodynamic alterations and subsequent uteroplacental perfusion; the position of the fetus; the woman's perception of her contractions, discomfort, and fatigue; and obstetric indications for confinement to bed for continuous fetal monitoring, medication, or care."[148]

Maternal Pushing Efforts During the Second Stage

There have been concerns regarding the effects of bearing down (i.e., prolonged Valsalva maneuver) and the Valsalva maneuver on maternal hemodynamics and fetal status.[59,90,149,198] A long Valsalva push increases maternal intrathoracic and intraabdominal pressure and decreases cardiac output, uterine blood flow, and blood in the intervillous space and thus fetal oxygenation.[59] Maternal hypotension and fetal hypoxia may develop more rapidly with supine position or epidural anesthesia. Maternal hemodynamic changes with bearing down and the Valsalva maneuver are mediated by sympathetic discharge and catecholamine release, which also increase maternal discomfort and, in combination with maternal acidosis, may decrease uterine activity.[149]

Investigations have compared the effects of open-glottis pushing (based on involuntary maternal urges to push) with those of the Valsalva maneuver accompanying directed bearing down.[46,153,194,195] Bearing down that lasts more than 5 to 6 seconds was associated with decreased maternal blood pressure and placental blood flow, alterations in maternal and fetal oxygenation, decreased fetal pH and PO_2, increased fetal PCO_2, an increased incidence of fetal heart rate pattern changes, and delayed recovery of the fetal heart rate with asphyxia; others have found shorter duration second stage with closed glottis pushing.[9,153,194,195] Open-glottis pushing was not associated with changes in maternal blood pressure (probably because intrathoracic pressure elevations were not sustained) or increased fetal pH.[2] Spontaneous involuntary pushing with minimal straining has been associated with fewer episiotomies, forceps deliveries, and second-degree to third-degree perineal tears, and a shorter second stage.[90,149,153] Roberts suggests that a semirecumbent position with bearing down efforts that are short and in accordance with involuntary urges to push is most conducive to favorable delivery outcomes.[149]

The second stage of labor is biphasic, with a latent phase (from complete dilation until a strong urge to push, during which the fetus passively descends into the vagina) and active phase with strong bearing down efforts as the fetal head nears the perineum.[59] Laboring down in women with epidurals involves no bearing down until the fetal head is visible or the woman has an urge to push. Laboring down increases the length of the second stage, but deceases the amount of time spent pushing in most studies.[146,165]

Preterm Labor

Infants born prematurely are at high risk for health alterations during the neonatal period and for later neurodevelopmental problems. As a result, much effort has been directed toward eliciting the causes for preterm labor and developing intervention strategies to prevent the onset of labor and to terminate uterine contractions that begin before term. Preterm labor is defined as the onset of regular contractions with progressive cervical effacement and dilation before 37 weeks.[150] Rates of preterm labor in the United States have been increasing until recently, but even with decreases in the past few years are still over 12%.[127] Preterm labor involves a group of factors that individually or in combination influence the various pathways involved in control of labor onset (see Figure 4-4). Preterm delivery may be due to maternal or fetal factors such as fetal growth restriction, placenta previa, preeclampsia, or placental abruption that results in early termination of the pregnancy (approximately 20% of all preterm labors); premature rupture of the membranes (PROM) (approximately 30%); intraamniotic infection (20% to

25%); or spontaneous, unexplained reasons (25% to 30%).[185] Many spontaneous preterm births are thought to be due to infection.[82]

Preterm birth also has a heritable basis in some women.[190] Labor onset is thought to be controlled by the fetal genome via several interrelated pathways involving endocrine and mechanical signaling.[22,131] Genetic factors may include individual genes, genes-environment interactions and gene-gene interaction.[119] Currently there are many ongoing studies examining the genetic basis of preterm birth. For example, Manuck et al. reported recently that spontaneous preterm birth in some African-American women may be mediated by a susceptibility locus on chromosome 7.[99] This locus has several possible genes that may play a role in preterm labor initiation including collagen type 1-α-2 gene and genes involved in calcium regulation. Polymorphisms in the TNF-α gene promoter region are associated with shorter gestation length and increased risk of spontaneous preterm birth.[60] Other work has focused on genetic variations in pro- and anti-inflammatory cytokine genes and their receptors.[7,199]

Four mechanisms have been proposed for preterm labor (Figure 4-7): (1) infection and inflammation (decidual, chorioamniotic, or systemic); (2) decidual hemorrhage or abruption; (3) maternal and fetal stress (activation of the maternal or fetal hypothalamic-pituitary-adrenal axis); and (4) uterine overdistention.[75,92,131,150] Inflammation activates a cytokine response, leading to increased matrix metalloproteinases (MMPs) and uterotonics. Initiation of preterm labor via infection/inflammation is due to release of proinflammatory cytokines such as IL-1β, platelet activating factor, TNF, and other mediators that increase production of prostaglandins (PG) by the fetal membranes and decidus.[150,189,200]

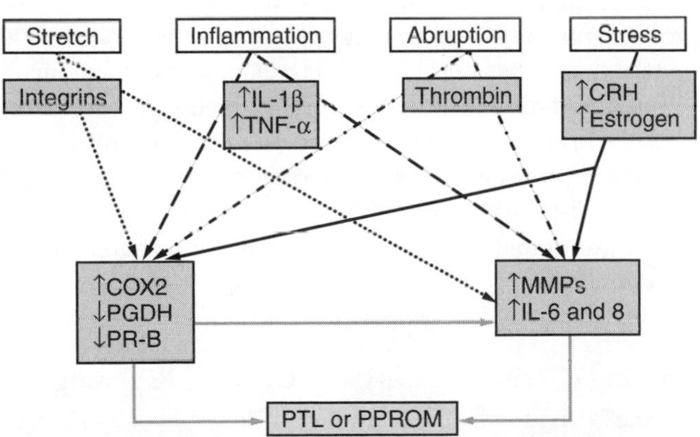

FIGURE 4-7 Principle biochemical mechanisms responsible for the main pathways of premature parturition. *COX2*, Cyclooxygenase-2; *CRH*, corticotrophin releasing hormone; *IL-1β*, interleukin -1β; *MMPs*, matrix metalloproteinases; *PGDH*, prostaglandin dehydrogenase; *PPROM*, preterm premature rupture of membranes; *PR-B*, progesterone receptor-B; *PTL*, preterm labor; *TNFα*; tumor necrosis factor-α. (From Romero, R. & Lockwood, C.J. [2009]. Pathogenesis of spontaneous preterm labor. In R.K. Creasy, et al. [Eds.]. *Creasy & Resnik's Maternal-fetal medicine: Principles and practice* [6th ed.]. Philadelphia: Saunders Elsevier, p. 525.)

Intrauterine (both clinical and subclinical) infections, including chorioamnionitis, bacterial vaginosis (BV), and extrauterine infections (including malaria, pyelonephritis, tuberculosis, pneumonia, and periodontal disease) have been implicated.[70,71,189,191,200] BV is "a pathologic state characterized by the loss of normal vaginal flora, particularly *Lactobacillus* species, and overgrowth of other microbes, including G *vaginalis*, *Bacteroides* sp, *Mobiluncus* sp, and *Mycoplasma hominis*."[143] Data regarding whether screening and prophylactic treatment with antibiotics for women with asymptomatic infection prevents preterm birth are conflicting, with reports of increased risks in some studies.[10,16,70,81,86,104,132,143,161,170,187] Although antibiotic therapy can eradicate BV, a Cochrane review found little evidence that treatment of asymptomatic women with antibiotics will prevent preterm birth.[143] Use of probiotics has also been investigated.[159] Treatment of periodontal disease has generally not been found in most trials to decrease the incidence of preterm birth, however care prior to rather than during pregnancy may be more effective.[49,142,197]

Both preterm labor and PROM may be adaptive events that occur when the intrauterine environment is "hostile." If the response to intrauterine infection is secretion of uterotonic agents, preterm labor results; if the response is protease (MMPs) production, PROM results.[170] A fetal inflammatory response syndrome (FIRS) has been described.[143,150] FIRS involves funisitis (umbilical cord inflammation) and chorionic vascularitis and is characterized by "systemic activation of the fetal immune system and defined by elevated IL-6 concentrations in neonatal cord blood."[143] Other biomarkers of FIRS include IL-β1, IL-8, and possibly C-reactive protein.[143]

Decidual hemorrhage, usually from placental abruption, with thrombin formation can activate phosphatidylinositol-signaling pathways that stimulate uterine contractions, release of plasminogen activators, and enhance activation of MMPs, neutrophil chemoattractants, and neutrophil activating chemokines.[14,41] Maternal or fetal stress may activate labor via increases in corticotropin-releasing hormone (CRH) leading to increased estriol production and increased PGs (Figure 4-8).[13,129] Uterine overdistention (polyhydramnios or multifetal gestation) or reduction in expansive capacity (uterine anomalies) activates cytokines (Figure 4-9).[98,150,170] The underlying mechanism may be myometrial stretch, which induces activation of integrin receptors and stretch-activated calcium channels, and phosphorylation of platelet-derived growth factors and G-proteins in the myometrium. These changes lead to increased MMPs, IL-8, PG, and nitric oxide (NO) in the cervix with cervical ripening and further stretching of the fetal membranes.[150]

A promising recent intervention to prevent preterm birth is use of 17-α-hydroxyprogesterone caproate for women with a risk for preterm labor or history of a previous preterm birth.[34,44,72,106-107,108,158,172] A meta-analysis of available studies found that use of 17-α-hydroxyprogesterone caproate decreased both preterm births (by 40% to 55%) and the incidence of infants weighing less than 2500 g.[157] Progesterone

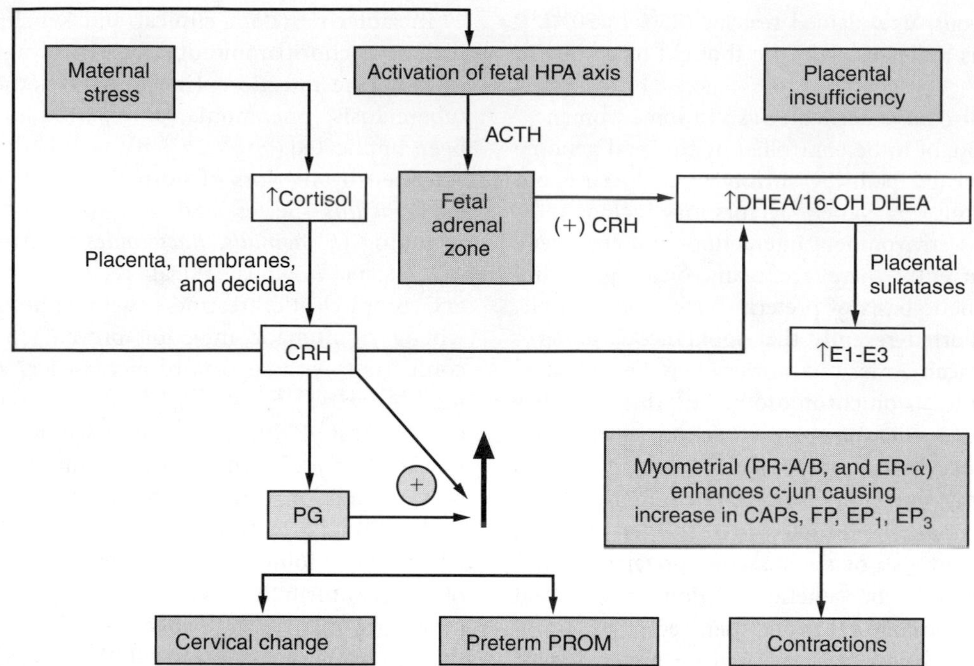

FIGURE 4-8 Proposed pathways by which stress can induce preterm labor. *ACTH*, Adrenocorticotropic hormone (corticotropin); *CAPs*, contraction-associated proteins; c-jun, a transcription factor; *CRH*, corticotropin-releasing hormone; *DHEA*, dehydroepiandrosterone; *E1-E3*, estrone, estradiol, estriol; *EP_1* and *EP_3*, prostaglandin E receptors types 1 and 3; *ER-α*, estrogen receptor-α; *FP*, prostaglandin f receptor; *HPA*, hypothalamic-pituitary-adrenal; *PG*, prostaglandins; *PR*, prostaglandin receptor; *PROM*, premature rupture of membranes. (From Romero, R. & Lockwood, C.J. [2009]. Pathogenesis of spontaneous preterm labor. In R.K. Creasy, et al. [Eds.]. *Creasy & Resnik's Maternal-fetal medicine: Principles and practice* [6th ed.]. Philadelphia: Saunders Elsevier, p. 530.)

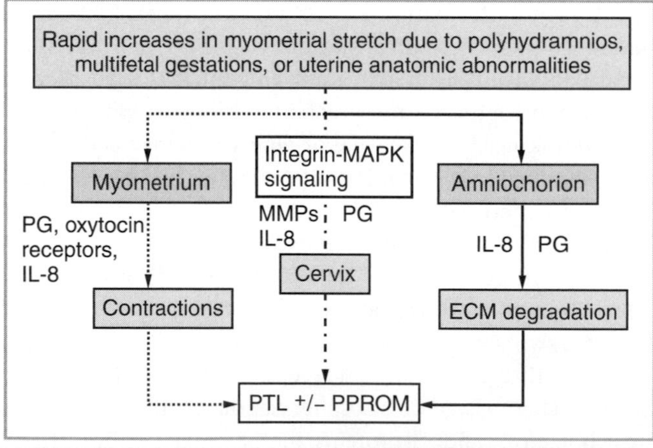

FIGURE 4-9 Proposed mechanism by which stretch can induce preterm labor. *ECM*, Extracellular matrix; *IL-8*, interleukin-8; *MAPK*, mitogen-activated protein kinase; *MMPs*, metalloproteinases; *PG*, prostaglandins; *PTL*, preterm labor; *PPROM*, preterm premature rupture of membranes. (From Romero, R. & Lockwood, C.J. [2009]. Pathogenesis of spontaneous preterm labor. In R.K. Creasy, et al. [Eds.]. *Creasy & Resnik's Maternal-fetal medicine: Principles and practice* [6th ed.]. Philadelphia: Saunders Elsevier, p. 531.)

supplementation may also enhance the tocolytic effects of β-adrenergic agonists.[157] Petrini and colleagues estimated that if all eligible women in the United States were treated, the prematurity rate would be reduced by 2% or by about 10,000 preterm births per year.[141] Neurodevelopmental follow-up at 48 months of offspring exposed to 17-α-hydroxyprogesterone caproate in utero showed no difference with control groups children.[130] The American College of Obstetricians and Gynecologists has recommended use of progesterone supplements for women with a history of previous spontaneous preterm birth.[5] 17-α-hydroxyprogesterone caproate is less effective with multiple gestation.[71]

Altering Uterine Motility and Cervical Ripening

Uterine activity can be controlled directly by blocking or stimulating specific hormonal receptors or altering electromechanical coupling, and indirectly via agents that interfere with the synthesis of enzymes and other mediators of myometrial contraction and relaxation. Use of these agents must take into consideration the physiologic properties of, as well as the pharmacologic actions on, both the cervix and the myometrium. A post term woman with altered myometrial contractility and an unripe (resistant) cervix needs an agent that increases and coordinates myometrial activity and decreases cervical resistance. On the other hand, agents used for women in preterm labor lead to myometrial relaxation and increase cervical resistance. This section examines pharmacology of labor related to control of cervical ripening, labor induction, and labor inhibition.

Control of Cervical Ripening

Cervical ripening is not dependent on myometrial contractions and occurs in the absence of regular uterine contractions. PGE_2 (Cervidil, Prepidil) and misoprostol (Cytotec), a PG analogue, are used most frequently for preinduction cervical ripening.[78,155,173,179] Use of vaginal PGs significantly increases the likelihood that delivery will occur within 24 hours.[76] Physiologic ripening is under the control of local mediators, in particular PGE_2, whose action is influenced by local mediators. Exogenous PGE_2 induces cervical ripening by relaxing cervical smooth muscle, enhancing enzymatic collagen degradation, and increasing hyaluronan and MMP.[173,179] Misoprostol is a synthetic PGE analogue that binds to EP_3 and EP_4 receptors and has a greater effect on the cervix than PGE_2 with a greater likelihood of vaginal delivery within 24 hours.[25,64,173] Antiprogesterone agents (RU-486, or mifepristone) have also been evaluated as alternative cervical ripening agents. RU-486 stimulates IL-8 release.[26,173,179]

Induction and Augmentation of Uterine Activity

Oxytocin (and synthetic forms such as Pitocin and Syntocinon) is usually the drug of choice to initiate uterine activity if the condition of the cervix is favorable.[33] Oxytocin is used for labor augmentation and induction and to promote uterine contraction following parturition.[164] Since oxytocin has little effect on the cervix, an unripe cervix may resist even forceful oxytocin-induced myometrial contractions. Oxytocin increases myometrial cell membrane spike activity, possibly by altering calcium flux through voltage-dependent calcium channels. Effects of oxytocin on uterine activity depend on the concentration of oxytocin receptors on the myometrial cells, number of available receptors, receptor affinity for oxytocin, and metabolic state of the myometrium. Oxytocin is a potent octapeptide synthesized in the hypothalamus and then transported along the neurons to the posterior pituitary gland via carrier proteins and released episodically. Oxytocin release can also be stimulated by nipple stimulation (similar to the mechanism with suckling described in Chapter 5).[168] Side effects include excessive uterine activity and uterine hyperstimulation with fetal hypoxia.[164]

Misoprostol has also been used for labor induction and there have been concerns regarding the risks of uterine hyperstimulation in women with a previous cesarean section.[8,55,173,179] Misoprostol has been reported to be less effective for third-stage labor than oxytocin and other uterotonics.[73] NO donors (isosorbide mononitrate, nitroglycerine, and sodium nitroprusside have also been investigated with outcomes similar to other agents but with an increase in maternal side effects.[77]

Inhibition of Labor

Inhibition of uterine smooth muscle contractions is used in the management of preterm labor. Uterine activity–inhibiting drugs (tocolytics) are most effective in stopping labor for 2 to 7 days and thus delay labor so glucocorticoids can be given to enhance fetal lung maturity (see Chapter 10). However, tocolytics do not decrease the overall rate of preterm delivery and there is little evidence that long-term prophylactic or maintenance use is effective.[10,17,36,69,70,131,156] Many tocolytic drugs have been investigated, including ethanol, β-adrenergic agonists, magnesium sulfate, calcium channel blockers, oxytocin receptor antagonists, cyclooxygenase inhibitors, and progestational agents.[12,29,57,58,70,131,152,178] Because each group of drugs has a different action, combinations of drugs may enhance their effectiveness because they act synergistically.[61]

Calcium antagonists (calcium channel blockers) are organic compounds such as nifedipine that act on the cell membrane to inhibit the influx of extracellular calcium through voltage-dependent channels, decreasing intracellular calcium and reducing release of stored calcium from intracellular sites.[17,57,61,71,125] These agents are less effective in blocking influx through receptor-operated channels that are less specific for calcium. Calcium antagonists may also act by altering calcium-calmodulin binding and thus inhibiting actin-myosin interaction. A Cochrane Review concluded that nifedipine can delay delivery for 2 to 7 days with a favorable risk-benefit ratio.[48] Although this drug crosses the placenta, no human studies of adverse fetal or neonatal effects have been published to date.[36] A recent meta-analysis of 26 trials ($n = 2179$ women) reported that nifedipine was superior to both magnesium sulfate and β-agonists for treatment of preterm labor.[30] Nifedipine may be associated with better neonatal outcomes and fewer maternal side effects and fetal side effects.[71] Calcium channel blockers are not recommended in combination with magnesium sulfate or β-agonists or with women with intrauterine infection, maternal hypertension, or cardiac disease.[71]

Magnesium affects smooth muscle excitation, excitation-contraction coupling, and the contractile apparatus by modulating calcium uptake, binding, and distribution in the cell; competitive blocking of Ca^{2+} influx across the cell membrane; and activation of adenyl cyclase and cAMP.[89] Magnesium regulates the voltage-gated calcium channels to prevent them from opening in response to the action potential. Thus magnesium sulfate acts on the myometrium, primarily by competitive antagonism to control calcium entry into the cell, reducing intracellular Ca^{2+} levels and thus contractility.[61] Magnesium sulfate has low tocolytic efficacy, but neuroprotective benefits with a decrease in moderate to severe cerebral palsy in offspring have been reported.[39,71,100,124,125,151]

β-Adrenergic agonists (β—sympathomimetics) are effective in postponing delivery for 24 to 48 hours but do not significantly reduce the rate of preterm birth or alter neonatal mortality or morbidity. Drugs in this class that have been used for inhibition of preterm labor include ritodrine, terbutaline, fenoterol, isoxsuprine, salbutamol, hexoprenaline, and orciprenaline.[85,192] Because significant side effects are common, these agents are used less commonly today and usually not as the first-line drug.[23,35,71] β-Adrenergic agonists act to relax myometrial cells by triggering intracellular formation of cAMP. These effects are mediated by β_2-receptors on the outer membrane of the myometrial cell.

Interaction of the β-adrenergic agonist and the β_2-receptor catalyzes the formation of cAMP by activating adenyl cyclase on the inner surface of the cell membrane. cAMP phosphorylates a protein kinase that decreases the affinity of medium light chain kinase for the calcium-calmodulin complex, thus promoting relaxation. cAMP also decreases intracellular calcium, possibly by interfering with the Na,K-ATPase exchange pump.[61] The myometrium contains both α- and β-receptors. When PGs or oxytocin stimulate the β-receptors, the uterus contracts. Stimulation of the β-receptors inhibits uterine contraction. Two subtypes of β-receptors may be present in the same organ or on the same cell. β_1-receptors dominate in the heart, small intestine, and adipose tissue; β_2-receptors predominate in the smooth muscle of the uterus, blood vessels, and bronchioles. Because β-adrenergic agonists are not specific for β_2- or β_1-receptors, use of these agents is associated with a number of systemic side effects.

Antioxytocic tocolytics such as atosiban are synthetic oxytocin analogues that competitively bind to myometrial oxytocin receptors, decreasing release of intracellular calcium and closing calcium voltage channels to prevent entry of extracellular calcium.[184] These agents act directly by blocking oxytocin receptors and indirectly by altering PG synthesis in the decidua. Atosiban has been used primarily in Europe and New Zealand. A Cochrane review of six trials found that atosiban delayed delivery for 2 to 7 days but did not find benefit over other agents and noted concerns about decreased birth weight and a possible association with later infant deaths (in one study).[137,138] These concerns have not been seen in other studies.[36] An international study found that atosiban was as effective as β-agonists with fewer maternal side effects, but in a recent meta-analysis neither agent was found to be as effective as nifedipine.[30,196]

Cyclooxygenase inhibitors reduce PG synthesis and include nonsteroidal anti-inflammatory agents such as indomethacin, Ketorolac, and Sulindac. These agents block PG synthesis by interfering with cyclooxygenase, the enzyme that regulates the production of PGs from arachidonic acid.[28,80] Because PGs are important in both initiation of myometrial activity and cervical ripening, the potential of this group of agents has generated considerable interest. Although their effectiveness has been documented, concerns remain over the potential risk for premature closure of the fetal ductus arteriosus and other side effects such as pulmonary hypertension and alterations in renal function.[61] The concern about ductal closure is that PG synthetase inhibitors act on both COX-1 (found primarily in fetal cardiovascular tissues) and cyclooxygenase-2 (COX-2) (found in the myometrium and fetal membranes). The risk for premature ductal closure is dose dependent and seems greatest in fetuses over 35 weeks' gestation and with long-term therapy. Generally indomethacin is used only for brief courses at ≤32 weeks' gestation.[71]

Dystocia

Dysfunctional labor can result from problems in the powers (alteration in myometrial function, expulsive forces, and contraction patterns), passage (obstruction of fetal descent by the maternal bony pelvis or soft tissues), or passenger (altered fetal size, position, or presentation). Functional dystocia due to alterations in the physiologic function (powers) results in inadequate contractility and failure of the cervix to dilate. The cellular and molecular basis for weak or ineffective myometrial contractions includes lack of adequate stimulation, depression or the presence of some form of strong inhibitory control, or a combination of these events.[46] Dystocia may have a genetic basis in some women.[3,4]

Understating of the usual duration and progression of labor is important in defining and identifying dystocia.[166] Cheng et al. found that with the use of epidurals, nulliparous women had longer first and second stage labors.[24] Neal et al. in their meta-analysis concluded that in nulliparous women with spontaneous active labor cervical dilation occurred at a mean of 1.2 cm/hour and lasted a mean of 6 hours.[128] At +2 S.D., this would be 0.6 cm/hour and a mean of 13.5 hours.[166]

Stimulation or inhibition of myometrial activity is influenced by myogenic, neurogenic, and hormonal control systems.[46] Dystocia secondary to alterations in myogenic properties arises from factors such as modifications in intracellular ion concentration (as a result of an inadequate supply of energy or calcium) with depression or absence of myometrial contractility, closure or inadequate function of gap junctions with modifications in the propagation of electrical events, and poor synchronization of contractions across the uterus. Abnormalities in gap junction structure or function may arise from alterations in regulatory hormones or their receptors. Dystocia can also arise secondary to alterations in neurogenic control (overstimulation by inhibitory neurons or understimulation by excitatory neurons) or in the hormonal control systems. These latter alterations arise directly from inadequate levels of hormones or their receptors or indirectly from alterations in gap junction function or structure.[46]

Supportive interventions with women experiencing dystocia are directed toward preventing or reducing maternal fatigue, providing calories for energy, maintaining hydration, monitoring fluid and electrolyte status, appropriate positioning, assessing maternal-fetal status at least every 15 minutes during induction and augmentation, and maintaining fetal homeostasis.[166] Energy (ATP) is essential for labor progression. If adequate calories and adenosine triphosphate (ATP) are not available, ketoacidosis may develop. With inadequate ATP, the effectiveness of uterine contractions is further impeded. Women with dystocia whose labor is not progressing and who are exhausted may be provided with a period of medicated therapeutic rest.[46]

Post Term Labor

Post term labor is the onset of labor after 42 weeks or 294 days from last menstrual period.[144] Fetal and neonatal morbidity increases after 42 weeks, often as a result of the effects of prolonged gestation on placental morphology and functional ability. Post term pregnancies are associated with

Table 4-1 Recommendations for Clinical Practice Related to Parturition and Uterine Physiology

Recognize usual changes in the uterine size and shape during pregnancy (p.116).
Know the usual changes in the myometrium during pregnancy and their bases (p.118).
Recognize factors involved in the initiation of labor and know how these may be altered (pp. 121-128).
Understand the physiologic basis for myometrial contraction and factors that may alter muscular contraction (pp. 116-118, 128-130 and Table 4-1).
Assess contractions and document their characteristics (pp. 129-130).
Monitor energy and oxygen needs of the laboring woman (pp. 128-129).
Understand the basis for cervical ripening and dilation and factors that may alter this process (pp. 119-120).
Avoid use of the supine position for prolonged periods during the first stage of labor (pp. 131-132).
Alternate supine and side-lying positions for a woman who prefers supine positions during the first stage (pp. 131-132).
Promote use of upright positions in first-stage (especially early) labor (pp. 131-132).
Assist the woman in selecting a position conducive to labor progress and maternal comfort (pp. 131-132).
Try side-lying position with a posterior fetus (p. 131).
Assist the woman in selecting a position at delivery to optimize alignment for fetal descent and maximize capacity of the pelvis and efficiency of maternal expulsive efforts (p.132).
Teach the woman to use open-glottis pushing (p.132).
Avoid supine positions during the second stage (p.132 and Chapter 9).
Recognize factors that increase the risk of preterm labor (pp. 132-134 and Figures 4-7, 4-8, and 4-9).
Understand the basis for pharmacologic agents used to control cervical ripening (pp. 134-135).
Understand the basis for pharmacologic agents used for induction or augmentation of labor (pp. 135-136).
Monitor the woman for side effects of agents used to induce or augment labor (pp. 135-136).
Understand the basis for pharmacologic agents used to inhibit labor (pp. 135-136).
Monitor the woman for side effects of agents used to inhibit labor (pp. 135-136).
Recognize and monitor for factors that can lead to dystocia (p. 136).
Monitor the woman with post-term labor for fetal distress (pp. 136-137 and Chapter 6).

an increased frequency of both IUGR (in 10% to 20% of post term pregnancies) and macrosomia (in most), fetal distress, meconium aspiration, congenital anomalies, and intrauterine death.[6,66,144]

Factors that may result in failure of initiation of spontaneous labor and postdate gestation include (1) lack of the normal increase in estrogen near term, perhaps due to anencephaly and associated adrenal hypoplasia, deficiency in placental sulfatase (necessary for production of estrogen), or fetal adrenal hypoplasia; (2) altered adrenocortical function, leading to reduction in cortisol levels (cortisol promotes hydroxylation of progesterone, reduction in progesterone levels, and increases in estrogen precursors); (3) alterations in local bioregulators of cervical ripening; and (4) decreased fetal adrenocorticotropic factors such as CRH and ACTH, which stimulate fetal cortisol and estrogen precursor production, perhaps related to delayed maturation of the fetal brain.[144,186] There may also be a genetic risk.[186] The result is delay in myometrial activation with failure of oxytocin receptor, PG receptor, or gap junction development, or delay in cervical ripening.[144]

SUMMARY

An understanding of physiologic processes during the intrapartum period is essential for recognition of the effects of parturition on the pregnant woman and the fetus and in optimizing maternal, fetal, and neonatal outcome. This knowledge provides the basis for assessment of functional and dysfunctional labor patterns and maternal responses to pharmacologic agents used to alter or control uterine activity, for recognition of preterm and post term labor, and for interventions such as positioning during the first and second stages of labor. Recommendations for clinical practice related to parturition and uterine physiology during parturition are summarized in Table 4-1.

References

1. Aguilar, H.N. & Mitchell, B.F. (2010). Physiological pathways and molecular mechanisms regulating uterine contractility. *Hum Reprod Update, 16*, 725.
2. Akerlund, M. (1997). Contractility in the nonpregnant uterus. *Ann N Y Acad Med, 828*, 213.
3. Algovik, M., et al. (2004). Genetic influence on dystocia. *Acta Obstet Gynecol Scand, 83*, 832.
4. Algovik, M., et al. (2010). Genetic evidence of multiple loci in dystocia-difficult labor. *BMC Med Genet, 11*, 105.
5. American College of Obstetricians and Gynecologists. (2008). ACOG Committee Opinion num 419. Use of progesterone to reduce preterm birth. *Obstet Gynecol, 112*, 963.
6. American College of Obstetricians and Gynecologists Committee on Practice Bulletins-Obstetrics. (2004). ACOG Practice Bulletin. Clinical management guidelines for obstetricians-gynecologists. Number 55, September 2004 Management of postterm pregnancy. *Obstet Gynecol, 104*, 639.
7. Anum, E.A., et al. (2009). Genetic contributions to disparities in preterm birth. *Pediatr Res, 65*, 1.
8. Arias, F. (2000). Pharmacology of oxytocin and prostaglandins. *Clin Obstet Gynecol, 43*, 453.

9. Berghella, V., Baxter, J.K., & Chauhan, S.P. (2008). Evidence-based labor and delivery management. *Am J Obstet Gynecol, 199,* 445.
10. Berkman, N.D., et al. (2003). Tocolytic treatment for the management of preterm labor: A review of the evidence. *Am J Obstet Gynecol, 188,* 1648.
11. Beshay, V.E., Carr, B.R. & Rainey, W.E. (2007). The human fetal adrenal gland, corticotropin-releasing hormone, and parturition. *Semin Reprod Med, 25,* 14.
12. Blumenfeld, Y.J. & Lyell, D.J. (2009). Prematurity prevention: The role of acute tocolysis. *Curr Opin Obstet Gynecol, 21,* 136.
13. Boggess, K.A. (2005). Pathophysiology of preterm birth: Emerging concepts of maternal infection. *Clin Perinatol, 32,* 561.
14. Buhimschi, C.S., et al. (2010). Novel insights into molecular mechanisms of abruption-induced preterm birth, *Expert Rev Mol Med, 12,* e35.
15. Buxton, I.L. (2004). Regulation of uterine function: A biochemical conundrum in the regulation of smooth muscle relaxation. *Mol Pharmacol, 65,* 1051.
16. Carey, J.C. & Klebanoff, M.A. (2005). Is a change in the vaginal flora associated with an increased risk of preterm birth? *Am J Obstet Gynecol, 192,* 1341.
17. Caritis, S.N. (2011). Metaanalysis and labor inhibition therapy. *Am J Obstet Gynecol, 204,* 95.
18. Challis, J.R. & Lye, S.J. (1994). Parturition. In E. Knobil & J. Neill (Eds.). *The physiology of reproduction* (2nd ed.). New York: Raven.
19. Challis, J.R. & Lye, S.J. (2004). Characteristics of parturition. In R.K. Creasy, R. Resnik, & J.D. Iams (Eds.). *Maternal-fetal medicine: Principles and practice* (5th ed.). Philadelphia: Saunders.
20. Challis, J.R., et al. (2002). Prostaglandins and mechanisms of preterm birth. *Reproduction, 124,* 1.
21. Challis, J.R., et al. (2005). Fetal signals and parturition. *J Obstet Gynaecol Res, 31,* 492.
22. Challis, J.R., Lye, S.J., & Dong, X.S. (2005). Transcriptional regulation of human myometrium and the onset of labor. *J Soc Gynecol Invest, 12,* 65.
23. Chan, J., et al. (2006). Pragmatic comparison of beta(2)-agonist side effects within the Worldwide Atosiban versus Beta Agonists Study, *Eur J Obstet Gynecol Reprod Biol, 128,*135.
24. Cheng, Y., et al. (2009). The second stage of labor and epidural use: A larger effect than previously suggested. *Am J Obstet* Gynecol, 201, S46.
25. Chong, Y.S., Su, L.L., & Arulkumaran, S. (2004). Misoprostol: A quarter century of use, abuse, and creative misuse. *Obstet Gynecol Surv, 59,* 128.
26. Chwalisz, K. & Garfield, R.E. (1997). Regulation of the uterus and cervix during pregnancy and labor: Role of progesterone and nitric oxide. *Ann N Y Acad Sci, 828,* 238.
27. Chwalisz, K. & Garfield, R.E. (1998). Role of nitric oxide in the uterus and cervix: Implications for the management of labor. *J Perinat Med, 26,* 448.
28. Cole, S., Smith, R., & Giles, W. (2004). Tocolysis: Current controversies, future directions. *Curr Opin Investig Drugs, 5,* 424.
29. Colombo, D.J. & Iams, J.D. (2000). Cervical length and preterm labor. *Clin Obstet Gynecol, 43,* 735.
30. Conde-Agudelo, A., Romero, R., & Kusanovic, J.P. (2011). Nifedipine in the management of preterm labor: A systematic review and metaanalysis, *Am J Obstet Gynecol, 204,* e1.
31. Conrad, K.P. (2010). Unveiling the vasodilatory actions and mechanisms of relaxin. *Hypertension, 56,* 2.
32. Cookson, V.J. & Chapman, N.R. (2010). NF-kappaB function in the human myometrium during pregnancy and parturition. *Histol Histopathol, 25,* 945.
33. Cunningham, G., et al. (2009). *Williams obstetrics* (23rd ed.). New York: McGraw-Hill.
34. da Fonseca, E.B., et al. (2003). Prophylactic administration of progesterone by vaginal suppository to reduce the incidence of spontaneous preterm birth in women at increased risk: A randomized placebo-controlled double-blind study. *Am J Obstet Gynecol, 188,* 419.
35. de Heus, R., et al. (2009). Adverse drug reactions to tocolytic treatment for preterm labour: Prospective cohort study, *BMJ, 338,* c744.
36. de Heus, R., Mulder, E.J., & Visser, G.H. (2010). Management of preterm labor: Atosiban or nifedipine? *Int J Womens Health, 2,* 137.
37. De Jonge, A., Teunissen, T.A., & Lagro-Janssen, A.L. (2004). Supine position compared to other positions during the second stage of labor: A meta-analytic review. *J Psychosom Obstet Gynaecol, 25,* 35.
38. Downe, S., Gerrett, D., & Renfrew, M.J. (2004). A prospective randomized trial on the effect of position in the passive second stage of labour on birth outcome in nulliparous women using epidural analgesia. *Midwifery, 20,* 157.
39. Doyle, L.W., et al. (2009). Magnesium sulphate for women at risk of preterm birth for neuroprotection of the fetus, *Cochrane Database Syst Rev, 1,* CD004661.
40. Ekman-Ordeberg, G., et al. (2003). Endocrine regulation of cervical ripening in humans—potential roles for gonadal steroids and insulin-like growth factor-I. *Steroids, 68,* 837.
41. El Khwad, M., et al. (2005). Term human fetal membranes have a weak zone overlying the lower uterine pole and cervix before onset of labor. *Biol Reprod, 72,* 720.
42. Enkin, M., Keirse, M.J.N.C., & Neilson, J. (2000). *A guide to effective care in pregnancy and childbirth* (3rd ed.). Oxford: Oxford University Press.
43. Estrada-Gutierrez, G. (2005). Initial characterization of the microenvironment that regulates connective tissue degradation in amniochorion during normal human labor. *Matrix Biol, 24,* 306.
44. Facchinetti, F. & Vaccaro, V. (2009). Pharmacological use of progesterone and 17-alpha-hydroxyprogesterone caproate in the prevention of preterm delivery. *Minerva Ginecol, 61,* 401.
45. Farina, L. & Winkelman, C. (2005). A review of the role of proinflammatory cytokines in labor and noninfectious preterm labor. *Biol Res Nurs, 6,* 230.
46. Garfield, R.E. (1987). Cellular and molecular basis for dystocia. *Clin Obstet Gynecol, 30,* 3.
47. Garfield, R.E., Blennerhassett, M.G., & Miller, S.M. (1988). Control of myometrial contractility: Role and regulation of gap junctions. *Oxf Rev Reprod Biol, 10,* 436.
48. Gaunekar, N.N. & Crowther, C.A. (2004). Maintenance therapy with calcium channel blockers for preventing preterm birth after threatened preterm labour. *Cochrane Database Syst Rev* 3, CD004071.
49. George, A., et al. (2011). Periodontal treatment during pregnancy and birth outcomes: A meta-analysis of randomised trials. *Int J Evid Based Healthc, 9,* 122.
50. Golay, J., et al. (1993). The squatting position for the second stage of labor: Effects on labor and on maternal and fetal well-being. *Birth, 20,* 73.
51. Goldsmith, L.T. & Weiss, G. (2009). Relaxin in human pregnancy. *Ann N Y Acad Sci, 1160,* 130.
52. Golightly, E., Jabbour, H.N., & Norman, J.E. (2011). Endocrine immune interactions in human parturition. *Mol Cell Endocrinol, 335,* 52.
53. Gomez-Lopez, N., et al. (2010). The role of chemokines in term and premature rupture of the fetal membranes: A review. *Biol Reprod, 82,* 809.
54. Grammatopoulos, D.K. (2007). The role of CRH receptors and their agonists in myometrial contractility and quiescence during pregnancy and labour. *Front Biosci, 12,* 561.
55. Gulmezoglu, A.M., et al. (2001). WHO multicentre randomized trial of misoprostol in the management of the third stage of labour. *Lancet, 358,* 689.
56. Gupta, J.K. & Hofmeyr, G.J. (2004). Position during second stage of labour. *Cochrane Database Syst Rev* 1, CD002006.
57. Haas, D.M., et al. (2011). A pilot study of the impact of genotype on nifedipine pharmacokinetics when used as a tocolytic. *J Matern Fetal Neonatal Med,* 2011 Jun 7. [Epub ahead of print.]
58. Han. S., Crowther, C.A., & Moore, V. (2010). Magnesium maintenance therapy for preventing preterm birth after threatened preterm labour, *Cochrane Database Syst Rev, 7,* CD000940.

59. Hanson, L. (2009). Second-stage labor care: Challenges in spontaneous bearing down. *J Perinat Neonatal Nurs, 23*, 31.
60. Harper, M., et al. (2011). Cytokine gene polymorphisms and length of gestation. Eunice Kennedy Shriver National Institute of Child Health and Human Development (NICHD) Maternal-Fetal Medicine Units Network (MFMU). *Obstet Gynecol, 117*, 125.
61. Hearne, A.E. & Nagey, D.A. (2000). Therapeutic agents in preterm labor: Tocolytic agents. *Clin Obstet Gynecol, 43*, 787.
62. Helliwell, R.J., et al. (2004). Nuclear prostaglandin receptors: Role in pregnancy and parturition? *Prostaglandins Leukot Essent Fatty Acids*, 70, 149.
63. Hillhouse, E.W. & Grammatopoulos, D.K. (2001). Control of intracellular signaling by corticotropin-releasing hormone in human myometrium. In R. Smith (Ed). *The endocrinology of parturition: Basic science and clinical application*. Basel, Switzerland: Karger.
64. Hofmeyr, G.J., Gulmezoglu, A.M., & Pileggi, C. (2010). Vaginal misoprostol for cervical ripening and induction of labour. *Cochrane Database Sys* 2010 Oct 6;(10):CD000941
65. Hofmeyr, G.J. & Kulier, R. (2005). Hands and knees posture in late pregnancy or labour for fetal malposition (lateral or posterior). *Cochrane Database Syst Rev 18*, CD001063.
66. Hollis, B. (2002). Prolonged pregnancy. *Curr Opin Obstet Gynecol, 14*, 203.
67. Hunter, S., Hofmeyr, G.J., & Kulier, R. (2007). Hands and knees posture in late pregnancy or labour for fetal malposition (lateral or posterior), *Cochrane Database Syst Rev, 4*, CD001063.
68. Hutchings, G., et al. (2009). Myometrial interstitial cells and the coordination of myometrial contractility. *J Cell Mol Med, 13*, 4268.
69. Iams, J.D., et al. (2003). What have we learned about uterine contractions and preterm birth? The HUAM Prediction Study. *Semin Perinatol, 27*, 204.
70. Iams, J.D., et al. (2008). Primary, secondary, and tertiary interventions to reduce the morbidity and mortality of preterm birth. *Lancet, 371*, 164.
71. Iams, J.D. & Romano, R. (2009). Preterm labor and birth. In R.K. Creasy, et al. (Eds.). *Creasy & Resnik's Maternal-fetal medicine: Principles and practice* (6th ed.). Philadelphia: Saunders Elsevier.
72. Jayasooriya, G.S. & Lamont, R.F. (2009). The use of progesterone and other progestational agents to prevent spontaneous preterm labour and preterm birth. *Expert Opin Pharmacother, 10*, 1007.
73. Joy, S.D., Sanchez-Ramos, L., & Kaunitz, A.M. (2003). Misoprostol use during the third stage of labor. *Int J Gynaecol Obstet, 82*, 143.
74. Kamel, R.M. (2010). The onset of human parturition. *Arch Gynecol Obstet, 281*, 975.
75. Kariminia, A., et al. (2004). Randomized controlled trial of effect of hands and knees posturing on incidence of occiput posterior position at birth. *BMJ, 328*, 490.
76. Kelly, A.J., et al. (2009). Vaginal prostaglandin (PGE_2 and $PGF_{2\alpha}$) for induction of labour at term. *Cochrane Database Syst Rev*, 2009 Oct 7;(4):CD003101.
77. Kelly, A.J., Munson, C., & Minden, L. (2011). Nitric oxide donors for cervical ripening and induction of labour, *Cochrane Database Syst Rev, 6*, CD006901.
78. Kelly, R.W. (2002). Inflammatory mediators and cervical ripening. *J Reprod Immunol, 57*, 217.
79. Khan, A.H., Carson, R.J., & Nelson, S.M. (2008). Prostaglandins in labor—a translational approach. *Front Biosci, 13*, 5794.
80. King, J., et al. (2005). Cyclo-oxygenase (COX) inhibitors for treating preterm labor, *Coch Database Syst Rev, 2*, CD001992.
81. Klein, L.L. & Gibbs, R.S. (2004). Use of microbial cultures and antibiotics in the prevention of infection-associated preterm birth. *Am J Obstet Gynecol, 190*, 1493.
82. Klein, L.L. & Gibbs, R.S. (2005). Infection and preterm birth. *Obstet Gynecol Clin North Am, 32*, 397.
83. Kruckier, I.I. (2003). Production of NO and oxidative destruction of proteins in the placenta during normal pregnancy and placental insufficiency. *Bull Exp Biol Med, 136*, 369.
84. Kumar, D., et al. (2006). Proinflammatory cytokines found in amniotic fluid induce collagen remodeling, apoptosis, and biophysical weakening of cultured human fetal membranes. *Biol Reprod, 74*, 29.
85. Lam, F. & Gill, P. (2005). beta-Agonist tocolytic therapy. *Obstet Gynecol Clin North Am, 32*, 457.
86. Lamont, R.F. (2005). Can antibiotics prevent preterm birth—the pro and con debate. *BJOG, 112*, 67.
87. Lawrence, A., et al. (2009). Maternal positions and mobility during first stage labour, *Cochrane Database Syst Rev, 2*, CD003934.
88. Lesny, P. & Killick, S.R. (2004). The junctional zone of the uterus and its contractions. *BJOG, 111*, 1182.
89. Lewis, D.F. (2005). Magnesium sulfate: the first-line tocolytic. *Obstet Gynecol Clin North Am, 32*, 485.
90. Liu, Y.C. (1989). The effects of the upright position during childbirth. *Image J Nurs Sch, 21*, 14.
91. Lockwood, C.J. (2004). The initiation of parturition at term. *Obstet Gynecol Clin North Am, 31*, 935.
92. López Bernal, A. (2007). Overview. Preterm labour: Mechanisms and management, *BMC Pregnancy Childbirth, 7*, S2.
93. López Bernal, A. (2007). The regulation of uterine relaxation. *Semin Cell Dev Biol, 18*, 340.
94. Lopez Bernal, A.L. (2003). Mechanisms of labour—biochemical aspects. *BJOG, 110*, 39.
95. Ludmir, J. & Sehdev, H.M. (2000). Anatomy and physiology of the uterine cervix. *Clin Obstet Gynecol, 43*, 433.
96. Lye, S.J. (1999). Myometrial physiology and parturition. In C.H. Rodeck & M.J. Whittle (Eds.). *Fetal medicine: Basic science and clinical practice*. London: Churchill Livingstone.
97. Lye, S.J., et al. (2001). Role of mechanical signals in the onset of term and preterm labor. In R. Smith (Ed.). *The endocrinology of parturition: Basic science and clinical application*. Basel, Switzerland: Karger.
98. Lyon, D., et al. (2010). Integrated review of cytokines in maternal, cord, and newborn blood: Part I—associations with preterm birth. *Biol Res Nurs, 11*, 371.
99. Manuck, T.A., et al. (2011). Admixture mapping to identify spontaneous preterm birth susceptibility loci in African Americans. Eunice Kennedy Shriver National Institute of Child Health and Human Development (NICHD) Maternal-Fetal Medicine Units Network (MFMU). *Obstet Gynecol, 117*, 1078.
100. Marret, S., et al. (2007). Magnesium sulphate given before very-preterm birth to protect infant brain: the randomised controlled PREMAG trial. PREMAG trial group. *BJOG, 114*, 310.
101. Maruyama, T., et al. (2010). Human uterine stem/progenitor cells: Their possible role in uterine physiology and pathology. *Reprod, 140*, 11.
102. Mastorakos, G. & Ilias, I. (2003). Maternal and fetal hypothalamic-pituitary-adrenal axes during pregnancy and postpartum. *Ann N Y Acad Sci, 997*, 136.
103. Maul, H., et al. (2003). The physiology of uterine contractions. *Clin Perinatol, 30*, 665.
104. McDonald, H., et al. (2007). Antibiotics for treating bacterial vaginosis in pregnancy. *Cochrane Database Syst Rev* 2007 Jan 24;(1):CD000262.
105. McGuane, J.T., et al. (2009). Role of relaxin in maternal systemic and renal vascular adaptations during gestation. *Ann N Y Acad Sci, 1160*, 304.
106. Meis, P.J., et al. (2003). Prevention of recurrent preterm delivery by 17 alpha-hydroxyprogesterone caproate. *N Engl J Med, 348*, 2379.
107. Meis, P.J. & Aleman, A. (2004). Drug treatment to prevent preterm birth. *Drugs, 64*, 2463.
108. Meis, P.J., et al. (2005). Does progesterone treatment influence risk factors for recurrent preterm delivery? *Obstet Gynecol, 106*, 557.
109. Mendelson, C.R. (2009). Minireview: Fetal-maternal hormonal signaling in pregnancy and labor. *Mol Endocrinol, 23*, 947.
110. Mendez-Bauer, C. & Newton, M. (1986). Maternal position in labor. In E. Phillip, J. Barnes, & M. Newton (Eds.). *Scientific foundations of obstetrics and gynecology*. London: Heinemann.

111. Menon, R. & Fortunato, S.J. (2004). The role of matrix degrading enzymes and apoptosis in rupture of membranes. *Soc Gynecol Invest, 11*, 427.
112. Mercer, B.M. (2009). Premature rupture of the membranes. In R.K. Creasy, et al. (Eds.). *Creasy & Resnik's Maternal-fetal medicine: Principles and practice* (6th ed.). Philadelphia: Saunders Elsevier.
113. Mesiano, S., et al. (2002). Progesterone withdrawal and estrogen activation in human parturition are coordinated by progesterone receptor A expression in the myometrium. *J Clin Endocrinol Metab, 87*, 2924.
114. Mesiano, S., Wang, Y., & Norwitz, E.R. (2011). Progesterone receptors in the human pregnancy uterus: Do they hold the key to birth timing? *Reprod Sci, 18*, 6.
115. Miller, F.C. (1983). Uterine motility in spontaneous labor. *Clin Obstet Gynecol, 26*, 78.
116. Monga, M. & Sanborn, B.M. (2004). Biology and physiology of the reproductive tract and control of myometrial contraction. In R.K. Creasy, R. Resnik, & J.D. Iams (Eds.). *Maternal-fetal medicine: Principles and practice* (5th ed.). Philadelphia: Saunders.
117. Moore, R.M., et al. (2006). The physiology of fetal membrane rupture: Insight gained from the determination of physical properties. *Placenta, 27*, 1037.
118. Moore, T.R. (1995). Patterns of human uterine contractions: Implications for clinical practice. *Semin Perinatol, 19*, 64.
119. Muglia, L.J. & Katz, M. (2010). The enigma of spontaneous preterm birth. *N Engl J Med, 362*, 529.
120. Myatt, L. & Lye, S.J. (2004). Expression, localization and function of prostaglandin receptors in myometrium. *Prostaglandins Leukot Essent Fatty Acids, 70*, 137.
121. Myatt, L. & Sun, K. (2010). Role of fetal membranes in signaling of fetal maturation and parturition. *Int J Dev Biol, 54*, 545.
122. Nagamatsu, T. & Schust, D.J. (2010). The contribution of macrophages to normal and pathological pregnancies. *Am J Reprod Immunol, 63*, 460.
123. Nagamatsu. T. & Schust, D.J. (2010). The immunomodulatory roles of macrophages at the maternal-fetal interface. *Reprod Sci, 17*, 209.
124. Nassar, A.H., et al. (2006). Adverse maternal and neonatal outcome of prolonged course of magnesium sulfate tocolysis. *Acta Obstet Gynecol Scand, 85*, 1099.
125. Nassar, A.H., Aoun, J., & Usta, I.M. (2011). Calcium channel blockers for the management of preterm birth: A review. *Am J Perinatol, 28*, 57.
126. Nathanielsz, P.W. (1998). Comparative studies on the initiation of labor. *Eur J Obstet Gynecol Reprod Biol, 78*, 127.
127. National Center for Health Statistics, final natality data. (2008). http://www.marchofdimes.com/peristats. Accessed June 21, 2011.
128. Neal, J.L., et al. (2010). "Active labor" duration and dilatation rates among low-risk, nulliparous women with spontaneous labor onset: A systematic review. *J Midwifery Womens Health, 55*, 308.
129. Newton, E.R. (2005). Preterm labor, preterm premature rupture of membranes, and chorioamnionitis. *Clin Perinatol, 32*, 571.
130. Northen, A.T., et al. (2007). Follow-up of children exposed in utero to 17 alpha-hydroxyprogesterone caproate compared with placebo. *Obstet Gynecol, 110*, 865.
131. Norwitz, E.R. & Lye, S.J. (2009). Biology of parturition. In R.K. Creasy, et al. (Eds.). *Creasy & Resnik's Maternal-fetal medicine: Principles and practice* (6th ed.). Philadelphia: Saunders Elsevier.
132. O'Brien, R.F. (2005). Bacterial vaginosis: Many questions—any answers? *Curr Opin Pediatr*, 17, 473.
133. Oh, S.Y., et al. (2005). Progesterone receptor isoform (A/B) ratio of human fetal membranes increases during term parturition. *Am J Obstet Gynecol, 193*, 1156.
134. Osman, I., et al. (2003). Leukocyte density and pro-inflammatory cytokine expression in human fetal membranes, decidua, cervix and myometrium before and during labour at term. *Mol Hum Reprod, 9*, 41.
135. Oyen, M.L., Cook, R.F., & Calvin, S.E. (2004). Mechanical failure of human fetal membrane tissues. *J Materials Science: Materials in Medicine, 15*, 651.
136. Page, E.W., Villee, C.A., & Villee, D.B. (1981). *Human reproduction: Essentials of reproductive and perinatal medicine* (3rd ed.). Philadelphia: Saunders.
137. Papatsonis, D., et al. (2005). Oxytocin receptor antagonists for inhibiting preterm labour, *Cochrane Database Syst Rev, 20*, CD004452.
138. Papatsonis, D., Flenady, V., & Liley. H. (2009). Maintenance therapy with oxytocin antagonists for inhibiting preterm birth after threatened preterm labour, *Cochrane Database Syst Rev, 21*, CD005938.
139. Parkington, H.C. & Coleman, H.A. (2001). Excitability in uterine smooth muscle. *Front Horm Res, 27*, 179.
140. Petraglia, F., Imperatore, A., & Challis, J.R. (2010). Neuroendocrine mechanisms in pregnancy and parturition. *Endocr Rev, 31*, 783.
141. Petrini, J.R., et al. (2005). Estimated effect of 17 alpha-hydroxyprogesterone caproate on preterm birth in the United States. *Obstet Gynecol, 105*, 267.
142. Polyzos, N.P., et al. (2010). Obstetric outcomes after treatment of periodontal disease during pregnancy: Systematic review and meta-analysis, *BMJ, 341*, c7017.
143. Randis, T.M. (2010). Progress toward improved understanding of infection-related preterm birth. *Clin Perinatol, 37*, 677.
144. Resnik, J.L. & Resnik R. (2009). Post-term pregnancy. In R.K. Creasy, et al. (Eds.). *Creasy & Resnik's Maternal-fetal medicine: Principles and practice* (6th ed.). Philadelphia: Saunders Elsevier.
145. Resnik, R. (1999). Anatomic alterations in the reproductive tract. In R.K. Creasy, et al. (Eds.). *Maternal-fetal medicine* (4th ed.). Philadelphia: Saunders.
146. Roberts, C.L., et al. (2004). Delayed versus early pushing in women with epidural analgesia: A systematic review and meta-analysis. *BJOG, 111*, 1333.
147. Roberts, C.L., et al. (2005). A meta-analysis of upright positions in the second stage to reduce instrumental deliveries in women with epidural analgesia. *Acta Obstet Gynecol Scand, 84*, 794.
148. Roberts, J.E. (1989). Maternal positioning during the first stage of labour. In I. Chalmers, M. Enkin, & M.J.N.C. Keirse (Eds.). *Effective care in pregnancy and childbirth.* Oxford, England: Oxford University Press.
149. Roberts, J.E. (2003). A new understanding of the second stage of labor: Implications for nursing care. *J Obstet Gynecol Neonatal Nurs, 32*, 794.
150. Romero, R. & Lockwood, C.J. (2009). Pathogenesis of spontaneous preterm labor. In R.K. Creasy, et al. (Eds.). *Creasy & Resnik's Maternal-fetal medicine: Principles and practice* (6th ed.). Philadelphia: Saunders Elsevier.
151. Rouse, D.J. (2009). Magnesium sulfate for the prevention of cerebral palsy. *Am J Obstet Gynecol, 200*, 610.
152. Sado, T., et al. (2011). Anticytokine therapy in preterm labor: Current knowledge and future perspectives, *Gynecol Obstet Invest, 71*, 1-10. Epub 2010.
153. Sampselle, C.M. & Hines, S. (1999). Spontaneous pushing during birth: Relationship to birth outcomes. *J Nurs Midwifery, 44*, 36.
154. Sanborn, B.M. (2000). Relationship of ion channel activity to control of myometrial calcium. *J Soc Gynecol Investig, 7*, 4.
155. Sanchez-Ramos, L. (2005). Induction of labor. *Obstet Gynecol Clin North Am, 32*, 181.
156. Sanchez-Ramos, L. & Huddleston, J.F. (2003). The therapeutic value of maintenance tocolysis: An overview of the evidence. *Clin Perinatol, 30*, 841.
157. Sanchez-Ramos, L., Kaunitz, A.M., & Delke, I. (2005). Progestational agents to prevent preterm birth: A meta-analysis of randomized controlled trials. *Obstet Gynecol, 105*, 273.
158. Schindler, A.E. (2005). Role of progestogens for the prevention of premature birth. *J Steroid Biochem Mol Biol, 97*, 435.
159. Senok, A.C., et al. (2009). Probiotics for the treatment of bacterial vaginosis, *Cochrane Database Syst Rev, 4*, CD006289.
160. Shennan, A. & Jones, B. (2004). The cervix and prematurity: Aetiology, prediction and prevention. *Semin Fetal Neonatal Med, 9*, 471.
161. Shennan, A., et al. (2006). A randomized controlled trial of metronidazole for the prevention of preterm birth in women positive for cervicovaginal fetal fibronectin: The PREMET Study. *BJOG, 113*, 65.

162. Sherwood, O.D. (2004). Relaxin's physiological roles and other diverse actions. *Endocrinol Rev, 25,* 205.
163. Shynlova, O., et al. (2009). Integration of endocrine and mechanical signals in the regulation of myometrial functions during pregnancy and labour, *Eur J Obstet Gynecol Reprod Biol, 144,* S2.
164. Simpson, K.R. (2011). Clinicians' guide to the use of oxytocin for labor induction and augmentation. *J Midwifery Womens Health, 56,* 214.
165. Simpson, K.R. & James, D.C. (2005). Effects of immediate versus delayed pushing during second-stage labor on fetal well-being: A randomized clinical trial. *Nurs Res, 54,* 149.
166. Simpson, K.R. & Miller, L. (2011). Assessment and optimization of uterine activity during labor. *Clin Obstet Gynecol, 54,* 40.
167. Sirianni, R., et al. (2005). Corticotropin-releasing hormone directly stimulates cortisol and the cortisol biosynthetic pathway in human fetal adrenal cells. *J Clin Endocrinol Metab, 90,* 279.
168. Sleep, J., Roberts, J., & Chalmers, I. (1989). Care during the second stage of labour. In I. Chalmers, M. Enkin, & M.J.N.C. Keirse (Eds.). *Effective care in pregnancy and childbirth.* Oxford, England: Oxford University Press.
169. Smith, R., Mesiano, S., & McGrath, S. (2002). Hormone trajectories leading to human birth. *Regul Pept, 108,* 159.
170. Snegovskikh, V., Park, J.S., & Norwitz, E.R. (2006). Endocrinology of parturition. *Endocrinol Metab Clin North Am, 35,* 173.
171. Snegovskikh, V.V., et al. (2011).Surfactant protein-A (SP-A) selectively inhibits prostaglandin F2alpha (PGF2alpha) production in term decidua: Implications for the onset of labor, *J Clin Endocrinol Metab, 96,* E624.
172. Spong, C.Y., et al. (2005). Progesterone for prevention of recurrent preterm birth: Impact of gestational age at previous delivery. *Am J Obstet Gynecol, 193,* 1127.
173. Stitely, M.L. & Satin, A.J. (2002). Cervical ripening agents and uterine stimulants. *Clin Obstet Gynecol, 45,* 114.
174. Stjernholm-Vladic, Y., et al. (2004). Differential regulation of the progesterone receptor A and B in the human uterine cervix at parturition. *Gynecol Endocrinol, 18,* 41.
175. Stjernholm-Vladic, Y., et al. (2004). Factors involved in the inflammatory events of cervical ripening in humans. *Reprod Biol Endocrinol, 2,* 74.
176. Strauss, J. & Barbieri, R. (2009). *Yen & Jaffe's reproductive endocrinology* (6th ed.). Philadelphia: Saunders Elsevier.
177. Stremler, R. (2005). Randomized controlled trial of hands-and-knees positioning for occipitoposterior position in labor. *Birth, 32,* 243.
178. Su, L.L., Samuel, M., & Chong, Y.S. (2010). Progestational agents for treating threatened or established preterm labour, *Cochrane Database Syst Rev, 1,* CD006770.
179. Tenore, J.L. (2003). Methods for cervical ripening and induction of labor. *Am Fam Phys, 67,* 2123.
180. Terzidou, V., et al. (2005). Mechanical stretch up-regulates the human oxytocin receptor in primary human uterine myocytes. *J Clin Endocrinol Metab, 90,* 237.
181. Timmons, B., Akins, M., & Mahendroo, M. (2010). Cervical remodeling during pregnancy and parturition. *Trends Endocrinol Metab, 21,* 353.
182. Tingåker, B.K. & Irestedt, L. (2010). Changes in uterine innervation in pregnancy and during labour. *Curr Opin Anaesthesiol, 23,* 300.
183. Tromp, G., et al. (2004). Genome-wide expression profiling of fetal membranes reveals a deficient expression of proteinase inhibitor 3 in premature rupture of membranes. *Am J Obstet Gynecol, 191,* 1331.
184. Tsatsaris, V., Carbonne, B., & Cabrol, D. (2004). Atosiban for preterm labour. *Drugs, 64,* 375.
185. Vadillo-Ortega, F. & Estrada-Gutierrez, G. (2005). Role of matrix metalloproteinases in preterm labour. *BJOG, 112,* 19.
186. Vaisanen-Tommiska, M., Nuutila, M., & Ylikorkala, O. (2004). Cervical nitric oxide release in women postterm. *Obstet Gynecol, 103,* 657.
187. Varma, R. & Gupta, J.K. (2006). Antibiotic treatment of bacterial vaginosis in pregnancy: Multiple meta-analyses and dilemmas in interpretation. *Eur J Obstet Gynecol Reprod Biol, 124,* 10.
188. Vidaeff, A.C. & Ramin, S.M. (2008). Potential biochemical events associated with initiation of labor. *Curr Med Chem, 15,* 614.
189. Vrachnis, N., et al. (2010). Intrauterine inflammation and preterm delivery. *Ann N Y Acad Sci, 1205,* 118.
190. Ward, K., et al. (2005). The heritability of preterm delivery. *Obstet Gynecol, 106,* 1235.
191. Wei, S.Q., Fraser, W., & Luo, Z.C. (2010). Inflammatory cytokines and spontaneous preterm birth in asymptomatic women: A systematic review. *Obstet Gynecol, 116,* 393.
192. Whitworth, M. & Quenby, S. (2008). Prophylactic oral betamimetics for preventing preterm labour in singleton pregnancies, *Cochrane Database Syst Rev, 23,* CD006395.
193. Wilczynski, J.R. (2005). Th1/Th2 cytokines balance—yin and yang of reproductive immunology. *Eur J Obstet Gynecol Reprod Biol, 122,* 136.
194. Woolley, D. & Roberts, J. (1995). Second stage pushing: A comparison of Valsalva-style with mini-pushing. *J Perinat Ed, 4,* 37.
195. Woolley, D. & Roberts, J. (1996). A second look at the second stage of labor. *J Obstet Gynecol Neonatal Nurs, 25,* 415.
196. Worldwide Atosiban versus Beta-Agonists Study Group. (2001). Effectiveness and safety of the oxytocin antagonist atosiban versus beta-adrenergic agonists in the treatment of preterm labour. The Worldwide Atosiban versus Beta-Agonists Study Group. *BJOG, 108,* 133.
197. Xiong, X., et al. (2006). Periodontal disease and adverse pregnancy outcomes: A systematic review. *BJOG, 113,* 135.
198. Yeates, D.A. & Roberts, J.E. (1984). A comparison of two bearing down techniques during the second stage of labor. *J Nurse Midwifery, 29,* 3.
199. Yılmaz, Y., et al. (2011). Maternal-fetal proinflammatory cytokine gene polymorphism and preterm birth, *DNA Cell Biol, 2011,* Jun 17. [Epub ahead of print.]
200. Zhou, X., et al. (2010). Recent advances in understanding the microbiology of the female reproductive tract and the causes of premature birth. *Infect Dis Obstet Gynecol, 12,* 737.
201. Zoumakis, E., Kalantaridou, S.N., & Makrigiannakis, A. (2009). CRH-like peptides in human reproduction. *Curr Med Chem, 16,* 4230.
202. Zwelling, E. (2010). Overcoming the challenges: Maternal movement and positioning to facilitate labor progress. *MCN Am J Matern Child Nurs, 35,* 72.

CHAPTER 5

The Postpartum Period and Lactation Physiology

Ilana R. Azulay Chertok

The postpartum period is a time of restoration and return to the nonpregnant state. This period is generally defined as the 6- to 8-week postpartum period from the delivery of the placenta to the involution and return of the reproductive organs to their nonpregnant state. The postpartum period is characterized by significant anatomic, physiologic, and endocrinologic changes related to the involution and lactation processes. It is also a time of major psychologic and social change as the new mother bonds with her infant, assumes responsibility for, and incorporates her infant into the family system. The focus of this chapter is on the physiologic and endocrinologic changes associated with return of the reproductive system to its nonpregnant state and with the anatomic, physiologic, and endocrinologic changes associated with initiation and maintenance of lactation. The physiologic and anatomic changes within other body systems as they return to the nonpregnant state are described in Chapters 8 to 20.

INVOLUTION OF THE REPRODUCTIVE ORGANS

The process of involution involves the gradual and progressive return of the reproductive system (i.e., uterus, cervix, vagina, and breasts in the nonlactating woman) to its nonpregnant state during the 6- to 8-week postpartum period.

Uterus

Immediately following delivery of the placenta, the uterus weighs approximately 1000 g and lies with its anterior and posterior walls in close approximation in midline about halfway between the umbilicus and symphysis pubis. Over the next 12 hours the fundus of the uterus is located approximately at the level of the umbilicus. Involution of the uterus involves uterine contraction, autolysis of myometrial cells, and epithelial regeneration and proliferation. The height of the fundus continues to decrease by about 1 cm per day so that by 3 days the fundus lies 2 to 3 fingerbreadths below the umbilicus (or slightly higher in multiparous women). By 1 week, the uterus weighs about 500 g and is 4 to 5 fingerbreadths below the umbilicus. By 2 weeks, the uterus weighs about 300 g and has descended into the true pelvis and the fundus can no longer be palpated abdominally. The size of the uterus gradually decreases over the next month so that by 6 weeks the uterus has nearly returned to its nonpregnant location and size.[69] Immediately following delivery of the infant, contractions of the uterine myometrium compress the blood vessels supplying the placental site, causing hemostasis and separation of the placenta from the uterine wall, leaving the basal portion of the decidua. Postpartum contractions ("afterpains") during the first few days of postpartum may be strong, especially with increasing parity, gradually diminishing in intensity and frequency within the first week. Infant suckling also stimulates oxytocin release resulting in uterine contractions.[17]

Subinvolution, slowed, delayed, and/or incomplete involution, is usually due to a lack of effective uterine contraction related to various causes including uterine atony (most common), retained placental fragments, uterine inversion, lacerations, or infection, which are usually responsive to early diagnosis and treatment.[17] There has been research indicating that uterine massage after placental delivery may prevent postpartum hemorrhage.[31] Signs and symptoms of infection may include fever, abdominal tenderness, and foul-smelling lochia. Signs and symptoms of hemorrhage include tachycardia, low blood pressure, boggy uterus, and excessive uterine bleeding with clots, consisting of a blood loss over 500 mL post-vaginal delivery and 1000 mL or more post-cesarean delivery. Postpartum hemorrhage is most commonly associated with coagulation disorders, infection, and subinvolution and its causes, as well as other risk factors including retained placenta, failure to progress in the second stage of labor, placenta accrete, lacerations, instrumental delivery, large for gestational age infant, hypertensive disorders, induction of labor, and oxytocin-augmented labor.[72] Assessment using the "four Ts" (tone of the uterus; trauma including lacerations, inversion, and rupture; tissue retention or invasion; and thrombin and coagulation disorders), along with prevention and early intervention are crucial. Management of uterine atony and hemorrhage is aimed at increasing uterine contractility by attempting bimanual uterine compression massage, and uterotonic medications such as uterotonic oxytocin, misoprostol, methylergonovine maleate, and other prostaglandins.[5,83] If uterine atony and hemorrhage persist, uterine suture compression or surgical intervention may be necessary.[17,37]

Under the influence of estrogens, the myometrium undergoes hypertrophy and hyperplasia during pregnancy with increases in cell cytoplasm and size. Following delivery, excess intracellular proteins (especially actin and myosin) and cytoplasm within the myometrial cells are eliminated by autolysis with degradation by proteolytic enzymes and macrophages. As a result, the size of individual myometrial cells is markedly reduced without a significant reduction in the total number of cells. Initially the endometrium resembles a large desquamating wound. The upper portion of the spongy endometrial layer is sloughed off with delivery of the placenta.

Regeneration of the uterine epithelial lining begins 2 to 3 days postpartum with differentiation of the remaining decidua into two layers, a superficial layer and a basal layer. The superficial layer of granulation tissue, which provides a barrier to infection, is formed as leukocytes invade the remaining decidua. This layer gradually degenerates, becoming necrotic, and is sloughed off in lochia. The basal layer, containing residual endometrial glands, remains intact and contributes to the new endometrium. By about 2 to 3 weeks, the endometrium has been restored and is similar to the nonpregnant endometrium in the proliferative phase of the menstrual cycle except for remnants of hyalinized decidua with areas of leukocyte infiltration.[69] Healing at the placental site takes longer with regeneration occurring gradually over 6 weeks. Following delivery, the placental site is a rough area 4 to 5 cm in diameter containing many thrombosed vessels. The large blood vessels that supplied the intervillous spaces are invaded by fibroblasts and their lumen is obscured. Some of these vessels recanalize later with smaller lumens. The placental site heals by decidual sloughing and exfoliation and by growth of endometrial tissue.[69]

Lochia

The process of involution and restoration of the endometrium is reflected in the characteristics of lochia, the postpartum vaginal discharge. Lochia varies in amount and color as healing progresses. Three forms of lochia are observed, generally in the following pattern: rubra, serosa, and alba. Lochia rubra is red or red-brown with a fleshy odor and is seen during the first few days or through the first week postpartum. Lochia rubra contains blood from the placental site; pieces of amnion and chorion; and cellular elements from the decidua, vernix, lanugo, and meconium. Lochia serosa is a pinkish-brown discharge lasting approximately 2 to 3 weeks. Lochia serosa contains some blood, wound exudate, erythrocytes, leukocytes, cervical mucus, microorganisms, and shreds of decidual tissue. The lochia becomes progressively lighter in color. Lochia alba is whitish-yellow in color because it primarily contains leukocytes and decidual cells which may continue for another few weeks. Overall lochia duration may last 4 to 6 weeks postpartum, which is a longer duration than traditionally described, and may vary according to breastfeeding practice and parity.[51,73,78]

Cervix, Vagina, and Perineum

Immediately following a vaginal delivery, the cervix hangs into the vagina and is dilated, bruised, and edematous, with possible lacerations. During the first 12 to 18 hours, the cervix shortens and becomes firmer ("forming up") and, as measured by magnetic resonance imaging, has a mean length of 5.6 cm by 30 hours (versus 2.9 cm by 6 months).[81] By the second or third day, the cervix is dilated 2 to 3 cm and by 1 week the cervix is approximately 1 cm dilated. By 4 weeks the external os appears as a small transverse slit, characteristic of multiparous women. Even by 6 weeks, there may still be evidence of stromal edema and round cell infiltrates, which may persist until 3 to 4 months.[69] Remodeling and involution of the cervix begin immediately postpartum and occurs rapidly with an increase in fibroblasts, which play a major role in remodelling, collagen, and proteoglycans. This process may be mediated by transforming growth factor-β (TGF-β) and other cytokines.[79] This process works to restore the cervical structure altered during cervical ripening and delivery.

After vaginal delivery, the vagina is edematous and relaxed, with decreased tone and absence of rugae. The vagina gradually decreases in size and regains tone, although it does not fully return to its prepregnancy state. By 3 to 4 weeks, rugae have begun to reappear, and edema and vascularity have decreased. The vaginal epithelium is generally restored by 6 to 10 weeks postpartum.[69] Decreased lubrication of the vagina during this period can lead to discomfort with sexual intercourse, especially in the lactating woman, as can perineal pain related to episiotomy, laceration, and trauma.[17]

The use of episiotomies has significantly decreased since the 1980s and 1990s when research documented risks associated with routine use and advocated for restrictive use of episiotomies. Systematic reviews have shown that restrictive use of episiotomies is associated with less severe perineal trauma, less suturing, fewer complications, and less pain.[10,27] While initial healing occurs in 2 to 3 weeks, the episiotomy site may take 4 to 6 months to completely heal. A strategy that has been found to protect the perineum and decrease the risk for performing an episiotomy is prenatal perineal massage.[6,19,20]

Urinary Function

Diuresis occurs during the postpartum period, reversing prenatal fluid retention. Overdistention of the bladder; prolonged labor; vulvar, urethral, or bladder trauma, may result in incomplete bladder emptying and urine retention, especially when analgesics were used in labor and delivery and following cesarean delivery.[44,87] Management of maternal reports of urine retention in the early postpartum period include providing privacy, positioning, and immersing the woman's hands in water, as least invasive measures, and catheterization and medication are more invasive options.[87] Urinary incontinence is associated with pregnancy and trauma during the delivery process. Research has found that pelvic floor exercises can be effective in preventing and treating prenatal and postpartum urinary incontinence.[28,39] Changes in postpartum urinary function are discussed further in Chapter 11.

Breasts

The breasts or mammary glands undergo marked changes during pregnancy with development of alveolar tissue and ductal system in preparation for lactation. Following delivery, further anatomic and physiologic changes occur in breastfeeding women (see "Physiology of Lactation").

In women who do not breastfeed, involution of the breasts occurs. Distention and stasis of the vascular and lymphatic circulation may result in primary engorgement by 2 to 4 days following delivery. The treatment of engorgement for nonlactating women includes abstaining from stimulation of milk production, abstaining from any breast stimulation, brief applications of cold compresses or cold packs, and administration of anti-inflammatory medication. Bromocriptine (Parlodel) is no longer approved by the Food and Drug Administration for lactation suppression due to numerous adverse maternal outcomes.[25] Without stimulation by suckling and removal of milk, secretion of prolactin decreases and milk production ceases. Glandular tissue gradually returns to a resting state over the next few weeks, although breasts do not completely return to their prepregnant state, as new alveoli formed during pregnancy do not completely disappear.

Physical Activity and Sexual Function

The postpartum period is often characterized by alterations in physical activity and function. Gradual resumption of safe physical exercise promotes postpartum maternal well-being, physically and psychologically, as well as facilitates postpartum weight management.[4,63] Fatigue, postpartum anatomic and physiologic changes, lochia, perineal trauma, pain, decreased perineal tone, leaking or engorged breasts, the presence and stress of the new baby, adaptation to the demands of the new parental role, and psychologic factors can modify physical and sexual function. Reduced vaginal lubrication associated with the decreased estrogen levels in the postpartum period, especially in lactating women, may contribute to an alteration in sexuality and sexual discomfort.[14] Masters and Johnson reported that orgasms in women for the first few months following birth tended to be shorter and less intense with greater latency of response and decreased vasocongestion of the labia majora and minora and decreased vaginal lubrication.[52] The timing of resumption of sexual intercourse should depend on maternal physical restoration (cessation of bleeding and absence of discomfort) and the emotional and psychologic readiness of both partners, while accounting for traditional and cultural beliefs, attitudes, and preferences. Health care providers should be aware of, respectful of, and sensitive to cultural and religious practices associated with sexuality during the postpartum period. Interventions include education and counseling regarding postpartum physical and sexual function, contraception, use of vaginal lubricants, alternate forms of intimacy, and pelvic floor exercises to strengthen and tone the perineal muscles.

ENDOCRINE CHANGES

Postpartum endocrine changes primarily occur secondary to fetoplacental hormonal withdrawal related to delivery of the infant and placenta and to increased production of prolactin. In general, most peptide hormones, enzymes, and other circulating proteins of placental origin reach nonpregnant levels by 6 weeks postpartum. Removal of placental hormones alters the physiologic function of many body systems, thus initiating return of those systems to their nonpregnant state. The rate at which placental hormones disappear from the maternal system depends on the half-life phases of the particular substance in maternal blood. There are two phases. The first half-life, which is relatively short, involves hormonal removal from the intravascular system; the second half-life involves the slower removal from extravascular and intracellular space.[77] For example, human placental lactogen (hPL) has a short second half-life and generally disappears by 1 to 2 days, whereas human chorionic gonadotropin (hCG) has a longer second half-life and can be detected for 3 to 4 weeks.[77] Substances of fetoplacental origin, such as pregnancy-associated proteins, also disappear soon after delivery, whereas other proteins such as alpha-fetoprotein, derived from both placental and maternal sources, are present in maternal plasma for several weeks postpartum.[77] Endocrine changes related to mammary development in lactating and nonlactating women are summarized in Figure 5-1.

Estrogens and Progesterone

During pregnancy, estrogen promotes development of the mammary ductal system and progesterone promotes lobular and alveolar growth. The elevated levels of these hormones inhibit prolactin action thereby inhibiting lactation. Because the placenta is the major source of estrogens and progesterone, these hormones disappear rapidly following delivery. Plasma estradiol (with a first half-life of 20 minutes and second half-life of 6 to 7 hours) reaches levels that are less than 2% of pregnancy values by 24 hours. By 1 to 3 days, estradiol levels are similar to those found during the follicular phase of the menstrual cycle (less than 100 pg/mL [367 pmol/L]), and unconjugated estriol is undetectable. Although the first and second half-lives of progesterone are short, progesterone levels do not fall as rapidly as estradiol levels because the corpus luteum continues progesterone secretion during the first days following delivery. Generally progesterone falls to levels similar to the luteal phase of the menstrual cycle (2 to 25 ng/mL [6.4 to 79.5 pmol/L]) by 24 to 48 hours and to the follicular phase (less than 1 ng/mL [3.2 pmol/L]) by 3 to 7 days.[77] Ovarian production of estrogens and progesterone is low during the first 2 weeks postpartum and gradually increases with resumption of gonadotropin secretion.

Pituitary Gonadotropin

The pituitary-hypothalamic-ovarian axis (see Chapter 2), along with production of pituitary gonadotropin, follicle-stimulating hormone (FSH), and luteinizing hormone (LH), is suppressed

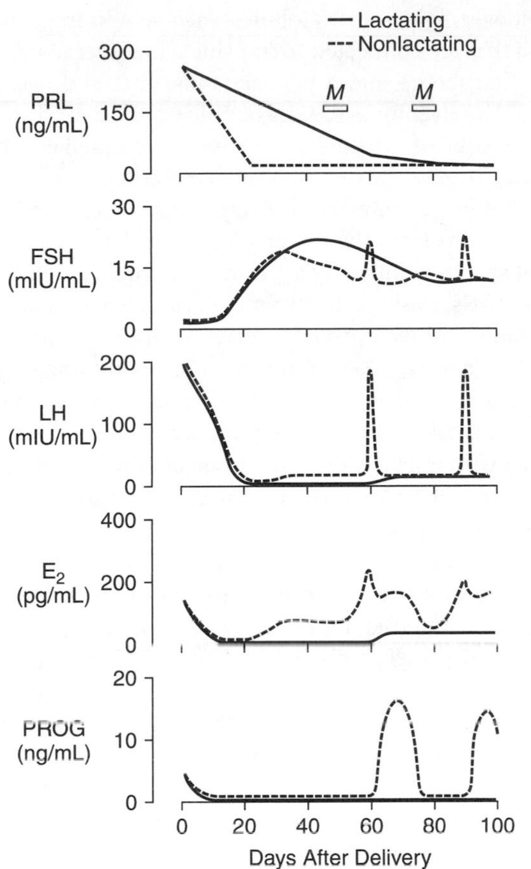

FIGURE 5-1 Changes in serum concentrations of pituitary and gonadal hormones in lactating and nonlactating women in the puerperium. In the top graph, the M boxes refer to menses in the nonlactating women. Changes in hormone levels associated with these menstrual periods are seen in the other graphs for the nonlactating woman. The lactating woman is still lactating and not menstruating. The elevated luteinizing hormone (LH) immediately postpartum is due to cross-reaction with assays of human chorionic gonadotropin and the estradiol (E_2) and progesterone (PROG) are of placental origin. *FSH*, Follicle-stimulating hormone; *PRL*, prolactin. (From Rebar, R.W. [2004]. The breast and the physiology of lactation. In R.K. Creasy, R. Resnik, & J.D. Iams. [Eds.]. *Maternal-fetal medicine: Principles and practice* [5th ed.]. Philadelphia: Saunders. Based on Rolland, R., et al. [1975]. The role of prolactin in the restoration of ovarian function during the early postpartum period in the human female. Part I: A study during physiological lactation. *Clin Endocrinol, 4,* 15.)

during pregnancy. Serum levels of follicle-stimulating hormone (FSH) and luteinizing hormone (LH) remain very low during the first 2 weeks postpartum in both lactating and nonlactating women, gradually increasing with resumption of pituitary function by 4 to 6 weeks. The basis for the initially sluggish pituitary response is unknown. Tulchinsky suggests that this phenomenon may be related to (1) suppression of the pituitary-hypothalamic-ovarian axis by the high levels of circulating estrogens during pregnancy, (2) need for time to reestablish adequate stores of follicle-stimulating hormone (FSH) and luteinizing hormone (LH) leading to a delay in secretion of gonadotropin-releasing hormone (GnRH) by the hypothalamus, and (3) possibly inhibition of luteinizing hormone (LH) release by human chorionic gonadotropin (hCG) and prolactin.[77]

Prolactin

Prolactin is a single-chain peptide hormone secreted in pulses by the anterior pituitary gland. Serum levels of prolactin dramatically increase during pregnancy (from 10 ng/mL to 200 ng/mL [434.8 to 8695.6 pmol/L]), working synergistically with other hormones to promote mammary development including lobular, alveolar, and nipple growth. Throughout pregnancy, secretion of prolactin by the anterior pituitary is controlled by hypothalamic prolactin-inhibiting factor (PIF), mainly dopamine.[55] A placental hormone, probably progesterone, inhibits the direct influence of prolactin on the breast during pregnancy, thereby suppressing lactation. With the expulsion of the placenta at delivery, and the significant drop in progesterone, lactogenesis II (copious milk secretion) is initiated.[61] Delayed lactogenesis may result from retained placental fragments with the potential to secrete progesterone.[61] Postpartum prolactin levels remain elevated due to frequent infant suckling and nipple stimulation.[55] In nonlactating women, prolactin levels fall into the high end of the nonpregnant range by 7 to 14 days.[77] Breastfeeding women experience a gradual decreasing trend in serum prolactin surges after 6 weeks postpartum, even with continued breastfeeding. Patterns of prolactin secretion associated with lactation are described in "Physiology of Lactation."

Oxytocin

Oxytocin is an octapeptide hormone produced in the hypothalamus and stored and secreted by the posterior pituitary gland. The uterus becomes increasingly sensitive to oxytocin throughout pregnancy, probably as a result of increasing estrogens that mediate an increase in oxytocin receptors. When the infant suckles, nerve impulses stimulate the release of oxytocin from the posterior pituitary into maternal blood. Oxytocin stimulates the electrical and contractile activity in the myometrium by causing the myoepithelial cells of the uterus to contract and involute. Oxytocin also causes contraction of the myoepithelial cells of the breast, resulting in milk ejection. Breastfeeding the infant after delivery enhances uterine contractions and promotes involution.[58]

RESUMPTION OF MENSTRUATION AND OVULATION

The early postpartum period tends to be a period of relative infertility for many women. Resumption of menstruation and ovulation varies among individual women regardless of whether or not the woman is lactating, although there is a greater tendency for exclusively breastfeeding women to experience a longer period of anovulation and amenorrhea. Menstruation usually resumes by 6 weeks postpartum in nonlactating women, although research has found even earlier resumption of menstruation.[35] The first postpartum menstrual cycle may be anovulatory, although nearly a third of these cycles are preceded by ovulation. That first cycle may also have inadequate luteal function, thereby decreasing fertility in the early postpartum period.[35] Considering the possibility of resumption of ovulation in the early postpartum period, discussion of contraceptive options should be initiated prenatally or immediately postpartum.

Lactation is associated with a delay in resumption of menstruation and ovulation. In response to infant suckling during breastfeeding, there is a disruption in the normal pattern of gonadotropin-releasing hormone (GnRH) secretion from the hypothalamus, resulting in lower levels of luteinizing hormone (LH) and follicle-stimulating hormone (FSH).[54] This relationship was demonstrated by a study whereby gonadotropin-releasing hormone (GnRH) infused every 90 minutes into amenorrheic lactating women resulted in stimulation of normal follicular growth.[88] Although pulsatile secretion of luteinizing hormone (LH) is seen by 8 weeks postpartum, levels are low and of variable frequency with no preovulatory surge. With regular suckling, luteinizing hormone (LH) remains suppressed.[58] With decreased lactation frequency, gonadotropin-releasing hormone (GnRH) secretion returns to normal and follicle-stimulating hormone (FSH) stimulates follicular growth, which in turn increases estradiol and results in luteinizing hormone (LH) release, causing follicular rupture, egg release, and formation of the corpus luteum.[54] Health care providers should discuss contraceptive options with lactating women, explaining the relationship between frequency of breastfeeding and fertility, in anticipation of contraceptive needs.

The duration of lactation-suppressed ovulation, known as *lactational amenorrhea,* depends upon the duration and frequency of breastfeeding and milk expression, with some evidence of longer duration in women who exclusively breastfeed than in those who partially breastfeed.[76] Therefore exclusive and frequent breastfeeding (often referred to as *on-demand*), at least 8 to 12 times per day with no supplementation, is a relatively reliable method for preventing pregnancy for the first 6 months postpartum, assuming the woman has not begun to menstruate. This method of family planning is called the *lactational amenorrhea method* (LAM) and has been studied and supported by research conducted since the 1988 Bellagio Consensus.[42,86]

ANATOMY OF THE MAMMARY GLANDS

The breasts or mammary glands are modified exocrine glands consisting of epithelial glandular tissue with an extensive system of branching ducts surrounded by adipose tissue and supported by the pectoralis major muscles and the fibrous bands of the Cooper's ligaments. Cooper's ligaments are suspensory and support the shape of the breast. The breasts are highly innervated with rich vascular and lymphatic systems. Each breast has been found to contain a range of 4 to 18 primary milk ducts arranged in a complex network and which converge at the nipple.[68] The basic glandular unit is a lobe consisting of 4 to 18 lobules, each containing clusters of alveoli that are connected to fine ducts that merge into larger ducts that merge into a primary milk duct and lead to the nipple. The alveolus is the site of milk synthesis and secretion and consists of clusters of mammary epithelial secretory cells (lactocytes) surrounded by myoepithelial cells to form smooth muscle contractile units responsible for ejecting milk into the ducts from the lumen of the alveoli.[67] The ducts and alveoli are surrounded by a stroma of fibroblasts, adipocytes, blood vessels, plasma cells (B lymphocytes capable of producing immunoglobulins, especially secretory immunoglobulin A), and a few nerves.[58] Research using ultrasound imaging demonstrated that there are not lactiferous sinuses under the areola rather that some women experience temporary duct dilation with milk ejection which subsides with milk flow.[67,68] Ducts serve to transport milk from the alveoli toward the nipple. The anterior and posterior medical branches of the internal mammary artery and the mammary branch of the lateral thoracic artery supply most of the blood to the breast. The internal thoracic, axillary, and cephalic veins drain the breast. Lymphatic drainage is conducted through the axillary and internal mammary nodes. The 2nd through 6th intercostal nerves innervate the breast. The structure of milk production and ejection portions of the mammary glands is illustrated in Figure 5-2. Figure 5-3 illustrates the mammary alveolus. The breast may be divided into four quadrants (lower inner, upper inner, lower outer, and upper outer quadrant with the adjacent Tail of Spence) for purposes of mapping and descriptive location.

The nipple is surrounded by the areola. Both the nipple and areola are elastic and darker in pigmentation than the

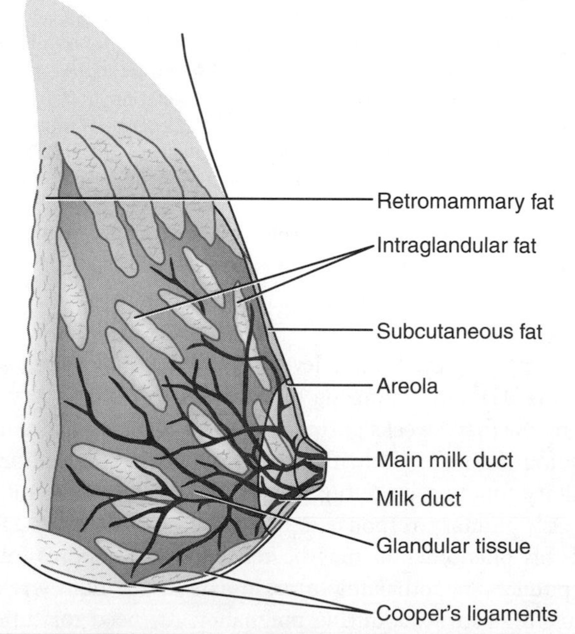

FIGURE 5-2 Side view of lactating breast. (From Ramsay, D.T., et al. [2005]. Anatomy of the lactating human breast redefined with ultrasound imaging. *J Anat, 206,* 531.)

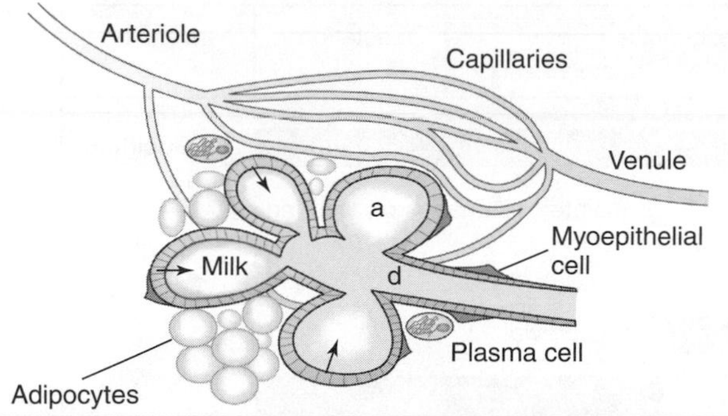

FIGURE 5-3 Model of mammary alveolus *(a)* with surrounding supporting structures that include a ductule *(d)* through which milk is ejected by contraction of the myoepithelial cells, vasculature, and a rich stroma composed of fibroblasts and adipocytes, some of them depleted of fat during lactation, and plasma cells. (From Neville, M.C. [1999]. Physiology of lactation. *Clin Perinatol, 26,* 252.)

rest of the breast, and become even darker during pregnancy and lactation, possibly providing a visual signal for the infant to latch. When not washed off, the mother's nipple and areola also attract the newborn infant immediately after delivery through the senses of taste and smell.[80] With suckling, the nipple and much of the areola are drawn into the infant's mouth, forming a teat. Milk is removed by the stripping action of the infant's tongue against the hard palate along with the infant's application of vacuum on the breast and the maternal milk ejection response.[23] Smooth muscle and elastic fibers in the areola and nipple form a sphincter to prevent milk loss when the infant is not suckling.[58]

Montgomery tubercles are sebaceous and lactiferous glands located around the areola. They are enlarged and elevated during pregnancy and lactation as they provide lubrication and antisepsis. Washing the nipples with soap or antiseptic is usually contraindicated as such action can remove the protective secretions of the Montgomery tubercles, leading to drying and cracking of the nipples and increasing the risk of infection.

PHYSIOLOGY OF LACTATION

Human milk is species-specific and promotes proper growth and development of nearly all infants. Lactation is a complex physiologic process involving integration of neuronal and endocrine mechanisms. Mammary development and lactation can be divided into phases: embryogenesis, mammogenesis (mammary growth during puberty and pregnancy), lactogenesis (I and II, initiation of milk secretion), lactogenesis III (maintenance of established milk secretion), and involution (cessation of lactation).[43,58] These phases are summarized in Table 5-1. Hormonal influences on lactation are summarized in Figure 5-4 and Table 5-2.

Embryogenesis

Mammary growth begins with development of the mammary band and streak in the fourth week of embryonic development, which progresses into the mammary ridge by the fifth week. The ectoderm continues to proliferate and undergo inward growth into the underlying mesoderm as the mammary bud is formed. From the sixth week, mammary glands, milk ducts, and lobular branching gradually develop throughout the

Table 5-1 Stages of Mammary Development

DEVELOPMENTAL STAGES	HORMONAL REGULATION	LOCAL FACTORS	DESCRIPTION
Embryogenesis	Unknown	Fat pad necessary for ductal extension	Epithelial bud develops in 18- to 19-week fetus, extending a short distance into mammary fat pad with blind ducts that become canalized; some milk secretion may be present at birth
Pubertal development prior to onset of menses	Estrogen, GH	IGF-1, HGF, TGF-β, unknown	Ductal extension into the mammary fat pad; branching morphogenesis
Pubertal development after onset of menses	Estrogen, progesterone, possibly PRL		Lobular development with formation of TDLU
Development in pregnancy	Progesterone, PRL, hPL	Herrugulin, unknown	Alveolus formation; partial cellular differentiation
Transition: lactogenesis	Progesterone withdrawal, PRL, glucocorticoid	Unknown	Onset of milk secretion: Stage I: Mid-pregnancy; Stage II: Parturition
Lactation	PRL, oxytocin	FIL, stretch	Ongoing milk secretion, milk ejection
Involution	Withdrawal of prolactin	Milk stasis, FIL	Alveolar epithelium undergoes apoptosis and remodeling and gland reverts to pre-pregnant state

Adapted from Neville, M.C. (2001). Anatomy and Physiology of lactation. *Pediatr Clin North Am*, 48, 16.
FIL, Feedback inhibitor of lactation; *GH*, growth hormone; *HGF*, hyperglycemic glyconeolytic factor; *hPL*, human placental lactogen; *IGF*, insulin-like growth factor; *TDLU*, terminal duct lobular unit.

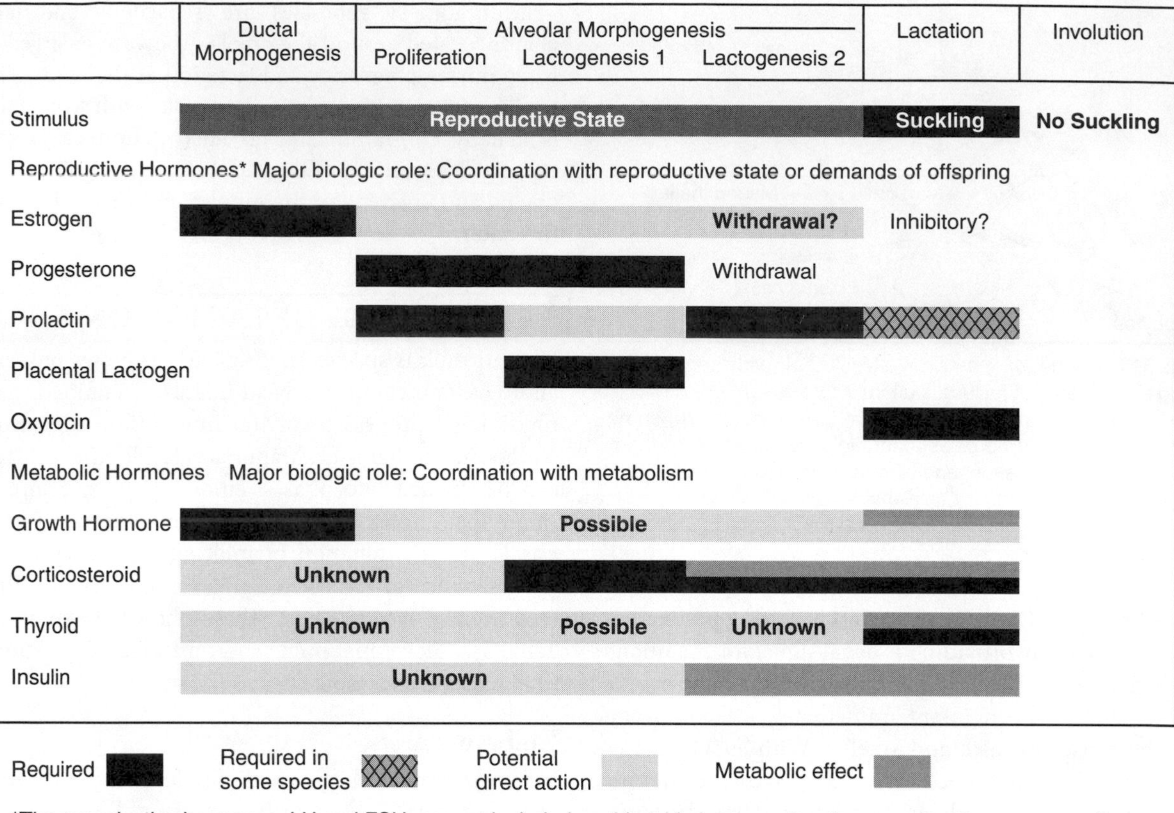

FIGURE 5-4 Hormones in mammary development. (From Neville, M.C., McFadden, T.B., & Forsyth, I. [2002]. Hormonal regulation of mammary differentiation and milk secretion. *J Mammary Gland Biol Neoplasia, 7,* 50.)

continued embryonic growth. The continued proliferation of ingrowing ectodermal cells leads to the development of the branching mammary duct system. By 18 to 19 weeks, a bulb-shaped mammary bud is evident and extends into the mesenchyme, where fat pads are developing. The bud forms secondary buds, which will form the duct system in the mature breast. The secondary buds elongate and invade the fat pads, then branch and canalize to form the rudimentary ductal system.[59] Occasionally the newborn may have transient secretions from the breast in the first few days after birth, probably due to maternal hormonal levels.

Mammogenesis

Mammogenesis involves mammary gland development that begins in fetal life, mediated by estrogen and growth hormone, and accelerates at puberty with ductal development, fatty tissue growth, lobuloalveolar development and further maturation of the breasts. Alveolar development continues under the influence of the luteal phase of the menstrual cycle and in early pregnancy. There is development of terminal duct lobular units and alveoli formation under the influence of progesterone secreted by the ovaries during the luteal phase, as well as under the influence of estrogen, and probably prolactin.[59]

During pregnancy, beginning soon after conception, and continuing through postpartum, breasts undergo additional changes, reaching full maturation. Lactogenesis I, characterized by mammary changes including secretory differentiation, occurs during pregnancy. External changes during pregnancy include increases in breast size and areolar pigmentation. The Montgomery tubercles enlarge and become more prominent, and the nipples become more erect. Toward the end of pregnancy, it is normal for some women to experience some leaking of colostrum while others may not (for most women, there is no special preparation of the nipples during pregnancy). The myoepithelial cells hypertrophy. The skin over the breasts appears thinner, the blood vessels are more prominent, and there is a twofold increase in blood flow to the breast. Much of the growth and development is a result of hormonal changes of the corpus luteum and placenta. During the first trimester, the ductal system proliferates and branches under the influence of estrogen and lobular formation is enhanced by progesterone. The glandular tissue of the alveoli proliferate under the influence of human placental lactogen (hPL), human chorionic gonadotropin (hCG), and prolactin (Figures 5-4 and 5-5). Growth hormone and adrenocorticotropic hormone (ACTH) act synergistically with prolactin and progesterone to promote mammogenesis.

As pregnancy progresses, the epithelial cells of the alveoli differentiate into secretory cells capable of milk production and the number of alveoli increases. Milk secretion is inhibited by the high levels of placental hormones including

Table 5-2 **Hormonal Contributions to Breast Development**

HORMONE	ORIGIN	FUNCTION BEFORE AND DURING PREGNANCY	FUNCTION AFTER DELIVERY
Prolactin (PRL)	Anterior pituitary	Serum levels rise but estrogen suppresses its effect during pregnancy	Stimulates alveolar cells to produce milk; important in initiating and maintaining lactation; may also cause lactation infertility by suppressing release of FSH and LH from pituitary or by causing ovaries to be unresponsive to various psychogenic factors, stress, an esthesia, surgery, high serum osmolality, exercise, nipple stimulation, and sexual intercourse
Prolactin-inhibiting factor (PIF)	Hypothalamus	Suppresses release of PRL into blood; release stimulated by dopaminergic impulses (i.e., catecholamines)	Suppresses release of PRL from anterior pituitary; agents that increase PRL by decreasing catecholamines and thus prolactin-inhibiting factor (PIF) include phenothiazides and reserpine
Oxytocin	Posterior pituitary	Generally no effect on mammary function; sensitivity of myoepithelial cells to oxytocin increases during pregnancy	Causes myoepithelial cells to contract, leading to milk ejection; release is inhibited by stresses such as fear, anxiety, embarrassment, distraction; also causes uterine contraction and postpartum involution of the uterus
Estrogen	Ovary and placenta	Stimulates proliferation of glandular tissue and ducts in breast; probably stimulates pituitary to secrete PRL but inhibits PRL effects on breasts	Blood level drops at parturition, which aids in initiating lactation; not important to lactation thereafter
Progesterone	Ovary and placenta	With estrogen, stimulates proliferation of glandular tissue and ducts in breast; inhibits milk secretion	Blood level drops at parturition, which aids in initiating lactation; probably unimportant to lactation thereafter
Growth hormone	Anterior pituitary		May act with PRL in initiating lactation but appears to be most important in maintaining established lactation
Adrenocorticotropic hormone (ACTH)	Anterior pituitary	Blood levels gradually increase during pregnancy; stimulates adrenal to release corticosteroids	High level is believed necessary for maintenance of lactation
Human placental lactogen (hPL)	Placenta	Like growth hormone in structure; stimulates mammary growth; associated with mobilization of free fatty acids and inhibition of peripheral glucose utilization and lactogenic action	
Thyroxine	Thyroid	Normally no direct effect on lactation	Appears to be important in maintaining lactation either through some direct effect on the mammary glands or by control of metabolism
Thyrotropin-releasing hormone	Hypothalamus	Normally no effect on lactation	Stimulates release of PRL; can be used to maintain established lactation

Adapted from Worthington-Roberts, B.S. & Williams, S.R. (1997). *Nutrition in pregnancy and lactation* (6th ed.). Madison, WI: Brown & Benchmark.
FSH, Follicle-stimulating hormone; *LH,* luteinizing hormone.

progesterone during pregnancy. Fat droplets accumulate in the secretory cells and concurrently breast interstitial tissue becomes infiltrated with lymphocytes, plasma cells, and eosinophils. During the second and third trimesters there is further lobular growth with formation of new alveoli and ducts and dilation of the lumens. Ductal arborization with development of extensive lobular clusters begins at midgestation. By the third month, prolactin stimulates production of colostrum, followed by the stimulation of its secretion by placental lactogen in the second trimester. Colostrum accumulates in the lumen. As such, a pregnant woman will produce colostrum as early as 16 weeks (see "Human Milk for the Preterm Infant"). Following birth, the alveolar epithelial cells continue to proliferate with synthesis of milk under the influence of increased levels of prolactin and the stimulus of suckling. Initial synthesis of milk components is preceded by an increase in required enzymes within the secretory cells.

Lactogenesis

Lactogenesis, or initiation of milk production, involves a complex neuroendocrine process with interaction of several hormones. Lactogenesis can be divided into three stages.

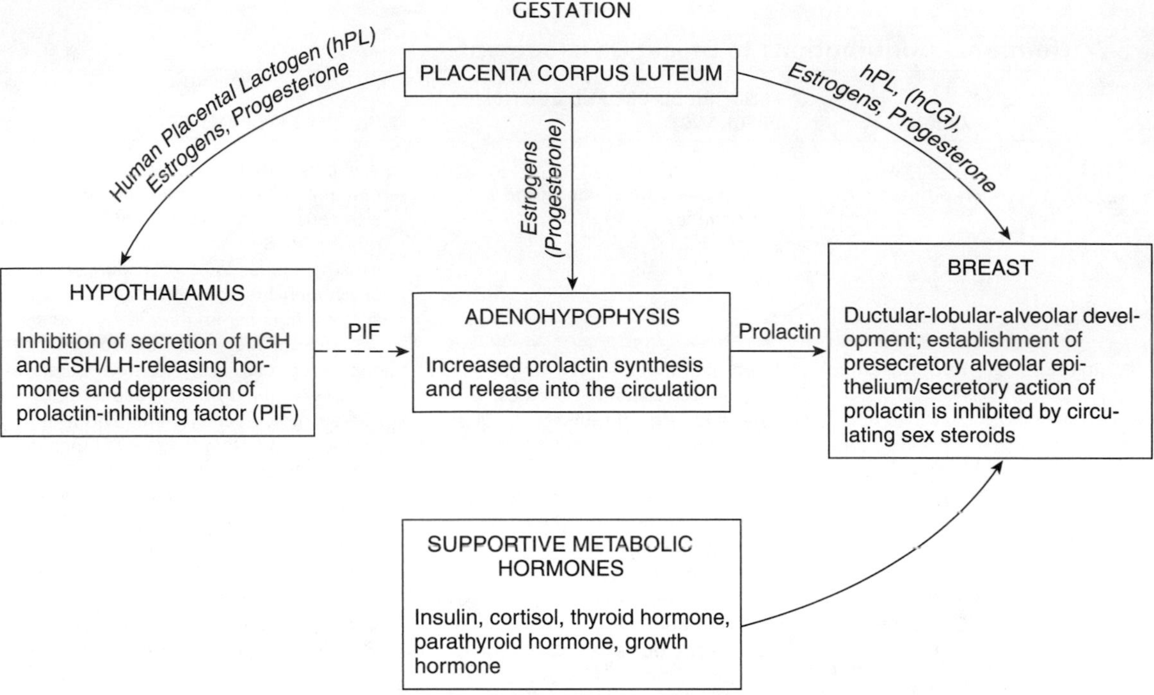

FIGURE 5-5 Hormonal preparation of breast during pregnancy for lactation. *hCG,* Human chorionic gonadotropin; *hGH,* human growth hormone. (Modified from Vorherr, H. [1974]. *The breast.* New York: Academic Press; and Lawrence, R.A. & Lawrence, R.M. [2005]. *Breastfeeding: A guide for the medical profession* [6th ed.]. Philadelphia: Mosby.)

Lactogenesis I occurs from early pregnancy to approximately the third postpartum day. This lactation initiation stage is not dependent upon suckling or milk removal, rather on the cascade of hormonal changes.[62] Only small amounts of milk are secreted, however, as a result of the inhibitory effects of the placental hormones. During lactogenesis I, secretory differentiation begins and there is a decrease in sodium, an increase in enzymes, proteins, and immunoglobulins and an increase in the size of fat droplets in the mammary cells.[61] During the first few postpartum days, colostrum has relatively high concentrations of immunoglobulin A, lactoferrin and oligosaccharide, which provide the newborn infant with protection against infection.

Lactogenesis II is the second stage, initiated by delivery of the placenta and a significant drop in progesterone along with the increasing level of prolactin. By days 2 to 4 postpartum, copious milk secretion begins, referred to as when a mother's "milk comes in," and plasma alpha-lactalbumin levels increase as there is a transformation in milk composition. During the first postpartum day, the infant receives less than 100 mL of breast milk which increases to approximately 500 mL by the fourth day.[61] The composition of milk changes as sodium and chloride concentrations decrease and the lactose concentration increases.[62] During this stage of lactogenesis II, junctions between mammary alveolar cells tighten. With frequent milk transfer, milk synthesis is increased and milk production rises. With increased vascularity and fluid congestion in the early postpartum period, many women feel breast fullness and heaviness, which resolves with efficient milk removal through infant sucking or pumping. Pathologic engorgement occurs when there is inadequate milk removal resulting in milk stasis, swelling, pain, tenderness, and inflammation. Research suggests that early and frequent suckling and pumping facilitates efficient milk production, especially as control of lactation changes from endocrine to autocrine, directed by milk removal.[18] Prolonged milk stasis triggers the feedback inhibitor of lactation (FIL), the autocrine inhibitory protein that controls and suppresses milk synthesis that may lead to decreased milk production.[38] Lactation research in Western populations points to the importance of early breastfeeding initiation, skin-to-skin contact, and lactation support to promote successful breastfeeding and extended breastfeeding duration, although breastfeeding may be successfully initiated and continued under many circumstances.[57] For the breastfeeding woman, prevention and early treatment with encouragement to continue adequate breastfeeding and/or pumping is recommended. For treatment recommendations, see Common Breastfeeding Problems later in the chapter.

By the end of the first or second week, during the next stage, lactogenesis III (or galactopoiesis), mature milk is established and milk supply is maintained through autocrine control. Milk production rate depends upon the milk removal rate, in a manner of supply-demand response through a feedback mechanism, and the hypothalamic-pituitary axis response regulating hormonal secretion including prolactin and oxytocin. Suckling stimulates sensory nerves in the nipple and areola, sending messages to the hypothalamus to secrete prolactin and oxytocin. Prolactin stimulates milk synthesis and oxytocin stimulates contraction of the myoepithelial cells causing milk ejection or "let-down." Other hormones enhancing lactogenesis include growth hormone, corticosteroids, thyroxine, and insulin, as demonstrated in Figures 5-5 and 5-6.[60] Growth hormone and insulin are important for survival of alveolar cells and for stimulating glucose entry in the mammary epithelial cells to accelerate lipogenesis.

Extended milk stasis causes increased pressure in the breast leading to inflammation and decreased milk synthesis, thereby inhibiting lactation. The introduction of supplements is associated with decreased breastfeeding duration.[33] Furthermore, the use of supplementation leads to decreased milk production as the demand placed on maternal milk production decreases. Breastfeeding on-demand and pumping when mother and infant are separated or unable to breastfeed are often effective means of maintaining adequate milk supply. If maternal milk supply is insufficient despite efforts of frequent breastfeeding or pumping, maternal use of galactagogues may augment milk production.[22]

Prolactin Patterns During Lactation

Milk production and release are controlled primarily by the effect of suckling on hormonal release via a complex neuroendocrine process. Suckling stimulates prolactin release from the anterior pituitary (Figure 5-7). Suckling also stimulates sensory nerve endings in the nipple and areola, sending impulses to the hypothalamus via the spinal cord. As a result, hypothalamic secretion of prolactin-inhibiting factor is suppressed, and adenohypophysis secretion of prolactin increases. Prolactin levels increase toward the end of a feeding, increasing the volume, fat, and protein content of milk in the next feeding.[77]

Prolactin, acting synergistically with insulin and cortisol, stimulates the alveolar secretory cells to produce milk proteins and fat. However, lactation must be preceded by a fall in progesterone and estrogens, removing an inhibitory effect and facilitating response to prolactin. The number of prolactin receptors in breast tissue increases markedly following delivery. The decrease in human placental lactogen (hPL) following expulsion or removal of the placenta may also facilitate prolactin action, in that human placental lactogen (hPL) competes with prolactin for the same breast tissue receptors.[77] Bromocriptine suppresses lactation by decreasing the number of specific prolactin receptors, and the FDA has withdrawn its approval for such use in postpartum women, even for medically-indicated lactation suppression, due to serious adverse outcomes.[25] New safer medications have been developed for lactation suppression although less medical interventions and abstaining from breast stimulation are preferred as initial efforts in indicated lactation suppression.

Serum prolactin levels are highest in the early postpartum period such that during the first month of pregnancy, baseline prolactin levels are 119 ± 19.1 μg/L and peak prolactin levels are 286 ± 22.6 μg/L in response to infant suckling stimulation.[15]

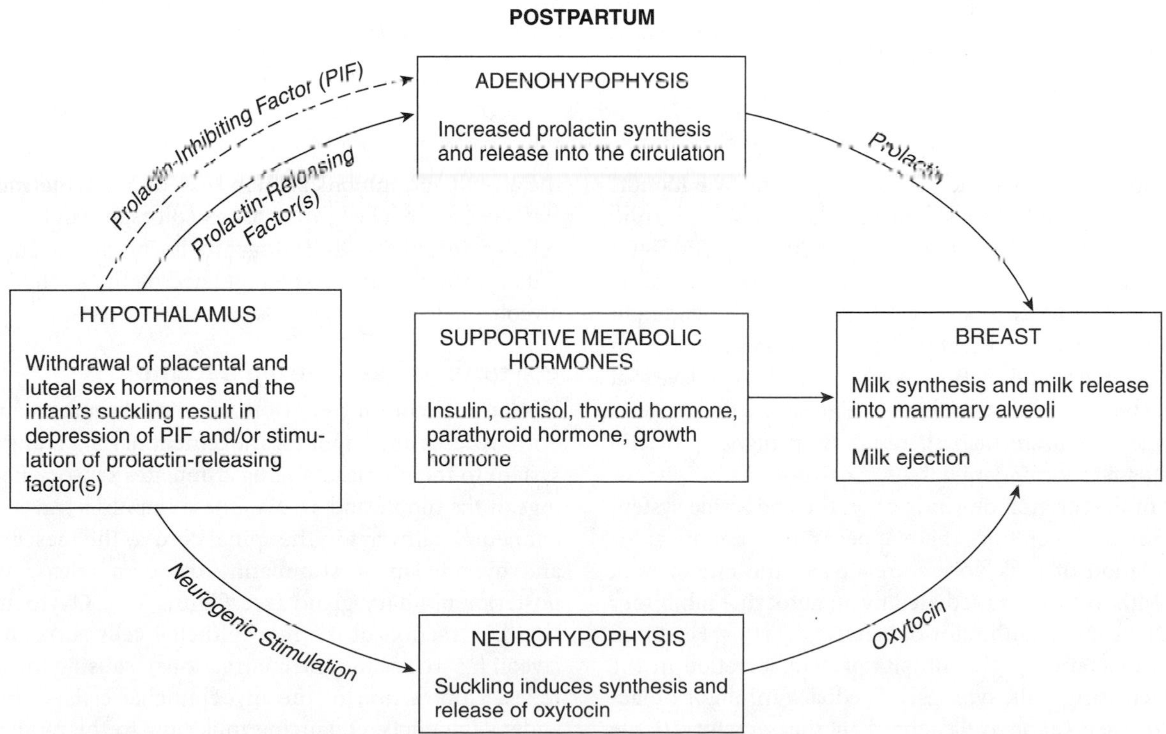

FIGURE 5-6 Hormonal preparation of the breast postpartum for lactation. (Modified from Vorherr, H. [1974]. *The breast.* New York: Academic Press; and Lawrence, R.A. & Lawrence, R.M. [2005]. *Breastfeeding: A guide for the medical profession* [6th ed.]. Philadelphia: Mosby.)

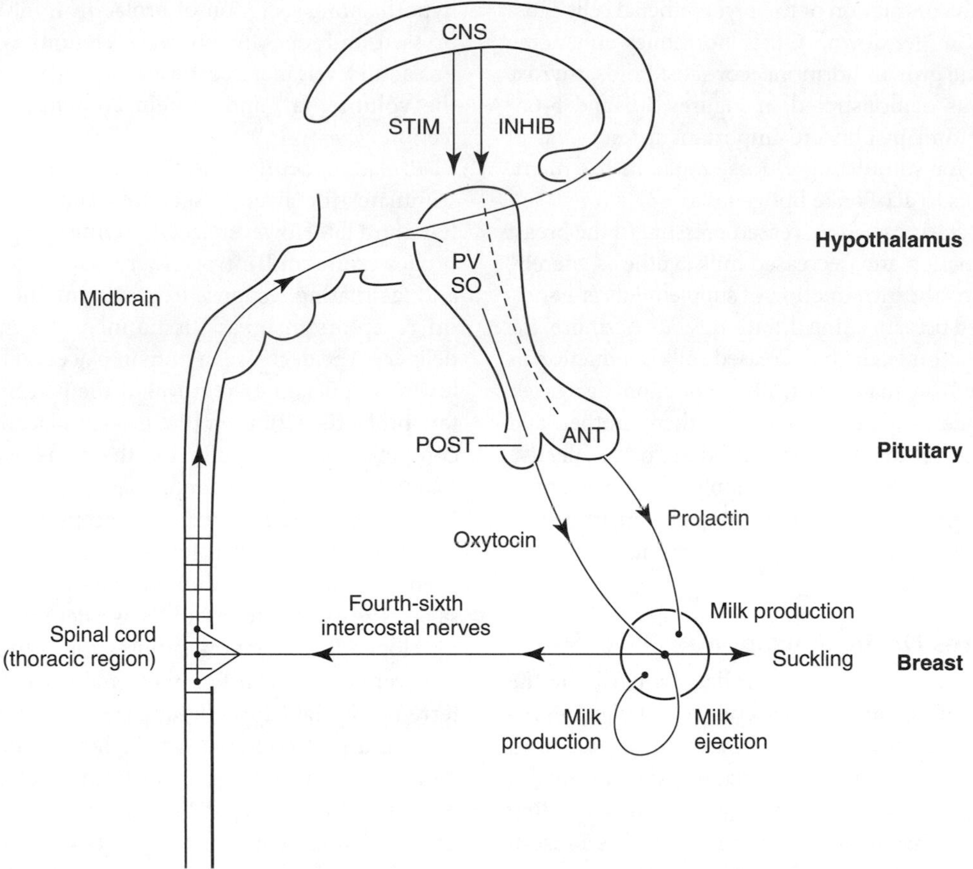

FIGURE 5-7 The neuroendocrine reflexes that are initiated by suckling. Stimulatory (STIM) as well as inhibitory (INHIB) influences leading to milk production are shown. *PV,* Paraventricular nucleus; *SO,* supraoptic nucleus. (From Tulchinsky, D. [1994]. Postpartum lactation and resumption of reproductive function. In D. Tulchinsky & A.B. Little [Eds.]. *Maternal-fetal endocrinology* [2nd ed.]. Philadelphia: Saunders.)

Baseline and peak prolactin levels steadily decline by 6 months postpartum although breastfeeding frequency and milk production may not be significantly different.[15] Prolactin peaks at approximately 45 minutes from the onset of suckling stimulus, and no difference was found between the left and right breasts in prolactin concentrations.[16] Prolactin circadian rhythm continues throughout lactation, manifesting higher levels at night when the rate of milk synthesis is highest and the prolactin levels in the alveoli are highest, resulting in higher prolactin levels in the first morning milk.[16]

While milk secretion depends upon the endocrine system such as prolactin secretion, there appears to be a more autocrine regulation of milk volume related to the rate of milk removal. Milk volume is mediated by an autocrine inhibitory protein, the feedback inhibitor of lactation (FIL).[38] Feedback inhibitor of lactation (FIL) inhibits protein secretion in the alveoli, decreasing milk synthesis. Feedback inhibitor of lactation (FIL) acts upon milk stored in the secretory tissue of the alveolar lumen, not upon milk moved to the sinuses. If milk is not completely or efficiently removed from the breast, feedback inhibitor of lactation (FIL) accumulates in the alveoli and inhibits protein secretion. Furthermore, milk stasis causes reduced prolactin receptors, possibly decreasing cellular sensitivity to lactogenic hormones.[38] The rate of milk synthesis may also be regulated by the stretching of the alveolar cells.[62]

Oxytocin Release During Lactation

The let-down or milk ejection reflex is a complex neuroendocrine process important for movement of milk along the duct system to the nipple. Suckling stimulates sensory nerve endings in the nipple and areola. These impulses travel via afferent neural pathways in the spinal cord to the mesencephalon and hypothalamus, stimulating oxytocin release from the posterior pituitary gland (see Figure 5-7). Oxytocin stimulates contraction of the myoepithelial cells surrounding the alveoli (as well as uterine contractions), causing the let-down reflex. Contraction of the myoepithelial cells shortens and widens the ducts, enhancing milk flow to the nipples.[58] As a result, milk is ejected into the duct system and propelled to the lactiferous ducts and sinuses. Oxytocin release and the let-down reflex may also be stimulated by thinking of the infant, hearing an infant crying, and experiencing orgasm, while it may be inhibited by stress through the HPA axis mechanism.[29]

Mammary Involution

Mammary involution upon cessation of lactation results from milk stasis and the absence of hormonal stimulus for lactation. Consequently, milk stasis and back-pressure of milk causes a buildup of feedback inhibitor of lactation (FIL) and possibly changes in the stretch response, thereby decreasing milk volume. The mammary epithelial cells undergo apoptosis. Involution of the breasts occurs over several months, although the breasts do not completely return to their prepregnancy state due to some retention of the mammary epithelium.

HUMAN MILK

Importance of Human Milk

Research around the world among different populations has demonstrated the benefits, health promotion, and health protection of human milk. It is superior and preferred for nearly all infants, with a few exceptions. The World Health Organization recommends exclusive breastfeeding for 6 months followed by continued breastfeeding until 2 years or mutually appropriate for the maternal-infant dyad.[85] The American Academy of Pediatrics' policy statement on breastfeeding provides an evidence-based approach to the recommendations for breastfeeding including: health promotional and beneficial for mother and infant, decreased acute and chronic diseases, promotion of infant neurodevelopment, and economic advantages.[3] Longer durations of breastfeeding have been associated with decreased risk of developing diabetes for both the mother and infant, helping to prevent an increasing chronic disease.[64,74] Discuss the importance of breastfeeding with the woman and her family during pregnancy and encourage continued breastfeeding during the postpartum period. Characteristics of women at risk for not breastfeeding have been noted and include cultural background and health practices, lack of health insurance, late prenatal care, lower level of maternal education, not being married, and smoking in pregnancy, to name a few.[13] For the woman who is smoking, providing clear messages about the importance of reducing and eliminating smoking along with practical advice and information about resources for assistance will promote healthier outcomes in both the mother and her infant. The prenatal and postpartum periods are motivating times, considered "teachable moments," for promoting modifiable lifestyle behaviors such as reduction of negative exposures and engagement in healthy, positive activities such as breastfeeding that are associated with improved maternal-infant health outcomes. Identify pregnant women who are at risk for not breastfeeding to target directed and appropriate messages regarding the importance of breastfeeding, barriers to breastfeeding, and resources for breastfeeding support.

Milk Production and Composition

The components of human milk are synthesized in the secretory cells of the alveoli (protein, fat, lactose) or extracted from maternal plasma (vitamins and minerals) by these same cells. The individual components of milk then pass into the alveolar lumen where the final milk is constituted. During lactation, milk synthesis constantly occurs at low levels and the milk is stored in the alveolar lumen until it is removed.[59] Active synthesis occurs at the highest rate during infant suckling or other areolar and nipple stimulation such as with pumping.

Milk synthesis depends upon four transcellular pathways and one paracellular pathway. The four transcellular pathways include exocytosis, fat synthesis and secretion, secretion of ions and water, and transcytosis of substances including immunoglobulins. The passage of substances via the paracellular pathway moves substances between epithelial cells (Figure 5-8).[59] The exocytosis process begins with mRNA synthesis in the nucleus for protein synthesis. The protein molecules are transported to the endoplasmic reticulum, where they undergo modification and transportation through the Golgi system. Calcium, phosphate, and citrate from the cytoplasm are transported into the Golgi system. Lactose is then synthesized and osmotically draws water into the Golgi system. Protein, lactose, and calcium undergo exocytosis in the Golgi secretory vesicles and are discharged into the alveolar lumen.[59]

Lipids, specifically triglycerides, are synthesized in the endoplasmic reticulum and cytoplasm. Milk fat is secreted in milk-fat globules (Figure 5-9). These globules have a core of triglycerides encased in a membrane containing phospholipids, preventing the individual fat globules from coalescing into large globules that would be difficult to secrete. The secretion of ions and water involve direct transport across the apical membrane. The small molecules transported by this route include sodium, potassium, chloride, some monosaccharides and water. Transcytosis, the fourth pathway, is the mechanism for movement of intact proteins from the interstitial space into milk. This mechanism is used for secretion of immunoglobulins, especially IgA, proteins, hormones, and growth factors from maternal plasma into milk.[59]

The paracellular pathway involves transport of substances between the tight junctions of adjacent epithelial cells. The tight junctions are gasket-like structures joining the cells together and preventing substances moving from the milk back to the mother. The junctions open and leak during pregnancy, mastitis, and following involution, allowing bidirectional movement: interstitial substances move into the milk and milk components move into the plasma. In mastitis, this route helps to provide entry for anti-inflammatory components and to clear the end products of the infectious process. With involution, this route allows removal of degraded components. Mammary sodium and chloride concentrations are higher when the junctions are open, such as during pregnancy, and may help in diagnosing breastfeeding problems.[59]

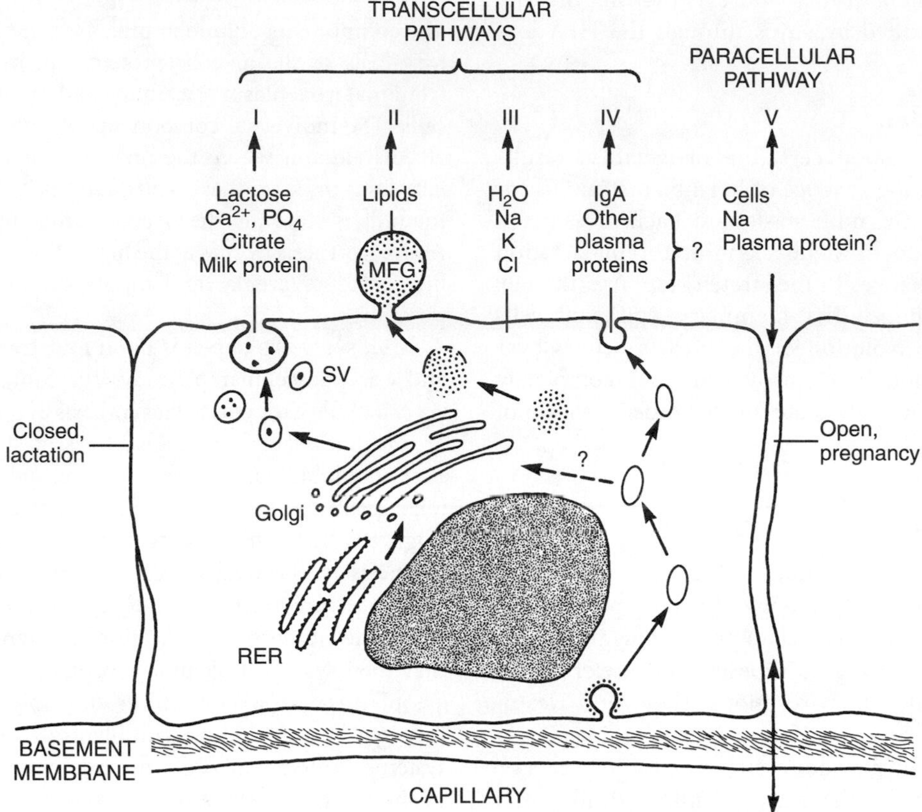

FIGURE 5-8 Pathways for milk synthesis and secretion in the mammary alveolus. *I.* Exocytosis of milk protein and lactose in Golgi-derived secretory vesicles. *II.* Milk fat secretion via milk fat globule. *III.* Secretion of ions and water across apical membrane. *IV.* Transcytosis of immunoglobulins. *V.* Paracellular pathway for plasma components and leukocytes. *MFG,* Milk fat globule; *RER,* rough endoplasmic reticulum; *SV,* secretory vesicle. (Modified from Neville, M.C. [1990]. The physiological basis of milk secretion. Part I: Basic physiology. *Ann NY Acad Sci, 586,* 1.)

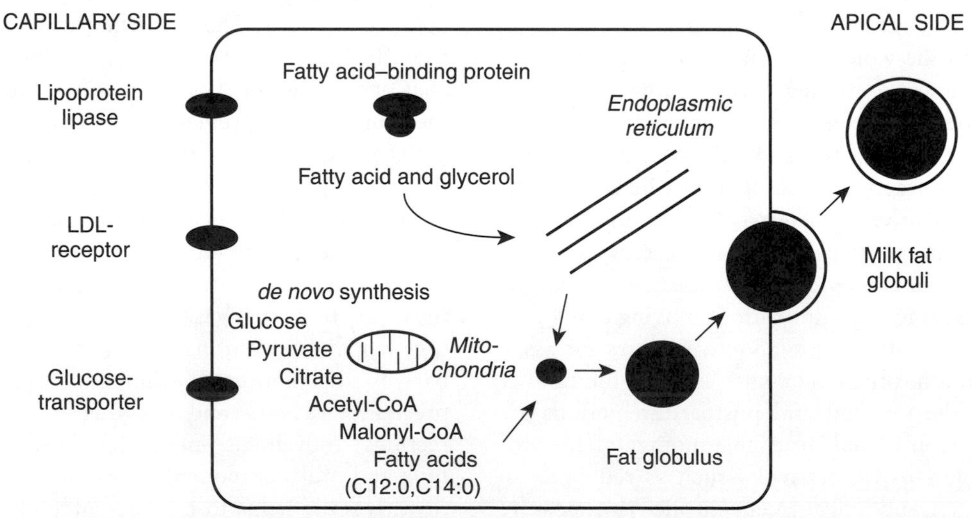

FIGURE 5-9 Formation of milk fat globule in the mammary alveolus. Substrates for milk fat synthesis are lipoprotein lipids taken up after hydrolysis by lipoprotein lipase activity or binding to low-density-lipoprotein (LDL) receptor, as well as glucose taken up by a glucose transporter. Fatty acids that are taken up from the circulation together with those synthesized de novo from glucose can be reesterified and incorporated into milk fat globules, which are surrounded by the milk fat globule membrane. (From Rodriguez-Palmero, M., et al. [1999]. Nutritional and biochemical properties of human milk. Part II. *Clin Perinatol, 26,* 336.)

Composition of Human Milk

In the first days following delivery, during lactogenesis I, the initial substance produced by the alveolar secretory cells is colostrum. Colostrum is a viscous, transparent yellowish fluid (high beta-carotene content causes the yellow color) that is produced in small quantities in the first postpartum days. Compared to mature milk, colostrum is lower in carbohydrate, fat, and calories and higher in sodium, chloride, potassium, and protein due to increased concentrations of globulins and lactoferrin. The high level of proteins and immunoglobulins in colostrum provides protective, anti-infective properties. As transition to lactogenesis II is underway, maternal milk gradually changes to mature milk and milk volume increases. There is a decrease in the concentration of immunoglobulins, total protein, lactoferrin, sodium, chloride, and carotenoids and an increase in lactose, fat, and calories.

The composition of human milk varies between women and for each woman due to gestation, stage of lactation, milk volume, and frequency of breastfeeding or milk expression, although the overall contents of human milk are fairly consistent. The primary components of mature human milk are water (87%), carbohydrates, fats, proteins, vitamins, and minerals. In a national sample of donor breast milk from 273 women at different stages of lactation, researchers found that the average mean energy content was 19 kilocalories per ounce (compared to many infant formula supplementation's energy content of 20 kilocalories per ounce).[84] The average volume of milk increases during exclusive breastfeeding from 500 mL/day by the end of the first week to at least 800 mL/day by 6 months.[58] Volume is higher with multiple breastfeeding infants due to increased frequency of suckling stimulation. Milk volume is 5% to 15% higher in women with very low body fat. This is thought to be due to the decreased milk fat content and caloric density, which leads to increased infant suckling stimulation.[59]

Human milk is isosmotic with human plasma. Lactose is the major osmotic component of milk and is highly concentrated in human milk. In order for milk to maintain isosmolarity with plasma, concentrations of other ions—sodium and chloride, in particular—must remain proportionately lower. Levels of protein, sodium, potassium, chloride, and other ions are lower in human milk than in bovine milk, thereby maintaining a lower renal solute load and placing less stress on the kidneys (see Chapter 11). Table 5-3 presents many of the representative values of the components of human milk.

Carbohydrate Synthesis and Release

The major carbohydrate found in human milk is lactose. Other carbohydrates found in small quantities include glucose, nucleotide sugars, glycolipids, glycoproteins, and oligosaccharides.[65] The oligosaccharides promote development of intestinal bacterial flora (such as bifidus) and inhibit bacterial adhesion, thereby reducing the risk of gastrointestinal infections. Immunologic properties of human milk are discussed further in Chapter 13.

The concentration of lactose in human milk is stable and independent of maternal nutritional status. Lactose acts as an osmotic compound to pull water into the Golgi apparatus, thereby regulating the amount of water in milk and the volume of milk produced. If less lactose is available, less milk will be produced, maintaining a constant lactose concentration. Lactose is synthesized in the Golgi apparatus from glucose and galactose. Glucose is obtained from maternal plasma and is necessary in metabolic processes including lactose synthesis. Lactose is an important source of energy for the developing infant brain. Alpha-lactalbumin, the most plentiful protein in human milk, plays an important role in lactose synthesis, as well as provides the osmotic force in the movement of water, and serves as a source of amino acids available for the infant.[34]

Fat Synthesis and Release

The largest portion of calories in human milk comes from fat. Fats comprise approximately 4% of milk, although their concentration varies between women and within each woman, based on individual characteristics. Variation of fat content is influenced by a host of factors including gestation (higher polyunsaturated fatty acids in very preterm and preterm delivery), stage of lactation (phospholipids and cholesterol higher in early lactation), milk volume (high volume associated with lower fat), maternal nutrition (low fat maternal diet associated with lower fat), and timing within breastfeeding session (fat progressively increases during breastfeeding session, called hindmilk).[65] The major constituents of milk fat are triglycerides (98%). The high proportion of lipids in human milk provides energy, short and long-chain fatty acids crucial in retinal and neural development. Human milk also contains enzymes to aid in fat digestion including lingual lipase, gastric lipase, bile salt-stimulated lipase, and pancreatic lipase that aids in fat digestion, enhancing release of energy and fat digestion and absorption.[65]

Most of the milk fat is derived from the maternal circulation resulting from nutrition and from stored lipids, while some of the fat is synthesized in the mammary gland from glucose metabolism.[40] Maternal nutrition affects the lipid components of milk, especially some essential fatty acids. Severe maternal caloric restriction alters the fatty acid composition as does the type of fat consumed by the mother, although changes are usually buffered by maternal lipid stores. For example, if the maternal diet is altered to include more polyunsaturated fatty acids, her milk will also contain more polyunsaturated fats. Likewise, a woman who consumes a high amount of fish or who takes fish oil supplements has an increased proportion of polyunsaturated fatty acids.[40]

Milk fat is synthesized in the endoplasmic reticulum (see Figure 5-9) from precursors available within the secretory cell or obtained from maternal blood. Insulin stimulates glucose uptake into the mammary cells. Short-chain fatty acids are synthesized from acetate, whereas long-chain fatty acids are obtained from maternal plasma. Triglycerides are

Table 5-3 **Representative Values for Constituents of Human Milk**

CONSTITUENT (PER LITER)*	EARLY MILK	MATURE MILK
Energy (kJ)		2730-2940
Carbohydrate		
Lactose (g)	20-30	67
Glucose (g)	0.2-1.0	0.2-0.3
Oligosaccharides (g)	22-24	12-14
Total nitrogen (g)	3.0	1.9
Nonprotein nitrogen (g)	0.5	0.45
Protein nitrogen (g)	2.5	1.45
Total protein (g)	16	9
Casein (g)	3.8	5.7
β-casein (g)	2.6	4.4
κ-casein (g)	1.2	1.3
α-lactalbumin (g)	3.62	3.26
Lactoferrin (g)	3.53	1.94
Serum albumin (g)	0.39	0.41
sIgA (g)	2.0	1.0
IgM (g)	0.12	0.2
IgG (g)	0.34	0.05
Total lipids (%)	2	3.5
Triglyceride (% total lipids)	97-98	97-98
Cholesterol† (% total lipids)	0.7-1.3	0.4-0.5
Phospholipids (% total lipids)	1.1	0.6-0.8
Fatty acids (weight %)	88	88
Total saturated	43-44	44-45
C12:0		5
C14:0		6
C16:0		20
C18:0		8
Monounsaturated		40
C18:1ω-9	32	31
Polyunsaturated	13	14-15
Total ω-3	1.5	1.5
C18:3ω-3	0.7	0.9
C22:5ω-3	0.2	0.1
C22:6ω-3	0.5	0.2

CONSTITUENT (PER LITER)*	EARLY MILK	MATURE MILK
Total ω-6	11.6	13.06
C18:2ω-6	8.9	11.3
C20:4ω-6	0.7	0.5
C22:4ω-6	0.2	0.1
Water-soluble vitamins		
Ascorbic acid (mg)		100
Thiamin (mcg)	20	200
Riboflavin (mcg)		400-600
Niacin (mg)	0.5	1.8-6.0
Vitamin B_6 (mg)		0.09-0.31
Folate (mcg)		80-140
Vitamin B_{12} (mcg)		0.5-1.0
Pantothenic acid (mg)		2.0-2.5
Biotin (mcg)		5-9
Fat-soluble vitamins		
Retinol (mg)	2	0.3-0.6
Carotenoids (mg)	2	0.2-0.6
Vitamin K (mcg)	2.5	2-3
Vitamin D (mcg)		0.33
Vitamin E (mg)	8-12	3-8
Minerals		
Major minerals		
Calcium (mg)	250	200-250
Magnesium (mg)	30-35	30-35
Phosphorus (mg)	120-160	120-140
Sodium (mg)	300-400	120-250
Potassium (mg)	600-700	400-550
Chloride (mg)	600-800	400-450
Trace minerals		
Iron (mg)	0.5-1.0	0.3-0.9
Zinc (mg)	8-12	1-3
Copper (mg)	0.5-0.8	0.2-0.4
Manganese (mcg)	5-6	3
Selenium (mcg)	40	7-33
Iodine (mcg)		150
Fluoride (mcg)		4-15

Data from Jensen, R.G. (1995). *Handbook of milk composition.* San Diego: Academic Press; Koletzko, B. & Rodriguez-Palermo, M. (1999). Polyunsaturated fatty acids in human milk and their role in early development. *J Mammary Gland Biol Neoplasia 4,* 269; Cuillere, M.L., Tregoat, V., Bene, M.C., et al. (1999). Changes in the kappa-casein and beta-casein concentrations in human milk during lactation. *J Clin Lab Anal 13,* 213; Picciano, M.F. (2001). Representative values for constituents of human milk. *Pediatr Clin North Am, 48,* 263.

*All values are expressed per liter of milk with the exception of lipids that are expressed as a percentage on the basis of milk volume or weight of total lipids.

†The cholesterol content of human milk ranges from 100 to 200 mg/L in most samples of human milk after day 21 of lactation.

either obtained from maternal plasma or synthesized from intracellular carbohydrates (primarily glyceride and glucose). Following delivery (and possibly due to prolactin), there is an increase in two enzymes, lipoprotein lipase which hydrolizes lipids and palmitoyl-coenzyme A transferase, involved in the production and utilization of triglycerides. Lipoprotein lipase acts in the capillaries to catalyze the lipolysis of triglycerides and the uptake of glycerol and fatty acids into the epithelial cells. Palmitoyl-coenzyme A transferase catalyzes intracellular synthesis of triglyceride from glyceride.[36] Fatty acids are esterified in the endoplasmic reticulum to form triglycerides. The triglycerides accumulate and coalesce to form larger fat droplets surrounded by a membrane rich in phospholipids and cholesterol. As fat droplets increase in size, they move to the membrane apex and become part of the milk fat globule.[53]

Protein Synthesis and Release

Protein components of human milk are critical to growth, development, and immunoprotection. Most proteins are synthesized in the mammary gland and some are transported from maternal circulation.[46] The primary means for protein secretion by alveolar cells is through the exocytotic pathway and processing in the Golgi bodies while the transcytotic pathway is also a mechanism for the transport of proteins into human milk although the transport mechanism for amino acids is unclear to date.[53] Human milk protein provides amino acids necessary for growth, protective factors such as immunoglobulins, bacteriostatic properties, bioactive factors and proteins to aid digestion and absorption, growth and promotion of beneficial gut flora, and development of a protective gastrointestinal mucosal barrier.[2]

Milk protein primarily consists of whey (alpha-lactalbumin; lactoferrin; serum albumin; and immunoglobulins sIgA, IgA, IgG, and IgM) and casein.[41] The concentrations of whey and casein in human milk are in a 60:40 ratio versus the 20:80 ratio in bovine milk. While human milk has less total protein than bovine milk, the protein content in human milk is more bioavailable to the infant. Whey protein is easily digested, forming soft, flocculent curds. Protein content slowly decreases during the first 6 months of lactation. The protein content of colostrum is approximately double that of mature milk due to the higher concentration of essential amino acids and the increased abundance of antibodies such as secretory IgA and lactoferrin (see Chapter 13). Lactoferrin promotes anti-inflammatory function, stimulates bactericidal and antiviral activity, and may inhibit tumor growth by activating natural killer cells.[26] Casein, the predominant bovine milk protein, is less easily digested and forms tough, rubbery curds. Casein requires greater energy expenditure to digest, and its digestion is more likely to be incomplete. Some casein is needed, however, to enhance the absorption of minerals by keeping them in solution in the gut. Casein may also promote the growth of beneficial gut flora and inhibit adherence of pathogenic organisms.[41]

Human milk also contains other nonprotein nitrogen components and other protein factors. These components are used to synthesize nonessential amino acids; enhance gut maturation, growth, and nutrient absorption; or contribute to the immunologic properties of human milk (see Chapter 13). The proteins in human milk are used for nutrition and growth as well as for other functions such as immunoprotection. The proteins in artificial formula do not contain all the proteins available in human milk and try to compensate by adding higher concentrations of total proteins, although the excess nitrogen resulting from protein metabolism may place an extra burden on the infant's kidneys.[2] Research and identification of some of the components of human milk motivates formula companies to augment their formula supplements, which implies that formula supplements cannot full copy human milk.[46] Examples of additional proteins and amino acids and their function in human milk include growth factors for gastrointestinal cellular development and tissue repair, lysozyme for destruction of gram-negative bacteria and amylase for digestion and absorption, carnitine for ketogenesis and thermogenesis, taurine involved in bile acid conjugation, neurotransmission, and neuromodulation, and glutamine and glutamic acid, providing energy substrates and neurotransmission in the brain.[1,2] Amino acid content is specific to the unique physiologic characteristics of the human newborn. For example, there are higher proportions of docosahexaenoic acid (DHA) in preterm mothers' milk than in term mothers' milk as it is needed for the less mature infants' neurodevelopment and function.[8]

Human milk is rich in immunologic substances that provide passive immunity and protect the infant from infections (especially gastrointestinal and respiratory infections) (Table 5-4). It serves as an important facilitator of the initiation and development of the microflora in the infant gastrointestinal system, such as bifidus factors.[24] Human milk may protect against the development of allergies—both by reducing exposure of the infant to bovine milk allergens and by supplying secretory IgA, which reduces intestinal absorption of potentially antigenic proteins before gut closure at 6 to 9 months. Cellular components of human milk include sloughed epithelial cells, macrophages, neutrophils, and lymphocytes.

Human milk also contains other components including enzymes, growth factors, hormones, resistance factors, macrophages, vitamins, minerals, and trace elements. While the amount of iron in human milk is lower than in bovine milk, it is more bioavailable to the infant because absorption is facilitated by lactose and ascorbic acid. Similarly, human milk's zinc is more bioavailable to the infant than the zinc in bovine milk. There are many components in human milk that have yet to be studied and their function yet to be understood. Considering this and the fact that human milk provides active protection and growth factors for nearly all newborn infants, human milk remains the gold standard for infant nutrition.

Human Milk for the Preterm Infant

By 16 weeks' gestation, the breast is prepared for lactation. The milk of a woman who delivers a preterm infant (less than 37 weeks) differs from that of a woman who delivers at term. Preterm breast milk has higher protein content and anti-infective properties, including secretory IgA and lactoferrin, higher fatty acids (such as docosahexaenoic acid [DHA]), oligosaccharides, fat, sodium, chloride, and iron content.[8,70] Research has found that proportions of fat and fatty acids were higher in milk from mothers of preterm infants born at earlier gestations.[56] The bioactive factors in human milk support the preterm infant's immature immune system. When fed human milk rather than formula, preterm infants better tolerate feedings and have lower rates of bacterial, viral, and protozoan infections.[11] Research has shown that preterm infants fed human milk have lower risk of infections including necrotizing enterocolitis (NEC), an especially threatening infection for preterm infants.[71,75]

Considering the high nutritional requirements of preterm infants and the lower presence of some components in preterm human milk, partially associated with the collection, storage, and delivery of human milk, it has been recommended to fortify human milk with iron, minerals, proteins, and fatty acids (to name a few fortifier components).[7,70] Recent research raises some concern about human milk fortification (HMF) since the source is usually bovine rather than human milk which has higher iron supplementation which may decrease lactoferrin antibacterial activity, potentially

Table 5-4 **Protective Components in Human Milk**

IMMUNE PROTECTION	FUNCTION
sIgA, G, M D, E nonspecific protection	Specific antigen targeted anti-infective activity Antibacterial, antiviral, and antimicrobial-toxin, enhancing newborn's immune system maturation
Lactoferrin (500-600 mg/dL [6025-7230 μmol/L]) colostrum (50 mg/dL in mature milk)	Iron chelation: bacteriostatic for siderophilic bacteria and fungi; lactoferrin: 18-amino-acid loop has broad-spectrum antimicrobial action; antiviral activity: (HIV, CMV, HSV) (probably by interfering with milk) the stage of virus adsorption and/or penetration; immunomodulating activity: reduced release of IL-1, IL-2, and IL-6 and TNF-α from monocytes and of PGE2 from macrophages; activation of NK cells, effect on complement activation and coagulation; antiadhesive for *Escherichia coli* and anti-invasive for *Shigella flexneri;* affects neonatal intestinal growth and recovery from injury; thereby reducing intestinal infection.
Lysozyme (5-25 mg/dL [0.5-2.5 g/L]), increases with prolonged lactation	Bacterial lysis: hydrolysis of β1-4 link between N-acetyl-glucosamine and N-acetylmuramic acid in bacterial walls; immunomodulating activity; muramyl dipeptide enhances IgA production, macrophase activation; binding to bacterial lipopolysaccharides: reduces endotoxic effect.
κ-casein (<100 mg/dL)	Antiadhesive: inhibits binding of *Helicobacter pylori* to human gastric mucosa and *Streptococcus pneumoniae* and *Haemophilus influenzae* to human respiratory tract epithelial cells; casein macropeptide is a strong growth promoting factor for *Bifodobacterium bifidum.*
MINOR NUTRIENTS	
Nucleotides	Enhance: T-cell maturation, NK cell activity, antibody response to certain vaccines, intestinal maturation and repair after diarrhea
VITAMINS	
A (β-carotene)	Anti-inflammatory (scavenging of oxygen radicals)
C (ascorbic acid)	Anti-inflammatory (scavenging of oxygen radicals)
E (α-tocopherol)	Anti-inflammatory (scavenging of oxygen radicals)
ENZYMES	
Bile salt dependent lipase	Production of FFA with antiprotozoan and antibacterial activity
Catalase	Anti-inflammatory (degrades H_2O_2)
Glutathione peroxidase	Anti-inflammatory (prevents lipid peroxidation)
PAF: acetylhydrolase	Protects against necrotizing enterocolitis (hydrolysis of PAF)
HORMONES	
Prolactin	Enhances the development of B and T lymphocytes, affects differentiation of intestinal lymphoid tissue
Cortisol, thyroxine, insulin and growth factors	Promote maturation of the newborn's intestine and development of intestinal host-defense mechanism
CELLS	
Macrophages, PMNs, and lymphocytes	Microbial phagocytosis, production of lymphokines and cytokines, interaction with and enhancement of other protective agents
Cytokines	Modulate functions and maturation of the immune system

Adapted from Hamosh, M. (2001). Bioactive factors in human milk. *Pediatr Clin North Am, 48,* 72.

CMV, Cytomegalovirus; *FFA,* free fatty acid; *HIV,* human immunodeficiency virus; *HSV,* herpes simplex virus; *IL,* interleukin, *NK,* natural killer; *PAF,* platelet activating factor; *PGE_2,* prostaglandin E_2; *PMN,* polymorphonuclear, *TNF-α,* tumor necrosis factor-α.

decreasing the anti-infective properties of human milk.[11] There is recent research supporting the use of human milk based human milk fortification (HMF) rather than bovine milk based human milk fortification (HMF) because of the increased risk of inhibition of antibacterial activity associated with bovine products added to human milk.[12,75] Use of human milk and human milk fortifiers for feeding low-birth-weight infants is discussed in Chapter 12.

During early lactation, increasing the frequency of feedings is important in establishing adequate milk production. This is especially true for the mother of a preterm infant because the infant is often transferred to the neonatal intensive care unit and is not located with the mother. Furthermore, the infant may be unable to tolerate enteral feedings or may have difficulty with the techniques needed for breastfeeding. Early and frequent breast stimulation and milk expression is recommended to help establish and maintain milk supply.[30] Researchers found that optimal milk production in mothers of preterm infants was associated with five or more milk expressions per day and pumping duration exceeding 100 min/day.[32] Skin-to-skin contact (kangaroo care) has been demonstrated to improve breastfeeding outcomes.[9]

NUTRITION DURING THE POSTPARTUM PERIOD AND LACTATION

Adequate nutrition is necessary to promote healing and restoration during the postpartum period. Lactation increases the nutritional demand on the breastfeeding woman. Maternal basal metabolic rate and cardiac output are greater with increased blood flow to the liver and gastrointestinal system to meet demands for specific nutrients and precursors as well as the redistribution of blood to augment the supply of nutrients and precursors to the mammary glands. For the healthy, well-nourished lactating woman, an additional 500 kcal is recommended to meet the energy requirements for milk production during the first 6 months of lactation. Approximately 100-150 kcal of the increased requirements are provided by maternal fat stores from pregnancy.[21] Additional nutrition may be required for the undernourished woman or the woman breastfeeding multiple children. Once lactation is established, an overweight or obese woman may restrict her caloric intake by 500 kcal per day to facilitate postpartum weight loss without negatively impacting growth of the breastfed infant.[47] Guidance and consultation on a healthy approach to postpartum weight loss in the breastfeeding woman is recommended.

Maternal diet influences water-soluble vitamins because they easily move from serum to milk.[82] Intake of water-soluble vitamins is increased, as are protein (65 g), calcium (1200 mg), vitamin D (10 mcg), vitamin E (12 mcg), and folate (280 mcg).[21] Fat-soluble vitamins are stored in fat and are more difficult to adjust by diet. Thus vitamin D supplementation is recommended for breastfed infants of women with insufficient vitamin D stores, especially those insufficiently exposed to ultraviolet light.[82] Cultural practices such as fasting may also affect the quality of a woman's milk and should be carefully considered and discussed in a respectful and health promotional manner.[66] Women who restrict their milk and dairy intake should be assessed for possible nutrient deficiencies, especially calcium and vitamin D.[50] Regarding fluid intake, lactating women should drink 600-700 mL additional healthy nutritional fluids and water per day, with extra attention to environmental and seasonal issues.[48] Changes in nutritional requirements during lactation are summarized in Table 5-5.

Table 5-5 Recommended Daily Dietary Allowances for Lactation

	FIRST 6 MONTHS	SECOND 6 MONTHS
Energy (kcal)	+500	+500
Protein (gm)	65	62
Vitamin A (RE*)	1300	1200
Vitamin D (mcg)	10	10
Vitamin E activity (mg αTE)†	12	11
Ascorbic acid (mg)	95	90
Folacin (mcg)	280	260
Niacin (mg)‡	20	20
Riboflavin (mg)	1.8	1.7
Thiamin (mg)	1.6	1.6
Vitamin B_6 (mg)	2.1	2.1
Vitamin B_{12} (mcg)	2.6	2.6
Calcium (mg)	1200	1200
Phosphorus (mg)	1200	1200
Iodine (mcg)	200	200
Iron (mg)	15	15
Magnesium (mg)	355	340
Zinc (mg)	19	16

Modified from Food and Nutrition Board, National Research Council. (1989). *Recommended dietary allowances* (10th ed.). Washington, DC: Government Printing Office; Worthington-Roberts, B.S. & Williams, S.R. (1997). *Nutrition in pregnancy and lactation* (6th ed.). Madison, WI: Brown & Benchmark.
* *RE,* Retinol equivalent.
†α-Tocopherol equivalents: 1 mg d-α-tocopherol = 1 αTE.
‡Although allowances are expressed as niacin, it is recognized that on average, 1 mg of niacin is derived from 60 mg of dietary tryptophan.

COMMON BREASTFEEDING PROBLEMS

Breastfeeding can be challenging, especially for primiparous and first-time breastfeeding women during the initial 2 weeks. Early education, support, and guidance may help prevent or minimize problems. Before lactation, it is advisable to discuss the importance of breastfeeding, plans and expectations of infant feeding, and to assess for potential problems or previous difficulties with breastfeeding to provide anticipatory guidance. Furthermore, minimizing the separation between the mother and her infant, whatever the mode of delivery, can help facilitate the breastfeeding process. For mothers whose infants have been transferred to the special care nursery, the provider should recommend and guide regular pumping with a hospital-grade breast pump from the first postpartum day.

Provided here are some common breastfeeding problems and their treatment, although oftentimes issues arise that require special attention by a trained professional. It is recommended to seek the advice of a health professional specializing in lactation.

Milk stasis, due to infrequent, insufficient, or missed feedings, may lead to *breast engorgement.* Frequent and sufficient suckling or milk expression such as by pumping reduces the congestion and provides relief, along with proper use of anti-inflammatory medication. Application of warm compresses prior to breastfeeding promotes milk flow. Brief milk expression immediately before breastfeeding reduces areolar distention related to engorgement, thereby facilitating infant latching. Milk expression between breastfeeding sessions causes overstimulation of milk production and is not recommended. Interventions such as application of cold packs and cabbage leaves have not been conclusively demonstrated to resolve engorgement or relieve symptoms and more research in the area is needed.[49] Untreated and extended milk stasis causes increased pressure in the breast and decreases capillary blood flow, decreasing milk synthesis and inhibiting lactation. Extended insufficient breast stimulation, by lack of either infant suckling or milk expression, will reduce milk synthesis and inhibit lactation. Increasing frequency of breast stimulation through increased breastfeeding frequency or pumping often resolves insufficient milk production, although some women require use of galactagogues to augment milk production.[22]

Mastitis, or breast infection, may be due to various causes including untreated or unresolved engorgement or plugged duct, milk stasis, breast or nipple trauma such as cracked nipples providing entry for infection, compromised immune status, or extreme fatigue. Common symptoms of mastitis are fatigue, general malaise, fever, and breast tenderness. The woman with mastitis should apply moist heat before breastfeeding and continue breastfeeding or expressing milk from the affected breast(s) to minimize milk stasis, preferably coordinated with the infant's feeding times. She should rest; drink fluids; and use anti-inflammatory, antibiotic, and probiotic medications for the full course of treatment as recommended by her health care provider.

Many women experience *sore nipples* during the first week of breastfeeding. It is important to address sore nipples as early and sufficiently as possible to mitigate the possibility of premature abandonment of breastfeeding. Sore nipples may be related to a host of maternal or infant factors including challenging infant anatomy (e.g., ankyloglossia), challenging maternal anatomy (e.g., inverted nipples), improper latching or positioning, dysfunctional infant suckling, infections (e.g., candidiasis), skin conditions (e.g., eczema), other conditions (e.g., Raynaud's syndrome), as well as other factors. It is crucial to identify the source of the problem and provide appropriate treatment, specific to the problem.

Consultation with expert resources regarding maternal medication during lactation is important because medication may transfer into milk (see Chapter 7). The amount of drug secreted into human milk depends upon the drug's lipid solubility, molecular weight, protein binding, ability to pass into the brain, and maternal plasma concentration.[25] Consideration of alternative, safer medications for the breastfeeding mother may preserve the breastfeeding relationship when a mother is required to take medication while breastfeeding. The safety of maternal ingestion of alcohol during lactation has not been verified and should be avoided.[45]

SUMMARY

The postpartum period is a time of rapid and complex change as the woman recovers from labor and delivery and undergoes reversal of the anatomic, physiologic, and endocrine changes of pregnancy, as well as changes to support lactation. These changes provide the background for the new mother's physical function, sense of well-being, and adaptation to her new role and her infant. Understanding of the physiologic basis of lactation is essential in intervening appropriately to support the lactating woman and in assisting with problems. Clinical recommendations related to postpartum involutional changes are summarized in Table 5-6.

Table 5-6 Summary of Recommendations for Clinical Practice Related to Involutional Changes and Lactation

Recognize and monitor the progress of normal postpartum involutional changes for each of the reproductive organs (pp. 142-144).
Observe for signs of uterine subinvolution, hemorrhage, and infection (pp. 142-143).
Monitor color and characteristics of lochia flow (p. 143).
Teach postpartum women the physiologic and anatomic changes to expect during the postpartum period (pp. 142-144).
Teach women signs and symptoms of complications and infection (pp. 142-143).
Provide comfort to postpartum women experiencing afterpains (p. 142).
Counsel women regarding urinary system changes postpartum (p. 143 and Chapter 11).
Counsel women and their partners regarding changes in vaginal tone and lubrication postpartum (p.144).
Counsel women and their partners regarding resumption of postpartum sexual activity (p. 144).
Counsel women regarding the expected timing for resumption of menstruation and ovulation (pp. 145-146).
Counsel women regarding methods and risks of family planning (including lactational amenorrhea method) to reduce risk of unplanned pregnancy (pp. 145-146).
Counsel women regarding the benefits of breastfeeding and human milk (pp. 153-158).
Teach women the physiology of lactation and milk production (pp.147-158).
Encourage and facilitate early initiation of breastfeeding after delivery (pp. 153-158).
Encourage frequent breastfeeding (on demand) or milk expression (pp.153-158).
Recognize breast engorgement and implement interventions appropriate for breastfeeding and non-breastfeeding women (pp. 150-151, 159-160).
Teach women interventions to reduce the risk of milk stasis, engorgement, and infection (pp. 150-151, 159-160).
Assist women who are pumping to increase their milk volume by increasing the frequency of pumping as well as other lactation promotional activities (pp. 158-160).
Counsel women to abstain from alcohol intake during lactation and to consult with health care provider regarding medication during lactation (p.160 and Chapter 7).
Know the composition of human milk and the factors that influence composition and volume (pp. 153-160).
Know the advantages and limitations of human milk for preterm infants (pp. 157-158 and Chapter 12).
Support breastfeeding in mothers of term and preterm infants (pp. 153-160).
Assess nutritional status and counsel women regarding nutritional needs postpartum (p. 159).
Counsel lactating women regarding nutritional requirements and effects of their nutritional status on milk production (p. 159).

References

1. Agostoni, C., et al. (2000). Free amino acid content in standard infant formulas: Comparison with human milk. *J Am Coll Nutr, 19*, 434.
2. Alvarez, M.J.L. (2007). Proteins in human milk. *Breastfeeding Review, 15*, 5.
3. American Academy of Pediatrics (AAP). (2005). Breastfeeding and the use of human milk. *Pediatrics, 115*, 496.
4. American College of Obstetrics and Gynecology. (2003). Exercise during pregnancy and the postpartum period. *Clin Obstet Gynecol, 46*, 496.
5. Anderson, J.M. & Etches, D. (2007). Prevention and management of postpartum hemorrhage. *Am Fam Physician, 75*, 875.
6. Beckmann, M.M. & Garrett, A.J. (2006). Antenatal perineal massage for reducing perineal trauma. *Cochrane Database Syst Rev*, CD005123.
7. Berseth, C.L., et al. (2004). Growth, efficacy, and safety of feeding and iron-fortified human milk fortifier. *Pediatrics, 114*, 699.
8. Bokor, S., Koletzko, B., & Decsi, T. (2007). Systematic review of fatty acid composition of human milk from mothers of preterm compared to full-term infants. *Ann Nutr Metab, 51*, 550.
9. Browne, J.V. (2004). Early relationship environments: Physiology of skin-to-skin contact for parents and their preterm infants. *Clin Perinatol, 31*, 287.
10. Carroli, G. & Mignini, L. (2009). Episiotomy for vaginal birth. *Cochrane Database Syst Rev*, CD000081.
11. Chan, G.M. (2003). Effects of powdered human milk fortifiers on the antibacterial actions of human milk. *J Perinatol, 23*, 620.
12. Chan, G.M., Lee, M.L., & Rechtman, D.J. (2007). Effects of a human milk-derived human milk fortifier on the antibacterial actions of human milk, *Breastfeeding Medicine, 2*, 205-208.
13. Chertok, I.R.A., Luo, J., & Culp, S. (2011). Intent to breastfeed: A population-based perspective. *Breastfeeding Medicine, 6*, 125.
14. Convery, K.M. & Spatz, D.L. (2009). Sexuality and breastfeeding: What do you know? *MCN Am J Matern Child Nurs, 34*, 218.
15. Cox, D.B., Owens, R.A., & Hartmann, P.E. (1996). Blood and milk prolactin and the rate of milk synthesis in women. *Experimental Physiology, 81*, 1007.
16. Cregan, M.D., Mitoulas, L.R., & Hartmann, P.E. (2002). Milk prolactin, feed volume and duration between feeds in women breastfeeding their full-term infants over a 24 h period. *Experimental Physiology, 87*, 207.
17. Cunningham, F.G., et al. (2009). *Williams Obstetrics* (23rd ed.). New York: McGraw-Hill.
18. Daly, S.E. & Hartmann, P.E. (1995). Infant demand and milk supply. Part 1: Infant demand and milk production in lactating women. *J Hum Lact. 11*, 21.
19. Davidson, K., Jacoby, S., & Brown, M.S. (2000). Prenatal perineal massage: Preventing lacerations during delivery. *J Obstet Gynecol Neonatal Nurs, 29*, 474.
20. Enkin, M., et al. (2000). *A guide to effective care in pregnancy and childbirth*. Oxford, England: Oxford University Press.
21. Food and Nutrition Board, National Research Council. (1989). *Recommended Dietary Allowances* (10th ed.). Washington, DC: National Academy Press.
22. Gabay, P.G. (2002). Galactogogues: Medications that induce lactation. *J Hum Lact, 18*, 274.
23. Geddes, D.T. (2007). Inside the lactating breast: the latest anatomy research. *J Midwifery & Women's Health, 52*, 556.
24. Gueimonde, M., et al. (2007). Breast milk: A source of bifidobacteria for infant gut development and maturation. *Neonatology, 92*, 64.
25. Hale, T.W. (2010). *Medications and mothers' milk* (14th ed.). Amarillo, TX: Pharmasoft Publishing.
26. Hamosh, M. (1998). Protective function of proteins and lipids in human milk. *Biol Neonate, 74*, 163.
27. Hartmann, K., et al. (2005). Outcomes of routine episiotomy: A systematic review. *JAMA, 293*, 2141.
28. Hay-Smith, J., et al. (2009). Pelvic floor muscle training for prevention and treatment of urinary and faecal incontinence in antenatal and postnatal women, *Cochrane Database Syst Rev, 4*, CD007471.
29. Heinrichs, M., Neumann, I., & Ehlert, U. (2002). Lactation and stress: Protective effects of breast-feeding in humans. *Stress, 5*, 195.
30. Hill, P.D., et al. (2005). Primary and secondary mediators' influence on milk output in lactating mothers of preterm and term infants. *J Hum Lact, 21*, 138.
31. Hofmeyr, G.J., Abdel-Aleem, H., & Abdel-Aleem, M.A. (2008). Uterine massage for preventing postpartum haemorrhage, *Cochrane Database Syst Rev, 3*, CD006431.
32. Hopkinson, J.M., Schanler, R.J., & Garza, C. (1988). Milk production by mothers of premature infants. *Pediatrics, 81*, 815.
33. Howard, C.R., et al. (2003). Randomized clinical trial of pacifier use and bottle-feeding or cup feeding and their effect on breastfeeding. *Pediatrics, 111*, 511.
34. Jackson, J.G., et al. (2004). A multinational study of alpha-lactalbumin concentrations in human milk. *J Nutr Biochem, 15*, 517.
35. Jackson, E. & Glasier, A. (2011). Return of ovulation and menses in postpartum non-lactating women. *Obstet Gynecol, 117*, 657.
36. Jensen, R.G., Bitman, J., & Carlson, S.E. (1995). Human milk lipids. In R.G. Jensen (Ed.). *Handbook of milk composition*. San Diego: Academic Press.
37. Kayem, G., et al. (2011). Uterine compression sutures for the management of severe postpartum hemorrhage. *Obstet Gynecol, 117*, 14.
38. Knight, C.H., Peaker, M., & Wilde, C.J. (1998). Local control of mammary development and function. *Rev Reprod, 3*, 104.
39. Ko, P.C., et al. (2011). A randomized controlled trial of antenatal pelvic floor exercises to prevent and treat urinary incontinence. *Int Urogynecol J Pelvic Floor Dysfunct. 22*, 17.
40. Koletzko, B., et al. (2001). Physiological aspects of human milk lipids. *Early Human Development, 65* (Suppl), S3.
41. Kunz, C., et al. (1999). Nutritional and biochemical properties of human milk: Part I. General aspects, proteins, and carbohydrates. *Clin Perinatol, 26*, 307.
42. Labbok, M.H., et al. (1997). Multicenter study of the lactational amenorrhea method (LAM): I. Efficacy, duration, and implications for clinical application. *Contraception, 55*, 327.
43. Lawrence, R.M. & Lawrence, R.A. (2009). The breast and the physiology of lactation. In R.K. Creasy, et al. (Eds.). *Creasy and Resnik's Maternal-fetal medicine: Principles and practice* (6th ed.). Philadelphia: Saunders.
44. Liang, C.C., et al. (2007). Postpartum urinary retention after cesarean delivery. *Int J of Gynecol & Obstet, 99*, 229.
45. Little, R.E., et al. (2002). Alcohol, breastfeeding, and development at 18 months. *Pediatrics, 109*, e72.
46. Lonnerdal, B. (2010). Novel insights into human lactation as a driver of infant formula development. *Nestle Nutr Workshop Ser Pediatr Program, 66*, 19.
47. Lovelady, C.A. (2004). The impact of energy restriction and exercise in lactating women. *Adv Exp Med Bio, 554*, 115.
48. Mahdavi, R., Nikniaz, L., & Arefhosseini, S. (2009). Energy, fluids intake and beverages consumption pattern among lactating women in Tabriz, Iran. *Pakistan J Nutr, 8*, 69.
49. Mangesi, L. & Dowswell, T. (2010). Treatment for breast engorgement during lactation, *Cochrane Database Syst Rev, 9*, CD006946.
50. Mannion, C.A., et al. (2007). Lactating women restricting milk are low on select nutrients. *J Am Coll Nutr. 26*, 149.
51. Marchant, S., et al. (1999). A survey of women's experienced vaginal loss from 24 hours to three months after childbirth (the BliPP Study). *Midwifery, 15*, 72.
52. Masters, W.H. & Johnson, V.E. (1966). *Human sexual response*. Boston: Little, Brown.
53. McManaman, J.L. & Neville, M.C. (2003). Mammary physiology and milk secretion. *Adv Drug Delivery Rev, 55*, 629.
54. McNeilly, A.S. (2001). Neuroendocrine changes and fertility in breast-feeding women. *Prog Brain Res, 133*, 207.
55. Molitch, M.E. (2009). Prolactin in human reproduction. In J.F. Strauss & R. Barbieri (Eds). *Yen & Jaffe's reproductive endocrinology: Physiology, pathophysiology, and clinical management* (6th ed.). Philadelphia: Saunders.

56. Molto-Puigmarti, C., et al. (2011). Differences in fat content and fatty acid proportions among colostrums, transitional, and mature milk from women delivering very preterm, preterm, and term infants. *Clin Nutr, 30*, 116.
57. Moore, E.R., Anderson, G.C., & Bergman, N. (2007). Early skin-to-skin contact for mothers and their healthy newborn infants, *Cochrane Database Syst Rev, 18*, CD003519.
58. Neville, M.C. (1999). Physiology of lactation. *Clin Perinatol, 26*, 251.
59. Neville, M.C. (2001). Anatomy and physiology of lactation. *Pediatr Clin North Am, 48*, 13.
60. Neville, M.C., McFadden, T.B., & Forsyth, I. (2002). Hormonal regulation of mammary differentiation and milk secretion. *J Mammary Gland Biol Neoplasia, 7*, 49.
61. Neville, M.C. & Morton, J. (2001). Physiology and endocrine changes underlying human lactogenesis II. *J Nutr, 131*, 3005S.
62. Neville, M.C., Morton, J., & Umemura, S. (2001). Lactogenesis: the transition from pregnancy to lactation. *Pediatr Clin North Am, 48*, 35.
63. Norman, E., et al. (2010). An exercise and education program improves well-being of new mothers: A randomized controlled trial. *Physical Therapy, 90*, 348.
64. Owen, C.G., et al. (2006). Does breastfeeding influence risk of type 2 diabetes in later life? A quantitative analysis of published evidence. *Am J Clin Nutr, 84*, 1043.
65. Picciano, M.F. (2001). Nutrient composition of human milk. *Pediatr Clin North Am, 48*, 53.
66. Rakicioglu, N., et al. (2006). The effect of Ramadan on maternal nutrition and composition of breast milk. *Pediatr Int, 48*, 278.
67. Ramsay, D.T., et al. (2004). Ultrasound imaging of milk ejection in the breast of lactating women, *Pediatrics, 113*, 361-367.
68. Ramsay, D.T., et al. (2005). Anatomy of the lactating human breast redefined with ultrasound imaging. *J Anat, 206*, 525.
69. Resnik, R. (2004). The puerperium. In R.K. Creasy, R. Resnik, & J.D. Iams (Eds.). *Maternal-fetal medicine: Principles and practice* (5th ed.). Philadelphia: Saunders.
70. Schanler, R.J. (2001). The use of human milk for premature infants. *Pediatr Clin North Am, 48*, 207.
71. Schurr, P. & Perkins, E.M. (2008). The relationship between feeding and necrotizing enterocolitis in very low birth weight infants. *Neonatal Netw, 27*, 397.
72. Sheiner, E., et al. (2005). Obstetric risk factors and outcome of pregnancies complicated by early postpartum hemorrhage: A population-based study. *J Matern Fetal Neonatal Med, 18*, 149.
73. Sherman, D., et al. (1999). Characteristics of normal lochia. *Am J Perinatol, 16*, 399.
74. Stuebe, A.M., et al. (2005). Duration and lactation and incidence of type 2 diabetes. *JAMA, 294*, 2601.
75. Sullivan, S., et al. (2010). An exclusively human milk-based diet is associated with a lower rate of necrotizing enterocolitis than a diet of human milk and bovine milk-based products. *J Pediatr, 156*, 562.
76. Tommaselli, G.A., et al. (2000). Using complete breastfeeding and lactational amenorrhea as birth spacing methods. *Contraception, 61*, 253.
77. Tulchinsky, D. (1994). Postpartum lactation and resumption of reproductive function. In D. Tulchinsky & A.B. Little (Eds.). *Maternal-fetal endocrinology* (2nd ed.). Philadelphia: Saunders.
78. Visness, C.M., Kennedy, K.I., & Ramos, R. (1997). The duration and character of postpartum bleeding among breast-feeding women. *Obstet Gynecol, 89*, 159.
79. Westergren-Thorsson, G., et al. (1998). Differential expressions of mRNA for proteoglycans, collagens, and transforming growth factor-beta in the human cervix during pregnancy and involution. *Biochem Biophys Acta, 1406*, 203.
80. Widstrom, A.M., et al. (2011). Newborn behavior to locate the breast when skin-to-skin: A possible method for enabling early self-regulation. *Acta Paediatr, 100*, 79.
81. Willms, A.B., et al. (1995). Anatomic changes in the pelvis after uncomplicated vaginal delivery: Evaluation with serial MR imaging. *Radiology, 195*, 91.
82. Wilson, P.R. & Pugh, L.C. (2005). Promoting nutrition in breastfeeding women, *J Obstet Gynecol Neonatal Nurs, 34*, 120.
83. Winikoff, B., et al. (2010). Treatment of post-partum haemorrhage with sublingual misoprostol versus oxytocin in women not exposed to oxytocin during labour: A double-blind, randomized, non-inferiority trial. *Lancet, 375*, 210.
84. Wojcik, K.Y., et al. (2009). Macronutrient analysis of a nationwide sample of donor breast milk. *J Am Dietetic Association, 109*, 137.
85. World Health Organization (WHO). (1998). *Evidence for the Ten Steps to Successful Breastfeeding* (revised). Geneva: World Health Organization.
86. World Health Organization (WHO). (1999). The WHO multinational study of breast-feeding and lactational amenorrhea: III. Pregnancy during breastfeeding. *Fertil Steril, 72*, 431.
87. Yip, S.K., et al. (2004).Postpartum urinary retention. *Acta Obstet Gynecol Scand, 83*, 881.
88. Zinaman, M.G., et al. (1995). Pulsatile GnRH stimulates normal cyclic ovarian function in amenorrheic lactating postpartum women. *J Clin Endocrinol Metab, 60*, 2088.

CHAPTER 6

Fetal Assessment

Tekoa L. King

Fetal growth and development are dependent upon adequate exchange of gases and nutrients within the placenta throughout the course of pregnancy. Fetal well-being in utero can be assessed via clinical measurement of the maternal fundal height, ultrasound measurement of fetal morphologic features, and tests of other biophysical parameters such as the fetal heart rate (FHR), amniotic fluid indices, and fetal movement. During labor, fetal oxygenation is monitored indirectly via assessment of FHR characteristics and FHR patterns. The status of fetal oxygenation can be measured directly via fetal scalp sampling and newborn umbilical cord gas analysis. This chapter reviews the physiology of fetal heart function, acid-base exchange, the fetal response to hypoxia, FHR patterns, and clinical implications for surveillance of the fetus during pregnancy, labor, and birth. First and second trimester genetic screening and diagnostic techniques are described in Chapter 3.

PHYSIOLOGY OF FETAL HEART FUNCTION

The average baseline FHR in a healthy fetus at 20 weeks is 155 beats per minute (range 110 to 180 beats per minute). This baseline rate is determined by the depolarization rate of the sinoatrial node, which is actively inhibited by tonic parasympathetic input. As the parasympathetic system matures with advancing gestational age, the resting heart rate decreases.[65] At term, the average FHR is 140 beats per minute and the normal range is 110 to 160 beats per minute.[65]

Autonomic Control of Fetal Heart Rate

The fetal heart has a pacemaker in the sinoatrial (SA) node that causes rhythmic contractions. The intrinsic pace is set by the SA node in the right atrium, which produces the fastest rate.[13] The average FHR is the result of several factors that modulate this intrinsic rate including: vagal stimulation at the SA node, sympathetic innervation, and feedback from baroreceptors and chemoreceptors. Vagal stimulation causes a decrease in the rate of firing of the SA node and slows the rate of transmission from the atria to the ventricles, which results in a slower heart rate. Although the fetal heart is innervated by the sympathetic system as well, parasympathetic (vagal) input maintains a baseline rate. The parasympathetic stimulation becomes dominant over sympathetic input as the fetus develops, which is why the FHR is initially faster when first detectable and slows as the fetus matures. The sympathetic nervous system innervates the heart muscle in the atria and ventricles and provides a reserve to improve the heart's pumping ability during intermittent stress. Other humoral factors, such as catecholamines, vasopressin, angiotensin II, and prostaglandins can also stimulate an increase or decrease in parasympathetic or sympathetic activity.[65]

Central Nervous System Influences

In addition to the tonic effect on the SA node that determines the baseline FHR, vagal stimulation induces variability in the time interval between each beat secondary to influences on the vagus in the central nervous system. These include baroreceptors, chemoreceptors, and other cortical influences. The central nervous system influences the FHR via an integrative center in the medulla oblongata where the vagus nerve originates (Figure 6-1). During fetal sleep, variation in the timing between each FHR diminishes and the variability has less amplitude. During fetal movement, the heart rate increases and a brief acceleration occurs. Because the medulla oblongata is near the respiratory center, the FHR may occasionally increase with inspiration and decrease with expiration.

Baroreceptors and Chemoreceptors

Baroreceptor reflexes in the aortic arch and carotid arteries are sensitive to changes in systemic arterial pressure (Figure 6-2). Baroreceptors are stimulated by the increase in blood pressure that occurs if umbilical cord circulation is occluded, which causes an increase in afterload.[6] This increase in pressure and baroreceptor stimulation initiates a rapid neural reflex to the midbrain which stimulates the vagus to slow the FHR, which results in fetal bradycardia.[64,81] Chemoreceptors are present in the carotid artery, carotid sinus, and aorta. When the chemoreceptors detect hypoxemia (a decrease in circulating oxygen) or hypercapnia (an increase in carbon dioxide), they stimulate a vagally mediated reflex bradycardia and a slight increase in blood pressure.[24,31] Baroreceptors and chemoreceptors are described further in Box 6-1 on page 165.

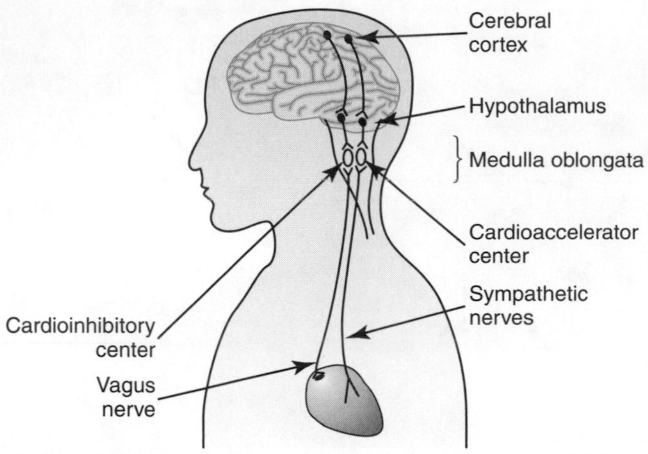

FIGURE 6-1 Cerebral influences on fetal heart rate. (From Parer, J.T. [1976]. Physiologic regulation of fetal heart rate. *J Obstet Gynecol Neonatal Nurs, 5,* 265.)

FETAL ACID-BASE PHYSIOLOGY

During aerobic or oxidative metabolism, the fetus forms carbonic acid (H_2CO_3) via hydration of CO_2. Carbonic acid dissociates into H_2O and CO_2, and CO_2 easily diffuses across the placental membranes into the maternal venous circulation in the intervillous space. During anaerobic metabolism, which occurs when there is insufficient oxygen for complete oxidation of glucose for production of adenosine triphosphate (ATP), noncarbonic metabolic acids such as lactic acid ($C_3H_6O_3$) are produced. These acids are not cleared quickly by the kidneys secondary to the immature renal function in the fetus and they also do not diffuse quickly across the placental membranes into the maternal circulation.[14] Under normal conditions, buffers such as bicarbonate (HCO_3) and hemoglobin maintain the pH within the fetal circulation within a narrow range.[8] If oxygen is not available and anaerobic metabolism continues, noncarbonic acids accumulate in the fetal compartment, bicarbonate is used up and metabolic acidosis develops. Normal metabolic activities fail when the pH falls below critical levels. Table 6-1 lists the definitions for respiratory physiology which state the importance important in understanding fetal acid-base physiology and abnormalities.

UTEROPLACENTAL CIRCULATION AND GAS EXCHANGE

Fetal "respiration" or transfer of oxygen and carbon dioxide between fetal and maternal circulations depends upon (1) adequate uterine blood flow into the intervillous space; (2) sufficient placental area available for gas and nutrient exchange; (3) efficient diffusion of oxygen, carbon dioxide, and nutrients across the membranes that separate fetal and maternal blood (see Chapter 3); and (4) unimpaired circulation within the umbilical vein that returns oxygenated blood to the fetus. It is important to remember that current knowledge about the fetal response to changes in placental function and gas exchange comes largely from studies of instrumented pregnant sheep, the animal in which gestational physiology most closely reflects human.[7]

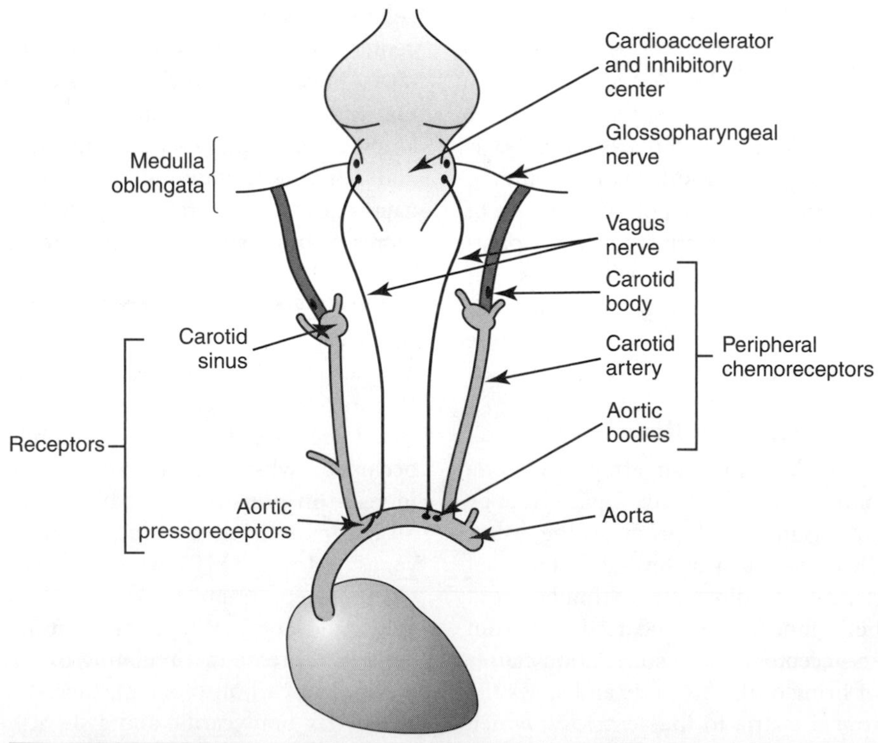

FIGURE 6-2 The peripheral chemoreceptors and baroreceptors and their input to the cardiac integrating center in the medulla oblongata. (From Parer, J.T. [1976]. Physiological regulation of fetal heart rate. *J Obstet Gynecol Neonatal Nurs, 5,* 265.)

BOX 6-1 Baroreceptors and Chemoreceptors

Baroreceptors and chemoreceptors are part of the homeostatic negative feedback mechanisms that regulate blood pressure. Chemoreceptors are also involved in regulating the respiratory rate.

Baroreceptors (see Figure 6-2) are sensory nerve endings located in the walls of most major arteries in the neck and chest. They are stimulated by changes in pressure. When arterial blood pressure increases and the walls of an artery stretch, the baroreceptors send signals to (1) the vasomotor center, which results in a reflex vasodilation; and (2) to the vagus nerve, which results in vagally mediated bradycardia. The combination of vasodilation and slower heart rate decreases blood pressure.

Chemoreceptors are sensory nerve endings located peripherally near the baroreceptors in the carotid sinus and aortic arch and centrally in the medulla oblongata. Chemoreceptors are stimulated by changes in blood oxygen and carbon dioxide tension. In the adult, when hypoxemia or hypercarbia is detected by the central chemoreceptors, a reflex is initiated that results in (1) vasomotor stimulation, which causes vasoconstriction and increased blood pressure; and (2) vagal inhibition, which results in tachycardia. In the fetus, central and peripheral chemoreceptor stimulation results in hypertension and bradycardia.

Table 6-1 Terms Related to Fetal Acid-Base Physiology

Term	Definition
Acidemia	Increased concentration of hydrogen ions in the blood.
Acidosis	Increased concentration of hydrogen ions in the tissue.
Aerobic metabolism	Metabolism of glucose using oxygen. The end products of aerobic metabolism are large amounts of energy (38 ATP molecules, H_2O, and CO_2).
Anaerobic metabolism	Metabolism of glucose without the use of oxygen. Glucose breaks down partially and the end products are a small amount of energy (2 ATP molecules) and lactic acid.
Asphyxia	From the Greek word for "pulseless." Asphyxia is characterized by profound acidemia that is both metabolic and respiratory in nature. Some authors say the diagnosis of asphyxia is based on evidence of ischemia and organ dysfunction, but this is not universal. In fact, discrimination between metabolic acidemia and asphyxia is not well defined.
Base	A substance that is capable of accepting hydrogen ions, thereby decreasing acidity.
Base excess (BE)	The amount of base or HCO_3^- that is left available for buffering. A BE of −8 means there is less BE available than a value of −4. The lower BE implies a greater degree of anaerobic metabolism and more production of acids.
Bicarbonate (bicarb)	HCO_3^- is the base or hydrogen acceptor that is part of the primary buffering system within the blood.
Buffer	A chemical substance that is both a weak acid and salt. Buffers can absorb or give up hydrogen ions, thereby maintaining a constant pH value. The primary buffer involved in fetal oxygenation is HCO_3^-.
Hypercapnia	Excessive carbon dioxide in blood.
Hypoxia	Decreased oxygen in tissue.
Hypoxemia	Decreased oxygen content in blood.
Metabolic acidosis	Low bicarbonate (low base excess) in the presence of normal PCO_2 values.
pH	pH refers to the concentration of hydrogen ions in blood. The term *pH* refers to "puissance hydrogen," which is French for strength (or power) of hydrogen. The term *pH* was devised by the Danish biochemist S.P. Sorenson in 1909. A pH of 7.0 is the same as 0.0000001 moles per liter of hydrogen ions, whereas 0.01 moles/liter is written as a pH of 2. How did the term develop? 0.0000001 can also be written as 1.0×10^{-7}. The exponent −7 refers to the number of zeros or number of times a particular number is multiplied by itself (e.g., 3^3 is the same as 3 x 3 x 3). When you read that pH is the "negative logarithm," this means a pH of 7.0 refers to the number of zero place markers (i.e., the number of times the number is multiplied by itself). Because small concentrations (fractions) are being multiplied, pH is actually referring to a negative number (number less than 1), which makes each multiplication a progressively smaller number. By convention, when assessing the pH or amount of hydrogen ions in blood, the place marker (logarithmic scale) zeros and the negative sign are dropped.
Respiratory acidosis	High PCO_2 with normal bicarbonate levels. Found in acute cord compression before anaerobic metabolism has started.

From King, T. & Parer, J. (2000). The physiology of fetal heart rate patterns and perinatal asphyxia. *J Perinat Neonatal Nurs, 14,* 19. Original table adapted from references 2, 7, 27, 28, and 65.

Uterine Blood Flow

Approximately 500 to 600 mL of blood flows to the uterus each minute. Seventy percent to 90% of the uterine blood flow circulates through the intervillous space and the volume of blood that reaches the intervillous space is dependent on adequate flow through the maternal spiral arteries. Maternal hypotension or hypertension and uterine contractions can decrease blood flow into the intervillous space. The maternal spiral arteries run perpendicular to uterine muscle and the maternal veins are usually parallel to the uterine wall, thus uterine contractions that occur during labor cause vasoconstriction, which temporarily interrupts blood flow in and out of the intervillous space. Both inflow and outflow tracts are affected. Thus, during uterine contractions, the volume of maternal blood in the intervillous space that is available for continued gas exchange remains the same or slightly more than the volume present during uterine quiescence.[9]

Because the spiral arteries are maximally dilated and have lost some of their ability to "autoregulate" or constrict if pressure in the vessel drops, there is very little that can increase uterine blood flow. However, maximal blood flow can be facilitated and events known to decrease blood flow can be avoided. For example, two interventions that maximize blood flow to the uterus are side-lying positions (prevents compression of the inferior vena cava) and administration of tocolytics (temporarily decreases uterine contractions).

Umbilical Blood Flow

The two umbilical arteries and one umbilical vein spiral through a matrix of a specialized connective tissue called *Wharton's jelly*. The umbilical cord is normally lighter than any of the fetal parts and generally moves freely within the amniotic fluid. However, the cord can be compressed during uterine contractions. Cord compression results in an increase in fetal blood pressure, which initiates the baroreceptor reflex and subsequent bradycardia, although occlusion of only the umbilical vein usually does not significantly change arterial pressure. Repetitive cord compression can cause the development of acidemia if oxygen and carbon dioxide transfer are significantly impeded enough to result in anaerobic metabolism and a build-up of lactic acid.[90] The FHR bradycardia response to cord compression depends on the baroreceptor detection of blood pressure or chemoreceptor detection of hypoxemia. The chemoreceptor response is slower than the baroreceptor response. In sudden, complete occlusion of the umbilical cord, there is an immediate rise in arterial pressure because of arterial occlusion, and bradycardia secondary to baroreceptor stimulation is instantaneous.[37,60] Following chemoreceptor detection of a decrease in the PO_2, the fall in FHR is slower.

Placental Area

The placental area available for exchange of gases and nutrients is approximately 1.8 m^2.[65] Several mechanisms can adversely affect the available villous surface. Abruptio placenta or uterine rupture causes an acute decrease in placental area. Fetal survival in these situations depends upon the percentage of placental tissue that remains, the reserve of the individual fetus, and the rapidity of clinical response. Chronic maternal conditions such as hypertension, preeclampsia, diabetes, and/or renal disease are characterized by small artery dysfunction, which can result in reduced placental growth, placental infarcts, and chronic intrauterine fetal growth restriction. Finally, infection within the placenta can cause a reduction in placental size and alter transfer of oxygen and nutrients.

Transfer of Oxygen and Carbon Dioxide

Diffusion of oxygen and carbon dioxide across the membranes that separate maternal and fetal blood in the intervillous space occurs quickly. Factors that affect the rate of maternal-to-fetal gas exchange in the intervillous space include maternal and fetal oxygen-hemoglobin dissociation curves, the Bohr effect (see Box 10-1 on p. 301 in Chapter 10), maternal and fetal hemoglobin concentrations, and the oxygen affinity of fetal hemoglobin (see Chapter 8). Carbon dioxide transfer is affected by hydrogen ion concentration and the Haldane effect.

Oxygen Transfer

The PO_2 in maternal arteries that supply the intervillous space is 30 to 35 mmHg (3.99 to 4.65 kPa), which is similar to the average PO_2 in maternal capillaries.[7] Thus the PO_2 in the fetal umbilical vein, which delivers oxygenated blood to the fetus, is approximately the same as the average PO_2 in maternal veins. Despite an arterial partial pressure of oxygen that is lower than the PO_2 in adult arteries, the fetus has several mechanisms that allow sufficient oxygenation.

The fetal oxygen-hemoglobin dissociation curve is to the left of the adult curve, because fetal hemoglobin (HbF) has a higher affinity for oxygen compared to adult hemoglobin. The pH of blood on the maternal side of the intervillous space drops (becomes more acidic) when oxygen is released and fetal metabolites are absorbed. This shifts the maternal oxygen-hemoglobin dissociation curve to the right (the Bohr effect), which further facilitates the transfer of oxygen from the mother to the fetus. As the fetus gives up carbon dioxide, the pH in the fetal compartment rises (becomes more alkaline), shifting the fetal dissociation curve to the left, which further aids oxygen uptake by the fetus. This movement of hydrogen ions results in a displacement of both dissociation curves, moving them further apart (double Bohr effect). As the distance between the two curves increases, oxygen transfers at a faster rate from maternal blood to fetal blood. This process is unique to the placenta.

In addition to a higher affinity for oxygen, the fetus has an increased number of red blood cells, more hemoglobin (approximately 15 g/dL [150 g/L] versus an average of 12 g/dL [120 g/L] in adults), and more capillaries per unit of tissue.[89] The combination of these factors results in a higher oxygen-carrying capacity when compared with the oxygen carrying capacity of the mother. Usual fetal blood gases are listed in Table 10-7.

Maternal hypoxia (especially a PO_2 below 60 mmHg [7.98 kPa]) can have significant consequences for the fetus. In this situation, the maternal oxygen-hemoglobin dissociation curve shifts to the left (toward the fetal curve), decreasing oxygen availability to the fetus.[12] Maternal hyperventilation, which results in decreased PCO_2, can also lead to decreased fetal oxygenation by shifting the maternal oxygen-hemoglobin dissociation curve to the left.

Carbon Dioxide Transfer

The rate at which the maternal compartment can take up carbon dioxide is dependent upon the amount of maternal hemoglobin that is not combined with oxygen. Uncombined hemoglobin is free to buffer the hydrogen ions formed by the dissociation of carbonic acid. This means that as maternal hemoglobin gives up oxygen, it is able to accept increased amounts of carbon dioxide (the Haldane effect). The fetus gives up carbon dioxide as oxygen is accepted, without altering the local $PaCO_2$ levels. This double Haldane effect is unique to the placenta and is probably responsible for half the transplacental carbon dioxide transfer.

In summary, uterine and umbilical blood flow are the most important components of uteroplacental gas exchange or fetal "respiration." Oxygen and carbon dioxide readily diffuse across the membranes separating fetal and maternal circulations. Rarely, an increased fetal need for oxygen as occurs in the presence of infection, fetal anemia, or the fetus is exposed to decreased maternal PO_2, which can occur if the mother experiences cardiopulmonary disease, severe anemia, or acute trauma.

FETAL RESPONSE TO HYPOXIA

The fetus is normally able to maintain aerobic metabolism during the transient decreases in oxygenation that are common when there is a temporary interruption in uterine or umbilical blood flow. Aerobic metabolism will be maintained until the available oxygen in the intervillous space falls to 50% of normal levels.[71] The fetus has several normal compensatory mechanisms for surviving transient hypoxic insults in addition to having more hemoglobin per cubic unit of whole blood and HbF, which has extra oxygen-carrying capacity. Transient hypoxemia initiates a redistribution of blood flow so that that blood is preferentially shunted to the heart, brain, and adrenal glands (increased twofold to threefold) and blood flow to the gut, spleen, kidneys, and limbs is decreased (Figure 6-3).[22,41] In addition, the FHR slows as a response to hypoxia, which decreases oxygen consumption. Together these physiologic mechanisms maintain blood flow and oxygenation in the organs that are critical for survival.

Acute Fetal Hypoxia and Asphyxia

If the normal compensatory mechanisms are not sufficient to allow the fetus to maintain aerobic metabolism, anaerobic metabolism will ensue.[10] Oxygen uptake by fetal hemoglobin becomes less efficient as the pH decreases.[76] The change from aerobic metabolism to anaerobic metabolism sets the stage for the development of a metabolic acidosis and metabolic acidemia. If normal fetal oxygenation does not resume, metabolic acidosis will progress to asphyxia, which interrupts metabolic processes. If this occurs, the adaptive mechanisms fail and arterial oxygenation will fall below critical levels, resulting in myocardial depression and loss of autoregulation in cerebral blood flow (see Chapter 15). The brain becomes ischemic in the presence of passive pressure circulation.[27,47,66,77]

Chronic Fetal Hypoxemia

Chronic reductions in uteroplacental perfusion stimulate hematopoiesis via renal production of erythropoietin. This leads to an increase in nucleated red blood cell counts that can be measured in the neonate.[82] Chronic hypoxia also causes the fetus to limit oxygen-consuming processes, which can result in growth and/or behavioral changes. Oxygen-consuming activities such as protein synthesis must be curtailed to direct limited resources to more vital functions. This may alter fetal growth. Metabolic normality may be maintained by the fetus, which suggests that the fetus is capable of rapid adaptation to limited substrate delivery by decreasing the growth rate. Over time, this adaptation results in clinically detectable fetal growth restriction. These alterations and restrictions in growth and development within specific organs can adversely influence subsequent extrauterine health.[38]

Along with growth restriction, changes in behavioral states can be seen during acute hypoxemia as well as in chronic hypoxemia. The development of well-defined behavioral states

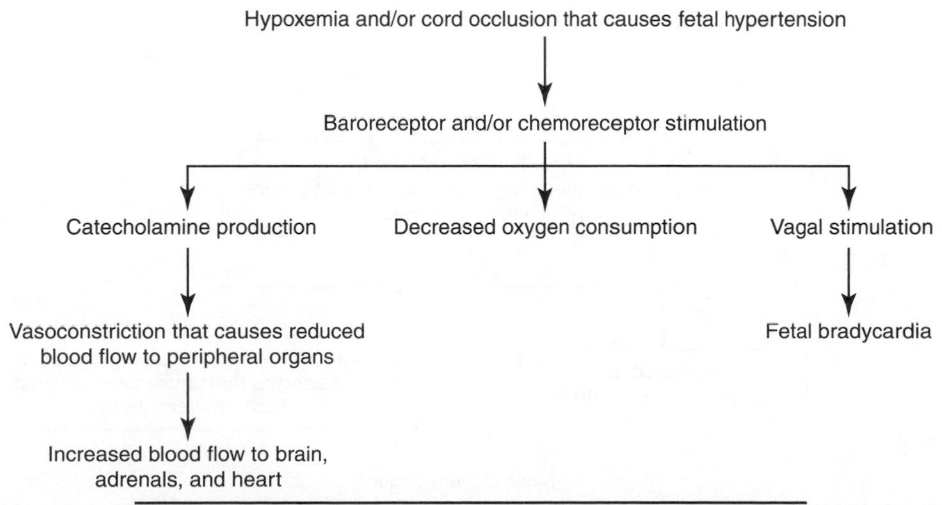

FIGURE 6-3 Fetal compensatory response to transient hypoxemia.

may be delayed in infants with fetal growth restriction compared to the behaviors observed in normal infants.[52] Rapid eye movement (REM) sleep states are decreased when the fetus experiences hypoxemia and may be indicative of changes in oxygen consumption.[48,76] In addition, when the fetus is hypoxemic, fetal movements are reduced. Acute asphyxia may result in a brief increase in extremity movement that falls off quickly if oxygenation is not restored. Cessation in fetal breathing movements and gross body movements can contribute to reducing fetal oxygen consumption and is an indication of decreased energy expenditure. The number and duration of general body movements are decreased in fetuses with fetal growth restriction. Although the fetus is capable of reducing its oxygen needs and compensating for limited substrate availability over a protracted period of time, this may end up being detrimental to organ development and functioning on a long-term basis.[38]

Hypoxic-Ischemic Encephalopathy

Because neurons have a high metabolic rate, severe asphyxia disproportionately damages the fetal brain. Oxygen deficiency in brain tissue results in both acidemia and ischemia. In addition, the brain does not store glucose so a disruption of blood flow quickly results in a depletion of both glucose and oxygen, which are needed for the production of ATP. Insufficient ATP sets off the final chain of events that result in cell death (Figure 6-4).[39]

Hypoxic-ischemic encephalopathy (HIE) is the term applied to the type of brain injury sustained by newborns who survive a severe asphyxial insult from oxygen deprivation.[42,51] When ATP is depleted, several critical cellular metabolic processes stop. Sodium-potassium pumps fail, which causes depolarization of the cellular membrane, cellular edema, and an influx of calcium into the cytosol of the cell.[19,42] Enzymatic processes are stimulated by the presence of free calcium, which produces a cascade of events that result in cellular death. First, calcium initiates a chain of reactions that leads to degradation of the phospholipid cell membrane, which results in release of free fatty acids into the intercellular spaces and production of thromboxane A. Thromboxane A causes further vasoconstriction. Neuronal cells that release the excitatory amino acid glutamate are activated by the influx of calcium. Glutamate accumulates outside the cell membrane and at toxic levels will cause seizures.[14,19,21,74]

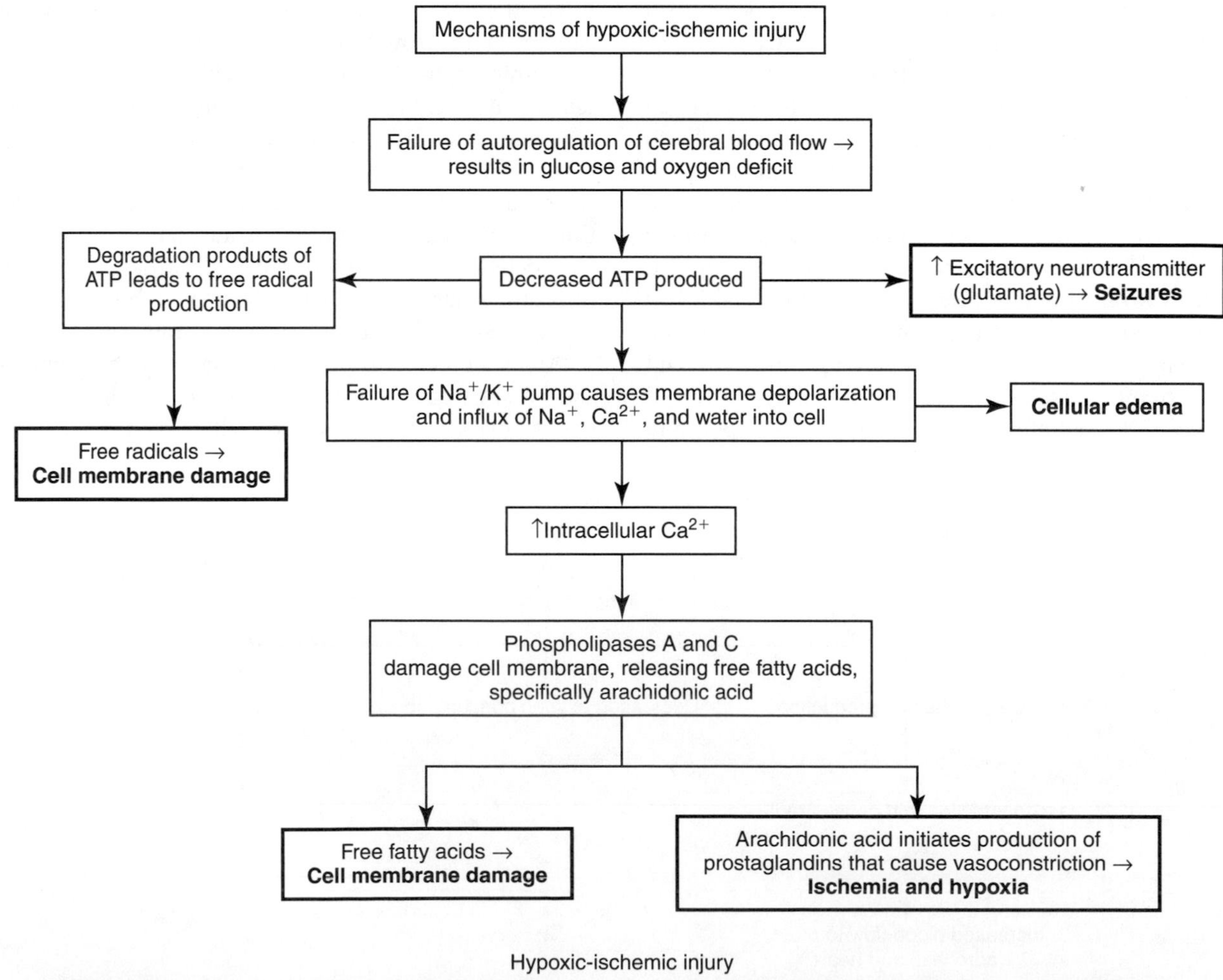

FIGURE 6-4 Hypoxic-ischemic injury. (From King, T. & Parer, J. [2000]. The physiology of fetal heart rate patterns and perinatal asphyxia. *J Perinat Neonatal Nurs, 14,* 19.)

HIE has a second phase of damage during reperfusion when the hypoxic event resolves. When oxygen is reintroduced, the oxygen-free radicals that are not inactivated by naturally occurring antioxidants cause further damage to the cell membrane and destruction of cellular DNA.[42]

The region of the brain affected by HIE is dependent on the gestational age of the fetus and the severity of the insult. Ischemic necrosis occurs most frequently in border zones that exist between the end branches of major cerebral vessels. Long-term outcomes of infants with HIE are in proportion to the severity of injury: Grade 1 HIE involves transient central nervous system (CNS) irritability that improves by 48 hours. Infants with grade 1 HIE generally develop normally without sequelae. Grade 2 HIE involves CNS suppression and possible injury producing lethargy, seizures, weak Moro reflex, and absent to weak suck. The infant's condition stabilizes and usually improves in 3 to 5 days; 80% develop normally. Grade 3 HIE involves CNS suppression with injury, coma, absent suck and absent Moro reflex, and seizures for several days; 50% do not survive.[30,78] HIE is discussed further in Chapter 15.

Cerebral Palsy Following Hypoxic-Ischemic Injury

Preterm infants who survive severe asphyxial insults characteristically develop intraventricular hemorrhage and/or periventricular white matter injury (see Chapter 15), which, if severe, ultimately manifests as the spastic diplegia type of cerebral palsy.[72] Infants born at 34 weeks' gestation or older who survive typically develop parasagittal injury, which will manifest as spastic quadriplegia if the insult was severe.[72] Because there are many nonasphyxial etiologies of cerebral palsy, criteria for determining that intrapartum asphyxia is the etiologic factor that has been developed (Table 6-2).[59,85]

CHARACTERISTICS OF THE FETAL HEART RATE

The FHR, general activity, and level of muscle tone are particularly sensitive to hypoxemia and acidemia. These responses are the basis of several clinical assessment techniques reviewed later in this chapter.[48,62] FHR patterns are categorized by the following: (1) baseline characteristics, variability, presence or absence of accelerations, and

Table 6-2 Criteria to Define Acute Intrapartum Hypoxic Event Sufficient to Cause Cerebral Palsy

ESSENTIAL CRITERIA (MUST MEET ALL FOUR)

1. Evidence of a metabolic acidosis in fetal umbilical cord arterial blood obtained at delivery (pH <7 and base deficit ≥12 mEq/L [mmol/L])
   a. pH of <7 is the pH at which acidemia is associated with adverse outcomes in the newborn.
   b. The metabolic component is the most important variable associated with subsequent neonatal morbidity.
   c. However, metabolic acidosis in and of itself does not infer the timing of the onset of injury.
2. Early onset of severe or moderate neonatal encephalopathy in infants born at 34 or more weeks' gestation
   a. Abnormalities appear in the first 24 hours.
3. Cerebral palsy of the spastic quadriplegic or dyskinetic type
   a. Spastic quadriplegia and less commonly dyskinetic cerebral palsy are the only types of cerebral palsy associated with acute hypoxic intrapartum events. Spastic quadriplegia is not specific to intrapartum hypoxia.
4. Exclusion of other identifiable etiologies such as trauma, coagulation disorders, infectious conditions, or genetic disorders

(This recommendation is controversial. Other etiologies do not preclude the presence of an intrapartum event as well.)

Criteria that collectively suggest intrapartum timing (within close proximity to labor and delivery, e.g., 0 to 48 hours) but are nonspecific to asphyxial insults

1. A sentinel (signal) hypoxic event occurring immediately before or during labor.
   a. Uterine rupture, massive hemorrhage, placental abruption, prolapsed cord, amniotic fluid embolism, maternal cardiopulmonary arrest
2. A sudden and sustained fetal bradycardia or the absence of fetal heart rate variability in the presence of persistent, late, or variable decelerations, usually after a hypoxic sentinel event when the pattern was previously normal.
   a. The best studies available on the event-to-delivery time and neonatal outcomes are in cases of uterine rupture.[44]
   b. Perinatal asphyxia occurs as soon as 10 minutes after onset of terminal bradycardia if preceded by repetitive late or variable decelerations.
   c. Perinatal asphyxia did not occur if the terminal deceleration to delivery time was less than 17 minutes if the previous FHR tracing was reassuring.
   d. FHR of less than 60 is an obstetric emergency.
   e. Loss of variability correlates better with subsequent neonatal outcome than the length of the bradycardia itself.
3. Apgar scores of 0 to 3 beyond 5 minutes.

Low Apgar score in infants with birth weight >2500 g and cerebral palsy at 7 yr.[57]

APGAR SCORES 0-3	CP AT 7 YR
At 1 min	0.7
At 5 min	4.7
At 20 min	57.1

4. Onset of multisystem involvement within 72 hours of birth.
5. Early imaging study showing evidence of acute nonfocal cerebral abnormality.

Adapted from Task Force on Neonatal Encephalopathy and Cerebral Palsy. (2003). *Neonatal encephalopathy and cerebral palsy: Defining the pathogenesis and pathophysiology.* American College of Obstetricians and Gynecologists (ACOG) and the American Academy of Pediatrics. Washington, DC: ACOG.

baseline rate, which is observed between uterine contractions; (2) periodic changes that are associated with uterine contractions; and (3) episodic changes that are not associated with uterine contractions. Definitions for fetal heart rate characteristics reviewed in this chapter are listed in Table 6-3.[58]

Beat-to-Beat Variability

The time interval between two heartbeats in a healthy fetus is seldom the same. This variability is secondary to changes in the timing between vagal impulses and effects of the sympathetic reflexes. Thus, the sources of variability in the FHR include input from the cerebral cortex, and midbrain via the vagus nerve, and to a lesser extent stimulation from sympathetic nerves that terminate in cardiac muscle.[65] Baseline variability is defined as fluctuations of 2 cycles/min or greater in the baseline FHR (Figure 6-5).[58] These fluctuations are irregular in both amplitude and frequency and involve short- and long-term changes.[67,71] Short-term variability is the beat-to-beat changes in timing. Vagal stimulation of the SA node is the primary driver of short-term variability. Long-term variability is the larger amplitude changes in several adjacent beats that rise above or below the averaged baseline. Long-term variability is also suppressed during fetal sleep and accentuated during fetal activity. Although short-term variability can exist without long-term variability, the reverse is not true. In practice, they exist together and are not separated in clinical assessments.[58] Factors that can affect the magnitude of FHR variability include gestational age, fetal breathing, fetal movement, fetal sleep state, hypoxia, and acidemia.

Absent variability can be idiopathic but absent variability in association with recurrent late or variable decelerations is the FHR characteristic most consistently associated with newborn acidosis and neonatal morbidity.[46,68,91]

The evolution of the FHR from normal variability and a normal baseline rate to absent variability in the presence of recurrent decelerations is believed to parallel the evolution from acidemia to acidosis and then asphyxia. However, the link between a specific FHR pattern and the actual acid-base status of the fetus has yet to be well demarcated. Therefore absent variability is an indication for obstetric evaluation and possible intervention. Absent variability in combination with recurrent late or variable decelerations is associated with metabolic acidemia frequently enough that delivery is recommended if this pattern is observed.[46]

Minimal variability can be seen in states of fetal sleep and/or following administration of opioids given for relief of labor pain. The use of local or general anesthetics as well as other maternal drugs (e.g., magnesium sulfate, meperidine,

Table 6-3 Fetal Heart Rate Characteristics: Definitions

TERM	DEFINITION
Baseline rate	Mean FHR rounded to increments of 5 beats per minute during a 10-minute segment excluding periodic or episodic changes, periods of marked variability, and segments of baseline that differ by more than 25 beats per minute. Duration must be ≥2 minutes.
Bradycardia	Baseline rate <110 beats per minute.
Tachycardia	Baseline rate >160 beats per minute.
Variability	Fluctuations in the baseline FHR of 2 cycles/min or greater.
Absent variability	Amplitude from peak to trough undetectable.
Minimal variability	Amplitude from peak to trough greater than undetectable and ≤5 beats per minute.
Moderate variability	Amplitude from peak to trough 6 to 25 beats per minute.
Marked variability	Amplitude from peak to trough >25 beats per minute.
Acceleration	Visually apparent abrupt increase (onset to peak <30 seconds) of FHR above baseline. Peak ≥15 beats per minute. Duration ≥15 beats per minute and <2 minutes. In gestations less than 32 weeks, peak of 10 beats per minute and duration of 10 seconds is an acceleration.
Prolonged acceleration	Duration of acceleration between 2 and 10 minutes.
Early deceleration	Visually apparent gradual decrease (onset to nadir ≥30 seconds) of FHR below baseline. Return to baseline associated with uterine contraction. Nadir of deceleration occurs at the same time as the peak of the contraction. Generally, the onset, nadir, and recovery of the deceleration occur at the same time as the onset, peak, and recovery of the contraction.
Late deceleration	Visually apparent gradual decrease (onset to nadir is ≥30 seconds) of FHR below baseline. Return to baseline associated with a uterine contraction. Nadir of deceleration occurs after the peak of the contraction. Generally, the onset, nadir, and recovery of the deceleration occur after same time as the onset, peak, and recovery of the contraction.
Variable deceleration	Visually apparent abrupt decrease (onset to nadir <30 seconds) in FHR below baseline. Decrease ≥15 beats per minute. Duration ≥15 seconds and <2 minutes.
Prolonged deceleration	Visually apparent abrupt decrease (onset to nadir <30 seconds) in FHR below baseline. Decrease ≥15 beats per minute. Duration ≥2 minutes but <10 minutes.

Adapted from National Institute of Child Health and Human Development Research Planning Workshop. (1997). Electronic fetal heart rate monitoring; Research guidelines for interpretation. *Am J Obstet Gynecol, 17,* 1385; and [No authors listed]. (1997). Electronic fetal heart rate monitoring: Research guidelines for interpretation. The National Institute of Child Health and Human Development Research Planning Workshop. *J Obstet Gynecol Neonatal Nurs, 26,* 635.

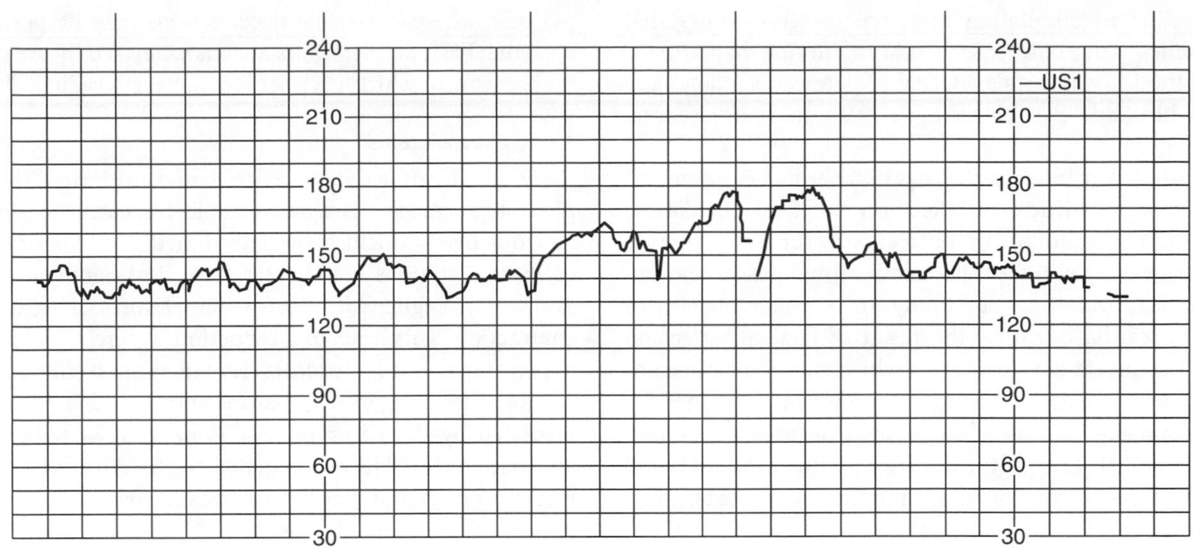

FIGURE 6-5 Fetal heart rate with moderate variability and accelerations.

methadone) can also depress beat-to-beat variability.[36,80] Moderate variability is the most important indicator of anatomic and functional integrity of the pathways regulating cardiac function and reflects adequate cerebral oxygenation.[68,71] Marked variability, which is sometimes called a *saltatory pattern,* is usually benign and thought to occur when sympathetic stimulation (α-adrenergic activity) overrides parasympathetic dominance in response to acute but temporary hypoxemia. This pattern is almost exclusively seen during labor. It can also occur following the administration of larger doses of ephedrine.[61]

Accelerations

Accelerations are visually apparent abrupt increases in the FHR above the baseline (see Figure 6-5). To qualify as an acceleration, the acme must be 15 beats per minute above the baseline and the acceleration must last at least 15 seconds in a term fetus.[58] In a fetus of gestational age less than 32 weeks, accelerations are less robust and diagnostic criteria are that the FHR increases 10 beats per minute above the baseline and will last a minimum of 10 seconds. Accelerations are associated with moderate variability and, like variability, are strongly prognostic of adequate fetal oxygenation.[11,46]

Alterations in Fetal Heart Rate

The baseline FHR at term normally ranges from 110 to 160 beats per minute.

Tachycardia

Fetal tachycardia (baseline more than 160 beats per minute for 10 minutes or more) can occur secondary to a host of fetal and maternal conditions. Tachycardia can be nonpathologic and is considered a normal rate in the premature fetus, in whom the sympathetic nervous system dominates control of cardiac function. Short periods of tachycardia are a normal compensatory response to transient hypoxemia and are often seen for a brief period following a prolonged FHR deceleration. These periods of tachycardia are probably due to a transient rise in catecholamine levels.[67]

The most common etiology of sustained tachycardia in the term fetus is maternal infection, specifically chorioamnionitis.[67] Fetal tachycardia can also be seen following sublethal hypoxic events that cause catecholamine release and sympathetic stimulation.

Other sources of fetal tachycardia are the use of β-sympathomimetic agents (to inhibit uterine contractions), ephedrine given to correct maternal hypotension following induction of epidural anesthesia, fetal anemia (Rh isoimmunization), acute fetal blood loss (placental abruption), or abnormal fetal conduction system (fetal arrhythmia).[67]

Bradycardia

Bradycardia is a sustained FHR of less than 110 beats per minute for longer than 10 minutes.[46] Bradycardia is the initial fetal response to acute hypoxemia or elevated blood pressure secondary to cord occlusion. Nonasphyxial causes of bradycardia include heart block and hypothermia. In addition, head compression during rapid descent in labor can stimulate a vagal response secondary to mild cerebral ischemia or increased intracranial pressure. These vagally stimulated bradycardias are nonasphyxial as long as the FHR remains higher than 80 to 100 beats per minute and has moderate variability.[68,71] End-stage bradycardia seen in the second stage of labor is probably a result of a vagal response to head compression as the fetus traverses the birth canal.[67]

A few otherwise normal fetuses have a heart rate below 110 that appear to be a normal variant.[67] A transient fetal bradycardia frequently follows administration of intrathecal opioids and/or local anesthetics for epidural analgesia during labor.[26] The etiology of this bradycardia is indirect in that the bradycardia is secondary to an interruption of uteroplacental circulation that occurs by one of two pathways: First, the rapid decline in circulating maternal catecholamines that accompanies pain relief can result in uterine hypertonus. Second, the induction of maternal hypotension following a regional blockade can cause a decrease in uteroplacental blood flow.

An acute severe bradycardia (below 80 beats per minute) is the response to an adverse effect on the fetal circulation, which would occur following a placental abruption or uterine rupture for example. Acute hypoxemia stimulates a chemoreceptor reflex, which causes bradycardia.[67] Alternatively, an acute bradycardia could be the result of fetal hypertension following complete cord occlusion which causes a baroreceptor reflex, which stimulates a vagal response and a fall in FHR. The duration and severity of the bradycardia are correlated to the length and severity of the interruption in umbilical blood flow or decreased oxygenation. In summary, an acute terminal bradycardia can be caused by (1) a decrease in umbilical blood flow (cord compression, cord prolapse), (2) decreased placental exchange area (abruptio placentae, uterine rupture), (3) impaired uterine blood flow (acute maternal hypotension or excessive uterine contractions), or (4) decreased maternal oxygenation (apnea secondary to seizures).[43,67]

Periodic and Episodic Fetal Heart Rate Decelerations

Periodic FHR decelerations are associated with uterine contractions. Episodic decelerations are those that are not associated with uterine activity. Late and early decelerations are periodic whereas variable decelerations may be periodic or episodic. FHR decelerations are characterized by the onset of the waveform, which is either "abrupt" or "gradual."[58]

Early Decelerations

Early decelerations have a gradual waveform. The exact physiologic mechanism responsible for early decelerations had not been conclusively determined. One theory is that early decelerations are the result of a physiologic chain of events that begins with head compression during a uterine contraction. This leads to a reduction in cerebral blood flow, hypercapnia, and hypoxemia. Hypercapnia results in hypertension that triggers the baroreceptors and a bradycardia mediated by the parasympathetic nervous system. The fall and rise of the FHR are matched to the rise and fall of the uterine contraction. Early decelerations may also be a benign variant of late reflex decelerations.[67] The nadir of the deceleration is rarely more than 40 beats per minute below the baseline and early decelerations are not indicative of fetal acidemia.[46,67]

Variable Decelerations

Variable decelerations may be inconsistent in timing when compared with uterine contractions (Figure 6-6). These decelerations have an abrupt onset (less than 30 seconds from onset to nadir) and they may be periodic (associated with a uterine contraction) or episodic (not associated with a uterine contraction). The clinical implications are related to the

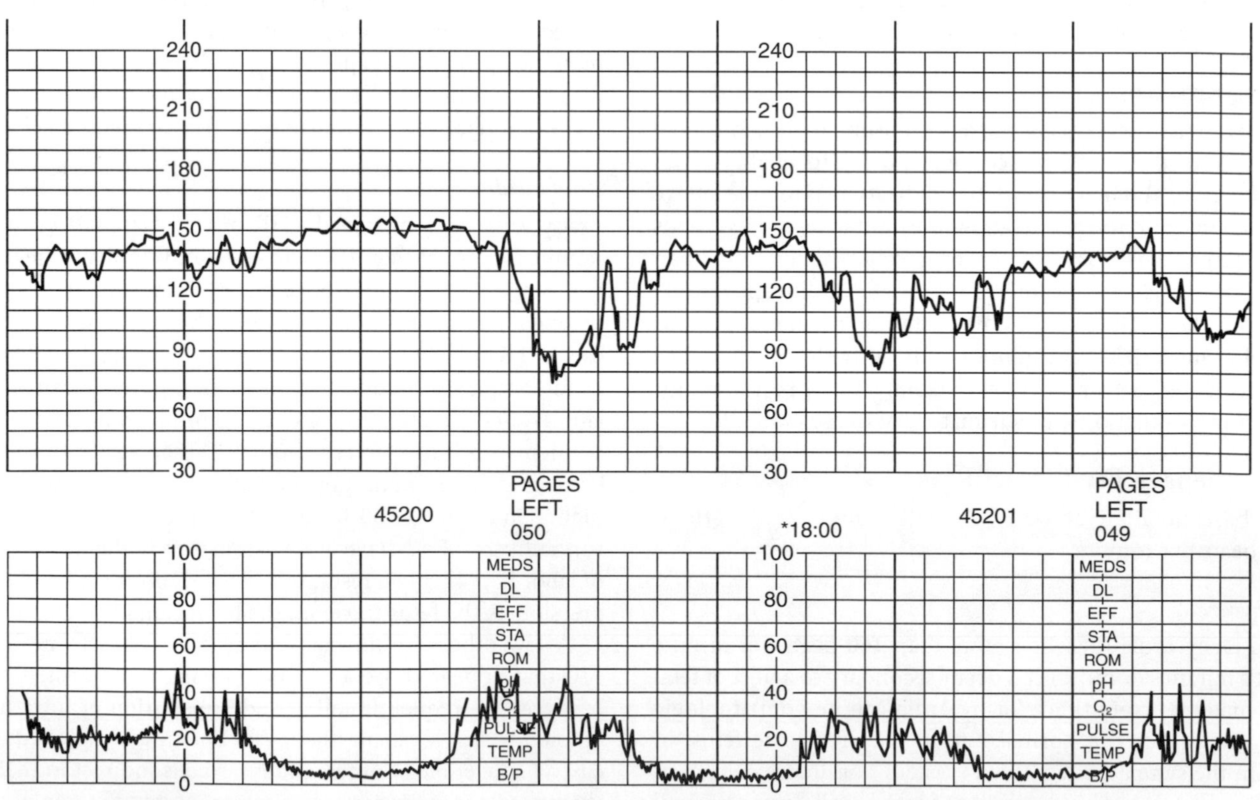

FIGURE 6-6 Variable decelerations. The upper graph is fetal heart rate; the lower graph is uterine pressure.

depth and duration of the deceleration.[68] The theorized physiology of variable decelerations is the following: partial compression of the umbilical cord results first in hypotension secondary to umbilical vein compression that causes a chemoreceptor-stimulated bradycardia.[6] The umbilical vein is larger and less protected by Wharton's jelly, thus it is more vulnerable to compression than the umbilical arteries.[15] Full compression results in fetal hypertension and a baroreceptor response that causes an abrupt bradycardia.[6] Head compression can also cause vagal stimulation and bradycardia.[6] These differing etiologic pathways may partially explain the wide variability in shape and duration of variable decelerations. Finally, recurrent severe variable decelerations can interrupt blood flow sufficiently to disallow normal exchange of oxygen and carbon dioxide, which can lead to metabolic acidosis and ultimately asphyxia. The FHR "pattern evolution" that is typically associated with developing metabolic acidosis in the fetus is a decrease in FHR baseline variability, a gradual rise in baseline rate (tachycardia) with increasing severity of variable decelerations (Figure 6-7).[68] In a previously healthy fetus, the development of significant metabolic acidosis occurs over a period of an hour to 90 minutes once this pattern starts to evolve.[68]

Late Decelerations

Late decelerations have a gradual waveform. They characteristically begin a few seconds after a contraction starts, reach their nadir 20 to 90 seconds later after the peak of the contraction, and have a slow recovery phase (Figure 6-8).[5,58] These decelerations can be recurrent, occurring with each contraction. Late decelerations are thought to be secondary to hypoxemia detected by chemoreceptors in the carotid artery, carotid sinus, and aortic arch. The nadir of the fetal bradycardia is "late" in that it follows the peak of the uterine contraction (see Figure 6-8) because the physiologic pathway that results in chemoreceptor stimulation takes time. An interruption in uteroplacental blood flow sufficient to impair oxygen transfer to the fetal compartment initiates this response (uterine contraction). Then the relatively deoxygenated blood circulates through the umbilical vein and fetal heart before reaching the chemoreceptors. In addition, the chemoreceptor reflex is slightly slower than the baroreceptor reflex. Thus the vagal stimulated bradycardia occurs "late."[65,67]

Late decelerations can occur in the presence of moderate variability or they can occur in the presence of minimal or absent variability.[71] Late decelerations with variability may be seen secondary to an acute insult, such as decreased uterine blood flow with maternal hypotension, in a previously well-oxygenated fetus and these late decelerations are not associated with significant fetal acidemia. Late decelerations with minimal or absent variability occur when the amount of oxygen in blood coming from the placenta cannot support fetal myocardial function. Thus late decelerations in the presence of absent or minimal variability may signify significant fetal acidemia.[46] A fetus with decreased placental reserve, such as in preeclampsia or fetal growth restriction, is more likely to exhibit late decelerations during labor.[67]

Sinusoidal Pattern

A true sinusoidal FHR pattern is rare. This is a smooth, wavelike baseline with a frequency of approximately 3 to 6 per minute, amplitude of up to 30 beats per minute, and an absence of short-term variability.[58] The pattern is associated with severe fetal anemia such as the anemia that occurs with

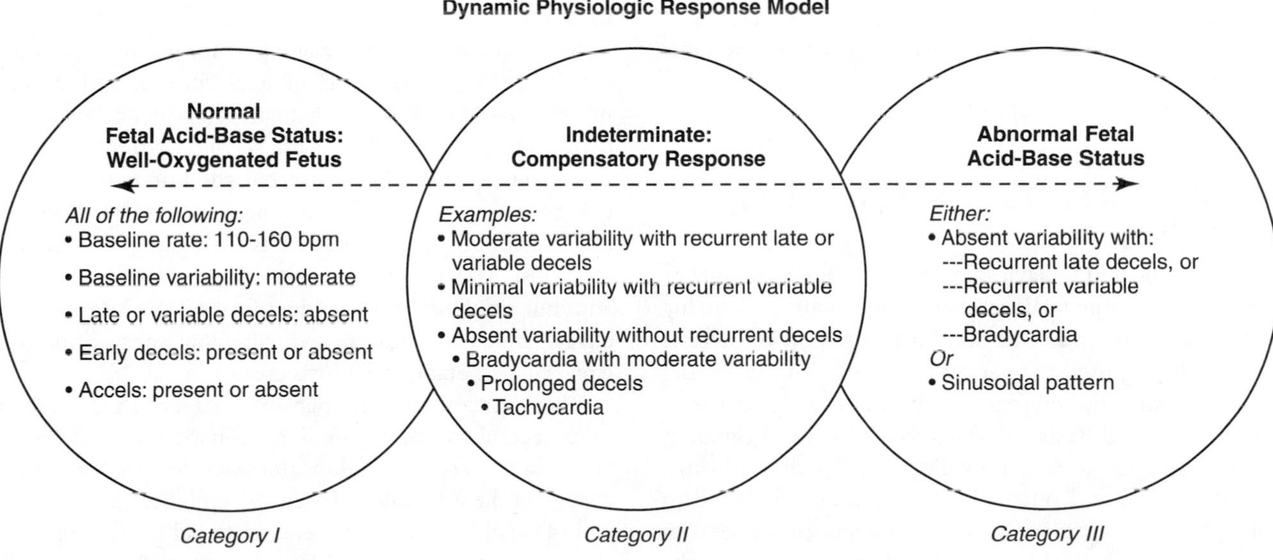

FIGURE 6-7 Continuum of fetal response to hypoxia that progresses to asphyxia. (From AWHONN. [2003]. *Fetal heart monitoring: Principles and practices* [3rd ed.]. Dubuque, IA: Kendall/Hunt Publishing.)

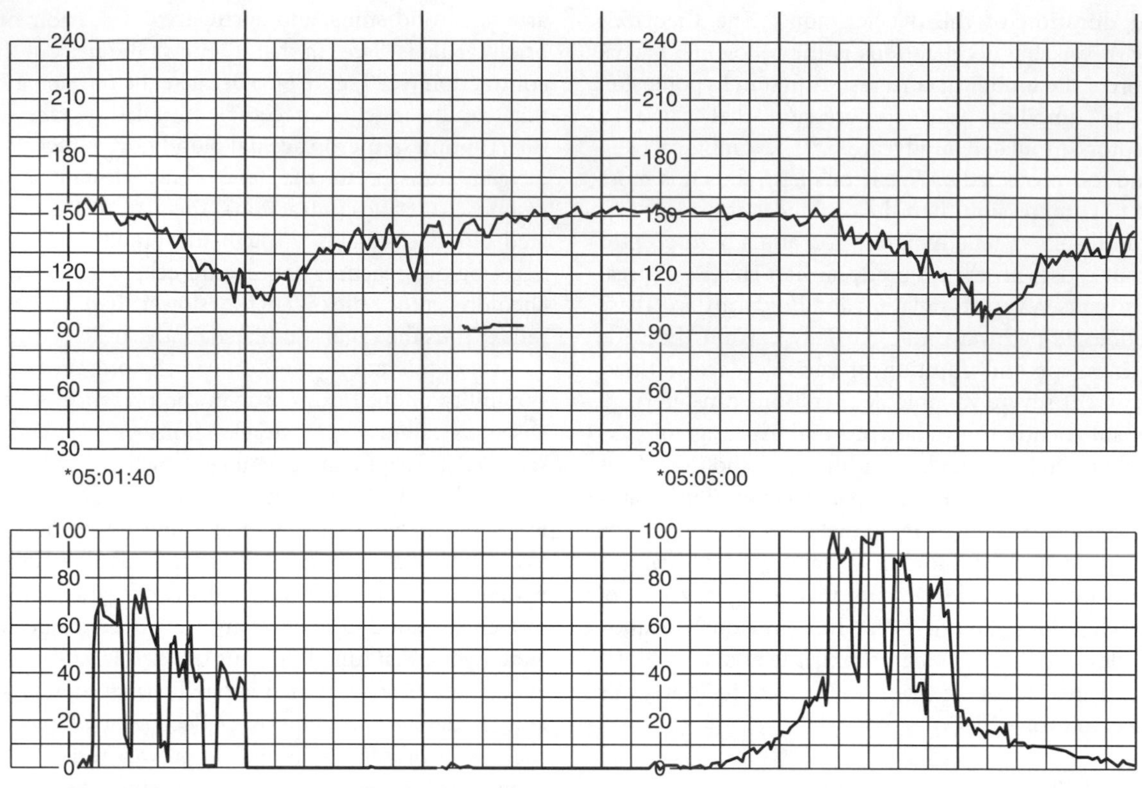

FIGURE 6-8 Late decelerations. The upper graph is fetal heart rate; the lower graph is uterine pressure.

Rh sensitization or fetal bleeding from a vasa previa. It is occasionally seen just before intrapartum demise and in fetuses with cardiac anomalies. A true sinusoidal pattern is an ominous sign indicating that the fetus is in marked jeopardy.[53] Pseudosinusoidal patterns have a similar wavelike look, but these patterns have short-term variability and are not associated with fetal compromise. They are often seen following maternal administration of intravenous opioids.[53]

CLINICAL IMPLICATIONS: THIRD TRIMESTER FETAL ASSESSMENT TECHNIQUES

Fetal physiologic and behavioral parameters are used in tests that seek to determine fetal well-being antenatally and during the intrapartum period. This section focuses on those tests conducted during the later part of pregnancy and/or during labor to determine the presence or absence of fetal acidemia. Maternal and fetal tests conducted earlier in pregnancy, which are designed to screen or diagnose Down syndrome, genetic disorders, and other birth defects, are discussed in Chapter 3. Many different pathophysiologic processes can cause fetal acidemia and intrauterine demise. Therefore the choice of an antenatal assessment technique for an individual woman is based on the presumed pathophysiologic mechanism and the biochemical parameters most likely to be prognostic for fetal compromise. Specific maternal conditions are associated with specific adverse effects on fetal health. For example, untreated diabetes with ketoacidosis can cause fetal demise, Rh sensitization can cause fetal anemia, and maternal autoimmune disorders can cause fetal heart block (see Chapter 13). This chapter focuses on those tests used to measure fetal acid-base balance.

The theoretical basis for antepartum testing is as follows: (1) the FHR pattern, level of fetal activity, and degree of muscle tone are all sensitive to hypoxemia and/or acidosis; (2) 20% to 40% of stillbirths are secondary to uteroplacental insufficiency; (3) certain maternal conditions have a higher risk of uteroplacental insufficiency; (4) fetal well-being or lack thereof can be evaluated by assessing biophysical parameters just as vital signs are used to assess well-being in an adult or child; and (5) identification of the fetus whose oxygen status is compromised will allow intervention before irreversible metabolic acidosis ensues.

The most common mechanisms that lead to fetal compromise secondary to impaired oxygenation or nutrition are (1) chronic uteroplacental insufficiency, (2) decreased gas exchange in the intervillous space, (3) umbilical cord accidents, and (4) fetal infection.[49] Several maternal conditions such as chronic hypertension, gestational hypertension, preeclampsia, maternal autoimmune disorders, and renal or vascular disease increase the likelihood of uteroplacental insufficiency, which can cause fetal growth restriction (Table 6-4).

Table 6-4 **Indications for Antenatal Testing***

MATERNAL CONDITIONS	PREGNANCY-RELATED CONDITIONS
Antiphospholipid syndrome	Gestational hypertension, preeclampsia
Hypertension	Decreased fetal movement
Type 1 diabetes	Oligohydramnios or polyhydramnios
Renal disease	Fetal growth restriction
Cyanotic heart disease	Postterm pregnancy
Hemoglobinopathies (hemoglobin SS, SC, or S-thalassemia)	Isoimmunization
Hyperthyroidism if poorly controlled	Previous unexplained fetal demise
Active substance abuse	Multiple gestation with growth discrepancy
Systemic lupus erythematosus and/or antiphospholipid syndrome	Elevated hCG value on maternal serum screen
	Cholestasis

Adapted from American College of Obstetricians and Gynecologists. (1999). Antepartum fetal surveillance. *Practice Bulletin #9,* October. Washington, DC: ACOG.
*Indications for antenatal testing in individual institutions may differ slightly.

Antenatal testing is a classic screening test. If the results are normal, well-being is ensured. If results are abnormal, further assessment or delivery is indicated. The tests most frequently used during the antepartum period to indirectly assess fetal acid-base balance include fetal movement counts, biophysical profile (BPP), non-stress tests, contraction stress tests, and umbilical artery Doppler velocimetry. Fetal acid-base status can be evaluated directly during the antepartum period by percutaneous umbilical blood sampling although this procedure is invasive and rarely performed. During labor, acid-base balance can be assessed indirectly via the use of FHR monitoring and directly via fetal scalp sampling. Vibroacoustic stimulation can be used as auxiliary assessments. Blood gas analysis of the umbilical artery and vein immediately after birth is a direct measure and accurate reflection of fetal acid-base balance during the time period immediately preceding birth.

The degree of hypoxemia or acidemia reflected in fetal physiologic or behavioral measures such as fetal movement, fetal breathing, and FHR changes cannot be predicted with precision. Nevertheless, these tests are clinically useful because their negative predictive value is 99% or greater.[63] Because the positive predictive values are much lower, clinical management of abnormal antenatal test results varies depending on other clinical factors. However, when abnormal fetal surveillance results have been compared to direct measurements of acid-base status in the newborn, some general correlations can be made that are helpful in guiding clinical practice. A detailed description of the full range of antepartum assessment techniques can be found in several recent reviews.[17,18,49]

Antepartum Fetal Assessment Techniques

Amniotic Fluid Index

In the second half of gestation, amniotic fluid is derived primarily from fetal urine, with a smaller contribution from fetal lung fluid. Urine production is dependent on renal perfusion. Renal perfusion may be decreased in states of hypoxemia secondary to a redistribution of cardiac output that favors the brain, heart, and adrenals. When the kidneys become underperfused, urine production decreases as well. Oligohydramnios (low fluid volume) is seen in postterm fetuses, in fetuses with growth restriction, and in fetuses with some congenital anomalies.[55]

Polyhydramnios (high fluid volume) is associated with some congenital anomalies, maternal diabetes, multiple pregnancies, and hydrops fetalis (see Chapter 3). Polyhydramnios can also be idiopathic. Amniotic fluid volume is measured during all prenatal ultrasound studies. It is an integral component of the BPP test. A low amniotic fluid index (0 to 5 cm) alone or in combination with other findings is a strong predictor of fetal intolerance of labor, cesarean delivery, and Apgar scores less than 7 at 5 minutes.[55] In women at term, the diagnosis of oligohydramnios is an indication for delivery or daily monitoring.[55]

Fetal Movement

Generalized fetal movements increase in frequency until approximately 32 weeks' gestation, then begin to occur less often.[16] The decrease is thought to be secondary to cerebral maturation not decreased amniotic fluid or space for movement. Fetal movement also decreases up to several days before fetal demise as the fetus presumably reduces activity in an effort to decrease oxygen requirements.[73] Because fetal movement is affected by many exogenous factors (e.g., sedating drugs, administration of corticosteroids, maternal position when counting the movements, amniotic fluid volume, normal fetal sleep periods, placental position), it is an inexact tool for prediction of fetal demise.[25,34] Prospective analyses of perinatal mortality in low-risk women randomly allocated to counting fetal movements (fetal kick counts) were unable to detect any differences in antepartum stillbirth between women who did fetal kick counts and those who did not formally monitor fetal movements.[25]

The fetal deaths that are most likely to be prevented via identification of decreased movement are those in which the fetus is experiencing chronic hypoxemia. Thus women who are at risk for fetal growth restriction and intrapartum fetal demise are often encouraged to perform formal fetal kick counts daily. Fetal kick counts have been shown to decrease perinatal mortality in studies that have evaluated perinatal mortality rates before and after fetal kick count protocols were initiated for select at-risk populations.[54]

Non-Stress Test

The physiologic basis of the non-stress test is that moderate variability and accelerations are highly predictive that the fetus is not acidemic.[63] The non-stress test is an evaluation of the FHR over 20 to 30 minutes conducted while the woman is sitting or semireclining. A fetus with an FHR between 110 and 160 beats per minute with moderate variability, accelerations, and no decelerations (see Figure 6-5) has a very low likelihood of adverse perinatal outcome within one week following a reactive test.[17] If the FHR does not have accelerations following an initial period of observation, vibroacoustic stimulation can be used to stimulate the fetus. A healthy full-term fetus will respond with FHR acceleration immediately following vibroacoustic stimulation.[17] The use of vibroacoustic stimulation decreases the incidence of nonreactive non-stress tests, and the generation of accelerations with vibroacoustic stimulation appears to be as valid as the observation of spontaneous accelerations in predicting fetal well-being.[50]

Contraction Stress Test

The contraction stress test (CST), also called the oxytocin challenge test (OCT), is an evaluation of the fetus' ability to maintain a normal heart rate baseline following the challenge of a uterine contraction. Contractions are initiated via nipple stimulation or a titrated dose of oxytocin given intravenously. When three contractions occur in a 10-minute window, the FHR pattern is assessed for baseline rate, variability, accelerations, and presence or absence of decelerations.[17] The fetus who develops decelerations in response to uterine contractions is presumed to be in a state of hypoxemia with deteriorating ability to compensate and thus may not withstand labor contractions without developing metabolic acidosis.[33] The CST is expensive, takes longer to conduct than less invasive forms of fetal testing, and has similar predictive value for perinatal mortality when compared to the non-stress test and BPP.[33] The positive predictive value for perinatal mortality is similar. In clinical practice, the CST is used when delivery is indicated and the fetal ability to withstand labor is in doubt.

Biophysical Profile (BPP)

The biophysical profile (BPP) is based on assessment of five fetal biophysical activities that are sensitive to hypoxia[48,63] (Table 6-5). Gross body movements, fetal breathing, fetal tone, and fetal heart rate variability both use oxygen and are not essential physiologic functions therefore they can be eliminated in the presence of acute hypoxia. Amniotic fluid volume is a measure of chronic hypoxemia that has resulted in decreased urine production over time. The BPP is conducted via ultrasound observation that includes a formal count of amniotic fluid index. Each variable is assigned a score of zero (not present) or 2 (present).[63] The relationship between the BPP score and fetal acidemia has been extensively evaluated.[87,88] Lower BPP scores are associated with lower mean pH values.[48,63] In a full-term fetus with a score of 8 to 10, the risk of fetal asphyxia occurring within a week following the test is approximately 1/1000, whereas the risk of fetal asphyxia for a fetus with a score of 1 to 4/10 is approximately 91 to 600/1000.[48,63]

Individual biophysical activities appear at different times during fetal development. Fetal tone appears first at approximately 8 gestational weeks, fetal movement appears at approximately 9 gestational weeks, fetal breathing appears

Table 6-5 Biophysical Profile

	NON-STRESS TEST	FETAL BREATHING MOVEMENTS	FETAL MOVEMENTS	FETAL TONE	AMNIOTIC FLUID VOLUME
Adequate Score (Score = 2)	2 Accelerations in 20 minutes, 15 beats above baseline lasting 15 seconds	One or more episodes of rhythmic fetal breathing of ≥20 seconds within 30 minutes	≥2 Discrete body/limb movements in 20 minutes of observation*	≥1 Episode of active extension with rapid return to flexion of fetal limb(s), trunk, or hand	Single pocket of fluid present measuring ≥2 cm in a vertical axis†
Inadequate Score (Score = 0)	<2 Accelerations in 20 minutes	<30 Seconds of sustained fetal breathing movements	<2 Episodes of fetal movement	Either slow extension with return to partial flexion or movement of limb in full extension or absent fetal movement	Evidence of decreased amniotic fluid oroligohydramnios†

*Simultaneous limb and trunk movements are considered one movement.
†Some protocols use a single pocket measurement, and some use the amniotic fluid index: ≤5.0 = oligohydramnios; 5.1-8 = low normal; 8.1-24 = normal; >24 = polyhydramnios.

at approximately 21 gestational weeks, and fetal heart rate reactivity is established by the late second trimester. The biophysical activity that appears first is the last to disappear in the presence of acidemia. Vintzileos et al. first observed this "gradual hypoxia concept" in early seminal studies on fetal activity observed via real-time ultrasound.[87] Thus the absence of fetal tone has a 100% positive predictive value for predicting fetal acidemia because by the time fetal tone disappears, acidemia is consistently present. The FHR variability is the biophysical activity that is the first to disappear.

Oligohydramnios is the one biophysical marker associated with chronic uteroplacental insufficiency. Oligohydramnios is also independently associated with an increased risk for perinatal mortality, particularly in the setting of fetal growth restriction.

Given the high sensitivity of FHR variability and the value of amniotic fluid volume as a reflection of chronic hypoxia, a modified BPP that uses just these two biophysical indices is often used in clinical practice for antenatal testing of women who are risk for fetal acidemia during pregnancy.[57]

Umbilical Artery Doppler Velocimetry

Doppler velocimetry assessment of the umbilical arteries, fetal aorta, and middle cerebral artery is an antepartum fetal surveillance method used to assess placental function in women who may have a growth restricted fetus. Normally, the end-diastolic velocity in the umbilical arteries increases with advancing gestation secondary to decreased resistance in the placenta as more tertiary vessels develop. The velocity of blood flow through the umbilical artery can be detected with Doppler waveform analysis. In animal studies, an increase in the ratio of velocity during systole versus diastole (S/D ratio) occurs when approximately 30% of the fetal vasculature in the placenta is abnormal.[56] Absent or reversed flow can occur when more of the vessels are abnormal. Currently, umbilical artery Doppler velocimetry is used to assess placental function in women with known or presumed fetal growth restriction and has been shown to decrease adverse perinatal outcomes for this population of women.[2] Absent or end-flow velocity is an indication for preparation for delivery in consideration with other clinical factors, and reversed end-flow velocity is usually considered an indication for immediate delivery.[35]

Intrapartum Fetal Assessment and Resuscitation

Electronic Fetal Monitoring

Continuous or intermittent electronic FHR monitoring is the primary method used for fetal surveillance during labor. Electronic fetal monitoring has been the subject of multiple randomized controlled trials and two large metaanalyses since it's introduction into clinical practice in the late 1960's.[68,71,86]

Electronic FHR monitoring can reliably predict the absence of acidemia when the FHR exhibits moderate variability and/or accelerations. However, the prevalence of variant FHR patterns during labor is high and the incidence of newborn asphyxia is rare, thus electronic fetal monitoring is not a sensitive predictor of newborn acidosis.[68] Although electronic FHR monitoring in unselected populations has not been found to decrease perinatal mortality, a consistent body of knowledge about the relationship between specific FHR patterns and newborn acidemia has emerged.[68]

Following a 2008 National Institute of Child Health and Human Development conference, FHR patterns have been divided into three interpretive categories (Table 6-6). Category I is a fetal heart rate pattern with a normal baseline rate, moderate variability, and no variable or late decelerations. This FHR pattern reliably predicts the absence of fetal hypoxemia. Conversely Category III FHR patterns are the four FHR patterns that reliably predict hypoxia or impending fetal asphyxia (see Table 6-3).[46,68] The positive predictive value of late decelerations with absent or minimal variability for predicting umbilical arterial base deficit greater than 16 mEq/L (mmol/L) is 18%.[45] Category II FHR patterns are all other patterns that are indeterminate with regard to their relationship to fetal acidemia.

When a Category II pattern is present, direct fetal scalp stimulation or vibroacoustic stimulation can be conducted to elicit an acceleration.[4] If the scalp stimulation or vibroacoustic stimulation results in a fetal heart acceleration, the likelihood that the fetus is acidemic is remote however if no acceleration is elicited, the test is inconclusive and does not indicate that fetal acidemia is present.[11,83]

Ongoing research is being conducted that subdivides Category II FHR patterns, and these subdivisions may be used in clinical practice as more knowledge is obtained about their relationship to fetal acidemia.[69,70]

Intrauterine Resuscitation Techniques

Intrauterine resuscitation techniques for improving fetal oxygenation in the presence of FHR patterns during labor include administration of an intravenous bolus, lateral positioning, oxygen therapy, tocolytic administration, any position other than supine, amnioinfusion, and pushing every other contraction during the second stage.

Amnioinfusion and lateral positioning may relieve cord compression. Administration of oxygen at 10 L/min with a nonrebreather facemask will increase the fetal oxygen saturation as measured with pulse oximetry.[84] Maternal oxygen therapy during the intrapartum period is useful in treating presumed fetal hypoxemia, even though the fetal PO_2 does not increase as dramatically as that of the mother given the differences in the oxygen-hemoglobin dissociation curve between the fetus and mother. Administration of oxygen to the mother increases maternal arterial PO_2, increasing the gradient between maternal and fetal values in the placenta. This increases oxygen transfer to the fetus, increasing fetal oxygen content and fetal cerebral oxygenation.[1,84]

Table 6-6 Fetal Heart Rate Patterns: Interpretive Categories

CATEGORY	DESCRIPTION
Category I Includes all of these:	Baseline rate 110-160 bpm Baseline FHR variability—moderate Late or variable decelerations—absent Early decelerations—present or absent Accelerations—present or absent
Category II All FHR tracings not categorized as Category I or Category III. Includes any of these:	Baseline rate Bradycardia not accompanied by absent baseline variability Tachycardia Baseline FHR variability Minimal baseline variability Absent baseline variability Marked baseline variability Accelerations Absence of induced accelerations after fetal stimulations Periodic or episodic decelerations Recurrent variable decelerations accompanied by minimal or moderate baseline variability Prolonged deceleration greater than 2 minutes but less than 10 minutes Recurrent late decelerations with moderate baseline variability Variable decelerations with other characteristics, such as slow return to baseline, "overshoots," or "shoulders"
Category III Includes either:	Absent baseline FHR variability and any of the following: Recurrent late decelerations Recurrent variable decelerations Bradycardia Sinusoidal pattern

Adapted from Macones, G.A., et al. (2008). The 2008 National Institute of Child Health and Human Development Research Workshop Report on Electronic fetal heart rate monitoring. *Obsetet Gyneocl, 112,* 661 and *JOGNN, 37,* 510.

Newborn Umbilical Cord Gas Analysis

At birth, analysis of umbilical cord blood gases can be used to determine the presence or absence of acidemia in the fetus just prior to the birth.[3] Umbilical artery blood flows from the fetus to the placenta and therefore blood gas analysis from one of the umbilical arteries best represents the status of the fetus. Umbilical venous blood flows from the placenta to the fetus so blood gas analysis from the umbilical vein best represents the status of the placenta and intervillous space (Table 6-7).[15,20,24]

The mean umbilical artery pH at birth at term is 7.26.[40] Pathologic acidemia can be present when the pH <7.00.[29] A low pH can be classified as respiratory, metabolic, or mixed acidemia. The amount of CO_2 determines the level of carbonic

Table 6-7 Guidelines for Interpretation of Umbilical Arterial Cord Gases in Term Newborns

DIAGNOSIS	pH	PCO_2 mmHg	BICARBONATE HCO_3 (mEq/L; mmol/L)	BASE DEFICIT* mEq/L (mmol/L)
Normal†	7.26 (±0.07)	53 (±10)	22.0 (±3.6)	4 (±3)
Respiratory academia	<7.20	>65	Normal	Normal
Metabolic acidemia‡	<7.20	Normal	≤17	≥15.9 ± 2.8
Mixed (metabolic-respiratory) acidemia‡	Low	>65	≤17	≥9.6 ± 2.5

From Fahey, J. & King, T.I. (2005). Intrauterine asphyxia: Clinical implications for providers of intrapartum care. *J Midwifery Women's Health, 50,* 498.
*May be reported as base excess (negative values) or base deficit (positive value); however, the numeric value is the same.
†Data from term infants with an Apgar of 7 or greater at 5 minutes.
‡There is a clinical association with adverse neonatal outcomes when the pH is less than 7 and the base deficit is greater than 12 mEq/L (mmol/L).

acid (H_2CO_3). The value of CO_2 reflects the respiratory (cord occlusion) component of acidosis. The amount of bicarbonate (HCO_3^-) represents the metabolic component. Lower levels of HCO_3^- indicate higher levels of lactic acid and acidosis. It is important to note that marked elevations in PCO_2 will result in a compensatory increase in bicarbonate ($CO_2 + H_2O \rightleftarrows H_2CO_3 \rightleftarrows H^+ + HCO_3^-$) so when an acute respiratory acidosis exists, there is more dissociation of carbonic acid and ultimately more HCO_3^- dissociated in fetal blood. In this situation, higher bicarbonate levels (HCO_3^-) can mask an underlying metabolic component. Therefore calculation of base excess best assesses the extent of a metabolic or mixed acidosis.[28,79] In human fetal umbilical arterial blood at the time of birth, the mean base excess is −4 mEq/L (mmol/L) and the 2.5th percentile is −11 mEq/L (mmol/L). These could be described as a mild metabolic acidemia in the case of the average value, and more substantial in the case of values below the 2.5th percentile.[32]

Respiratory Acidosis

Most infants born vaginally have some degree of respiratory acidosis that is physiologic for a newborn (Figure 6-9). The mean pCO_2 value found in umbilical arterial blood in the healthy newborn at the time of birth is 53 mmHg (7.04 kPa). Two standard deviations above the mean (which is the 97th percentile) is 73 mmHg (9.7 kPa). This cutoff using the percentile definition could be described as a substantial respiratory acidemia.[32] Respiratory acidosis is characterized by pH less than 7.20, high PCO_2, and normal bicarbonate in the umbilical artery. In a fetus, this implies an inability to clear CO_2 at the placenta but a continuation of aerobic metabolism without acidosis. For example, cord compression will cause respiratory acidosis in the fetus. In this scenario, the blood in the umbilical arteries (carrying blood with higher PCO_2) cannot get to the placenta to exchange the CO_2 for O_2. Because blood within the intervillous space is normally oxygenated, the gases in the umbilical vein sample will be normal. A simple respiratory acidosis is common in newborns with tight nuchal cords and/or second stage bradycardias in a previously well-oxygenated fetus. These infants usually clear the CO_2 rapidly after birth and do well. If the cord occlusion occurs too frequently or is severe (complete versus partial occlusion), metabolic acidosis can develop.

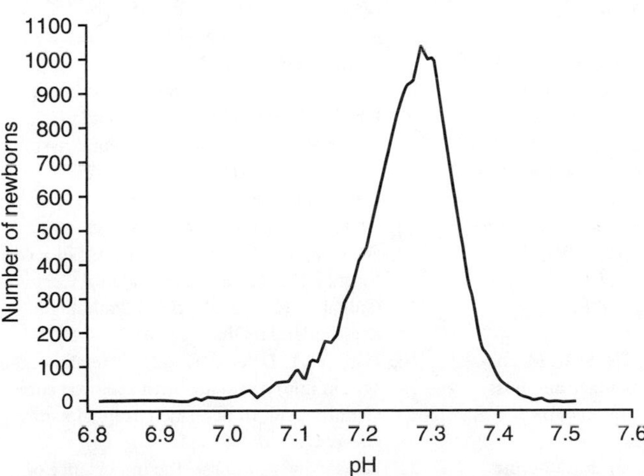

FIGURE 6-9 Frequency distribution of umbilical arterial blood pH in babies with Apgar scores of 7 or greater at 5 minutes. (From Helwig, J.T., et al. [1996]. Umbilical cord blood acid-base state: What is normal? *Am J Obstet Gynecol, 174*, 1807.)

Metabolic Acidosis

When the fetus experiences a real deficit of oxygen, the switch to anaerobic metabolism occurs, and lactic acid is generated. Unlike CO_2, lactic acid does not cross the placenta quickly.[75] A pH less than 7.20, low bicarbonate level, and normal PCO_2 characterize metabolic acidosis. As lactic acid accumulates in the fetal compartment, the amount of bicarbonate buffer decreases, the pH decreases, and the base excess decreases. Acidosis can progress to asphyxia if uncorrected.

Mixed Acidemia

Mixed acidemia is a metabolic acidosis that develops when respiratory acidosis is prolonged. This is the most common pattern seen after prolonged end-stage bradycardias.

SUMMARY

The fetal response to an oxygen deficit is the result of interaction between the degree of the stress and the responsiveness and reserve of the individual fetus.[75] Some fetuses are more intolerant to hypoxic stress than others. Fetuses with less placental reserve (e.g., fetal growth restriction, maternal hypertension, postdates) are less able to maintain normal oxygenation during hypoxemia.[52] This maxim is the basis for the screening criteria for antepartum fetal surveillance. However, the concept of a continuum of causality in the sense that a small amount of asphyxia causes a small amount of damage and a larger amount causes more severe damage is not certain.[44] Rather, there appears to be a degree of hypoxia that can be tolerated without adverse effects over a varied period of time and when this degree or duration is exceeded, the threshold for metabolic acidemia is reached and the chain of adverse physiologic effects will proceed.[23] Given this wide biologic variability in the fetal response to hypoxia, the biochemical indexes that signal decompensation from physiologic adaptation to pathologic consequences has not been determined.[66] In clinical terms, the degree of metabolic acidemia that causes irreversible damage has not been defined. Antepartum and intrapartum fetal assessment techniques designed to assess the presence or absence of fetal acidemia, continue to be developed as knowledge of fetal physiology and the fetal response to hypoxia is discovered. Recommendations for clinical practice related to fetal assessment are summarized in Table 6-8.

Table 6-8 Recommendations for Clinical Practice Related to Fetal Assessment

Understand that the fetal heart rate is highly sensitive to changes in oxygenation and blood pressure (p. 163).
Recognize the fetal response to hypoxemia: bradycardia and a decrease in beat-to-beat variability (p. 173).
Understand that fetal heart rate variability is the key reflection of intact cerebral oxygenation (p. 171).
Recognize the normal baseline rate, moderate variability, and accelerations and understand that these features are highly predictive of fetal well-being (p. 177)
Monitor minimal fetal heart rate variability, which may be secondary to fetal sleep, maternal administration of opiates, corticosteroids and other drugs, idiopathic, or developing metabolic acidosis (p. 172).
Identify periodic fetal heart rate patterns that are most likely to be associated with fetal acidosis (late decelerations [mild or severe] and severe variable decelerations in the presence of absent variability), which are a significant risk for newborn acidemia (p. 173).
Recognize typical fetal heart rate pattern evolutions that are associated with the development of metabolic acidosis (tachycardia with decreased variability and increasing severity of variable or late decelerations) (p. 173).
Identify the criteria necessary to determine an intrapartum etiology for neonatal encephalopathy (p. 169, Table 6-2).
Collect umbilical cord gases on any newborn who might be at risk for intrapartum asphyxia (p. 178).
Understand the efficacy and indications for antenatal surveillance tests: non-stress test, contraction stress test, biophysical profile, umbilical artery Doppler velocimetry (p. 178).
Identify appropriate intrapartum resuscitation techniques that are efficacious in improving fetal oxygen saturation in the presence of periodic fetal heart rate decelerations (p. 177).

References

1. Aldrich, C.J., et al. (1994). The effect of maternal oxygen administration on human fetal cerebral oxygenation measured during labor by near infrared spectroscopy. *Br J Obstet Gynecol, 101,* 509.
2. Alfirevic, Z., Stampalija, T., & Gyte, G.M.L. (2010). Fetal and umbilical Doppler ultrasound in high-risk pregnancies. *Cochrane Database of Systematic Reviews* 1, CD007529.
3. American College of Obstetricians and Gynecologists. (1996). Umbilical artery blood acid-base analysis. Technical Bulletin #216. *Int J Gynaecol Obstet, 52,* 305.
4. American College of Obstetricians and Gynecologists. (2010). Management of Intrapartum Fetal Heart Rate Tracings. Practice Bulletin Number 116 (November) *Obstet Gynecol, 116,* 1232.
5. Association of Women's Health, Obstetric, and Neonatal Nurses. (2003). *Fetal heart monitoring: Principles and practices* (3rd ed.). Dubuque, IA: Kendall/Hunt Publishing.
6. Ball, R.H. & Parer, J.T. (1992). The physiologic mechanisms of variable decelerations. *Am J Obstet Gynecol, 166,* 1683.
7. Bennet, L.A. & Gunn, A.J. (2009). The fetal heart rate responses to hypoxia: Insight from animal models. *Clinics in Perinatology, 36,* 655.
8. Blechner, J.N. (1993). Maternal fetal acid base physiology. *Clin Obstet Gynecol, 36,* 3.
9. Bleker, O.P., et al. (1975). Intervillous space during uterine contractions in human subjects: An ultrasonic study. *Am J Obstet Gynecol, 123,* 697.
10. Carter, B.S., Havercamp, A.D., & Merenstein, G.B. (1993). The definition of acute perinatal asphyxia. *Clin Perinatol, 20,* 287.
11. Clark, S.L., Gimovsky, M.L., & Miller, F.C. (1982). Fetal heart rate response to scalp sampling. *Am J Obstet Gynecol, 144,* 706.
12. Cousins, L. (1999). Fetal oxygenation, assessment of fetal well-being, and obstetric management of the pregnant patient with asthma. *J Allergy Clin Immunol, 103,* S34.
13. Dalton, K.J., et al. (1983). The autonomic nervous system and fetal heart rate variability. *Am J Obstet Gynecol, 146,* 456.
14. de Haan, H.H. & Hasaart, T.H. (1995). Neuronal death after perinatal asphyxia. *Eur J Obstet Gynecol, 61,* 123.
15. de Laat, M.W., et al. (2005). The umbilical coiling index, a review of the literature. *J Matern Fetal Neonatal Med, 17,* 93.
16. D'Elia, A., et al. (2001). Spontaneous motor activity in normal fetuses. *Early Hum Dev, 65,* 139.
17. Devoe, L.D. (2008). Antenatal fetal assessment: Contraction stress test, nonstress test, vibroacoustic stimulation, amniotic fluid volume, biophysical profile, and modified biophysical profile—An overview. *Seminars in perinatology, 32,* 247.
18. East, C.E., et al. (2005). Vibroacoustic stimulation for fetal assessment in labour in the presence of a nonreassuring fetal heart rate trace. *Cochrane Database Syst Rev 18,* CD004664.
19. Espinoza, M.F. & Parer, J.T. (1991). Mechanisms of asphyxial brain damage and possible pharmacologic interventions. *Am J Obstet Gynecol, 164,* 1582.
20. Fahey, J. & King, T.L. (2005). Intrauterine asphyxia: Clinical implications for providers of intrapartum care. *J Midwifery Women's Health, 50,* 498.
21. Flavin, N.E. (2001). Perinatal asphyxia: A clinical review, including research with brain hypothermia. *Neonatal Netw, 20,* 31.
22. Fox, H.A. (1979). The effects of catecholamines and drug treatment on the fetus and newborn. *Birth Fam J, 6,* 157.
23. Freeman, J.M. (1985). Prenatal and perinatal factors associated with brain disorders. National Institute of Child Health and Human Development. *NIH Publication 85-1149.* Washington, DC: National Institutes of Health.
24. Friedman, A.H. & Fahey, J.T. (1993). The transition from fetal to neonatal circulation: Normal responses and implications for infants with heart disease. *Semin Perinatol, 17,* 106.
25. Froen, J.F., et al. (2008). Fetal movement assessment. *Seminars in Perinatology, 32,* 243.
26. Gaiser, R.R., et al. (2005). Predicting prolonged fetal heart rate deceleration following intrathecal fentanyl/bupivacaine. *Int J Obstet Anesth, 14,* 208.
27. Gilstrap, L.C., et al. (1989). Diagnosis of birth asphyxia on the basis of fetal pH, Apgar score, and newborn cerebral dysfunction. *Am J Obstet Gynecol, 161,* 825.
28. Gilstrap, L.C. & Cunningham, G. (1994). Umbilical cord blood acid-base analysis. *Supplement #4 Williams' obstetrics* (19th ed.). Raritan, NJ: Ortho Pharmaceutical Corp.
29. Goldaber, K.G., et al. (1991). Pathologic fetal acidemia. *Obstet Gynecol, 78,* 1103.
30. Hankins, G.D., et al. (2002). Neonatal organ system injury in acute birth asphyxia sufficient to result in neonatal encephalopathy. *Obstet Gynecol, 99,* 688.
31. Hanson, M.A. (1988). The importance of baro- and chemo-reflexes in the control of the fetal cardiovascular system. *J Dev Physiol, 10,* 491.
32. Helwig, J.T., et al. (1996). Umbilical cord blood acid base state: What is normal? *Am J Obstet Gynecol, 174,* 1807.

33. Huddleston, J.F. (2002). Continued utility of the contraction stress test? *Clin Obstet Gynecol, 45,* 1005.
34. Jackson, J.R., et al. (2003). The effect of glucocorticosteroid administration on fetal movements and biophysical profile scores in normal pregnancies. *J Matern Fetal Neonatal Med, 13,* 50.
35. Jang, D.G., et al. (2011). Perinatal outcomes and maternal clinical characteristics in IUGR with absent or reversed end-diastolic flow velocity in the umbilical artery. *Arch Gynecol Obstet, 284,* 73.
36. Jansson, L.M., Dipietro, J., & Elko, A. (2005). Fetal response to maternal methadone administration. *Am J Obstet Gynecol, 193,* 611.
37. Jensen, A., et al. (1999). Dynamics of fetal circulatory responses to hypoxia and asphyxia. *Eur J Obstet Gynecol Reprod Biol, 84,* 155.
38. Kaaja, R.J. & Greer, I.A. (2005). Manifestations of chronic disease during pregnancy. *JAMA, 294,* 2751.
39. King, T. & Parer, J. (2000). The physiology of fetal heart rate patterns and perinatal asphyxia. *J Perinat Neonatal Nurs, 14,* 19.
40. Kitlinski, M.L., Kallen, K., & Marsal, K. (2003). Gestational age-dependent reference values for pH in umbilical cord arterial blood at term. *Obstet Gynecol, 102,* 338.
41. Lagercrantz, H. & Slokin, T.A. (1986). The "stress" of being born. *Sci Am, 254,* 100.
42. Lai, M.C. & Yang, S.N. (2011). Perinatal hypoxic-ischemic encephalopathy. *J Biomed Biotechnol, 2011,* 609813.
43. Leung, A.S., Leung, E.K., & Paul, R.H. (1993). Uterine rupture after previous cesarean delivery: Maternal and fetal consequences. *Am J Obstet Gynecol, 169,* 945.
44. Low, J.A., et al. (1988). Motor and cognitive deficits after intrapartum asphyxia in the mature fetus. *Am J Obstet Gynecol, 158,* 356.
45. Low, J.A., Victory, R., & Derrick, E.J. (1999). Predictive value of electronic fetal monitoring for intrapartum fetal asphyxia with metabolic acidosis. *Obstet Gynecol, 93,* 285.
46. Macones, G.A., et al. (2008). The 2008 National Institute of Child Health and Human Development Research Workshop Report on Electronic fetal heart rate monitoring. *Obsetet Gyneocl, 112,* 661 and *JOGNN, 37,* 510.
47. Mallard, E.C., et al. (1995). Neuronal death in the developing brain following intrauterine asphyxia. *Reprod Fertil Dev, 7,* 647.
48. Manning, F.A. (2002). Fetal biophysical profile: A critical appraisal. *Clin Obstet Gynecol, 45,* 975.
49. Manning, F.A. (2009). Antepartum fetal testing: A critical appraisal. *Current Opinion in Obstetrics and Gynecology, 21,* 348.
50. Marden, D., et al. (1997). A randomized controlled trial of a new fetal acoustic stimulation test for fetal well-being. *Am J Obstet Gynecol, 176,* 1386.
51. McLean, C. & Ferriero, D. (2004). Mechanisms of hypoxic ischemic injury in the term infant. *Semin Perinatol, 28,* 425.
52. Miller, J., Turan, S., & Baschat, A.A. (2008). Fetal growth restriction. *Seminars in Perinatology, 32,* 274.
53. Modanlou, H.D. & Murata, Y. (2004). Sinusoidal heart rate pattern: Reappraisal of its definition and clinical significance. *J Obstet Gynaecol Res, 30,* 169.
54. Moore, T.R. & Piacquadio, K. (1989). A prospective evaluation of fetal movement screening to reduce the incidence of antepartum fetal death. *Am J Obstet Gynecol, 160,* 1075.
55. Moore, T.R. (2011). The role of amniotic fluid assessment in evaluating fetal well-being. *Clin Perinatol, 38,* 33.
56. Morrow, R.J., et al. (1989). Effect of placental embolization on the umbilical arterial velocity waveform in fetal sheep. *Am J Obstet Gynecol, 161,* 1055.
57. Nageotte, M.P., et al. (1994). Perinatal outcome with the modified biophysical profile. *Am J Obstet Gynecol, 170,* 1672.
58. National Institute of Child Health and Human Development Research Planning Workshop. (1997). Electronic fetal heart rate monitoring: Research guidelines for interpretation. *Am J Obstet Gynecol, 17,* 1385.
59. Nelson, K.M. & Elenberg, J.H. (1981). Apgar scores as predictors of chronic neurologic disability. *Pediatrics, 68,* 36.
60. Nordstrom, L. (2001). Lactate measurements in scalp and cord arterial blood. *Curr Opin Obstet Gynecol, 13,* 141.
61. O'Brien-Abel, N.E. & Benedetti, T.J. (1992). Saltatory fetal heart rate pattern. *J Perinatol, 12,* 13.
62. Odegard, R.A., et al. (2000). Preeclampsia and fetal growth. *Obstet Gynecol, 96,* 950.
63. Oyelese, Y. & Vintzileos, A.M. (2011). The uses and limitations of the fetal biophysical profile. *Clin Perinatol, 38,* 47.
64. Parer, J.T. (1976). Physiological regulation of fetal heart rate. *J Obstet Gynecol Neonatal Nurs, 5,* 265.
65. Parer, J.T. (1997). *Handbook of fetal heart rate monitoring* (2nd ed.). Philadelphia: Saunders.
66. Parer, J.T. (1998). Effects of fetal asphyxia on brain cell structure and function: Limits of tolerance. *Comp Biochem Physiol, 199A,* 711.
67. Parer, J.T. (2004). Fetal heart rate. In R.K. Creasy, R. Resnik, & J.D. Iams (Eds.). *Maternal-fetal medicine: Principles and practice* (5th ed.). Philadelphia: Saunders.
68. Parer, J.T., et al. (2006). Fetal acidemia and electronic fetal heart rate patterns: Is there evidence of an association? *J Matern Fetal Neonatal Med, 19,* 289.
69. Parer, J.T. & Ikeda, T. (2007). A framework for standardized management of intrapartum fetal heart rate patterns. *Am J Obstet Gynecol, 197,* 26e.1.
70. Parer, J.T., Ikeda, T., & King, T.L. (2009). The 2008 National Institute of Child Health and Human Development report on fetal heart rate monitoring. *Obstet Gynecol, 114,* 136.
71. Parer, J.T.P. & King, T.L. (1999). Whither fetal heart rate monitoring? *Obstet Gynecol Fertil, 22,* 149.
72. Pearlman, M. & Shah, P.S. (2011). Hypoxic-ischemic encephalopathy: Challenges in outcome and prediction. *J of Pediatrics, 158,* e51.
73. Pearson, J.F. & Weaver, J.B. (1976). Fetal activity and fetal wellbeing: An evaluation. *Br Med J, 6021,* 1305.
74. Perlman, J.M. (2004). Brain injury in the term infant. *Semin Perinatol, 28,* 415.
75. Reece, E.A. (1986). The fetus as the final arbitrator of intrauterine stress/distress. *Clin Obstet Gynecol, 29,* 23.
76. Richardson, B.S. (1989). Fetal adaptive responses to asphyxia. *Clin Perinatol, 16,* 595.
77. Rivkin, M.J. (1997). Hypoxic-ischemic brain injury in the term newborn. *Clin Perinatol, 24,* 607.
78. Robertson, C.M.T. (2003). Long-term follow-up of term infants with perinatal asphyxia. In D.K. Stevenson, W.F. Benitz, & P. Sunshine. (Eds.). *Fetal and neonatal brain injury* (3rd ed.). Cambridge: Cambridge University Press.
79. Ross, M.G. & Gala, R. (2002). Use of umbilical artery base excess: Algorithm for the timing of hypoxic injury. *Am J Obstet Gynecol, 187,* 1.
80. Rotmensch, S., et al. (2005). Effect of beta methasone administration on fetal heart rate tracing: A blinded longitudinal study. *Fetal Diagn Ther, 20,* 371.
81. Rudolph, A.M., et al. (1988). Fetal cardiovascular responses to stress. In G.H. Wiknjosastro, W.H. Prakoso, & K. Maeda (Eds.). *Perinatology.* New York: Elsevier.
82. Silva, A.M., et al. (2006). Neonatal nucleated red blood cells and the prediction of cerebral white matter injury in preterm infants. *Obstet Gynecol, 107,* 550.
83. Simpson, K.R. (2007). Intrauterine resuscitation during labor: Review of current methods and supportive evidence. *J Midwifery Women's Health, 52,* 229.
84. Simpson, K.R. (2008). Intrauterine resuscitation during labor: Should maternal oxygen administration be a first-line measure? *Semin Fetal Neonatal Med, 13,* 362.
85. Task Force on Neonatal Encephalopathy and Cerebral Palsy. (2003). *Neonatal encephalopathy and cerebral palsy: Defining the pathogenesis and pathophysiology.* American College of Obstetricians and Gynecologists (ACOG) and the American Academy of Pediatrics. Washington, DC: ACOG.
86. Thacker, S.B., Stroup, D., & Chang, M. (2001). Continuous electronic heart rate monitoring for fetal assessment during labor. *Cochrane Database Syst Rev 2,* CD000063.
87. Vintzileos, A.M., et al. (1987). The relationship between fetal biophysical profile and cord pH in patients undergoing cesarean section before the onset of labor. *Obstet Gynecol, 70,* 196.

88. Vintzileos, A.M., et al. (1991). Relationship between fetal biophysical activities and umbilical cord blood gas values. *Am J Obstet Gynecol, 165,* 707. Erratum in: *Am J Obstet Gynecol* 1992 Feb;166(2):772. *Am J Obstet Gynecol* 1992 Apr;166(4):1313.
89. Walker, J. & Trunbull, E.P.N. (1953). Haemoglobin and red cells in the human foetus and their relation to the oxygen content of the blood in the vessels of the umbilical cord. *Lancet, 2,* 312.
90. Westgate, J.A., et al. (2007). The intrapartum deceleration in center stage: A physiologic approach to the interpretation of fetal heart rate changes in labor. *Am J Obstet Gynecol, 197,* 236.e1.
91. Williams, K.P. & Galerneau, F. (2003). Intrapartum fetal heart rate patterns in the prediction of neonatal acidemia. *Am J Obstet Gynecol, 188,* 850.

Pharmacology and Pharmacokinetics During the Perinatal Period

CHAPTER

Pharmacologic therapy for the pregnant woman, fetus, neonate, and lactating woman is one of the most challenging therapies in health care. Pharmacologic treatment during pregnancy is unique in that a drug taken by one person (pregnant woman) may significantly affect another (embryo or fetus). Maternal handling of drugs may be altered by the normal physiologic changes of pregnancy, such as increased plasma volume, altered gastrointestinal (GI) motility, and changes in plasma components and renal function. These changes influence plasma levels, half-lives, and distribution and elimination of many drugs, and may increase the risk of subtherapeutic or toxic drug levels.

Fetal drug exposure may be inadvertent (secondary to maternal treatment) or intended (treatment of fetus via treatment of mother). For many years it was believed that the placental barrier shielded the fetus from many drugs and other potentially harmful substances. However, the placenta provides little protection for the fetus from many drugs. The placenta and fetus are able to metabolize some agents; however, postmenstrual age and maturation of hepatic enzyme systems influence the efficiency of these processes. Many maternal drugs are present in the fetus in lower levels than seen in the mother, but some drugs may be found at higher levels in the fetus. Fetal effects of maternal drugs can range from no effect to pregnancy loss to teratogenesis with structural or functional changes, to alterations in later growth and development.

Pharmacologic therapy of the neonate is complex because hepatic metabolism and renal elimination change rapidly over the first weeks after birth. This challenge is magnified in preterm infants in whom maturation of hepatic and renal systems is changing based on both postmenstrual age and postbirth age. This can lead to significant changes in drug handling, sometimes within a few days or weeks.

Many drugs cross the blood-milk barrier in the lactating woman and have the potential to affect the infant. The amount of drug reaching the nursing infant is influenced by maternal drug handling, mode of administration, and maternal serum levels at time of feeding. However, drugs generally reach breast milk in significantly lower quantities than drugs reach the fetus across the placenta.

Pharmacokinetics refers to the processes involved in drug absorption, distribution, metabolism, and biotransformation and excretion (Figure 7-1). Site of absorption depends on route of administration (e.g., oral, intramuscular, intravenous, topical, inhaled). Drugs are carried in the blood, either bound to plasma proteins or as free drug. Protein-bound drugs provide a reservoir for future use, whereas free drug is the active component available to interact with the target cell. Biotransformation occurs primarily in the liver with a series of enzymatic reactions to modify and convert the drug into more polar (water-soluble) compounds. Intermediary steps in biotransformation may result in active metabolites. For example, codeine is demethylated to morphine, and in the neonate theophylline is methylated to caffeine.[32] Biotransformation also takes place in the lungs, intestinal mucosa, and kidneys. Hepatic biotransformation occurs in two phases. Phase I (nonsynthetic reactions) takes place primarily in the microsomes, although some occurs in the mitochondria and cytosol. Phase I reactions modify the activity of a drug. Phase I enzymes include the cytochrome P450 (CYP450) monooxygenase system. Phase II (synthetic) reactions require adenosine triphosphate (ATP) and, except for glucuronidation, are extramicrosomal.[37] Phase II reactions generally inactivate the drugs by converting them to more polar substances. Table 7-1 provides examples of drugs metabolized by various phase I and phase II reactions. Not all drugs undergo hepatic metabolism before elimination; some drugs are excreted directly via the kidneys.

Variations in drug pharmacokinetics and pharmacodynamics occur among individuals at all ages, even with similar doses of a given medication, due to extrinsic (diet, environment, other therapies) and intrinsic (development, genetic constitution, diseases) factors.[95] Currently much research focuses on understanding these factors, especially the contributions of individual genetic polymorphisms (see Chapter 1). This has led to new fields of study such as pharmacogenetics and pharmacogenomics. Pharmacogenetics is the study of "genetic variations that give rise to interindividual responses to drugs,"[95, p.256] while pharmacogenomics integrates pharmacology and genomics into "the broader application of genome-wide technologies and strategies to identify both disease processes that represent new targets for drug development

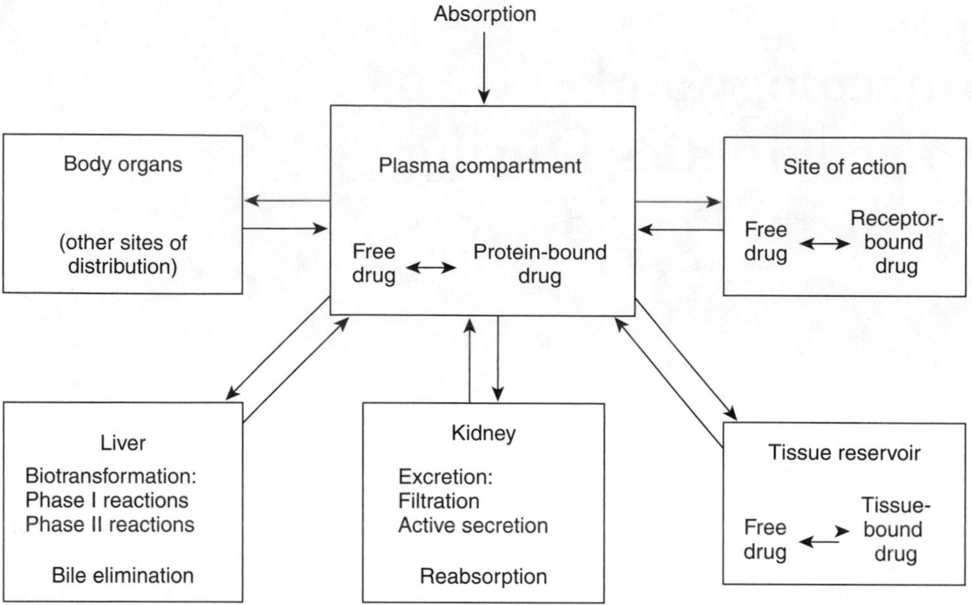

FIGURE 7-1 Schema of possible disposition of drugs throughout various compartments in the body. (From Chemtob, S. [2004]. Basic pharmacologic principles. In R.A. Polin, W.W. Fox, & S.H. Abman [Eds.]. *Fetal and neonatal physiology* [3rd ed.]. Philadelphia: Saunders.)

Table 7-1 Biotransformation Reactions

REACTION	EXAMPLES OF DRUG SUBSTRATES
PHASE I (NONSYNTHETIC REACTIONS)	
Oxidation	Phenytoin, phenobarbital, ibuprofen, acetaminophen, morphine, codeine, diazepam, cimetidine
Reduction	Prontosil, chloramphenicol, ethanol
Hydrolysis	Acetylsalicylic acid, indomethacin
PHASE II (SYNTHETIC REACTIONS: CONJUGATIONS)	
Glucuronide conjugation	Morphine, acetaminophen
Glycine conjugation	Salicylic acid
Sulfate conjugation	Acetaminophen, α-methyldopa
Glutathione conjugation	Ethacrynic acid
Methylation	Dopamine, epinephrine
Acetylation	Sulfonamides, clonazepam

Adapted from Chemtob, S. (2004). Basic pharmacologic principles. In R.A. Polin, W.W. Fox, & S.H. Abman (Eds.). *Fetal and neonatal physiology* (3rd ed.). Philadelphia: Saunders.

and factors predictive of therapeutic efficacy and risk of adverse drug reactions."[95, p.256] Genetic polymorphisms are small variations in an individual's genome that may either be nonfunctional (have no effect on the individual) or modify expression of a protein that may alter the effects of exposures to environmental health hazards or result in individual differences in responses to drugs (changing efficacy, risk of adverse effects, or therapeutic dosing regimens).[76,95] Understanding these variations, which is just beginning, can individualize pharmacologic management. During pregnancy, these individual differences may occur in the other, fetus and/or placental, or in any combination of these to influence the expression of specific genes involved in biotransformation, amount and activity of enzymes produced and thus levels of the drug and potential risks.[76]

The term *drug* is used generically in this chapter to refer to prescription and nonprescription pharmacologic agents, herbal agents, and vitamins, as well as drugs of abuse. In addition, the principles that govern placental transfer of drugs are also applicable to transfer of chemicals, food additives, and environmental agents. Definitions of common terms used in pharmacokinetics are summarized in Box 7-1 on p. 185.

PHARMACOKINETICS DURING PREGNANCY

Drug Use During Pregnancy

A survey of drug utilization by 14,000 pregnant women in 22 countries found that 86% of these women took some medication during pregnancy, with an average woman taking 2.9 medications (range, 1 to 15).[73] A longitudinal survey from the United States surveyed 578 women throughout pregnancy. These women took a mean of 1.14 prescribed drugs per person, excluding iron and vitamins, with the most frequent being antibiotics, respiratory agents, gastrointestinal (GI) agents, and opioids. Of these women, 59.7% used at least one prescribed drug; 3.1% used more than five. In addition, these women took a mean of 2.95 over-the-counter drugs per person (92.6% of the women studied used at least one; 20.8% used more than five), with the most frequent being analgesics and agents for gastrointestinal or upper respiratory symptoms. Herbal agents

BOX 7-1 Definitions of Selected Terms Used in Pharmacokinetics

Pharmacokinetics is the study of drug disposition over time and includes absorption, distribution, metabolism, and excretion.

Volume of distribution (Vd) is the distribution of a drug in the body. The greater the Vd, the longer it will take the drug to be cleared from the body. Drugs can be distributed in body water and fat compartments, or bound to plasma proteins or tissue.

Half-life is the time for blood concentration of a drug to decline by 50%. There may be two half-lives calculated for drugs given intravenously: the initial or distribution half-life and the terminal or elimination half-life.

Oral bioavailability is the ability of a drug taken orally to reach the systemic circulation. A drug with high oral bioavailability moves readily from the GI tract to the systemic circulation.

Protein binding is the percentage of the drug that is normally bound to plasma proteins. The two main drug-binding proteins are albumin and α1-acid glycoprotein.

Free drug is the fraction of drug that is unbound in plasma. Free drug can move across the placenta or blood-milk barrier; bound drug cannot.

Clearance is the amount of a drug that is cleared from the plasma by hepatic and renal systems in a given unit of time. Hepatic and renal clearance can be calculated separately.

Molecular weight (MW) is the weight of the drug in daltons. The smaller the MW, the more readily a substance can cross cell membranes. Very small substances (MW less than 100 to 200 daltons) may be able to move though pores in the cell membrane.

pKa is the pH at which a drug is 50% ionized. Ionized drugs do not cross cell membranes (including the placenta and the blood-milk barrier) as readily.

were used by 45.2% of study participants, with a mean of 0.77 herbal agents per person; most frequently used were peppermint tea, cranberry juice, aloe, and other herbal teas.[49] A retrospective chart review of eight U.S. health maintenance organizations (n = 152,531 women) from 1996 to 2000 found that 59% of the women received drugs other than vitamin or mineral supplements after their first prenatal care visit (39% in the first, 34.4% in the second, and 37.9% in the third trimester). Approximately one third of the women were on prescribed drugs for which there is evidence of some fetal risk (FDA category C, D, or X).[8] More recently Mitchell and associates reviewed drug use during pregnancy between 1976 and 2008. They found that (1) average use of prescribed and over the counter drugs increased over these years from 2.5 to 4.2; (2) use of prescribed drugs increased 63% during the first trimester and by 2008, 94% of women took at least one prescribed drug; and (3) <1% of pregnant women took an antidepressant in 1988-90 versus 7.5% in 2006-08.[89] Petersen et al. reported a four-fold increase in use of antidepressants during pregnancy from 1992 to 2006.[104]

Adherence to prescribed drug regimens is a problem during pregnancy, with up to 50% of women either not taking a prescribed drug or stopping before receiving a full course of the drug.[27,72,104] This can lead to maternal risks, especially in women with chronic diseases.[72,104] Peterson et al. found that antidepressants were more likely to be discontinued by pregnant than nonpregnant women, often leading to increased depression and other complications.[104] Problems with adherence stem primarily from concerns about teratogenic effects. Most women overestimate the teratogenic risks of common agents.[69] For example, in one study women personally estimated that the risk of having a baby with a birth defect was 25% (which is the risk associated with a potent teratogen such as thalidomide). After counseling, however, they more correctly estimated the risk at 5%.[69] The background risk of a birth defect for the general population is 3% to 5%. However, the risk may be higher or lower for an individual woman depending on factors such as her health status, teratogen exposures, and genetic makeup.

Several principles have been identified to guide drug therapy during pregnancy: (1) avoid medications in the first trimester whenever possible; (2) anyone prescribing drugs for a woman of childbearing age must consider a potential pregnancy before prescribing; (3) women receiving long term drug therapy require counseling before pregnancy of the potential implications and risks; (4) a necessary treatment should not be stopped without good reason; (5) drugs may have altered effects during pregnancy (e.g., the increased metabolism of methicillin or increased renal elimination of digoxin may result in decreased levels, resulting in the need for higher doses); (6) use single action, short-acting medications rather than long-acting or combination drugs; (7) use the lowest effective dose of the safest available medication; (8) use drugs only if the benefits outweigh the risks; (9) use alternate routes of administration if available (i.e., topical or inhaled rather than systemic agents); (10) select drugs that have a history of use during pregnancy without adverse effects, rather than the "latest" drug; and (11) use doses at the low end of the normal dose range while recognizing that for some drugs (e.g., digoxin, phenytoin, lithium), the woman's usual dose may need to be increased due to increased volume of distribution (Vd) and clearance of these agents during pregnancy.[73,109] These principles also apply to all women of childbearing age and to preconceptional and interconceptional use of drugs, in that approximately half of all pregnancies are unplanned and critical developmental processes occur before most women realize they are pregnant.[73]

Alterations in Drug Absorption, Distribution, Metabolism, and Excretion During Pregnancy

Maternal responses to drugs during pregnancy are influenced by both maternal physiology and the presence of the placental-fetal unit.[81] Variations in handling of specific drugs by the pregnant woman may occur due to effects of the normal physiologic changes of pregnancy on drug absorption, distribution, metabolism, and excretion (Table 7-2). The presence of the placental-fetal compartment can also

Table 7-2 Influence of Pregnancy on Physiologic Aspects of Drug Disposition

PHARMACOKINETIC PARAMETER	CHANGE IN PREGNANCY
ABSORPTION	
Intestinal motility	Decreased
Ventilation	Increased
Cardiac output	Increased
Blood flow to skin	Increased
DISTRIBUTION	
Plasma volume	Increased
Total body water	Increased
Plasma proteins	Decreased
Body fat	Increased
METABOLISM	
Hepatic metabolism	±
Extrahepatic metabolism	±
EXCRETION	
Uterine blood flow	Increased
Renal blood flow	Increased
Glomerular filtration rate	Increased
Ventilation	Increased

From McClary, J., Blumer, J.L., & Aranda, J.V., et al. (2011). Developmental pharmacology. In R.J. Martin, A.A. Fanaroff, & M.C. Walsh (Eds.). *Fanaroff and Martin's neonatal-perinatal medicine: Diseases of the fetus and infant* (9th ed.). Philadelphia: Mosby Elsevier, p. 711.

alter maternal kinetics.[81] For example, many antibiotics are lipid-soluble and may readily cross the placenta and become sequestered in the fetal compartment and thus be unavailable to the mother. This can lead to lower maternal levels.

Evidence regarding effects, effectiveness, and safety of most pharmacologic agents during pregnancy is limited.[69,80,87] Pharmacokinetic data on specific drugs during pregnancy is often minimal because pregnant women are excluded from drug trials. As a result, many drugs are not labeled for use in pregnancy, because the effects of the drug on the fetus are unknown.[70,131] This is protective for the fetus but may also limit benefits to the pregnant women from these drugs. The net result of changes in drug handling during pregnancy depends on the individual drug, with both increases in levels (with need for a lower dose or less frequent dosing) and decrease in levels (with a need for a higher dose or more frequent dosing) seen.[78] In general, both peak and steady-state serum concentrations are lower or unchanged in the pregnant woman.[20] Although changes may not be clinically significant the efficacy and toxicity of drugs can be harder to predict, because of the physiologic changes during pregnancy that have the potential to alter pharmacokinetics.[20,57]

Little analyzed data on pharmacokinetics of drugs in pregnancy and found that across all agents (1) drug oral bioavailability decreased during pregnancy in 47% of studies of different agents; (2) Vd increased in 39%, with no change in 48%; (3) peak plasma levels decreased in 33%, with no change in 57%; (4) steady-state plasma levels decreased in 45%, with no change in 45%; (5) half-life decreased in 41%, with no change in 44%; (6) clearance increased in 55%, with no change in 34%; and (7) protein binding decreased in 86%.[78] Therefore during pregnancy, there are considerable variations in the direction of pharmacokinetic changes among different drugs. This increases the complexity for the practitioner in choosing a specific pharmacologic agent and monitoring its effects. Many studies have significant methodologic problems, for example, sample sizes may be small, the composition of the control group may vary (e.g., the group may include nonpregnant women, adult males, or the same subjects postpartum), women of various gestational ages may be grouped together, and dosing methods may vary.[36,78] Pregnancy drug registries have been established to collect experiences with specific drugs or groups of drugs (such as antiepileptic agents) during pregnancy and fetal and neonatal outcomes (see Box 7-2). Three types of drug registries have been established: individual academic sites; pharmaceutical drug company sites; and population-based sites (from individual countries or a group of countries).[24,128]

Drug Absorption

Pulmonary, GI, and peripheral blood flow changes during pregnancy can alter absorption of drugs from the lungs, gut, and skin (see Chapters 9, 10, and 12). The increased minute ventilation that occurs in pregnancy can increase the rate of drug uptake across the alveoli.[81,86] As a result, the pulmonary system may have a greater role in drug and metabolite excretion during pregnancy.[91] Alveolar uptake of inhalation agents is also influenced by changes in cardiac output, which leads to increased pulmonary blood flow and thus increased alveolar uptake. As a result, doses of volatile anesthetics (e.g., halothane, isoflurane, methoxyflurane) may need to be decreased to compensate for these changes in the pregnant women.[81,102] Inhaled aerosols such as anti-inflammatory and bronchodilators may have enhanced absorption.[106]

Absorption of oral medications is influenced by gastric acidity, gastric motility, presence of bile acids or mucus, nausea and vomiting of pregnancy, and intestinal transit time. During pregnancy there is decreased gastric acid (hydrochloric acid [HCl]) secretion, altered intestinal emptying time, increased mucus, and decreased gastric and intestinal motility.[36,106] Decreased gastric motility can increase the oral bioavailability of slowly absorbed drugs (such as digoxin) by prolonging transit time, and can decrease peak plasma levels of rapidly absorbed drugs. Factors altering GI function in pregnancy may initially delay, then prolong absorption of oral medications. Peak plasma levels may be lower, and the time to peak levels may be later than in nonpregnant women. These changes tend to peak in the third trimester.[68] Changes in pH affect ionization, and

BOX 7-2 Resources for Information on Drugs and Teratogens During Pregnancy and Lactation

BOOKS

Briggs, G., Freeman, R.K., & Yaffe, S.J. (2011). *Drugs in pregnancy and lactation* (9th ed.). Philadelphia: Lippincott Williams & Wilkins.

Hale, T.W. (2010). *Medications and mother's milk* (14th ed.). Amarillo, Texas: Pharmasoft Medical Publishing.

Weiner, C. & Buhimschi, C. (2009). Drugs for Pregnant and Lactating Women (2nd ed.). London: Churchill Livingstone.

INTERNET

American College of Occupational and Environmental Medicine (ACOEM) Reproductive and Developmental Hazard Management Guidance (http://www.acoem.org/Reproductive_Developmental_Hazard_Management.aspx)

The Effects of Workplace Hazards on Female Reproductive Health (http://www.cdc.gov/niosh/docs/99-104/)

The Effects of Workplace Hazards on Male Reproductive Health (http://www.cdc.gov/niosh/malrepro.html)

FDA List of pregnancy exposure registries. Available at http://www.fda.gov/scienceresearch/specialtopics/womenshealthresearch/ucm134848.htm. Accessed August 10, 2011.

InfantRisk Center (http://www.infantrisk.com/) Information on risks of medications use during pregnancy and breastfeeding (Thomas W. Hale, Director) online or via the InfantRisk Helpline (806)-352-2519.

March of Dimes Professional Resources (http://www.marchofdimes.com/professionals)

Organization of Teratology Information Services (http://www.otis-pregnancy.org) (links to teratology information services in each state and in Canada).

Teratology Information System (TERIS) (http://depts.washington.edu/terisweb/teris/)

absorption of drugs.[36,81] For example, decreased gastric pH slows the rate at which weak acids (e.g., aspirin) are absorbed and increases absorption of weak bases (e.g., narcotic analgesics).[102] Decreased GI motility may alter initial absorption of oral antibiotics and lead to unpredictable patterns of intestinal absorption. Absorption of hydrophilic drugs may be enhanced due to the longer intestinal transit time (from delayed intestinal emptying and decreased motility).[83] Increased cardiac output and peripheral blood flow may increase the rate of absorption of drugs from the stomach and small intestine.[78] Iron chelates with some drugs taken concurrently, preventing absorption. However, even with these changes in GI function, the clinical effect for most drugs is not significant. This is because therapeutic windows are usually wide enough for drugs administered orally that these factors do not significantly alter therapeutic effects.[91]

Cardiovascular and integumentary changes during pregnancy may lead to more rapid absorption of agents delivered via transdermal, intranasal, intravascular, epidural, and subcutaneous routes.[102] The increased extracellular water and peripheral blood flow to the skin during pregnancy may enhance absorption and alter distribution of topical agents. For example, topical and vaginal iodine-based preparations are not recommended during pregnancy because of the increased absorption of iodine. Iodine is of concern because it is actively transported across the placenta to the fetus, whose thyroid gland has a high avidity for this substance (see Chapter 19). Increased peripheral perfusion secondary to decreased peripheral vascular resistance and vasodilation may increase absorption of intramuscular drugs.[36]

Drug Distribution

The distribution of drugs within the body depends on many factors, including the amount of body water, which affects Vd; degree to which a drug is bound to plasma proteins or body tissues; and the presence of the fetal-placental unit. For many drugs the Vd is increased during pregnancy because of the increased plasma volume, blood volume, cardiac output, total body water, and body mass.[20,36,91] The increased plasma and blood volumes, and thus Vd, may result in decreased drug levels in the central compartment, reduce serum levels of drugs, and necessitate larger loading doses.[83,103] Increases in total body water during pregnancy affect primarily water-soluble (polar) drugs that tend to stay in the extracellular space. Initial doses may need to be increased to achieve therapeutic concentrations; however, maternal doses for most drugs are not significantly altered since drug steady state is influenced by bioavailability and clearance as well as Vd.[68] Due to changes in the Vd, some pregnant women may notice that their prepregnancy dose of a drug taken regularly, such as digoxin or phenytoin, may not achieve the same therapeutic effect during pregnancy.

Some lipid-soluble drugs (e.g., caffeine, diazepam, thiopental) have a longer half-life in the pregnant woman, whereas polar drugs (e.g., oxazepam, ampicillin) tend to have a shorter half-life.[52,130] The Vd for lipophilic drugs is increased during pregnancy because of the accumulation of fat, which may serve as a reservoir for some drugs via tissue binding.[36,78] Tissue binding is a mechanism by which a drug is removed from circulation and stored in tissue such as hair, bone, teeth, and adipose tissue. This mechanism can result in storage of significant quantities of a drug, because tissue storage sites may need to be saturated before there is sufficient free drug to be effective at receptor sites. Factors reducing maternal serum drug levels increase the risk of subtherapeutic drug levels. When the drug is discontinued, tissue deposits may give up their stores slowly, resulting in persistent drug effects. Because lipid-soluble drugs are stored in adipose tissue, the increased adipose tissue during pregnancy can lead to a slight decrease in the amount of free lipid-soluble drugs, such as sedatives and hypnotics, and persistence of drug effects ("hangover") after the drug has been discontinued.

Drugs in plasma are either unbound (free) or bound to plasma proteins, primarily albumin or α1-acid glycoprotein. The reduction in plasma proteins, especially albumin, during pregnancy may increase plasma levels of free (active) drug. Albumin is the major binding protein for acidic drugs such as salicylates, anticonvulsants, nonsteroidal anti-inflammatory agents, and some neutral drugs such as warfarin and diazepam.[81] Serum albumin levels fall during pregnancy, increasing the unbound or free drug fraction. Total plasma drug concentration stays the same during pregnancy, but the unbound fraction of albumin-bound drugs is greater; therefore the drug may be cleared faster or transported more rapidly across the placenta.[81] Increases in free drug do not necessarily lead to an increase in plasma levels of that drug if the increase in free drug is balanced by more rapid hepatic biotransformation or renal elimination.[36,81,102] However, with regard to doses of some drugs that are bound to albumin (such as many antiepileptic drugs), total and free drug concentrations may be altered, and doses may need to be adjusted during pregnancy. For example, phenytoin total plasma concentration is decreased by 55% to 65% and levels of free drug by 18% to 31% during pregnancy; carbamazepine total concentration is reduced 0% to 43% and free drug 0% to 28%; phenobarbital total concentration is reduced by 50% to 55%.[102] Thus when monitoring serum concentrations of drugs such as phenytoin during pregnancy, free versus total levels should be evaluated (many laboratories report free levels if specified when ordering).[36]

Free fatty acids and steroid hormones, both of which are increased in pregnancy, may compete with drugs for albumin binding sites, further increasing levels of unbound drug. The decrease in albumin, coupled with increases in free fatty acids and steroid hormones, are most prominent in late pregnancy. This change can result in unpredictable transient increases in free levels of some drugs, such as phenytoin, valproate acid, carbamazepine, sulfisoxazole, theophylline, and phenobarbital as well as the potential for more rapid elimination increases the risk of subtherapeutic maternal levels.[36,46] α1-Acid glycoprotein is the major protein for binding basic drugs such as local anesthetics, most opioids, and β-blockers. α1-Acid glycoprotein is decreased slightly during pregnancy.[6,106]

Changes in protein binding during pregnancy not only influence availability of free drug in the mother but also the amount of drug available to cross the placenta. This may alter fetal-to-maternal drug ratios, thus further altering placental transfer. Drugs with hepatic blood flow–limited biotransformation (e.g., propranolol, lidocaine) are rapidly eliminated in their first pass through the liver, regardless of whether they are bound or unbound.[20,103] Therefore even with the decreased protein binding in pregnancy, hepatic clearance and total drug concentration generally are not significantly altered, although concentrations of free drug, Vd, and half-life may increase. Conversely, with drugs whose hepatic biotransformation is independent of hepatic blood flow (e.g., warfarin, phenytoin), only the unbound fraction is removed by the liver. For these drugs, total drug concentrations may be lower than usual, with a decreased half-life and greater fluctuations in peak and trough levels.

Hepatic Drug Metabolism

The hepatic changes during pregnancy (see Chapter 12) can alter biotransformation of drugs by the liver and clearance of drugs from the maternal serum. Drugs that are primarily (greater than 70%) metabolized in their first pass through the liver (high extraction ratio) are usually cleared rapidly by the liver, because clearance of these drugs is dependent on hepatic blood flow. Hepatic elimination of drugs with high extraction ratios is generally unchanged in pregnancy. Drugs with low (less than 30%) first-pass hepatic clearance (low extraction ratio) are more dependent on liver enzyme systems. The rate of elimination of these drugs (e.g., theophylline, caffeine, and diazepam) is related to free drug levels and tends to be decreased in pregnancy with increased half-lives. Hepatic elimination of other drugs—including many antibiotics, pancuronium, phenytoin, and acetaminophen—is increased in the pregnant woman.

Some liver enzymatic processes may be slower during pregnancy, delaying drug metabolism and degradation; other processes have increased activity. The cytochrome P450 (CYP450) monooxygenase system is a group of phase I enzymes essential for hepatic metabolism of drugs. The enzymes of this system are indicated by the prefix CYP (cytochrome) followed by a series of numbers and letters, (e.g., CYP1A2, CYP3A4, CYP2D6). Activity of the following are increased during pregnancy: CYP3A4 (50% to 100%), CYP2A6 (54%), CYP2D6 (50%), and CYP2C9 (20%).[5,57,72,123] Up regulation of CYP2C9 decreases plasma concentrations and increases clearance of phenytoin, nonsteroidal anti-inflammatory agents and some oral antidiabetic agents.[57,68] Changes to CYP3A4 may increase the metabolism of methadone, nifedipine, and indinavir during pregnancy.[102,123] However, activity of CYP1A2, which is responsible for hepatic elimination of many drugs, is decreased (33% in the first, 50% in the second, and 65% in the third trimester); activity of CYP2C19 is also decreased (50%).[5,6,78,123] CYP1A2 is also involved in clearance of caffeine so decreased activity may lead to slower clearance and enhance effects during pregnancy.[72,102]

Activity of phase II enzymes is also altered during pregnancy, including some of the uridine 5′-diphosphatase glucuronosyltransferase (UGT) enzymes.[5,102,106] For example, UGT1A4 is increased 200% in the first and second trimesters and 300% in the third trimester; UGT2B7 is increased 50% to 200% by the third trimester.[6,123] Some extrahepatic enzymes, particularly cholinesterase, are also decreased, which may alter the woman's response to neuromuscular agents.[28,36,131] For example, the decrease in pseudocholinesterase during pregnancy has been enough to impair breakdown of suxamethonium with subsequent prolonged paralysis after anesthesia in some women. The relative increase in hepatic metabolism and blood flow during pregnancy (as a consequence of the increased cardiac output), may increase clearance of polar drugs.[36] In general, slowly metabolized drugs that are cleared primarily by the liver tend to be cleared more slowly in pregnancy due to decreased enzymatic activity and the net decrease in liver blood flow. This may also increase the length of time potentially teratogenic intermediary metabolites remain in circulation.

Clearance and metabolism of drugs by the liver during pregnancy may also be influenced by the increases in steroid hormones that stimulate hepatic microsomal enzyme activity. For example, progesterone may induce enzyme activity for phenytoin clearance, whereas progesterone and estradiol alter hepatic elimination of caffeine and theophylline by competitive inhibition of microsomal oxidase.[36,81] Estrogens have cholinergic effects and may interfere with clearance of drugs such as rifampin that are excreted into the biliary system.[81] Smoking and alcohol may also induce hepatic enzymes.

Renal Drug Excretion

Many drugs are excreted primarily by the kidneys. Thus the increased glomerular filtration rate (GFR) in pregnancy (see Chapter 11) alters renal excretion of drugs, especially water-soluble drugs such as penicillin G, digoxin, aminoglycosides, lithium, and pancuronium. These drugs are eliminated more rapidly, leading to lower and potentially subtherapeutic blood and tissue levels.[36,78,91] These effects are most prominent in late pregnancy.[77] In many cases the changes are not clinically significant enough to require alteration in drug dose.[36] However, this is not always the case. For example, pregnant women with paroxysmal atrial tachycardia may experience an increased frequency of attacks when taking usual doses of digoxin. These women may require up to a 50% increase in their digoxin dose during pregnancy.[81] In addition, shorter dosage intervals are recommended for nifedipine and labetalol due to a threefold increase in clearance in the pregnant woman.[81] The half-life of atenolol, digoxin, and peripheral myorelaxants is shorter during pregnancy.[102] Because lithium is eliminated entirely by GFR, the pregnant woman may require a higher dose of this drug, especially during the third trimester.[99] More rapid clearance and shorter half-lives are also seen with many penicillins, cephalosporins, aminoglycosides, and sulfonamides as a consequence of the changes in renal function during pregnancy.[102] Morphine metabolites may be cleared more quickly in late pregnancy and may lead to a lowered analgesic effect.[72]

Alterations in Drug Absorption, Distribution, Metabolism, and Excretion During the Intrapartum and Postpartum Periods

Drug handling is further altered during the intrapartum period. GI absorption may decrease to a greater extent than seen in pregnancy. Gastric emptying is reported to decrease during labor (see Chapter 12), although this may be secondary to use of opiate agents such as meperidine and pentazocine. Administration of antacids to decrease the risk of acid aspiration with anesthesia can alter ionization by altering gastric pH, prolonging gastric emptying, or complexing with drugs, reducing their absorption. Cardiac output increases in the intrapartum period further increase the Vd and may transiently alter hepatic and renal blood flow.[101] Blood flow to the lower extremities may be reduced, especially if the woman is in a supine position. This may result in a slower and more unpredictable rate of absorption of drugs given intramuscularly in the buttock or thigh.[101] Plasma nonesterified fatty acids rise during labor and may compete for albumin binding sites, with an increase in free drug levels.[101] Both supine positioning and oxytocin may reduce renal blood flow and delay renal excretion of drugs and drug metabolites during labor. Most analgesics and anesthetics used in labor, especially opioids, tend to be low-molecular-weight, lipid-soluble, weak bases that enhance movement across the placenta to the fetus once they enter maternal circulation. The clinical effects depend on the timing of the dose, half-life, drug physicochemical characteristics, placental blood flow, and maternal and fetal drug metabolism and excretion.[79]

During the immediate postpartum period, the pattern of pharmacokinetics and drug distribution is similar to that of late pregnancy and remains so until the pregnancy-induced physiologic alterations of each system return to nonpregnant status.[42] During this transition, drug handling by the woman may remain altered to some extent for some drugs. Transfer of drugs to nursing infants is discussed later in this chapter in "Drugs and Lactation."

Transfer of Drugs Across the Placenta

Dancis suggested that in thinking of placental transfer one should "Ask not whether a maternal [substance] crosses the placenta. Ask rather, how, how much, and how fast. Ask also as to fetal need."[35] There are few compounds, endogenous or exogenous, that are unable to cross the placenta in detectable amounts given sufficient time and sensitivity of detection.[20,23,35,87,91] Drugs with similar physiodynamic properties can differ in placental transfer.[87,105] Plonait and Nau suggest that if no other information is available and a group of drugs is not known to have teratogenic effects, then a comparison of lipid solubility, molecular weight (MW), ionization, and degree of protein binding might assist the clinical selection of an appropriate drug for more efficient transfer (fetal drug therapy) or least efficient transfer (limited fetal exposure).[105] For example, drugs that are lipid soluble have an extremely low (50 daltons) or low (51 to 599 daltons) MW, and are nonionized with low protein binding in maternal plasma cross the placenta more rapidly and in higher concentrations than drugs that are water soluble (polar), have a high MW (greater than 600 daltons), and are ionized and highly bound to protein in maternal plasma. Transfer of drugs across the placenta varies with developmental changes in the placental, and thus gestational age.[121]

Patterns of Transfer Kinetics

Three major patterns of transfer pharmacokinetics are seen: (1) complete transfer (drugs rapidly equilibrate between mother and fetus, with blood flow being the rate limiting step); (2) exceeding transfer (levels are higher in the fetus than in the mother); and (3) incomplete transfer (levels are higher in the mother than the fetus).[99] These patterns are illustrated in Figure 7-2. Examples of drugs with each pattern are listed in Table 7-3.

There is a great deal of variability even among drugs with similar pharmacokinetic characteristics. However, in general, complete transfer tends to be seen with drugs that have a high pKa and MW less than 600 daltons, whereas incomplete transfer is seen with drugs that have a high pKa and MW greater than 600 daltons. Strongly ionized drugs generally have incomplete transfer, although exceptions occur. For example, ampicillin and methicillin are strongly ionized but have lipophilic side groups, so they have a complete transfer pattern.[98,101] Valproate and salicylates are ionized at the normal (physiologic) pH level but rapidly cross the placenta.[81]

Factors Influencing Placental Transfer

Most drugs cross the placenta by diffusion. Diffusion of a substance across the placenta can be expressed as follows:

$$\text{Diffusion} = \frac{\text{Substance characteristics} \times \text{Surface area} \times \text{Concentration gradient}}{\text{Distance}}$$

Placental transfer is influenced by the following: (1) maternal and fetal drug handling; (2) surface area of the placenta; (3) diffusing distance between maternal and fetal blood; (4) physicochemical characteristics of the drug; (5) gradients (drug concentration, electropotential [normally 20 mV], and pH) between mother and fetus; (6) degree of binding of a substance to proteins in maternal and fetal circulations; (7) concentrations of binding proteins and protein binding gradients between mother and fetus; (8) permeability of the placental barrier (primarily the syncytiotrophoblast); (9) rates of maternal and fetal blood flow through the intervillous space and villi; and (10) placental influx and efflux transporters (Table 7-4).[58,68,86,98,99,102,126]

Diffusing Distance and Surface Area. Increased surface area for exchange, increased concentration gradient, and decreased diffusing distance enhance transfer across the placenta. With increasing gestation and placental growth, efficiency of the placental transfer increases as a result of the increased surface area. As the placenta matures, the distance between maternal and fetal blood decreases due to thinning of the syncytiotrophoblast and connective tissue and increases in the size and number of capillaries in the villi (see Chapter 3). Thus more drug passes to the fetus in the third trimester than in the first trimester. Transfer may be reduced with decreased surface area (small placenta, placental infarcts) or increased diffusing distance (placental edema, infection). Edema with fetal hydrops increases the diffusing distance and decreases transfer so drugs such as digoxin may be less effective in treating arrhythmias in the fetus with hydrops.[71]

Physiochemical Characteristics and Concentration Gradients. Physiochemical characteristics that influence movement across the placenta include lipid solubility, MW, degree of ionization, and protein binding. These characteristics can increase, decrease, or deter movement of potentially harmful drugs and other substances from the maternal to the fetal circulation.[105] For example, placental transfer may be increased or enhanced if a substance is lipid soluble (e.g., diazepam, lipoproteins, most sedatives) or nonionized (e.g., phenobarbital), has a low MW (e.g., alcohol), or has a lower albumin binding (e.g., ampicillin). A substance will have reduced, slower, or no transport across the placenta if it has a certain charge or molecular configuration (e.g., heparin) or certain size (e.g., heparin, IgM), is altered or bound by enzymes within the placenta (e.g., amines, insulin), or is firmly and highly bound to the maternal red blood cell (e.g., carbon monoxide) or plasma proteins (e.g., dicloxacillin).

Lipid-soluble substances cross the placenta more readily than water-soluble substances, because cell membranes are made primarily of lipids that enhance diffusion. Lipid-soluble substances dissolve in the lipid membranes of the tissues separating maternal and fetal blood, primarily the syncytiotrophoblast. Polar substances cross slowly unless they have low MW and can move through pores. If the syncytiotrophoblast has a high lipid affinity for a drug (e.g., buprenorphine), the drug may be sequestered in the placenta with decreases in both maternal and fetal concentrations.[120]

The exact MW limit for placental transfer is unknown, although transfer of substances with MW >500 to 600 daltons is limited.[105] Insulin (with an MW of more than 6000) does not cross the placenta because of its size and configuration and because of the effects of placental insulinase enzymes.[36,99] Substances with higher MW tend to cross more slowly and are influenced by maternal concentrations; for example, if maternal concentrations are high, the substance is

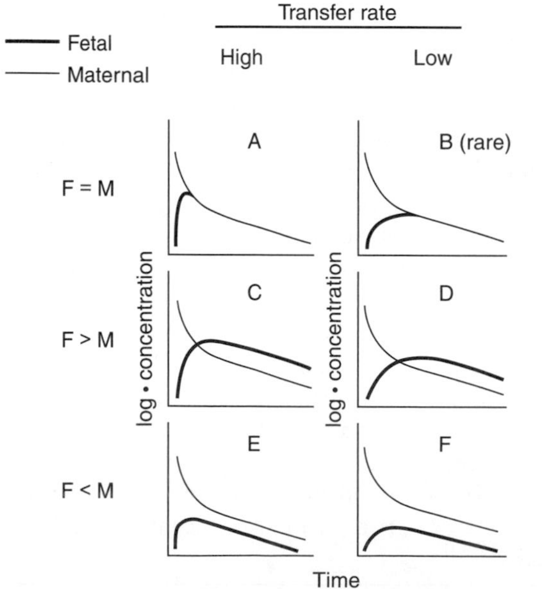

FIGURE 7-2 Simulation of maternal and fetal plasma concentrations time curves from various transplacental pharmacokinetic models. Examples of drugs that fit each curve *(A to F)* are in Table 7-3. (From Plonait, S.L. & Nau, H. [2012]. Physiochemical and structural properties regulating placental drug transfer. In R.A. Polin, W.W. Fox, & S.H. Abman [Eds.]. *Fetal and neonatal physiology* [4th ed.]. Philadelphia: Saunders.)

Table 7-3 Examples of Drugs with Transplacental Kinetics*

MODEL A OR B	MODEL C	MODEL D	MODEL E	MODEL F
Some barbiturates:	Some benzodiazepines:	Ascorbate	Amide-type local anesthetic agents:	Heparin
Thiopental	Diazepam	Colistimethate†	Lidocaine	Quaternary ammonium compounds:
Pentobarbital	Lorazepam	Furosemide	Bupivacaine	Tubocurarine
Secobarbital	Desmethyl-diazepam	Meperidine	Some β-adrenoceptor blockers:	Succinylcholine
Antipyrine	Oxazepam	Some cephalosporins:	Propranolol	Vecuronium
Promethazine	Valproate	Cephalothin	Sotalol	Pancuronium
Ritodrine	Salicylate	Cefazolin	Labetalol	Elementary ions:
Magnesium sulfate	Nalidixic acid	Cephapirin	Dexamethasone	Chlorthalidone
Digoxin	Nicotine	Cephalexin	Cimetidine	Dicloxacillin
	Urea	Some aminoglycosides:	Ranitidine	Erythromycin
	Some penicillins:	Gentamycin	Methadone	Nitrofurantoin
	Ampicillin	Kanamycin	Some sulfonamides‡	
	Penicillin G			
	Methicillin			

Modified from Plonait, S.L. & Nau, H. (2012). Physiochemical and structural properties regulating placental drug transfer. In R.A. Polin, W.W. Fox, & S.H. Abman (Eds.). *Fetal and neonatal physiology* (4th ed.). Philadelphia: Saunders.

*According to models A through F in Figure 7-2. Differentiation between models A and B, C and D, and E and F is often uncertain because of incomplete data on the initial phase of drug distribution across the placenta. Model B is rarely applied.

†Polypeptide antibiotic, with a molecular weight of 1200 daltons.

‡First and second trimester.

Table 7-4 Factors Influencing the Distribution of Drugs and Other Substances in the Fetus

FACTOR	POSSIBLE INFLUENCES
Type of drug	Factors that increase transfer include lipid solubility, low molecular weight (less than 500 to 600 daltons for lipid soluble and less than 100 daltons for polar substances), nonioinized, and unbound.
Amount of drug	Transfer is increased by greater maternal-to-fetal gradient, especially for drugs transferred by diffusion.
Membrane permeability	Diffusion of substances increases with increasing gestation and greater placental efficiency. Some drugs have greater affinity for specific fetal tissues (e.g., tetracycline in teeth, warfarin in bones, phenytoin in the fetal heart [because this is a highly lipid organ in the fetus, whereas in adults the central nervous system has a high lipid content owing to myelin sheaths], streptomycin in the optic nerve).
Fetal body water compartment	Drug distribution and dilution change as the total body water compartment decreases with increasing gestation. With an increased volume of distribution, peak volumes of drugs are reduced and excretion may be delayed.
Fetal circulation	Maternal and fetal blood flow rates will influence transfer. Upon reaching the fetal circulation, drugs may be shunted by the ductus venosus past the liver (thus missing an opportunity for detoxification), with highest concentrations of these substances in blood going to the heart and upper body.
Serum protein binding	Protein binding of a drug in the maternal system limits the amount of free drug available for transfer to the fetus. Binding of drugs to macromolecules in the fetal circulation may increase the maternal-to-fetal transfer by maintaining a concentration gradient from the mother to the fetus.
Receptor function	Functional ability of receptors on cell membranes increases with gestation, leading to increased specificity to respond to or exclude certain drugs.
Placental enzymes	Enzymes produced by the placenta (e.g., insulinase) may detoxify drugs and reduce transfer to the fetus.
Gestational age	Many of the factors identified above are altered with advancing gestation and maturity of the fetus and placenta. The size and efficiency of the placental exchange area increase with increasing gestational age.
Fetal pH during labor	The fetal pH is usually 0.1 to 0.15 units below that of the mother. A decrease in the fetal pH may increase the transfer of acidophilic agents from the mother to fetus. Hypoxia alters blood flow and thus drug distribution, metabolism, and excretion. For example, with hypoxia, blood flow to the liver and kidneys may be reduced with preferential flow to the brain. Albumin binding of drugs may also be reduced, resulting in more free drug in the fetal circulation.

more likely to cross. These substances may also cross via active transport if a carrier is present. Immunoglobulin G (IgG) with an MW of 150,000 daltons is transported across the placenta via endocytosis and exocytosis (see Chapters 3 and 13).[37] Water-soluble substances with an MW of less than 100 daltons diffuse readily; those with an MW greater than 100 diffuse more slowly. Small lipid-soluble substances (MW less than 500 to 600 daltons) cross rapidly and are blood flow–dependent; those with an MW of more than 500 to 600 daltons cross more slowly and may have incomplete transfer.[20,91,120] However, MW is of limited value clinically in that most drugs have MWs less than 600 daltons. Exceptions include thyroid hormones (MW 889), insulin (MW greater than 5000), heparin (MW 20,000 to 40,000), and low-MW heparin (MW 3000 to 5000).[52,68,99,102]

Maternal-to-fetal concentration or electrochemical gradients also influence transfer. The maternal-fetal pH gradient influences transfer of drugs and can result in "ion trapping," with higher concentrations of some drugs in the fetus than in the mother. Nonionized substances cross the placenta more efficiently than ionized substances.[36] Normally the fetus and amniotic fluid are slightly more acidotic than the mother by 0.1 to 0.15 pH units.[99] As a result of this difference, basic drugs may accumulate in the fetus and amniotic fluid with levels higher than in the mother. In the mother, a weak base tends to remain nonionized in her plasma and cross the placenta rapidly. As this weak base comes into contact with the more acidic fetal blood, the drug becomes more ionized, increasing the flow gradient from mother to fetus. The now-ionized drugs cannot return across the placenta to the mother as readily, thus becoming trapped in the fetus.[20,81,99,120] For example, most opioids are weak bases that may accumulate in the fetus, which is one reason that effects of these drugs may persist in the neonatal period. The opposite effect is seen with acidic drugs: that is, these drugs are more likely to be ionized in the mother and thus not cross the placenta as readily.[20] For nonionized, lipophilic drugs, the rate-limiting step for placental transfer is blood flow; for polar drugs, the rate-limiting step is diffusion.[81] Hypoxia and acidosis in the fetus can influence transplacental passage of drugs. For example, local anesthetics are weak bases whose degree of ionization depends on pH. If the fetus becomes acidotic, ionization of these drugs increases with accumulation ("ion trapping") in the fetus and neonate.[47,99,102]

Drug metabolites also cross the placenta to the fetus and vice versa. The majority of fetal drug elimination is by transfer back to the mother across the placenta. However, some elimination may occur by fetal metabolism, placental metabolism, or excretion into amniotic fluid.[91] This transfer is also based on physicochemical characteristics, primarily ionization and lipid solubility. Most drug metabolites are polar, because polarity enhances biliary and renal elimination. Once polar substances are transferred to the fetus, elimination back across the placenta is slow and may result in accumulation in the fetus or amniotic fluid.[91] In addition the fetus may metabolize a drug producing polar metabolites. These metabolites can also become trapped and accumulate in the fetus or be excreted into amniotic fluid and reswallowed by the fetus. Examples of drugs that tend to concentrate in amniotic fluid are the β-lactams, such as penicillin G, dicloxacillin, and amiodarone.[36,91]

If a drug is transferred slower than the maternal elimination rate, then a significant portion of the drug may be eliminated by the mother before it can be transferred to the fetus. A single dose of a drug given to the mother by intravenous administration tends to cross more quickly to the fetus until concentrations are equalized. As the mother clears the drug from her blood, transfer is reversed as the drug crosses from fetus back to mother. With drugs given repeatedly to reach steady-state concentrations in the mother, protein binding and fetal drug elimination are more critical in determining fetal exposure.

Protein Binding. Drugs that are protein bound, usually to albumin or α1-acid glycoprotein, in the mother or fetus do not cross the placenta. Therefore plasma protein gradients between mother and fetus can also influence transfer. For example, ampicillin has a lower protein binding to albumin, thus increasing the amount of free drug that can cross to the fetus, and resulting in decreased maternal levels. Protein binding of dicloxacillin is 96%. Therefore dicloxacillin would be an appropriate choice to treat maternal infections, but not to treat intrauterine or fetal infection. Another example is propranolol, which is highly protein bound so it crosses much slower than atenolol, which has minimal binding.[71]

Maternal albumin levels fall during pregnancy and are about 15% to 20% lower than those in the fetus at term; α1-acid glycoprotein levels in the fetus are only about 37% to 40% of maternal levels.[91,99,120] Thus at term, albumin (or fetal albumin macromolecule) bound drugs may be more highly bound in the fetus, whereas α1-acid glycoprotein drugs are more highly bound in the mother.[91] Binding to proteins in the fetus may increase transfer of the drug by maintaining a concentration gradient across the placenta. Plasma protein binding and thus concentrations of drugs in the mother versus the fetus changes with increasing gestational age for some drugs. The decreased maternal albumin with increasing gestation increases the amount of free drug in the mother available for placental transfer. For example, diazepam binds to albumin. Albumin binding of diazepam is low in the fetus in the first half of gestation. However, in late gestation, as maternal serum albumin levels decrease, more free diazepam is present in maternal serum and, because this is a lipophilic drug, readily crosses the placenta. Thus by term, fetal diazepam levels are greater than maternal levels (Table 7-5).[105] This may increase the risk of neonatal hyperbilirubinemia in that diazepam competes with bilirubin for albumin binding (see "Neonatal Pharmacokinetics").

Placental Blood Flow. The rate of maternal blood flow to and through the intervillous space and fetal blood flow to and through the villi influence placental transfer, particularly of nonionized, lipophilic substances such as anticonvulsants, alcohol, and opioid derivatives. Contractions decrease transfer

Table 7-5 Fetal and Maternal Protein Binding and Total Concentration Ratios of Selected Drugs During Late Human Gestation

DRUG	PRIMARY BINDING PROTEIN	BOUND IN MOTHER (%)	BOUND IN FETUS (%)	FETUS/MOTHER TOTAL PLASMA CONCENTRATION RATIO
Betamethasone	AGP	60	41	0.33
Bupivacaine	AGP	91	51	0.27
Diazepam	ALB	97	98.5	1.6
Lidocaine	AGP	64	24	0.66
Mepivacaine	AGP	55	36	0.71
N-desmethyl diazepam	ALB	95	97	1.7
Phenobarbital	ALB	41	36	1.0
Phenytoin	ALB	87	82	1.0
Salicylate	ALB	43	54	1.2
Valproic acid	ALB	73	88	1.7

From Plonait, S.L. & Nau, H. (2012). Physiochemical and structural properties regulating placental drug transfer. In R.A. Polin, W.W. Fox, & S.H. Abman (Eds.). *Fetal and neonatal physiology* (4th ed.). Philadelphia: Saunders.
AGP, α1-Acid glycoprotein; *ALB,* albumin.

so drugs that cross rapidly and are given during a contraction may demonstrate decreased transfer to the fetus. Contractions may also delay clearance of drugs from the fetus.[120] In addition to uterine contractions, factors that may alter uteroplacental blood flow include maternal position; anesthesia; nicotine, β-lactams, ototoxics and other drugs; emotional or physical stress; and degenerative changes within the placenta that are seen with hypertension, prolonged pregnancy, diabetes, or renal disease.[71]

Route of Administration. The route of administration can also affect placental transfer. For example, nalbuphine that is given intramuscularly results in fetal blood levels that are 80% of maternal venous levels; if it is given intravenously, fetal levels are three to six times greater than maternal levels.[81,99] Peak drug concentrations in the fetus (and the infant, if delivered after maternal administration) do not necessarily occur at the same time as in the mother. For example, meperidine peaks at 30 to 50 minutes in the mother, but 90 minutes to 3 hours after maternal administration in the fetus as a result of transfer kinetics across the placenta. Therefore meperidine levels are highest in the infant if given to the mother 90 minutes to 3 hours before delivery; on the other hand, fentanyl is higher in the neonate than mother if given shortly before delivery. Therefore it is reasonable to give meperidine if birth is expected within the hour.

Antibiotics are some of the most commonly prescribed drugs in pregnancy. Because antibiotics cross the placenta primarily by simple diffusion, rate-limiting factors include maternal-fetal concentration gradients, MW, and other physicochemical characteristics of the drug, placental surface area, diffusing distance, and the degree to which the drug is bound to maternal plasma proteins (see Table 7-5). A general pattern of antibiotic distribution to the fetus has been described. After an intravenous dose, peak maternal serum concentrations are seen within 15 minutes then fall exponentially. Peak umbilical cord values are seen in 30 to 60 minutes followed by an exponential fall. Peak amniotic fluid levels are seen in 4 to 5 hours. This lag results from slow excretion in fetal urine due to fetal renal immaturity.[114]

Placental Transporters. Although many drugs cross the placenta by simple diffusion, some drugs use placental influx or efflux transporters. These transporters are located along the apical membrane of the microvillus brush border facing maternal blood in the intervillous space and on the syncytiotrophoblast basal membrane (facing the fetal connective tissue matrix and blood vessels in the villi) or fetal capillary epithelium to facilitate movement of nutrients and other physiologic substances across the placenta.[44,58,91,98,102,106,120,126] Some drugs may also be transferred across the placenta by nutrient (influx) transporters, including glucose, carnitine, monoamine, and organic ion carriers.[102] Nonphysiologic substances—some drugs, environmental pollutants, and toxins—if structurally similar to nutrients, may compete for nutrient transporters. The drugs that seem to be particularly able to use this method to cross the placenta include amphetamines, cocaine, cannabinoids, and nicotine and other substances from cigarettes.[44,129] By successfully competing with nutrients for these transporters, nutrient transfer is reduced and fetal growth and development altered. In addition, cephalosporins, ganciclovir, and corticosteroids cross by facilitated diffusion, probably by using carriers that normally transport dipeptides, hormones, and steroids.[98]

The placenta also contains a variety of efflux transporters whose role is to remove steroids and other potentially toxic substances and thus protect the fetus.[68,71,102,120,129,135] Originally most of the transporters were identified in studies of multidrug resistance in tumors as is reflected in some of their names. Examples of drug efflux transporters in the placenta include members of the APT-binding cassette (ABC) group such as multidrug-resistant gene protein (MRP) 1, commonly called P-glycoprotein (P-gp), MRP-2, MRP-3, and breast cancer resistance protein (BCRP).[58,68,102,121,126,129,135] P-gp, MRP-2, and

BCRP are located on the apical membrane of the syncytiotrophoblast cells facing maternal blood; MRP-1 and MRP-3 are on the basal or fetal side of the trophoblast (see Figure 7-3).[47,68,126] Efflux transporters are also found on the gut, lung, and blood brain barrier and help protect entry of substances into the body and brain. Efflux transporters are under hormonal regulation, for example, BCRP by estradiol, and progesterone and P-gp by glucocorticoids.[126] Inflammation and infection may alter regulation of these transporters.[89]

Each transporter appears to have specific substrates for which they provide protection. For example, studies of P-gp suggest that it exports cations, steroids, cytotoxic drugs, some antibiotics, opioids, phenobarbital, erythromycin, phenytoin, verapamil, and other substances that enter the placenta back into maternal blood, thus reducing fetal exposure.[20,58,102,135] BCRP is involved in efflux of flavinoids, zidovudine, cimetidine, glyburide, nitrofurantoin, and the food-borne chemical carcinogen PhiP.[58,68,102] MRP 1 and 3 prevent entry of organic anions and promote excretion and reduce entry of glutathione/glucuronide metabolites into the fetus.[47] Some transporters may have bidirectional flow which can allow xenobiotics to be transported across the placenta to the fetus.[68] Thus BCRP and P-gp cannot only decrease the amount of drug reaching the fetus but enhance removal of any drug reaching the fetal circulation.[129] A drug that is a P-gp or BCRP substrate would be preferred for treating a maternal disorder with minimal fetal drug exposure, whereas a drug that is not a P-gp or BCRP substrate would be preferred for fetal pharmacotherapy.[120]

Deficiency of these transporter proteins increases the risk of teratogenesis from fetal drug and chemical exposure.[58,135] Gene polymorphisms for the ABC efflux transporters may increase or decrease placental transfer of these substances and thus alter fetal susceptibility to effects of maternal drugs.[58]

Placental Metabolism of Drugs

The placenta has many enzyme systems, including various peptidases that can metabolize drugs, thus influencing transfer of specific substances from mother to fetus or fetus to mother.[120] Both phase I and phase II drug metabolizing enzymes are present.[106,129] Several isoforms of the CYP450 system (phase I reactions) are found in the placenta, although at levels about half of those seen in the liver. The primary CYP450 isoforms seen in the placenta are CYP1A1/1A2, although other isoforms, including CYP2E1, CYP3A4, CYP3A7, and CYP4B1, have also been reported, although with low activity.[20,55,91,101,106,112,120] Expression of placental CYP1A1 increases with exposure to polychlorinated biphenyls (PCBs) or maternal cigarette smoking.[120] Phase II reactions including UGTs are also present during most of gestation.[102,129] UGT has a role in detoxifying endogenous and exogenous substances and in regulating steroid hormones produced in the trophoblast.[129] Glutathione S-transferase may

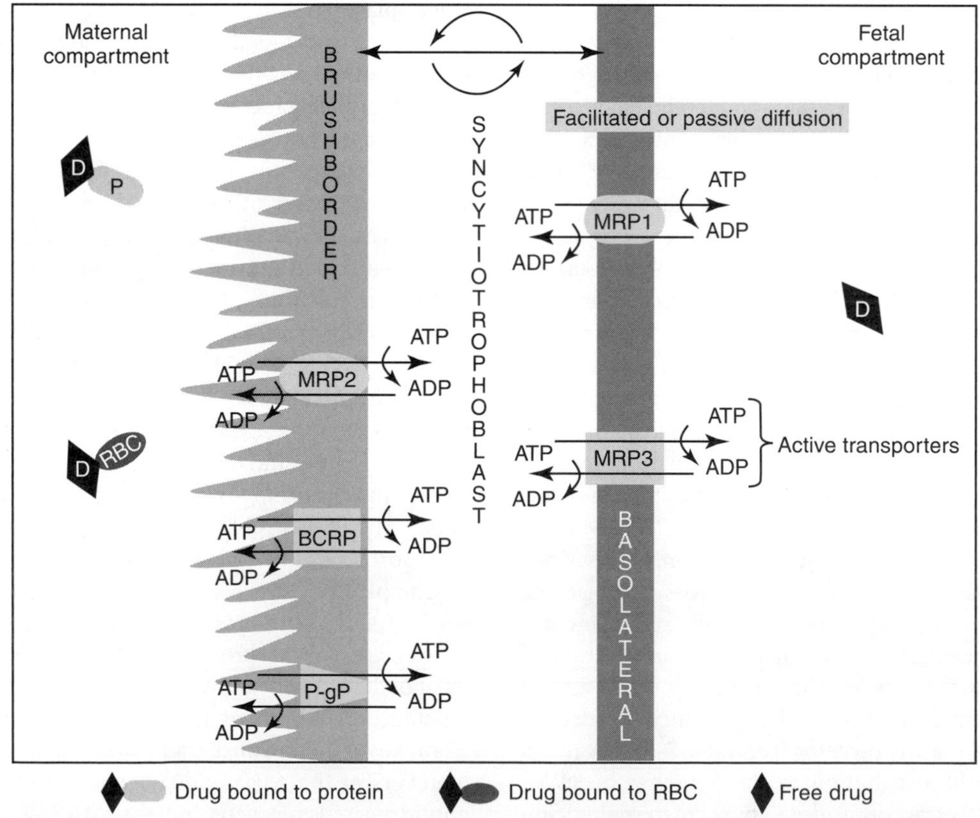

FIGURE 7-3 Transport across the placental barrier. (From Gedeon, C. & Koren, G. (2006). Designing pregnancy centered medications: Drugs which do not cross the human placenta. *Placenta, 27*, p. 862.)

help protect the placenta and fetus from oxidative stress and is also involved in placenta hormone metabolism.[129] These enzymes may increase with maternal nicotine or alcohol use, although alcohol dehydrogenase (a phase I reactant) is seen in low concentrations and is not inducible.[20,106,120,129]

SUMMARY

The impact of maternal physiologic alterations on fetal drug transfer can be illustrated by examining pharmacokinetics and distribution of several drug classes, namely hypoglycemic agents, antibiotics, and anticonvulsants. For example glyburide, which has been used as an adjunct to insulin therapy in treating gestational diabetes, has minimal placental transfer because it is >99.8% protein bound with a short elimination half-life, rapid clearance, and rapid transfer from the placenta back to the mother by placental ABC efflux transporters thus minimizing fetal exposure.[47,129]

Serum levels and the half-life of many antibiotics are reduced during pregnancy, primarily because of a more rapid excretion associated with the increased GFR and expanded plasma volume.[96] Most cephalosporins have a shorter half-life in late pregnancy, except for cefoperazone, which is excreted in bile rather than by the kidneys, so it has a similar half-life in pregnant and nonpregnant women.[96] Penicillins have decreased serum levels and increased renal clearance.[96]

The increased GFR augments renal clearance of antibiotics, thus further reducing serum levels. Most antibiotics are lipid soluble and readily cross the placenta. As a result, dosages of some antibiotics may need to be increased or the dosing interval reduced.[96,116] With most local infections the reduction in maternal serum concentrations probably does not alter therapeutic efficacy of the antibiotic. Pregnant women with acute infections or who need high serum concentrations may require higher doses than nonpregnant women. In these situations, maternal antibiotic levels must be carefully monitored to ensure that the mother is receiving an adequate therapeutic dose and to avoid maternal or fetal toxicity.

Drugs with lower protein binding such as ampicillin and penicillin are associated with increased levels of free drug that readily crosses into the fetal compartment.[96] As a result, fetal and amniotic fluid levels are elevated and maternal serum and plasma levels decreased. The Vd and renal clearance are increased and the half-life of ampicillin in particular is reduced in the pregnant woman.[96] Decreased maternal serum and plasma levels of aminoglycosides are also found in some women, increasing the likelihood of subtherapeutic levels. If aminoglycosides are used, drug blood levels (to evaluate the risk of subtherapeutic levels) and maternal renal function (to evaluate the risk of nephrotoxicity) require careful monitoring.[96]

Higher maternal serum levels and lower fetal and amniotic fluid levels are seen with the use of antibiotics with increased protein binding such as dicloxacillin (96%). As noted earlier, a drug such as dicloxacillin would be appropriate for treating a maternal infection but not effective in treating an intrauterine infection.[131] Dicloxacillin and erythromycin (base or stearate) have limited placental transfer, so fetal levels are low. Maternal absorption, serum levels, and tissue levels of erythromycin may be somewhat erratic and unpredictable.[96,131] Higher concentrations of antibiotics are found in the fetus and amniotic fluid after bolus administration versus continuous drip infusion to the mother and after multiple versus single doses.

A major factor affecting the pregnant epileptic is the effect of the usual physiologic changes of pregnancy on the metabolism of antiepileptic drugs (AEDs).[26,54] As a result of these changes, the apparent plasma clearance of AEDs decreases with subtherapeutic plasma concentrations and increased risk of seizures. However, these changes vary between women and with different AEDs, leading to unpredictability in dosing regimens.[103] The pregnant woman on AEDs may need to have the dosages of some medications increased by 30% to 50% above prepregnant levels.[4] These changes occur predominantly during the second half of pregnancy and reverse by 6 weeks postpartum. As the physiologic alterations of pregnancy are reversed following delivery, drug levels may fluctuate rapidly, leading to toxicity. Drug levels are monitored regularly during pregnancy to ensure therapeutic dosages, with monitoring continuing after delivery until drug levels have stabilized. Phenytoin, phenobarbital, carbamazepine, valproic acid, primidone, and other AEDs have also been associated with teratogenic effects (see Teratogenesis).[24] Valproic acid in particular appears to have a higher risk of major fetal anomalies than carbamazepine and possibly phenytoin and lamotrigine.[53] Fetal anticonvulsant drug syndrome is multifactorial in etiology and characterized by various combinations of symptoms including an increased risk of congenital malformations, microcephaly, cognitive dysfunction (especially with valproic acid), and fetal growth restriction.[48,53,103,128] In addition, some AEDs, including carbamazepine, valproic acid, and phenytoin, have been associated with an increase in facial dysmorphisms. The risks increase with increasing numbers of AEDs used, so monotherapy is recommended during pregnancy.[48,53,103,128] Some agents may also interfere with folic acid increasing the risk of neural tube defects (see Chapter 15).[54] The risks of AED therapy must be balanced against the risks to the mother and fetus of increased seizure activity.[128]

PHARMACOKINETICS IN THE FETUS

Drug Distribution, Metabolism, and Excretion in the Fetus

Distribution, metabolism, and elimination of drugs are altered in the fetus. Factors that influence the effects of drugs in the fetus include individual drug characteristics, dosage, duration of use of the drug, genetic makeup of the mother and fetus (genetic susceptibility), maternal handling and elimination of the drug, timing in relation to stage of embryonic or fetal development, maternal physiology, and placental transfer. Placental transfer is affected by drug physicochemical characteristics (described in the previous section), blood flow, maturation, and metabolic activity. Placental transfer was discussed in the previous section (see "Transfer of Drugs Across the Placenta").

Fetal Drug Distribution

Fetal drug distribution is influenced by individual drug characteristics, specificity of individual agents for certain fetal tissues, and receptor function. Some drugs have a greater affinity for a specific fetal tissue that is not necessarily the agent's expected target tissue. Examples include the high affinity of tetracycline for fetal teeth, warfarin for the fetal bones, and phenytoin for fetal heart tissue. Receptor function of fetal cells increases with increasing gestational age.[86] Receptors become more specific in their ability to respond to or exclude certain drugs, whereas in the embryo and young fetus, these receptors are less discriminating in excluding drugs, increasing the likelihood of teratogenic effects. Other factors influencing drug distribution in the fetus are gestational age, degree of serum protein binding, and fetal body water compartment and pH.[86,102] Fetal pH is slightly lower than maternal, so weak bases (such as anesthetics, cocaine, meperidine, codeine, hydrocodone, erythromycin, barbiturates, and iodine) become more ionized in the fetus and may accumulate in the relatively more acidotic fetus ("ion trapping").[47,102] This phenomenon is more likely during the intrapartum period when fetal pH is further decreased.

The fetus has lower levels of serum proteins, increasing the amount of free drug. Fetal proteins may bind some drugs with greater affinity than in the mother (salicylates) and others (ampicillin, benzyl penicillin) with less affinity.[81] Levels of α1-acid glycoprotein are up to three times lower in the fetus than in the mother with a fetal-to-maternal concentration ratio at term of 0.37.[47,91,99,102] The maternal-to-fetal serum concentration ratio of albumin increases to term as fetal albumin concentrations increase and maternal levels decrease (due to hemodilution). Thus this ratio increases from 0.38 at 12 to 15 weeks to 0.66 at 16 to 25 weeks, 0.97 at 26 to 35 weeks and 1.2 after 35 weeks.[102] Even as serum binding proteins increase with advancing gestational age, levels of free drug tend to remain high because of the lowered protein binding affinity. The fetus has an increased Vd due to increased total body water. This results in a reduction in peak volume of drugs, but also wider distribution of drugs in the body and delayed excretion. Factors influencing distribution of drugs and other substances within the fetus are summarized in Table 7-4.

Fetal Drug Metabolism and Elimination

Once a drug reaches the fetal circulation, the drug can (1) be metabolized by the fetal liver, (2) bypass the fetal liver via the ductus venosus to enter specific fetal tissues or body compartments, (3) be eliminated by the fetal kidney into amniotic fluid, or (4) return to the maternal circulation via the umbilical arteries and placenta. Drugs and metabolites in amniotic fluid may diffuse across the fetal membranes and decidua to maternal blood or be swallowed by the fetus. Swallowed drugs or their metabolites are reabsorbed into the fetal blood from the gut and cleared via the placenta.

Drug metabolites are also excreted by the liver into bile and thus into meconium. Polar metabolites may accumulate in amniotic fluid, reaching levels higher than in either the mother or fetus. Examples of drugs that may accumulate in amniotic fluid are ampicillin, amoxicillin, cefuroxime, and cephalothin.[99] Because most drug metabolites are more polar than the original drug, substances that cross the placenta to the fetus may not return across the placenta to the mother as readily. Therefore, these substances can accumulate in fetal tissues and at levels that may be higher than in the mot her.[36,47,81,102] Metabolites of some drugs that the fetus is exposed to in the third trimester, such as opiates and cocaine may also be found in fetal hair.

Fetal Hepatic Metabolism.Immature phase I and II metabolism is present by about 8 weeks' postconception.[36] By the end of the first trimester, the fetal liver can oxidize some substances via the CYP450 system (phase I biotransformation) (see Table 7-1).[112] The major fetal isoform is CYP3A7, a form found primarily in the fetal and neonatal liver, although it can also be found in the placenta and endometrium.[17,86,102] CYP3A7 accounts for about 50% of the total fetal CYP450 content.[55] Levels peak at 20 weeks, then decrease to term, decreasing rapidly after birth.[102] CYP3A7 may protect the fetus by detoxifying steroids and retinoic acid derivatives and is involved in estriol biosynthesis.[17,66,112] Fetal CYP3A7 has a lower catalytic activity than in adults; levels decrease markedly after birth.[99,112] Other isoforms reported in the fetal liver (although in low quantities) include CYP1A1 (involved in metabolism of endogenous toxins) and probably CYP2E1 (found by the second trimester and involved in prenatal alcohol metabolism), CYP1B1 and CYP2D6.[31,55,91,102,112] By term, CYP450 enzyme activity is about 30% to 60% that of adults, primarily due to CYP3A7 activity.[55,102]

Phase II hepatic biotransformation reactions (see Table 7-1) mature at different rates.[85,112] Glucuronyl transferase activity is low at term, so substances dependent on this mechanism for elimination (e.g., salicylates or lorazepam) are metabolized much more slowly than in the adult. On the other hand, morphine can be glucuronidated in the first trimester, whereas sulfate conjugation is well developed at birth. Sulfation activity increases with gestational age and activity in infancy eventually exceeds that of adults.[76,112]

Lipophilic drugs are more dependent on hepatic metabolism for elimination than are polar (water soluble) substances. The reduced hepatic metabolism in the fetus may be an advantage because drug metabolites are polar and thus tend to slowly cross back to the mother. Lipophilic drugs that remain in that form for longer periods without being metabolized are more likely to cross back to the mother for elimination. Phase I metabolites from the CYP450 system generally slowly cross the placenta to the mother for elimination. Phase II metabolites are more polar, an advantage after birth because these are primarily eliminated by biliary excretion or renal elimination. In the fetus these metabolites have decreased placental transfer, so they tend to accumulate in the fetus and amniotic fluid.[112]

Fetal hepatic metabolism of drugs is limited by a decreased first-pass effect, because some of the blood coming to the fetus from the placenta via the umbilical vein bypasses the liver through the ductus venosus. Biochemically, the left and right lobes of the fetal liver function independently of each other. The more highly oxygenated blood in the umbilical vein coming from the placenta supplies the left lobe, whereas less oxygenated portal vein blood supplies the right lobe. CYP450 activity is higher in the right lobe.[112]

Thus the fetal liver has the ability to metabolize drugs but at a decreased rate due to lower enzyme activity. Metabolism of drugs by the fetal liver may not be an advantage because the intermediary metabolites in these reactions may be toxic, tend to be more polar, and are cleared more slowly than the original drug, thus prolonging exposure.[112] Heroin is a lipophilic drug that readily crosses the placenta, where it is converted by the fetal liver to morphine and other metabolites. These substances are less lipid-soluble than heroin and may be "trapped" on the fetal side of the placenta.[36]

Fetal Renal Elimination. Although polar substances cross the placenta slowly, they are rapidly eliminated by the fetal kidney into amniotic fluid. These drugs may be recycled as the fetus swallows amniotic fluid. Because renal blood flow is low (about 5% of cardiac output), renal elimination in general is not a significant mechanism in the fetus.[91]

Fetal Drug Therapy

Planned fetal drug exposure may occur as a method of treating fetal disorders by administration of drugs to the mother. The most common fetal treatment is administration of glucocorticoids to induce surfactant synthesis and reduce the risk of respiratory distress syndrome in preterm infants (see Chapter 10). Not all glucocorticoids are equally effective, because some are metabolized by the maternal-fetal-placental unit and thus rendered inactive. Inactivation of betamethasone and dexamethasone is limited, so these glucocorticoids are more effective in enhancing surfactant synthesis than drugs such as hydrocortisone, which are rapidly metabolized in the placenta.

Glucocorticoids may prevent development of ambiguous genitalia in female fetuses in families with a history of congenital adrenal hyperplasia. If begun prior to onset of adrenal androgen secretion, these drugs suppress excessive adrenal androgen production and may prevent virilization of the external female genitalia.[71,97] Glucocorticoids act by crossing the placenta and suppressing ACTH production by the fetal pituitary, which reduces adrenal cortex output. Ideally therapy is begun based on family history soon after conception and at least before 6-7 weeks from conception (~9th week of pregnancy).[16] Maternal adverse effects include Cushing syndrome, hypertension, hyperglycemia, gastric irritation, excess weight gain, and pedal edema.[16,97] Drugs may also be given to the mother to treat several specific inborn errors of metabolism.[16,71,110]

Anti-infective agents are given to the mother as prophylaxis against group B streptococcal infection, to treat congenital syphilis (penicillin) or toxoplasmosis (pyrimethamine and sulfadiazine), listeria (ampicillin usually in combination with an aminoglycoside), or to prevent infection with human immunodeficiency virus (HIV).[16,47,71,129] In prophylaxis to prevent HIV transmission, zidovudine with protease inhibitors (such as lamivudine) are not substrates for placental drug efflux transporters. Thus these drugs achieve higher fetal blood concentrations and have greater efficacy than other agents whose transfer across the placenta is reduced by these efflux transporters.[47,129] Administration of antibiotics to the mother with the purpose of protecting the fetus is probably reasonably effective for protection of the GI (swallowing of amniotic fluid) and renal (adequate blood flow) systems. The fetal circulation shunts blood away from the lungs, however, which limits delivery of antibiotics to the respiratory tract for protection against congenital pneumonia in the presence of chorioamnionitis. Because amniotic fluid levels of antibiotics are dependent on excretion of the drug in fetal urine, therapeutic levels of antibiotics in amniotic fluid are attained only with a live fetus. This limits the effectiveness of this treatment for chorioamnionitis after intrauterine death.[114]

Fetal pharmacotherapy has also been used to treat fetal arrhythmias (most often for supraventricular tachycardia, atrial flutter, and fibrillation), hydrops, and congestive heart failure.[129] Examples of drugs used include digoxin, procainamine, quinidine, propanolol, flecainide, amiodarone, and sotalol.[16,129] Fetal therapy has also been used to treat polyhydramnios (indomethacin), hypothyroidism (intraamniotic thyroxine), hyperthyroidism (propylthiouracil and thiamazole), and severe anemia or thrombocytopenia (blood transfusions).[71] Another example of a preventive fetal drug therapy is the use of folic acid for prevention of neural tube defects (see Chapter 15).

NEONATAL PHARMACOKINETICS

Absorption, distribution, metabolism, and excretion of drugs are developmentally different in newborns than in adults. Pharmacokinetic changes in the neonate are dependent on both postmenstrual age and postbirth age. Changes in absorption, distribution, metabolism, and elimination of drugs occur at different rates; there may be marked individual differences as well as day-to-day differences. Postbirth age changes are especially marked in the first month. In terms of pharmacokinetics, the neonatal time is the "period of life when most profound and rapid physiologic changes occur."[60]

There are relatively few pharmacokinetic studies for most agents used in neonates. The majority of studies involve relatively heterogeneous samples (in terms of age, weight, disease state) of infants being treated with the specific drug rather than randomized studies.[60] Alterations in drug absorption, distribution, hepatic metabolism, and renal elimination in the neonate affect pharmacokinetics of drugs used in the neonatal period. Often an individual drug is influenced by multiple pharmacokinetic factors. For example, the prolonged diuretic response to furosemide seen in newborns is due to both an increased plasma half-life (which is eight times greater than in adults and may be up to 24 hours in infants younger than 3 weeks of age), and an increase in volume of distribution (Vd) (four times greater than adults), probably because of decreased protein binding.[62] Drug half-lives are almost always longer in the fetus and neonate than in older individuals (Table 7-6). Physiologic differences affecting drug pharmacokinetics in neonates are summarized in Table 7-7.

Drug Absorption

Oral Agents

Absorption of oral medications in the neonate is altered by the following: (1) decreased bile salts and pancreatic enzymes; (2) slower gut transit time due to delayed gastric emptying and decreased motility; (3) mucus in the stomach; (4) differences in gastric and duodenal pH; (5) high levels of β-glucuronidase in the duodenum; and (6) intestinal surface area.[31,32,66,86,93,106] These alterations are more pronounced in preterm and intrauterine growth–restricted (IUGR) infants.[32,93] Oral drug absorption matures by 4 to 5 months of age.[31] Decreased bile salts and pancreatic enzymes can result in poorer absorption of lipid-soluble substances such as vitamin K, or drugs that must be hydrolyzed for absorption. Slower gut transit time due to delayed gastric emptying and decreased motility initially delays then prolongs absorption. Mucus in the stomach may also delay absorption. Differences in gastric and duodenal pH may partially or totally inactivate some drugs. Absorption of oral drugs by the neonate is also influenced by the drug's physicochemical characteristics. Drugs such as phenytoin, acetaminophen, and chloramphenicol are absorbed slowly and erratically, whereas penicillin and ampicillin are absorbed more efficiently than in adults because of the higher gastric pH in the neonate.[105] Other drugs such as theophylline, digoxin, and diazepam have oral absorption patterns that are more similar to those in adults.

Gastric and duodenal pH influences drug solubility and ionization. An acid pH increases the absorption of acidic drugs (low pKa) because these drugs tend to stay in a nonionized, lipid-soluble form. A higher pH enhances alkaline drug absorption and slows absorption of acidic drugs. Gastric pH is higher for the first 12 to 24 hours after birth, gradually reaching adult values by 2 years.[7] Preterm infants who are less than 32 weeks' gestational age have decreased gastric acid secretion with a more alkaline pH and thus poorer absorption of weak acids and bases.[19,32,93] Gastric emptying is delayed for up to 6 to 8 hours in immature infants and is slower in all infants before 6 to 8 months. This may delay absorption and prolong the time to reach peak drug concentration.[19,66] Oral absorption is also influenced by drug efflux transporter expression on the intestinal lining and type of bacterial flora.[86,95]

The neonate's duodenum has higher levels of β-glucuronidase, an enzyme that unconjugates drugs (e.g., indomethacin, chloramphenicol) that the liver has metabolized via glucuronyl conjugation.[32,66,93] These drugs reenter the blood via the enterohepatic circulation (see Chapter 18) and must be remetabolized by the liver. This increases the half-life and prolongs activity of these drugs.[31,93] Intestinal absorption of drugs, gut transit time, and motility depend on perfusion and food intake. Better gastrointestinal (GI) absorption occurs with drugs of low molecular weight (MW) that are nonionized and lipid-soluble.[93] An ill infant who is not being fed may have further impairment of gut function and erratic absorption of oral medications. Intestinal surface area is decreased with genetic disorders such as cystic fibrosis and disorders such as short bowel syndrome and necrotizing enterocolitis, thus reducing absorption.[19,93]

Table 7-6 Comparative Plasma Half-Lives of Miscellaneous Drugs in Newborns and Adults

DRUG	PLASMA HALF-LIFE (hours) IN NEWBORNS	PLASMA HALF-LIFE (hours) IN ADULTS
Acetaminophen	3.5	2.2
Phenylbutazone	21-34	12-30
Indomethacin	7.5-51	6
Meperidine	22	3.5
Phenytoin	21	11-29
Carbamazepine	8-28	21-36
Phenobarbital	82-199	24-140
Caffeine	100	6
Theophylline	30	6
Chloramphenicol	14-24	2.5
Salicylates	4.5-11.5	2.7
Digoxin	52	31-40

Data from Aranda, J.V., et al. (1980). Drug monitoring in the perinatal patient: Uses and abuses. *Ther Drug Monit, 2,* 39; Morselli, P.L., et al. (1980). Clinical pharmacokinetics in newborns and infants: Age-related differences and therapeutic implications. *Clin Pharmacokinet, 5,* 485; and Morselli, P.L. (1976). Clinical pharmacokinetics in neonates. *Clin Pharmacokinet, 1,* 81.

Intramuscular and Rectal Absorption

The infant's small muscle mass and alterations in peripheral perfusion influence intramuscular medications. Decreased muscle mass may limit use of intramuscular administration in very low-birth weight (VLBW) infants. Drugs given intramuscularly may have slower, more erratic absorption, depending on the infant's gestational age and health status. In the first few days after birth, muscle blood flow is decreased, slowing absorption.[19] Variations in muscle blood flow last for 2 to 3 weeks after birth.[14] Infants with respiratory problems or low cardiac output have decreased peripheral perfusion, leading to even slower and more erratic absorption of drugs given intramuscularly.[66] On the other hand, rectal administration may be more effective in neonates than in adults.[66]

Skin Absorption

Percutaneous absorption of substances occurs via the cells of the stratum corneum (transepidermal route) or via the hair

Table 7-7 **Summary of Developmental Dependent Changes in Drug Disposition**

PHYSIOLOGIC SYSTEM	AGE-RELATED TRENDS	PHARMACOKINETIC IMPLICATIONS	CLINICAL IMPLICATIONS
Gastrointestinal tract	Neonates and young infants: reduced and irregular peristalsis with prolonged gastric emptying time. Neonates: greater intragastric pH (>4) relative to infants. Infants: enhanced lower GI motility.	Slower rate of drug absorption (e.g., increased Tmax) without compensatory compromise in the extent of bioavailability. Reduced retention of suppository formulations.	Potential delay in the onset of drug action following oral administration. Potential for reduced extent of bioavailability from rectally administered drugs.
Integument	Neonates and young infants: thinner stratum corneum (neonates only), greater cutaneous perfusion, enhanced hydration and greater ratio of total BSA to body mass.	Enhanced rate and extent of percutaneous drug absorption. Greater relative exposure of topically applied drugs as compared to adults.	Enhanced percutaneous bioavailability and potential for toxicity. Need to reduce amount of drugs applied to skin.
Body compartments	Neonates and infants: decreased fat, decreased muscle mass, increased extracellular and total body water spaces.	Increased apparent volume of distribution for drugs distributed to body water spaces and reduced apparent volume of distribution for drugs that bind to muscle and/or fat.	Requirement of higher weight-normalized (i.e., mg/kg) drug doses to achieve therapeutic plasma drug concentrations.
Plasma protein binding	Neonates: decreased concentrations of albumin and α_1-acid glycoprotein with reduced binding affinity for albumin bound weak acids.	Increased unbound concentrations for highly protein-bound drugs with increased apparent volume of distribution and potential for toxicity if the amount of free drug increases in the body.	For highly bound (i.e., >70%) drugs, need to adjust dose to maintain plasma levels near the low end of the recommended "therapeutic range."
Drug metabolizing enzyme (DME) activity	Neonates and young infants: immature isoforms of cytochrome P450 and phase II enzymes with discordant patterns of developmental expression. Children 1-6 years: apparent increased activity for selected DMEs over adult normal values. Adolescents: attainment of adult activity after puberty.	Neonates and young infants: decreased plasma drug clearance early in life with an increase in apparent elimination half-life. Children 1-6 years: increased plasma drug clearance (i.e., reduced elimination half-life) for specific pharmacologic substrates of DMEs.	Neonates and young infants: increased drug dosing intervals and/or reduced maintenance doses. Children 1-6 years: for selected drugs, need to increase dose and/or shorten dose interval in comparison to usual adult dose.
Renal drug excretion	Neonates and young infants: decreased glomerular filtration rates (first 6 months) and active tubular secretion (first 12 months) with adult values attained by 24 months.	Neonates and young infants: accumulation of renally excreted drugs and/or active metabolites with reduced plasma clearance and increased elimination half-life, greatest during first 3 months of life.	Neonates and young infants: increased drug dosing intervals and/or reduced maintenance doses during the first 3 months of life.

From Rakhmanina, N.Y. & van den Anker, J.N. (2006). Pharmacological research in pediatrics: From neonates to adolescents. *Adv Drug Deliv Rev, 58*, 10.

follicle–sebaceous gland complex (transappendageal route). The major pathway is most likely transepidermally, with diffusion of a substance through the stratum corneum and epidermis into the dermis and microcirculation. The subepidermal circulation is also readily accessible, enhancing rapid absorption. Preterm infants have greater skin absorption because their skin is thinner than that of the term infant. VLBW infants have minimum to no stratum corneum and higher dermal water content.[66,93]

Neonates are at increased risk for toxic reactions from absorption of topically applied substances. Skin metabolism is different in neonates, so drugs applied topically may result in the release of metabolites different from those that would occur if the drugs were given by other routes. This increases the risk of toxicity.[19,66] Occlusion of the skin (e.g., placement against the mattress) permits more complete absorption, with longer contact enhancing absorption of the substance. In preterm infants, percutaneous absorption occurs even more rapidly and completely as a result of the markedly increased skin permeability. Topical analgesic agents are more easily absorbed, increasing the risk of toxicity (see Chapter 14). Permeability of these agents, such as EMLA cream (lidocaine and prilocaine) is further increased in preterm infants in the first few weeks after birth.[93]

Neonatal toxicity secondary to the use of topical agents such as hexachlorophene, pentachlorophenol-containing laundry detergents, isopropyl alcohol, and povidone-iodine has been well documented.[19,23,28,66] Practices can lead to detrimental effects if not monitored carefully. Topical application of povidone-iodine (Betadine) yields significantly elevated levels of iodine in blood plasma if not removed completely from the skin after completion of invasive procedures (e.g., chest tube insertion, percutaneous line insertion).[19] Gentle cleansing of the skin with water reduces this risk.

Isopropyl alcohol is also absorbed through the skin. Alcohol use can result in dry skin, skin irritation, and skin burns. The concentration of the solution, duration of exposure, and condition of the exposed skin determine the effects of alcohol use. Tissue destruction occurs with the deesterifying of the skin and the disruption of the cell structure. Exposure, pressure, and decreased perfusion can contribute to the development of burns from alcohol, complicating fluid management and providing portals for infection.

Drug Distribution

The distribution of drugs is influenced by the infant's large extracellular fluid space, increased total body water, decreased fat, and decreased plasma protein content and binding. The blood-brain barrier is less well developed, which may result in increased amounts of drugs (especially lipid-soluble substances) reaching and being deposited in the brain.[95,119] The greater total body water and lower fat content in neonates increases the apparent Vd, especially for water-soluble substances.[14,93,116,122]

The altered Vd in the neonate may reduce peak volumes of drugs and delay excretion. Because of the increased extracellular water, higher doses per kilogram may be needed in the neonate for water-soluble drugs distributed in extracellular fluid. For example, an increased Vd is seen with drugs such as theophylline, caffeine, phenobarbital, phenytoin, digoxin, and aminoglycosides such as gentamicin.[93,116,122] The Vd is further increased with decreasing gestational age, because more immature infants have a greater total body water percentage. VLBW infants may need higher loading doses and a longer dosing interval of some drugs because of their even greater apparent Vd and immature hepatic and renal function. Other factors that alter total body water include those that alter drug distribution by increasing (congestive heart failure, patent ductus arteriosus, syndrome of inappropriate antidiuretic hormone secretion) or decreasing (diuretic use) extracellular water.[31,32]

Decreased fat in the newborn, especially preterm and IUGR infants, decreases the apparent Vd for lipophilic drugs.[31,93] Body fat content increases from 1% to 3% at 28 weeks' gestation to 15% to 28% by term, thus increasing the deposition and distribution of lipid-soluble drugs with increased gestational age.[32,93] In addition, neonatal adipose tissue is more than 50% water (versus approximately 25% in adults), further altering tissue distribution of lipid-soluble drugs.[32]

APT-binding cassette (ABC) drug efflux transporters (that prevent specific toxins from crossing the blood brain barrier or moving into hepatic, renal tubular or intestinal cells) appear to have decreased activity in the newborn.[66,95] This may increase central nervous system permeability to drugs, and alter rates of hepatic and renal clearance.[19,66,95,119] Examples of the transporters are P-glycoprotein (P-gp)/multidrug-resistant gene protein (MRP)-1, MRP-2, MRP-3, and breast cancer resistance protein (BCRP).[86,95] P-gp increases rapidly in the first 3 to 6 months and reaches adult levels by 2 years.[95]

Protein binding is lower in the neonate due to decreased concentrations of binding proteins; altered binding affinity, especially in the presence of fetal albumin, which has a poorer binding capacity; and increased levels of nonesterified fatty acids and bilirubin, which compete for protein binding sites.[19] The major drug-binding proteins are albumin, which generally binds acidic drugs, and α1-acid glycoprotein, which along with lipoproteins generally binds basic drugs.[31,105] Levels of both albumin and α1-acid glycoprotein are low in the neonate, reaching adult levels by about 1 year, resulting in increased free drug levels of substances such as theophylline, digoxin, phenytoin, and many analgesic compounds.[7,31,32,93,116]

In addition to lower plasma protein levels, the newborn tends to have fewer binding sites and a lower affinity of these sites for drugs such as phenobarbital, phenytoin, penicillin, and theophylline. As a result, the newborn tends to saturate protein binding sites at lower drug concentrations with increased free drug, longer half-lives, and risk of toxicity.[66,93] However, increased levels of free drug can also lead to lower drug levels because the free drug may be more rapidly eliminated by the kidneys.[32,93] Drugs can also bind to albumin outside the vascular space in sites such as cardiac and skeletal muscle. Newborns tend to have more binding to the myocardium than adults, which can result in an increased volume of distribution for drugs such as digoxin.[31]

Protein binding of drugs may also be reduced by acidosis, free fatty acids, maternal drugs from placental transfer before birth, and indirect bilirubin. Drugs and bilirubin compete with each other for binding sites. Bilirubin is displaced from albumin by sulfonamides, ceftriaxone, and chloral hydrate, leading to increased free indirect bilirubin levels. However, bilirubin is more likely to displace drugs than to be displaced. Drugs that may be displaced from albumin by bilirubin include ampicillin, penicillin, phenobarbital, and phenytoin, leading to higher free drug concentrations of these agents.[93] Other drugs, such as furosemide and indomethacin, if given together, compete against each other for albumin binding sites.[93]

Hepatic Drug Metabolism

Neonates and infants have immature organ systems, especially the lungs (see Chapter 10), kidney (see Chapter 11), and liver (see Chapter 12), which are typical routes for drug excretion. The large surface-to-mass ratio and high metabolic rate of the neonate and infant affect drug metabolism.

Liver enzyme systems necessary for metabolism of many drugs are depressed in the newborn. In the mature liver, oxidation and conjugation result in water-soluble metabolites that are readily excreted into bile. In the fetus, depression of these processes may be an advantage, because lipid-soluble metabolites are more readily transferred across the placenta where they can be handled by the maternal system. The liver smooth endoplasmic reticulum (SER) is the location of many hepatic microsomal enzymes. The neonatal liver has little SER, and activities of many microsomal enzymes are reduced or undetectable at birth, altering drug metabolism.[85] As a result, drug metabolism may be characterized by slower biotransformation and elimination and increased individual variability.[93] The reduced activity of hepatic microsomal enzymes extend the half-life of drugs dependent on them for metabolism and increase the risk of drug intolerance.

Phase I (see Table 7-1) biotransformation reactions are reduced in the fetus and newborn, impairing degradation and increasing half-lives of drugs such as phenytoin, phenobarbital, diazepam, mepivacaine, lidocaine, caffeine, theophylline, phenylbutazone, salicylate, indomethacin, furosemide, and sulfa drugs.[32,86]

Both microsomal enzyme (e.g., CYP450 system, NADPH-cytochrome reductase) and extramicrosomal enzyme (e.g., deaminases, esterases) activity are decreased in the newborn, with a rapid increase in activity over the first few weeks after birth.[32,66] CYP3A7 is predominant at birth, peaking shortly after birth, then decreases to low levels within 1 to 2 weeks.[17,55,56,66,102,108] CYP3A4 activity is low at birth but increases 3-fold in the first 3 months, reaching 20% of adult activity by 1 month and around 70% by 1 year.[7,56,108] CYP2E1 surges within a few hours after birth.[108] Levels of CYP1A1, the isoform responsible for degradation of over half of all drugs in adults, has low activity until 1 to 3 months after birth.[17,31,56] By 2 to 3 weeks of age, liver enzyme systems are maturing at varying rates.[17] Maturation of some enzyme activity may be rapid; other systems mature more slowly. Activity of CYP1A2 and CYP2B6 are minimal at birth and reach 50% of adult activity around a year.[7,56,108] CYPC9 has 20% of adult activity at birth reaching 50% of adult activity by 3 months; CYP2C19 has 30% of adult activity reaching adult activity by 1 year.[7,56,108] Alternative pathways of biotransformation are seen for some drugs in the neonate. For example, methylxanthine metabolism is different in neonates versus adults. In the neonate, theophylline is methylated, some is converted to caffeine, and its clearance is 50% of adults; whereas in adults, theophylline is metabolized to 1,3 dimethyluric acid and other metabolites.[7,31,93,108]

There are marked variations in maturation rates of processes for specific drugs and within individual infants. This increases elimination half-lives and the risk of both underdosing and overdosing.[31,32] Maturation is correlated with both postmenstrual age and postbirth age. For example, midazolam and phenytoin are both metabolized by CYP2C9 and CYP2C19. Midazolam clearance increases up to five-fold from 1 to 3 months; low activity of these enzymes in preterm infants increases bioavailability.[7,14,108] Phenytoin biotransformation increases and half-life decreases in early infancy with a half-life of approximately 75 hours in preterm infants, decreasing to about 20s by term and 8 hours by 2 weeks post term.[7,108]

Phase II reactions (see Table 7-1), particularly glucuronidation, are also altered in the newborn. Glucuronic acid conjugation (via uridine 5′-diphosphatase glucuronosyltransferase or UGT enzymes), needed for metabolism of drugs such as morphine, acetaminophen, phenytoin, sulfonamides, chloramphenicol, salicylic acid, and indomethacin, is reduced at birth and does not reach adult levels until 24 to 30 months.[31] An example of maturation of the ability to metabolize drug via glucuronidation is seen with morphine. Morphine glucuronidation is found in preterm infants by 24 weeks' gestation. Morphine metabolism increases with increasing postmenstrual (PMA), due to maturation of UGT isoforms, so that clearance quadruples from 27 to 40 weeks' PMA, requiring increased dosages for pain management.[53,95] Zidovudine is also metabolized by glucuronidation and its plasma clearance in infants <2 weeks of age is half that of infants over 2 weeks.[108] Acetaminophen is metabolized by UGT1A6 and UGT1A9. These enzymes are low at birth and reach full activity by 9 to 12 months; bioavailability increases with age due to an increased first pass effect and enzyme maturation.[14,108] UGT1A1 is the major enzyme for bilirubin glucuronidation. Variants of this enzyme lead to reduced activity and prolonged neonatal jaundice. Mutations in the gene for this enzyme occur with Criglar-Najjar syndrome.[95]

Chloramphenicol is eliminated by the kidney after conjugation in the liver. The hepatic glucuronyl transferase system responsible for conjugation of this drug is immature in the neonate (especially in preterm infants), and free (unconjugated) chloramphenicol is eliminated by glomerular filtration, which is reduced in neonates. The result is higher and prolonged peak serum chloramphenicol concentrations. Half-life of chloramphenicol is approximately 20 hours in the neonate and longer in preterm infants, falling to about 10 hours by 21 days (versus 4 to 5 hours in adults).[75] This results in increased risk of toxicity ("gray baby syndrome") with aplastic anemia, shock, and cardiovascular collapse.[31,86]

Other phase II reactions (sulfate and glycine conjugation) are somewhat decreased but more similar to those in adults.[93] Methylation reactions may be more important in infants than in adults for drugs such as theophylline.[93] Decreased hydrolysis and increased Vd may prolong the effect of local anesthetic agents. Ligandin (carrier protein Y) needed for hepatocyte uptake of substances including bilirubin and many drugs is low for 5 to 10 days after birth, further altering hepatic clearance of some drugs.

Thus immaturity of liver enzyme systems can delay metabolism and clearance of drugs and increase their serum levels and half-lives. McClary et al. concluded that in terms of drug metabolism and disposition in the neonate:

"1. The rate of drug metabolism is generally low at birth in full-term babies and even lower in premature infants regardless of the specific route of metabolism. Decreased clearance and a prolonged drug half-life require drug administration with longer dosing intervals.

2. Many of the enzymes responsible for metabolism exhibit significant development during the first month of life. Dosing regimens appropriate during the first few days of postnatal life may not be appropriate 3 to 4 weeks after birth because dose requirements may increase and dosing intervals decrease.

3. The development of individual drug-metabolizing enzymes varies widely among neonates and may be delayed in premature infants. Predicting clearance is difficult, and dosing regimens must be individualized for patients based on the careful observation of the patient's response and tolerance; monitoring of plasma drug concentration may be useful for selected drugs."[86,p.727]

Renal Drug Excretion

Because of the decreased hepatic metabolism in neonates, the infant is more reliant on renal elimination. However, renal elimination is reduced compared to adults and correlated with both postmenstrual and postbirth ages. Alterations in renal function in neonates can markedly alter the infant's ability to eliminate drugs and drug metabolites, increasing the half-life and risk of toxic effects and the need for longer dosing intervals. Any pathologic event that alters renal function (e.g., congestive heart failure, respiratory distress syndrome, hypovolemia, ischemia, or hypoxemia) further compromises the ability of the infant to eliminate drugs. In addition, drugs such as indomethacin may decrease glomerular filtration rate (GFR), further impeding excretion.[31] Renal processes involved in drug handling are GFR, tubular secretion, and, to a lesser extent, tubular reabsorption.

The GFR is significantly lower in the neonate than in adults (see Chapter 11), although partially compensated by an increase in tubular reabsorption. The reduced GFR delays clearance of drugs that are eliminated by the kidneys, leading to prolonged half-lives and longer dosing intervals.[62,127] For example, clearance of indomethacin and many aminoglycosides is 10% to 30% lower than in adults. The GFR is particularly low in the first week after birth, increasing susceptibility to nephrotoxic drugs such as aminoglycosides. Plasma half-lives of many drugs used in the neonate—including penicillin, aminoglycosides, methicillin, furosemide, barbiturates, and digoxin—vary inversely with creatinine clearance (which is a measure of GFR).

Renal maturation progresses at variable rates after birth depending on postmenstrual and post birth ages. The most rapid changes in GFR are seen in the first 7 to 10 days after birth.[31] The increased half-life of drugs such as digoxin, vancomycin, and indomethacin correlate with both postmenstrual and postbirth age and may be significantly longer in preterm infants.[62,127] Drug levels must be carefully and regularly monitored. Use of drugs such as vancomycin in combination with indomethacin (which decreases GFR) can further decrease vancomycin elimination.[93] Renal elimination of drugs is further altered in preterm infants who are younger than 34 weeks' gestational age. In these infants, GFR increases at birth, but then tends to plateau or increase slowly until about 34 weeks, when nephron maturation is complete (see Chapter 11). As a result, some antibiotics and other drugs are given less frequently to VLBW infants. Serum half-lives of antibiotics change rapidly over the first few weeks after birth as renal function matures. Therefore dosages of these drugs or dosing intervals may need to be increased.[66] For example, gentamicin dosing intervals range from 24 to 48 hours in more immature infants to every 8 to 12 hours in the term newborn.[31]

Elimination of drugs by tubular secretion is reduced in the neonate for the first 6 months as a result of decreased renal blood flow to the peritubular area, shorter tubular length, decreased energy for carriers, and reduced number of carriers to transport drugs from the blood into the tubule.[62] This affects drugs such as furosemide and penicillin G, which are therefore more dependent on GFR than tubular secretion for clearance during early infancy. In older children and adults, tubular secretion is the most important mechanism for penicillin excretion (versus GFR in neonates). As a result, penicillin clearance is nearly one fifth that of adults, and penicillin blood levels may persist for three times as long. Urine flow rates can also influence elimination of drugs such as chloramphenicol, phenobarbital, and theophylline by decreasing the concentration gradient due to formation of dilute urine or reducing the time for drug diffusion.[62]

SUMMARY

Specific physiologic alterations that influence handling of drugs by the neonate include changes in the Vd, liver and renal function, and protein binding. The functional immaturity of the neonate's body systems alters drug distribution and pharmacokinetics and renders the infant more susceptible to adverse reactions. The ability to metabolize and excrete a given agent varies with postmenstrual age, health status, and postbirth age. Individual infants often have unique responses to drugs, so infants with similar postmenstrual and postbirth ages may vary in their ability to metabolize and excrete a specific drug.

The Vd is altered in the neonate because of the increased total body water and increased proportion of extracellular water. As a result, peak volumes of some drugs are reduced and excretion delayed. Immaturity of liver enzyme systems can delay metabolism and clearance of drugs. The reduced GFR seen in neonates increases serum concentrations and prolongs the half-life of many drugs and may result in longer dosing intervals. Doses of some drugs may be higher per weight in neonates than adults due to an increased Vd, reducing plasma levels. Doses may also need to be altered because of increased or decreased sensitivity of neonatal tissue to some drugs. Digoxin doses are relatively higher in the neonate due to increased Vd and decreased sensitivity of the myocardium to both therapeutic and toxic effects.[116]

Because of these physiologic limitations, serum concentrations and drug dosages of drugs such as aminoglycosides, phenytoin, phenobarbital, digoxin, and theophylline must be carefully monitored. Monitoring of peak and trough levels of drugs such as aminoglycosides (e.g., gentamicin) is particularly important, because levels associated with toxicity are close to therapeutic levels. Peak (highest drug concentration) plasma levels are measured approximately 30 minutes after administration, whereas trough (lowest drug concentration) levels are measured immediately before an ordered dose. If peak levels are not within therapeutic ranges (i.e., subtherapeutic or in the toxic range), the dose should be altered. Trough levels can be used to determine how frequently a drug should be given. Drug doses cannot be determined on infant size alone, but must also take into account postbirth age, maturity, and health status.

CLINICAL IMPLICATIONS FOR THE PREGNANT WOMEN, FETUS, AND NEONATE

Teratogenesis

Embryonic and fetal development can be altered by internal events, external events and teratogens, which result in structural and functional defects. Fetal defects can result from malformation, deformation, or disruption. A malformation is an embryonic alteration in morphogenesis due to an intrinsically abnormal developmental process such as may occur with a chromosome or multifactorial disorder (see Chapter 1).[64] Deformation defects are the abnormal form, shape, or position of a body part arising from extrinsic mechanical forces (e.g., clubfoot due to fetal restraint or lung hypoplasia with congenital diaphragmatic hernia); a disruption is caused by an external force that alters a previously normal tissue (e.g., teratogenic effects or amputation of a fetal part by an amniotic band).[64] Birth defects may be major or minor abnormalities. Minor abnormalities may be normal variations, family traits, or isolated defects, or may provide clues to the presence of internal malformations, genetic disorders, or chromosomal problems. Three or more minor abnormalities are associated with an increased risk for a major birth defect.[64] Information about human teratogens can be found in a variety of on-line and print resources (see Box 7-2 on p. 187).[23-25,30,86,130]

Drugs administered to the mother during pregnancy can affect the fetus in a variety of ways ranging from no effect to major structural or functional deficits. Drugs administered during labor affect the fetus primarily by exaggerating the degree of fetal asphyxia and influencing the rate and quality of infant recovery from birth, adaptation to extrauterine life, and neurobehavioral status. A teratogen is any substance, organism, physical agent, or deficiency state present during gestation that is capable of inducing abnormal postnatal structure or function (biochemical, physiologic, or behavioral) by interfering with normal embryonic and fetal development. Thus many substances can act as teratogens including infectious agents (such as toxoplasmosis, cytomegalovirus, syphilis), ionizing radiation, hyperthermia, pesticides, metal (e.g., mercury and lead), organic solvents, excess or deficient nutrients, effects of maternal chronic disorders (such as diabetes and phenylketonuria), as well as over-the-counter, prescribed, and abused drugs. Some herbal agents are also contraindicated in pregnancy, including those that have the potential to act as abortifacients and/or uterine stimulants (black cohash, chamomile, chasteberry, goldenseal, white horehound, licorice, mistletoe, nettle, pennyroyal, rue, tansy, and yarrow).[33]

Fewer than 30 drugs are proven teratogens and fewer still are in current clinical use.[67,80] Most women exposed to these known teratogens have normal offspring.[80] The FDA categories consider both the potential risks of and benefits from the drug and are based largely on preapproval animal studies.[100] The category is assigned via structured regulatory process and negotiation with drug sponsors and is not meant to provide estimates of teratogenic risk, although the information is widely used that way in clinical practice.[30,40,80,87] There have been efforts in recent years to revise these categories for pregnancy labeling. One proposal is that the revised categories address clinical considerations, summarize risk assessment, and provide data to support this assessment.[109] Very few drugs are classified as FDA category A or B or as X (contraindicated during pregnancy). Category X drugs include thalidomide, isotretinoin, acitretin, radioactive iodine, oral contraceptives, and diethylstilbesterol.[24] Most drugs are in category C (risk cannot be determined).[87] Category D drugs are those for which there are known risks but there may be no safer alternative and the risks outweigh the potential benefits. Examples of drugs in category D include paroxetine, angiotensin converting enzyme inhibitors (captopril, enalapril, and lisinopril), valproic acid, phenytoin, carbamazepine, diazepam, carbimazole, and lithium.[24]

Lo and Friedman examined 468 drugs approved by the Food and Drug Administration between 1980 and 2000.[80] The teratogenic risk was undetermined in 91.2%. Eleven drugs (2.4%) were demonstrated to pose "some" to "high" teratogenic risk, with a mean of 6 years (SD ± 4.1) to determine risk. Only 30 drugs (6.1%) were proven to pose no risk, with a mean of 9 years to recognize apparent safety of these drugs in literature (the longer time was probably due to the fact that studies showing no risk are often not published).[80] Lo and Friedman also found poor agreement between TERIS risk rating and the FDA pregnancy categories (A, B, C, D, X) for 163 drugs. TERIS is a teratogenic resource complied via consensus of teratology experts based on published data and does not consider potential risk and benefit to the mother. Recently this group examined 172 drugs approved by the FDA between 2000 and 2008 using the TERIS risk rating system (data were rated by an expert advisory panel).[1] They found that 168 (97.7%) of these drugs had "undetermined" teratogenic risk and 126 (73.3%) had no data available regarding safety during pregnancy. The authors also relooked at the 468 drugs from the earlier 1980-2000 study to see if the risk had been revised in the past 10 years.[80] Twenty-three drugs (5%) had a change in risk category (some from unknown to risk; some from unknown to no risk). The mean time for drugs classed as undetermined risk to having a more precise risk assignment was 27 years.[1]

Teratogenesis is often difficult to prove. To detect a defect due to a specific agent, an increase in a specific anomaly or group of anomalies over what would be expected by chance must be documented. Thalidomide was recognized as a teratogen sooner than some other agents because it produced significant malformations, with small doses given once or twice in early pregnancy with a malformation rate of 20% to 30%.[70] Documentation of teratogenesis is often difficult to do in a single location, especially with rare anomalies. Koren and colleagues note the following:

"Most congenital malformations occur rarely, and many teratogens, even when known to be associated with an increased risk of a given malformation, do not affect the great majority of exposed fetuses. In fact, very few drugs increase the malformation rate by a factor of more than two (isotretinoin and thalidomide are two such drugs). If, for example, the risk of malformations in a given population is 3%, then at least 220 pregnancies with a specific exposure and a similar number of control pregnancies will be required to show a risk that is increased by a factor of 2.5 with a power of 80%."[70, p. 1133]

Other common methodologic issues in establishing teratogenesis, in addition to sample size, are recall bias in retrospective studies, use of nonrandomized observational studies, limitations in voluntary reporting, issues in choosing the right animal model, and the effects of maternal disease.[22,37,70,100,131] An example of the difficulty with recall bias occurred with Bendectin in which women whose infants had defects recalled taking this drug, which was commonly used, in early pregnancy. Subsequent studies did not confirm a link between Bendectin and malformations.[11,94] Maternal pharmacologic therapy may be administered for an illness that itself leads to a defect or malformations or may produce maternal symptoms requiring treatment with a specific drug; several agents may interact with each other so that the combination is teratogenic rather than either individual drug; or the mother may be taking multiple drugs for different problems.[70] Problems with human studies include difficulty studying cause and effect, lack of random sampling, lack of control over dosing and timing, and expense.

Animal studies can also be problematic. Drug studies with animals may involve administration of large doses that exceed the usual therapeutic dose in humans. Selecting the appropriate animal model can be difficult. Drug kinetics and metabolism may differ between different species and between humans and animals.[22,70] For example, thalidomide, a potent teratogen in humans, did not produce limb reduction anomalies in the animal models used to study the drug before its release; subsequently, similar anomalies were seen in macaque monkeys. On the other hand, benzodiazepines cause oral clefts in some animal models but not in humans given clinically appropriate doses. Similarly, salicylates cause cardiac defects in some animal species but not humans. Most human teratogens have been discovered by either epidemiology studies or by health care professionals, not animal studies.[22] Dicke noted, "We will never be in a position to state that an environmental agent has no teratogenic potential. The most we can say is that an agent poses no measurable risk."[38]

Principles of Teratogenesis

General principles that govern the action of teratogens include the following:

1. *Susceptibility to a teratogenic agent is dependent upon the genotype of the embryo and the manner in which the agent interacts with environmental factors.*[38,133] The genetic makeup of the developing embryo is the environmental programmer to which the teratogenic agent is introduced. This programming means that the genes and extrinsic factors interact in varying degrees with varied responses in different individuals and species. Because individual sensitivity is dependent upon the biochemical and morphologic makeup of that particular individual, data from animal models and sometimes even from studies on other individuals cannot always be applied. For example, individuals with a gene mutation that reduces levels of an enzyme needed to detoxify anticonvulsant drugs such as phenytoin are at greater risk of having a child with defects.[30]
2. *Susceptibility to teratogenic agents is dependent on the timing of the exposure and the developmental stage of the embryo.*[38,89,133] A basic precept of biology is that the more immature an organism is, the more susceptible that organism is to change.[133] This suggests that there is a critical period where teratogenic events have the greatest impact. The period of greatest susceptibility is during the first trimester, when cell differentiation and organogenesis are occurring. Structural and functional maturation continues after birth, and therefore many systems remain susceptible to alterations in later development. Sometimes the specific period of vulnerability can be identified. For example, the hypoplastic limb defects seen with thalidomide occur only with exposure at 21 to 36 days after fertilization; valproic acid exposure results in a neural tube defect only with exposure between 14 and 27 days.[87,117]

The most likely period for structural defects to occur is during organogenesis, because exposure of the embryo to a teratogenic agent either during or before a critical stage in development of that organ can lead to anomalies.[29,90] The time of greatest susceptibility during development is defined as the time when the highest incidence of defects occurs (usually gross anatomic defects). Other defects, especially neurobehavioral and other functional defects, have peaks in sensitivity at different times during development. These periods of sensitivity vary depending on the timing and duration of the period of cell proliferation (e.g., brain growth and development extend into early childhood and thus are vulnerable for a longer period of time).[90,133]

Malformations resulting from incomplete morphogenesis within an organ usually originate before organ structure is complete. The exact time at which a specific defect occurs cannot be determined; it can be said only that a defect occurred at some time before a particular point. For example, anencephaly must occur before closure of the anterior neural tube (25 to 26 days); meningomyelocele before closure of the posterior neural tube (27 to 28 days); cleft palate before fusion of the maxillary palatal shelves (10 weeks); cleft lip before closure of the lip (36 days); tracheoesophageal fistula before separation of the foregut into the trachea and primitive esophagus (30 days); ventricular septal defect before closure of the ventricular septum (6 weeks); transposition of the great vessels before development of the aorticopulmonary septum (34 days); diaphragmatic hernia before closure of the pleuroperitoneal canal (6 weeks); omphalocele before or during return of the gut to the abdomen (10 to 10.5 weeks); and imperforate anus before perforation of the anal membrane (8 weeks).

3. *Teratogenic agents act in specific ways on cells or tissues to cause pathogenesis.*[38,133] Unfavorable factors within the environment are able to trigger changes in developing cells that alter their subsequent development. These changes are not specific to the type of causative factor, and initial changes may result in a variety of alterations within the embryo. These early changes may not be discernible because they occur subcellularly at the molecular level. Pathogenesis is the visible sign of cellular damage and may occur from cell necrosis or by secondary interference with cellular interactions—that is, by induction, adhesion, and migration; reduced biosynthesis of macromolecules; or accumulation of foreign materials, fluids, or blood.[38,133]
4. *The final manifestations of abnormal development are death, malformation, growth restriction, and functional disorders.*[38,133] For the early embryo a teratogenic event will most likely result in death. Once organogenesis begins, teratogenic events lead to malformation in the organs or organ systems. The teratogenic insult might also make the embryo more susceptible to death or general cell necrosis, resulting in a reduced cell mass and slower overall rate of growth. Functional defects may be diagnosed throughout infancy and childhood.

Before conception, damage can occur to the chromosomes of one or both parents, or new gene mutations may arise. Alterations in spermatogenesis; in seminal fluid or sperm transport in the male; or in oogenesis or the environment of the vagina, cervix, or uterus of the female may also alter development.[124]

The preembryonic stage (conception to 14 days) is a time of little morphologic differentiation in specific organ systems. Exposure to teratogens during this period usually has an all-or-nothing effect; that is, either the damage is so severe that the zygote is aborted or there are no apparent effects.[24,87,109] However, this may be the time that syndromes affecting multiple organ systems arise. Teratogens or environmental disturbances may interfere with implantation of the blastocyst or cause death and early abortion. However, most congenital anomalies probably do not arise during this period, possibly due to the lack of cell differentiation, at least in the early part of this period. Many cells within the inner cell mass are not yet programmed to become specific structures. Thus damage to a few cells does not alter development if the preembryo is able to produce sufficient cells to restore the lost volume.[133] If a teratogen is potent or the dosage is high, the effect is death or possibly mitotic disjunction during cleavage, with chromosomal alterations that subsequently cause malformation syndromes rather than local defects.[64,107] If only a few cells are damaged, development continues, although the genetically programmed schedule may be delayed.[90]

The period of organogenesis (15 to 60 days after conception) is a period of extreme sensitivity to teratogens; it is the period when many congenital malformations develop. Insults early in this period (15 to 30 days) are likely to result in death if the embryo is damaged. Early events in organ formation are generally most sensitive to external forces, although in some systems (e.g., the sensory organs), critical periods occur during relatively late stages. The more specialized the metabolic requirements of a group of cells, the more sensitive they are to deprivation and damage.[90,107,133]

From 11 weeks to term, the fetus becomes increasingly resistant to structural damage from toxic agents as the ability to produce major structural deviations is reduced as organ systems become organized. Thus once the definitive form and relationships within a system are established, gross anatomic defects are no longer possible. However, histogenesis continues and the function of organ systems can still be altered.[90,133] Defects can occur at the microscopic level, or neurobehavioral or other functional abilities can be altered, resulting in physiologic defects and delayed growth. Insults during fetal life can lead to dysfunction such as brain damage or deafness, prematurity, growth restriction, stillbirth, infant death, or malignancy.

5. *Access to the embryo by environmental teratogens depends on the nature of the agent.*[38,133] There are several routes by which agents reach the embryo or fetus. Agents such as ultrasound, ionizing radiation, and microwaves pass directly through maternal tissue without modification. Chemical agents or their metabolites reach developing tissues indirectly via transmission across the placenta. Whether these agents reach toxic or teratogenic concentrations depends on maternal dosage, rate of absorption, and maternal homeostatic capabilities as well as physical properties of the agent and the placenta. Pathogenic organisms may also reach the fetus by an ascending route via the vaginal canal and cervix.
6. *As the dosage increases, manifestations of deviant development increase.*[38,133] There appears to be a threshold at which embryotoxicity occurs and damage is initiated. When the effect threshold is exceeded, cell damage or death exceeds restoration. For example, diagnostic x-rays with a dose lower than 5 rads (dosage for most common

procedures) is not thought to have teratogenic effects. Exposure to 5 to 10 rads is of concern, whereas exposure to more than 10 rads (e.g., with radiation therapy) is associated with significant risk.[30] Valproic acid increases the risk of neural tube defects and the risk increases with increased dosage levels.[30] Sometimes the specific threshold cannot be determined, as is the case with alcohol. Different types of embryotoxicity exist for different thresholds.

A given teratogenic effect may be induced by a variety of agents. For example, a specific defect may result from infection, drugs, genetic alteration, an environmental toxin, or a combination of these factors.[38,133]

Mechanisms of Teratogenesis

Proposed mechanisms of teratogenesis include the following:

1. *Gene mutation.* Mutation is the basis of heritable developmental defects and is the result of a change in the sequence of nucleotides. If the change appears in the germinal cell line (i.e., oocytes and spermatocytes), it is likely to be heritable. A mutation in a somatic cell will be passed to daughter somatic cells but cannot be transferred to the next generation. Gene mutations can result in biochemical or structural disorders or later development of malignancies (see Chapter 1).[133]
2. *Chromosome breaks and nondisjunction.* These alterations lead to excesses, deficiencies, or rearrangements of chromosomes or parts of chromosomes and can be transmitted to offspring. For example, sperm of men exposed to radiation or chemotherapy have increased numbers of chromosomal aberrations for at least 3 to 4 months (chemotherapy) to up to 36 months (ionizing radiation).[124]
3. *Mitotic interference and cell death.* Interference with mitosis can result from inhibition of deoxyribonucleic acid (DNA) synthesis, prevention of spindle formation, or failure of chromosome separation. For example, aminopterin and methotrexate inhibit an enzyme needed during the cell cycle (see Chapter 1), leading to cell death during the S (DNA synthesis) phase.[30] Viruses and other infectious agents may also interfere with mitosis.
4. *Altered nucleic acid integrity or function.* These alterations occur secondary to biochemical changes that interfere with nucleic acid replication, transcription, natural base incorporation, or ribonucleic acid (RNA) translation and protein synthesis. Because processes such as protein synthesis are essential for survival of the embryo, interference usually results in death rather than malformation. Diethylstilbestrol (DES) acts on estrogen-responsive tissue by altering RNA, protein, and DNA synthesis with development of columnar epithelium not normally found in the vaginal area. This "foreign" tissue is at risk for later malignant degeneration.[30]
5. *Lack or excess of precursors, substrates, or coenzymes needed for biosynthesis.* These deficiencies result in slowed or altered growth and differentiation and occur because of dietary deficiencies, placental transfer failure, maternal absorption failure, or the presence of specific analogues or antagonists. Some agents, such as amphetamines, cocaine, cannabis, and nicotine, may occupy receptors for nutrient, thus decreasing transfer of critical substances and altering fetal growth and development.[44] Retinoic acid regulates expression of one of the developmental genes involved in craniofacial and axial skeleton development. Excess levels—as occurs with isotretinoin—leads to malformations in these systems. Coumadin inhibits formation of substances needed for proteins to bind to calcium and can alter bone ossification with craniofacial and other skeletal anomalies.[30]
6. *Altered energy sources.* As a result of interference with energy pathways (glucose sources, glycolysis, citric acid cycle, terminal electron transport systems), the energy needs of the rapidly proliferating and synthesizing tissues of the embryo are not met. For example, biotin deficiency—seen with an inborn error of metabolism—decreases activity of a mitochondrial biotin-dependent enzyme.[30]
7. *Enzyme and growth factor inhibitions.* Inhibition of critical enzymes interferes with cell functioning, cellular repair, differentiation, and growth. Inadequate folic acid increases the risk of neural tube defects, especially if the deficiency occurs in women with an enzyme defect in folic acid metabolism. Thalidomide may inhibit angiogenesis and thus limb growth by decreasing critical growth factors such as insulin-like growth factor-I and fibroblast growth factor.[117] Inhibition of alcohol dehydrogenases, needed to detoxify alcohol, alters retinoic acid metabolism similarly to the action of isotretinoin (which also leads to craniofacial and skeletal defects).[30]
8. *Osmolar imbalance.* These imbalances lead to pathogenesis by causing edema that impinges upon the embryo.[133]
9. *Altered membrane characteristics.* These changes can result in abnormal membrane permeability and lead to osmolar imbalances and edema.[133]
10. *Altered cell and neuronal migration or CNS organization.* These processes are influenced by neurotransmitters, especially monoamines (dopamine, serotonin, and norepinephrine). Inborn errors of metabolism—especially those involved with amino acid metabolism—alter CNS organization. Drugs, such as cocaine, that increase or reduce levels of neurotransmitters may alter migration or later organization of cortical neurons (see Chapter 15).[133]

Specific proposed teratogenic mechanisms associated with drugs are folate antagonism, oxidative stress, angiotensin-converting enzyme inhibition, angiotensin II receptor antagonism, cyclooygenase-1 and -2 inhibition, 5-hydroxytryptamine-reuptake inhibition, and placental drug transporters.[132]

Effects of Drug Exposure in Utero

The fetus is a passive recipient of all drugs entering the mother's system. Drug use in pregnancy is common. From laxatives and antacids to cocaine and heroin, all of these substances are chemicals that may have an effect on the fetus and newborn. Medications are not "approved" for use in pregnancy; rather, medications are "presumed safe" for use in pregnancy. Some classes of drugs are more significant to CNS development and function after birth than are others. Examples of drugs known to produce significant effects are ethanol, tobacco smoke, narcotics, amphetamines, and cocaine.

Cigarette Smoking

Smoking during pregnancy and its metabolites are "one of the leading preventable causes of adverse maternal and fetal outcomes."[92,p.75] Cigarette smoke contains many chemicals. Nicotine a particularly important in adverse pregnancy outcomes.[18,92] Nicotine and cotinine readily cross the placenta with fetal levels often exceeding maternal levels.[92] Animal data suggest that one mechanism by which nicotine may influence offspring is by binding to cholinergic receptors, leading to premature onset of cell differentiation and disrupting cell replication.[92,115]

The effects of smoking include an increased risk of low birth weight and prematurity.[11,18,21,30,92] Smoking increases pregnancy and placental complications (e.g., ectopic pregnancy, placental abruption, and miscarriage) and may alter fertility in both female and males.[30,92] Nicotine exposure increases the risk of altered cognitive and learning skills, sudden infant death syndrome, and altered respiratory function and increased respiratory infections.[92] Chronic exposure to secondhand smoke also reduces fetal growth and increases the risk of low birth weight. The effects of smoking on birth weight and other effects are dose-dependent so that the fewer cigarettes a woman smokes, the less likely her infant will be affected.[30]

Alcohol

Ethanol is one of the most common abused drugs during pregnancy with specific teratogenic effects of fetal alcohol syndrome seen in 0.5 to 2/1000 births.[130] Infants who were exposed to alcohol in utero are at increased risk for a range of alcohol-related damage including fetal alcohol syndrome (FAS) and other forms of alcohol-related damage.[13,65,81] These differential effects may be due in part to variations in the metabolism of alcohol in the placenta by CYP2E1 and alcohol dehydrogenases.[129] Diagnosis of FAS requires the presence of prenatal or postnatal growth restriction, CNS involvement, and specific craniofacial features. Other forms of alcohol-related damage seen in infants of women with a history of substantial alcohol intake during pregnancy include physical defects (e.g., congenital heart defects) without the characteristic facial features or mental and behavioral abnormalities without defects or facial features.[65]

Damage from ethanol may be due to chromosomal damage or acetyldehydrate (the placenta deoxidizes ethanol to this substance), which reaches 50% of maternal levels. Acetyldehydrate effects cell membranes and cell migration altering embryonic tissue organization with dysmorphic changes.[43] Alcohol interferes with transport of amino acids across the placenta and incorporation into proteins. This may limit the number of fetal cells and lead to fetal growth restriction.[43] Decreased placental transfer of linoleic and docosahexanoic acid may also alter fetal growth and development.[129]

No level of drinking alcohol has been proven safe in that drinking alcohol at any stage of pregnancy can affect the brain and other areas of development.[43] Current studies do not support identifying a "safe level" of alcohol consumption by pregnant women. FAS usually occurs in offspring of chronic alcohol abusers, although it has occurred in women who drink less. Mild to moderate alcohol consumption during pregnancy has been associated with a range of later neurobehavioral effects, although the effects of moderate and light drinking are not yet well understood.[21]

Opiods

The fetus is not immune from developing chemical dependency. Neonatal abstinence syndrome (NAS) refers to particular withdrawal behaviors (CNS hypersensitivity, respiratory distress, autonomic dysfunction, and GI disturbances) observed in neonates exposed to dependency-producing drugs in utero.[67] NAS is seen most commonly with maternal heroin or methadone use, but can also occur with drugs such as oxycodone, hydrocodone, and codeine. The timing and severity of withdrawal are based on the type of drug, the mother's drug dosage, the length of time since the mother's last dose, the duration of exposure, the neonate's degree of immaturity, and the neonate's general health status. Symptoms usually appear within 72 hours after birth but can be seen as late as 2 to 4 weeks of age. The neonate's withdrawal responses may last from 6 days to 8 weeks.

Methadone has a long elimination half-life, which minimizes fluctuations in maternal serum levels and the risk of drug withdrawal in the fetus, reduces infant morbidity and mortality, and leads to less fetal growth restriction.[11] Withdrawal symptoms may be more frequent and severe in infants exposed to methadone, possibly because methadone accumulates in fat tissue and is released slowly. Until the late 1990s, the widespread recommendation was to reduce a pregnant woman's daily methadone intake to $\leq$20 mg/day in order to prevent NAS, however, the pregnant woman's volume of distribution is increased so many women need higher doses to prevent withdrawal.[11,34] Buprenorphine is a potent long acting (72 h) synthetic opioid with partial mu-receptor agonist and κappa-receptor antagonist properties that is being used with increased frequency as an alternative to methadone for the treatment of opiate-dependency. A recent multicenter international double-blinded study comparing buprenorphine with methadone treatment (n = 191) reported that neonates from mothers in the buprenorphine group required significantly less morphine, shorter hospital stay, and shorter duration of treatment for NAS. No significant differences were reported between groups in other outcomes or in rates of adverse events.[63]

The responses to drug withdrawal in the neonate are similar to those in the adult, but because of the nature of neurologic organization, the implications are more severe in neonates.

NAS includes both physiologic and behavioral responses. Several scales have been developed to aid observation and measurement of the responses to neonatal abstinence. Interventions are initiated based on the severity of withdrawal as assessed by these scales. Withdrawal may be treated pharmacologically with drugs such as phenobarbital and morphine.[67]

Cocaine and Amphetamines

Cocaine, amphetamine, and methamphetamine are central and peripheral stimulants that produces their effects by interfering with the reuptake of monoamines such as dopamine, norepinephrine, and serotonin at presynaptic adrenergic nerve terminals, thus increasing levels of these neurotransmitters at the neuronal junction (these transporters are inhibited by many antidepressants such as selective serotonin receptor reuptake inhibitors).[2,11,45,48,134] The excess monoamines result in prolonged neuronal activation, leading to characteristic neurobehavioral responses (due to binding to central receptors) and cardiovascular and motor effects (due to binding to peripheral receptors located in tissues innervated by the sympathetic nervous system).[9] Monoamines have a trophic role in CNS cell proliferation, neural migration, and organization. Thus exposure to elevated levels of monoamines may alter CNS organization, increasing the risk for later alterations in arousal and attention. Serotonin and norepinephrine receptors are found on the maternal facing side of the placental syncytium. Inhibition increases serotonin and norepinephrine in the intervillous space, which may lead to uterine contractions, vasoconstriction, and decreased placental blood flow, thus increasing the risk of preterm labor and fetal growth restriction.[11,45,50,61]

The actions of cocaine and amphetamines are similar, causing intense sympathetic nervous system activity. Cocaine produces vasoconstriction, tachycardia, and elevation of blood pressure in addition to a sense of excitement and euphoria. Cocaine is lipid-soluble, easily crossing the placenta. In the fetus, it produces increased motor activity and tachycardia; cocaine crosses the fetal blood-brain barrier. Cocaine competes with nutrients for monoamine transporters in the placenta.[44] By successfully competing with nutrients for these transporters, cocaine reduces nutrient transfer, which can lead to fetal growth restriction. Levels of cocaine are high in amniotic fluid, resulting in a reservoir that prolongs fetal exposure.

Vasoconstrictive effects with reduction in placental blood flow to the placenta are associated with a high incidence of placental abruption.[50] Blood flow to the fetus through the placenta is also reduced. In addition, the umbilical arteries constrict in response to cocaine. The resultant placental ischemia has been attributed as the cause of low birth weight, decreased body length, and smaller head circumference found among infants of cocaine-abusing mothers. Cocaine also increases uterine irritability and results in contractions. Cocaine may have teratogenic effects via damage to developing tissue either by vascular disruption and placental vascular insufficiency or production of reactive oxygen species during biotransformation of cocaine in the liver by P450 enzymes.[9] Cocaine may cause cerebral infarcts in the fetus. Cocaine use during pregnancy also poses risks to the mother, including an increased risk of stroke, seizure, and uterine rupture.[113]

After birth, cocaine does not produce withdrawal behaviors, per se, but its effect appears to be related to an alteration of neurobehavioral organization that probably results from its direct influence on the developing brain. Neonates exposed to cocaine in utero are irritable, tremulous, and difficult to soothe and have rapid respiratory and heart rates; these infants exhibit excessive motor activity, altered sleep-wake patterns, poor feeding and feeding intolerance, and diarrhea.[9,12,61] No increase in anomalies has been found in recent studies.[77] Later outcomes of prenatal cocaine exposure include catch-up growth by 1-2 years in many but not all studies and an increased risk of behavior, attention, language development, information processing alterations in many studies of 4- to 14-year-olds.[61,77] Outcomes are related to cumulative effects of cocaine, environment and possibly alcohol or other drug use.[77]

The half-life of cocaine is longer in the fetus and neonate than in the adult since the enzyme systems governing the drug's metabolism are not mature; thus cocaine may persist in the neonate for several days after birth. Cocaine passes easily into breast milk; active use of cocaine by a lactating mother may produce severe reactions and possibly death in the neonate. Cocaine has been found in breast milk as late as 36 hours after maternal use.

Neonatal symptoms from methamphetamine exposure are similar to those with cocaine, with neurobehavioral alterations (decreased arousal, increased stress, altered movements) reported.[61,77] Animal and human studies demonstrate an increased risk of adverse pregnancy outcome with isolated anomalies reported.[61] These infants are at increased risk of fetal distress, placental abruption, preterm birth, and a 2.5 fold increased risk of fetal growth restriction.[61,129] Children usually achieve catch up growth by 2 years, depending on environment.[77] While few studies have been done on older children, available studies suggest similar findings to cocaine exposure.[77]

Drugs and Lactation

The majority of breastfeeding women take at least one drug during lactation.[51,118] Many pharmacologic agents and environmental pollutants (as well as alcohol, nicotine, and other abused drugs) can be found in human milk, although usually at levels lower than those in the mother. Drugs cross into breast milk across the milk-blood barrier via the following mechanisms: (1) transcellular diffusion of low molecular weight (<100 to 200 daltons), nonionized, lipid soluble substances such as ethanol, which are pulled across by water flow; (2) intercellular movement of large molecules through spaces between alveolar cells; (3) passive diffusion across a concentration gradient; (4) carrier mediated diffusion of polar substances; and (5) active movement via specific drug transporters.[15,111] A few drugs—nitrofurantoin, acyclovir, ranitidine, and iodine—are actively transported across the blood-milk barrier into human milk by influx transporters.[51]

Often, breastfeeding is interrupted or discontinued for maternal therapy even though there are relatively few maternal medications that are not compatible with breastfeeding.[39,41] Even if the mother is on drugs with potential risks, careful monitoring and strategies to minimize infants' exposure can be often used so that the mother can decide to continue breastfeeding if she chooses. In general, serious side effects in infants are uncommon.

The use of any pharmacologic agent in the breastfeeding woman should be carefully evaluated. Most drugs enter breast milk in some quantity, although few drugs are contraindicated during lactation.[24] Often little is known about side effects of less commonly used agents. Some drugs should be used with caution and only as absolutely needed in the lactating woman, with careful monitoring of both infant and mother. The nurse and the mother should be aware of potential hazards of any drug, for both mother and infant. There are many reviews of drugs used during breastfeeding and concerns or potential hazards of specific agents[3,4,23-25,33,41,51,52,59,87] as well as textbooks and online sites (see Box 7-2 on p. 187).

Drugs taken by a nursing mother reach infants in much smaller amounts through breast milk than drugs from the pregnant woman reach the fetus across the placenta.[62,111] Figure 7-4 illustrates transfer of milk from mother to infant. Drugs from the pregnant woman to the fetus move directly from maternal blood to fetal blood, whereas drugs from the nursing mother to infant pass from mother's blood into milk and then to the infant's gut. In the infant's gut, the drug may be destroyed or absorption reduced due to limitations in GI absorption in infants, especially in the early months. In addition, there are more tissue layers between maternal blood and milk than between maternal and fetal blood across the placenta. This increases the diffusing distance and reduces the efficiency of transfer. Calculated doses of maternal drug received by the infant are generally significantly less than the standard therapeutic doses tolerated by infants without toxicity for most drugs.[111] Therefore, some drugs that are not recommended during pregnancy may pose little risk during lactation.

Factors influencing the amount and rapidity of drug excretion into milk include drug dosage and duration; route of administration; drug physicochemical characteristics; blood level in maternal circulation; oral bioavailability; protein binding in maternal circulation; maternal physiology and drug handling; blood-milk barrier (Figure 7-4); and infant physiology, drug handling, and maturity (see Table 7-7). Other infant factors to consider include the age of the infant, drug oral bioavailability, amount of milk intake, and the record of the drug's use as a therapeutic agent in infants.[15,51,75,86,123] Characteristics of drugs most likely to cross into milk are agents that are lipid-soluble, have low molecular weight (MW), have a long half-life in the mother, have low protein binding, are given to the mother in large doses, or are used for chronic conditions or are used long term so that plasma levels are maintained at steady-state conditions.[5,51,81,86]

Infant drug exposure can be calculated by the milk-to-plasma ratio of a drug, percentage of maternal dose, infant dosage (drug concentration in milk times the volume of milk ingested), and estimated infant serum concentration (using oral bioavailability/clearance in the infants).[82] The milk-to-plasma (M/P) ratio is the most common index and ranges from 0.01 to 6.5 (averaging 0.5 to 1 for most drugs used during lactation).[10,74] This value may be calculated as a single value, but the M/PAUC (where AUC is the area under the curve), which is based on concentration time curves, provides a better estimate of the ratio over a dosing interval. Highly lipid-soluble and water-soluble substances with MW lower than 200 daltons generally have an M/P ratio near 1. High M/P ratios (greater than 1) are seen with weak bases and actively transported substances; a low M/P ratio (less than 1) is generally found with drugs that are weak acids or highly protein bound substances.[75] Drugs with a low (less than 1) M/P ratio and high maternal and infant clearance rates generally have low risk of infant side effects.[39] M/P and M/PAUC ratios are available in several resources.[10,15,52,74]

Most drugs cross by passive or facilitated diffusion from higher to lower concentrations between maternal plasma and milk.[51] Some low MW drugs may also cross via membrane pores, while other substances such as immunoglobulins may pass between alveolar cells.[111] The blood-milk barrier consists of the maternal capillary epithelium, mammary alveolar cell membrane, intracellular structures (including protein micelles and lipid vesicles), and the apical membrane of the mammary alveolar cell (Figure 7-5). The alveolar cell is a lipid barrier that reduces transfer of water-soluble and ionized drugs.[15] Therefore, lipid-soluble drugs cross into milk more readily than water-soluble drugs, although this is somewhat

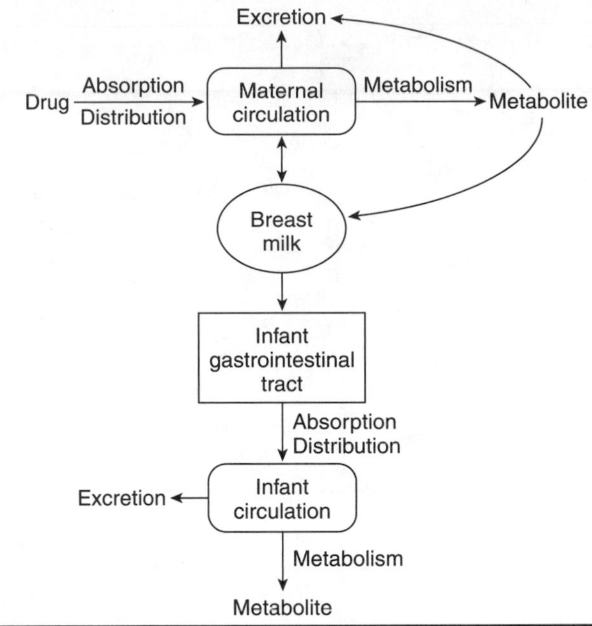

FIGURE 7-4 Steps involved in transfer of drugs from lactating mothers to nursing infants via breast milk. (From Reider, M.J. [1998]. Drug excretion during lactation. In R.A. Polin, W.W. Fox, & S.H. Abman [Eds.]. *Fetal and neonatal physiology* [3rd ed.]. Philadelphia: Saunders.)

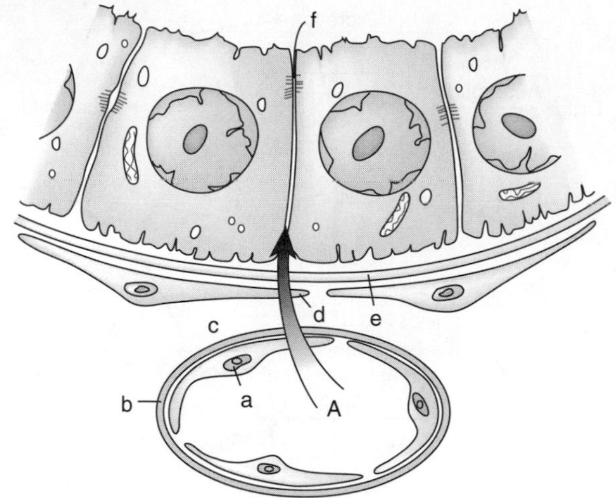

FIGURE 7-5 Milk-blood barrier of mammary gland alveolus. The arrow *(A)* shows passive diffusion of material in lumen of blood vessel into lumen of alveolus. All nonionized molecules must cross the endothelial cell of the blood vessels *(a)*, basement membrane of blood vessel *(b)*, interstitial breast space *(c)*, myoepithelial cell of alveolus *(d)*, basement membrane alveolus *(e)*, and intraalveolar space *(f)*. (From George, D.I. & O'Toole, T.J. [1983]. A review of drug transfer to the infant by breast-feeding: Concerns for the dentist. *J Am Dent Assoc, 106,* 204. Copyright © 1983 American Dental Association. All rights reserved.)

influenced by MW. Concentration of drugs in milk may change with time from birth or during a feeding. For example, drugs such as diazepam and phenobarbital that are highly lipid-soluble may be more concentrated in hindmilk, which has four to five times greater lipid content than foremilk.[10,51] Lipid content is higher in mature milk versus colostrum; thus concentrations of lipid-soluble drugs may be reduced initially after birth.[82] Efflux transporters such a P-gp may transport some substances out of milk back to maternal plasma.[51]

Low MW substances such as ethanol rapidly diffuse across the tissue layers between maternal blood and milk. Water-soluble drugs with an MW of less than 200 daltons can move across the blood-milk barrier via water-filled membrane pores.[82] Molecules greater than 200 daltons cannot pass through these pores and are transferred more slowly because they must first dissolve in the outer lipid membrane of the alveolar cell, diffuse across the cell, then dissolve in the apical membrane to reach milk. Substances with MWs larger than 800 daltons, such as insulin and heparin, generally do not cross into milk or do so very minimally.[51,75] Larger substances may cross in the first 4 to 10 days after delivery due to larger gaps between alveolar cells during this time.[37,87,98,111]

The major milk protein (α-lactalbumin) does not significantly bind drugs. One of the main serum drug-binding proteins (α1 acid-glycoprotein) is not present in milk. Therefore the major milk drug-binding proteins are albumin and lactoferrin, which have markedly decreased binding compared to plasma proteins. Drugs that are highly bound in maternal blood (such as warfarin which is 99% bound) are less likely to cross, because plasma levels of free drug are lower. If a drug is at least 85% bound in maternal blood, measureable concentrations of the drug are unlikely to be found in the infant.[5] Conversely a drug such as lithium which has no protein binding and a low MW can reach high levels in milk.[5] Free drug levels may be increased in the mother in the first 5 to 7 weeks postpartum as the lower albumin levels of pregnancy gradually return to nonpregnant values.[82]

Milk pH (mean of 7.08 with a range of 6.35 to 7.35) is lower than blood pH.[111] Weak acids are highly ionized in maternal plasma and less likely to cross into milk. However, weak bases (e.g., erythromycin, iodides, antihistamines, barbiturates) tend to be transferred and are at equal or higher concentrations in milk than in maternal plasma.[82] Colostrum has a mean pH of 7.45, so it is more likely to have higher levels of basic drugs than mature milk.[111] Ion trapping may occur in milk. Weak bases are generally nonionized and readily cross into milk. As these drugs encounter the low milk pH, they become ionized. This creates a gradient toward movement of more of the drug into milk and reduces the ability of the drug to return across the blood-milk barrier to maternal blood.[15,51,82] Drugs with a pKa greater than 7.2 are most likely to be sequestered in milk.[51]

Steady-state concentrations of drugs in the infant are influenced by drug oral bioavailability, dose, and infant clearance. Drugs given to the mother via methods other than oral administration often have a low oral bioavailability. Drugs with high oral bioavailability may be sequestered in milk at high levels. Drugs with low oral bioavailability have only minimal milk transfer.[51,82] This reduces infant exposure since the infant receives these drugs via milk into the gut. The amount of drugs reaching the nursing infant is also influenced by non–steady-state conditions. Milk is supplied on a continuous basis during sucking, so milk drug concentrations at time of feeding tend to reflect maternal plasma levels at that time. Concentrations of drugs in milk (including most narcotics) are independent of volume of milk.

Drugs may also affect lactation via either central or peripheral mechanisms to increase or reduce milk output.[39,51,111] Central mechanisms include increased or decreased oxytocin, prolactin, or CNS dopamine release. Increased dopamine depresses prolactin. Peripheral mechanisms act directly on the breast to alter milk production. Exogenous substances that increase milk production include thyrotropin-releasing hormone, domperidone, metoclopramide, and psychotropic agents such as reserpine, imipramine, and phenothiazine derivatives that interfere with dopamine release.[39,51] Nicotine, estrogens, and possibly pseudoephedrine may also depress lactation.[51,59]

Use of combination oral contraceptives by lactating women is controversial, with many differing opinions. Estrogen-containing oral contraceptives should be avoided as they suppress lactation probably through inhibition of prolactin by estrogen.[51] These agents have been associated with decreases in milk production, shorter overall length of time of breastfeeding, and slower infant weight gain, although this is not well documented and the available studies are limited and have significant methodologic limitations.[15,51,111,124] Truitt and colleagues conducted a systematic review of randomized controlled studies and concluded that existing trials were "insufficient to establish an effect of hormonal contraception, if any, on milk quality and quantity."[125] The effects on breast milk production are reportedly most prominent in the first 4 to 6 weeks postpartum.[39,111] Although progestin only or combination agents have been thought to be safer,[39,111] Hale recommends that mothers be advised to avoid progestin agents for 4 to 6 weeks postpartum and that even with use after 6 weeks some mothers report decreased milk synthesis.[51]

Minimizing Infant Drug Exposure

A drug with a high dose may be safe if given after feeding or before the infant's longest predictable sleep period. However, a normally safe drug may be problematic if given in a high dose or over a long duration.[39] Most data on drug levels in milk are with mature milk, with minimal data on milk from mothers of preterm infants. These infants may be at greater risk for adverse effects from exposure to drugs in breast milk due to their immature hepatic and renal function. In addition, these infants are more likely to absorb large macromolecules across their immature ("open") gut (see Chapter 13).[10] Although the major concern is that the infant will receive a pharmacologically significant concentration of drug, other possible effects are allergic sensitivities and altered gut flora with antibiotics.[39]

Suggestions for reducing the effects of drugs in breast milk on the infant include: (1) using alternative forms of drugs within the same drug class that pass more poorly into milk, have shorter half-lives, or can be given via alternate routes (topical or inhaled); (2) using single components rather than compound drugs (e.g., a decongestant for allergy rather than a multisymptom drug); and (3) feeding the infant before taking the medication, thus avoiding feeding during peak plasma levels, which tend to occur 1 to 3 hours after a maternal oral dose.[13,37,39,52,75,82,87,98,111] Use of a short-acting form of the drug may reduce the risk of accumulation for drugs with concerns at high levels, however use of preparations that can be given at longer intervals (once versus three to four times per day) may be a useful strategy for other agents.[13,37,39,52,75,82,87,98,111]

If the mother is taking a drug for which there are concerns about the potential for elevated infant plasma levels, drug levels may need to be monitored periodically. Monitor the infant closely (growth pattern, sleep patterns, activity, alertness, behaviors, responsiveness, and general health). Breastfeeding may need to be temporarily discontinued when mothers are taking medication for diagnostic procedures or are taking drugs with a high potential for toxicity that are given once. In such cases, previously expressed milk or formula may be used. The timing for reinstitution of breastfeeding varies with the toxicity of the agent. For mild toxicity, resumption of nursing may be as soon as 1 to 2 maternal half-lives (50% to 75% elimination); for high toxicity, it may be necessary to wait for 4 to 5 maternal half-lives (94% to 97% elimination) or longer.[82,111] Rarely, breastfeeding may need to be discontinued if a highly toxic drug is necessary for maternal health such as chemotherapy.

SUMMARY

Drug therapy of the pregnant woman, fetus, neonate, and lactating woman is a complex health challenge. Both pregnant women and neonates have alterations in drug absorption, distribution, metabolism, and elimination that increase the risk of subtherapeutic or toxic levels of individual drugs. An understanding of the principles influencing transfer of drug across the placenta and into breast milk is critical to reducing risk in the fetus and young infant. Drug therapy of the lactating woman generally poses fewer risks to the infants than therapy of the pregnant woman. However, the use of any pharmacologic agent for either the pregnant and breastfeeding woman must be carefully evaluated and drugs used with caution. Neonates present a unique challenge for pharmacologic therapy, not only because of their physiologic immaturity but also because their systems continue to undergo maturation during early infancy, so drug handling can change within a relatively short period of time. Recommendations for clinical practice related to perinatal pharmacology are listed in Table 7-8. Box 7-2 on p. 187 lists print and online resources for information about drugs in pregnancy and lactation.

Table 7-8 Recommendations for Clinical Practice Related to Perinatal Pharmacology

Know the effects of physiologic alterations during pregnancy on pharmacokinetics (pp. 185-189 and Table 7-2).
Recognize the effects of altered gastrointestinal and hepatic function during pregnancy on drug absorption and metabolism (pp. 185-189).
Recognize the effects of altered body water, fat, and plasma proteins on drug distribution and binding during pregnancy (pp. 187-188).
Recognize the effects of altered renal function on drug elimination during pregnancy (p. 189).
Counsel women regarding the side effects of drugs and potential toxicity to mother, fetus, and neonate (pp. 185, 203-208).
Counsel women regarding planned fetal drug therapy (p. 197).
Monitor and evaluate maternal responses to drugs for evidence of subtherapeutic doses (pp. 185-189, 195).
Know or verify the usual doses for medications given during pregnancy (pp. 184-189).
Recognize the effects of maternal physiologic adaptations on the pharmacokinetics potential toxicity to the woman and fetus (pp. 185-189, 195). of antibiotics (p. 195).
Counsel women regarding the side effects of drugs used to treat specific chronic conditions and potential toxicity to the woman and fetus (pp. 185, 203-208).
Counsel women with chronic disorders regarding the impact of their disorder and its pharmacologic treatment during pregnancy and of treatment alternatives (pp. 185-189, 195).
Know the factors that influence distribution of drugs and other substances in the fetus (pp. 195-197 and Table 7-4).
Recognize critical periods of development and principles of teratogenesis (pp. 203-206 and Chapter 3).
Recognize risks associated with fetal exposure to drugs and other environmental agents during pregnancy (pp. 203-208).
Provide appropriate counselling and health teaching to promote optimal fetal development and health (pp. 203-208 and Chapter 3).
Provide counselling and health teaching to reduce exposure of the fetus to adverse environmental influences (pp. 203-208 and Chapter 3).
Counsel women regarding the use of drugs or exposure to other environmental agents during pregnancy (pp. 203-208).
Know the effects of neonatal physiology on pharmacokinetics (pp. 197-202 and Table 7-7).
Recognize the effects of immature gastrointestinal and hepatic function in the neonate on drug absorption and metabolism (pp. 199, 200-202).
Recognize the effects of altered body water, fat, and plasma proteins on drug distribution and binding in the neonate (p. 200).
Recognize the effects of maturation of liver enzyme systems on drug metabolism and risks of side effects in the neonate (pp. 200-202).
Recognize the effects of immature renal function on drug elimination and risks of side effects in the neonate (p. 202).
Know or verify the usual doses for drugs given during the neonatal period (pp. 197-202).
Recognize the side effects of drugs and potential toxicity to the neonate (pp. 197-202).
Monitor and evaluate neonatal responses to drugs, including peak and trough and serum levels (pp. 200-203).
Know the factors that place neonates at risk for toxic responses to topically applied substances (pp. 198-200).
Provide care to reduce the risk of topically applied substances (pp. 198-200).
Counsel women regarding the use of medications during lactation (pp. 208-211).
Recognize the risks associated with use of pharmacologic agents in breastfeeding women (pp. 208-211).
Evaluate the need for use of specific drugs and counsel women regarding side effects (pp. 208-211).
Monitor and evaluate maternal and neonatal responses to drugs taken by the breastfeeding woman (pp. 208-211).
Institute interventions as appropriate to reduce the risks associated with specific drugs (p. 211).
Assess infants for signs of intrauterine drug exposure from maternal substance abuse (pp. 206-208).
Know resources for obtaining information about risks of specific drugs during pregnancy and lactation (Box on p. 187).

References

1. Adam, M.P., Polifka, J.E. & Friedman, J.M. (2011). Evolving knowledge of the teratogenicity of medications in human pregnancy. *Am J Med Genet C Semin Med Genet, 157,* 175.
2. Alwan, S. & Friedman, J.M. (2009). Safety of selective serotonin reuptake inhibitors in pregnancy. *CNS Drugs, 23,* 493.
3. American College of Radiology (ACR) Committee on Drugs and Contrast Media. (2010). ACR Bulletin available at: http://www.acr.org/SecondaryMainMenuCategories/quality_safety/contrast_manual/BreastFeeding Mothers.aspx; Accessed August 10, 2011.
4. Aminoff, M.J. (2009). Neurologic disorders In R.K. Creasy, et al. (Eds.). *Creasy & Resnik's Maternal-fetal medicine: Principles and practice* (6th ed.). Philadelphia: Saunders Elsevier.
5. Anderson, G.D. (2005). Pregnancy-induced changes in pharmacokinetics: A mechanistic-based approach. *Clin Pharmacokinet, 44,* 989.
6. Anderson, G.D. & Carr, D.B. (2009). Effect of pregnancy on the pharmacokinetics of antihypertensive drugs. *Pharmacokinet, 48,* 159.
7. Anderson, G.D. & Lynn, A.M. (2009). Optimizing pediatric dosing: A developmental pharmacologic approach. *Pharmacotherapy, 29,* 680.
8. Andrade, S.E., et al. (2004). Prescription drug use in pregnancy. *Am J Obstet Gynecol, 191,* 398.
9. Askin, D.F. & Diehl-Jones, B. (2001). Cocaine: Effects on the fetus and neonate. *J Perinat Neonatal Nurs, 14,* 83.
10. Atkinson, H.C., Begg, E.J., & Darlow, B.A. (1988). Drugs in human milk: Clinical pharmacokinetic considerations. *Clin Pharmacokinet, 14,* 217.
11. Bandstra, E.S. & Accornero, VH. (2010). Infants of substance-abusing mothers. In R.J. Martin, A.A. Fanaroff, & M.C. Walsh (Eds.). *Fanaroff and Martin's neonatal-perinatal medicine: Diseases of the fetus and infant* (9th ed.). Philadelphia: Mosby Elsevier.
12. Bandstra, E.S., et al. (2010). Prenatal drug exposure: Infant and toddler outcomes. *J Addict Dis, 29,* 245.
13. Banta-Wright, S. (1997). Minimizing infant exposure to and risks from medications when breastfeeding. *J Perinat Neonat Nurs, 11,* 71.
14. Bartelink, I.H., et al. (2006). Guidelines on paediatric dosing on the basis of developmental physiology and pharmacokinetic considerations. *Clin Pharmacokinet, 45,* 1077.
15. Berlin, C.M., Jr. (2011). The excretion of drugs and chemicals in human milk. In S.J. Yaffe & J.V. Aranda (Eds.). *Neonatal and pediatric pharmacology: Therapeutic principles in practice* (4th ed.). Philadelphia: Lippincott Williams & Wilkins.
16. Blackburn, S. (2008). Fetal pharmacotherapy. *J Perinatal and Neonatal Nursing, 22,* 264.
17. Blake, M.J., et al. (2005). Ontogeny of drug metabolizing enzymes in the neonate. *Semin Fetal Neonatal Med, 10,* 123.
18. Blood-Siegfried, J. & Rende, E.K. (2010). The long-term effects of prenatal nicotine exposure on neurologic development. *J Midwifery Womens Health, 55,* 143.

19. Blumer, J.L. & Reed, M.D. (2011). Principles of neonatal pharmacology. In S.J. Yaffe & J.V. Aranda (Eds.). *Neonatal and pediatric pharmacology: Therapeutic principles in practice* (4th ed.). Philadelphia: Lippincott Williams & Wilkins.
20. Boskovic, R. & Koren, G. (2005). Placenta transfer of drugs. In S.J. Yaffe & J.V. Aranda (Eds.). *Neonatal and pediatric pharmacology: Therapeutic principles in practice* (3rd ed). Philadelphia: Lippincott Williams & Wilkins.
21. Boskovic, R., Kopecky, E., & Koren, G. (2012). Maternal drug abuse: Effects on the fetus and neonate. In R.A. Polin, W.W. Fox, & S.H. Abman (Eds.). *Fetal and neonatal physiology* (4th ed.). Philadelphia: Saunders.
22. Brent, R.L. (2004). Utilization of animal studies to determine the effects and human risks of environmental toxicants (drugs, chemicals, and physical agents). *Pediatrics, 113,* 984.
23. Briggs, G., Freeman, R.K., & Yaffe, S.J. (2011). *Drugs in pregnancy and lactation* (9th edition). Philadelphia: Lippincott Williams & Wilkins.
24. Buhimschi, C.S. & Weiner, C.P. (2009). Medications in pregnancy and lactation: Part 1. Teratology. *Obstet Gynecol, 113,* 166. Erratum in: *Obstet Gynecol.* 2009 Jun;113(6):1377.
25. Buhimschi, C.S. & Weiner, C.P. (2009). Medications in pregnancy and lactation: Part 2. Drugs with minimal or unknown human teratogenic effect. *Obstet Gynecol, 113,* 417.
26. Burakgazi, E., Pollard, J., & Harden, C. (2011). The effect of pregnancy on seizure control and antiepileptic drugs in women with epilepsy. *Rev Neurol Dis, 8,* 16.
27. Butters, L. (1990). Awareness among pregnant women of the effect on the fetus of commonly used drugs. *Midwifery, 6,* 146.
28. Capparelli, E.V. (2011). Clinical pharmacotherapeutics in infants and children. In S.J. Yaffe & J.V. Aranda (Eds.). *Pediatric pharmacology: Therapeutic principles in practice* (4th ed.). Philadelphia: Saunders.
29. Carlson, B.M. (2008). *Human embryology & developmental biology* (4th ed.). St. Louis: Mosby.
30. Chambers, C. & Weiner, C.P. (2009). Teratogenesis and environmental exposure. In R.K. Creasy, et al. (Eds.). *Creasy & Resnik's Maternal-fetal medicine: Principles and practice* (6th ed.). Philadelphia: Saunders Elsevier.
31. Chemtob, S. (2012). Basic pharmacologic principles. In R.A. Polin, W.W. Fox, & S.H. Abman (Eds.). *Fetal and neonatal physiology* (4th ed.). Philadelphia: Saunders.
32. Chemtob, S. & Aranda, J.V. (2005). Pharmacology in the fetus & newborn. In A.R. Spitzer (Eds.). *Intensive care of the fetus and neonate* (2nd ed.). St. Louis: Mosby.
33. Conover, E.A. (2003). Herbal agents and over-the-counter medications in pregnancy. *Best Pract Res Clin Endocrinol Metab, 17,* 237.
34. Cleary, B.J., et al. (2010). Methadone dose and neonatal abstinence syndrome—systematic review and meta-analysis. *Addiction, 105,* 2071.
35. Dancis, J. (1981). Placental transport of amino acids, fats and minerals. In Placental transport. *Mead Johnson Symposium on Perinatal and Developmental Medicine* (No. 18). Evansville, IN: Mead Johnson.
36. Dawes, M. & Chowienczyk, P.J. (2001). Drugs in pregnancy. Pharmacokinetics in pregnancy. *Best Pract Res Clin Obstet Gynaecol, 15,* 819.
37. Della-Giustina, K. & Chow, G. (2003). Medications in pregnancy and lactation. *Emerg Med Clin North Am, 21,* 585.
38. Dicke, J.M. (1989). Teratology: Principles and practice. *Med Clin North Am, 73,* 567.
39. Dillon, A.E., et al. (1997). Drug therapy in the nursing mother. *Obstet Gynecol Clin North Am, 24,* 675.
40. Feibus, K.B. (2008). FDA's proposed rule for pregnancy and lactation labeling: Improving maternal child health through well-informed medicine use. *J Med Toxicol, 4,* 284.
41. Fortinguerra, F., Clavenna, A., & Bonati, M. (2009). Psychotropic drug use during breastfeeding: A review of the evidence. *Pediatrics, 124,* e547.
42. Frederiksen, M.C. (2001). Physiologic changes in pregnancy and their effect on drug disposition. *Semin Perinatol, 25,* 120.
43. Frost, E.A., Gist, R.S., & Adriano, E. (2011). Drugs, alcohol, pregnancy, and the fetal alcohol syndrome. *Int Anesthesiol Clin, 49,* 119.
44. Ganapathy, V. (2000). Placental transporters relevant to drug distribution across the maternal-fetal interface. *J Pharmacol Exp Ther, 294,* 413.
45. Ganapathy, V. (2011). Drugs of abuse and human placenta. *Life Sci, 88,* 926.
46. Garland, M. (2012). Drug distribution during fetal life. In R.A. Polin, W.W. Fox, & S.H. Abman (Eds.). *Fetal and neonatal physiology* (4th ed.). Philadelphia: Saunders.
47. Gedeon, C. & Koren, G. (2006). Designing pregnancy centered medications: Drugs which do not cross the human placenta. *Placenta, 27,* 861.
48. Gentile, S. (2010). Neurodevelopmental effects of prenatal exposure to psychotropic medications. *Depress Anxiety, 27,* 675.
49. Glover, D.D., et al. (2003). Prescription, over-the-counter, and herbal medicine use in a rural, obstetric population. *Am J Obstet Gynecol, 188,* 1039.
50. Gouin, K., et al. (2011). Effects of cocaine use during pregnancy on low birthweight and preterm birth: Systematic review and metaanalyses. *Am J Obstet Gynecol, 204,* 340.
51. Hale, T.W. (2010). Breastfeeding mothers. In T.L. King & M.C. Brucker, M. C. (eds.). *Pharmacology for women' health.* Boston: Jones & Bartlett.
52. Hale, T.W. (2010). *Medications and mother's milk* (13th Ed). Amarillo, Texas: Pharmasoft Medical Publishing.
53. Harden, C.L., et al. (2009). Practice parameter update: Management issues for women with epilepsy—focus on pregnancy (an evidence-based review): Teratogenesis and perinatal outcomes: Report of the Quality Standards Subcommittee and Therapeutics and Technology Assessment Subcommittee of the American Academy of Neurology and American Epilepsy Society. *Neurology, 73,* 133.
54. Harden, C.L., et al. (2009). Practice parameter update: Management issues for women with epilepsy—focus on pregnancy (an evidence-based review): Vitamin K, folic acid, blood levels, and breastfeeding: Report of the Quality Standards Subcommittee and Therapeutics and Technology Assessment Subcommittee of the American Academy of Neurology and American Epilepsy Society. *Neurology, 73,* 142.
55. Hines, R.N. (2007). Ontogeny of human hepatic cytochromes P450. *Biochem Mol Toxicol, 21,* 169.
56. Hines, R.N. (2008). The ontogeny of drug metabolism enzymes and implications for adverse drug events. *Pharmacol Ther, 118,* 250.
57. Hodge, L.S. & Tracy, T.S. (2007). Alterations in drug disposition during pregnancy: Implications for drug therapy. *Expert Opin Drug Metab Toxicol, 3,* 557.
58. Hutson, J.R., Koren, G., & Matthews, S.G. (2010). Placental P-glycoprotein and breast cancer resistance protein: Influence of polymorphisms on fetal drug exposure and physiology. *Placenta, 31,* 351.
59. Ito, S. & Lee, A. (2003). Drug excretion into breast milk—Overview. *Adv Drug Deliv Rev, 55,* 617.
60. Jacqz-Aigrain, E. & Burtin, P. (1996). Clinical pharmacokinetics of sedatives in neonates. *Clin Pharmacokinet, 31,* 423.
61. Jansson, L.M. & Velez, M.L. (2011). Infants of drug-dependent mothers. *Pediatr Rev, 32,* 5.
62. John, E.G. & Guignard, J.P. (1998). Development of renal excretion of drugs during ontogeny. In R.A. Polin & W.W. Fox (Eds.). *Fetal and neonatal physiology* (2nd ed.). Philadelphia: Saunders.
63. Jones, H.E., et al. (2010). Neonatal abstinence syndrome after methadone or buprenorphine exposure. *N Engl J Med, 363,* 2320.
64. Jones, K.L. (2005). *Smith's recognizable patterns of human malformation* (6th ed.). Philadelphia: Saunders.
65. Jones, K.L. (2011). The effects of alcohol on fetal development. *Birth Defects Res C Embryo Today, 93,* 3.
66. Kearns, G.L., et al. (2003). Developmental pharmacology—Drug disposition, action, and therapy in infants and children. *N Engl J Med, 349,* 1157.
67. Kenner, C. & Amlung, S. (2000). *Nursing management of substance-dependent neonates: A continuing education module.* Des Plaines, IL: National Association of Neonatal Nurses.

68. Klieger, C., et al. (2009). Hypoglycemics: Pharmacokinetic considerations during pregnancy. *Ther Drug Monit, 31,* 533.
69. Koren, G., et al. (1989). Perception of teratogenic risk by pregnant women exposed to drugs and chemicals during the first trimester. *Am J Obstet Gynecol, 160,* 1190.
70. Koren, G., Paturszack, A., & Ito, S. (1998). Drugs in pregnancy. *N Engl J Med, 228,* 1128.
71. Koren, G., Klinger, G., & Ohlsson, A. (2002). Fetal pharmacotherapy. *Drugs, 62,* 757.
72. Koren, G. (2011). Pharmacokinetics in pregnancy: Clinical significance. *J Popul Ther Clin Pharmacol, 18,* e523.
73. Larrimore, W.L. & Petrie, K.L. (2000). Drug use during pregnancy and lactation. *Prim Care, 27,* 35.
74. Larsen, L.A., Ito, S., & Koren, G. (2003). Prediction of milk/plasma concentration ratio of drugs. *Ann Pharmacother, 37,* 1299.
75. Lawrence, R.A. (2011). *Breastfeeding: A guide for the medical profession* (7th ed.). Philadelphia: Saunders..
76. Leeder, J.S. (2009). Developmental pharmacogenetics: A general paradigm for application to neonatal pharmacology and toxicology. *Clin Pharmacol Ther, 86,* 678.
77. Lester, B.M. & Lagasse, L.L. (2010). Children of addicted women. *J Addict Dis, 29,* 259.
78. Little, B.B. (1999). Pharmacokinetics during pregnancy: Evidence-based maternal dose formulation. *Obstet Gynecol, 93(5, Pt 2),* 858.
79. Littleford, J. (2004). Effects on the fetus and newborn of maternal analgesia and anesthesia: A review. *Can J Anesth, 51,* 6.
80. Lo, W.Y. & Friedman, J.M. (2002). Teratogenicity of recently introduced medications in human pregnancy. *Obstet Gynecol, 100,* 465.
81. Loebstein, R., Lalkin, A., & Koren, G. (1997). Pharmacokinetic changes during pregnancy and their clinical relevance. *Clin Pharmacokinet, 33,* 328.
82. Logsdon, B.A. (1997). Drug use during lactation. *J Am Pharm Assoc (Wash), NS37,* 407.
83. Manns-James, L. (2010). Pregnancy. In T.L. King & M.C. Brucker (eds.). *Pharmacology for women' health.* Boston: Jones & Bartlett.
84. Manzo-Avalos, S. & Saavedra-Molina, A. (2010). Cellular and mitochondrial effects of alcohol consumption. *Int J Environ Res Public Health, 7,* 4281.
85. McCarver, D.G. & Hines, R.N. (2002).The ontogeny of human drug-metabolizing enzymes: Phase II conjugation enzymes and regulatory mechanisms. *J Pharmacol Exp Ther, 300,* 361.
86. McClary, J., Blumer, J.L., Aranda, J.V., et al. (2011). Developmental pharmacology. In R.J. Martin, A.A. Fanaroff, & M.C. Walsh (Eds.). *Fanaroff and Martin's Neonatal-perinatal medicine: Diseases of the fetus and infant* (9th ed.). Philadelphia: Mosby Elsevier.
87. Mehta, N. & Larson, L. (2011). Pharmacotherapy in pregnancy and lactation. *Clin Chest Med, 32,* 43.
88. Menon, S.J. (2008). Psychotropic medication during pregnancy and lactation. *Arch Gynecol Obstet, 277,* 1.
89. Mitchell, A.A., et al. (2011). Medication use during pregnancy, with particular focus on prescription drugs: 1976-2008. National Birth Defects Prevention Study. *Am J Obstet Gynecol, 205,* e1.
90. Moore, K.L., Persaud, T.V.N., & Torchia, M.G. (2011). *The developing human: Clinically oriented embryology* (9th ed.). Philadelphia: Saunders.
91. Morgan, D.J. (1997). Drug disposition in mother and foetus. *Clin Exp Pharmacol Physiol, 24,* 869.
92. Murin, S., Rafii, R., & Bilello, K. (2011). Smoking and smoking cessation in pregnancy. *Clin Chest Med, 32,* 75.
93. Nagourney, B.A. & Aranda, J.V. (1998). Physiologic differences of clinical significance. In R.A. Polin & W.W. Fox (Eds.). *Fetal and neonatal physiology* (2nd ed.). Philadelphia: W.B. Saunders.
94. Neutel, C.L. & Johnson, H.L. (1995). Measuring drug effectiveness by default: The case of Bendectin. *Can J Public Health, 68,* 66.
95. Neville, K.A., et al. (2011). Developmental pharmacogenomics. *Paediatr Anaesth, 21,* 255.
96. Niebyl, J.R. (2003). Antibiotics and other anti-infective agents in pregnancy and lactation. *Am J Perinatol, 20,* 405.
97. Nimkarn, S. & New, M.I. (2007). Prenatal diagnosis and treatment of congenital adrenal hyperplasia. *Horm Res, 67,* 53.
98. Ostrea, E.M., Jr, Mantaring, J.B., 3rd, & Silvestre, M.A. (2004). Drugs that affect the fetus and newborn infant via the placenta or breast milk. *Pediatr Clin North Am, 51,* 539.
99. Pacifici, G.M. & Nottoli, R. (1995). Placental transfer of drugs administered to the mother. *Clin Pharmacokinet, 28,* 235.
100. Parisi, M.A., et al. (2011). We don't know what we don't study: The case for research on medication effects in pregnancy. *Am J Med Genet C Semin Med Genet, 157,* 247.
101. Pasanen, M. (1999). The expression and regulation of drug metabolism in the human placenta. *Adv Drug Del Rev, 38,* 81.
102. Pavek, P., Ceckova, M., & Staud, F. (2009). Variation of drug kinetics in pregnancy. *Curr Drug Metab, 10,* 520.
103. Pennell, P.B. (2003). Antiepileptic drug pharmacokinetics during pregnancy and lactation. *Neurology, 1,* S35.
104. Petersen, I., et al. (2011). Pregnancy as a major determinant for discontinuation of antidepressants: An analysis of data from The Heath Improvement Network. *J Clin Psychiatry, 72,* 979.
105. Plonait, S.L. & Nau, H. (2012). Physiochemical and structural properties regulating placental drug transfer. In R.A. Polin, W.W. Fox, & S.H. Abman (Eds.). *Fetal and neonatal physiology* (4th ed.). Philadelphia: Saunders.
106. Poggesi, I., et al. (2009). Pharmacokinetics in special populations. *Drug Metab Rev, 41,* 422.
107. Polifka, J.E. & Friedman, J.M. (2002). Medical genetics: 1. Clinical teratology in the age of genomics. *CMAJ, 167,* 265.
108. Rakhmanina, N.Y. & van den Anker, J.N. (2006). Pharmacological research in pediatrics: From neonates to adolescents. *Adv Drug Deliv Rev, 58,* 4.
109. Rayburn, W.F. & Amanze, A.C. (2008). Prescribing medications safely during pregnancy. *Med Clin North Am, 92,* 1227.
110. Reed, M.D. & Blumer, J.L. (2006). Pharmacologic treatment of the fetus. In R.J. Martin, A.A. Fanaroff, & M.C. Walsh (Eds.). *Fanaroff and Martin's Neonatal-perinatal medicine: Diseases of the fetus and infant* (8th ed.). Philadelphia: Saunders.
111. Reider, M.J. (2012). Drug excretion during breast feeding. In R.A. Polin, W.W. Fox, & S.H. Abman (Eds.). *Fetal and neonatal physiology* (4th ed.). Philadelphia: Saunders.
112. Ring, J.A., et al. (1999). Fetal hepatic drug elimination. *Pharmacol Ther, 84,* 429.
113. Schiller, C. and Allen, P.J. (2005). Follow-up of infants prenatally exposed to cocaine. *Pediatric Nurs, 31,* 427.
114. Schwartz, R.H. (1981). Considerations of antibiotic therapy during pregnancy. *Obstet Gynecol, 58(Suppl),* 95.
115. Slikker, W., et al. (2005). Mode of action: Disruption of brain cell replication, second messenger, and neurotransmitter systems during development leading to cognitive dysfunction-developmental neurotoxicity of nicotine. *Critical Rev Toxicol, 35,* 703.
116. Steinberg, C. & Notterman, D.A. (1994). Pharmacokinetics of cardiovascular drugs in children: Inotropes and vasopressors. *Clin Pharmacokinet, 27,* 345.
117. Stephens, T.D., et al. (2000). Mechanism of action in thalidomide teratogenesis. *Biochem Pharmacol, 59,* 1489.
118. Stultz, E.E., et al. (2007). Extent of medication use in breastfeeding women. *Breastfeed Med, 2,* 145.
119. Suggs, D.M. (2000). Pharmacokinetics in children: History, considerations, and applications. *J Am Acad Nurse Pract, 12,* 236.
120. Syme, M.R., Paxton, J.W., & Keelan, J.A. (2004). Drug transfer and metabolism by the human placenta. *Clin Pharmacokinet, 43,* 487.
121. Tomi, M., Nishimura, T., & Nakashima, E. (2011). Mother-to-fetal transfer of antiviral drugs and the involvement of transporters at the placental barrier. *J Pharm Sci, 100,* 3708.
122. Touw, D.J., Westerman, E.M., & Sprij, A.J. (2009). Therapeutic drug monitoring of aminoglycosides in neonates. *Clin Pharmacokinet, 48,* 71.
123. Tracy, T.S., et al. (2005). Temporal changes in drug metabolism (CYP1A2, CYP2D6 and CYP3A Activity) during pregnancy. National Institute for Child

Health and Human Development Network of Maternal-Fetal-Medicine Units. *Am J Obstet Gynecol, 192,* 633.

124. Trasler, J.M. & Doerksen, T. (1999). Teratogen update: Paternal exposures—reproductive risks. *Teratology, 60,* 161.
125. Truitt, S.T., et al. (2003). Hormonal contraception during lactation. Systematic review of randomized controlled trials. *Contraception, 68,* 233.
126. Vähäkangas, K. & Myllynen, P. (2009). Drug transporters in the human blood-placental barrier. *Br J Pharmacol, 158,* 665.
127. van den Anker, J. & Allegaerti, K. (2011). Renal function and excretion of drugs in the newborn. In S.J. Yaffe & J.V. Aranda (Eds.). *Neonatal and pediatric pharmacology: Therapeutic principles in practice* (4th ed.). Philadelphia: Lippincott Williams & Wilkins.
128. Walker, S.P., Permezel, M., & Berkovic, S.F. (2009). The management of epilepsy in pregnancy. *BJOG, 116,* 758.
129. Weier, N., et al. (2008). Placental drug disposition and its clinical implications. *Curr Drug Metab, 9,* 106.
130. Weiner, C. & Buhimschi, C. (2009). *Drugs for pregnant and lactating women* (2nd edition). London: Churchill Livingstone.
131. Weller, T.M. & Rees, E.N. (2000). Antibacterial use in pregnancy. *Drug Saf, 22,* 335.
132. Wilffert, B., et al. (2011). Pharmacogenetics of drug-induced birth defects: What is known so far? *Pharmacogenomics, 12,* 547.
133. Wilson, J.G. (1977). Current status of teratology: General principles and mechanisms derived from animal studies. In J.G. Wilson & F.C. Fraser (Eds.). *Handbook of teratology: General principles and etiology.* New York: Plenum.
134. Wisner, K.L., et al. (2009). Major depression and antidepressant treatment: Impact on pregnancy and neonatal outcomes. *Am J Psychiatry, 166,* 557.
135. Young, A.M., Allen, C.E., & Andus, K.L. (2003). Efflux transporters of the human placenta. *Adv Drug Deliv Res, 21,* 125.

CHAPTER 8

Hematologic and Hemostatic Systems

The hematologic system encompasses blood and plasma volume, the constituents of plasma, and the formation and function of blood cellular components. Hemostasis involves mechanisms that result in the formation and removal of fibrin clots. Pregnancy and the neonatal period are associated with significant changes in these processes, increasing the risk for anemia and alterations in hemostasis such as thromboembolism and consumptive coagulopathies. This chapter examines alterations in the hematologic system and hemostasis during the perinatal period and their implications for the mother, fetus, and neonate.

MATERNAL PHYSIOLOGIC ADAPTATIONS

The significant changes in the hematologic system and hemostasis during pregnancy have a protective role for maternal homeostasis and are important for fetal development. These changes are also critical in allowing the mother to tolerate blood loss and placental separation at delivery. The maternal adaptations also increase the risk for complications such as thromboembolism, iron deficiency anemia, and coagulopathies.

Antepartum Period

Most hematologic parameters, including blood and plasma volume, cellular components, plasma constituents, and coagulation factors, are altered during pregnancy. These changes are reflected in progressive changes in many common hematologic laboratory values. As a result, it is essential to recognize the normal range of laboratory values and usual patterns of change during pregnancy and to evaluate findings in conjunction with clinical data and previous values in order to distinguish between normal adaptations and pathologic alterations (Table 8-1).

Changes in Blood and Plasma Volume

Among the most significant hematologic changes during pregnancy are increases in blood and plasma volume (Figure 8-1). These changes result in the hypervolemia of pregnancy, which is in turn responsible for many of the alterations in blood cellular components and plasma constituents. Circulating blood volume increases by 30% to 40% (approximately 1 ½ L), with a usual range of 30% to 45%.[46,87,128,179] The increased blood volume is due to an increase in plasma volume that is followed by an increase in the total red blood cell (RBC) volume. Blood volume changes begin at 6 to 8 weeks, peak at 28 to 34 weeks at values about 1200 to 1600 mL higher than in nonpregnant women, then reach a plateau or decrease slightly to term.[87,128]

Plasma volume increases progressively from 6 to 8 weeks by approximately 45% to 50% (range, 40% to 60%) or about 1200 to 1600 mL above nonpregnant values.[54,87,128,158,188] Plasma volume increases rapidly during the second trimester, followed by a slower but progressive increase that reaches its maximum of 4700 to 5200 mL around 32 weeks.[87,128] The enlarged plasma volume is accommodated by the vasculature of the uterus, breasts, muscles, kidneys, and skin. The increased volume leads to hemodilution with a net decrease in RBC volume and total circulating plasma proteins.

Plasma volume, placental mass, and birth weight are positively correlated.[54,73] Fetal growth correlates more closely with maternal plasma volume increases than with changes in RBC volume. Alterations in the usual increase in plasma volume are associated with pregnancy complications. A greater than normal increase in plasma volume has been observed in multiparous women (probably related to a tendency for higher weight infants) and with maternal obesity, large for gestational age infants, prolonged pregnancy, and multiple gestation.[54]

In twin pregnancies, plasma volume increases up to 70% over nonpregnant values, with further elevations seen in women with triplets and other multiple pregnancies.[38,54] The lower than expected hematocrit seen in these women may be due to hemodilution from excessive plasma volume and may not indicate a problem with erythropoiesis per se. Preeclampsia is associated with a reduction in the expected increase in plasma volume in most studies (see Chapter 9).[6,10,29,62,100,108,128] This may be due to vasoconstriction altering the intravascular compartment or a more "leaky" vasculature.[10]

The etiology of plasma volume changes in pregnancy is thought to be related to the effects of nitric oxide–mediated vasodilation on the renin-angiotensin-aldosterone system and subsequent sodium and water retention (see Chapter 11).[32,128] These changes are also influenced by hormonal effects and are closely linked with the alterations seen in fluid balance and in the renal and cardiovascular systems. Hormonal influences,

Table 8-1 Normal Laboratory Values in Nonpregnant and Pregnant Women

	NONPREGNANT	PREGNANT
GENERAL SCREENING ASSAYS		
Hemoglobin	12-16 g/dL (120.0-160.0 g/L)	11-14 g/dL (110.0-140.0 g/L)
Packed cell volume (PCV)	37%-47%	33%-44%
Red blood cell count (RBC)	4.2-5.4 million/mm^3	3.8-4.4 million/mm^3
Mean corpuscular volume (MCV)	80-100 fl	70-90 fl
Mean corpuscular hemoglobin (MCH)	27-34 fl	23-31 fl
Mean corpuscular hemoglobin concentration (MCHC)	32-35 fl	32-35 fl
Reticulocyte count	0.5%-1%	1%-2%
SPECIFIC DIAGNOSTIC TESTS		
Serum ferritin	25-200 ng/mL (56.1-449.4 pmol/L)	15-150 ng/mL (33.7-337.0 pmol/L)
Serum iron	135 mcg/dL (24.2 μmol/L)	90 mcg/dL (16.1 μmol/L)
Iron binding capacity	250-460 mcg/dL (44.8-82.3 μmol/L)	300-600 mcg/dL (53.7-107.4 μmol/L)
Transferrin saturation	25%-35%	15%-30%
Iron	135 mcg/dL (24.2 μmol/L)	90 mcg/dL (16.1 μmol/L)
Red blood cell folate	150-450 ng/mL cells (339.9-1019.7 nmol/L cells)	100-400 ng/mL cells (226.6-906.4 nmol/L cells)
Serum vitamin B_{12}	70-85 ng/dL (51.7-62.7 pmol/L)	70-500 ng/dL (51.7-369.0 pmol/L)

Adapted from Morrison, J.C. & Pryor, J.A. (1990). Hematologic disorders. In R.D. Eden & F.H. Boehm (Eds.). *Assessment and care of the fetus.* Norwalk, CT: Appleton & Lange; Burrow, G.N., Duffy, T.P., & Copel, J.A. (2004). *Medical complications during pregnancy* (6th ed.). Philadelphia: Saunders.

especially the effects of progesterone, on the vasculature of the venous system lead to decreased venous tone, increased capacity of the veins and venules, and decreased vascular resistance. These changes allow the vasculature to accommodate the increased blood volume. Estrogen and progesterone influence plasma renin activity and aldosterone levels, resulting in retention of sodium and an increase in total body water.[73] Most of this extra water is extracellular and available to contribute to the increased plasma volume. Changes in plasma volume have also been linked to a mechanical effect, with the low-resistance uteroplacental circulation acting as an arteriovenous shunt. This shunt provides physical space to accommodate the increased cardiac output and corresponding change in plasma volume.[38,73]

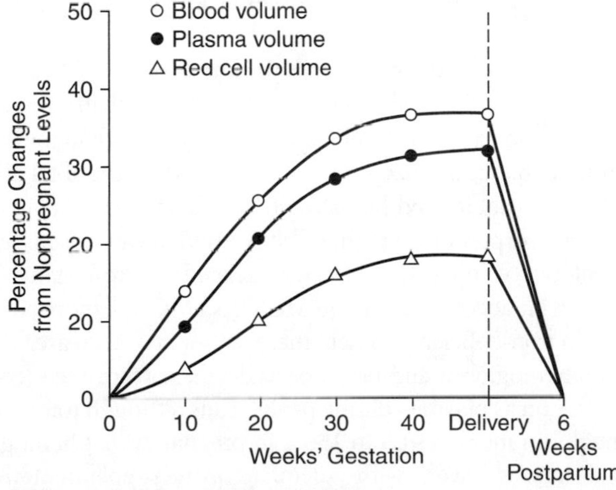

FIGURE 8-1 Changes in blood volume, plasma volume, and red blood cell volume during pregnancy and postpartum. (From Peck, T.M. & Arias, F. [1979]. Hematologic changes associated with pregnancy. *Clin Obstet Gynecol, 22,* 788.)

Increased plasma volume and hypervolemia reduce blood viscosity. Hypervolemia also leads to hemodilution and changes in plasma protein and blood cellular components, which further reduce viscosity. Blood viscosity decreases approximately 20% during the first two trimesters. During the third trimester, viscosity may increase slightly. The decreased viscosity reduces resistance to flow and the cardiac effort needed, thus conserving maternal energy resources.[38]

Changes in Blood Cellular Components

The principal change in blood cellular components during pregnancy is an increase in RBC volume (Table 8-2). This alteration, in conjunction with changes in plasma volume, is reflected in changes in the hemoglobin and hematocrit.

Changes in Red Blood Cells. The total RBC volume increases by 20% to 30% (250 to 450 mL) during pregnancy.[54,128,158] Changes in RBC volume are due to increased circulating erythropoietin (Epo), which stimulates erythropoiesis and accelerated RBC production. The rise in Epo in the last two trimesters is due to progesterone, possibly prolactin, and human placental lactogen rather than to a decrease in oxygen-carrying capacity, which is the usual stimulus for Epo production.[54,128] The magnitude of change in RBC volume varies and is influenced by the woman's iron stores.[38] The increase in RBCs reflects the increase in oxygen demands (which rise 15%) during pregnancy.[178,179]

Table 8-2 **Changes in Blood Cellular Components During Pregnancy**

COMPONENT	CHANGE	PATTERN OF CHANGE	BASIS FOR CHANGE	INTRAPARTUM CHANGES	POSTPARTUM CHANGES
Red blood cells (RBCs)	Increases 20%-30% (250-450 mL)	Slow, continuous increase beginning in first trimester; may accelerate slightly in third trimester	Erythropoietin stimulated by human placental lactogen, progesterone, and prolactin	Slight increase due to slight hemoconcentration; 50% of increased RBCs lost at delivery	RBC production ceases temporarily; remainder of increased RBCs lost via normal catabolism
Hematocrit	Decreases 3%-5% to 33.8% at term (range, 33%-39%)	Decreases from second trimester as plasma volume peaks	Hemodilution		Returns to nonpregnant levels by 4-6 weeks as a result of RBC catabolism
Hemoglobin	Decreases 2%-10% to 12.1-12.5 g/dL (range, 11-13 g/dL) at term	If iron and folate are adequate, little change to 16 weeks; lowest values at 16-22 weeks; slowly increases to term	Hemodilution; total body hemoglobin increases by 65-150 g	Slight increase as a result of stress and dehydration	Initial decrease; stabilizes at 2-4 days; nonpregnant values by 4-6 weeks
Reticulocytes	Increase 1%-2%	Gradual increase to third trimester	Increased RBC production		Increases slightly; nonpregnant values by 4-6 weeks
White blood cells	Increase 8% to 5000-12,000/mm^3 (up to 15,000/mm^3 seen)	Begins in second month; increase involves primarily neutrophils	Estrogen	Increase to 25,000-30,000/mm^3	Decrease to 6000-10,000/mm^3; normal values by 4-7 days
Eosinophils Basophils	Probably increases slightly Decreases slightly	Variable	Hemodilution	Disappear from peripheral blood	By 3 days return to peripheral blood
Platelets	May decrease slightly but within normal adult ranges; usual range 150,000-400,000/mm^3	Variable		20% decrease with placental separation	Increase by 3-5 days with gradual return to nonpregnant levels
Erythrocyte sedimentation rate	Increases	Progressive	Increased plasma globulin and fibrinogen	Increases	Initially 55-80 mm/hr; peaks 1-2 days postpartum

The increase in erythropoiesis and total RBC volume begins during the first trimester.[54,87] The increase occurs at a relatively constant rate, but slower than changes in plasma volume, and may accelerate slightly during the third trimester.[54,73] Hemodilution is maximal at 28 to 34 weeks and leads to a lower hemoglobin, hematocrit and RBC count.[87] The increased RBC production results in a moderate erythroid hyperplasia of the bone marrow and an increase in the reticulocyte count.

RBC 2,3-diphosphoglycerate (2,3-DPG) rises beginning early in pregnancy and leads to a gradual shift to the right of the maternal oxygen-hemoglobin dissociation curve (see Chapter 10). This reduces the affinity of maternal hemoglobin for oxygen (see box on p. 301) and favors release of oxygen in the peripheral tissues, including the intervillous space, which facilitates oxygen transfer from mother to fetus and fetal growth.[54,73,128] Alterations in placental function that occur with maternal disorders such as preeclampsia, chronic renal disease, diabetes, and severe anemia can decrease oxygen transfer across the placenta. The fetus may develop chronic hypoxia, with stimulation of erythropoietin (Epo) production, increased erythropoiesis, polycythemia, and increased neonatal morbidity.

The mean cell diameter and thickness of the RBCs also change, resulting in a cell that is more spherical in shape. Because the increase in plasma volume is three times greater than the RBC volume increase, the net result is a decrease in the total RBC count, hemoglobin, and hematocrit (see Table 8-2). Changes in the mean corpuscular volume (MCV) and mean corpuscular hemoglobin volume (MCHV) are related to iron status. In women with adequate iron, the MCV and MCHV are relatively stable; in iron-deficient women, these values may decrease.[87,179]

The hemoglobin and hematocrit decrease from the second trimester on as plasma volume peaks. Thus although total body hemoglobin increases 85 to 150 g in pregnancy, net hemoglobin decreases. Even with adequate iron supplementation, the hemoglobin decreases about 2 g/dL (20 g/L) to a mean of about 11.6 g/dL (116 g/L) in the second trimester as a result of hemodilution.[74] At term the hemoglobin averages 12.1 to 12.5 g/dL (121 to 125 g/L), with a range of 11 to 13 g/dL

(110 to 130 g/L) versus a mean of 14 ± 2 (140 ± 20 g/L) for nonpregnant females. The Centers for Disease Control and Prevention (CDC) suggests values of 11 g/dL (110 g/L) (first and second trimesters) and 10.5 g/dL (105 g/L) (third trimester) as the lowest acceptable values for screening pregnant women.[36,54] The mean hematocrit is 33.8% (range, 33% to 39%) at term.[54,87] The fall in the hematocrit may help protect the woman from thromboembolism by decreasing blood viscosity and enhancing perfusion.[128] A high hematocrit in a pregnant woman may indicate a low plasma volume and a relative hypovolemia. Changes in the hemoglobin and hematocrit in pregnant women are illustrated in Figure 8-2.

Changes in White Blood Cells. Total white blood cell (WBC) volume increases slightly beginning in the second month and levels off during the second and third trimesters (see Table 8-2). The total WBC count in pregnancy varies with individual women, ranging from 5000 to 12,000/mm³, with values as high as 15,000/mm³ reported.[87,128] The increased WBC count is due to a neutrophilia with an elevation in mature leukocyte forms. A slight shift to the left may occur with occasional myelocytes and metamyelocytes seen on the peripheral smear.[87] Changes in other WBC forms are minimal (see Table 8-2), with a possible slight increase in eosinophils and slight decrease in basophils and no systematic changes in monocytes.[87] Leukocyte alkaline phosphatase activity rises during pregnancy, falling several days before to delivery. Changes in leukocytes accompanying pregnancy are similar to changes that occur with physiologic stress, such as vigorous exercise, with return to the circulation of mature leukocytes that were previously shunted out of the circulatory system.[46] The basis for these changes is unclear but is probably related to hormonal changes.[54,87] The neutrophil count normally increases slightly with the estrogen peak during the menstrual cycle. In women who become pregnant, the neutrophils continue to increase after fertilization, peaking around 30 weeks then remaining stable to term. The total lymphocyte count is unchanged, as are numbers of circulating B and T lymphocytes (see Chapter 13).

Changes in Platelets. In general, platelet values do not change significantly during pregnancy.[71,87] A slight decrease in platelet count, probably due to hemodilution, and an increase in platelet aggregation during the last 8 weeks of pregnancy has been reported, suggesting a low-grade activation and consumption of platelets.[69,71,87] In healthy pregnant women, platelet counts have generally not been reported at values below lower limits for normal nonpregnant women.[87,117] Mild to moderate thrombocytopenia (less than 150,000/mm³) has been reported in late pregnancy in 7% of healthy pregnant women.[26,87,181] This may be due to hemodilution, decreased platelet production, or increased turnover.[24] The acceptable range for platelet values in pregnancy is 150,000 to 400,000/mm³.

Changes in Plasma Components

Many components of plasma—including plasma proteins, electrolytes, serum iron, lipids, and enzymes—change during pregnancy (Table 8-3). Total plasma proteins decrease

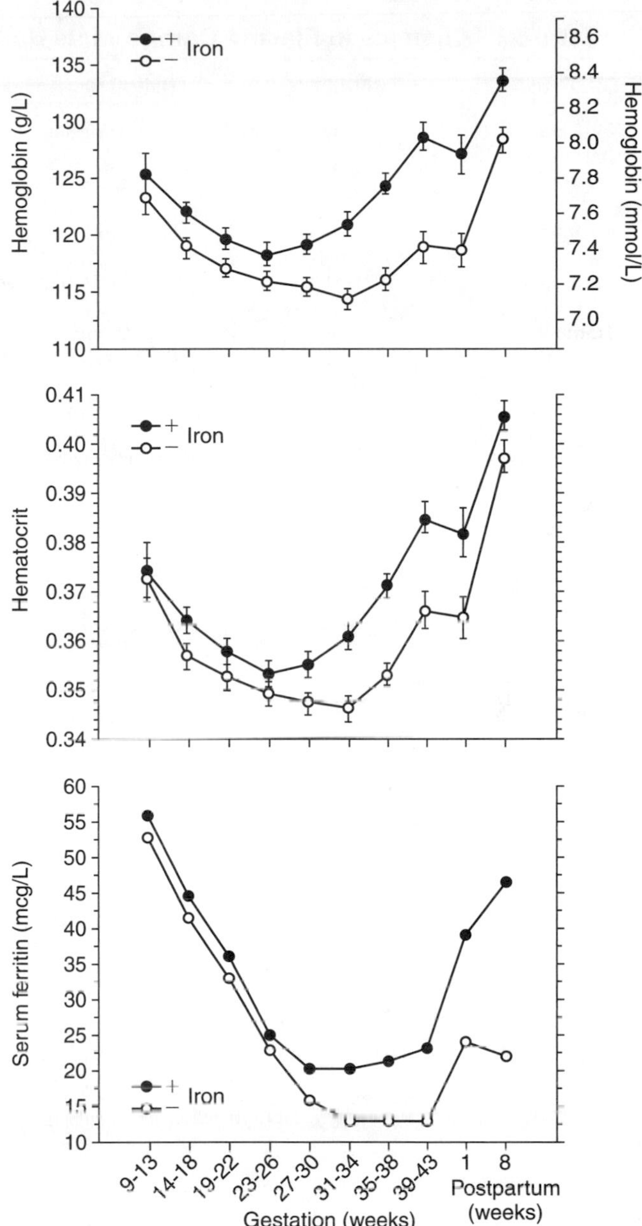

FIGURE 8-2 Variations in hemoglobin and hematocrit (mean ± SEM) and serum ferritin (median) in normal pregnancy and postpartum in placebo-treated and iron-treated women taking 66 mg ferrous iron daily. (From Milman, N., et al. [1999]. Iron status and iron balance during pregnancy: A critical reappraisal of iron supplementation. *Acta Obstet Gynecol Scand, 78,* 749.)

10% to 14%, with much of the change occurring in the first trimester. Although there is an absolute increase in albumin concentration during the first trimester, there is a relative decrease due to increased blood volume and hemodilution. Decreased albumin leads to a net decrease in colloid osmotic (oncotic) pressure, reducing the normal forces counteracting edema formation. Although edema formation in pregnancy is primarily due to alterations in venous hydrostatic pressure, decreased oncotic pressure from the relative decrease in albumin is an important contributory factor.[15]

Table 8-3 **Changes in Plasma Components During Pregnancy**

COMPONENT	CHANGE	TIMING	BASIS	SIGNIFICANCE
Total plasma proteins	↓10%-14%	First trimester	Estrogen/progesterone	↓ Colloid osmotic pressure (edema formation) Altered protein binding of calcium, drugs, and so on
Albumin	Total: 144 g Serum: 3.5 g	First trimester	Estrogen/progesterone	See above
Fibrinogen	↑50%-80%	First to third trimesters	Hemodilution	Alterations in hemostasis ↓ Erythrocyte sedimentation rate
Globulin	↑	First to third trimesters	Estrogen/progesterone	↓ Erythrocyte sedimentation rate
α- and β-globulin	↓	Progressive throughout pregnancy	Estrogen/progesterone	See individual globulins Facilitate transport of carbohydrates and lipids to placenta and fetus
γ-Globulin	↓	Third trimester		Transplacental passage of IgG
Thyroxin-binding globulin	↑	First trimester		↑Plasma T_3 and T_4
α_1-Antitrypsin	Doubles			Protects lungs from deported trophoblast tissue
α_2-Macroglobulin	↑20%			Antiplasmin effect, which may predispose to DIC
Total serum lipids	↑40%-60%	Continuous to term	Human placental lactogen and altered metabolism	
Cholesterol	↑40%	Continuous to term		Essential precursor for steroid hormones (e.g., estrogen, progesterone)
Phospholipids	↑37%	Continuous to term		Major component of cell membranes needed for maternal and fetal growth
β-Lipoprotein	↑Up to 180%			Possible ↑ risk of thrombosis
Serum electrolytes	↓ 5-10 mg/L	First trimester		↓ Plasma osmolarity
Serum ferritin	↓ 30%	To 28 weeks (with adequate iron) or 30-32 (without)	Hemoglobin synthesis (early) Fetal uptake (late)	Reflects decreasing iron stores
Transferrin	↑ 70%	Linear rise	Altered liver function	Facilitates Fe absorption and transport
Iron-binding capacity	↓ 15%			

DIC, Disseminated intravascular coagulation; *Fe,* iron; *IgG,* immunoglobulin G.

Globulin concentration demonstrates both absolute and relative increases, leading to progressive falls in the albumin-to-globulin ratio. Both α- and β-globulin increase progressively during pregnancy; γ-globulin decreases slightly. Fibrinogen also demonstrates both absolute and relative increases of 50% to 80%.[15,46] The erythrocyte sedimentation rate (ESR) increases progressively during pregnancy, probably due to the elevation in plasma globulin and fibrinogen levels. Alterations in other plasma proteins are summarized in Table 8-3.

The alterations in plasma proteins alter protein binding of substances such as calcium, drugs, and anesthetic agents. Because many drugs are transported in the blood bound to albumin, doses of some drugs may need to be altered during pregnancy (see Chapter 7). Increased binding of substances such as calcium reduces the level of free calcium in the maternal plasma. As a result, calcium must be actively transported across the placenta to the fetus (see Chapter 17).

Decreases in serum electrolytes (anions, cations, and buffer base) reduce plasma osmolarity by 8 to 10 mOsm/L during the first trimester.[15] These changes are due to both hypervolemia and the effects of respiratory system alterations, particularly hyperventilation with increased CO_2 loss (see Chapter 10).[38]

Serum iron decreases during pregnancy, especially after 28 weeks and in women without adequate iron stores. Iron needs during pregnancy are summarized in Table 8-4. Serum ferritin is a more precise indicator of reticuloendothelial iron stores. 1 mcg/L (2.5 pmol/L) serum ferritin is equal to 8 mg of stored iron in the adult. Serum ferritin levels in pregnancy are 15 to 150 ng/mL (33.7 to 337 pmol/L).[54] In women

Table 8-4 Iron Requirements for Pregnancy

REQUIRED FOR	AVERAGE (mg)	RANGE (mg)
External iron loss	170	150-200
Expansion of red blood cell mass	450	200-600
Fetal iron	270	200-370
Iron in placenta and cord	90	30-170
Blood loss at delivery	150	90-310
Total requirement	980	580-1340
Requirement less red blood cell expansion	840	440-1050

From Kilpatrick, S.J. & Laros, R.K. (2004). Maternal hematologic disorders. In R.K. Creasy, R. Resnik, & J.D. Iams (Eds.). *Maternal-fetal medicine: Principles and practice* (5th ed.). Philadelphia: Saunders.

without adequate iron, serum ferritin levels fall until 30 to 32 weeks and then stabilize. The greatest decrease in serum ferritin is between 12 and 25 weeks due to the rapid expansion of maternal RBC volume during this time (see Figure 8-2).[189] With adequate iron, serum ferritin levels stabilize by 28 weeks or slightly earlier, and may even rise near term.[15,54] Decreases in serum ferritin in early pregnancy are due to mobilization of iron stores for maternal hemoglobin synthesis; later decreases are due to increased fetal iron uptake. In multiparous women the decrease in serum ferritin occurs earlier and may be greater.

Levels of serum lipids rise with marked elevations in cholesterol and phospholipids. Cholesterol is an essential precursor for steroid hormone production by the placenta; phospholipids are major components of cell membranes. The rise in serum lipids begins in the first trimester, increasing to 40% to 60% at term (see Table 8-3). Increases in serum alkaline phosphatase are due to increased placental production. As a result, alkaline phosphatase levels are not useful in evaluating liver disorders during pregnancy. Serum cholinesterase activity decreases by 30%. Increased cholinesterase activity may lead to longer periods of paralysis if substances such as succinylcholine are used during surgical procedures.[15]

Changes on Coagulation Factors and Hemostasis

Pregnancy has been called an acquired hypercoagulable state, reflecting an increased risk for thrombosis and consumptive coagulopathies such as disseminated intravascular coagulation (DIC). Pregnancy is associated with increased clotting potential, decreased anticoagulants, and decreased fibrinolysis.[7,103] Hemostatic changes during pregnancy are thought to result in an ongoing low-grade activation of the coagulation system in the uteroplacental circulation, beginning as early as 11 to 15 weeks. This state of compensated intravascular coagulation is characterized by thrombin formation and local consumption of clotting factors in which component synthesis equals or exceeds consumption.[69,169] Figures 8-3 to 8-5 summarize coagulation and fibrinolysis.

Intravascular and extravascular fibrin deposits are found in the uteroplacental circulation, intervillous spaces, and placental bed. Tissue factor is found in amniotic fluid, placenta, decidua, and endometrial stroma.[93,103] Tissue factor (previously called thromboplastin) may play a nonhemostatic role in angiogenesis, cell signaling and embryogenesis.[63] Circulating high-molecular-weight, soluble fibrin-fibrinogen complexes—which are indicative of uteroplacental fibrin formation—also increase. During pregnancy, smooth muscle and elastic tissue within the uterine spiral arteries are replaced by a fibrin matrix (see Chapter 3). These changes allow for expansion of the vessels to accommodate increased blood flow to the placenta and to facilitate collapse of the terminal portion of the vessel with placental separation.[69,129,133,178] Elevated levels of plasminogen-activated inhibitors may assist with the deposition of fibrin in the maternal blood vessels.[65] Increased fibrinogen, thrombin generation, and inhibition of fibrinolysis during pregnancy may interact to ensure integrity of uteroplacental vessels.[103] During late pregnancy, accumulation of mural thrombi in the vessel walls decreases the diameter of the lumen, reducing blood flow, which may result in the placental infarcts and small areas of ischemia often seen at term.

Alterations are seen in coagulation (procoagulant) factors, coagulation inhibitors, and fibrinolysis. Contact factors involved in initiation of the clotting cascade and many coagulation factors are elevated in pregnancy.[69,103,129] Factors I (fibrinogen), VII, VIII, IX, XII, and X; as well as von Willebrand factor (vWF), which is important in platelet adhesion, are markedly increased.[26,42,71,103,129,179] Factors II and V are generally unchanged.[103] Factor XIII increases initially then decreases to about 50% of nonpregnant values in late pregnancy.[26,65] Factor XI decreases to term.[103] These changes increase thrombin generating potential.[103] A concurrent increase in fibrinogen and decrease in factor XIII (fibrin stabilizing factor) alters the process of clot stabilization and subsequent lysis during pregnancy.[69] Thrombin-antithrombin complexes double by the third trimester, indicating increased thrombin generation.[26,133]

Changes in coagulation factors during pregnancy are reflected in the activated partial thromboplastin time (aPTT) and prothrombin time (PT), which decrease slightly from midpregnancy to term.[26] D-dimer concentrations increase progressively, which is consistent with the hypercoagulable state of pregnancy.[42,133] Bleeding times are normally unchanged.[71]

Coagulation inhibitors form an endogenous anticoagulant system that inhibits hemostasis (see Figure 8-4). Absolute levels of antithrombin are generally unchanged during pregnancy or may be slightly decreased by term.[71] Both free and total protein are decreased.[103,128] Free protein S decreases by 60% to 70%, with the lowest levels seen at delivery.[103] This decrease is due to an increase in its carrier protein (complement 4β-binding protein).[103] Activated protein S may be decreased by up to 40% during pregnancy.[65,103] Levels of protein C, which is complexed to protein S, do not change; however, resistance to activated protein C increases, particularly in

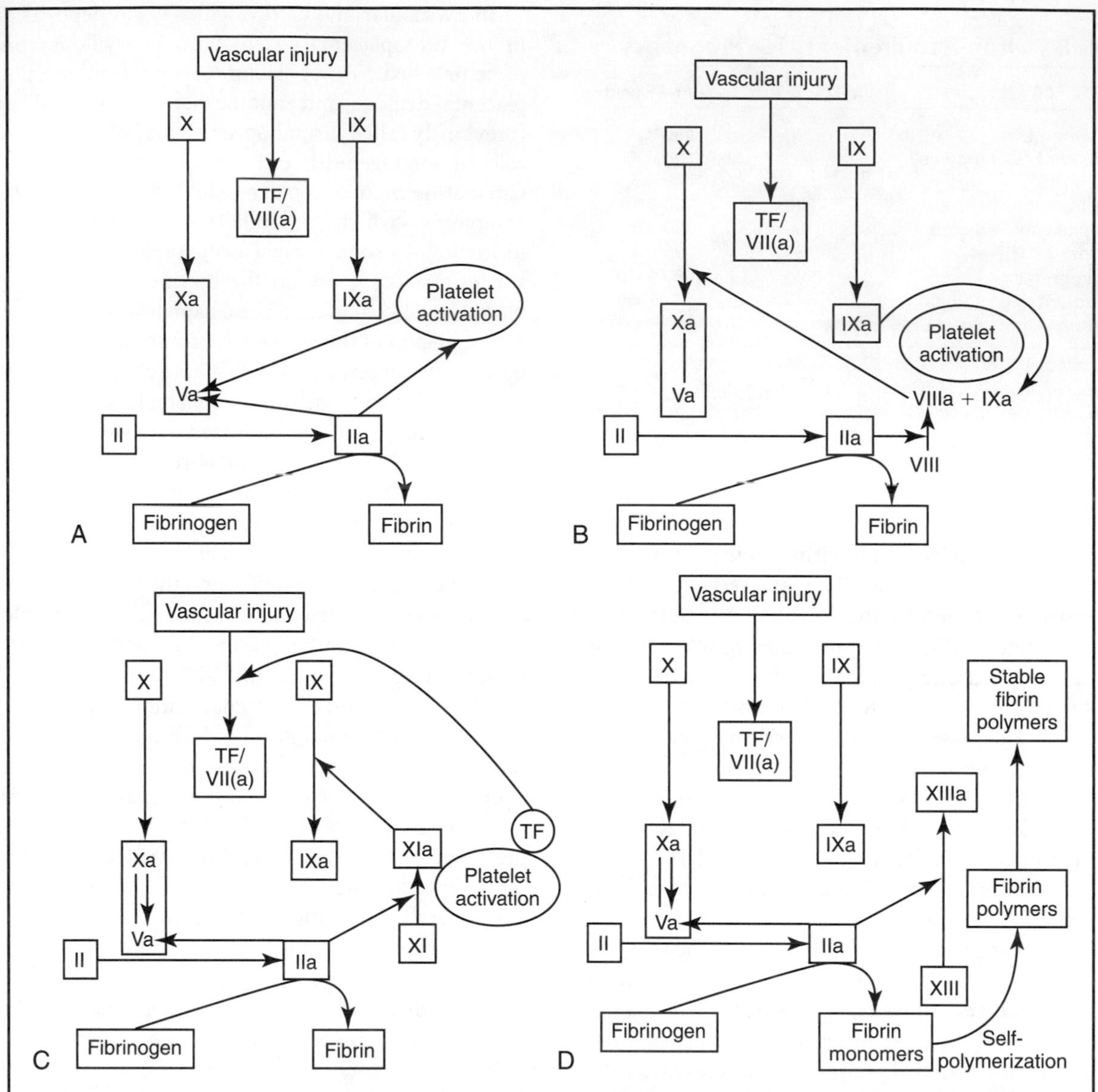

FIGURE 8-3 Fibrin plug formation. **A,** After vascular disruption, plasma factor VII binds to tissue factor (TF) to form the TF/VII(a), which activates both factor X and factor IX. Factor Xa binds to factor Va, which has been activated by thrombin factor (Factor IIa) or released from platelet α-granules. The Xa/Va complex catalyzes the conversion of prothrombin (factor II) to thrombin, which, in turn converts fibrinogen to fibrin and activates platelets. **B,** The clotting cascade is amplified by clotting reactions that occur on adjacent activated platelets. Locally generated factor IXa binds to factor VIIIa, which is activated by thrombin. The factor IXa/VIIIa complex them generates factor Xa. **C,** Coagulation is further boosted by the thrombin-mediated activation of factor XI to XIa, which also activates factor IX. Circulating TF-bearing microparticles may also bind to activate platelets at sites of vascular injury. **D,** The stable hemostatic plug is finally formed when fibrin monomers self-polymerize and are cross-linked by thrombin-activated factor XIIIa. (From Lockwood, C.J. & Silver, R. [2009]. Coagulation disorders in pregnancy. In R.K. Creasy, et al. [Eds.]. *Creasy & Resnik's Maternal-fetal medicine: Principles and practice* [6th ed.]. Philadelphia: Saunders Elsevier, p. 827.)

the second and third trimesters, due to the changes in protein S.[103] Thrombomodulin, a marker of endothelial damage, which activates protein C, is increased.[27,102] Tissue factor pathway inhibitor increases while heparin cofactor II and α_1-macroglobulin are generally unchanged.[26,71]

Fibrinolytic activity (see Figure 8-5) increases early in pregnancy, then decreases to term.[42,71,133] Type 1 and type 2 plasminogen activator inhibitors (PAI-1 and PAI-2) inhibit fibrinolysis. PAI-1 is produced by the decidua and increases 3 to 5 fold during pregnancy.[103,115] PAI-2 is produced by the placenta and increases to term impairing maternal fibrinolytic activity.[27,65,103,115] PAIs also regulate local fibrin deposition in the uteroplacental vessels and have been reported to be further increased with preeclampsia.[102]

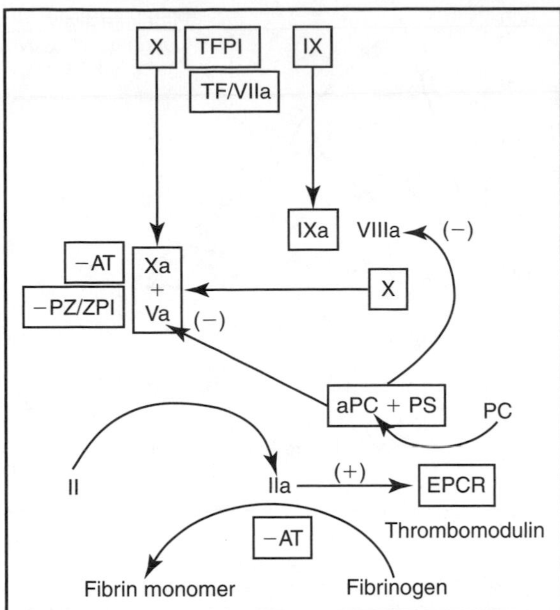

FIGURE 8-4 The anticoagulant system. Tissue factor pathway inhibitor (TFPI) binds with tissue factor (TF), factor VIIa, and factor Xa to form the prothrombinase complex. Thrombin, after binding to thrombomodulin, can activate protein C (PC) when bound to the endothelial protein C receptor (EPCR). Activated protein C (aPC) then binds to its co-factor, protein S (PS), to activate factors VIIIa and Va. Factor Xa is inhibited by the protein Z-dependent protease inhibitor (ZPI) when complexed to its cofactor, protein Z (PZ). Antithrombin (AP) potently inhibits both factor Xa and thrombin. (From Lockwood, C.J. & Silver, R. [2009]. Coagulation disorders in pregnancy. In R.K. Creasy, et al. [Eds.]. *Creasy & Resnik's Maternal-fetal medicine: Principles and practice* [6th ed.]. Philadelphia: Saunders Elsevier, p. 828.)

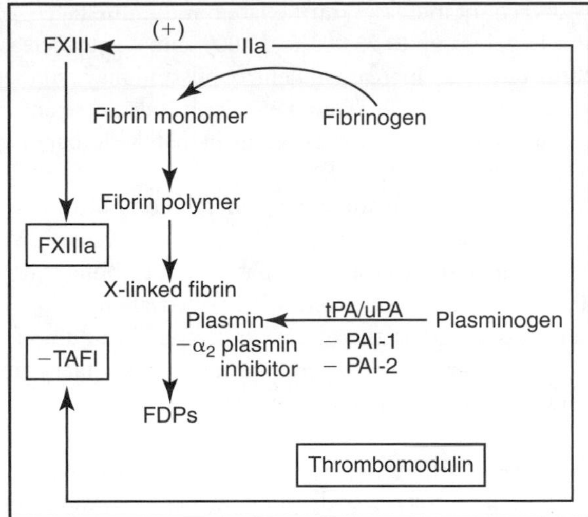

FIGURE 8-5 Fibrinolysis. The cross-linked fibrin polymer (x-linked fibrin), which was stabilized by thrombin (factor IIa)-activated factor XIIIa, is degraded to fibrin degradation products (FDPs) by the action of plasmin, which is generated by the proteolysis of plasminogen via tissue-type plasminogen activator (tPA) and urokinase-type plasminogen activator (uPA). To prevent excessive fibrinolysis, plasmin is inhibited by α_2-plasmin inhibitor, and tPA and uPA are inhibited by plaminogen activator inhibitor type-(PAI-1) and type 2 (PAI-2). In addition, thrombin-activated fibrinolytic inhibitor (TAFI), which is activated by thrombin-activated thrombomodulin complex, cleaves terminal lysine residues from fibrin to render it resistant to plasmin. (From Lockwood, C.J. & Silver, R. [2009]. Coagulation disorders in pregnancy. In R.K. Creasy, et al. [Eds.]. *Creasy & Resnik's Maternal-fetal medicine: Principles and practice* [6th ed.]. Philadelphia: Saunders Elsevier, p. 828.)

Circulating fibrin degradation products are increased, possibly due to increased fibrin generation and degradation in the placenta.[42] Since D-dimer values, a marker of fibrinolysis, are increased, this laboratory test must be used with caution for clinical evaluation in pregnancy.[65,133]

The net effect of changes in hemostasis during pregnancy is increased activity of most procoagulant proteins and a lowering of factors that inhibit coagulation, resulting in increased thrombin generation. The result is a hypercoagulable state that promotes clot formation, extension, and stability.[103,129] The hypercoagulable state of pregnancy is balanced to some extent by changes in plasminogen. Plasminogen is elevated and tissue plasmin inhibitors are decreased, which helps retain the dynamic equilibrium between clotting and clot lysis and thus overall hemostatic balance during pregnancy.[65,69] The increased tendency toward coagulation during pregnancy may also be partly balanced by pregnancy-specific proteins, which act similarly to heparin to facilitate neutralization of thrombin. Many clotting factors are synthesized by the liver and influenced by estrogen, and many of the changes seen in pregnancy are similar to those seen with oral contraceptives.[42] Estrogen may also alter uptake of coagulation proteins by the uterus and increase uterine tissue factor production in preparation for rapid onset of coagulation after placental separation.[18,42,165]

Intrapartum Period

Changes in the hematologic system and hemostasis during pregnancy are crucial in preparing the woman to tolerate the normal blood loss at delivery and prevent significant bleeding with placental separation. The amount of blood loss with delivery is up to 500 mL (vaginal delivery) or 1000 mL (cesarean section or a vaginal delivery of twins) and occurs with minimal changes in blood pressure or pulse.[15,46,54,128] This loss at delivery may be underestimated by up to 50%.[107] Blood loss at delivery and in lochia over the first few postpartum days account for about half of the increased RBC volume acquired during pregnancy.[46]

Changes in Hematologic Parameters

Hemoglobin levels tend to increase slightly during labor due to hemoconcentration. The degree of hemoconcentration is related to increases in erythropoiesis (as a stress response), muscular activity, and dehydration.[46] Leukocyte alkaline phosphatase activity increases with the onset of labor. Increases in this enzyme are often associated with inflammatory responses.

The WBC count increases during labor and immediately postpartum to values up to 25,000 to 30,000/mm^3. This increase is primarily due to an increase in neutrophils and may represent a response to stress.[149] Circulating eosinophils decrease and may disappear.[179] Intrapartum changes in hematologic parameters are summarized in Table 8-2.

Changes in the hematologic system can complicate diagnosis of infection during this period. The usual increase in WBC count may include release of immature neutrophils, which is similar to findings associated with bacterial infection. The ESR also rises and is therefore less useful. In addition, the laboring woman may experience a relative tachycardia, dehydration, and elevated temperature.

Changes in Hemostasis

The coagulation system undergoes further activation during the intrapartum period both before and after placental separation. The placenta and decidua are rich in tissue factor, the primary initiator of coagulation. Tissue factor is a membrane-bound protein expressed on the surface of cells that are normally not in direct contact with plasma.[133] With cellular injury, such as with placental separation, tissue factor is released and activates coagulation (see Figure 8-3). Concentrations of clotting factors increase during labor. PT shortens significantly, especially during the third stage of labor with clotting at the placental site. Levels of fibrinogen and plasminogen may also decrease as a result of their increased utilization after placental separation.[69] Factor VIII complex increases during labor and delivery. Factor V increases after placental separation, which contributes to activation of clotting.

Fibrinolytic activity decreases further during labor and delivery, enhancing formation of clots at the placental site following separation.[15,69,94] This promotes development of a hemostatic endometrial fibrin mesh over the wound. About 5% to 10% of the total body fibrin is deposited at this site.[69]

Fibrin levels and fibrin-fibrinogen degradation products (FDP) reach their nadir with placental separation.[42] FDP and D-dimer both increase after delivery.[42,71,133] This change may increase the risk of coagulation disorders in the immediate postpartum period by interfering with formation of firm fibrin clots.[15,69] The number of platelets falls about 20% with placental separation due to clotting at the placental site. Platelet activation and fibrin formation are maximal at delivery (Figure 8-6). Thus the hypercoagulable state of pregnancy is further magnified during the intrapartum period. This state protects the woman from hemorrhage and excessive blood loss at delivery by providing for rapid hemostasis following removal of the placenta.

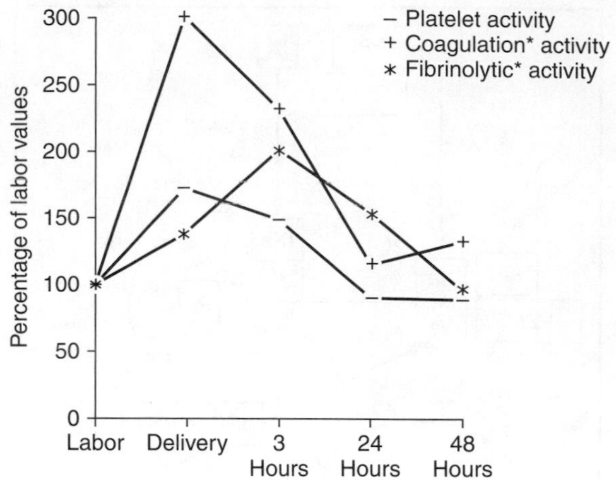

FIGURE 8-6 Platelet, coagulation, and fibrinolytic activity in labor, delivery, and postpartum. Hemostasis activity is calculated from β-thromboglobulin, platelet factor 4 (platelet), fibrinopeptide A (clotting), and fibrin-fibrinogen degradation product (fibrinolysis) values. (From Gerbasi, F.R., et al. [1990]. Changes in hemostasis during delivery and the immediate postpartum period. *Am J Obstet Gynecol, 162,* 1158.)

Postpartum Period

Changes in Blood Volume

The decrease in blood and plasma volume during the immediate postpartum period corresponds to the amount of blood loss with delivery. This loss usually accounts for over half of the RBC volume accumulated during pregnancy.[38] During the first few days after delivery, plasma volume decreases further as a result of diuresis. After 3 to 4 days, mobilization of interstitial fluid leads to a slight increase in plasma volume. This hemodilution decreases hemoglobin, hematocrit, and plasma protein by the end of the first postpartum week.[38] The volume change may contribute to circulatory embarrassment in women with cardiac problems (see Chapter 9). Plasma volume continues to decrease after the first week, reaching nonpregnant values by 6 to 8 weeks or earlier.

Accurate and consistent assessment of blood loss is essential at delivery and postpartum. Blood losses during these periods are reported to be both underestimated and overestimated. Unit and product-specific standards for estimating losses increase accuracy of these assessments.[155]

Changes in Hematologic Parameters

Increased RBC production ceases early in the postpartum period due to suppression of Epo.[38,157] Mean hemoglobin levels decrease slightly in the first 24 hours after delivery, then plateau for 4 days, followed by a slow rise to day 14.[54,87] Hematocrit values follow a similar pattern. A 500-mL blood loss such as may occur with vaginal delivery will usually result in a 1-g reduction in hemoglobin. The hematocrit returns to nonpregnant levels by 4 to 6 weeks with the normal catabolism of RBCs. The reticulocyte count is increased by the end of pregnancy, with a further increase during the first 1 to 2 postpartum days, followed by a rapid decrease. The initial increase may be a result of Epo stimulation because of decreased RBC oxygen-carrying capacity from blood loss at delivery.[54,87]

Excess circulating hemoglobin is catabolized, and the iron released is stored in the reticuloendothelial system. During the first 2 weeks, there is little change in serum ferritin levels, with a decrease in transferrin and increase in serum iron, and marked decrease in C-reactive protein.[54,87] Serum ferritin levels increase by 5 to 8 weeks to levels seen early in pregnancy. This increase occurs regardless of whether or not the woman received supplemental iron during pregnancy and is more marked after vaginal delivery.[54,74]

The WBC count, which increases in labor and immediately postpartum, falls to 6000 to 10,000/mm^3, then returns to normal values by 6 days.[87,170] Eosinophils, which tend to disappear from the peripheral blood during delivery, return by 3 days postpartum; basophils and monocytes remain unchanged.[178,179] The number of platelets, which falls following placental separation, increases beginning 3 to 4 days postpartum and gradually returns to nonpregnant levels. It is unclear whether this change is due to stimulation of platelet production or is secondary to changes in blood volume.[54,87] Postpartum changes are summarized in Table 8-2.

Changes in Hemostasis

Fibrin degradation products increase after placental delivery.[42] Fibrinolytic activity returns to normal ranges as early as 1 hour after delivery and fibrinolysis to nonpregnant levels by 24 to 48 hours.[26,71] Return to normal activity reflects removal of the fibrinolytic inhibitors produced by the placenta. PAI-1 and PAI-2 decrease after separation of the placenta. PAI-1 reaches non-pregnant values by 5 weeks.[26] PAI-2 that was originally produced by the placenta can be detected for up to 8 weeks.[71] Secondary increases in fibrinogen, factor V, and factor VIII complex occur during the first week, followed by a return to predelivery levels by 1 to 7 days, and a slow decrease to nonpregnant levels.[42] Clotting factors, which increase during labor, slowly decrease, reaching their lowest levels by 7 to 10 days. Factors VII and X return to normal levels by 2 weeks. The hemostatic system usually returns to nonpregnant status at 4 to 6 weeks postpartum, although levels of free protein S may remain low for up to 8 weeks.[71] Activated protein C resistance decreases to nonpregnant values by 1 to 7 days.[42] Changes in the flow velocity and diameter of the deep veins may take up to 6 weeks to return to prepregnant levels.[115] Thus the postpartum period continues to be a time of increased risk for thromboembolism.

CLINICAL IMPLICATIONS FOR THE PREGNANT WOMAN AND HER FETUS

The changes in the hematologic system and in hemostasis during pregnancy are important for maternal and fetal homeostasis but also increase the woman's need for iron and other nutrients and place her at risk for developing anemia, thromboembolic disorders, and coagulopathies. This section examines maternal-fetal implications related to hypervolemia, hemodilution, and the hypercoagulable state, along with implications for women with pathophysiologic states affecting the hematologic system.

The increased blood and plasma volume during pregnancy results in a physiologic hypervolemia that allows the woman to tolerate many of the changes associated with pregnancy and delivery and helps to (1) meet the demands of an enlarged uterus and hypertrophied vascular system while maintaining normal systemic blood pressure; (2) allow the woman to tolerate blood loss at delivery; (3) protect the woman from impaired venous return and hypotension with position changes late in the third trimester (when a significant proportion of her fluid volume may be sequestered within the venous system of the lower extremities) and thus reduce the risk of supine hypotension; (4) enhance maternal-fetal exchange of gases and nutrients; and (5) increase cutaneous blood flow by fourfold to sevenfold, thus assisting with heat dissipation via the skin.[15,38,46,54]

The increased red blood cell (RBC) volume helps offset hemodilution and maintain blood oxygen-carrying capacity and availability of oxygen for the fetus. The increased volume allows for adequate blood flow within the expanding uteroplacental circulation, thus ensuring adequate nutrient availability for the fetus throughout gestation. These changes alter evaluation of hematologic variables in the pregnant woman (see Table 8-1).

Iron Requirements During Pregnancy

Iron stores in nonpregnant women are generally marginal due to menstrual blood, and thus iron, loss. The usual menses loss is 12 to 15 mg of elemental iron (1 mL blood is equal to 0.5 mg of iron).[87] Most women have a daily iron intake of about 9 mg/day, below the recommended 12 to 18 mg.[128] Worldwide, an estimated 20% of fertile women have iron reserves greater than 500 mg, the minimum iron requirement in pregnancy; 40% have reserves between 100 and 500 mg; and 40% have reserves less than 100 mg.[128] In the United States, pregnant women have an average of 300 mg of iron stored at the beginning of pregnancy. So, to meet the iron demands of pregnancy, women must absorb an additional 500 to 700 mg (or 2 to 8 mg/day more than normal).[109] The World Health Organization estimates that the prevalence of anemia in pregnant women worldwide is 41.8%.[203,204] However, the prevalence varies by geographic area with estimates of 55.8% of pregnant women in Africa, 41.6% in Asia, 31.1% in Latin America and the Caribbean, 30.4% in Oceania, 18.7% in Europe, and 6.1% in North America.[203]

Iron requirements increase during pregnancy by about 1 g over the usual body iron stores of 2 to 2.5 g in adult women.[109] Table 8-4 summarizes how this additional iron is used during pregnancy. The need for iron begins early in the second trimester and peaks in the second half of pregnancy (increasing from an additional 0.8 mg/day in early pregnancy to 7.5 mg/day by term).[109,128]

The amount of iron needed by the fetus and placenta and to replace usual maternal losses is an obligatory requirement that is met regardless of the cost to maternal iron stores. Even if the mother is has low iron levels and is anemic, the fetus will usually not suffer, because the placenta continues to transport iron to meet fetal needs. If adequate iron is not available for synthesis of additional maternal RBCs, her RBC volume will not increase to the usual levels and the hematocrit and hemoglobin will decrease further as plasma volume increases.[46,87]

Low iron levels in low income countries have been associated with an increase in maternal and neonatal morbidity and mortality.[181] Iron-folic acid supplementation during pregnancy has been reported to increase hemoglobin levels by 1.17 g/dL in high income countries and 1.13 g/dL in low income countries.[160] In low income countries, use of these supplements were estimated to decrease maternal anemia by ⅓ to ½ over 10 years.[160] However, routine use of prophylactic iron supplementation in pregnancy continues to be controversial in the United States with little evidence documenting significant improvements in perinatal outcomes.[5,75,87,145,189] A Cochrane meta-analysis of 49 trials (n = 23,300 pregnant women) found that daily iron or iron plus folate supplementation increased hemoglobin levels before birth and decreased the risk of anemia at term, however no significant reduction in low birth weight infants, delayed development, preterm birth, infection, or postpartum hemorrhage was found.[145] A beneficial effect on neonatal iron stores and a risk of hemoconcentration (hemoglobin levels >130 g/dL) with daily supplementation were suggested.[145]

Although intestinal iron absorption increases in the second half of pregnancy (probably as a compensatory mechanism in response to increased iron demand), dietary sources and maternal stores alone may not be adequate to meet the increased demands of pregnancy. Iron stores affect iron absorption. Women who have good iron stores have minimal increases in absorption during the first trimester, then increase absorption during the second trimester. By later pregnancy, iron stores may be exhausted and iron needs met primarily from absorption.[109] Thus if a woman has good iron stores before pregnancy and a diet high in bioavailable iron, most of these women will not develop anemia if they are not supplemented.[87] However, iron stores in young, healthy nonpregnant women may be marginal to nonexistent.[34]

Iron supplementation increases iron reserves, hemoglobin levels, and decreases the risk of iron deficiency anemia during pregnancy and postpartum, even in women with good iron stores at the beginning of pregnancy.[128] Even with adequate nutrition, 10% to 20% of pregnant women will develop an iron deficiency.[74,75] General recommendations made by the Institute of Medicine (IOM) for iron supplementation during pregnancy are 30 mg ferrous iron (which is provided by 150 mg ferrous sulfate, 300 mg ferrous gluconate, or 100 mg ferrous fumarate) daily beginning at 12 weeks' gestation along with a well-balanced diet.[75] The need for iron can also be met with supplementation of 60 to 85 mg/day of elemental iron beginning at 20 to 28 weeks.[75,87] Although the IOM recommended supplementation only if serum ferritin levels were <20 μg/L, the high cost of this screening has limited applicability.[75,87] Iron supplementation does not prevent or correct the normal decline in hemoglobin seen in pregnancy but it can prevent depletion of stores, the first stage of iron deficiency anemia.[74]

Severe Anemia and Pregnancy

Anemia during pregnancy is defined as a hemoglobin <11 g/dL by the World Health Organization and <10.5 g/dL in the second trimester and <11.1 g/dL in the third trimester by the Center for Disease Control.[188] The most common anemias encountered in pregnancy are iron deficiency anemia, megaloblastic anemia of pregnancy (folic acid deficiency), sickle cell disorders, and α- and β-thalassemia.[54] Changes in the hematologic system may influence the course of these disorders during pregnancy and alter fetal outcome. Anemia caused by iron or folate deficiency is due to underproduction of RBCs and is associated with decreased reticulocytes. The normal hematologic changes along with altered nutritional needs during pregnancy increase the risk for these nutritional anemias.

In women with severe anemia (hemoglobin less than 6 to 8 mg/dL [60 to 80 g/L]), maternal arterial oxygen content and oxygen delivery to the fetus are decreased. The fetus attempts to adapt through increased placental blood flow, redistribution of blood within the fetal organs, increased RBC production (to increase the total oxygen-carrying capacity), and a decrease in the diffusing distance for oxygen across the placenta. Because fetuses have predominantly fetal hemoglobin, they cannot readily increase the availability of oxygen to the tissues by further altering the affinity of hemoglobin for oxygen. Although the fetus adapts, the cost may be high, with decreased growth and an increased mortality due to the lack of an adequate oxygen supply and nutrients. Several meta-analyses have found significant relationships between maternal anemia (hemoglobin less than 8.5 g/dL [85 g/L]) in early pregnancy and preterm birth, but not with small-for-gestational-age infants.[165] Conversely, an elevated hemoglobin (greater than 14.5 [145 g/L]) in early pregnancy is associated with stillbirth and small-for-gestational-age infants, perhaps because the increased hemoglobin is due to a reduction in the usual increase in plasma volume and thus reduced blood flow to the intervillous space.[179]

Iron Deficiency Anemia

The most common cause of anemia during pregnancy is iron deficiency anemia.[36,87] Generally this form of anemia is preventable or easily treated with iron supplements. Hematologic changes in pregnancy can make diagnosis of iron deficiency difficult.[54] Total iron binding capacity and serum iron often fall during pregnancy, as well as with iron deficiency anemia. A useful test for iron deficiency in the pregnant woman is measurement of serum ferritin levels, which correlate well with iron stores during pregnancy.[54] Serum ferritin levels lower than 12 mcg/L with a low hemoglobin indicate iron deficiency, which can be treated with ferrous sulfate until the hemoglobin returns to levels normal for the stage of gestation.[54,74] Because ferritin is an acute phase reactant, falsely high levels may occur with infection. Therefore serum ferritin levels less than 60 to 100 mcg/L may indicate deficiency if infection is present.[54]

In general, even with significant maternal iron deficiency, the fetus will often be protected and receive adequate stores at cost to the mother. However, if the mother is severely iron deficient and anemic, the fetus may have decreased RBC volume, hemoglobin, iron stores, and cord ferritin levels and an increased risk of iron deficiency during infancy.[38,54,87] Iron deficiency anemia before midpregnancy is associated with an increased risk of low birth weight, preterm birth, and perinatal mortality.[54,74,128]

Megaloblastic Anemia

Megaloblastic anemia in the nonpregnant woman is usually due to folic acid or vitamin B_{12} deficiency. Folic acid deficiency is the most common cause of megaloblastic anemia encountered during pregnancy.[54] Vitamin B_{12} deficiency with pregnancy is less common because (1) stores of vitamin B_{12} are normally large (most women have a 2- to 3-year store in their liver), so deficient states take years to develop; (2) vitamin B_{12} is used for DNA replication, so a severe deficiency usually leads to infertility; and (3) vitamin B_{12} deficiency is usually due to pernicious anemia, a disorder seen primarily in older women.[54,87] Vitamin B_{12} dietary deficiency in pregnancy most often occurs with a vegan diet. Vitamin B_{12} deficiency may be misdiagnosed in a pregnant woman, because serum vitamin B_{12} levels fall with the expanded plasma volume and consequent hemodilution.[54]

Folate demands increase threefold during pregnancy from 50 μg/day to 300 to 500 μg/day during pregnancy.[87] Because folic acid is essential for DNA synthesis and cell duplication, folate is needed for growth of the fetus and placenta as well as for maternal RBC production. Folate requirements increase throughout pregnancy and are higher in multiple pregnancy.[54] Maternal serum folate levels fall during pregnancy, and women with an inadequate dietary intake need supplements. Prenatal vitamins generally contain 1 g of folate; increased levels are needed for individuals with hematolytic disorders. The changes in folate metabolism during pregnancy are due to decreased serum folate and RBCs, increased plasma clearance, increased urinary excretion, and altered histidine metabolism.[121]

Severe folic acid deficiency has been associated with fetal malformations, preeclampsia, abruptio placenta, prematurity, and low birth weight.[54] Maternal folate deficiency increases the risk of neural tube defects (NTDs) and has been associated with a increased risk of cleft lip and palate and preterm birth.[35,54,87,114,121] A recent Cochrane meta-analysis (5 trials; n = 6105) confirmed that daily folic acid supplementation reduced the risk of neural tube defects, but did not find evidence for a role in preventing cleft lip and palate, congenital heart disease, miscarriage, or other defects.[52] Supplementation is recommended for all women of childbearing age to reduce the risk of neural tube defects. Supplementation should begin before pregnancy because NTDs occur early in the first trimester (see Chapter 15).[35] During pregnancy, folate is included in prenatal vitamins.[111] In later pregnancy, the fetus has higher levels of folate and elevated folate-binding protein, which protects against fetal folate deficiency; even with low maternal folate levels, neonatal cord levels are usually within normal limits.

Sickle Cell Disease

Sickle cell disease is a group of disorders that involve mutations in the genes that determine hemoglobin β-chain structure. In women with sickle cell anemia, tissue deoxygenation or acidosis triggers structural changes in the sickle hemoglobin (HbS), so the RBCs take on a half-moon or sickle appearance. The sickled cells can obstruct blood flow in the microvasculature. The areas most susceptible to obstruction are those characterized by slow flow and high oxygen extraction such as the spleen, bone marrow, and placenta. Obstruction leads to venous stasis, further deoxygenation, platelet aggregation, hypoxia, acidosis, further sickling, and eventually infarction.[54,87]

A woman with sickle cell anemia normally has a lower hemoglobin level (7 to 8 g/dL [70 to 80 g/L]) and oxygen-carrying capacities, to which her system has adjusted. Pregnancy places both the woman and her infant at greater risk for complications due in part to the effects of hematologic, cardiovascular, renal, and respiratory changes during pregnancy.[158] As plasma volume increases during pregnancy, the woman may become slightly more anemic. In addition, she may experience an increased risk of sickling attacks. Sickle cell crises are triggered by physical or emotional stress, which may be caused by infection, trauma, hypoxia, and pregnancy. Crises in pregnancy and postpartum may be related to the hypercoagulable state, increased susceptibility to infection, or vascular stress.[158] The rapid hemodynamic changes postpartum often precipitate crises, especially if associated with a long or difficult labor and delivery.[87] Fetal and neonatal complications such as prematurity and fetal growth restriction may arise due to placental infarction and fetal hypoxia. Fetal hypoxia results from decreased oxygen transport due to the abnormal biochemistry of the maternal hemoglobin and the loss of functional placental tissue for gas and nutrient exchange caused by the infarctions.[54,87]

Thalassemias

Thalassemia is a disorder in the synthesis of either the α or β peptide chains of the hemoglobin molecule. This leads to alterations in the RBC membrane and decreased RBC life span. α-Thalessemia is an alteration in the production of α chains, in which one or more of the four genes on chromosome 16 that are involved in α-chain production are altered or deleted. Phenotype and severity depend on how many genes are involved and whether the genes are deleted (nonfunctional) or present but with altered function.[194] Most pregnant women with α-thalessemia have one or two genes affected and have either a silent presentation or mild anemia.[87,194] If all four α-chain genes are missing, the fetus cannot synthesize either normal fetal hemoglobin (composed of two α- and two γ-chains) nor adult hemoglobin (composed of two α- and two β-chains). Infants develop high output cardiac failure, hydrops fetalis, and are often stillborn or die shortly after birth. Intrauterine transfusions are associated with decreased perinatal mortality and morbidity. These infants currently require lifelong transfusion therapy; however, stem cell transplants have been reported to be effective in treating this disorder.[194]

β-Thalassemia minor is a frequently encountered β-thalassemia during pregnancy. Many females with thalassemia major (Cooley anemia) die in childhood or adolescence; those who survive are often amenorrheic and infertile.[54,87] Some pregnancies have occurred in these women, with an increased risk of fetal loss.[54] Women with β-thalassemia minor have a mild hypochromic, microcytic anemia, but are usually healthy otherwise and generally do not have increased maternal or infant morbidity if their condition is stable.[87] With the plasma volume expansion that accompanies pregnancy, they may develop a more pronounced anemia, but they generally require only supportive care.[188] Women with β-thalassemia intermedia may develop a more severe anemia during pregnancy, especially in the second and third trimesters, and may require transfusion therapy.[25]

Thromboembolism and Pregnancy

The hypercoagulable state of pregnancy is crucial in protecting the mother against excessive blood loss with delivery and placental separation. However, the hypercoagulable state is also a disadvantage because it significantly increases the risk of thromboembolic disorders during pregnancy and postpartum. Venous thromboembolism (VTE) is a leading cause of maternal mortality in the United States.[102]

The risk of VTE increases up to sixfold during pregnancy (0.76 to 1.723 per 1000 pregnant women).[115] The risk increases with parity and age, and is nine times higher among women with cesarean deliveries than among women who give birth vaginally.[102,196] VTE includes both deep vein thrombosis (DVT) and pulmonary emboli.[102] Pulmonary embolism occurs in 1 in 2000 pregnancies and is a major cause of maternal mortality.[69,102] Pulmonary emboli usually result from dislodged deep venous thrombi in the lower extremities.

The three factors (Virchow triad) that predispose to thromboembolic disorders (stasis, altered coagulation, and vascular damage) are all present or potentially present during pregnancy.[102] Ninety-eight percent of DVTs arise in the lower extremities.[102] During pregnancy, increased venous capacitance (due to the effects of progesterone and local endothelial production of prostacyclin [PGI_2] and nitric oxide) leads to increased distensibility, decreased flow in the lower extremities, and venous stasis. By late pregnancy, the velocity of venous blood flow in the lower extremities has been reduced by half, and venous pressure has risen an average of 10 mmHg (1.33 kPa).[69,102,115] The blood flow velocity decreases by early in the second trimester, with a nadir from 34 weeks to term that does not return to prepregnant values until 6 or more weeks after delivery. In addition, the diameter of the major leg veins increases, more so on the left than the right. During pregnancy, greater than 80% of DVTs occur on the left (versus 55% in nonpregnant women).[102,133,156] This is because of compression of the left iliac vein by the right iliac and ovarian veins. About three fourths of DTVs occur during the antepartum period, and one fourth occur postpartum.[102,156,196] Most pulmonary emboli develop postpartum and are associated with cesarean section.[102]

The hypercoagulable state during pregnancy increases the risk of clot formation. The increased fibrinogen, coagulation factors, and decreased protein S and resistance to activated protein C increased thrombin generation, decrease endogenous anticoagulants and impair fibrinolysis. If a clot develops, the decreased fibrinolytic activity and increased PAI-1 and PAI-2 (which inhibit clot lysis) impedes fibrin removal and clot lysis.[102] An increase in the incidence of VTEs is seen during the third trimester when fibrinolytic activity decreases. Finally, the potential for localized vascular damage and release of tissue factor exists with delivery and particularly with cesarean section. Further decreases in protein S after cesarean delivery or with infection may increase the risk of pulmonary emboli postpartum.[102] VTE is also increased with obesity, increased parity, maternal age, prolonged bed rest, and in women with thrombophilia, antiphospholipid syndrome, anemia, artificial heart valves, or preeclampsia (due to exaggeration of the hypercoagulable state).[102,115,125] Once a thrombus develops, it is more likely that it will extend if the predisposing factors persist over time, as occurs with pregnancy. Women with a history of VTE either before or during pregnancy, especially if associated with thrombophilia, have an increased risk of developing a similar disorder in subsequent pregnancies. Ambulation soon after delivery decreases venous stasis and the risk of VTE.

In pregnant women with VTEs the anticoagulant therapy of choice is usually either unfractionated or low molecular weight heparin. Heparin is considered the drug of choice for thromboembolic disorders during pregnancy because the molecular weight of both of these forms of heparin prevents placental transfer.[58,102,119] Heparin doses may need to be increased as pregnancy progresses, particularly during the third trimester. Changes in heparin requirements have been related to increasing plasma volume and renal clearance and to the presence of a placental heparinase enzyme. Heparin doses may need to be decreased in women who develop significant alterations in renal function or in whom plasma volume changes are reduced.[102,119] Coumarin derivatives (warfarin sulfate) inhibit vitamin K–dependent coagulation factors. These agents cross the placenta, whereas vitamin K–dependent coagulation factors do not, impairing fetal coagulation and increasing the risk of fetal and neonatal hemorrhage.[119] The risk of fetal bleeding and intracranial hemorrhage is especially high during labor. Warfarin has also been associated with an increased risk of abortion and with a specific syndrome of fetal anomalies involving the face, eyes, bones, and central nervous system, if given in the first 11 to 13 weeks of gestation.[119,122] These abnormalities may be due to inhibition of vitamin K–dependent proteins (osteocalcins) involved in bone development.

Coagulation Disorders During Pregnancy

Thrombophilias are being increasingly regarded as having potential roles in the pathophysiology of preeclampsia, fetal growth restriction, and miscarriage due to the effects of thrombotic changes in the placental bed.[65,70] Changes in pregnancy may exacerbate the effects of inherited thrombophilias such as the factor V Leiden and prothrombin gene variants and deficiencies of protein C and S and increase the risk of pregnancy complications.[103] Women with these disorders may develop clinical signs for the first time during pregnancy.[65] The most common acquired thrombophilic disorder is antiphospholipid syndrome (APS), an autoimmune disorder seen in 0.2% to 2% of pregnant women.[103,159] In this disorder, antibodies are produced that promote thrombosis. APS involves activation of endothelial cells, monocytes, and platelets by the APL antibodies.[159] Women with APS have an increased risk of arterial and venous thrombosis, autoimmune thrombocytopenia, miscarriage, and fetal loss.[96,159] Pregnancy or use of estrogen-containing birth control pills increase the risk of thrombosis in women with APS, who are treated with heparin with or without low-dose aspirin.[159]

Antiphospholipid antibodies such as lupus anticoagulant and anticardiolipin are also seen in pregnancies complicated by preeclampsia, fetal growth restriction, placental insufficiency, placental abruption, and preterm birth.[65,103] The increase in fetal loss with antiphospholipid antibodies is thought to be due to an increase in the thromboxane to prostacyclin ratio in the decidua and placenta, leading to increased platelet activation, vasoconstriction, placental thrombosis and infarct, and subsequent fetal death.[103]

Pregnancy is characterized by increases in fibrinolytic activity, plasminogen and plasminogen activators in the uterus, and an ongoing low-grade activation of the coagulation system within the uteroplacental circulation. As a result, events such as extravasation of blood into the myometrium or rupture of blood vessels in the area can activate the fibrinolytic system and lead to a consumptive coagulopathy.[15] The risk of coagulopathies such as disseminated intravascular coagulation (DIC) is higher during pregnancy, particularly in association with placental abruption, severe preeclampsia, eclampsia, intrauterine fetal death, amniotic fluid embolism, or septic abortion.[87] These events result in one or more of the processes commonly associated with intravascular coagulation: release of tissue factor and activation clotting (preeclampsia, eclampsia), endothelial injury with activation of coagulation (placental abruption, fetal death), or shock and stasis (amniotic fluid embolism, gram-negative sepsis).[87,191] Many of these complications trigger the formation of tissue factor or endotoxins, thus inducing thrombin formation. The resulting activation of the coagulation pathway (see Figure 8-3) leads to depletion of fibrinogen and increased fibrinolytic activity.[69]

DIC arises from inappropriate activation of normal clotting processes within the circulation with intravascular consumption of procoagulant proteins, clotting factors and platelets, formation of fibrin clots within the vascular bed, production of anticoagulants, and activation of fibrinolysis. As a result, the normal balance between the coagulation and fibrinolytic systems is disrupted. Consumption of the clotting factors can lead to hemorrhage and shock. As clots are formed and fibrin is deposited in the microcirculation, further cell (tissue) injury occurs, triggering further coagulation and eventual depletion of plasma clotting factors. These fibrin clots may also cause intravascular obstruction and infarction. Activation of clotting also activates the fibrinolytic system, which leads to formation of fibrin-fibrinogen degradation products or fibrin split products. These fibrin degradation products further inhibit coagulation and decrease platelet function.[202]

SUMMARY

The hematologic and hemostatic systems undergo significant alterations during pregnancy that promote maternal adaptation but also influence interpretation of laboratory values and increase the risk of thromboembolic insults and coagulopathies. Because of the significant risks associated with these events, appropriate measurement, observation, data gathering, and evaluation are essential. Changes in the hematologic system during pregnancy are also critical for fetal homeostasis. Maternal hypervolemia promotes delivery of oxygen and nutrients to the fetus; changes in serum albumin concentration may influence the availability of both nutrients and potentially harmful substances. The fetus can, in turn, affect maternal status, as is the case with iron metabolism and needs. Clinical recommendations for nurses working with pregnant women based on changes in the hematologic system are summarized in Table 8-5.

DEVELOPMENT OF THE HEMATOLOGIC SYSTEM IN THE FETUS

The hematologic system arises early in gestation and along with the primitive cardiovascular system is one of the earliest systems to achieve some functional capacity. The hematologic system is critical for the well-being of the fetus through transport of nutrients and oxygen and removal of waste products. Fetal red blood cells (RBCs), white blood cells (WBCs), and platelets are often found in the maternal circulation. Fetomaternal transfusion occurs in an estimated 50% of pregnancies, although this generally involves a small volume. RBCs can pass as early as 4 to 6 weeks. Later, antigens on some of these cells may stimulate maternal antibody production against the fetal cells, which can lead to fetal anemia, neutropenia, or thrombocytopenia.[30] Fetal iron requirements were discussed in the previous section.

Formation of Blood Cells

Blood cells first appear in the yolk sac and can be found as early as 2 weeks, gestation.[106] By about 6 weeks' gestation, hematopoietic stem cells are found in the developing liver and migrate from there to the bone marrow.[209] Hematopoiesis in the fetus can be divided into three periods: mesoblastic, hepatic, and myeloid. In all sites, cells arise from stem cells derived from mesoderm tissues. Primitive cells arise first,

Table 8-5 Recommendations for Clinical Practice Related to Changes in the Hematologic System of Pregnant Women

Recognize usual hematologic values and patterns of change during pregnancy and postpartum (pp. 216-225 and Tables 8-1 to 8-3).
Recognize that isolated laboratory values must be evaluated in light of clinical findings and previous values (pp 216-225).
Assess maternal nutritional status in relation to iron, folate, and vitamins, and provide nutritional counselling (pp. 225-227).
Monitor hematocrit and hemoglobin values throughout pregnancy (pp. 218-219, 225-227).
Know the patterns of change in plasma and blood volume during pregnancy and the postpartum period (pp. 216-217, 223-224).
Monitor and counsel women with cardiac problems, paying particular attention to periods when blood and plasma volume increases significantly (pp. 216-217, 223-224 and Chapter 9).
Monitor for and teach pregnant woman to recognize the signs of thromboembolism and consumptive coagulopathy (pp. 228-229).
Recognize risk factors for the development of thromboembolism (p. 228).
Encourage ambulation soon after delivery to reduce the risk of thromboembolism (p. 228).
Recognize risk factors for development of consumptive coagulopathies (p. 229).
Evaluate maternal responses to prescribed drugs for signs of subtherapeutic levels or side effects (p. 220 and Chapter 7).
Counsel women regarding the effects of plasma volume increases and decreased plasma proteins on drug levels during pregnancy (pp. 216-217, 220 and Chapter 7).
Recognize factors that may alter signs of infection during the intrapartum and early postpartum period (pp. 223-224).
Note the timing of cord clamping (pp. 234-235).

followed by definitive cells. Embryonic and fetal hematopoietic stem cells are pluripotent cells that can reproduce and repopulate in adults better than adult stem cells. Thus these fetal cells have greater potential for transplant with lower risk of graft failure.[33,47,209] Embryonic and fetal stem cells also have the ability to differentiate into cells of different tissues types, not just hematopoietic cells, depending on environment.[141]

During the mesoblastic period (from 14 to 19 days to a peak at 6 weeks' gestation), blood cells are formed in blood islands in the secondary yolk sac. The secondary yolk sac arises at 12 to 15 days and is a site of early protein synthesis, nutrient transfer, and hematopoiesis. Peripheral cells in these islands form primitive blood vessels; central cells develop into hematoblasts (primitive RBCs).[33,148] Although only RBCs and macrophages are produced in the yolk sac, the yolk sac stem cells are all multipotential.[67,81] Blood formation in the yolk sac is maximal from 2 to 10 weeks and disappears by the third month.[3,48] Another site of early blood formation during this period is the ventral aspect of the aorta in the periumbilical area. Hematopoiesis occurs in this area until 28 to 40 days' gestation.[33,81,187]

The hepatic period begins during the fifth to sixth week, shortly after the onset of circulation during weeks 4 to 5. This period peaks from 6 to 18 weeks. Thus from 3 to 5 months the liver is the major source of fetal blood cells, although some blood formation continues in this site through the first week after birth. Liver mass increases 40-fold after liver hematopoiesis begins, and at 11 to 12 weeks' gestation, hematopoietic cells make up 60% of the liver.[47,81] The predominant cells produced by the liver are normoblastic erythrocytes, although megakaryocytes, granulocytes, and lymphocytes are also produced.[148] Hematopoiesis can be detected in the spleen, omentum, and thymus during the third month and shortly thereafter in the lymph nodes. Blood formation in the spleen, initially producing erythrocytes and later lymphocytes, declines after 4 to 5 months' gestation.[207]

Extramedullary erythropoiesis may continue in the liver and spleen and develop in other organs, including the adrenal glands, pancreas, thyroid, endocardium, skin, and brain, after bone marrow is established.[81] This may occur with any event resulting in reduced bone marrow function, as can occur with rubella or parvovirus B19 infection. When this occurs in the skin, it can been seen as the "blueberry muffin" rash.[81]

The thymus and lymph nodes become seeded with stem cells by the fourth month. These structures are primarily involved in lymphopoiesis but are also involved in maturation and activation of the immature WBCs that develop from myeloid stem cells.[33,140]

The myeloid period begins at about 18 weeks, with eventual production of all types of blood cells.[3,47,81] The bone marrow is the major site for blood production after 30 weeks' gestation.[3,81] Centers for blood formation arise in mesenchymal tissues and invade cavities produced during bone formation (see Chapter 17). Initially bone marrow produces granulocytes and megakaryocytes. After liver erythropoiesis declines, bone marrow erythropoiesis increases. The major area of blood production is the fatty marrow in the core of the long bones. Large fat cells are not found in fetal marrow as they are in adults, suggesting that fetal marrow is functioning at full hematopoietic capacity under homeostatic conditions.

The long bones of the fetus and newborn are cartilaginous, and their relative marrow volume is smaller than in older individuals. As a result, the only way the fetus or newborn can significantly increase production of blood cells is by either reactivation or persistence of extramedullary hematopoiesis in the abdominal viscera, such as the liver and spleen. This extramedullary erythropoiesis is responsible for much of the hepatosplenomegaly seen in infants with erythroblastosis fetalis.[53]

All blood cells arise from pluripotent stem cells under the influence of various cytokines and growth factors for specific cell lineages (Figure 8-7). Fetal and post birth hematopoiesis are mediated by hematopoietic growth factors and cytokines, including stem cell factors, interleukin(IL)-1, IL-4, IL-6, IL-9, erythropoietin (Epo), macrophage colony-stimulating factor (M-CSF), granulocyte colony-stimulating factor (G-CSF), thrombopoietin, and possibly insulin and insulin-like growth factors.[31,47,81,106,148] Hematopoietic growth factors are either non–cell-lineage– or cell-lineage–specific. Non–cell-lineage–specific growth factors—such as IL-3 and granulocyte-macrophage colony-stimulating factor (GM-CSF)—stimulate a variety of progenitor cells. Cell-lineage–specific growth factors stimulate differential maturation of granulocytes (G-CSF), monocytes (M-CSF), or erythrocytes.[81,106] Epo and other hematotpoietic growth factors also appear to be important in development of other systems (including cardiovascular, gastrointestinal, and brain) both before and after birth.[67,79,80,92,186,205]

Development of Red Blood Cells

Fetal RBC production is independent of the mother. The initial RBCs are primitive nucleated megaloblasts that appear at 3 to 4 weeks' gestation, followed by normative megaloblastic erythropoiesis at 6 weeks. The primitive cells contain embryonic hemoglobin and are not dependent on Epo. The definitive fetal RBC, produced initially in the liver, contains primarily fetal hemoglobin (HbF) and is regulated by Epo.[47,148] By 10 weeks, the latter cells constitute 90% of the RBC volume. The early cells are large nucleated cells with increased deformability. With increasing gestation, hemoglobin, hematocrit, and total RBC count increases, whereas numbers of nucleated RBCs, mean corpuscular volume, cell diameter, mean corpuscular hemoglobin volume, reticulocytes, and proportion of immature cell forms decrease.[81,140] Yolk sac cells differentiate intravascularly, while erythoblasts in the liver and bone marrow mature attached to macrophages in blood islands.[142]

Epo does not cross the placenta, so fetal erythropoiesis is endogenously controlled.[33,81] Fetal Epo increases from 19 weeks to term and is produced primarily in the liver, and also in the spleen, rather than in the kidneys. Increasing amounts of Epo are produced in the kidneys from 20 weeks, and especially from 30 weeks to term as the kidneys mature.[47,81] The shift from liver to renal Epo production after 30 weeks is thought to be due to increased Epo expression in interstitial cells along with renal growth and maturation. Epo inhibits the death of erythroid precursors and stimulates development and differentiation of these precursors. Epo levels are elevated with fetal hypoxia, anemia, and placental insufficiency and in infants of insulin-dependent diabetic mothers.[47]

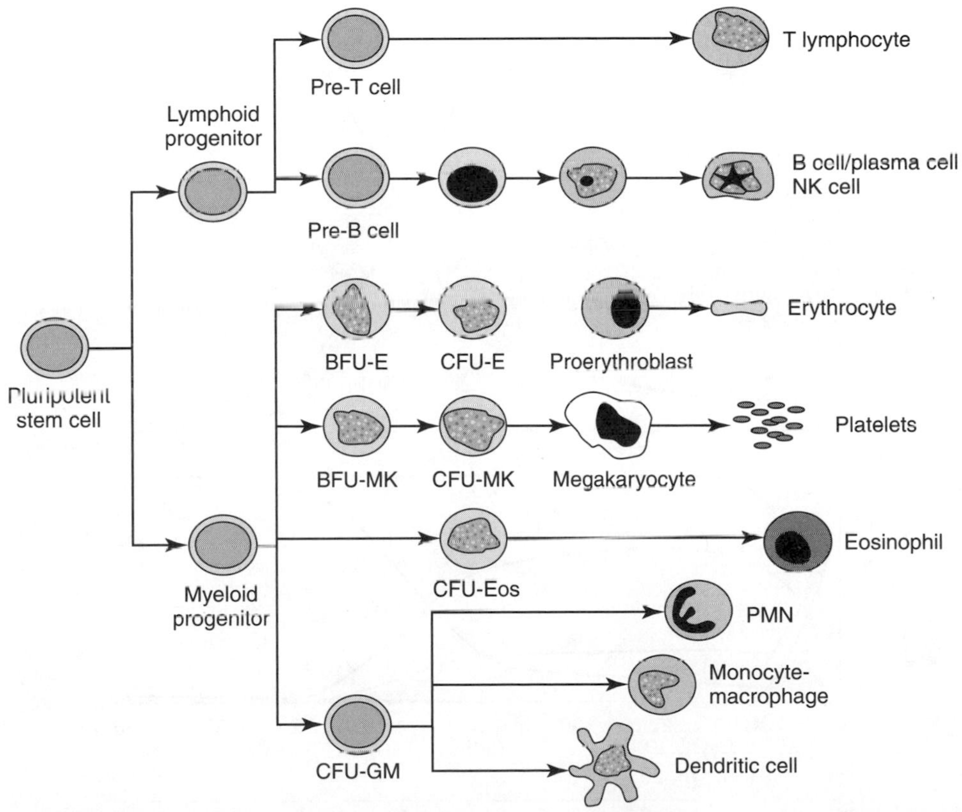

FIGURE 8-7 Overview of hematopoiesis. Hematopoietic lineages are outlined. *BFU*, Burst forming unit; CFU, colony forming unit; E, erythroid; MK, megakaryocyte; GM, granulocyte-macrophage; Eos, eosinophil; NK, natural killer cell; PMN, polymorphonuclear. (From Nguyen-Vermillion, A. & Juul, S. [2012]. Developmental biology of the hematologic system. In C.A. Gleason & S. Devaskar [Eds.]. *Avery's diseases of the newborn* [9th ed.]. Philadelphia: Saunders.)

Development of White Blood Cells and Platelets

Formation of WBCs begins in the liver at 5 weeks, although a few macrophages are produced in the yolk sac, followed by the thymus (8 to 9 weeks), spleen (11 weeks), and lymph nodes (12 weeks).[81] Significant numbers are not produced until the myeloid period. Initially, erythropoiesis is greater than granulopoiesis; however, by 10 to 12 weeks, granulopoiesis predominates, and by 21 weeks the adult ratio of granulopoiesis to erythropoiesis is seen.[208] Circulating granulocytes increase rapidly during the third trimester. The neutrophil count doubles from 14 to 18 weeks, gestation and increases four-fold from 24 to 32 weeks.[110] At birth, numbers of WBCs are equal to or greater than those found in adults. Eosinophils appear by 10 weeks, increasing to 5% of total marrow cells by 21 weeks. Basophils also appear by 10 weeks, but levels remain low. Monocytes are found in the yolk sac by 3 to 4 weeks and initially are the most prominent cells in liver hematopoietic tissue, then decrease to birth. Circulating monocytes are seen at 5 to 6 months, gestation.[89] Macrophage levels peak at 10 to 16 weeks; monocyte levels peak by 12 to 16 weeks.[208]

Lymphocytes are formed in the fetal liver and lymphoid plexuses initially, then in the thymus (7 to 10 weeks), and spleen and bone marrow (10 to 12 weeks).[81] The numbers of circulating lymphocytes increase rapidly to peak at 20 weeks (10,000 mm^3), then decline to 3000/mm^3 by term.[140] Megakaryocytes are found at 5 to 6 weeks in the yolk sac, by 8 to 9 weeks in the circulation, in the liver and spleen by 10 weeks, and reach adult levels by 18 weeks.[148,177] Platelets increase from a mean of 187,000/mm^3 at 15 weeks to a mean of 274,000 by term.[143,175] Thrombopoietin, produced primarily in the liver and kidneys, is the major factor controlling platelet production.[81]

Formation of Hemoglobin

Hemoglobin synthesis begins around 14 days' gestation. Several forms of hemoglobin (Hb) are found in the embryo and fetus (Figure 8-8). Two pairs of polypeptide chains form each of the different hemoglobin types (Table 8-6). All forms have two α or α-like globulin chains (controlled by genes on chromosome 16). The primitive embryonic varieties formed in the yolk sac are Gower 1 (seen at less than 5 weeks' gestation), followed by Gower 2 and Hb Portland (seen between 5 and 10 to 12 weeks' gestation).[47,148] Two points of hemoglobin switching occur during development, the first is the switch from embryonic hemoglobin to fetal hemoglobin (HbF); the second is the switch from HbF to adult hemoglobin (HbA).[16]

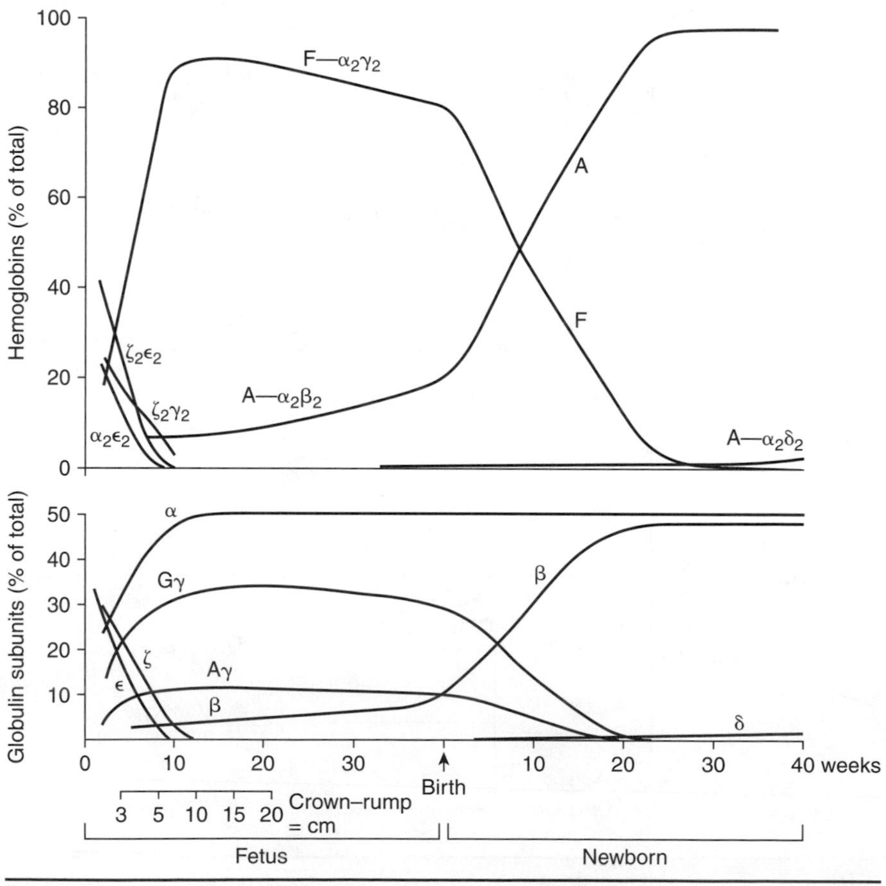

FIGURE 8-8 Development of hemoglobin in the fetus and newborn. The relative proportions of each globulin chain produced at each stage of gestation are shown. Refer to Table 8-7 for descriptions of the different types of hemoglobin. (Adapted from Bunn, H.F., et al. [1986]. *Hemoglobin: Molecular, genetic and clinical aspects.* Philadelphia: Saunders.)

Table 8-6 **Human Hemoglobins Expressed During Development**

HEMOGLOBIN (Hb)	GLOBULIN CHAIN COMPOSITION	STAGE OF EXPRESSION	PRIMARY SITE OF PRODUCTION
Hb Gower 1	Zeta$_2$ epsilon$_2$ ($\zeta_2\epsilon_2$)	Embryonic	Yolk sac
Hb Gower 2	Alpha$_1$ epsilon$_2$ ($\alpha_1\epsilon_2$)	Embryonic	Yolk sac
Hb Portland	Zeta$_2$ gamma$_2$ ($\zeta_2\gamma_2$)	Embryonic	Yolk sac
HbF	Alpha$_2$ ^{A} gamma$_2$ or alpha$_2$^{G} gamma$_2$	Fetal	Liver
HbA_2	Alpha2 delta2 ($\alpha_2\delta_2$)	Adult	Bone marrow
HbA	Alpha2 beta2 ($\alpha_2\beta_2$)	Adult	Bone marrow

From Luchtman-Jones, L., Schwartz, A.L., & Wilson, D.B. (2006). Hematological problems in the fetus and neonate. In R.J. Martin, A.A. Fanaroff, & M.C. Walsh (Eds.). *Fanaroff & Martin's Neonatal-perinatal medicine: Diseases of the fetus and infant* (8th ed.). Philadelphia: Mosby.

The predominant hemoglobin from 10 to 12 weeks to term is HbF, which consists of a pair of α chains and a pair of γ chains. HbA, which consists of pairs of α and β chains (controlled by genes on chromosome 11), appears after 6 to 8 weeks and increases rapidly after 16 to 20 weeks' gestation.[140] By 30 to 32 weeks, 90% to 95% of the hemoglobin is HbF. After this point, the amount of HbF begins to slowly decline to 84% at 34 weeks and 60% to 80% by term.[146] Simultaneously, levels of HbA increase along with the total body hemoglobin mass.[140] The switch from fetal to adult hemoglobin synthesis is related to postmenstrual, not post birth, age. Synthesis of HbA and HbF is not significantly affected by intrauterine transfusions or exchange transfusions after birth.

All forms of hemoglobin have similar functions but vary in their oxygen affinity, with earlier forms having greater affinity.[14,47] HbF has a greater affinity for oxygen because HbF does not bind 2,3-diphosphoglycerate (2,3-DPG) as effectively as does HbA. Increased affinity facilitates oxygen transfer across the placenta but reduces oxygen release to the tissues. Fetal hemoglobin has several other unique properties. HbF is more resistant to acid elution and can be oxidized to methemoglobin more readily, increasing the susceptibility of newborns to methemoglobinemia.

The resistance of fetal hemoglobin to acid elution is the basis for tests such as the Kleihauer-Betke techniques used to detect fetal cells in maternal blood. These tests may be unreliable as a measure of fetal cells if maternal HbF is elevated or with ABO incompatibility. In the presence of ABO incompatibility, fetal cells may be destroyed by maternal antibody and cleared from the mother's circulation. Altered levels of HbF are seen in women with sickle cell anemia, thalassemia minor, hydatidiform mole, and leukemia and in a pregnancy-induced elevation of HbF. Fetal cells may still be identified, because with elevated maternal HbF there tend to be many cells with varying amounts of HbF and the fewer fetal cells have consistently high HbF concentrations.[53]

Fetal Iron Requirements

Fetal iron content is 75 mg/kg by the third trimester.[153] The majority (75%) of fetal iron is found in hemoglobin, with about 7 mg/kg in tissues and 10 mg/kg stored in the liver and spleen.[152] The stored iron doubles during the last few weeks of gestation. Iron passes rapidly against a concentration gradient from mother to fetus via transferrin. Maternal transferrin releases its iron in the intervillous space. The iron is taken up by transferrin receptors located on the surface of syncytiotrophoblast cells and is actively transported across the syncytiotrophoblast and cytotrophoblast by a series of iron transporters.[87,152,210] Iron transported across the placenta enters fetal blood and attaches to fetal serum transferrin. Fetal transferrin is synthesized by the fetal liver beginning about 29 to 30 days' gestation.[140]

By the end of pregnancy, 90% of the mother's transferrin-bound iron is delivered to the placenta.[152] Placental transferrin receptor density is thought to be the major determinant of placental iron transfer.[210] Increased expression of placental transferrin receptors is seen with low maternal stores, low fetal stores, and with adolescents (who have increased iron needs due to their own growth and development).[210] This compensatory mechanism enhances uptake of iron by the placenta. Other mechanisms to decrease the risk of fetal iron deficiency are increased maternal intestinal iron absorption and increased placental iron transport.[87]

With fetal growth the rate of iron transfer across the placenta increases. Thus transport of iron from mother to fetus is greatest during the last few months of gestation (up to 4 mg/day at term).[152] Serum iron and ferritin levels in cord blood are higher than in maternal blood and have been related to maternal hemoglobin or ferritin in most but not all studies. Cord blood serum ferritin levels are lower (but usually still within normal limits) in infants of iron-deficient mothers, reflecting lower fetal iron stores. These infants are reported to have reduced iron stores and an increased risk of anemia in the first year.[152]

Development of the Hemostatic System

The hemostatic and fibrinolytic systems develop simultaneously. Most coagulation proteins are present in measurable quantities by 5 to 10 weeks' gestation.[56,91] Fetal blood demonstrates clotting ability by 11 to 12 weeks.[69] Fibrinogen synthesis in the liver begins at 5 weeks. Fibrinogen can be found in the plasma by 12 to 13 weeks, reaching adult values by 30 weeks.[180]

The placenta is rich in tissue factor (TF), which also plays a role in angiogenesis, cell signaling, and embryogenesis. Thus the placenta is able to respond rapidly to insults with initiation of the clotting cascade.[18,63,69,166] This helps protect the fetus from significant blood loss. Vitamin K levels are 30% of adult values by the end of the second trimester and 50% by term.[180]

Fibrinolytic activity can be demonstrated at 12 to 13 weeks' gestation. The whole blood clotting time in the fetus is relatively short, and the fetus is in a hypercoagulable state during the first and second trimesters. Fibrinolytic activity in the fetus is increased even though levels of blood plasminogen are low, due to increased tissue plasminogen activator (tPA) or decreased inhibitor or both.[69] The elevated fibrinolytic activity may help protect and maintain the extensive fetal capillary circulation within the placental villi.

NEONATAL PHYSIOLOGY

The neonate experiences significant alterations in the hematologic system and hemostasis. Among the more striking differences are the structural and functional alterations in the neonatal red blood cell (RBC) and the potential impact of fetal hemoglobin (HbF) on oxygen delivery to the tissues. Variations are also seen in blood volume and blood cellular components and in hemostasis parameters. These alterations increase the risk for anemia, thromboembolism, and coagulopathies in the neonate.

Transitional Events

A major transitional event for the neonate is removal of the placental circulation with clamping of the umbilical cord. The timing of umbilical cord clamping influences the amount of placental transfusion and subsequent plasma and RBC volume of the neonate. At term, fetal blood volume is approximately 70 to 80 mL/kg; placental blood volume accounts for 30% of this volume.[123] At 30 weeks' gestation, about one half of this volume is in the fetal circulation, increasing to two thirds by term; the remainder is in the placenta.[44,197]

The umbilical arteries constrict at birth in response to the increasing PaO_2. Therefore blood does not flow from the infant back into the placenta via these vessels. The umbilical vein remains dilated, however, so blood flows from the placenta to the infant via gravity.[39,123,206] If the newly delivered infant is kept at or below the level of the placenta, transfer of blood from the placenta to the fetus will occur for about 3 minutes after birth. If the newborn is significantly elevated above the placenta, blood in the umbilical vein can flow back into the placenta.[39]

The timing of cord clamping and the position of the infant in relation to the placenta influence placental transfusion. Yao and Lind reported that, if the infant's position was maintained at the level of the introitus (± 10 cm) until the cord was clamped, or held 40 cm below the introitus for no more than 30 seconds, the infant received a placental transfusion of approximately 80 mL.[206] The amount of placental transfusion was negligible if the infant was held 50 to 60 cm above the introitus. With the infant held at the level of the introitus or slightly below, if the cord was clamped 30 to 60 seconds after delivery, placental transfusion increased the newborn's blood volume by 15% to 20%; clamping at 60 to 90 seconds resulted in a 25% increase; and clamping at 3 minutes produced a 50% to 60% increase.[206] No disadvantage was found for term infants placed on the mother's abdomen with delay of clamping until cessation of pulsations. However, no clinical trials have systematically evaluated the influence of gravity of placental transfusion.[4]

The timing of umbilical cord clamping and the magnitude of placental transfusion has physiologic and clinical effects on many body systems. The significance of these changes in healthy infants is unclear; however, concerns have been raised that early clamping may deprive infants of blood that has an important role in opening the lungs, increasing pulmonary perfusion, enhancing lung fluid clearance, and improving oxygen delivery to the infant's tissues.[124,197] Mercer, Nelson, and Skovgaard note that early cord clamping may interfere with completion of normal physiologic transition at birth, resulting in a 25% to 30% decrease in blood volume.[123] With birth the amount of cardiac output going to the lungs must increase up to 45% for transition to air breathing.[44] In preterm infants, early cord clamping may lead to hypovolemia, with reduction in RBCs and thus decreased oxygen-carrying capacity, oxygen delivery, and pulmonary blood flow, limiting lung expansion.[197] Optimizing placental-fetal transfusion in preterm infants may enhance lung expansion, reduce need for later transfusions and thus blood donor exposure, and increase autologous stem cells (especially rich in blood of infants 25 to 31 weeks of age), which have long-term hematologic and immunologic benefits.[197]

Although timing of cord clamping has been controversial, recent analyses have demonstrated advantages to delayed cord clamping in both term and preterm infants. Delayed cord clamping (between 30 and 180 seconds) in term and preterm infants has been found to decrease the need for blood transfusions, increase the post birth hematocrit, improve tissue oxygenation, and reduce the incidence of intraventricular hemorrhage (IVH) in preterm infants.[9,11,44,57,72,84,90,97,131,150,172,183,190,206] For example, Hutton & Hassan conducted a meta-analysis of early versus late clamping in term infants and concluded that delayed clamping for ≥ 2 minutes was beneficial and that although there were a greater number of infants who were polycythemic, this was benign requiring no treatment.[72] Rabe et al. in a meta-analysis of 10 randomized clinical trials ($n = 454$ infants <37 weeks' gestational age) comparing early (<20 seconds) to delayed (30 to 120 seconds) clamping found that delayed cord clamping in preterm infants decreased the number of blood transfusion (3/10 studies) and total number of transfusions (4/10 studies), led to higher hematocrits at birth and 1 hour of age (5/10 studies), and decreased the incidence of IVH (7/10).[150] Others have reported that delayed clamping in preterm infants reduced exogenous surfactant needs, improved cerebral oxygenation and fewer days on ventilator support.[183,190] The risks of delayed cord clamping reported in recent studies have been a slight increase in polycythemia, which was generally not symptomatic and required no treatment, and a slight increase in the need for phototherapy in some studies.[44,57,72,118] Neonatal resuscitation guidelines recommend that cord clamping be delayed for at least one minute after the infant is completely delivered for newborns not requiring resuscitation, but note that "evidence is insufficient to recommend a time for clamping in those who require resuscitation."[21,147]

Changes in Hematologic Parameters

Hematologic parameters differ in neonates as compared with adults and change rapidly during the first week after birth. Considerable variation may be noted between individual infants and within the same infant over time.[215] Values for infants of varying gestational and post birth ages can be found in neonatology texts.[106,116,209]

Blood Volume

Blood volume averages about 80 to 100 mL/kg in term infants and 90 to 105 mL/kg in preterm infants.[134] Variations in blood volume at birth are due primarily to placental transfusion and gestational age. Total combined fetal and placental blood volume in term infants is 115 mL/kg and 150 mL/kg at 26 weeks.[84] The higher blood volume of the preterm infant is due to increased plasma volume. Plasma volume decreases with gestation.[134]

Red Blood Cells

RBC counts are 4.6 to 5.2 million/mm^3 at birth, increasing by about 500,000 in the initial hours after birth, then falling to cord blood levels by the end of the first week.[116,140,209] Red blood cell mass is lower with decreasing gestational age.[148] Nucleated RBCs are seen in most newborns during the first 24 hours, perhaps as a response to the stresses of delivery, disappearing by 3 to 4 days in term infants and by one week in most preterm infants.[148] Increased numbers of nucleated RBCs are found in more immature infants (and may persist beyond the first week) and in infants with Down syndrome or congenital anomalies.[140] Nucleated RBCs are also seen in the neonate as an acute stress response to asphyxia, with anemia, and following hemorrhage. In older individuals, these cells are rare and associated with abnormal erythropoiesis.[215] The erythrocyte sedimentation rate (ESR) is decreased in neonates due to alterations in plasma viscosity, protein content, and hematocrit. The RBC of the neonate differs from that of the adult. These differences and their implications are summarized in Table 8-7.

Hemoglobin and Hematocrit

Hemoglobin levels are higher in newborns, ranging from 13.7 to 20.1 g/dL (137 to 201 g/L), with most in the 16.6 to 17.5 g/dL (166 to 175 g/L) range.[116,140,209] Hemoglobin levels increase by up to 6 g/dL (60 g/L) within the first hours after birth. This increase results from a shift in fluid distribution after birth—with a decrease in plasma volume and a net

Table 8-7 Characteristics of Neonatal Red Blood Cells and Their Implications

RBC CHARACTERISTIC	CLINICAL IMPLICATION
Macrocytosis with increased mean cellular diameter and mean corpuscular volume	More susceptible to damage in small capillaries; increased RBC turnover
Increased permeability to sodium and potassium	Increased risk of cell lysis as a result of osmotic changes
Altered enzyme activity with increased glucose utilization	Risk of hypoglycemia, especially in infants with low glucose stores or altered glucose metabolism with a tendency toward polycythemia (i.e., cases of IDM, SGA)
Increased ATP utilization	Higher energy (glucose) needs and oxygen consumption
Decreased survival time (80 to 100 days for term infants and 60 to 80 days for preterm infants versus 35 to 50 days for ELBW infants versus 120 days for adults)	Increased RBC turnover rate; proportionately greater amounts of bilirubin produced
Increased receptor sites for substances such as insulin and digoxin	Insulin receptor sites facilitate increased glucose uptake; digoxin sites contribute to greater tolerance for digoxin
Increased fetal hemoglobin and less adult hemoglobin	Increased affinity of hemoglobin for oxygen with less ready release to tissues
Increased RBC count at birth (4.6 to 5.2 million/mm^3, falling to 3 to 4 million/mm3 by 2 to 3 months of age)	Increased RBC turnover rate and bilirubin production
Increased phospholipid, cholesterol, and total lipid content	Increased risk of lipid peroxidation and hemolysis (cholesterol may provide protection against hemolysis)
Decreased catalase glutathione peroxidase	Increased susceptibility to oxidative injury and decreased RBC life span
Increased fragility, decreased deformability, and increased variety and frequency of morphologic abnormalities	Increased susceptibility to damage, especially in microcirculation; increased RBC turnover
Increased free intracellular iron	May lead to decreased RBC survival

Data compiled from references 48, 53, 116, 135, 140.

ATP, Adenosine triphosphate; *ELBW,* extremely low birth weight; *IDM,* infant of a diabetic mother; *RBC,* red blood cell; *SGA,* small for gestational age.

increase in RBCs—and partially compensates for placental transfusion.[1,99] Levels peak at four to six hours, then slowly decrease over the next 12 to 18 hours and are similar to birth values by 24 hours of age.[1]

The hemoglobin concentration decreases by the end of the first week to values similar to cord blood levels. Higher hemoglobin levels are seen in infants with severe hypoxia, in some infants with fetal growth restriction, and in postterm infants, possibly as a compensatory mechanism to increase oxygen availability to the tissues. Lower hemoglobin levels are found in preterm infants. An elevation of either the reticulocyte count or the number of nucleated RBCs above normal values in any infant, regardless of the hemoglobin level, suggests a compensatory response and may indicate anemia.[116,140,209]

Cord blood at term contains 60% to 80% HbF, 15% to 40% HbA, and less than 1.8% hemoglobin A_2 (a minor normal adult form). A fourth type, Hb Bart (less than 0.5%), is seen in small amounts in some infants. Cord blood hemoglobin levels vary with gestational age. Preterm infants have a greater percentage of HbF than term infants.

HbF does not bind 2,3-DPG as readily as does adult hemoglobin (HbA), shifting the oxygen-hemoglobin dissociation curve of the fetus and newborn to the left (see box on p. 301). Increased concentrations of HbF are seen in infants that are small for gestational age (SGA) and other infants who have experienced chronic hypoxia in utero, probably due to a delay in the normal switch to synthesis of HbA at about 32 weeks' gestation.[53,180] Alterations in HbF are usually not seen in infants with acute intrapartal hypoxia, because the more recent onset of this condition does not allow the infant sufficient time to compensate.[140] The increased HbF seen in infants with trisomy 13 during the first two years of life is also thought to be due to a delay in HbA synthesis. Decreased HbF is also seen in infants with Down syndrome. Increased HbA is found in infants with erythroblastosis fetalis due to rapid destruction of older RBCs containing HbF and replacement by new cells containing higher concentrations of HbA.[140]

Hematocrit levels at birth normally range from 51.3% to 56%. The hematocrit increases in the first few hours or days due to the movement of fluid from intravascular to interstitial spaces. The hematocrit falls again to levels near cord blood values by the end of the first week.[39]

2,3-DPG

Although 2,3-DPG levels at birth in term infants are similar to those in adults, the 2,3-DPG of infants is less stable than that of adults. Concentrations of 2,3-DPG may fall the first week but increase by the time the infant is 2 to 3 weeks of age.[135] The P_{50} (the PO_2 at which 50% of the hemoglobin is saturated with oxygen) is decreased at birth but gradually increases during the first week after birth.[215] This change in the P_{50} is due primarily to an increase in 2,3-DPG rather than in the percentage of HbF. In comparison with term infants, the preterm infant has a lower P_{50}, decreased concentrations of 2,3-DPG, and increased amounts of HbF. Therefore in the initial few weeks after birth, the functioning DPG fraction in the preterm infant is significantly reduced.[51,135,215]

Erythropoietin

Erythropoietin (Epo) levels are higher at birth in term infants than in preterm infants. After the first day, Epo levels fall and plasma levels in healthy term infants reach a nadir at 4 to 6 weeks of age. Stimulation of Epo production at that point coincides with the resumption of bone marrow activity and RBC production (see "Physiologic Anemia of Infancy"). Epo levels remain low for longer periods in the preterm infant. In the preterm infant, the liver is still the main site of Epo production, because the switch to renal Epo production is related to postmenstrual age rather than post birth age.[184] Hepatocyte production of Epo in response to hypoxic stimulation is only 10% of that produced by renal cells. In addition, the liver requires more prolonged hypoxic stimulation to produce Epo. In preterm infants, this increases the risk of anemia, but it may also protect from polycythemia.[47]

Elevated levels of Epo are found at birth in infants with Down syndrome, growth restriction, or anemia secondary to erythroblastosis fetalis and those born to women with diabetes or preeclampsia.[198] In the first 24 hours, Epo is elevated in infants with severe anemia or cyanotic congenital heart defects. The increased levels result from decreased oxygen-carrying capacity (anemia) or low arterial oxygen saturations (congenital heart defects), which stimulate continued production of Epo. Epo is also thought to be important in maturation of the gut and neurologic development.[79-81,92,120,205,211]

Reticulocytes

The reticulocyte count is elevated at birth, ranging from 3% to 7% (absolute values of 200,000 to 400,000/μL [200 to 400 10^9/L]) in term infants and up to 8% to 10% (absolute values of 400,000 to 500,000/μL [400 to 500 10^9/L]) in preterm infants.[39] The reticulocyte count decreases markedly to 0% to 1% (absolute values of 0 to 50,000/μL [0 to 50 10^9/L]) by 1 week of age.[39]

Iron and Serum Ferritin

Maturity, birth weight, and hemoglobin level determine iron status of the neonate. Cord serum ferritin levels at term are higher than maternal values and rise further in the first 24 hours with RBC catabolism and release of hemoglobin iron. Cord serum ferritin levels increase with increasing gestational age, from a mean of 63 mμg/L at 23 weeks to 171 at 41 weeks.[173] Cord hemoglobin and serum ferritin levels are inversely related. At birth the serum folate level of the neonate is also higher than that in maternal blood. Stores in preterm infants are lower and more rapidly depleted in the first months due to rapid growth.

White Blood Cells

There are two pools of WBCs in the body, a circulating pool and marginated cells. Cells usually circulate in blood for about 6 to 8 hours and survive for another 24 hours in tissues.[178] The

WBC count ranges from 10,000 to 26,000/mm^3 in term infants and from 6000 to 19,000/mm^3 in preterm infants. The number of cells increases during the first 12 to 24 hours, then gradually decreases to 6000 to 15,000/mm^3 (mean of 12,000/mm^3) by 4 to 5 days in both term and preterm infants.[140] The initial increase in WBCs is due to displacement of cells from the margins of larger vessels or bone marrow mobilization of the existing neutrophil pool (similar to changes seen in adults following strenuous exercise) due to the stress of labor and delivery rather than an increase in WBC production rate.[69,148]

Initially, up to 60% of the WBCs may be neutrophils with a variety of immature forms. During the first 3 to 4 days, the neutrophil count is higher in preterm than in term infants. Reference limits for neutrophil counts in neonates were published by Manroe et al. and Mouzinho et al.[113,130] In term infants, neutrophils peak at 8 to 12 hours at 7800 to 14,500 cells/mm^3, although individual variations can be seen in otherwise healthy infants.[89,130,148] Values less than 3000 in the first 48 hours and less than 1500 after that are abnormal.[89] Very low-birth weight (VLBW) infants show a similar peak but the peak occurs later (at 18 to 20 hours). In preterm infants, the lower limit for normal values is 2200 in the first 12 to 24 hours and less than 1100 after 60 hours.[89] Immature forms of neutrophils (e.g., bands, metamyelocytes, myelocytes) may be seen in healthy neonates during the first 2 to 3 days.[113] The number of monocytes increases slightly during the first 12 hours, then gradually decreases. A study done at altitude found similar findings in the first 70 hours after birth, but with slightly higher upper and lower limits at both birth and 72 hours and peak values at 8 hours.[167]

Eosinophil counts in the neonate show great individual variation, with reported values ranging from 19 to 851 cells/mm^3 in term infants in the first 12 hours and increasing during the first 4 to 5 days of life to 100 to 2500 cells/mm^3.[53] Eosinophilia (more than 700/mm^3) is more common in preterm infants during the first few weeks, with 75% having values greater than 700/mm^3. Disappearance of eosinophils from the peripheral circulation has been noted before death.

Monocytes range from 0 to 2000 cells/mm^3 at birth, peaking at 12 to 24 hours, then falling to 450 to 600 in the first week.[89] After circulating in the blood for about 72 hours, monocytes migrate into the tissues and become macrophages.

Platelets

In term and healthy preterm infants, platelet counts are similar to those in adults, ranging from 150,000 to 450,000/mm^3. Age-related reference ranges are available.[126] Preterm infants tend to have values slightly lower than term infants, but still within normal range.[39,91,177] Platelet counts increase by the end of the first month in both term and preterm infants. Higher levels may persist for the first 3 months in preterm infants. Platelet counts below 150,000/mm^3 are abnormal in neonates.[53,180] Neonatal megakaryocytes are small and generate fewer platelets than in adults. The normal (i.e., similar to adult values) platelet count in neonates is probably due to the increased proliferative rate by these smaller cells.[91,163,176] The platelet life span in healthy infants is similar to that of adults.[91] Thrombopoitin levels are three to four times higher than in adults, increasing on day 2, then decreasing to cord blood levels by 1 month.[177] The response of thrombopoietin to thrombocytopenia is reduced with decreasing gestational age.[91]

Neonatal platelets have a decreased functional reserve capacity and hypoactive response to stimuli in the first few days. Platelet aggregation, adhesion, and release of substances that enhance the clotting cascade, may also be altered.[66,77,143,163] Platelet function tends to be generally normal however due to enhanced von Willebrand factor (vWF) activity.[193] Platelet hypoactivity tends to resolve by about 10 days.[91] However, if the infant is ill or immature, these limitations increase the risk of bleeding and coagulopathy. Coagulation in the neonate may be impaired by maternal drugs such as aspirin that alter platelet aggregation and factor XII (contact factor) activity.[176]

Alterations in Hemostasis

Neonatal hemostasis is altered and characterized by a low reserve capacity. Values for all components are related to gestational age and change gradually after birth, necessitating use of post birth- and gestational age–dependent reference tables for accurate assessment of individual parameters.[56,91,127]

Coagulation

Vitamin K–dependent clotting factors II (prothrombin), VII, IX, and X are approximately 50% of adult plasma values at birth and in the early weeks after birth.[55,56,66,91] This reduction is greater in preterm infants, because concentrations of vitamin K–dependent factors are related to gestational age. Contact factors involved in the initiation of the clotting cascade are at less than 50% of adult plasma values at birth.[66,91] This leads to the prolonged activated partial thromboplastin time seen in neoantes.[66] Neonatal fibrinogen levels are similar to those in adults or slightly increased at birth.[143] Plasma concentrations of vWF and factor VIII are increased in the first week.[66,91] Factors V and XIII levels are greater than 70% of adult values or are indistinguishable from adult values.[56] As a result of these changes, thrombin generation is 50% of adult capacity, resulting in resistance to heparin and an increased risk of hemorrhage.[91] Activity is further diminished with decreasing gestational age and in severely ill neonates. The clotting cascade is illustrated in Figure 8-3.

Inhibitors of coagulation are also altered (see Figure 8-4). Levels of antithrombin (a protease inhibitor that neutralizes activated clotting factors) and heparin cofactor II (HCII) are at 50% of adult values.[56,91] Protein C and S (inhibitors of factors VII and V and the vitamin K–dependent factors) are also decreased. Protein C is decreased to 35% (17% to 53%) and protein S to 36% (12% to 60%) of adult values.[86] Protein C is found in a fetal form in neonatal circulation. Protein S is found primarily in a free form in neonates (versus protein bound as in adults) because of absence of its binding protein. This is an advantage for the neonate, because the increased levels of free protein S result in net activity that is 75% of adult values even though absolute values are closer to one-third of adult levels.[56,86] Levels of another inhibitor, α_1-macroglobin, are elevated to twice adult values, which may help compensate for the alterations in antithrombin, protein C, protein S, and heparin cofactor II.[56,66,91,143] Possible mechanisms for these alterations in coagulation include decreased factor synthesis, accelerated clearance (due to the accelerated basal metabolic rate), and activation and increased consumption of coagulation components at birth.[8,56] These changes increase the risk for hypercoagulable states and thrombi formation.[69,180] Inhibition of thrombin is slower in the newborn, but it is balanced by increased binding of thrombin by the elevated α_1-macroglobin. Edstrom and colleagues note that "thrombin generation in neonates is similar to that in adults receiving therapeutic doses of warfarin or heparin."[56, p. 243]

Prothrombin time (PT), thrombin clotting time (TT), and activated partial thromboplastin time (aPTT) are prolonged, more so with decreasing gestational age. However, specific values for these tests vary between laboratories and with differences in cord versus neonatal samples, reagents used, and assay conditions. Reference values are available for term and preterm infants of varying post birth ages.[56,91] The difference in PT time reflects the decrease in vitamin K dependent factors in the newborn; whereas the altered aPTT is a reflection of decreases in both contact factors and vitamin K dependent factors.[85] PT greater than 17 seconds at any gestational age or aPTT greater than 45 to 50 seconds in a term infant is of concern. aPTT is generally not a useful parameter in preterm infants. aPTT measures all coagulation factors except VII and XIII and is abnormal if any one factor is 20% to 40% of normal. aPTT is influenced unduly by decreases in the contact factors, such as are seen in many healthy preterm infants. Despite the prolonged aPTT, PT, and TT, newborn whole blood clotting times are slightly shorter than adult values (mean of 80 ± 5.1 in term infants).[50,91,143] The mechanism for this paradoxical finding may represent a slight overbalance of the tendency toward thrombosis (decreased antithrombin and proteins C and S) in comparison with the physiologic hypocoagulability (low levels of factors II, VII, IX, and X) as well as increased vWF levels and function and the increased size and number of RBCs.[8,85,143]

Fibrinolysis

Activity of the fibrinolytic system is (see Figure 8-5) transiently increased at birth with a decrease in plasmin generation.[66,91] In general, fibrinolysis is less effective in the newborn due to the presence of fetal plasminogen, low plasminogen and tissue plasminogen activator, and increased inhibitors of fibrinolysis (plasminogen activator inhibitor-1 and α_2-antiplasmin).[66,91,143] Levels of plasminogen activator inhibitor (PAI-1) and tPA are twice adult levels, decreasing by 5 days; PAI-1 increases again after 5 days to twice adult values by 6 months.[56] Fetal fibrinogen may also be more resistant to lysis than adult fibrinogen.[143] In addition, clearance of collagen debris, fibrin, and injured cells is delayed secondary to immaturity of the reticuloendothelial activating system and low levels of fibronectin (glycoprotein involved in clearance of debris from tissue injury and inflammation). Alterations in healthy preterm infants are similar to or slightly less than those in term newborns. However, activity of the fibrinolytic mechanism may be significantly depressed in some infants—especially preterm infants with severe respiratory distress syndrome or in infants following a hypoxic-ischemic insult—for at least the first 24 hours after birth and possibly longer. Plasminogen levels are 60% to 70% of adult values at birth and are decreased even further in SGA infants and some preterm infants, increasing the risk for hemostatic disorders.[56,91]

CLINICAL IMPLICATIONS FOR NEONATAL CARE

Alterations in the hematologic system and hemostasis in the neonate have a significant impact on neonatal adaptations to extrauterine life. These alterations, along with the changes that occur during the first few months of life, can influence interpretation of laboratory test results, lead to alterations such as physiologic anemia or hemorrhagic disease of the newborn, and increase the risk of thromboembolism and consumptive coagulopathies. This section discusses these implications and two areas of controversy related to the hematologic system: the role of vitamin K and decisions regarding transfusion of preterm infants.

Factors Influencing Hematologic Parameters

Factors that influence blood values and their interpretation in the neonate include the timing, site, and amount of blood sampled; placental transfusion; and infant growth rate.[53] The timing of blood sampling in relation to changes in hemoglobin and hematocrit during the first week of postnatal life and effects of placental transfusion are discussed earlier in this chapter. The detection of hemolysis can be more difficult due to the unique characteristics of the neonate's hematologic system.[53,215]

Site of Sampling

The site of sampling can result in significant variations in values. Capillary hemoglobin values average 2 to 4 g/dL higher than venous values (with differences up to 8 g/dL reported); arterial values average 0.5 g/dL above venous values and are probably of less clinical significance.[53,187] Hematocrits, hemoglobins, and red blood cell (RBC) counts from heel capillaries are 5% to 25% higher than venous or arterial values.[1,39] Differences are greatest with decreasing gestational age. The neonate's hematocrit does not reflect RBC mass as accurately as in an adult, with a correlation of 0.63 versus 0.78 in adults.[47] Poorer correlations are reported in ill and preterm infants who are growing rapidly and thus have increased circulating blood volumes.

Both sampling site and physical activity can alter white blood cell (WBC) counts. A mean capillary difference of 1.8 X 10^9/L has been found in neutrophil counts between capillary and arterial samples.[187] Using simultaneously drawn blood samples, arterial WBC counts were reported to be 75% of venous or capillary values.[39] These differences may be due to the pulsatile nature of arterial flow that moves larger cells to the periphery.[39] Intense crying or other events such as chest physiotherapy has been associated with an increase in WBC counts of up to 146% and a shift to the left in the differential count, with the appearance of more immature forms of WBCs in the peripheral circulation.[39] No differences were noted in platelet counts between umbilical artery catheter, venipuncture, and capillary heel stick samples.[187]

Differences between capillary and venous blood samples are due to poorer circulation and venous stasis in the peripheral circulation. Differences between arterial and venous samples are thought to be due to passage of plasma to the interstitial spaces in the capillary bed with later return to circulation via the lymphatic system.[187] Capillary and venous differences are more marked with decreasing gestational age; after a large placental transfusion; and in infants with acidosis, hypotension, or severe anemia.[53] The site of sampling is critical in interpreting hematologic values in the neonate and should be recorded for all samples. Unfortunately, site-related differences are most marked in those infants for whom accurate determination of hematologic values is most critical.[140]

Iatrogenic Losses

Hematologic parameters are also influenced by iatrogenic losses. In the first 6 weeks after birth, infants in intensive care nurseries had a mean iatrogenic blood loss equivalent to 22.9 ± 10 mL of packed cells; 46% of these infants had cumulative losses that exceeded their circulating RBC mass at birth.[53] Iatrogenic blood losses were greater in ill than in healthy preterm infants (26.9 ± 9 mL versus 14.6 ± 5 mL). In VLBW infants, these losses were equivalent to a significant proportion of their circulating RBC mass (32.2 to 45.5 mL/kg in the preterm infant). Another study reported significant overdraws of blood (19% ± 1.8% above that required by the laboratory) for laboratory testing of neonatal intensive care unit infants.[98] The greatest overdraws were in the smallest and most critical infants. Removal of 1 mL of blood from a 1000-g infant is estimated to be equivalent to removing 70 mL from the average adult.[53,136] Accurate determination of true anemia versus "anemia" due to blood loss is often dependent on accurate recording of the amount of blood that has been previously drawn for sampling.[53] Iatrogenic losses can be reduced by microsampling, careful monitoring of losses, avoiding overdraws, and use of bedside or point of care sampling.[105,184,188]

Growth Influences

Rapid weight gain results in an obligatory increase in total blood volume that often precedes any change in RBC mass.[140] The ensuing hemodilution can lead to a static or falling hemoglobin even with active erythropoiesis as evidenced by reticulocytosis. The correlation between RBC mass and hemoglobin is low during the first 6 weeks due to the effects of this hemodilution, so hemoglobin levels may not accurately reflect RBC mass.[53]

Alterations in Hemoglobin-Oxygen Affinity

The increased affinity of hemoglobin for oxygen is an advantage to the fetus in facilitating oxygen transfer across the placenta but may be a liability for the neonate. Preterm infants who have higher levels of HbF and lower concentrations of 2,3-diphosphoglycerate (2,3-DPG) are more vulnerable. With increased affinity, oxygen is unloaded less rapidly and efficiently in the peripheral tissues. Therefore the newborn may be less able to respond to hypoxia by significantly increasing oxygen delivery to the tissues. The newborn is also lacking in some of the protective responses seen in adults. For example, in adults, but not in neonates, hypoxia tends to stimulate increased production of 2,3-DPG, a response that further facilitates oxygen release to the tissues.[140]

The measurement of arterial hemoglobin saturation (SaO_2) by pulse oximetry is generally as reliable in neonates (who have high levels of HbF) as it is in adults (whose hemoglobin is predominantly HbA). This occurs because pulse oximetry is a direct measure of percent saturation, whereas calculating saturation from PaO_2 requires consideration of the percent concentrations of HbA and HbF in the blood.[49] Pulse oximetry works on the principle of light absorbance. The light absorbed by the hemoglobin molecule is absorbed primarily by the heme portion (which is similar in both HbA and HbF) and not by the globulin chains (which are different in HbA and HbF). Infants with significant amounts of HbF can have an SaO_2 greater than 85% even with a low PaO_2; therefore infants on pulse oximeters must also have their PaO_2 levels regularly evaluated. Even if an infant is well saturated, PaO_2 levels must be kept within normal ranges, because this is the driving force for movement of oxygen from the blood to the tissues. In preterm infants with a higher percentage of HbF, a PaO_2 of 41 to 53 (5.46 to 7.06 kPa) is often high enough to provide an SaO_2 of 88% to 92%.[49,51]

Because the P_{50} (see box on p. 301) of preterm infants is lower than that of term infants, the progressive shift to the right of the oxygen-hemoglobin dissociation curve is more gradual in preterm infants and related to postmenstrual rather than post birth age.[140] As a result, the oxygen-unloading capacity in the preterm infant who has not been transfused is reduced for at least the first 3 months.[215] In some circumstances, the shift to the left in the oxygen-hemoglobin dissociation curve may be an advantage to the infant by helping maintain oxygen delivery with severe hypoxemia and low cardiac output.[139]

Vitamin K Deficiency Bleeding

The newborn has reduced levels of all the vitamin K–dependent clotting factors (II, VII, IX, X) at birth, leading to a physiologic hypoprothrombinemia. The reduction in these factors is the consequence of poor placental transport of vitamin K to the fetus as well as lack of intestinal colonization by bacteria that normally synthesize vitamin K. The low vitamin K levels in the fetus may be a mechanism to control levels of other (noncoagulation-related) vitamin K–dependent proteins, which act as ligandins for cutaneous receptor enzymes that regulate growth in the fetus. Because normal fetal growth is carefully regulated within a narrow range, vitamin K levels may be kept low to prevent growth dysregulation.[76]

Neonatal vitamin K deficiency is characterized by low plasma vitamin K_1 (phylloquinone), low liver K_1, and a near absence of K_2 (menaquinone), the major vitamin K component in the liver.[64,76,216] Unless the infant is given vitamin K at birth, the deficiency intensifies in the first few days after birth as maternally acquired vitamin K is catabolized (half-life is about 24 hours). This decline is more marked in infants who are breastfed, have a history of perinatal asphyxia, or are born to mothers on coumarin derivative anticoagulants. Neonatal liver stores are one fifth those of adults because placental transport of K is low. In addition, neonatal stores are composed primarily of K_1, which has a rapid turnover, especially with a diet such as breast milk that is low in vitamin K.[216] Stores gradually increase in the first month, more rapidly in infants who are formula fed rather than breastfed. This is due both to the increased levels of vitamin K in formula (40 to 50 mcg [88.8 to 111 nmol/L] versus less than 5 mcg/L [11 nmol/L]) and differences in intestinal colonization. Formula-fed infants are colonized with bacteria that can produce K_2, whereas lactobacillus, the primary organism colonizing the intestine of breastfed infants, cannot. Vitamin K recycling by the liver is lower in preterm than term infants due to lower enzyme activity in the preterm.[43]

Because this decline in vitamin K after birth leads to a bleeding tendency in some newborns, prophylactic vitamin K is given after birth to prevent hemorrhagic disease of the newborn (HDN) also known as vitamin K deficiency bleeding (VKDB). VKDB involves bleeding from the gastrointestinal tract, umbilical cord, or circumcision site; oozing from puncture sites; and generalized ecchymosis. Although it is likely that many newborns do not need vitamin K at birth, VKDB usually occurs in infants without specific risk factors.[216] Therefore it is difficult to identify which infants need this prophylaxis and which do not, and clinical and research evidence clearly demonstrates the risk of hemorrhage in some infants. In countries where routine use of vitamin K was eliminated, the incidence of VKDB increased.[216] Thus prophylaxis at birth is recommended.

Three forms of VKDB have been described: early, classic , and late.[101,164,216] The early form occurs within 24 hours of birth and is seen primarily in infants of women on certain medications.[101] Vitamin K–dependent clotting factors may be further reduced in infants of women taking antiepileptic drugs such as carbamazepine, barbiturates, and phenytoin diphenylhydantoin (Dilantin) during pregnancy.[101] These agents tend to concentrate in the fetal liver and inhibit the action of vitamin K in the formation of precursor proteins for factors II, VII, IX, and X.[91] The incidence of bleeding in these infants has been reported as 6% to 12%.[101] Women on antiepileptic drugs have been given vitamin K in the last weeks of pregnancy to reduce the risk of neonatal bleeding. However, a recent review of evidence for management of women with epilepsy concluded that there was insufficient evidence to determine if mothers on antiepileptic drugs were actually at risk of increased bleeding, nor was there adequate evidence to determine if maternal prenatal vitamin K supplementation reduced neonatal hemorrhage.[68] Vitamin K–dependent clotting factors may also be reduced in infants of women on anticoagulants (warfarin) and long-term antibiotic therapy, especially antituberculosis medications (e.g., isoniazid, rifampin).[101] In addition to receiving the usual dose of vitamin K following birth, these infants must be assessed for signs of bleeding throughout the neonatal period.[91,143]

The classic form of VKDB is seen at 24 hours to 7 days as the vitamin K deficiency intensifies.[101] The prevalence of VKDB is 0.4 to 1.7 per 100 if no vitamin K is given.[91,143] Laboratory findings include reduction in the vitamin K–dependent clotting factors, decreased prothrombin activity, and prolonged clotting time and PT.[91,143,216] Breastfed infants with delayed or insufficient intake are at higher risk if no prophylaxis is given because breast milk has low levels of vitamin K. VKDB is rarely seen when prophylactic vitamin K is given.[101,149]

The late form of VKDB is uncommon (incidence of 1/15000 to 1/20,000) and usually seen at 2 to 12 weeks in infants who did not receive vitamin K at birth or who received an inadequate oral dose and were breastfed, or in infants with hepatobiliary problems.[91,101,149] This form is also sometimes seen in infants with gastrointestinal disorders leading to fat malabsorption. Prophylactic vitamin K may be given to preterm and ill infants who are on prolonged antibiotic therapy (particularly with use of third-generation cephalosporins). Antibiotics may significantly reduce the normal intestinal bacterial flora essential for vitamin K synthesis and compete for vitamin K in the liver.

Vitamin K is not required for the synthesis of clotting factors per se but rather for the conversion of precursor proteins synthesized in the liver to activated proteins with coagulant properties.[48] This process (posttranslational γ-carboxylation) is needed for calcium binding, which is critical for activation of these factors. The hypoprothrombinemia commonly present at birth is secondary to decreased levels of the precursor proteins. Term neonates respond to prophylactic vitamin K administration at birth by achieving normal or near normal PTs, although actual values of individual clotting factors may not reach adult values for several weeks or more. The response in preterm infants is less predictable, with minimal response to vitamin K seen in some VLBW infants due to an inability of the immature liver to synthesize adequate amounts of the precursor proteins.[140]

Neonatal Polycythemia and Hyperviscosity

Factors that increase RBC production or decrease neonatal blood volume can lead to polycythemia and hyperviscosity. Neonatal polycythemia is generally defined as a venous hematocrit $\geq$65% or hemoglobin greater than 22 g/dL

(220 g/L).[99,162,200] Infants with polycythemia usually have increased RBC mass with increased or normal plasma volume, leading to increased total blood volume. Hyperviscosity can occur in infants with hematocrits below 65%, although rarely with those below 60% because blood viscosity is not only proportional to the hematocrit but also influenced by increases in mean cell volume and decreases in deformability. Blood viscosity increases with acidosis as more fluid enters the RBC, altering its shape.[162] Polycythemia and hyperviscosity arise from prenatal, intrapartal, and post birth factors and are uncommon in infants born at <34 weeks, gestation.[162,199]

Infants who experience chronic hypoxia before birth—including infants with IUGR and cyanotic heart disease; those born at high altitudes or to mothers who smoke or have hypertension syndromes, and possibly infants of diabetic mothers (especially with poor maternal diabetic control during pregnancy)—respond to decreased tissue oxygenation by increasing erythropoietin (Epo) production.[162,200] Polycythemia is also sometimes seen in infants with trisomy 13, 18, or 21; congenital adrenal hyperplasia; and Beckwith-Wiedemann syndrome.[162,200] Epo increases erythropoiesis and fetoplacental blood volume. Infants with acute hypoxemia during the intrapartum period may also develop polycythemia due to fluid shifts from the intravascular to interstitial space and hemoconcentration. Fluid transudation within the lungs can produce respiratory distress, and the increased RBC mass leads to hypoglycemia (due to the high glucose utilization of the neonatal RBC), hypocalcemia (possibly due to alterations in vitamin D metabolism or increased levels of calcitonin gene-related peptide) and hyperbilirubinemia.[162,184]

Infant with a Hemoglobinopathy

Disorders such as β-thalassemia and sickle cell anemia usually do not cause difficulty in the neonatal period because of the neonate's increased levels of HbF (which consists of two α and two γ chains) in relation to HbA (two α and two β chains). The neonate with a higher proportion of HbF has an increased number of γ chains, fewer β chains, and similar percentage of α chains to those of the adult. Thus disorders of β-chain structure (sickle cell anemia) or synthesis (β-thalassemia) do not manifest themselves until the infant is 1 to 2 months of age and usually not before 3 to 6 months.[16,87] On the other hand, α-chain disorders such as α-thalassemia may be apparent in the neonate, depending on the clinical severity and number of affected genes (with α-thalassemia, the affected gene is either deleted or altered). Because α-chain production is controlled by two pairs of genes, infants may have one to four deleted or altered genes on chromosome 16. Phenotype and severity depend on how many genes are involved and whether the genes are deleted (nonfunctional) or present but with altered function.[194] If all four α-chain genes are missing, the fetus cannot synthesize either normal fetal hemoglobin (composed of two α- and two γ-chains) nor adult hemoglobin (composed of two α- and two β-chains). These infants develop high output cardiac failure, hydrops fetalis, and are often stillborn or die shortly after birth. These fetuses do produce hemoglobin Bart, which does not have α-chains, however this form of hemoglobin has a very high oxygen affinity and so releases little oxygen into the tissues. As a result, the infant becomes hypoxic and, if not transfused in utero, usually develops hypoxia-induced central nervous system injury. Intrauterine transfusions are associated with decreased perinatal mortality and morbidity. These infants currently require lifelong transfusion therapy, however stem cell transplants have been reported to be effective in treating these children.[194]

Infant at Risk for Altered Hemostasis

High-risk neonates are at increased risk for both thromboembolism and consumptive coagulopathies such as disseminated intravascular coagulation (DIC) as a result of the imbalance between procoagulant, anticoagulant, and fibrinolytic factors. The preterm infant, in particular, is at risk for hemostatic problems as a result of significant decreases in clotting factors, platelet function, and factors protecting against excessive clot formation. Although clotting factors are also decreased in term infants, these infants, unless severely ill, generally do not have impaired hemostasis, because only 20% to 30% of the usual levels of most coagulation factors are normally needed for clot formation. Thus even with the significant alterations in concentrations of procoagulant, anticoagulant, and fibrinolytic factors, these factors are still at physiologic levels in the neonate.

The increased risk for DIC is secondary to decreased levels of antithrombin and protein C, which normally protect against accelerated coagulation by neutralizing or inhibiting activated clotting factors. Other limitations that make the newborn more susceptible to DIC are a decreased capacity of the reticuloendothelial system to clear intermediary products of coagulation (which stimulate further coagulation and consumption of clotting factors), difficulty in maintaining adequate perfusion of small vessels (resulting in local accumulation of clotting factors and delayed clearance), hepatic immaturity (with delay in compensatory synthesis of essential clotting factors), and vulnerability to pathologic problems known to initiate DIC.[69,91] Even in preterm infants, the major risks for bleeding disorders or thrombosis are not the infant's physiologic limitations per se but rather the presence of other pathologic problems (for DIC) and trauma or indwelling lines (for thrombosis).[55,193]

Respiratory distress, sepsis, necrotizing enterocolitis, and other severe diseases are all associated with one or more of the processes that usually lead to intravascular coagulation: (1) release of tissue factor (sepsis; severe perinatal asphyxia; and other hypoxic-ischemic events such as severe respiratory distress syndrome, necrotizing enterocolitis, and central nervous system hemorrhage), (2) endothelial injury (viral infections), and (3) shock and venous stasis (severe disease that promotes local accumulation of clotting factors and decreased clearance by the liver of activated factors).[55,69,91,193]

Altered hemostasis in the ill VLBW infant—with release of tissue factor secondary to ischemic events in the germinal matrix microcirculation—may increase the risk of both intraventricular hemorrhage and extension of earlier hemorrhages.[69] Fibrinolytic activity in the periventricular area and germinal matrix is increased, leading to more rapid destruction of fibrin clots that might prevent further hemorrhage.

Thrombosis is also a risk during the neonatal period. The three factors that predispose to thromboembolism (stasis, altered coagulation, and vascular damage) are present in some neonates. Infants with polycythemia and hyperviscosity have alterations in blood flow with increased platelet adhesion as well as thrombi formation in the microcirculation, especially in the bowel, kidneys, and extremities. This may explain the increased risk of renal vein thrombosis in infants of diabetic women, who also have a high incidence of polycythemia. The infant with shock or perinatal asphyxia also has altered flow with hypotension and stasis.[53] Vascular damage can occur before birth within placental vessels in association with maternal complications such as preeclampsia or after birth secondary to trauma from indwelling catheters.[55,140] The most common cause of thromboembolism in the newborn is central venous lines; thrombotic lesions are found with umbilical catheters.[53,91,161,164] Catheters act as foreign bodies along which fibrin is deposited and thrombi form. Infants with catheters require close observation for vasospasm or emboli formation, especially in the extremities or buttocks.

The newborn is also at risk for thrombi caused by alterations in hemostasis such as the shorter whole blood clotting time, increased levels of factors V and VIII, and altered function along with decreased levels of major naturally occurring anticoagulants (antithrombin and proteins C and S).[66,69,91] Antithrombin levels are further reduced in SGA infants, increasing their risk of thrombosis. The neonatal period is also characterized by decreased fibrinolytic activity, so that once clots develop the infant is less able to remove fibrin and lyse the clots, and increased plasminogen activator inhibitor in plasma.[193]

Physiologic Anemia of Infancy

Both term infants and preterm infants experience a decline in hemoglobin during the first few months after birth. This process has been termed *physiologic anemia of infancy* in term infants because the infant tolerates the change without any clinical difficulties. Preterm infants experience a similar phenomenon that leads to anemia of prematurity (see next section). Physiologic anemia of infancy results from postnatal suppression of hematopoiesis (Figure 8-9). Hematopoiesis is controlled by Epo, which increases when oxygen delivery to the tissues is reduced. This hormone stimulates the bone marrow to increase production of RBCs. The low fetal arterial oxygen tension stimulates Epo release, which leads to production of RBCs.

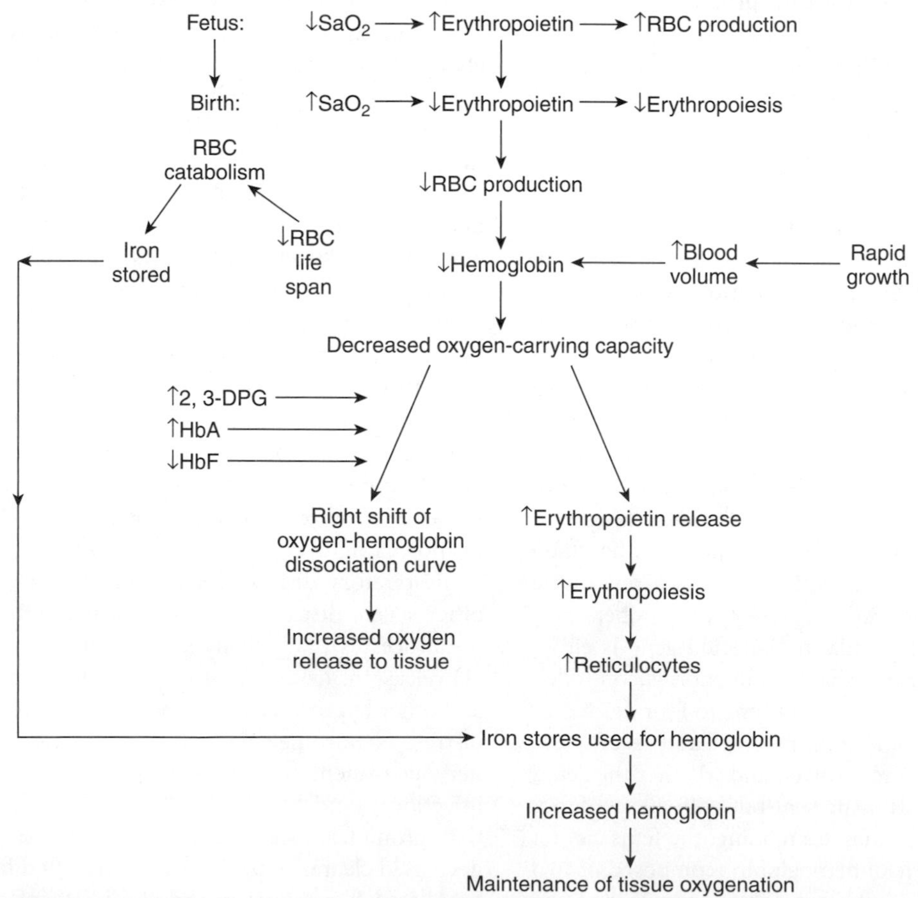

FIGURE 8-9 Physiologic anemia of infancy.

At birth, the arterial oxygen saturation rapidly increases, Epo is down-regulated and disappears from the plasma, and production of new RBCs is supressed.[3] Little Epo is found in the infant's blood from the second day of life to 6 to 8 weeks of age.[195] Because of the shorter life span of neonatal RBCs, the turnover of these cells is more rapid. Iron released from the destroyed cells is stored in the reticuloendothelial system. With rapid expansion of blood volume due to the infant's rapid growth, hemoglobin levels progressively decrease to 2 to 3 months of age in the term infant.

Although the decrease in hemoglobin reduces the oxygen-carrying capacity of the blood in early infancy, this is balanced by the gradual shift to the right in the oxygen-hemoglobin dissociation curve caused by increasing concentrations of 2,3-DPG and HbA. As a result, the actual amount of oxygen capable of being released to the tissues increases. Eventually hemoglobin levels fall to a point where tissue oxygen needs stimulate Epo and resumption of erythropoiesis (see Figure 8-9). Adult levels of Epo are reached by 10 to 12 weeks.[81]

In the term infant, the lowest hemoglobin level (11.4 ± 0.9 g/dL [114 ± 9 g/L]) is reached at 6 to 12 weeks, then slowly increases by 4 to 6 months.[3,53] Administration of iron during this period will not increase the hemoglobin to the level necessary to stimulate erythropoiesis nor diminish the rate of hemoglobin decrease.[151,215] With resumption of erythropoiesis, the reticulocyte count increases to 2% to 8%, followed by a decrease to 1% to 2% after 5 to 6 months. Total body hemoglobin levels also rise. Blood hemoglobin levels may not increase significantly if RBC production only keeps up with growth and the increase in blood volume. In older individuals, the combination of increased production of RBCs (as evidenced by a reticulocytosis) with no change in hemoglobin levels would indicate either hemorrhage or hemolysis. However, during early infancy the infant is growing so rapidly that, although total body hemoglobin is increasing, blood hemoglobin values decrease because of hemodilution.[140,215]

Once erythropoiesis is resumed, iron stores are used to produce new RBCs. The reticuloendothelial system of the term infant has adequate iron stores at this point for another 6 to 12 weeks.[153] After this time, hemoglobin levels will again decrease if adequate iron (about 1 mg/kg/day) is not available from dietary sources or as a supplement (see "Iron Supplementation").[215]

The resumption of Epo production and erythropoiesis may be delayed in infants who have had exchange transfusion or multiple blood transfusions during the first few weeks after birth. These infants have increased HbA, which releases oxygen more readily to the tissues, providing less stimulation for Epo production.[215] Infants with hemolytic disorders due to isoimmunization may experience a late and often severe anemia that is not physiologic but the result of continued hemolysis. Infants with severe hemolysis who never required an exchange transfusion are at greatest risk for this form of late anemia because of the presence in the infant's blood of maternal antibodies that continue to hemolyze the infant's RBCs. Maternal antibodies are normally removed during an exchange transfusion, reducing the risk of late anemia. The normal hemoglobin decrease after birth is often not seen in infants with cyanotic heart disease, who maintain higher Epo levels (because of their low PaO_2 levels) and thus higher hemoglobin levels in an attempt to increase oxygen delivery to their tissues.

Anemia of Prematurity

Preterm infants also experience a decline in hemoglobin during the first few months after birth secondary to postnatal suppression of hematopoiesis; this decline is similar to that described in "Physiologic Anemia of Infancy" (see Figure 8-9). However, preterm infants experience a greater decline in hemoglobin, and their hemoglobin levels remain low for a longer period of time. This phenomenon, termed *anemia of prematurity,* is a normocytic, normochromic anemia characterized by low Epo levels.

Anemia of prematurity is seen most often in infants of less than 32 weeks' gestational age with the lowest hemoglobin levels seen in the most immature infants. These levels may be as low as 7 to 10 g/dL (70 to 100 g/L) even without significant loss from blood draws.[184] The hemoglobin nadir is reached by 3 to 12 (usually 4 to 6) weeks and hemoglobin levels remain low for 3 to 6 months.[184] The level of the nadir is inversely related to gestational age.[195] Despite this decrease, tissue oxygenation actually gradually increases because HbA and 2,3-DPG are also increasing during this time, thus shifting the oxygen-hemoglobin dissociation curve to the right. As a result, oxygen is bound less tightly to hemoglobin and is more readily released to the tissues.[12] The decrease in hemoglobin cannot be prevented by nutritional supplements (i.e., iron, folate, vitamin B_{12}, vitamin E) and is not associated with hematologic abnormalities.[3,140,186] However, deficiencies of folate, vitamin E and Vitamin B_{12} can aggravate anemia of prematurity in extremely low birth-weight infants.[3] In addition, RBC transfusions increasing the proportion of HbA may, by improving oxygen availability to the tissues, lower the stimulus for Epo production, thus inadvertently contributing to anemia of prematurity.[195]

The lower hemoglobin values in preterm versus term infants are due to decreased iron stores; an altered response of Epo; a net decrease in RBC mass, RBC survival time, and marrow erythroid elements; and rapid postnatal growth and concomitant increase in circulating blood volume.[3,12,140,184,195,215] The drop in hemoglobin may be intensified in sick infants who have had repeated blood sampling. Preterm infants do not readily increase serum Epo levels in the face of hypoxia, as occurs in term infants and older individuals. This may be because Epo production in the preterm infant occurs primarily in the liver. The time for the switch from liver to primarily renal Epo production is based on postmenstrual age and does not change with preterm birth.[184] Hepatocytes require a more prolonged hypoxic stimulus to produce Epo because the hepatic oxygen sensor is relatively insensitive to hypoxic stimuli.[3,184] Hepatic production of Epo in response to hypoxic stimulation is only 10% of that seen in renal cells.[47] However, once Epo is released, the erythroid progenitor cells respond readily.[168] The decreased

Epo release by the liver may be a preventative mechanism in the fetus so that the normal low fetal PO_2 does not stimulate excessive erythropoiesis and hyperviscosity in utero.[168] Epo levels are also low due to accelerated metabolism and clearance.[184]

Although administration of iron does not prevent anemia of prematurity, once erythropoiesis resumes, the infant uses the stored iron. In preterm infants or infants who experienced early blood losses, iron stores are reduced and may be depleted by 2 to 3 months of age. Therefore iron supplementation is critical to ensure adequate stores for RBC production once erythropoiesis is resumed (see "Iron Supplementation").

Infants with anemia of prematurity may be symptomatic or asymptomatic. Clinical findings include tachycardia, tachypnea, lethargy, poor feeding, fatigue with feeding, poor weight gain (less than 25 g/day), pallor, increased serum lactate, increased oxygen requirements, and episodes of apnea or bradycardia.[22,106] The appropriate time to transfuse the preterm infant has been an area of controversy because none of these clinical signs have been consistently useful either by themselves or as a group in determining when to transfuse an infant with low hemoglobin secondary to a combination of (physiologic) anemia of prematurity and iatrogenic losses.[3,12,19,184] The goal of transfusion in infants with anemia of prematurity is to "restore or maintain oxygen delivery without increasing oxygen consumption."[28] Transfusion practices vary markedly across different units and there is a lack of evidence-based studies to guide practice.[3,12,184]

Most institutions have implemented more restrictive transfusion guidelines in recent years to reduce the numbers of transfusions and donor exposures (see "Blood Transfusions").[22,184] Use of these restrictive guidelines, which use specific hematocrit levels, clinical status, and sometimes infant age to determine when to transfuse, has reduced both the number of transfusions and donor exposures by 70% to 80% without an increase in length of stay or morbidity.[3,28,200] The lower hematocrit levels at which infants are currently being transfused do not appear to alter respiratory outcomes, length of hospitalization, or growth parameters. Donor exposure has also been reduced by use of small-volume RBC transfusions with multiple aliquots from the same unit.[3,81,112]

Administration of recombinant human erythropoietin (rEpo) has used for treatment of anemia of prematurity, although less frequently in recent years. rEpo increases the hematocrit and reticulocyte count, however, it does not appear to decrease the number of blood donor exposures.[112] Vamvakas and Strauss conducted a meta-analysis of 21 rEpo trials, all using conservative transfusion guidelines. Although there were considerable variations in findings from these studies, Vamvakas and Strauss calculated that the use of rEpo reduced the amount of blood transfused over the course of the infant's hospital stay by an average of 11 mL/kg ($p < - 0.001$).[192] Cochrane meta-analyses examined later, early and late versus early use of rEpo.[1,2,138] These analyses concluded that early use of rEpo (prior to 8 days) had limited benefits and increased the risk of retinopathy of prematurity (ROP), while late rEpo (given at 8 days or later) reduced the number of RBCs transfusions but did not reduce donor exposure since most infants received transfusions prior to treatment with rEpo.[1,2,138]

The use of restrictive transfusion guidelines appears to have similar results in terms of numbers of transfusions as use of rEpo.[22,60,112,184] Although findings are inconsistent, concerns have been raised that transfusion guidelines are too restrictive and may increase the risk of neurologic injury and altered outcomes, wheras more liberal transfusions may be neuroprotective.[17,19,37,82,88,132,184,201]

Rates of common morbidities such as chronic lung disease, necrotizing enterocolitis, and intraventricular hemorrhage were found to be similar in control and experimental (rEpo) groups.[2] As noted above, early rEpo may increase the risk of severe ROP, especially at high doses.[2,171] Some studies have reported improved scores on neurodevelopmental outcomes in infants who received rEpo.[137,205] Epo is currently being investigated as a neuroprotectant.[59,92,112,205,211] Epo has anti-inflammatory, antioxidant, angiogenic, antiepileptic, and neurotropic effects.[92,205] Neural tissues have Epo receptors which when activated lead to cell division, maturation, and inhibition of apoptopsis.[92,205] Endogenous Epo is produced in the brain, primarily by astrocytes, but also by oligodendrocytes, endothelial cells, neurons, and microglia.[92] Production is up regulated by hypoxia, so Epo may have a protective role with hypoxic- ischemic encephalopathy (HIE), periventricular leukomalacia, and hyperoxic brain injury.[92] Although much of the work to date have been with animal models, trials of rEpo with term infants with HIE have demonstrated potential efficacy in improving neurodevelopmental outcomes.[59,211] Additional clinical trials are ongoing. Epo receptors are found in the fetal and neonatal small intestine, and human milk contains Epo, thus Epo may play a role in maturation of the gut.[95]

Iron Supplementation

Iron supplementation is generally begun before the point of depletion to maintain and build up the infant's iron stores. Breast milk is low in iron, although the available iron is more readily absorbed. The American Academy of Pediatrics (AAP) recently revised guidelines recommend that breastfed infants receive 1 mg/kg oral iron beginning at 4 months of age, until iron containing foods such as iron-fortified infant cereal are started.[13] This recommendation has been controversial.[61,166] Rates of iron-deficiency anemia in unsupplemented term breast fed infants are only 3%.[213] Once the infant is started on solids, iron fortified cereals have been reported to be as effective as medicinal iron for breast fed infants.[212,214] Formula-fed infants should be fed with an iron-fortified formula for the first 12 months. Iron deficiency in infancy may alter neurocognitive development since iron is essential for neurotransmission, energy metabolism, myelinization, and synaptogenesis.[13,45,153]

Preterm infants are at increased risk of inadequate iron.[20,153,154] The AAP recommends that preterm infants should receive at least 2 mg/kg/day of iron through 12 months, plus introduction of iron-containing foods after 4 to 6 months corrected age, and in breast fed preterm infants iron supplementation should start by 1 month of age.[13] The exception is if the infant has received an iron load from multiple transfusion of packed RBCs. Iron overload can also alter neurodevelopment.[12,20,45,173]

Blood Transfusions

As discussed above, decisions regarding whether or not to transfuse an infant, especially VLBW infants, are often difficult.[3,19,184] Although transfusions are still a frequent procedure in the neonatal intensive care unit, the average number of transfusions each VLBW infant receives has decreased over the past 15 years, from 10 to between 1 and 5.[12,83,185] This decrease is due to many factors, including improved outcomes with newer therapies (e.g., surfactant replacement and ventilator management strategies) reducing the number of blood draws, more restrictive transfusion criteria, and improved blood sampling techniques.[3,12,83,185] The usual cause of anemia in VLBW infants is a combination of iatrogenic losses, immaturity of the hematopoietic system, RBC characteristics (e.g., a shorter RBC life span), and decreased erythropoiesis due to anemia of prematurity.[3,12,83,182] Because the cardiovascular system of the newborn can usually tolerate an increase in intravascular volume of 10% to 15%, and because the total blood volume of the newborn is estimated at 80 to 100 mL/kg, the usual transfusion is 10 to 20 mL/kg.[184] A recent feasibility trial suggested that drawing blood for initial baseline testing from the placenta versus the infant in VLBW infants may delay the time of the initial transfusion.[41] However, there are many issues associated with this technique.[3,19,184] As noted in the section on Transitional Events, delayed cord clamping has also been found to reduce the number of blood transfusions needed in preterm infants.[150]

The advantages of transfusion must be balanced against the consequences and potential risks. Risks of transfusion include infection (especially from cytomegalovirus; hepatitis A, B, C, and G; human immunodeficiency virus; and parvovirus B19), metabolic and cardiovascular complications (volume overload, arrhythmias, and thromboembolism), hypothermia, exposure to multiple donors, and graft-versus-host disease.[60,174] Following transfusions, particularly exchange transfusions with adult blood, there may be rapid alterations in the oxygen-hemoglobin dissociation curve. This shift is an advantage to the infant because it improves oxygen release to the tissues; however, it may result in rapid changes in PaO_2, increasing the risk of ROP. Following an exchange transfusion or after multiple transfusions, a portion of the infant's HbF will have been replaced by HbA, which has a greater ability to unload oxygen. This change can lead to a rapid improvement in the amount of oxygen delivered to the tissues at a given PaO_2 and possible hyperoxia. Some studies have reported an association between packed red blood cell transfusion and necrotizing enterocolitis (NEC) in preterm infa nts.[23,40,78,144,192] It is uncertain if the transfusion per se increased the risk of NEC or if the need for transfusion was indicative of other factors that might lead to NEC.[144] The interaction of NEC and transfusion may be due to a transfusion-related acute reaction in the intestines, impaired blood flow to the intestines (and thus intestinal injury) from an anemia that led to the need for transfusion, or injuries to stored RBCs used for the transfusion that could increase the risk of vasoconstriction and ischemia in the intestinal microcirculation.[23,40,144]

MATURATIONAL CHANGES DURING INFANCY AND CHILDHOOD

Most of the maturational changes in the hematologic system occur during the first 6 to 12 months. The most significant changes are related to the decline in hemoglobin, with the resulting physiologic anemia of infancy, accumulation of higher concentrations of 2,3-diphosphoglycerate (2,3-DPG), and shift of the oxygen-hemoglobin dissociation curve to the right. An awareness of these changes in infancy is necessary for an appropriate evaluation and treatment of anemia and hypoxia.

Changes in Hematologic Parameters

Blood volume values per unit weight are higher than adult values for the first month or two, increasing the risk of hypovolemia.[140] The mean red blood cell (RBC) corpuscular volume and mean diameter decrease rapidly during the first week, followed by a gradual decrease to diameters similar to those of adult cells by 3 to 4 months, declining further to lower than adult by 4 to 6 months, then increasing to adult volumes by about 1 year.[39] RBC fragility also decreases and is similar to that of adults by 3 months. During the first 2 to 3 months, blood and total body hemoglobin levels decrease secondary to decreased RBC production, resulting in the physiologic anemia of infancy discussed previously.

Erythropoietin (Epo) production reaches adult levels by 10 to 12 weeks and the switch from hepatic to renal Epo production is probably completed by several months of age.[47,81] Differences between capillary and venous hemoglobin levels persist until 3 months of age.[140] The hematocrit decreases to around 30% by 2 months, then increases to 35% by 1 year and to adult values in adolescence. Reticulocyte levels reach adult values by 2 years. Serum ferritin levels rise after birth and remain high for 4 to 6 weeks, with a mean of 356 ng/mL (800 pmol/L). After this time, levels fall to 30 ng/mL (67.4 pmol/L)—versus 39 ng/mL [87.6 pmol/L] in female adults and 140 ng/mL [314.6 pmol/L] in male adults—by 6 months and remain stable until early to mid-adolescence.[104,140] RBC membrane characteristics are similar to those of adults by 4 to 6 weeks.[81]

With the occurrence of hypoxia, congestive heart failure, or other physiologic stressors, the liver and spleen in early childhood can resume active hematopoiesis and serve as alternative sites for RBC production.[104] During early childhood, blood cells are found in the bones of the tibia, femur, ribs, sternum, and vertebrae rather than in the axial skeleton as seen in adults. Blood tissue in long bones is gradually replaced by adipose tissue beginning at 3 years. By puberty the red marrow in these bones is found only in the upper ends of the humerus and femur and has disappeared by adulthood.

Production of WBCs in the thymus ceases in early childhood. Megakaryocytes reach adult size by 2 years.[81]

Activity of coagulation factors gradually increases during infancy and early childhood with the gradual evolution of hemostasis to adult parameters by adolescence.[8] Most values approach adult levels by 2 weeks to 12 months depending on the individual factor.[143] However, vitamin K–dependent factors remain 15% to 20% below adult values until childhood.[8] Levels of antithrombin, heparin cofactor II, and protein S reach adult ranges by 6 months; protein C does not reach adult values until early childhood.[56,66,86,91,174] α_1-Macroglobulin is twice adult values at 6 months and remains high throughout childhood.[8,91] Contact factors also reach adult levels by 6 months.[66] During childhood, bleeding times remain longer than in adults.[8]

Changes in Oxygen-Hemoglobin Affinity

During the first 3 months after birth, the P_{50} gradually increases, and by 4 to 6 months the P_{50} and the oxygen-hemoglobin dissociation curve is similar to that of the adult.[215] From 8 to 11 months, the curve may actually be shifted slightly to the right of the adult curve due to increased blood organic phosphates along with changes in the concentrations of HbA and 2,3-DPG.[140] HbF concentrations decrease 3% to 4% per week during the first 6 months. By 4 months, HbF accounts for only 5% to 10% of the hemoglobin. Levels of HbF gradually decrease to adult levels (less than 2%) by 2 to 3 years. HbA_2 concentrations increase to adult levels of 2% to 3% by 5 to 6 months.

The gradual shift of the oxygen-hemoglobin dissociation curve during the first 6 months after birth is determined by the relative proportions of HbF to HbA and concentrations of 2,3-DPG. Infants with similar concentrations of HbF may have different P_{50} values if they have significantly different levels of 2,3-DPG. Similarly, infants with similar levels of 2,3-DPG may have different P_{50} values if concentrations of HbF are significantly different. Thus an infant with elevated levels of HbA and low levels of 2,3-DPG may have a P_{50} that is similar to that of another infant with high levels of HbF and 2,3-DPG.[53,140] This seeming paradox is explained by what Delivoria-Papadopoulous and colleagues called the functioning DPG fraction: the gradual decrease in affinity of hemoglobin for oxygen during the first 6 months after birth correlates with a fraction derived from multiplying the total RBC 2,3-DPG content by the percentage of HbA.[51] Thus two critical factors in determining the position of the oxygen-hemoglobin dissociation curve during infancy are the amount of HbA and the amount of 2,3-DPG. The rate of postnatal decline in fetal hemoglobin concentrations is generally not affected by persistent cyanosis secondary to cyanotic heart disease.[140]

SUMMARY

The hematologic and hemostatic systems undergo significant alterations during the neonatal period. Because of these changes, the infant is at risk for anemia, thromboembolic insults, and coagulopathies. Many of the changes in the hematologic system encountered in the neonate occur progressively over time. Therefore gestational and post birth age, as well as health status must be considered in evaluating and managing individual infants. Clinical recommendations for nurses working with neonates based on changes in the hematologic system are summarized in Table 8-8.

Table 8-8 Recommendations for Clinical Practice Related to the Hematologic System in Neonates

Know normal parameters for hematologic values in the preterm and term neonate and patterns of change during the neonatal period (pp. 235-238).
Recognize changes in hematocrit during the first few days post birth due to fluid shifts (versus changes indicating pathologic processes) (pp. 234-236).
Monitor for problems for which the newborn is at increased risk due to alterations in the neonate's red blood cells (p. 235 and Table 8-7).
Recognize the effects of sampling site and physical activity (especially crying) on hematologic values (pp. 238-239).
Record the sampling site and infant activity each time blood is drawn (pp. 238-239).
Record the amount of blood drawn and other iatrogenic blood loss (pp. 238-239).
Evaluate the amount of iatrogenic blood loss in light of infant's blood volume (pp. 238-239).
Ensure that vitamin K is given following birth (pp. 239-240).
Monitor for signs of vitamin K deficiency bleeding, especially in infants of mothers on anticonvulsants, anticoagulants, or long-term antibiotic therapy and in infants on long-term antibiotic therapy (pp. 239-240).
Recognize laboratory and clinical signs associated with anemia in preterm and term neonates and with anemia is infancy (pp. 242-244).
Monitor for clinical signs of anemia, anemia of prematurity, and hemolysis (pp. 242-244).
Recognize and monitor for signs of bleeding and disseminated intravascular coagulation, especially in infants at risk (pp. 241-242).
Recognize transfusion complications (p. 245).
Monitor PO_2 values regularly in infants on pulse oximetry and maintain within normal limits (p. 239).
Monitor PO_2 and for hyperoxia in infants following transfusions (especially with fresh blood, after multiple or exchange transfusions) (pp. 239, 244-245).
Recognize and monitor for signs of thromboembolism in infants with indwelling lines or who are hypotensive, polycythemic, or in shock (pp. 241-242).
Recognize and monitor infants at risk for polycythemia and hyperviscosity (pp. 240-241).
Ensure that term and preterm infants receive iron supplementation at recommended time points (pp. 244-245).

References

1. Aher, S. & Ohlsson, A. (2006). Late erythropoietin for preventing red blood cell transfusion in preterm and/or low birth weight infants. *Cochrane Database Syst Rev,* 3, CD004868.
2. Aher, S.M. & Ohlsson, A. (2006). Early versus late erythropoietin for preventing red blood cell transfusion in preterm and/or low birth weight infants. *Cochrane Database Syst Rev,* 3, CD004865.
3. Aher, S., Malwatkar, K., & Kadam, S. (2008). Neonatal anemia. *Semin Fetal Neonatal Med, 13,* 239.
4. Airey, R.J., Farrar, D., & Duley, L. (2010). Alternative positions for the baby at birth before clamping the umbilical cord. *Cochrane Database Syst Rev, 10,* CD007555.
5. Allen, L. (1997). Pregnancy and iron deficiency: Unresolved issues. *Nutr Rev, 55,* 91.
6. Amburgey, O.A., et al. (2009). Maternal hemoglobin concentration and its association with birth weight in newborns of mothers with preeclampsia. *J Matern Fetal Neonatal Med, 22,* 740.
7. Anderson, J.A. & Weitz, J.I. (2010). Hypercoagulable states. *Clin Chest Med, 31,* 659.
8. Andrew, M. (1995). Developmental hemostasis: Relevance to hemostatic problems during childhood. *Semin Thromb Hemost, 21,* 341.
9. Arca, G., et al. (2010). Timing of umbilical cord clamping: New thoughts on an old discussion. *J Matern Fetal Neonatal Med, 23,* 1274.
10. August, P. (2004). Hypertensive disorder in pregnancy. In G.N. Burrows, T.P. Duffy, & J.A. Copel, (Eds.). *Medical complications during pregnancy* (6th ed.). Philadelphia: Saunders.
11. Baenziger, O., et al. (2007). The influence of the timing of cord clamping on postnatal cerebral oxygenation in preterm neonates: A randomized, controlled trial. *Pediatrics, 119,* 455.
12. Bain, A. & Blackburn, S. (2004). Issues in transfusing preterm infants in the NICU. *J Perinat Neonatal Nurs, 18,* 170.
13. Baker, R.D. & Greer, F.R. (2010). Committee on Nutrition American Academy of Pediatrics. Diagnosis and prevention of iron deficiency and iron-deficiency anemia in infants and young children (0-3 years of age). *Pediatrics, 126,* 1040.
14. Bard, H. (2000). Hemoglobin synthesis and metabolism during the neonatal period. In Christenson, R.D. (Ed.). *Hematologic problems of the neonate.* Philadelphia: Saunders.
15. Bassell, G.M. & Marx, G.F. (1981). Physiologic changes of normal pregnancy and parturition. In E.V. Cosmi (Ed.). *Obstetrical anesthesia and perinatology.* New York: Appleton-Century-Crofts.
16. Bauer, D.E. & Orkin, S.H. (2011). Update on fetal hemoglobin gene regulation in hemoglobinopathies. *Curr Opin Pediatr, 23,* 1.
17. Bell, E.F., et al. (2005). Randomized trial of liberal versus restrictive guidelines for red blood cell transfusions in preterm infants. *Pediatrics, 115,* 1685.
18. Bell, E.F. (2008). When to transfuse preterm babies. *Arch Dis Child Fetal Neonatal Ed, 93,* F469.
19. Bell, E.F. (2011). When to transfuse preterm babies. *Arch Dis Child Fetal Neonatal Ed, 93,* f469.
20. Berglund, S., Westrup, B., & Domellöf, M. (2010). Iron supplements reduce the risk of iron deficiency anemia in marginally low birth weight infants. *Pediatrics, 126,* e874.
21. Biban, P., et al. (2011). New cardiopulmonary resuscitation guidelines 2010: Managing the newly born in delivery room. *Early Hum Dev, 87,* S9.
22. Bishara, N. & Ohls, R.K. (2009). Current controversies in the management of anemia of prematurity. *Semin Perinatol, 33,* 29.
23. Blau, J., et al. (2011). Transfusion-related acute gut injury: Necrotizing enterocolitis in very low birth weight neonates after packed red blood cell transfusion. *J Pediatr, 158,* 403.
24. Boehlen, F., et al. (2000). Platelet count at term pregnancy: A reappraisal of the threshold. *Obstet Gynecol, 95,* 29.
25. Borgna-Pignatti, C., Marsella, M., & Zanforlin, N. (2010). The natural history of thalassemia intermedia. *Ann N Y Acad Sci, 1202,* 214.
26. Bremme, K.A. (2003). Haemostatic changes in pregnancy. *Best Pract Res Clin Haematol, 16,* 153.
27. Brenner, B. (2004). Haemostatic changes in pregnancy. *Thromb Res, 114,* 409.
28. British Committee for Standards in Haematology (BCSH), Transfusion Task Force. *Transfusion guidelines for neonates and older children.* (2003). Available at: www.bcshguidelines.com/ guidelines.asp.
29. Brosens, J.J., Pijnenborg, R., & Brosens, I.A. (2002). The myometrial junctional zone spiral arteries in normal and abnormal pregnancies: A review of the literature. *Am J Obstet Gynecol, 187,* 1416.
30. Calhoun, D.A. (2000). Hematologic aspects of the maternal-fetal relationship. In R. Christensen (Ed.). *Hematologic problems of the neonate.* Philadelphia: Saunders.
31. Calhoun, D.A. & Christensen, R.D. (2004). Hematopoietic growth factors in neonatal medicine: the use of enterally administered hematopoietic growth factors in the neonatal intensive care unit. *Clin Perinatol, 31,* 169.
32. Carbillon, L., Uzan, M., & Uzan, S. (2000). Pregnancy, vascular tone, and maternal hemodynamics: A crucial adaptation. *Obstet Gynecol Surv, 55,* 574.
33. Carlson, B.M. (2008). *Human embryology and developmental biology* (4th ed.). Philadelphia: Mosby.
34. Cavil, J.L. (2000). Iron requirements in adolescent females. *J Nutr, 12,* 440.
35. Centers for Disease Control and Prevention. (1991). Use of folic acid for prevention of spina bifida and other neural tube defects. *MMWR, 40,* 531.
36. Centers for Disease Control and Prevention. (1998). Recommendations to prevent and control iron deficiency anemia in the United States. *MMWR 47,* 1.
37. Chen, H.L., et al. (2009). Effect of blood transfusions on the outcome of very low body weight preterm infants under two different transfusion criteria. *Pediatr Neonatol, 50,* 110.
38. Chesley, L.C. (1972). Plasma and red cell volumes during pregnancy. *Am J Obstet Gynecol, 112,* 440.
39. Christensen, R.D. (2000). Expected hematologic values for term and preterm neonates. In R. Christensen (Ed.). *Hematologic problems of the neonate.* Philadelphia: Saunders.
40. Christensen, R.D. (2011). Association between red blood cell transfusions and necrotizing enterocolitis. *J Pediatr, 158,* 349.
41. Christensen, R.D., et al. (2011). Postponing or eliminating red blood cell transfusions of very low birth weight neonates by obtaining all baseline laboratory blood tests from otherwise discarded fetal blood in the placenta. *Transfusion, 51,* 253.
42. Clark, P. (2003). Changes of hemostasis variables during pregnancy. *Semin Vasc Med, 3,* 13.
43. Clarke, P. (2010). Vitamin K prophylaxis for preterm infants. *Early Hum Dev, 86,* 17.
44. Coggins, M. & Mercer, J. (2009). Delayed cord clamping: Advantages for infants. *Nurs Womens Health, 13,* 132.
45. Collard, K.J. (2009). Iron homeostasis in the neonate. *Pediatrics, 123,* 1208.
46. Cunningham, G., et al. (2009). *Williams obstetrics* (23rd ed.). New York: McGraw-Hill.
47. Dame, C. & Juul, S. (2000). The switch from fetal to adult erythropoiesis. *Clin Perinatol, 27,* 507.
48. de Alarcón, P. & Werner, E. (2005). *Neonatal hematology.* Cambridge, England: Cambridge University Press.
49. Deckardt, R. & Steward, D.J. (1984). Noninvasive arterial oxygen saturation versus transcutaneous oxygen tension monitoring in the preterm infant. *Crit Care Med, 12,* 935.
50. Del Vecchio, A. & Sola, M.C. (2000). Performing and interpreting the bleeding time in the neonatal intensive care unit. *Clin Perinatol, 27,* 643.
51. Delivoria-Papadopoulous, M., Roncevic, N.P., & Oski, F.A. (1971). Postnatal changes in oxygen transport of term, preterm, and sick infants: the role of 2,3-DPG and adult hemoglobin. *Pediatr Res, 5,* 235.
52. De-Regil, L.M., et al. (2010). Effects and safety of periconceptional folate supplementation for preventing birth defects. *Cochrane Database Syst Rev, 10,* CD007950.
53. Doyle, J.J., et al. (1999). Hematology. In G.B. Avery, M.A. Fletcher, & M.G. Macdonald (Eds.). *Neonatology: Pathophysiology and management of the newborn* (5th ed.). Philadelphia: J.B. Lippincott.

54. Duffy, T.P. (2004). Hematologic aspects of pregnancy. In G.N. Burrows, T.P. Duffy, & J.A. Copel (Eds.). *Medical complications during pregnancy* (6th ed.). Philadelphia: Saunders.
55. Edstrom, C.S. & Christensen, R.D. (2000). Evaluation and treatment of thrombosis in the neonatal intensive care unit. *Clin Perinatol, 27,* 623.
56. Edstrom, C.S., Christensen, R.D., & Andrew, M. (2000). Developmental aspects of blood hemostasis and disorders of coagulation and fibrinolysis in the neonatal period. In R. Christensen (Ed.). *Hematologic problems of the neonate.* Philadelphia: Saunders.
57. Eichenbaum-Pikser, G. & Zasloff, J.S. (2009). Delayed clamping of the umbilical cord: A review with implications for practice. *J Midwifery Womens Health, 54,* 321.
58. Eldor, A. (2002). The use of low-molecular-weight heparin for the management of venous thromboembolism in pregnancy. *Eur J Obstet Gynecol Reprod Biol, 104,* 3.
59. Elmahdy, H., et al. (2010). Human recombinant erythropoietin in asphyxia neonatorum: Pilot trial. *Pediatrics, 125,* e1135.
60. Fasano, R. & Luban, N.L.C. (2011). Blood component therapy for the neonate. In R.J. Martin, A.A. Fanaroff, & M.C. Walsh (Eds.). *Fanaroff and Martin's Neonatal-perinatal medicine: Diseases of the fetus and infant* (9th ed.). Philadelphia: Mosby Elsevier.
61. Furman, L.M. (2011). Exclusively breastfed infants: Iron recommendations are premature. *Pediatrics, 127,* e1098.
62. Ganzevoort, W., et al. (2004). Plasma volume and blood pressure regulation in hypertensive pregnancy. *J Hypertens, 22,* 1235.
63. Girardi, G. (2011). Role of tissue factor in feto-maternal development: A xiphos. *J Thromb Haemost, 9,* 250.
64. Greer, F.R. (2010). Vitamin K the basics—what's new? *Early Hum Dev, 86,* S43.
65. Greer, I.A. (2003). Thrombophilia: Implication for pregnancy outcome. *Thromb Res, 109,* 73.
66. Guzzetta, N.A. & Miller, B.E. (2011). Principles of hemostasis in children: Models and maturation. *Paediatr Anaesth, 21,* 3.
67. Halvorsen, S. & Bechensteen, A.G. (2002). Physiology of erythropoietin during mammalian development. *Acta Paediatr Suppl, 91,* 17.
68. Harden, C.L., et al. (2009). Practice parameter update: Management issues for women with epilepsy—focus on pregnancy (an evidence-based review): Vitamin K, folic acid, blood levels, and breastfeeding: Report of the Quality Standards Subcommittee and Therapeutics and Technology Assessment Subcommittee of the American Academy of Neurology and American Epilepsy Society. *Neurology, 73,* 142.
69. Hathaway, W.E. & Bonnar, J. (1987). *Hemostatic disorders of the pregnant woman and newborn infant.* New York: Elsevier.
70. Heller, C. & Nowak-Gotti, U. (2003). Maternal thrombophilia and neonatal thrombosis. *Best Pract Res Clin Haematol, 16,* 333.
71. Hellgren, M. (2003). Hemostasis during normal pregnancy and puerperium. *Semin Thromb Hemost, 29,* 125.
72. Hutton, E.K. & Hassan, E.S. (2007). Late vs early clamping of the umbilical cord in full-term neonates: Systematic review and meta-analysis of controlled trials. *JAMA, 297,* 1241.
73. Hytten, F. (1985). Blood volume changes in normal pregnancy. *Clin Hematol, 14,* 601.
74. Institute of Medicine. (1990). *Nutrition during pregnancy.* Washington, DC: National Academy Press.
75. Institute of Medicine. (1993). *Iron deficiency anemia: Guidelines for prevention, detection, and management among U.S. children and women of childbearing age.* Washington, DC: National Academy Press.
76. Israels, L.G., et al. (1997). The riddle of vitamin K1 deficit in the newborn. *Semin Perinatol, 21,* 90.
77. Israels, S.J. (2009). Diagnostic evaluation of platelet function disorders in neonates and children: An update. *Semin Thromb Hemost, 35,* 181.
78. Josephson, C.D., et al. (2010). Do red cell transfusions increase the risk of necrotizing enterocolitis in premature infants? *J Pediatr, 157,* 972.
79. Juul, S. (2000). Nonerythropoietic roles of erythropoietin in the fetus and neonate. *Clin Perinatol, 27,* 527.
80. Juul, S. (2004). Recombinant erythropoietin as a neuroprotective treatment: In vitro and in vivo models. *Clin Perinatol, 31,* 129.
81. Juul, S.E. (2000). Nonhematopoietic aspects of hematopoietic growth factors in the fetus and newborn. In R. Christensen (Ed.). *Hematologic problems of the neonate.* Philadelphia: Saunders.
82. Juul, S.E., et al. (2008). A phase I/II trial of high-dose erythropoietin in extremely low birth weight infants: Pharmacokinetics and safety. *Pediatrics, 122,* 383.
83. Kabra, N.S. (2003). Blood transfusion in preterm infants. *Arch Dis Child Fetal Neonatal Ed, 88,* F78.
84. Kakkilaya, V., et al. (2008). Effect of placental transfusion on the blood volume and clinical outcome of infants born by cesarean section. *Clin Perinatol, 35,* 561.
85. Kenet, G., et al. (2010). Bleeding disorders in neonates. *Haemophilia, 16,* 168.
86. Khor, B. & Van Cott, E.M. (2009). Laboratory evaluation of hypercoagulability. *Clin Lab Med, 29,* 339.
87. Kilpatrick, S.J. (2009). Anemia and pregnancy. In R.K. Creasy, et al. (Eds.). *Creasy & Resnik's Maternal-fetal medicine: Principles and practice* (6th ed.). Philadelphia: Saunders Elsevier.
88. Kirpalani, H., et al. (2006). The Premature Infants in Need of Transfusion (PINT) study: A randomized, controlled trial of a restrictive (low) versus liberal (high) transfusion threshold for extremely low birth weight infants. *J Pediatr, 149,* 301.
89. Koenig, J.M. & Yoder, M.C. (2005). White blood cell disorders in the neonate. In A.R. Spitzer (Ed.). *Intensive care of the fetus & neonate* (2nd ed.). Philadelphia: Mosby.
90. Kugelman, A., et al. (2007). Immediate versus delayed umbilical cord clamping in premature neonates born <35 weeks: A prospective, randomized, controlled study. *Am J Perinatol, 24,* 307.
91. Kuhne, T. & Imbach, P. (1998). Neonatal platelet physiology and pathophysiology. *Eur J Pediatr, 157,* 87.
92. Kumral, A., et al. (2011). Erythropoietin in neonatal brain protection: the past, the present and the future. *Brain Development, 33,* 632.
93. Lanir, N., Aharon, A., & Brenner, B. (2003). Haemostatic mechanisms in human placenta. *Best Pract Res Clin Haematol, 16,* 183.
94. Lanir, N., Aharon, A., & Brenner, B. (2003). Procoagulant and anticoagulant mechanisms in human placenta. *Semin Thromb Hemost, 29,* 175.
95. Ledbetter, D.J. & Juul, S.E. (2000). Erythropoietin and the incidence of necrotizing enterocolitis in infants with very low birth weight. *J Pediatr Surg, 35,* 178.
96. Levine, J.S., Branch, D.W., & Rauch, J. (2002). The antiphospholipid syndrome. *N Engl J Med, 346,* 752.
97. Levy, T. & Blickstein, I. (2006). Timing of cord clamping revisited. *J Perinat Med, 34,* 293.
98. Lin, J.C., et al. (2000). Phlebotomy overdraw in the neonatal intensive care nursery. *Pediatrics, 106,* e19.
99. Lindeman, R. & Haga, P. (2000). Evaluation and treatment of polycythemia in the neonate. In R. Christensen (Ed.). *Hematologic problems of the neonate.* Philadelphia: Saunders.
100. Lindheimer, M.D. & August, P. (2009). Aldosterone, maternal volume status and healthy pregnancies: A cycle of differing views. *Nephrol Dial Transplant, 24,* 1712.
101. Lippi, G. & Franchini, M. (2011). Vitamin K in neonates: Facts and myths. *Blood Transfus, 9,* 4.
102. Lockwood, C.J. (2009). Thromboembolic disease in pregnancy. In R.K. Creasy, et al. (Eds.). *Creasy & Resnik's Maternal-fetal medicine: Principles and practice* (6th ed.). Philadelphia: Saunders Elsevier.
103. Lockwood, C.J. & Silver, R. (2009). Coagulation disorders in pregnancy. In R.K. Creasy, et al. (Eds.). *Creasy & Resnik's Maternal-fetal medicine: Principles and practice* (6th ed.). Philadelphia: Saunders Elsevier.
104. Lowrey, G.H. (1986). *Growth and development of children.* Chicago: Year Book.
105. Luban, N.L. (2008). Management of anemia in the newborn. *Early Hum Dev, 84,* 493.

106. Luchtman-Jones, L. & Wilson, D.B. (2011). Hematological problems in the fetus and newborn. In R.J. Martin, A.A. Fanaroff, & M.C. Walsh (Eds.). *Fanaroff and Martin's Neonatal-perinatal medicine: Diseases of the fetus and infant* (9th ed.). Philadelphia: Mosby Elsevier.
107. Luegenbiehl, D.L., et al. (1990). Standardized assessment of blood loss. *MCN Am J Matern Child Nurs, 15,* 241.
108. Luft, F.C., Gallery, E.D.M., & Lindheimer, M.D. (2009). Normal and abnormal volume homeostasis. In M.D. Lindheimer, J.M. Roberts, & F.G. Cunningham (Eds.). *Chesley's hypertensive disorders in pregnancy* (3rd ed.). San Diego: Elsevier.
109. Lynch, S.R. (2000). The potential impact of iron supplementation during adolescence on iron status in pregnancy. *J Nutr, 120,* 448.
110. Maheshwari, A. & Christensen, R. D. (2012). Developmental granulocytopoiesis. In R.A. Polin, W.W. Fox, & S.H. Abman (Eds.). *Fetal and neonatal physiology* (4th ed.). Philadelphia: Saunders.
111. Mahomed, K. (2000). Iron and folate supplementation in pregnancy. *Cochrane Database Syst Rev, 2,* CD001135.
112. Mainie, P. (2008). Is there a role for erythropoietin in neonatal medicine? *Early Hum Dev, 84,* 525.
113. Manroe, B.L., et al. (1979). The neonatal blood count in health and disease. I. Reference values for neutrophil cells. *J Pediatr, 95,* 89.
114. March of Dimes. (2002). Folic acid supplementation and prevention of birth defects. *J Nutr, 12,* 507.
115. Marik, P.E. (2010). Venous thromboembolism in pregnancy. *Clin Chest Med, 31,* 731.
116. Matthews D.C. & Glader, B.E. (2012). Erythrocyte disorders in infancy. In C.A. Gleason & S. Devaskar (Eds.). *Avery's diseases of the newborn* (9th ed.). Philadelphia: Saunders.
117. McCrae, K.R. (2010). Thrombocytopenia in pregnancy. *Hematology Am Soc Hematol Educ Program, 2010,* 397.
118. McDonald, S.J. & Middleton, P. (2008). Effect of timing of umbilical cord clamping of term infants on maternal and neonatal outcomes. *Cochrane Database Syst Rev, 2,* CD004074.
119. McPhedren, P. (2004). Venous thromboembolism during pregnancy. In G.N. Burrows, T.P. Duffy, & J.A. Copel (Eds.). *Medical complications during pregnancy* (6th ed.). Philadelphia: Saunders.
120. McPherson, R.J. & Juul, S.E. (2010). Erythropoietin for infants with hypoxic-ischemic encephalopathy. *Curr Opin Pediatr, 22,* 139.
121. Medical Research Counsel Vitamin Study Research Group. (1991). Prevention of neural tube defects. Results of the Medical Research Counsel Vitamin Study, *Lancet, 338,* 131.
122. Mehndiratta, S., et al. (2010). Fetotoxicity of warfarin anticoagulation. *Arch Gynecol Obstet, 282,* 335.
123. Mercer, J.S., Nelson, C.C., & Skovgaard, R.L. (2000). Umbilical cord clamping: Beliefs and practices of American nurse-midwives. *J Midwifery Womens Health, 45,* 58.
124. Mercer, J.S. & Skovgaard, R.L. (2002). Neonatal transitional physiology: A new paradigm. *J Perinat Neonatal Nurs, 15,* 56.
125. Mitic, G., et al. (2011). Clinical characteristics and type of thrombophilia in women with pregnancy-related venous thromboembolic disease. *Gynecol Obstet Invest, 72,* 103
126. Monagle, P., Ignjatovic, V. & Savoia, H. (2010). Hemostasis in neonates and children: Pitfalls and dilemmas. *Blood Rev, 24,* 63.
127. Monagle P. & Hagstrom, J.N. (2012). Developmental hemostasis. In R.A. Polin, W.W. Fox, & S.H. Abman (Eds.). *Fetal and neonatal physiology* (4th ed.). Philadelphia: Saunders.
128. Monga, M. (2009). Maternal cardiovascular, respiratory and renal adaptation to pregnancy. In R.K. Creasy, et al. (Eds.). *Creasy & Resnik's Maternal-fetal medicine: Principles and practice* (6th ed.). Philadelphia: Saunders Elsevier.
129. Montagnana, M., et al. (2010). Disseminated intravascular coagulation in obstetric and gynecologic disorders. *Semin Thromb Hemost, 36,* 404.
130. Mouzinho, A., et al. (1994). Revised reference ranges for circulating neutrophils in very-low-birth-weight neonates. *Pediatrics, 94,* 76.
131. Nicholl, R.M., et al. (2010). Question 1. Is delayed clamping of the umbilical cord in moderately preterm babies beneficial? *Arch Dis Child, 95,* 235.
132. Nopoulos, P.C., et al. (2011). Long-term outcome of brain structure in premature infants: Effects of liberal vs. restricted red blood cell transfusions. *Arch Pediatr Adolesc Med, 165,* 443.
133. O'Riordan, M.N. & Higgins, J.R. (2003). Haemostasis in normal and abnormal pregnancy. *Best Pract Res Clin Obstet Gynaecol, 17,* 385.
134. Ohls, R.K. (2000). Evaluation and treatment of anemia in the neonate. In R. Christensen (Ed.). *Hematologic problems of the neonate.* Philadelphia: Saunders.
135. Ohls, R.K. (2012). Developmental erythropoiesis. In R.A. Polin, W.W. Fox, & S.H. Abman (Eds.). *Fetal and neonatal physiology* (4th ed.). Philadelphia: Saunders.
136. Ohls, R.K., et al. (2001). Effects of early erythropoietin therapy on the transfusion requirements of preterm infants below 1250 grams birth weight: A multicenter, randomized, controlled trial. *Pediatrics, 108,* 934.
137. Ohls, R.K., et al. (2004). Neurodevelopmental outcome and growth at 18 to 22 months' corrected age in extremely low birth weight infants treated with early erythropoietin and iron. *Pediatrics, 114,* 1287.
138. Ohlsson, A. & Aher, S.M. (2006). Early erythropoietin for preventing red blood cell transfusion in preterm and/or low birth weight infants. *Cochrane Database Syst Rev, 3,* CD004863.
139. Oski, F.A. (1979). Clinical implications of the oxygen-hemoglobin dissociation curve in the neonatal period. *Crit Care Med, 7,* 412.
140. Orkin, S.H. & Nathan, D.G. (2008). *Nathan and Oski's Hematology of infancy and childhood* (7th edition). Philadelphia: Saunders Elsevier.
141. Orkin, S.H. & Zon, L.I. (2008). Hematopoiesis: An evolving paradigm for stem cell biology. *Cell, 132,* 631.
142. Palis, J. (2008). Ontogeny of erythropoiesis. *Curr Opin Hematol, 15,* 155.
143. Parker, R.I. (2005). Neonatal thrombosis, hemostasis and platelet disorders. In A.R. Spitzer (Ed.). *Intensive care of the fetus & neonate* (2nd ed.). Philadelphia: Mosby.
144. Paul, D.A., et al. (2011). Increased odds of necrotizing enterocolitis after transfusion of red blood cells in premature infants. *Pediatrics, 127,* 635.
145. Peña-Rosas, J.P. & Viteri, F.E. (2009). Effects and safety of preventive oral iron or iron+folic acid supplementation for women during pregnancy. *Cochrane Database Syst Rev, 4,* CD004736.
146. Peri, K.G., et al. (1998). Quantitative correlation between globulin mRNAs and synthesis of fetal and adult hemoglobin during hemoglobin switchover in the perinatal period. *Pediatr Res, 43,* 504.
147. Perlman, J.M., et al. (2010). Part 11: Neonatal resuscitation: 2010 International Consensus on Cardiopulmonary Resuscitation and Emergency Cardiovascular Care Science With Treatment Recommendations. *Circulation, 122,* S516.
148. Proytcheva, M.A. (2009). Issues in neonatal cellular analysis. *Am J Clin Pathol, 131,* 560.
149. Puckett, R.M. & Offringa, M. (2000). Prophylactic vitamin K for vitamin K deficiency bleeding in neonates. *Cochrane Database Syst Rev, 4,* CD002776.
150. Rabe, H., Reynolds, G., & Diaz-Rossello, J. (2008). A systematic review and meta-analysis of a brief delay in clamping the umbilical cord of preterm infants. *Neonatology, 93,* 138.
151. Rao, R. & Georgieff, M.K. (2001). Neonatal iron nutrition. *Semin Neonatol, 6,* 425.
152. Rao, R. & Georgieff, M.K. (2002). Perinatal aspects of iron metabolism. *Acta Paediatr Suppl, 91,* 124.

153. Rao, R. & Georgieff, M.K. (2007). Iron in fetal and neonatal nutrition. *Semin Fetal Neonatal Med, 12,* 54.
154. Rao, R. & Georgieff, M.K. (2009). Iron therapy for preterm infants. *Clin Perinatol, 36,* 27.
155. Rath, W.H. (2011). Postpartum hemorrhage—update on problems of definitions and diagnosis. *Acta Obstet Gynecol Scand, 90,* 421.
156. Ray, J.G. & Chan, W.S. (1999). Deep vein thrombosis during pregnancy and the puerperium: A meta-analysis of the period of risk and the leg of presentation. *Obstet Gynecol Surv, 54,* 265.
157. Richter, C., et al. (1995). Erythropoiesis in the perinatal postpartum period. *J Perinat Med, 23,* 51.
158. Rogers, D.T. & Molokie, R. (2010). Sickle cell disease in pregnancy. *Obstet Gynecol Clin North Am, 37,* 223.
159. Ruiz-Irastorza, G., et al. (2010). Antiphospholipid syndrome. *Lancet, 376,* 1498.
160. Sanghvi, T.G., Harvey, P.W., & Wainwright, E. (2010). Maternal iron-folic acid supplementation programs: Evidence of impact and implementation. *Food Nutr Bull, 31,* S100.
161. Saracco, P., et al. (2009). Management and investigation of neonatal thromboembolic events: Genetic and acquired risk factors. *Thromb Res, 123,* 805.
162. Sarker, S. & Rosenkranz, T.S. (2008). Neonatal polycythemia and hyperviscosity. *Semin Fetal Neonatal Med, 13,* 248.
163. Saxonhouse, M.A. & Sola, M.C. (2004). Platelet function in term and preterm neonates. *Clin Perinatol, 31,* 15.
164. Saxonhouse, M.A. & Manco-Johnson, M.J. (2009). The evaluation and management of neonatal coagulation disorders. *Semin Perinatol, 33,* 52.
165. Scanlon, K.S., et al. (2000). High and low hemoglobin levels during pregnancy: Differential risks for preterm birth and small for gestational age. *Obstet Gynecol, 96,* 741.
166. Schanler, R.J., et al. (2011). Concerns with early universal iron supplementation of breastfeeding infants. *Pediatrics, 127,* e1097.
167. Schmutz, N., et al. (2008). Expected ranges for blood neutrophil concentrations of neonates: the Manroe and Mouzinho charts revisited. *J Perinatol, 28,* 275.
168. Sehgal, A. & Francis, J.V. (2011). Hemodynamic alterations associated with polycythemia and partial exchange transfusion. *J Perinatol, 31,* 143.
169. Sere, K.M. & Hackeng, T.M. (2003). Basic mechanisms of hemostasis. *Semin Vasc Med, 3,* 3.
170. Setaro, J.F. & Caulin-Glaser, T. (2004). Pregnancy and cardiovascular disease. In G.N. Burrows, T.P. Duffy, & J.A. Copel (Eds.). *Medical complications during pregnancy* (6th ed.). Philadelphia: Saunders.
171. Shah, N., et al. (2010). The effect of recombinant human erythropoietin on the development of retinopathy of prematurity. *Am J Perinatol, 27,* 67.
172. Shirvani, F., et al. (2010). Effect of timing of umbilical cord clamp on newborns' iron status and its relation to delivery type. *Arch Iran Med, 13,* 420.
173. Siddappa, A.M., et al. (2007). The assessment of newborn iron stores at birth: A review of the literature and standards for ferritin concentrations. *Neonatology, 92,* 73.
174. Sloan, S.R. (2011). Neonatal transfusion review. *Paediatr Anaesth, 21,* 25.
175. Sola, M.C. (2000). Fetal megakaryocytopoiesis. In R. Christensen (Ed.). *Hematologic problems of the neonate.* Philadelphia: Saunders.
176. Sola, M.C. & Rimsza, L.M. (2002). Mechanisms underlying thrombocytopenia in the neonatal intensive care unit. *Acta Paediatr Suppl, 91,* 66.
177. Sola-Viisner M. & Poterjoy, B.S. (2012). Developmental megakaryocytopoiesis. In R.A. Polin, W.W. Fox, & S.H. Abman (Eds.). *Fetal and neonatal physiology* (4th ed.). Philadelphia: Saunders.
178. Stables, D. (1999). *Physiology in childbearing with anatomy and related biosciences.* Edinburgh: Balliere Tindall.
179. Stephansson, O., et al. (2000). Maternal hemoglobin concentration during pregnancy and risk of stillbirth. *JAMA, 284,* 2611.
180. Stockman, J.A. (1990). Fetal hematology. In R.D. Eden & F.H. Boehm (Eds.). *Assessment and care of the fetus.* Norwalk, CT: Appleton & Lange.
181. Stoltzfus, R.J. (2011). Iron interventions for women and children in low-income countries. *J Nutr, 141,* 756S.
182. Strauss, R.G. (1995). Red blood cell transfusion practices in the neonate. *Clin Perinatol, 22,* 641.
183. Strauss, R.G., et al. (2008). A randomized clinical trial comparing immediate versus delayed clamping of the umbilical cord in preterm infants: Short-term clinical and laboratory endpoints. *Transfusion, 48,* 658.
184. Strauss, R.G. (2010). Anaemia of prematurity: Pathophysiology and treatment. *Blood Rev, 24,* 221.
185. Strauss, R.G. & Widness, J.A. (2010). Is there a role for autologous/placental red blood cell transfusions in the anemia of prematurity? *Transfus Med Rev, 24,* 125.
186. Strunk, T., Hartel, C., & Schultz, C. (2004). Does erythropoietin protect the preterm brain? *Arch Dis Child Fetal Neonatal Ed, 89,* F364.
187. Thurlbeck, S.M. & McIntosh, N. (1987). Preterm blood counts vary with sampling site. *Arch Dis Child, 62,* 74.
188. Tsatalas, C., et al. (2009). Pregnancy in beta-thalassemia trait carriers: An uneventful journey. *Hematology, 14,* 301.
189. U.S. Preventive Services Task Force. (1993). Routine iron supplementation during pregnancy. *JAMA, 270,* 2848.
190. Ultee, C.A., et al. (2008). Delayed cord clamping in preterm infants delivered at 34-36 weeks' gestation: A randomized controlled trial. *Arch Dis Child Fetal Neonatal Ed, 93,* F20.
191. Uszyński, M. & Uszyński, W. (2011). Coagulation and fibrinolysis in amniotic fluid: Physiology and observations on amniotic fluid embolism, preterm fetal membrane rupture, and pre-eclampsia. *Semin Thromb Hemost, 37,* 165.
192. Vamvakas, E.C. & Strauss, R.G. (2001). Meta-analysis of controlled clinical trials studying the efficacy of rHuEPO in reducing blood transfusions in the anemia of prematurity. *Transfusion, 41,* 406.
193. Veldman, A., et al. (2010). Disseminated intravascular coagulation in term and preterm neonates. *Semin Thromb Hemost, 36,* 419.
194. Vichinsky, E. (2010). Complexity of alpha thalassemia: Growing health problem with new approaches to screening, diagnosis, and therapy. *Ann N Y Acad Sci, 1202,* 180.
195. Von Kohorn, I. & Ehrenkranz, R.A. (2009). Anemia in the preterm infant: Erythropoietin versus erythrocyte transfusion—it's not that simple. *Clin Perinatol, 36,* 111.
196. Walker, I.D. (2003). Venous and arterial thrombosis during pregnancy: Epidemiology. *Semin Vasc Med, 3,* 25.
197. Wardrop, C.A. & Holland, B.M. (1995). The roles and vital importance of placental blood to the newborn infant. *J Perinat Med, 23,* 139.
198. Watts, T. & Roberts, I.A.G. (1999). Hematological abnormalities in the growth restricted infant. *Semin Perinatol, 4,* 41.
199. Werner, E.J. (1995). Neonatal polycythemia and hyperviscosity. *Clin Perinatol, 23,* 693.
200. Westcamp, E., et al. (2002). Blood transfusion in anemic infants with apnea of prematurity. *Biol Neonate, 82,* 228.
201. Whyte, R.K., et al. PINTOS Study Group. (2009). Neurodevelopmental outcome of extremely low birth weight infants randomly assigned to restrictive or liberal hemoglobin thresholds for blood transfusion. *Pediatrics, 123,* 207.
202. Widmaier, G.P., Raff, H., & Stang, K.T. (2010). *Vander's human physiology: the mechanism of body function* (12th ed.). New York: McGraw-Hill.
203. World Health Organization. (2008). *Worldwide prevalence of anaemia 1993-2005.* Geneva: World Health Organization.
204. World Health Organization. (2009). *Global health risks. Mortality and burden of disease attributable to selected major risk factors.* Geneva: World Health Organization.
205. Xiong, T., et al. (2011). Erythropoietin for neonatal brain injury: Opportunity and challenge. *Int J Dev Neurosci, 29, 583*

206. Yao, A.C. & Lind J. (1982). *Placental transfusion.* Springfield, IL: Charles C Thomas.
207. Yoder, M.C. (2000). Embryonic hematopoiesis. In R. Christensen (Ed.). *Hematologic problems of the neonate.* Philadelphia: Saunders.
208. Yoder, M.C. (2002). Embryonic hematopoiesis in mice and humans. *Acta Paediatr Suppl, 91,* 5.
209. Young, G. (2012). Hemostatic disorders of the newborn In C.A. Gleason & S. Devaskar (Eds.). *Avery's diseases of the newborn* (9th ed.). Philadelphia: Saunders.
210. Young, M.F., et al. (2010). Impact of maternal and neonatal iron status on placental transferrin receptor expression in pregnant adolescents. *Placenta, 31,* 1010.
211. Zhu, C., et al. (2009). Erythropoietin improved neurologic outcomes in newborns with hypoxic-ischemic encephalopathy. *Pediatrics, 124,* e218.
212. Ziegler, E.E., Nelson, S.E., & Jeter, J.M. (2009). Iron status of breastfed infants is improved equally by medicinal iron and iron-fortified cereal. *Am J Clin Nutr, 90,* 76.
213. Ziegler, E.E., Nelson, S.E., & Jeter, J.M. (2009). Iron supplementation of breastfed infants from an early age. *Am J Clin Nutr, 89,* 525.
214. Ziegler, E.E., et al. (2011). Dry cereals fortified with electrolytic iron or ferrous fumarate are equally effective in breast-fed infants. *J Nutr, 141,* 243.
215. Zipursky, A. (1987). Hematology of the newborn infant. In L. Stern & P. Vert (Eds.). *Neonatal medicine.* New York: Masson.
216. Zipursky, A. (1999). Prevention of vitamin K deficiency bleeding in newborns. *Br J Haematol, 104,* 430.

CHAPTER 9

Cardiovascular System

The circulatory system is the transport system that supplies body cells with substrates absorbed from the gastrointestinal tract and oxygen from the lungs and returns carbon dioxide to the lungs for disposal; other by-products of metabolism are routed to the kidneys for elimination. The cardiovascular system (CVS) is also involved in the regulation of body temperature and the distribution of hormones and other substances that regulate cellular functioning.

During pregnancy the maternal cardiovascular system must meet the demands of both the mother and the dynamically changing fetus. The constant ebb and flow of nutrients and by-products via the uteroplacental system creates a sensitive interdependence between the mother and the fetus. At birth the infant undergoes significant changes in the CVS that may, if altered, compromise extrauterine existence and postnatal adaptation. This chapter examines alterations in the CVS during the perinatal period and implications for the mother, fetus, and neonate.

MATERNAL PHYSIOLOGIC ADAPTATIONS

Pregnancy is associated with physiologically significant but reversible changes in maternal hemodynamics and cardiac function. These changes are mediated by increased levels of circulating estrogens; progesterone; prostaglandins (PG), especially PGE_1 and PGE_2; and other vasoactive substances, as well as by the increased load on the cardiovascular system. The increased circulating maternal blood mass, fetal nutritional requirements, and placental circulatory system place increased demands on the maternal cardiovascular system. In most women these demands are met without compromising the mother. However, when superimposed upon an existing disease state, in which hemodynamics are already compromised, pregnancy may prove to be a dangerous situation for maternal homeostasis.

Conversely, if maternal hemodynamics do not change, adverse effects on the uteroplacental circulation can lead to fetal compromise, which may be manifested as fetal malformations (including congenital heart disease), fetal growth restriction, or pregnancy loss. Therefore the maternal cardiovascular system must achieve a balance between fetal needs and maternal tolerance.

The maternal cardiovascular system is further altered during the intrapartum period. During the second stage of labor, expulsive efforts lead to an increase in muscle tension and intrathoracic and intraabdominal pressure, all of which affect the functioning of the heart and the hemodynamics of the maternal system. Intraabdominal pressure is abruptly decreased upon delivery and blood pools in the abdominal organs, thereby affecting cardiac return. Blood loss during delivery may also affect hemodynamics.

Antepartum Period

The major hemodynamic changes that occur during pregnancy are outlined in Table 9-1. These changes begin as early as 4 to 5 weeks of gestation and tend to plateau during the second or early third trimester.[48] Cardiovascular and hemodynamic changes are due to hormonal influences, changes in other organ systems, and mechanical forces. The hemodynamic changes are partly the result of hormonal influences as well as of the development of the placental circulation and alterations in systemic vascular resistance (SVR). These changes include increases in total blood volume, plasma volume, red blood cell (RBC) volume, and cardiac output. Anatomic changes, such as the upward displacement of the diaphragm by the gravid uterus, shift the heart upward and laterally. There is slight cardiac enlargement on radiograph, and the left heart border is straightened. The size and position of the uterus, the strength of the abdominal muscles, and the configuration of the abdomen and thorax determine the extent of these changes.[34]

Hemodynamic Changes

Hemodynamic alterations in pregnancy include changes in blood volume, cardiac output, heart rate, systemic blood pressure, vascular resistance, and distribution of blood flow. Stroke volume, heart rate, and cardiac output increase significantly, whereas SVR, pulmonary vascular resistance (PVR), and colloid osmotic pressure decrease. Changes in blood, plasma, and RBC volume are discussed further in Chapter 8.

Table 9-1 Physiologic Changes of Pregnancy on the Cardiovascular System

PARAMETER	MODIFICATION	MAGNITUDE	TIME OF PEAK INCREASE OR DECREASE
Oxygen consumption (VO_2)	Increase	+20% to 30%	Term
Blood volume:			
Plasma	Increase	+40% to 60% (usually 45% to 50%)	32 weeks
Red blood cells	Increase	+20% to 30%	30 to 32 weeks
Total body water	Increase	+6 to 8 L	Term
Resistance changes:			
Systemic circulation	Decrease	–20% to 30%	16 to 34 weeks
Pulmonary circulation	Decrease	–30%	34 weeks
Blood pressure (SVR X CO):*			
Systolic	Slight or no decrease		
Diastolic	Decrease	10 to 15 mmHg (1.33 to 1.99 kPa)	24 to 32 weeks
Myocardial contractility:			
Chronotropism (HR)	Increase	+0% to 20%	28 to 32 weeks
Inotropism (SV)	Increase	+25% to 30%	16 to 24 weeks
Cardiac output (HR X SV)*	Increase	+30% to 50%	28 to 32 weeks
Uteroplacental circulation	Increase	Greater than 1000%	Term

Adapted from Gei, A.F. & Hankins, G.D. (2001). Cardiac disease and pregnancy. *Obstet Gynecol Clin North Am, 28,* 469.
CO, Cardiac output; *HR,* heart rate; *SV,* stroke volume, *SVR,* systemic vascular resistance.
*Position dependent.

Total Blood Volume. Total blood volume (TBV) is a combination of plasma volume and RBC volume, each of which increases during pregnancy. Circulating blood volume increases begin by at least 6 weeks' gestation.[111] Circulating blood volume increases by 30% to 40% (approximately 1½ L), with a usual range of 30% to 45%.[40,111,115] TBV increases rapidly until mid-pregnancy and then more slowly during the latter half, peaking at 28 to 34 weeks, then plateaus or decreases slightly to term.[27,81,111,135] Changes in blood volume are due to the increased steroid hormones, plasma renin activity, aldosterone, human placental lactogen, atrial natriuretic factor, and other mediators.[18,48] Figure 8-1 illustrates changes in total blood volume and its component parts, plasma volume, and RBC volume.

The rise in blood volume correlates directly with fetal weight, supporting the concept of the placenta as an arteriovenous shunt in the maternal vascular compartment. Although the degree of hypervolemia varies from woman to woman, subsequent pregnancies in the same woman result in similar increases in circulating volume. Twin and other multiple pregnancies, however, result in greater increases in blood volume, imposing substantially greater demands on the cardiovascular system.[111,135]

Plasma Volume. About 75% of the TBV increase is in plasma volume. Plasma volume increases progressively from 6 to 8 weeks by approximately 45% to 50% (range, 40% to 60%) or about 1200 to 1600 mL above nonpregnant values [27,111] This change begins at 6 to 8 weeks and increases rapidly during the second trimester, followed by a slower but progressive increase that reaches its maximum of 4700 to 5200 mL at about 32 weeks.[22,81,111] Alterations in blood and plasma volume are influenced by hormonal effects, nitric oxide mediated vasodilation, mechanical factors (blood flow in uteroplacental vessels) (see Chapter 8), and changes in the renal system and in fluid and electrolyte homeostasis (see Chapter 11).

Nitric oxide mediated vasodilation induces changes in the renin-angiotensin-aldosterone system, with increased sodium and water retention (see Chapter 11).[111] Plasma renin activity and blood aldosterone levels are increased due to the action of estrogens, progesterone, and prostaglandins. An increase in plasma renin activity enhances sodium retention, thereby stimulating aldosterone secretion. Progesterone inhibits the action of aldosterone on the renal tubular cells, thus contributing to sodium retention and an increase in total body water. The degree of fluid retention is influenced by the increased distensibility of the vascular system and the uterine vein capacity present during pregnancy.[27]

Fluid distribution changes depending on body position. For example, the standing position or prolonged sitting is associated with the development of dependent edema. This is probably due to the trapping of blood in the legs and pelvis as the gravid uterus creates a mechanical impedance to blood flow through the inferior vena cava. This causes an increase in venous pressure in the lower extremities and a sharp rise in hydrostatic pressure in the microcirculation, with subsequent leakage of fluid from the vascular bed into the interstitium. The result is edema of the feet and ankles. Venous distensibility contributes to the decreased venous return to the heart.[112]

Red Blood Cell Volume. Red blood cell (RBC) production and thus volume increases throughout pregnancy to a level 20% to 30% higher than nonpregnant values.[27,111] Intravascular expansion is mainly due to an increase in plasma volume;

therefore hemodilution occurs. This physiologic anemia of pregnancy is reflected in a lower hematocrit and hemoglobin. These changes cannot be prevented with iron supplementation; however, women who are provided exogenous sources of iron do have higher hemoglobin levels in the third trimester than women not receiving supplements (see Figure 8-2). Changes in RBC volume are due to increased circulating erythropoietin and accelerated RBC production. The rise in erythropoietin in the last two trimesters is stimulated by progesterone, prolactin, and human placental lactogen.[111] Changes in RBC volume and the role of iron are described further in Chapter 8.

Cardiac Output and Stroke Volume. Cardiac output, which is the product of heart rate times stroke volume, is one of the most significant hemodynamic changes encountered during pregnancy. Fifty percent of the increase occurs by 8 weeks' gestation, mediated by changes in SVR.[22,111] Cardiac output continues to rise more slowly until the third trimester to values, as measured in the left lateral recumbent position, 30% to 50% (usually 40% to 45%) greater than in nonpregnant women.[1,18,25,27,111,115] A slight decline in cardiac output may be seen in late pregnancy due to the decrease in stroke volume near term.[111] The increase in cardiac output is associated with an increase in venous return and greater right ventricular (RV) output, especially in the left lateral position.[158]

The increased cardiac output is due to changes in both stroke volume and heart rate. Changes in heart rate and stroke volume are reported by 5 weeks' and 8 weeks' gestation, respectively.[111] The rise in cardiac output early in pregnancy is due primarily to an increase in stroke volume.[1,60,111] Stroke volume increases progressively during the first and second trimesters, to a peak value of approximately 25% to 30% above nonpregnant values, peaking at 16 to 24 weeks.[27,110] Stroke volume declines during the latter stages of pregnancy, and returns to values that are within the prepregnant range by term.[22,27,111,158,162] The changes in stroke volume are likely due to increased ventricular muscle mass and end-diastolic volume changes.[111] As pregnancy advances, the heart rate (see section on Heart Rate), which increases more slowly, becomes a more dominant factor in determining cardiac output.[111] Figure 9-1 compares the changes in heart rate and stroke volume over gestation.

During pregnancy (especially the third trimester), the resting cardiac output fluctuates markedly with changes in body position.[110,111,160] For example, a change from the left lateral recumbent position to supine can lead to a 25% to 30% decrease in cardiac output.[160,162] Compression of the inferior vena cava by the uterus in the third trimester results in decreased venous return, stroke volume, and cardiac output.[111] Heart rate changes do not necessarily occur with positional changes; therefore these changes in cardiac output are more likely due to a decrease in stroke volume.[111,160]

Twin, triplet, and other multiple pregnancies have a greater increase in cardiac output than do singleton pregnancies, possibly due to an increase in inotropy.[78] The peak is greater, and the decline in cardiac output seen in late pregnancy is smaller. The cardiac output in multiple pregnancies

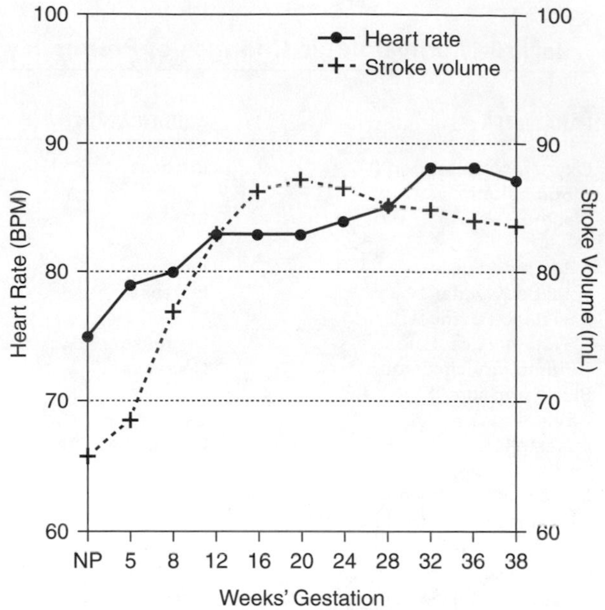

FIGURE 9-1 Alteration of stroke volume and heart rate during pregnancy. Stroke volume increases maximally during the first half of gestation. There is a slight decrease in stroke volume toward term. The mild increase in heart rate begins early in gestation and continues until term. (Adapted from Robson, S.C., et al. [1989]. Serial study of factors influencing changes in cardiac output during human pregnancy. *Am J Physiol, 256,* H1060 by Monga, M. [2004]. Maternal cardiovascular and renal adaptation to pregnancy. In R.K. Creasy, R. Resnik, J.D. Iams [Eds.]. *Maternal-fetal medicine: Principles and practice* [5th ed.]. Philadelphia: Saunders.)

is higher than that encountered in a singleton pregnancy by 20 weeks' gestation and remains higher for the remainder of gestation.[78,122]

The increase in cardiac output during pregnancy is not related to the metabolic requirements of the mother or the fetus, or to the increase in maternal body mass. At the time the increase in cardiac output occurs, the fetus is relatively small. When fetal growth is accelerated (late in gestation), there is an actual decline in maternal cardiac output. There is, however, a progressive increase in maternal oxygen consumption, which may be due to the rising metabolic needs of the fetus as well as the demands of the maternal heart and respiratory muscles. Pregnancy at high altitudes is associated with less of an increase in cardiac output accompanied by a reduction in the usual expansion of maternal intravascular volume.[79]

The increased oxygen requirements are most likely the result of the contractility-promoting influences of estrogen and progesterone on heart and respiratory muscles and the development of the placental circulation. The placenta functions much like an arteriovenous shunt, with a concomitant decrease in peripheral vascular resistance. Therefore, despite the increase in cardiac output, there is a decrease in mean blood pressure due to a decrease in diastolic pressure. The concomitant increase in blood volume (either in time or magnitude) probably explains the increase in cardiac output. Both begin to rise as early as 6 to 8 weeks' gestation, peaking toward the end of the second trimester, around 30% to 50% higher than prepregnant levels.[110,111]

Changes in uterine blood flow might also contribute to the increased cardiac output. Progesterone, estrogens, and prolactin may cause changes in hemodynamics by directly affecting the myocardium. For example, estrogens may alter the actomyosin-adenosine triphosphatase (ATP) relationship in the myocardium, thereby increasing the contractility of the heart and altering the stroke volume. Similar effects can be seen with oral contraceptive use.

Heart Rate. Heart rate is the determinant of cardiac output that has the widest range of values. This wide range provides stability to the circulatory system under a variety of circumstances (e.g., from rest to maximal exercise). Heart rate can be altered in order to maintain blood pressure if changes in vascular resistance or stroke volume are encountered. However, an increased heart rate is insufficient to increase cardiac output; it must be accompanied by an increase in venous return. Both heart rate and venous return are increased in pregnancy, contributing to the increase in cardiac output seen throughout gestation.[110,111] The increased heart rate compensates for the decreased SVR and is due to increased myocardial α receptors due to estrogen.[25,68]

The maternal heart rate increases progressively during pregnancy, averaging 10 to 20 beats per minute higher (10% to 20% increase) by 32 weeks (see Figure 9-1).[18,27,65,68,111] At term, the heart rate may return to near baseline levels in some women. Twin pregnancies have an earlier acceleration in heart rate, with a maximum increase 40% above the nonpregnant level near term.[34]

The increased heart rate results in an elevated myocardial oxygen requirement, which is probably not important in women without cardiac disease, but may become significant in pregnant women with underlying cardiovascular pathology. Beyond this, the increased resting heart rate decreases the maximal work capacity by diminishing the output increment that can be achieved during maximal exercise.[110]

Blood Pressure. Although there are substantial increases in both blood volume and cardiac output during pregnancy, these changes are not associated with increases in either venous or arterial pressure since the increase in intravenous volume is balanced by the decreased SVR.[18,111] In fact, blood pressure, especially diastolic pressure, is generally reported to decrease, reaching a nadir by midpregnancy.[18,111] The initial decrease is thought to be due to a lag in compensation for changes in peripheral vascular resistance.[111] The diastolic blood pressure decrease reaches a nadir at 24 to 32 weeks and then gradually returns to nonpregnant baseline values by term (Figure 9-2).[23,27,111] The magnitude of blood pressure changes vary with the position of the woman during measurement. For example, arterial blood pressures are about 10 mmHg higher in sitting or standing than in a left lateral recumbent or supine position.[111] Serial observations in a sitting or standing position show that as women advance through their pregnancies, systolic blood pressure remains either stable or decreases slightly, whereas diastolic pressure decreases an average of 10 to 15 mmHg (1.33 to 1.99 kPa).[27,111] Mean arterial pressure decreases until midpregnancy, then

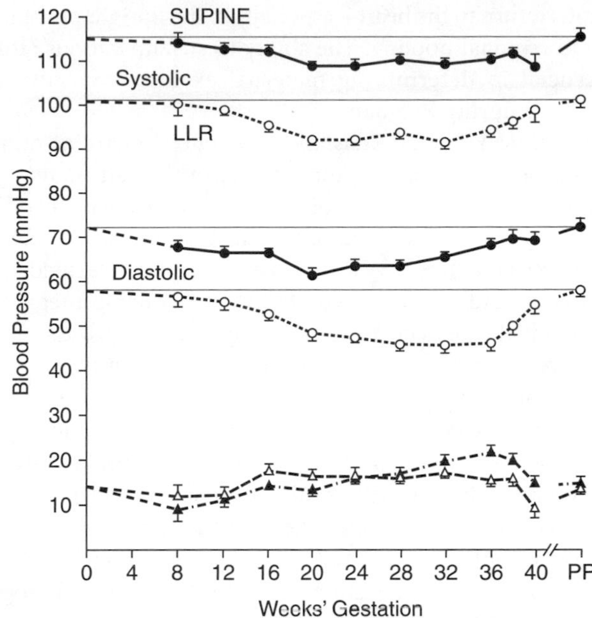

FIGURE 9-2 Sequential changes in blood pressure throughout pregnancy with subjects in supine and left lateral recumbent (LLR) positions. The change in systolic *(open triangles)* and diastolic *(closed triangles)* blood pressures produced by movement from the left lateral recumbent to the supine position is illustrated in the bottom part of the figure. (From Wilson, M., et al. [1980]. Blood pressure, the renin-aldosterone system, and sex steroids throughout normal pregnancy. *Am J Med, 68,* 97.)

increases to term.[23] The reduction in blood pressure may be secondary to the vasodilatory effects of nitric oxide, which increases in pregnancy, as well as hormonal and other factors such as prostacyclin and relaxin that mediate a decrease in peripheral vascular resistance.[123] Some investigators, have not found this midtrimester fall in blood pressure, but instead reported either no change or a slight rise from the first trimester until late pregnancy.[116,151,165]

Techniques and differences in the diastolic measurement point also influence blood pressure measurement. Therefore it is important to use a consistent method and maternal position to evaluate blood pressure.[111,166] Conventional blood pressure techniques often lack standardization in terms of use of appropriate cuff size, equipment calibration, rounding off (to nearest 5 to 10 mmHg [0.66 to 1.33 kPa] versus the recommended 2 mmHg [0.26 kPa]), and method.[57,66]

Venous pressures during pregnancy also do not change significantly. Given the large increase in blood volume during pregnancy, an increase in venous pressure would be expected. The increased vascular capacitance and compliance seen during pregnancy explain this lack of change. These alterations are thought to be due to the effects of progesterone and endothelial-derived relaxant factors such as nitric oxide on blood vessel smooth muscle and collagen.[4,111] Venous pressure below the uterus is increased, which may be caused by the increased capacitance encountered in the large pelvic veins and the veins distal to the uterus. The latter may affect venous return to the heart—especially in the upright position—due to regional pooling. The ability to sustain venous return is crucial in determining maternal exercise capacity (see "Exercise during Pregnancy").[110]

Systemic Vascular Resistance. Changes in cardiac output during pregnancy are accomplished without an increase in arterial pressures because of the marked decrease in SVR, especially in peripheral vessels (reduction in peripheral vascular resistance).[24,158] SVR (mean arterial pressure divided by cardiac output) is decreased 20% to 30% during pregnancy and parallels the decrease in blood pressure.[65] SVR decreases by 5 weeks and usually reaches its lowest level by 16 to 34 weeks, then progressively increases to term (Figure 9-3).[22,111]

The decreased vascular resistance is due to softening of collagen fibers and hypertrophy of smooth muscle, systemic vasodilation due to the vasodilatory effects of progesterone and prostaglandins, remodeling of the maternal spiral arteries (see Chapter 3), fluid retention (leading to blood volume expansion), and the addition of the low-resistance uteroplacental circulation, which receives a large proportion of cardiac output.[26,48,111] The decline in resistance is not limited to the uteroplacental circulation; rather, it is seen throughout the body.[90] The decreased SVR is also mediated by endothelial prostacyclin, and endothelial-derived relaxant factors (e.g., nitric oxide) that enhance vasodilation.[24,48,65,111,144] Decreased systemic and renal vascular tone occur very early in pregnancy and precede changes in blood volume.[24] Thus the decrease in SVR may be the stimulus for changes in heart rate and stroke volume, and thus cardiac output, in early pregnancy, as well as sodium and water retention (see Chapter 11), and alterations in blood pressure.[24,25,48,111] The hormonal activity of pregnancy also has a role in the reduction of SVR and contributes to changes in regional blood flow. Along with this, the increased heat production (from maternal, fetal, and placental metabolism) stimulates vasodilation of vessels (especially in heat-losing areas such as the hands) and further reductions in resistance.

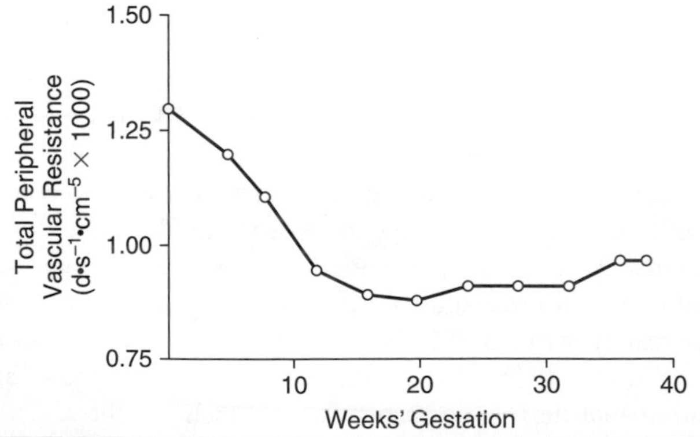

FIGURE 9-3 Total peripheral vascular resistance drops dramatically over the course of pregnancy. (From Thornburg, K.L., et al. [2000]. Hemodynamic changes in pregnancy. *Semin Perinatol, 24,* 12.)

Regional Blood Flow. Much of the increased maternal cardiac output is distributed to the uteroplacental circuit. The increase in cardiac output above the needs of the uteroplacental circulation leads to increased flow to other organ systems, particularly the mammary glands, skin, and kidneys. This creates a reservoir that can be tapped as pregnancy progresses. Blood flow to the splanchnic bed and skeletal muscle perfusion may decrease.[68]

Mammary blood flow is increased. Clinically increased flow is evident by the engorgement that occurs early in pregnancy and the dilation of veins on the surface of the breasts. This dilation is usually accompanied by a sensation of heat and tingling. The effect of pregnancy on coronary artery blood flow is unknown. With the increased workload of the left ventricle (LV) (because of the increased cardiac output, blood volume, fetal growth, uterus enlargement, and body weight gain), it can be assumed that the coronary blood flow is increased to meet the cardiac myometrial demands. Cerebral blood flow is not significantly altered during pregnancy.[111,123] Although absolute blood flow to the liver does not change significantly, the percentage of the cardiac output perfusing the liver decreases.[111]

Uterine Blood Flow. The decline in uterine vascular resistance allows blood flow to the uterus to increase during gestation. At 10 weeks' gestation the blood flow is approximately 50 mL/min, increasing to 200 mL/min by 28 weeks and 500 to 800 mL/min at term.[111,115] Thus by term the uterus is receiving between 10% and 20% of the maternal cardiac output, versus 2% in nonpregnant women.[111] The uterine spiral arteries undergo marked changes during pregnancy (see Chapter 3) that disrupt their muscular and elastic elements. As a result, the uteroplacental arteries are almost completely dilated and are no longer responsive to circulating pressor agents or influences of the autonomic nervous system.[136] This results in a large pool of blood within the uterus to maintain fetoplacental blood flow and oxygenation.

Renal Blood Flow. Renal blood flow (RBF) increases by the end of the first trimester and then decreases to term (see Chapter 11). The percentage of the cardiac output perfusing the kidneys does not change and remains around 18%. The glomerular filtration rate (GFR) increases 40% to 50% over nonpregnant levels and is due in large part to the increased RBF. The decrease in renal vascular resistance may be mediated by nitric oxide, prostacyclin (PGI_2), and atrial natriuretic factor.[90]

Skin Perfusion. Skin perfusion increases significantly during pregnancy, with a slow but steady rise in perfusion up to 18 to 20 weeks' gestation. This slow rise is followed by a sharp increase between 20 and 30 weeks, with no significant increase after that. The increased flow is measurable for up to 1 week postpartum.[90] Clinically this increased flow may be accompanied by an increase in skin temperature and clammy hands, which are the result of dermal capillary dilation. Vascular spiders and palmar erythema can be seen in many women during pregnancy (see Chapter 14). The vasodilation may facilitate the dissipation of excessive heat created by fetal metabolism. Increased peripheral flow can also be seen in the mucous membranes of the nasal passages, explaining the nasal congestion that is common in pregnancy (see Chapter 15).[90,123]

Pulmonary Blood Flow. Pulmonary blood flow increases secondary to increased circulating blood volume and increased cardiac output. This can be demonstrated on x-ray by increased vascular markings. The increase in pulmonary blood flow is balanced by a decrease in PVR.[35] The 30% decrease in PVR is probably in response to hormonal stimulation, and is reflected in a lowered mean pulmonary artery pressure.[35,65]

Oxygen Consumption

Oxygen consumption is a reflection of metabolic rate. During pregnancy there is a progressive increase in resting oxygen consumption, with a peak increase of 20% to 30% by term (Figure 9-4). This increase in oxygen consumption is due to the increased metabolic needs of the mother and the growing fetus.[158] Oxygen consumption increases gradually over gestation, whereas cardiac output increases dramatically in the first and second trimesters. Because the resting cardiac output increases before there is a significant rise in maternal oxygen consumption, the arteriovenous oxygen difference decreases in early pregnancy, then gradually increases as oxygen consumption rises during pregnancy. This provides the uterus with well-oxygenated blood flow during the first trimester, before the completed development of the fetoplacental circulation.[22,158]

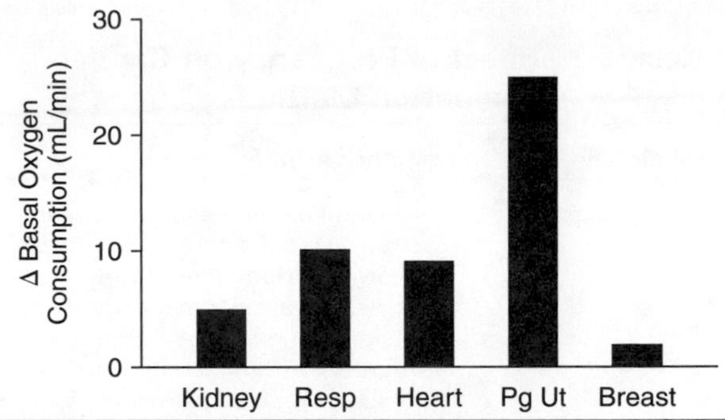

FIGURE 9-4 The maximal increase in basal oxygen consumption (mL/min) during pregnancy. *Pg Ut,* Pregnant uterus. (From Thornburg, K.L., et al. [2000]. Hemodynamic changes in pregnancy. *Semin Perinatol, 24,* 12.)

Physical Changes

The physiologic hypervolemia of pregnancy results in alterations in the cardiac silhouette, chamber size, pressures, and electrocardiogram (ECG). These changes—along with the hemodynamic alterations lead to changes in the physical findings encountered during cardiovascular assessment of the pregnant woman (Figure 9-5 and Table 9-2).

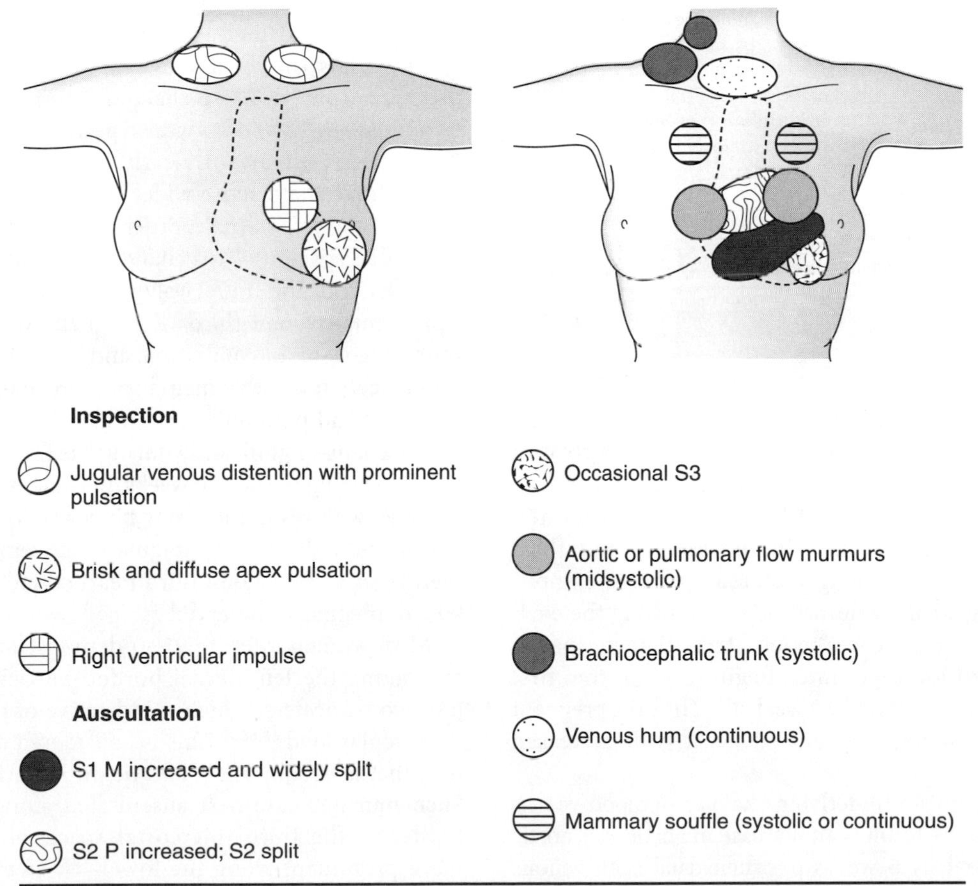

FIGURE 9-5 Normal cardiac examination findings in the pregnant woman. *M,* Mitral; *P,* pulmonary; *S1,* first sound; *S2,* second sound. (From Gei, A.F. & Hankins, G.D. [2001]. Cardiac disease and pregnancy. *Obstet Gynecol Clin North Am, 28,* 472.)

Table 9-2 Effect of Pregnancy on Cardiac Evaluation Methods

PARAMETER	MODIFICATIONS
Chest radiography	Apparent cardiomegaly (enlarged transverse diameter) Enlarged atrium (lateral view) Increased vascular markings Straightening of left-sided heart border Postpartum pleural effusion (right-sided)
Electrocardiography	Rate: Right axis deviation Right branch bundle block ST-segment depression of 1 mm on left precordial leads (14%) Rhythms: Q wave in lead III* T-wave inversion in III*, V2, and V3 (14%) Intervals: Small decrease of PR and QT (heart rate dependent) Axis: Rotation of ±15 degrees (QRS axis)
Echocardiogram	Trivial tricuspid regurgitation Pulmonary regurgitation Increased left atrial size by 12% to 14% Increased left ventricle end-diastolic dimensions by 6% to 10% Inconsistent increase in left ventricle thickness Mitral regurgitation at term (28%) Pericardial effusions (40% postpartum)

From Gei, A.F. & Hankins, G.D. (2001). Cardiac disease and pregnancy. *Obstet Gynecol Clin North Am, 28*, 473.
*Decrease or normalize with deep inspiration.

The heart and blood vessels undergo remodeling during pregnancy.[68,158] All four chambers enlarge, with the greatest change seen in the left atrium.[68] Cardiac ventricular wall muscle mass increases by 10% to 15% in the first trimester; end-diastolic volume increases in the second and third trimesters.[27,111,158] These changes increase cardiac compliance, augmenting stroke volume and maintaining the ejection fraction.[27,111,158] Increases in left atrial diameter parallel increases in blood volume, beginning in the first trimester and peaking around 30 weeks.[111] Thus the pregnant woman has a physiologically dilated heart with increased compliance.[111,158]

The exact mechanism underlying changes in blood vessels is also unclear, but the result is an increase in aortic size, aortic compliance (evident by 5 weeks postmenstrual age), venous blood volume, and venous compliance.[111,158] Compliance of the entire vasculature is increased due to softening of the collagen and smooth muscle hypertrophy.

As the uterus grows, the diaphragm is displaced upward and the heart shifts to a more horizontal position (see Figure 9-5).[34,68,111] The LV point of maximum impact is easily palpated and may be shifted to the left. A right ventricle (RV) impulse can usually be palpated at the middle- to lower-left sternal border; this is the pulmonary trunk. Difficulty in localizing this point may be caused by the enlarged breast tissue.

Pulse pressure increases slightly in the third trimester due to changes in the differences between systolic and diastolic pressures.[111] The arterial pulse is full, becoming sharp and jerky between 12 and 15 weeks. This finding remains until one week after delivery. Jugular vein pulsations are more readily seen, because vein distention appears around 20 weeks' gestation. A venous hum may be associated with the rapid downward flow through the jugular veins. This is indicative of a rapid circulation and high cardiac output state.

Edema of the ankles and legs is a frequent finding during the latter part of pregnancy (see Chapter 14). As maternal age increases, edema is more common. An increase in capillary permeability and the fall in plasma colloid osmotic pressure, along with the increase in femoral venous pressure, are implicated in edema formation.[125] Thigh-high support hose may reduce this edema by increasing SVR and reducing venous pooling.

Heart Sounds. Auscultation of the heart reveals an exaggerated split and loudness of both components of the first heart sounds (mitral and tricuspid valve closure) in most pregnant women. These changes can be heard for the first time between 12 and 20 weeks' gestation and continue until 2 to 4 weeks postpartum. Nearly 90% of pregnant women will have a louder and more widely split first sound that is best heard at the left sternal border between the third and fifth intercostal spaces.[111] This change is primarily due to the earlier closure of the mitral valve along with increased flow.[111] Approximately one third of pregnant women have minor mitral regurgitation; pulmonic and tricuspid valve regurgitation is seen in most women during pregnancy.[68]

Aortic and pulmonic elements of the second heart sound do not change significantly during the first 30 weeks of gestation.[111] During the last 10 weeks, persistent splitting that does not vary with respiration may be heard. This change may be due to the reduced diaphragmatic movement secondary to uterine size.[90,125] A loud third heart sound is heard in up to 90% of pregnant women.[53,111]

Most women (92% to 95%) demonstrate a systolic murmur along the left sternal border, particularly during the last two trimesters, which is indicative of the increased cardiovascular load.[18,68,90] This is considered an innocent murmur that is usually short and heard in early to mid-systole. Such murmurs are best auscultated along the left sternal border in the third intercostal space, although some are more prominent along the lower-left sternal border at the apex or in the aortic area. These murmurs have a musical quality and represent audible vibrations caused by ejection of blood from the RV into the pulmonary trunk or from the

LV into the brachiocephalic arteries at the point of branching from the aortic arch.[125] A systolic precordial murmur due to functional tricuspid regurgitation may also be heard.[111] Systolic murmurs louder than grade 2/4 or any diastolic murmurs require further investigation. A third heart sound, venous hum, or mammary soufflé may be misinterpreted as a diastolic murmur.[68,125]

About 14% of women have murmurs of mammary vessel origin.[111] Of these, 70% are continuous, whereas the other 30% are heard only during diastole. They are more common in lactating women but can be auscultated during pregnancy as well. Often unilateral and high pitched, these murmurs are best heard at the second to fourth intercostal space lateral to the left sternal border.[68,125] They can be changed or obliterated by varying the pressure applied by the stethoscope. The mammary soufflé is an indication of the increased blood flow in the mammary vessels. The murmur disappears after the termination of lactation.[125] An increase in arrhythmias is reported during pregnancy (see Arrhythmias on p. 260).[45,56]

Electrocardiograph and Echocardiograph Changes. Changes in the ECG occur as the position of the heart shifts with the enlarging uterus and elevated diaphragm.[27] These changes are usually minor and are summarized in Table 9-2. A small Q wave and inversion of the P wave are not uncommon. T-wave and ST-segment changes can also be seen.[18,53] With descent of the fetus into the pelvis in late pregnancy, a right axis shift may be noted.[18] As the heart size increases, the incidence of arrhythmias—usually in the form of supraventricular tachycardias—increases. Benign arrhythmias that were present before pregnancy may intensify or progress.

Echocardiography demonstrates an increase in left end-diastolic dimensions during the second and third trimesters. This is probably due to the expanded blood volume and increased filling during diastole. The increased stroke volume that accompanies this added volume maintains the end-systolic dimensions of the LV at nonpregnant levels. These findings are supported by cardiac catheterization data. The right ventricular diastolic pressure is slightly increased over the nonpregnant values. On the other hand, the RV systolic pressure is just below the nonpregnant values (25 to 30 mmHg [3.32 to 3.99 kPa]). This is probably due to the diminished mean pulmonary artery pressure and decreased PVR.[53,111]

Lack of understanding of these changes in clinical signs and symptoms during pregnancy may lead to inappropriate diagnosis of heart disease. A complete cardiac history; careful physical assessment; and an understanding of the changes, differential diagnosis, and norms related to pregnancy should limit cardiac referrals to those women who warrant specialized evaluation and monitoring.

Intrapartum Period

During the intrapartum period, the repetitive, forceful contractions of the uterus as well as pain, anxiety, and apprehension can affect the cardiovascular system.[90] Significant hemodynamic changes can be attributed to the pain and anxiety associated with labor and delivery (see Chapter 15), especially in primiparous women. This is due to the release of catecholamines and the increased systemic vascular tone. Each contraction contributes approximately 300 to 500 mL of additional volume to the circulation.[27,60,111] This results in a significant increase in cardiac output, with a cumulative effect over the course of labor.[1] A progressive rise in cardiac output is seen during the first stage of labor. Cardiac output rises further during the second stage and peaks immediately after delivery.[111] Cardiac output increases 10% to 15% above pregnancy values during the first stage and is up to 50% greater in the second stage of labor.[27,65,111,160] These increases in cardiac output are due to increases in both stroke volume and heart rate. Hemodynamic changes during a contraction lead to an improved venous return, transient tachycardia, and an increased circulating volume. The increase in pulmonary arterial-venous oxygen difference also supports this hypothesis, suggesting that there is a sudden influx of blood from the maternal vascular bed into the systemic circulation.

Other factors that contribute to the increase in cardiac output include sympathetic nervous system stimulation by pain and anxiety, position, method of delivery, and anesthesia.[22,27] Pain and anxiety can be reduced by psychoprophylactic strategies as well as analgesia and anesthesia. Epidural or spinal anesthesia results in a sympathetic blockade that can lead to decreased blood pressure, hypotension, and decreased uteroplacental perfusion if maternal intravascular volume is not maintained.

In general, both systolic and diastolic blood pressure increase during contractions, returning to baseline levels between contractions, with greater increase seen in systolic (35 mmHg or 4.66 kPa) than diastolic values (25 mmHg or 3.32 kPa).[111] Oxygen consumption gradually increases approximately 23%.[22] Heart rate changes are variable, with increases or decreases occurring. SVR does not change.[22] Labor may lead to an increase in not only the number but also the variety of arrhythmias. Arrhythmias seen during labor may include premature ventricular contractions, atrial premature beats, premature nodal contractions, sinus bradycardia, sinus tachycardia, and supraventricular tachycardia.[122,138]

Postpartum Period

Delivery of the fetus, placenta, and amniotic fluid results in dramatic maternal hemodynamic alterations that can result in cardiovascular instability during the immediate postpartum period. These changes are due to the loss of blood at delivery and the body's compensatory mechanisms. Up to 500 mL (10%) of blood may be lost in vaginal deliveries and 1000 mL (15% to 30%) with cesarean sections, although average loss is less. Despite this blood loss, cardiac output is significantly elevated above prelabor levels for 1 to 2 hours postpartum.[128,129] The loss of blood is compensated for by an autotransfusion (influx of up to 500 mL of blood from the uteroplacental system into the maternal systemic circulation due to splanchnic vasoconstriction after placental delivery), increased central venous pressure, increased ventricular preload and increased cardiac output.[60]

Immediately after delivery, cardiac output is 60% to 80% higher than prelabor levels. However, within 10 to 15 minutes there is a sharp decline that stabilizes at prelabor values by 1 hour.[111] Several factors may contribute to this transient increase in maternal cardiac output. These include reduction in gravid uterus pressure and improved venacaval blood flow, autotransfusion of uteroplacental blood back into maternal circulation, and decreased SVR and vascular capacitance due to contraction of the muscular uterus and absence of placental blood flow.[90] Mobilization of extracellular fluid improves venous return to the heart, and is reflected in an increase in left atrial size at 1 to 3 days.[111] The increased return to the heart contributes to the higher central venous pressure seen postpartum. Maternal hypervolemia acts as a protective mechanism for excessive blood loss at delivery (see Chapter 8).

During the first week after delivery, up to 2 L of body fluid is mobilized and excreted. This results in a 3-kg weight loss. Diuresis (in order to dissipate the increased extracellular fluid) occurs between day 2 and day 5.[132] Without the diuresis of mobilized extracellular fluid, increased pulmonary wedge pressures and pulmonary edema can result.[34,90] The latter may be encountered in women with preeclampsia or heart disease who do not undergo normal diuretic patterns.

Stroke volume and thus cardiac output remain elevated for at least 48 hours after delivery.[132] This increase is probably due to increased venous return with loss of uterine blood flow and mobilization of interstitial fluid (see Chapter 11).[111,132] Left atrial size increases over the first 1 to 3 days postpartum probably due to the increased venous return with mobilization of fluid.[111] Cardiac output decreases by 30% by 2 weeks postpartum then gradually decreases to nonpregnant values by 6 to 12 weeks in most women but may last up to 24 weeks in some women.[24,111,132]

Most of the other cardiovascular system changes resolve by 6 to 8 weeks postpartum. Left atrial size and heart rate reach prepregnancy values by 10 days postpartum and LV size by 4 to 6 months.[111] However in some women, stroke volume, cardiac output, end diastolic volume, and SVR may remain elevated for up to 12 to 24 weeks or longer.[111,132] LV wall muscle mass gradually decreases over the first 6 months postpartum.[68] The audible vibrations caused by ejection of blood from the RV into the pulmonary trunk or from the LV into the brachiocephalic arteries at the point of branching from the aortic arch usually disappear by postpartum day 8. For approximately 20% of women, the systolic murmur persists beyond 4 weeks postpartum. The intensity of the murmur does, however, decrease by day 8, even if it does not disappear.[122,132]

CLINICAL IMPLICATIONS FOR THE PREGNANT WOMAN AND HER FETUS

The effects of pregnancy on the cardiovascular system can result in alterations in the ability of the woman to carry on the activities of daily living, exercise, or be comfortable in various positions. Because the maternal circulatory system is the lifeline for the fetus to receive oxygen and nutrients, hemodynamic alterations can affect the well-being of the fetus. Some of the changes experienced are exaggerations of normal and have little impact on the fetus; however, disease states may result in significant growth alterations or potentiate hypoxic episodes.

Arrhythmias

Many pregnant women experience rhythm disruptions that become more intense during the second and third trimesters.[45,56] It is unclear how much of the reported increase is due to closer monitoring versus an actual change in frequency with pregnancy.[27] Most of these arrhythmias are benign and are not indicative of heart disease. The most common (seen in 50% to 60%) are simple ventricular or atrial ectopy.[45] The woman may describe skipped beats, momentary pressure in the neck or chest, or extra beats. These are usually representative of premature ventricular contractions and require no further treatment. Extra systoles or supraventricular tachycardia may also be seen in some women.[18] The reason for the increase in arrhythmias may be related to the electrophysiologic effects of hormones, increased sympathetic nervous system activity, hemodynamic alterations, increased potassium, or in some cases, underlying cardiac disease.[56] In addition, atrial stretching and estrogen may lower the threshold for arrhythmias.[68] Most arrhythmias are neither life-threatening nor due to structural defects.[27]

Occasionally cardiac problems may present during pregnancy, so arrhythmias should be evaluated and managed in a manner similar to that in nonpregnant women. Awareness of the increased heart rate can be uncomfortable for some women. True tachycardia, such as paroxysmal atrial tachycardia or paroxysmal atrial fibrillation, may be evident for the first time during pregnancy. This may be frightening for the woman. Taking a deep breath, coughing, or the Valsalva maneuver may result in a slowing or conversion of the heart rate into a more normal pattern.

Supine Hypotensive Syndrome

Orthostatic stress generated by changes in position (from recumbent to sitting to standing) is associated with acute hemodynamic changes. Blood pools in dependent vessels, which reduces venous return and decreases cardiac output and blood pressure with increasing orthostatic stress. Heart rate and systemic vascular resistance (SVR) increase; mean arterial pressure changes, however, are not significant. In addition, decreased baroreflex sensitivity during pregnancy leads to blunted reflex activation of the sympathetic nervous system and inadequate peripheral vasoconstriction.[23]

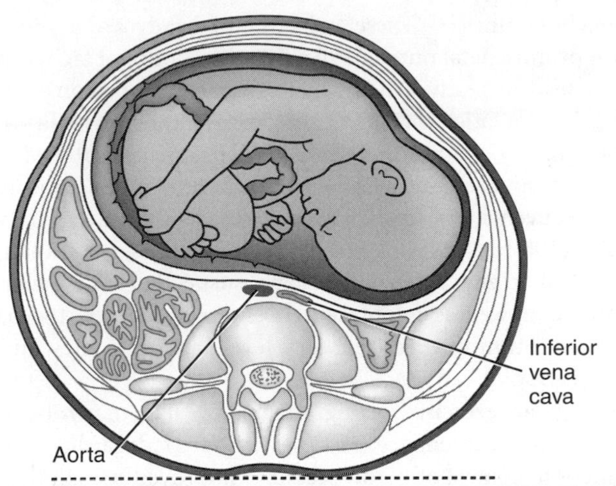

FIGURE 9-6 The pregnant uterus compressing the aorta and the inferior vena cava (aortocaval compression). Patient in supine position. (From Cohen, W.R., Acker, D.B., & Friedman, E.A. [Eds.]. [1989]. *Management of labor* [2nd ed.]. Rockville, MD: Aspen.)

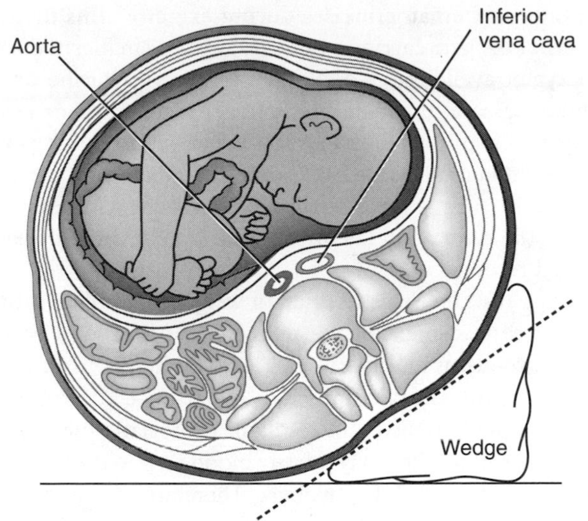

FIGURE 9-7 Uterine displacement with wedge under hip to relieve aortocaval compression. (From Cohen, W.R., Acker, D.B., & Friedman, E.A. [Eds.]. [1989]. *Management of labor* [2nd ed.]. Rockville, MD: Aspen.)

The gravid uterus is also associated with a significant amount of caval blood flow obstruction in the supine position. Approximately 90% of gravid women experience obstruction of the inferior vena cava in the supine position in late pregnancy, but rarely does this lead to hypotension or other symptoms. Late in pregnancy, but before the fetal presenting part becomes engaged, the uterus is mobile enough to fall back against the inferior vena cava in the supine position (Figure 9-6). This results in vena caval tamponade. Vascular compression may also be applied to the aorta and its branches. In most women, paravertebral collateral circulation develops during pregnancy. This, along with the dilated utero-ovarian circulation, permits blood flow from the legs and pelvis to bypass the vena cava.[90] These changes are reversed in the left lateral position (see Figure 9-7), which displaces the uterus to the left and off the vena cava. In the supine position the aorta may also be compressed (Figure 9-6), which can also alter arterial blood pressure.[34]

Usually the fall in cardiac output due to a posture change is compensated for by an increase in peripheral resistance. This allows systemic blood pressure and heart rate to remain unchanged. However, up to 8% of pregnant women in the supine position may experience a significant decrease in heart rate and blood pressure, leading to symptoms of weakness, lightheadedness, nausea, dizziness, or syncope.[111] This is referred to as supine hypotensive syndrome of pregnancy and is usually corrected when position is changed.[34,111] These women may be more vulnerable due to inadequate paravertebral collateral blood supply.[111]

Exercise During Pregnancy

Exercise has significant benefits for the mother and fetus. Regular aerobic exercise done two to three times per week maintains or improves maternal fitness during pregnancy.[87] Fit women have been shown to have shorter labors and fewer perinatal complications.[58,133] Concerns regarding exercise during pregnancy include the effects on the fetus and mother, including the risks of hyperthermia (see Chapter 20) and increased cardiac workload.

Physiologic responses to exercise include increased oxygen consumption, redistribution of blood, altered venous pooling, and changes in cardiac output and stroke volume. With submaximal exercise, minute ventilation, cardiac output, and heart rate are greater in the pregnant versus nonpregnant woman.[65,107,121] Both exercise and pregnancy increase oxygen consumption and the need for energy substrate by different tissues. Respiratory system responses to exercise during pregnancy are discussed in Chapter 10.

Blood flow is redistributed during exercise, moving blood away from the viscera and to the skin and skeletal muscles. This leads to a reduction in utero-ovarian blood flow.[28,169] Greater intensity and duration of exercise is associated with increased redistribution of blood from the uterus to the skin and muscles.[62] The limitation in substrate delivery to the fetus could potentially have adverse effects resulting in fetal hypoxia; however, to cause such changes, the reduction in uterine blood flow has to exceed 50%. In healthy pregnant women, these occurrences would be rare, being most likely during strenuous, prolonged exercise.[29,110]

Therefore under normal conditions enough oxygen is thought to be available to the uterus to meet and exceed uterine and fetal demands. Compensatory mechanisms help maintain oxygen availability during maternal exercise.[62] The decrease in placental blood flow is significantly less than the decrease in uterine blood flow.[62] Blood flow is selectively distributed to the placenta at the expense of the myometrium.[62] Regular sustained exercise during pregnancy has been reported to increase placental villous size and volume.[121] The significance of this change is uncertain.

Maternal hematocrit rises during exercise. This increases maternal oxygen-carrying capacity, with a smaller reduction in oxygen availability–to–blood flow ratio. Uterine oxygen uptake increases during exercise in order to maintain a stable oxygen consumption level.[62] Maternal ventricular performance is maintained with exercise. In response to strenuous exercise in early pregnancy, the LV adapts by increasing its contractile reserve; in late pregnancy, it adapts by increasing preload reserve.

Along with the redistribution of weight that occurs with the anterior displacement of the uterus, the progressive enlargement of the fetus and uterus can lead to alterations in venous blood return. The woman may experience dizziness due to poor venous return and resultant orthostatic hypotension. Altered cardiac return may modify blood flow to the uterus and place the fetus at risk for hypoxia. Therefore certain positions and activities may need to be modified in exercise regimens.

Pregnancy increases the workload of the heart, although in most pregnancies the cardiac reserve is adequate to meet these demands. During early pregnancy, exercise is associated with further increases in stroke volume and cardiac output.[65] As pregnancy progresses, the cardiac output changes with exercise are lower.[121] These changes in later pregnancy may be due to increased peripheral pooling rather than a progressive decline in circulatory reserve as pregnancy progresses. Decreased exercise tolerance with fatigue and dyspnea is also noted in later pregnancy. Most studies show no change in the maximum heart rate during exercise with pregnancy, although some suggest the heart rate change may be slightly reduced due to a blunted sympathetic response.[121]

Exercise results in changes in epinephrine, norepinephrine, glucagon, cortisol, prolactin, and endorphin levels. Maternal exercise is also associated with a significant increase in circulating catecholamines. Under normal circumstances, the placenta is very efficient in metabolizing catecholamines, and only 10% to 15% reach the fetus. Elevated catecholamine levels could have an additional restrictive effect on the fetal circulation.[110,121]

The usual fetal response to maternal exercise is an increase in heart rate by 5 to 25 beats per minute.[58,107,133] This increase may be due to decreased placental blood flow, stimulation of maternal vasoactive hormones, or exercise-induced uterine contractions.[58,133] These changes are independent of either gestational age or intensity of maternal exercise. Immediately after exercise and during the next 5 minutes, the fetal heart rate (FHR) remains elevated regardless of the type of exercise. Within 15 minutes, the FHR drops to preexercise values in women engaged in mild to moderate exercise activities. For women engaged in strenuous activities, the FHR may not return to baseline for up to 30 minutes.[58,110,133,164] The elevated FHR seen following exercise may also be a normal physiologic response to compensate for short periods of mild hypoxia.

In some women, transient fetal bradycardia has been reported after maximal exercise (heart rate greater than 180 beats per minute), possibly due to a rapid increase in catecholamines.[144] These episodes of bradycardia did not compromise fetal outcome. An initial response of tachycardia may lead to bradycardia if hypoxia becomes prolonged and vagal stimulation occurs. There is also the possibility that these brief occurrences are within the normal realm of fetal reflex responses to major maternal hemodynamic and hormonal events.[80,110] In most situations, fetal bradycardia was mild (100 to 119 beats per minute). Fetal reserve should be assessed if any abnormalities are suspected, and maternal cardiac as well as fetoplacental reserve should be the basis for determining exercise, work levels and activities during pregnancy.[154]

Regular exercise during pregnancy has many benefits including maintenance of fitness; improved cardiovascular function; control of blood pressure; improved metabolic efficiency, decreased backaches, fatigue, and shortness of breath; shorter labors; decreased clot formation and varicosities; feelings of wellness; prevention of excessive weight gain and fat deposition; decreased leg cramps; decreased leg edema; and more rapid postpartum recovery.[4,27,28,30,58,62,74,107,113,133,156] Fetal benefits may include better growth, improved stress tolerance, and enhanced neurobehavioral maturation, with a leaner body composition at 5 years of age.[30,31,107] Women with conditioning before pregnancy demonstrate improved metabolic effects with exercise during pregnancy compared to unconditioned women.[28] Mild to moderate aerobic exercise (to 50% to 85% of maximum) has not been demonstrated to increase spontaneous abortions, but does decrease length of labor, number of cesarean births, fetal fat mass (and thus mean birth weight), and number of episodes of fetal distress.[4,28,58,169] Non–weight-bearing exercise and low-intensity exercise do not appear to affect fetal growth.[91] Maternal risks of exercise include musculoskeletal injury, risk of cardiovascular complications, hypoglycemia, and uterine contractions.[62,107]

The American College of Obstetricians and Gynecologists (ACOG) recommends moderate exercise of 30 minutes or more on most days of the week in the absence of complications.[4] Sedentary women are encouraged to begin an exercise program; women with complications may begin an exercise program after medical evaluation.[4] Suggested activities include swimming, biking, aerobic walking, stretching, and normal walking if the women cannot tolerate aerobic exercise. Weight-bearing exercises increase energy expenditure during pregnancy, whereas weight-supported exercises (biking, swimming) do not.[121] Swimming and other aquatic exercises have particular benefits during pregnancy. Changes in heart rate and vital capacity are less while stroke volume is increased during exercise in water.[80] Hydrostatic pressure moves extravascular fluid back into the vascular space, reducing fluid retention and enhancing diuresis.[62] The water reduces thermal changes with exercise by acting as a thermoregulatory buffer around the woman.[62]

Vigorous exercise should not be performed in hot, humid weather or during a period of febrile illness, and body temperature should never exceed 40° C (104° F).[4] Jumping, jerky movements, or deep flexion or extension of joints should be avoided because of the joint instability that occurs during pregnancy. Women should avoid sports with a high risk of blunt abdominal trauma.[4] Gradual changes in position should be undertaken to avoid orthostatic stress and hypotension. Heart rate should be self-monitored during peak activity and should not exceed 70% of maximum. Heart rate and respiratory rate should return to resting rates within 15 minutes after exercise. Strenuous activity should be limited to 15 minutes. Caloric intake needs to be high enough to meet not only the demands of exercise but also of pregnancy.[4]

Studies on elite athletes with high-intensity exercise during pregnancy are limited, but there is some evidence of an increase in lighter (but not low-birth-weight) infants.[4,91,127] However, after reviewing current studies, Pivarnik concluded that "data supporting adverse effects are suppositional. Data supporting the safety of training during pregnancy, although limited in quantity, are reassuring."[127]

Maternal anatomic changes (weight gain, relaxation of ligaments and joints, progressive lordosis, and changes in center of gravity) of pregnancy often interfere with standard training routines in these athletes by the second trimester.[58] ACOG guidelines state that "recreational and competitive athletes with uncomplicated pregnancies can remain active during pregnancy and should modify their usual routines as medically indicated" and recommend close medical supervision.[4] Aerobic fitness during pregnancy does not decline significantly if women continue to exercise.[107,127] Endurance trained athletes experience an increased blood volume expansion with increases in both RBC and plasma volume during pregnancy.[127] Pregnancy-related changes in submaximal capacities may alter the woman's athletic performance. The pregnant athlete may need to adjust her usual training heart rate upward to achieve the same amount of work as when she was not pregnant.[127] If the woman continues resistance training, she should avoid supine exercises due to concerns about vena cava compression.[127]

At no time should exercise be continued if pain or contractions are experienced. The primary health care provider should be contacted if bleeding, dizziness, shortness of breath, palpitations, faintness, tachycardia, back pain, pubic pain, or difficulty in walking is experienced. Women designated as high risk for preterm labor need to receive special counseling regarding not only appropriate activity levels but also signs and symptoms of labor.[4] Exercise programs for women with gestational diabetes mellitus have been shown to be a useful adjunct therapy and may also decrease the risk of developing this disorder.[4,8,20,36,38] Exercise is also being examined as an intervention to reduce the risk of preeclampsia.[43,106,170,171]

Multiple Pregnancy

The woman with a multiple pregnancy is subject to a higher risk of morbidity and mortality. There is an increased production of estriol, progesterone, and human chorionic somatomammotropin or placental lactogen (hPL) that results in an increased volume expansion and weight gain. Whereas plasma volume is increased by about 50% in single pregnancies, in twins there is an increase of up to 65%, with further elevations seen in women with higher order multiples.[111] There is also a higher RBC volume, increased hemodilution of iron and folate, and an exaggerated physiologic anemia. The hemodilution may be due to a greater increase in total body volume or a greater demand for iron or folic acid.[122]

The increase in maternal cardiac output, stroke volume and heart rate are also greater in multiple pregnancies than that found in singletons.[100] The change in cardiac output suggests decreased cardiovascular reserve. Characteristic changes in blood pressure with multiple pregnancy include a lowered diastolic pressure at 20 weeks (74% of women with twins have a diastolic pressure less than 80 mmHg [10.6 kPa]), which is followed by a greater rise in diastolic pressure between midpregnancy and delivery (95% experience a rise in diastolic pressure of 15 mmHg [1.99 kPa] or more).[27,100,122]

Mothers with multiple pregnancies are at greater risk for preterm labor, preeclampsia, placenta previa, placental abruption, anemia, hyperemesis gravidarum, and postpartum hemorrhage. The length of labor is similar in twin and single pregnancies, although with twins the active phase is longer and the latent phase is shorter. Labor may be more difficult, possibly due to uterine overdistention and an increased incidence of malpresentation. Blood loss is about double that in a single delivery, and hemorrhage is more frequent due to uterine atony and sudden decompression of the overdistended uterus. There is also a slightly higher incidence of vasa previa and placenta previa, increasing the possibility of hemorrhage at delivery. The risk of preeclampsia is greater in twin than in single pregnancies, possibly related to the larger placental mass found with twin pregnancies.[122]

Cardiac Disease and Pregnancy

Cardiac disease affects about 1% (range 0.1% to 4%) of pregnant women and accounts for 15% of pregnancy related to maternal morbidity.[27,167] The incidence of pregnant women with cardiac disease is slowly increasing as improved management and technical capabilities for both the mother and fetus make it possible to sustain pregnancy in those who previously would have been advised to terminate or avoid pregnancy.[173] Corrective surgery for infants and children with congenital heart disease has increased the number of these women who are now of childbearing age. In addition, the incidence of heart disease increases in women who wait until their forties or later to have children.

The profound alterations in the cardiorespiratory system and hemodynamics during pregnancy can result in death or disability to women who have underlying heart disease. Many early symptoms of cardiac disease, such as fatigue, dyspnea on exertion, dependent edema, presyncope (due to pressure on the inferior vena cava), and palpitations are normal findings in pregnancy. Thus the diagnosis of cardiac disease may be delayed in women who present with symptoms of cardiac disorders for the first time during pregnancy.

Some women may actually benefit somewhat from the increase in cardiac output, decrease in SVR, and increased heart rate. On the other hand, cardiac diseases associated with fixed lesions do not tolerate the volume increase because the stenotic area cannot accommodate the increased flow. When blood volume reaches its peak, the potential for congestive heart failure (CHF) increases. The increased heart rate shortens the diastolic filling time, thereby preventing adequate filling of the heart. This combined with the decrease in SVR may result in a drop in blood pressure, increased fatigue, dizziness, and reduced uterine blood flow.

At delivery the risk for CHF is further increased by the increase in blood volume. Acute pulmonary edema may occur. Applying pressure to the abdomen can slow the blood return to the heart and facilitate cardiovascular stabilization. If the heart is unable to compensate for the decrease in SVR, the blood pressure falls. Maintenance of blood pressure can be attempted by administration of chronotropic and alpha pressor agents. Epidural and spinal anesthesia may further decrease SVR and should be used with caution in these patients. The increased cardiac load with the marked increase in cardiac output immediately after delivery may significantly increase ventricular filling pressures and stroke volume increasing the risk of clinical deterioration.[35]

Pregnancy is particularly dangerous and may be contraindicated for women who have Eisenmenger syndrome, peripartum cardiomyopathy, severe primary pulmonary hypertension, aortic stenosis, coarctation of the aorta, Marfan syndrome, and hemodynamically significant mitral stenosis (Table 9-3).[18] The presence of a cardiac lesion involving pulmonary hypertension during pregnancy carries a risk of maternal mortality somewhere between 30% and 50%. Pregnancy may also aggravate preexisting cardiac conditions such that damage is extensive and recovery to prepregnancy levels is not possible. In addition, pregnancy may result in maternal heart disease (e.g., peripartum cardiomyopathy).[18,27,35,67,119]

The fetus must also be monitored closely during pregnancy in a woman with cardiac disease. Fetal well-being and growth are dependent upon a continuous flow of well-oxygenated blood to the uterus. When this supply is reduced or interrupted or oxygenation is decreased, the fetus is at risk for altered growth and development and for increased mortality.[35,54] In addition, the fetus is at increased risk (3% to 12% depending on the defect versus 0.8% in the general population) of being born with a congenital heart defect if either parent has congenital heart disease since this can be a multifactorial disorder (see Chapter 1).[35] If the mother is the affected parent, she adds an environmental risk (altered hemodynamics during pregnancy) as well as a genetic risk for her infant.

All of these factors and the risk to the mother and fetus should be discussed in depth with couples before pregnancy. Preconception counseling allows the potential problems and treatment options to be explored and the woman's current health status to be characterized. Surgical correction or palliative procedures are generally recommended to be done before pregnancy, followed by several months to a year of recovery time.[18]

Table 9-3 High Risk Maternal Cardiovascular Conditions

DISORDER	ESTIMATED MATERNAL MORTALITY RATE (%)
Aortic valve stenosis	10-20
Coarctation of the aorta	5
Marfan syndrome	10-20
Peripartum cardiomyopathy	15-60
Severe pulmonary hypertension	50
Tetralogy of Fallot	10

From Blanchard, D.G. & Shabetal, R. (2009). Cardiac disease. In R.K. Creasy, et al. (Eds.). *Creasy & Resnik's Maternal-fetal medicine: Principles and practice* (6th ed.). Philadelphia: Saunders Elsevier, p. 798.

Obstructive Lesions

These lesions are basically stenotic in nature. The main concern is an obstruction of flow causing an elevation of pressure proximal to the obstructive lesion and a decrease in flow distal to the stenotic area. Pulmonary stenosis without septal defect, coarctation of the aorta, aortic stenosis, mitral stenosis, and tricuspid stenosis are included in this group. Mitral valve stenosis, regurgitation and prolapse are presented as examples.

Mitral Stenosis. This lesion is caused almost exclusively by rheumatic heart disease. The stenotic valve restricts cardiac output, resulting in fatigue, which is the most common symptom. The obstruction of left atrial outflow leads to pressure elevations in the left atrium, pulmonary veins, and pulmonary capillaries, causing severe pulmonary congestion. Risk of death is greatest in the third trimester and postpartum.[18] About one fourth of women experience their first symptoms with pregnancy.[27]

The increased blood volume, cardiac output, and heart rate of pregnancy, along with the fluid retention, may lead to an increase in symptoms, especially after 20 weeks.[27] Signs of pulmonary congestion usually occur by 20 to 24 weeks as intravascular volumes begin to peak and stabilize around 30 weeks.[27] The increase in cardiac output, plasma volume, and heart rate peak by this time, decrease diastolic filling time in the LV, and increase the pressure gradient across the mitral valve.[27] An exacerbation may occur at the time of delivery due to increased pulmonary wedge pressure if there is prolonged tachycardia. The first 24 hours after delivery is a time of increased vulnerability in these women due to intravascular fluid shifts.[27] The risk of maternal and neonatal complications is higher in women with abnormal functional capacity, cyanosis, or left-sided valve obstruction and is increased with maternal smoking, maternal age younger than 20 or older than 35 years, multiple pregnancy, and anticoagulant therapy.[152]

Management includes avoidance of the supine position and prophylaxis against rheumatic disease during pregnancy and against endocarditis during labor and delivery. If severe mitral stenosis is diagnosed, mitral commissurotomy is advised before conception.[18] If symptoms develop during the course of pregnancy, activity restrictions to reduce the strain on the heart, sodium intake restrictions, diuretics, and digitalis may be considered. If symptoms of pulmonary congestion persist despite medical therapy, surgical intervention (either a balloon valvuloplasty or valve replacement) may be necessary. If thromboembolism occurs, anticoagulation therapy is needed.[18,27]

Mitral Regurgitation. Mitral regurgitation may be due to rheumatic heart disease; however, there are numerous other conditions that can lead to its development, including congenital heart disease, hypertension, ischemia, and idiopathic myocardial disease.[18] Prolapse of the mitral valve during systole allows for regurgitation of blood back into the left atrium. Fatigue is the result. If severe, pulmonary congestion can occur. These women have a propensity for atrial fibrillation and left atrial thrombus formation. Individuals with mitral regurgitation may be asymptomatic for extended periods of time. In the woman with mild regurgitation, pregnancy is usually well tolerated, and the development of congestive heart failure (CHF) is rare.

Mitral Valve Prolapse. Mitral valve prolapse (MVP) is one of the most common congenital heart lesions. Most women with MVP are asymptomatic and tolerate pregnancy well; in fact, there is evidence that pregnancy may actually improve hemodynamics and symptoms in some women. Although rare, complications associated with MVP (arrhythmias, infective endocarditis, and cerebral ischemic events) may result in serious complications during pregnancy. MVP can be both a primary disease function and a secondary pathology associated with connective tissue diseases or cardiac disease that reduces the size of the LV. The latter includes syndromes such as Marfan syndrome, pseudoxanthoma elasticum, and osteogenesis imperfecta.

The hemodynamic changes of pregnancy can reduce the clinical signs of MVP by decreasing audible murmurs (usually a late systolic murmur associated with a click), possibly by increasing the LV end-diastolic volume and favorably realigning the mitral valve complex. The decrease in peripheral vascular resistance relieves the mitral insufficiency, thereby reducing the murmur. Once these parameters return to normal in the postpartum period, the auscultatory findings of MVP return. These changes are also reflected on echocardiography.

In most situations, pregnancy is tolerated well in women with MVP, especially if there is no mitral valve regurgitation, with good maternal and fetal outcomes. The woman may experience an increase in palpitations, lightheadedness, dizziness, fainting with prolonged standing, arrhythmias, or chest pains that may require medical intervention with the use of β blockers.[18]

Left-to-Right Shunts

Left-to-right shunts are characterized by recirculation of oxygenated blood through the lungs, bypassing the peripheral circulation. This can occur through an atrial septal defect (ASD), ventricular septal defect (VSD), or a patent ductus arteriosus (PDA). In most patients born with these defects, the defect has either closed on its own during childhood or corrective surgery has been performed to reduce the defect. A residual defect may remain, however.

The magnitude of the left-to-right shunt is dependent upon the ratio of resistance in the systemic and pulmonary vascular circuits. During pregnancy, both circuits have a decline in resistance (see Table 9-1) so that there is usually no significant change if shunting occurs. If pulmonary vascular disease exists, the normal fall in pulmonary vascular resistance (PVR) may not occur. Cyanosis rarely occurs with these defects unless significant pulmonary hypertension or RV failure develops. Pregnancy does not seem to precipitate these events, however.

Atrial Septal Defect. An uncorrected ASD is usually asymptomatic but may become symptomatic for the first time in pregnancy.[18,27] The most common complications are arrhythmias, pulmonary hypertension, and heart failure. The hypervolemia of pregnancy increases the left-to-right shunt through the ASD, thereby creating an additional burden on the RV. This additional load is usually tolerated well by most women, although up to 15% fetal loss has been reported.[27] If the additional load is not well tolerated, which usually occurs if the woman has pulmonary hypertension, chronic atrial fibrillation or RV dysfunction, RV failure occurs, leading to marked peripheral edema, atrial arrhythmias, pulmonary hypertension, and paradoxical systemic emboli across the septal defect.[18,35]

Ventricular Septal Defect. A VSD can occur either as an isolated lesion or in conjunction with other congenital cardiac anomalies (such as tetralogy of Fallot, transposition of the great vessels, or coarctation of the aorta). The size of the defect determines the degree of shunting, tolerance to the additional burden of pregnancy, and prognosis. Small defects are usually tolerated well.[18,27] Large VSDs often lead to CHF, arrhythmias, or development of pulmonary hypertension or Eisenmenger syndrome with increased maternal and fetal mortality.[18,27] These women are often counseled to avoid becoming pregnant.[18] A large VSD is often associated with some degree of aortic regurgitation, which contributes to the risk of CHF during pregnancy.

Patent Ductus Arteriosus. A PDA is usually identified during infancy and is surgically corrected at that time. Therefore it is uncommon to find this type of defect in childbearing women. However, if it does exist, it is usually well tolerated during gestation, labor, and delivery, although closure before pregnancy is usually recommended.[18] If the PDA is complicated by pulmonary hypertension, the prognosis is poorer.[18]

Right-to-Left Shunts

Right-to-left shunts are characterized by shunting of blood from the systemic venous circulation to the arterial circulation without oxygenation. Right-to-left shunting occurs through an ASD, VSD, or PDA when the PVR rises so that it exceeds the SVR or when an obstruction to RV outflow exists. These women present with cyanosis, clubbing of the fingers, and RV hypertrophy. Conditions include Eisenmenger syndrome, tetralogy of Fallot, and primary pulmonary hypertension.

Eisenmenger Syndrome. This syndrome combines the presence of a congenital communication between systemic and pulmonary circulations with progressive pulmonary hypertension that leads to shunt reversal or bidirectional flow. It is often associated with VSD or PDA. During pregnancy the increased plasma volume increases the burden on the compromised heart.[18] The decreased SVR increases the degree of right-to-left shunting, which reduces pulmonary perfusion, leading to hypoxemia and maternal and fetal compromise.[18,35,60] Systemic hypotension leads to decreased RV filling pressures, which may be insufficient to perfuse the pulmonary bed, when high PVR exists. The result may be the onset of sudden and profound hypoxemia. Hemorrhage or complications of conduction anesthesia (hypovolemia) may precipitate hypoxemia and lead to death during the intrapartum period.[18]

The fetal and maternal mortality rate for pregnant women with Eisenmenger syndrome can be 50% when pulmonary hypertension is associated with a VSD.[27] Death is usually from right ventricular failure with cardiogenic shock.[27] Maternal mortality is greatest during parturition and early postpartum.[18,169] Because of the high mortality rate, women are usually discouraged from becoming pregnant and pregnancy termination is usually recommended. If gestation continues, hospitalization, continuous oxygen administration, and the use of pulmonary vasodilators are recommended. During labor it is essential to maintain an adequate fluid load to maintain venous return and right ventricular filling.[27] However, maintaining a preload edge to protect against unexpected blood loss may risk tipping the scales toward pulmonary edema. Only about one fourth of pregnancies in women with this disorder are term and approximately one third of the infants are growth restricted.[169]

Tetralogy of Fallot (TOF). This defect is the most common cause of right-to-left shunting. TOF includes a combination of VSD, pulmonary valve stenosis, RV hypertrophy, and rightward displacement of the aortic root. PVR is normal. Surgical correction usually occurs during infancy, although there may be residual shunting following correction. Pregnancy outcome is relatively good for those individuals who have undergone surgical correction who have good ventricular function and no significant right ventricular outflow tract obstruction.[18,60,159] In pregnant women with uncorrected VSDs, the decrease in systemic vascular resistance (SVR) leads to increases in right-to-left shunting and cyanosis.[27] This can be complicated by intrapartum blood loss, leading to systemic hypotension. Therefore careful monitoring of fluid status is warranted.[18]

Pulmonary Artery Hypertension. Severe pulmonary hypertension associated with pregnancy carries a 50% maternal mortality rate and a 40% fetal mortality rate if the mother survives, although a recent study found a lower maternal mortality rate of 25%.[16,18,27] Deterioration of cardiac function with right heart failure usually begins in the second trimester.[35] Significant pulmonary hypertension is a contraindication to pregnancy, and pregnancy should be prevented or termination recommended if it occurs. If termination is not possible, physical activity should be curtailed and supine positioning avoided during late gestation. Careful monitoring of oxygenation and fluid status at the time of labor and delivery is essential in order to identify problems early and intervene appropriately.[27]

Marfan Syndrome

Marfan syndrome is an autosomal dominant disorder of connective tissue whose clinical manifestations include skeletal, ocular, and cardiovascular abnormalities. Aortic dilation is one of these manifestations. Complications that can result include aneurysm formation and rupture, aortic dissection, and aortic regurgitation. Structural changes in the aortic wall due to high estrogen levels predispose pregnant women to aortic dissection. Rupture is more likely to occur in the third trimester or in the first stage of labor.[18,159] Counseling regarding the risk of inheritance and the potential maternal complications should be given before conception if possible. If pregnancy occurs, the use of long-acting β blockers to decrease pulsatile pressure on the aortic wall is indicated, along with limitations on physical activity and preventing hypertensive complications.[18]

Peripartum Cardiomyopathy

Peripartum cardiomyopathy is a form of dilated cardiomyopathy seen in women without a previous history of heart disease, which develops during the last month of pregnancy or up to 5 months postpartum.[18,35] In dilated cardiomyopathy the cardiac chambers become significantly dilated with a hypokinetic LV and progressive decrease in LV function. Peripartum cardiomyopathy has a frequency of 1/3000 to 1/4000 live births with recurrence risk in subsequent pregnancies of up to 50%.[18,35] This disorder has a variable and unpredictable clinical course. Generally 30% to 50% of women demonstrate partial recovery with persistence of some cardiac dysfunction; 20% develop deteriorating cardiac function to the point of needing a heart transplant.[18,96] In women with partial recovery, cardiac function may improve over time.[33] The cause of peripartum cardiomyopathy is unknown. It is not clear if the pregnancy/postpartum state causes the disorder or aggravates an underlying cardiomyopathic process.[18,35,67] The risk of developing peripartum cardiomyopathy is higher with increased maternal age, chronic hypertension, multiple gestation, multiparity, and preeclampisa.[35,67]

Hypertensive Disorders

Hypertensive disorders are one of the most common complications of pregnancy and a leading cause of maternal mortality.[94,95] Hypertension during pregnancy is classified as (1) chronic hypertension, (2) preeclampsia, (3) preeclampsia superimposed on chronic hypertension, and (4) gestational hypertension. Definitions of each form are in Table 9-4.

Chronic hypertension occurs in 2% to 5% of pregnant women. Maternal-fetal complications of chronic hypertension

Table 9-4 Classification of Hypertensive Disorders of Pregnancy

CLASSIFICATION	DEFINITION AND DIAGNOSTIC CRITERIA
Preeclampsia	Hypertension with proteinuria Hypertension: blood pressure >140 mmHg (18.62 kPa) systolic or 90 mmHg (11.97 kPa) diastolic after 20 weeks' gestation in a woman normotensive before 20 weeks' gestation Proteinuria: 300 mg/L (30 mg/dL) protein in a random specimen and excretion of 300 mg/24 hours Hypertension with other systemic symptoms of preeclampsia in the absence of proteinuria is highly suspicious of preeclampsia
Chronic hypertension	Blood pressure 140/90 mmHg (18.62/11.97 kPa) or greater before the twentieth week of gestation or, if only diagnosed during pregnancy, persisting 6 weeks after pregnancy
Preeclampsia superimposed on chronic hypertension	Highly likely in women who develop new proteinuria or with preexisting hypertension and proteinuria who develop sudden increases in blood pressure or proteinuria, thrombocytopenia, or increases in hepatocellular enzymes
Gestational hypertension	Development of hypertension without other signs of preeclampsia

Adapted from National High Blood Pressure Education Program. (2000). Report of the National High Blood Pressure Education Program Working Group on high blood pressure in pregnancy. *Am J Obstet Gynecol, 183,* 1.

include superimposed preeclampsia (in 15% to 20%), abruptio placentae, stroke, preterm delivery, stillbirth, low birth weight, and neonatal loss. Perinatal mortality is two to four times higher.

Nonpregnant women with chronic hypertension generally have decreased renal plasma flow (RPF) and GFR, with an exaggerated excretion of sodium in response to a salt load. During early pregnancy, RPF and GFR increase, but the total increase by late pregnancy is less than in normotensive pregnant women. With increased blood pressure, fluid moves from the vascular to the extravascular spaces, and the blood becomes hemoconcentrated with further reductions in RPF and GFR. The pregnant woman with chronic hypertension also has a 20% to 30% decrease in sodium excretion. Vasoconstriction may reduce uteroplacental perfusion, with alterations in fetal growth.

Preeclampsia

Preeclampsia is a hypertensive, multisystem disorder characterized by hypertension and proteinuria that complicates 3% to 6% of all pregnancies.[39,52,66,137] Other features may include central nervous system irritability and, at times, coagulation or liver function abnormalities. Changes in different organ systems with preeclampsia are summarized in Table 9-5. Women with preeclampsia may develop seizures (eclampsia) or a variant with abnormal liver function and thrombocytopenia known as the HELLP syndrome. The term HELLP comes from this syndrome's characteristic clinical findings: hemolysis (H), elevated liver enzymes (EL), and a low platelet (LP) count. This syndrome occurs in 0.5% to 0.9% of all pregnancies, and in 10% to 20% of women with severe preeclampsia.[82,150] Women with preeclampsia may be at risk of later cardiovascular disease.[172]

"Placental and maternal factors interact to develop preeclampsia. Originating in the placenta as a result of decreased trophoblast invasion, ischemia leads to oxidative stress and a continuum of events which adversely affect the maternal vasculature leading to hypertension and proteinuria."[115,p. 380] Preeclampsia is characterized by increased SVR, enhanced platelet aggregation, activation of the coagulation system, endothelial cell dysfunction, pathologic changes and decreased perfusion to most organ systems, especially the liver, kidney, brain, and placenta secondary to vasoconstriction; increased sensitivity to pressors, including angiotensin II; and a reduction in the usual increase in plasma volume due to loss of fluid from the vascular space.[50,72,137,147,148] Factors predisposing to preeclampsia include conditions in which oxygen demand is increased (multiple pregnancy, molar pregnancy, or an edematous placenta) or conditions with decreased oxygen transfer (primipara, microvascular disease, chronic hypertension, diabetes, collagen disorders, or abnormal placentation).[72,134,137,149] The net result of these factors is a direct or relative placental hypoperfusion. This suggests altered uteroplacental perfusion as an early event in the pathogenesis of preeclampsia, possibly due to oxidative stress and ischemia-reperfusion. In addition, many of these factors are also associated with increased fetal antigen load (i.e., multiple pregnancy, hydrops, molar pregnancy, or other increased placental mass) or inflammatory response (rheumatoid disease, infection) supporting an immunologic basis for preeclampsia.[149] An immunologic basis is also supported by the greater frequency of preeclampsia in first pregnancies with limited exposure of the mother's system to paternal sperm, and thus the paternal antigens expressed on fetal tissues, or in mutigravida women with new partners (see Chapter 13).[138,147]

Although the exact pathogenesis of preeclampsia is still unclear, "relative ischemia or hypoxia of the placenta resulting from defective progression of spiral artery remodeling and placental angiogenesis is thought to underlie preeclampsia."[115,p. 380] This is followed by maternal multisystem involvement with endothelial dysfunction.[92,131,135,147] Thus inadequate remodeling of maternal uterine spiral arteries is an early pathogenic event.[24,39,134,135,148,149] Normally extravillous trophoblast cells from the placenta migrate into the uterine spiral arteries in both

Table 9-5 Findings and Clinical Manifestations of Preeclampsia

VASCULATURE OR SYSTEM	FINDINGS	CLINICAL MANIFESTATIONS
Cardiovascular	Increased cardiac output (CO) and systemic vasoconstriction	Systemic hypertension
	Increased hydrostasis present	Generalized edema
	High CO and hypertension	Increased hemolysis
Uteroplacental	Uteroplacental insufficiency	Fetal somatic growth deficiency; fetal hypoxemia and distress
	Decidual ischemia	Abruptio placentae; placental infarcts
	Decidual thrombosis	Thrombocytopenia
Renal	Decreased renal blood flow and glomerular filtration rate; endothelial damage	Proteinuria; elevated creatinine and decreased creatinine clearance; oliguria
	High angiotensin II responsiveness in tubular vasculature	Elevated uric acid
	All of the above	Renal tubular necrosis and renal failure
Cerebrovascular	Cerebral motor ischemia	Generalized grand mal seizures (eclampsia)
	High cerebral perfusion pressure with regional edema	Cerebral hemorrhage
	Cerebral edema	Coma
	Regional ischemia	Central blindness; loss of speech
Hepatic	Ischemic and hepatic cellular injury	Elevated liver enzymes
	Mitochondrial injury	Intracellular fatty deposition
Hematologic	Intravascular hemolysis	Schistocyte burr cells; elevated free hemoglobin and iron-decreased haptoglobin levels
	Decidual thrombosis, release of fibrin degradation products	Thrombocytopenia; antiplatelet antibodies

From Shah, D.M. (2011). Hypertensive disorder of pregnancy. In R.J. Martin, A.A. Fanaroff, & M.C. Walsh (Eds.). *Fanaroff and Martin's Neonatal-perinatal medicine: Diseases of the fetus and infant* (9th ed.). Philadelphia: Mosby Elsevier, p. 280.

the decidua and myometrium. These trophoblast cells remodel the maternal spiral arteries so that little vascular smooth muscle tissue, neural elements, and elastic matrix are left.[10,147] The spiral arteries become large, flaccid uteroplacental vessels establishing a low-resistance circuit that enhances blood supply to the fetus and placenta. This remodeling process is described in Chapter 3. In preeclampsia the remodeling is incomplete and often confined to the decidual portion of the blood vessels (see Chapter 3), with 30% to 50% of the vessels in the myometrium and their adrenergic nerve supply left intact.[46,134] The result is that the spiral arteries remain thick walled and muscular, leading to inadequate placental flow and thus reduced oxygen delivery to the placenta.

Alterations in implantation and remodeling of maternal spiral arteries may be secondary to maternal-fetal immune maladaptation at the maternal-fetal interface (see Chapter 13) due to ischemia-reperfusion leading to oxidative stress and vascular disease.[147] An immunologic basis is supported by the increased incidence of classic preeclampsia in primiparous women or multiparous women with new partners.[147,149] A similar lack of spiral artery change is seen without preeclampsia in some forms of fetal growth restriction and in some women with preterm labor. Development of preeclampsia seems to require decreased placental perfusion, with oxidative stress and endothelial activation. This may be due to genetic factors or maternal disease that alters maternal antioxidant enzymes or increases sensitivity to oxidative stress.

These changes within the placenta are thought to be linked to a maternal multisystem syndrome with endothelial dysfunction via "increased release of antiangiogenic factors sflt-1, endoglin, and syncytiotrophoblast membrane fragments into the maternal circulation. These may interact with or damage the maternal vasculature resulting in an inflammatory response and increased maternal vasculature resistance and vascular dysfunction in preeclampsia. Heightened oxidative/nitrative stress is seen in maternal vasculature and particularly in the placenta in preeclampsia."[115,p. 380] Oxidative stress secondary to hypoxia (due to altered perfusion) occurs at the maternal-fetal interface. Plasma lipoproteins, nonesterified fatty acids, and low-density lipoproteins are elevated in women with preeclampsia.[157] These provide increased substrate for lipid peroxidation. Decreased placental perfusion may also increase lipid peroxidation with release of oxygen radicals without adequate counteracting antioxidant enzymes.[39] This damages maternal vascular endothelium with activation of neutrophils and macrophages (inflammatory response). Women with preeclampsia have a greater rate of lipid peroxidation, release of reactive oxygen species (free radicals), and lower levels of antioxidants that may contribute to endothelial dysfunction.[135,147]

Release of antiangiogenic factors into maternal circulation by the oxidatively stressed placenta stimulate a generalized systemic inflammatory response leading to endothelial dysfunction.[131] These antiangiogenic factors include sflt1, which is the soluble receptor for vascular endothelial growth factor (VEGF), and soluble endoglin, which is a co-receptor for transforming growth factor-β.[72,115] These substances bind VEGF and placental growth factors, decreasing free levels of these factors, thus preventing their action on systemic endothelium, leading to endothelial dysfunction.[3,72,84,103,115,131,149]

Alterations in implantation and spiral artery remodeling decrease uteroplacental perfusion, placental ischemia, and alterations in maternal vascular.[137] Placental ischemia stimulates release of cytokines that disrupt endothelial function by inducing structural and functional changes in endothelial cells, enhancing endothelin production and decreasing acetylcholine-induced vasodilation. The endothelium is a single layer of epithelium lining the blood vessels and in direct contact with blood. The endothelium releases factors to maintain vascular tone, enhance permeability, control plasma lipids, inhibit white blood cell adhesion and migration, inhibit platelet activation and aggregation, and inhibit smooth muscle proliferation and migration (to prevent atherosclerotic changes).[1] Normally antithrombic, antiproliferative, vasodilating substances (e.g., nitric oxide, prostacyclin [or PGI_2]) are in a homeostatic balance with vasoconstrictive, prothrombic, proliferative factors (e.g., thromboxane A^2, endothelin, platelet-activating factor, superoxide, angiotensin II).

The balance within the uteroplacental circulation normally favors vasodilation. In women with preeclampsia, this balance is disrupted. Endothelial dysfunction leads to altered control of vascular tone (hypertension), increased glomerular permeability (proteinuria), altered procoagulant/anticoagulant ratio (coagulopathy), endothelial injury, and vasoconstriction (liver dysfunction).[92] Markers of endothelial dysfunction found in women with preeclampsia include alteration in the procoagulant/anticoagulant ratio; increased fibronectin; enhanced platelet activation; alterations in vasomediators such as nitric oxide, endothelin, prostaglandins, and cytokines; factor VIII antigen; thrombomodulin; and VEGF.[92]

Substances such as cellular fibronectin, growth factors, vascular cell adhesion molecules, factor VIII, antigen, and other peptides released after endothelial injury are elevated in preeclampsia.[115] The woman with preeclampsia has increased responsiveness to angiotensin II, leading to increased vascular resistance and eventually vasoconstriction, hypoxemia, and cell damage in various organs (see Table 9-5).[147] This leads to further endothelial damage aggravated by oxidative stress.

Genetics plays a role in preeclampsia, but the exact pattern of inheritance is unclear. Preeclampsia is more common in daughters of women who had preeclampsia and in pregnancies fathered by sons of women with preeclampsia.[72,135,137] Models of inheritance that have been proposed include a maternal dominant gene with reduced penetrance, maternal and fetal gene interaction, mitochondrial inheritance, or a gene-environment interaction increasing susceptibility.[160] Preeclampsia has been associated with loci on chromosomes 2p, 2q, 4q, 9, and 10 in various studies.[137,160]

SUMMARY

The cardiovascular changes associated with pregnancy are significant although well tolerated by most women. Maternal and fetal risks occur when underlying cardiovascular or pulmonary disease processes are compounded with the changes incurred during pregnancy. Cardiovascular problems increase maternal morbidity and mortality and can compromise the health and well-being of the fetus. Careful assessment and ongoing monitoring of cardiovascular status throughout the prenatal, intrapartum, and postpartum periods are essential for early identification and prompt intervention, thereby improving maternal and neonatal outcomes. Table 9-6 summarizes clinical implications related to the cardiovascular system during pregnancy.

Table 9-6 Recommendations for Clinical Practice Related to the Cardiovascular System in Pregnant Women

Recognize usual cardiovascular and hemodynamic patterns of change during pregnancy (pp. 252-259, Table 9-1).
Assess maternal cardiovascular changes throughout pregnancy (pp. 252-259).
Counsel women on normal cardiovascular changes and anticipated symptoms associated with those changes (pp. 252-259).
Counsel women in the third trimester to use the lateral recumbent position (pp. 261-262 and Figures 9-6 and 9-7).
Assess and closely monitor women at risk for and with preeclampsia throughout pregnancy (pp. 267-269).
Encourage moderate exercise on a regular basis during pregnancy (pp. 261-263).
Encourage sedentary women to begin an exercise program (pp. 261-263).
Counsel women with complications to be medically evaluated before beginning an exercise program (pp. 262-263).
Recommend interval-type exercises rather than long continuous exercise (p. 263).
Provide counseling and regularly evaluate pregnant women who start a progressive exercise program during pregnancy (pp. 262-263).
Teach women self-uterine palpation to assess for uterine contractions during exercise (p. 263).
Advise cessation of exercise if contractions, pain or bleeding occurs (p. 263).
Recognize usual changes in heart sounds and rhythms during pregnancy. (pp. 258-260).
Monitor vascular volume status carefully during the intrapartum and postpartum periods (pp. 259-260).
Evaluate blood loss and fundal tone postpartum (pp. 260-261).
Monitor for signs of congestive heart failure in women with cardiac disease, especially in the second half of pregnancy and during the intrapartum and immediate postpartum periods (pp. 255, 264-266).
Assess maternal activity tolerance in women with cardiac disease and discuss management of daily activities (pp. 263-266).
Teach women with cardiac disease the signs and symptoms of cardiovascular decompensation (pp. 263-266).

DEVELOPMENT OF THE CARDIOVASCULAR SYSTEM IN THE FETUS

The cardiovascular system is the first system in the embryo to begin to function. The need for substrates to support the rapid growth and development of the embryo necessitates the early development of a system that transports nutritional elements and metabolic by-products to and from the cells of the body. Initially the embryo is small enough that diffusion of nutrients can meet the demands of the cells; however, this is short lived because of the exponential growth of the embryo. Blood can be seen circulating through the embryonic body as early as the end of the third week.[112] Each of the developing regions of the embryo requires different amounts of circulatory support at various times throughout gestation; therefore the pattern of vessel development is markedly different from one region to the next, depending on the demand.[26]

The cardiovascular system is comprised of the heart and the blood vessels. Their development is both independent and contiguous, with the final product being a closed system that continuously circulates a given blood volume. Although considered separately here, development of the two elements of the system (heart and vessels) occurs simultaneously. Major landmarks in the development of the cardiovascular system are summarized in Table 9-7.

Table 9-7 Timelines in Normal and Abnormal Cardiac Development

NORMAL TIME	DEVELOPMENTAL EVENTS	MALFORMATIONS ARISING DURING PERIOD
18 days	Horseshoe-shaped cardiac primordium appears.	Lethal mutations
20 days	Bilateral cardia primordial fuse. Cardiac jelly appears. Aortic arch is forming.	Cardia bifida (experimental)
22 days	Heart is looping into S shape. Heart begins to beat. Dorsal mesocardium is breaking down. Aortic arches I and II are forming.	Dextrocardia
24 days	Atria are beginning to bulge. Right and left ventricles act like two pumps in series. Outflow tract is distinguished from right ventricle.	
Late in week 4	Sinus venosus is being incorporated into right atrium. Endocardial cushions appear. Septum primum appears between right and left atria. Muscular interventricular septum is forming. Truncoconal ridges are forming. Aortic arch I is regressing. Aortic arch III is forming. Aortic arch IV is forming.	Venous inflow malformations Persistent atrioventricular canal Common atrium Common ventricle Persistent truncus arteriosus
Early in week 5	Endocardial cushions are coming together, forming right and left atrioventricular canals. Further growth of interatrial septum primum and muscular interventricular septum occurs. Truncus arteriosus is dividing into aorta and pulmonary artery. Atrioventricular bundle is forming; there is possible neurogenic control of heart beat. Pulmonary veins are being incorporated into the atrium. Aortic arches I and II have regressed. Aortic arches III and IV have formed. Aortic arch VI is forming.	Persistent atrioventricular canal Muscular ventricular septal defects Transposition of the great vessels; aortic and pulmonary stenosis or atresia Aberrant pulmonary drainage
Late in week 5 to early in week 6	Endocardial cushions fuse. Interatrial foramen secundum is forming. Interatrial septum primum is almost contacting endocardial cushions. Membranous part of interventricular septum starts to form. Semilunar valves begin to form.	Low atrial septal defects Membranous interventricular septal defects Aortic and pulmonary vascular stenosis
Late in week 6	Interatrial foramen secundum is large. Interatrial septum secundum starts to form. Atrioventricular valves and papillary muscles are forming. Interventricular septum is almost complete. Coronary circulation is becoming established.	High atrial septal defects Tricuspid or mitral valve stenosis or atresia Membranous interventricular septal defects
8 to 9 weeks	Membranous part of interventricular septum is complete.	Membranous interventricular septal defect

From Carlson, B.M. (2004). *Human embryology and developmental biology* (3rd ed.). St. Louis: Mosby.

Anatomic Development

Cardiogenesis is a complex process that is controlled by many factors including members of the transforming growth factor-β (TGF-β) and fibroblast growth factor families, retinoic acid and many transcriptional and signaling factors.[114] The GATA family of zinc finger probes is also critical for cardiac formation.[61] Hypoxia inductible factor 1 and vascular endothelial growth factor (VEGF) are important in signaling fetal heart formation, development of the outflow tract and coronary vessel growth.[124] Septation of the heart involves signaling between myocardial and endothelial cells by growth factors such as TGF-β, VEGF, extracellular matrix molecules, and homeobox genes (see Chapter 3).[168]

Development of the Primitive Heart

The cardiovascular system arises from mesenchyme cells known as the angioblastic tissue, which appears early in the third week. These cells appear as scattered, small masses at the anterior margin of the embryonic disk cranial to the neural plate (see Figure 15-4). The cells coalesce to form a plexus of endothelial vessels that fuse to form two longitudinal cellular strands called *cardiogenic cords.* These cords can be seen ventral to the coelomic cavity at the end of the third week. These cords canalize to form two thin-walled tubes—the endocardial heart tubes. As the embryo undergoes lateral folding, the tubes come into proximity and fusion occurs in a cranial-to-caudal direction (Figure 9-8, *A* through *C*). Fusion results in a single tube that will eventually form the endocardium.[26,101,112]

At this stage the mesenchymal tissue around the endocardial tube thickens to form the myoepicardial mantle. An extracellular matrix separates the inner endothelial tube from the thicker outer mesenchymal tube, resulting in the appearance of a tube within a tube (see Figure 9-8, *C*). The inner tube becomes the endothelial lining of the heart (endocardium), and the myoepicardial mantle develops into the myocardium.[112,168] The outflow tract and sinus venosus form later at the distal end of this tube.[11,141] The epicardium appears after septation of the heart has begun. The epicardium forms from epithelial tissue that spreads over the myocardium. Epicardial cells invade the myocardium to give rise to fibroblast cells, smooth muscle cells, and the coronary vasculature.[114,168] The epicardium also has a role in signaling cardiomyocytes and differentiation of Purkinje fibers.[61]

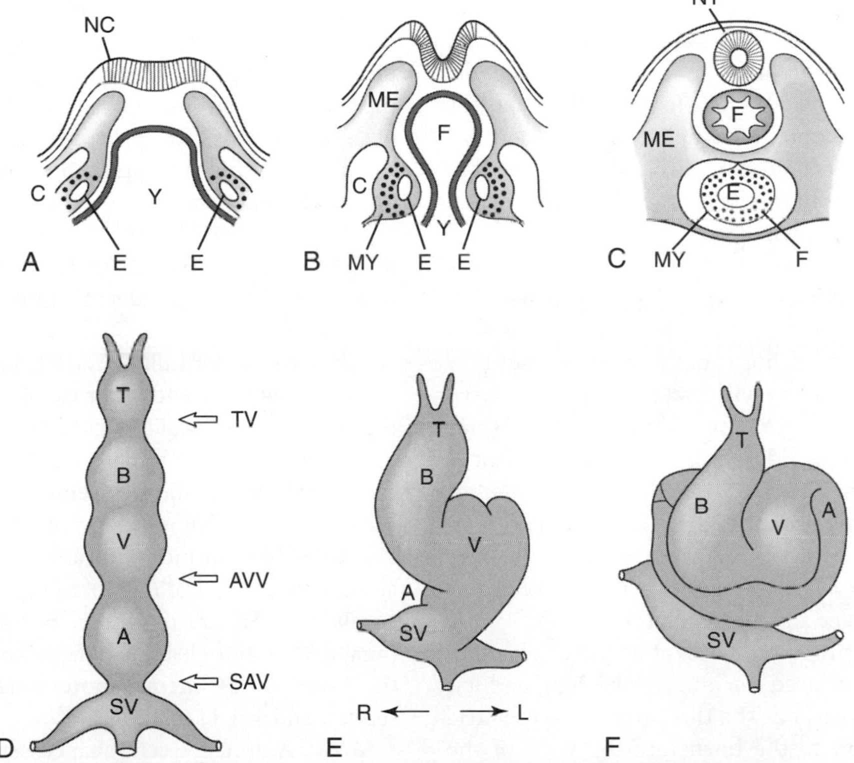

FIGURE 9-8 Development of the heart. Upper figures (**A** through **C**): transverse sections **(A)** showing that fusion of the paired endocardial and myoepicardial tubes **(B)** results in a single straight cardiac tube **(C)**. *C,* Coelomic cavity; *E,* endocardial tubes; *F,* foregut; *ME,* mesoderm; *MY,* myocardium; *NC,* neural crest; *NT,* neural tube; *Y,* yolk sac. Lower figures (**D** through **F**): **D,** Simple tubular heart; **E,** early looping to the left side; and **F,** established looping with definition of unseptated cardiac chambers. The *open arrows* indicate the valve sites. *A,* Atrium; *AVV,* atrioventricular valve; *B,* bulbus cordis; *SAV,* sinoatrial valve; *SV,* sinus venosus; *T,* truncus arteriosus; *TV,* truncal valve. (From Reller, M.D., et al. [1991]. Cardiac embryology: Basic review and clinical correlations. *J Am Soc Echocardiogr, 4,* 519.)

With cranial folding, the pericardial cavity and heart rotate on the transverse axis almost 180 degrees to lie ventral to the foregut and caudal to the oropharyngeal membrane. The septum transversum is therefore positioned between the pericardial cavity and the yolk sac (see Figure 12-5), and the heart is then situated in a definitive pericardial cavity.[26,112] The primitive heart, consisting of the endothelial tube and myoepicardial mantle, passes cranially-caudally through the pericardial cavity and is fixed to the pericardial wall only at the venous entrance (caudal end) and at the arterial outlet (cranial end). The cardiac tube begins to beat around 20 to 22 days, moving blood from the caudal venous end to the cranial arterial end. At this time, fetal vascular genesis also begins.

Differentiation of the heart regions begins and alternating dilations and constrictions can be identified (see Figure 9-8, *D* through *F*). The first areas to appear include the bulbus cordis, ventricle, and atrium. The truncus arteriosus and sinus venosus follow.[112] The truncus arteriosus lies above and is connected to the bulbus cordis. The aortic sac from which the aortic arches arise is included in the truncus arteriosus. The large sinus venosus receives the umbilical, vitelline, and common cardinal veins from the primitive placenta, yolk sac, and embryo, respectively.[26,112]

During this differentiation stage, there is rapid growth of the cardiac tube as well. Because the ends are held fixed and the bulboventricular portion of the tube grows more rapidly (doubling its length from day 21 to day 25) than the surrounding cavity, the tube bends upon itself and forms a U-shaped loop that has its convexity directed forward and to the right. Continued growth results in an S-shaped curve that nearly fills the pericardial cavity (see Figure 9-8, *E* and *F*).

The separation of the atrium and sinus venosus from the septum transversum positions the atrium dorsal and to the left of the bulboventricular loop; the sinus venosus lies dorsal to the atrium. The right and left horns of the sinus venosus now partially fuse to form a single cavity that opens into the atrial cavity via the sinoatrial orifice. The right horn of the sinus venosus becomes incorporated into the right atrium. Most of the wall of the left atrium is derived from the primitive pulmonary vein. The vein develops to the left of the septum primum (see "Septation of the Heart") and is an outgrowth of the dorsal atrial wall. However, as the atrium expands, the vein is progressively incorporated into the wall of the atrium.[26,112]

The heart is still a single tube except at the caudal end, where the remaining unfused portions of the right and left horns of the sinus venosus lie. The three pairs of symmetric veins that return blood to the horns are the veins of the placenta (umbilical), yolk sac (vitelline), and embryonic body (cardinal). The vitelline vessels soon develop asymmetrically, with the left vein undergoing retrogression. At 33 to 34 days, the right umbilical vein atrophies and disappears. The left horn of the sinus venosus also becomes much smaller as the veins in the septum transversum rearrange. Eventually the left sinus venosus becomes the coronary sinus.[26,112]

During the rearrangement of vessels, the ductus venosus (DV) is formed. This shunt between the left umbilical vein and the right hepatocardiac channel allows some of the blood from the developing placenta to bypass the liver sinusoids and flow directly into the heart via the inferior vena cava (see "Fetal Circulation"). This results in an enlargement of the right horn of the sinus venosus and a change in the position of the sinoatrial orifice. The latter is positioned to the right side of the dorsal surface and is converted to a vertical alignment. The margins are now projected into the atrium and compose the right and left venous valves.[26]

The atrium, ventricle, and bulbus cordis continue to expand rapidly with changes in position. The atrium expands transversely, extending laterally and ventrally, and appears on either side of the bulbus cordis. This results in the atria being deeply grooved. Further growth results in the right and left auricular appendages being formed. At the same time, the bulboventricular sulcus dissipates with the growth of these structures. Eventually the caudal portion of the bulbus becomes part of the ventricle. The ventricle gradually moves to the left and ends up on the ventral surface of the heart. This change defines the atrioventricular canal.[26]

Septation of the Heart

Septation of the atrioventricular canal, the atrium, and the ventricle begins in the middle of the fourth week and is complete by the sixth week. The changes in shape and position of the heart tube, as described earlier, facilitate the partitioning of these structures. The process of septation takes place while the heart continues to pump and blood continues to move unidirectionally through the tube. The subdivision of the heart into right and left compartments occurs simultaneously in the various regions of the heart; however, all of the processes must be integrated so that normal functional development occurs.

Atrioventricular Canal. The atrium leads into the ventricle via a narrow atrioventricular canal. During the fourth week the endocardium proliferates to produce dorsal and ventral bulges in the wall of the atrioventricular canal (Figure 9-9). These swellings are the atrioventricular endocardial cushions. Mesenchymal cells invade the swellings, which results in the growth of the cushions toward each other. Fusion of the cushions occurs, leading to right and left atrioventricular canals.[101,112] Failure of septation results in atrioventricular canal defects and Ebstein anomaly and can alter formation of the heart valves, membranous portion of the ventricular septum and atrial septation.[61,168]

Atria. A thin, crescent-shaped septum (septum primum) begins to grow downward from the roof of the atrium during the fourth week. Initially a large opening exists between the caudal free edge of the septum and the endocardial cushions; this is the foramen primum. This allows oxygenated blood that is returned to the right atrium from the placenta to pass to the left atrium and be distributed to the systemic circulation. The opening progressively gets smaller and is eventually obliterated when the septum primum fuses with the

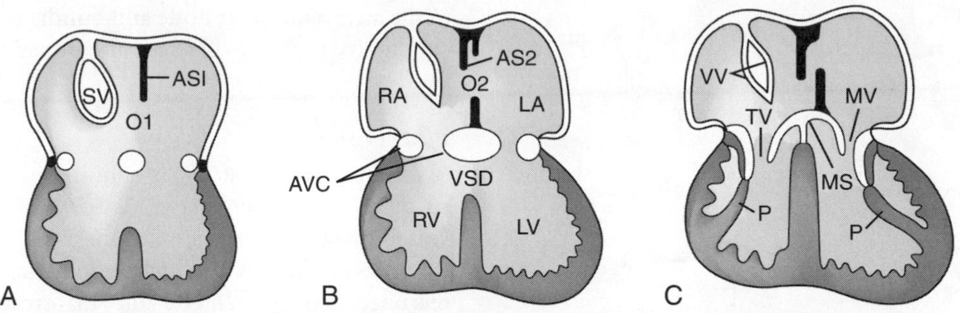

FIGURE 9-9 Changes in cardiac chamber septation. The diagrams represent coronal sections of the heart: **A,** Early stage, commencing atrial and ventricular septation; **B,** atrial ostium primum closed, ostium secundum forming, and ventricular septum incomplete; and **C,** septation complete and membranous septum formed. The atrioventricular valves have been formed by atrioventricular (endocardial) cushion tissue and delamination of myocardium. *AS1,* Atrial septum primum; *AS2,* atrial septum secundum; *AVC,* atrioventricular cushion; *LA,* left atrium; *LV,* left ventricle; *MS,* membranous septum; *MV,* mitral valve; *O1,* atrial ostium primum; *O2,* atrium ostium secundum; *P,* papillary muscles; *RA,* right atrium; *RV,* right ventricle; *SV,* sinus venosus; *TV,* tricuspid valve; *VSD,* ventricular septal defect; *VV,* venous valves. (From Reller, M.D., et al. [1991]. Cardiac embryology: Basic review and clinical correlations. *J Am Soc Echocardiogr, 4*[5], 519.)

endocardial cushions. Before the septum primum reaches the atrioventricular cushions, however, a second interatrial communication forms as the result of multiple perforations that coalesce in the upper part of the septum. This is the foramen secundum.[101,112]

A second, thicker septum (septum secundum) begins to develop just to the right of the septum primum. This septum is also crescent shaped, but it grows only until it overlaps the foramen secundum. The partition is incomplete, and an oval opening, the foramen ovale, is left.[26,112] The upper portion of the septum primum regresses, whereas the lower segment (attached to the endocardial cushions) remains, serving as a flap valve for the foramen ovale. Before birth this valve allows directed blood to move freely from the right to the left atrium. However, flow from the left to the right is prevented by apposition of the thin flexible septum primum to the rigid septum secundum after birth. This results in fusion of the septa and eventual anatomic closure of the foramen ovale. Atrial septation is illustrated in Figure 9-9.

Ventricles. The interventricular septum consists of muscular and membranous portions. Division of the bulboventricular cavity is first indicated by a sagittal muscular ridge appearing on the floor of the ventricle near the apex; this is the interventricular septum. At first the septum appears to lengthen as a result of the dilation of the lateral halves of the ventricle. Later there is active proliferation of the septal tissue as the muscular portion of the interventricular septum forms.[26,112] Communication between the right and left sides of the ventricle is maintained until the bulbar ridges fuse. This closure is the result of fusion of subendocardial tissue from the bulbar ridges with the atrioventricular cushions.[112]

The membranous portion of the ventricular septum is derived from tissue that extends from the right side of the endocardial cushions. This eventually fuses with the aorticopulmonary septum of the truncus arteriosus and the muscular interventricular septum. Closure of the interventricular foramen results in the pulmonary trunk being in communication with the right ventricle (RV) and the aorta with the left ventricle (LV) (see Figure 9-9).[112]

Bulbus Cordis and Truncus Arteriosus. Before the interventricular septum has developed completely, spiral subendocardial thickenings appear in the distal part of the bulbus cordis. These are the bulbar ridges, which can be seen during the fifth week of gestation. Initially these ridges are composed of cardiac jelly, but they are later invaded by mesenchymal cells. In the proximal part of the bulbus, the ridges are located on the ventral and dorsal walls, whereas in the distal portion they are attached to the lateral walls. The distal portion of the bulbus is continuous with the truncus arteriosus, which develops truncal ridges that match those of the bulbus cordis. The growth and fusion of these ridges during the eighth week results in the spiral aorticopulmonary septum (Figure 9-10). The spiral effect may be due to the streaming of blood from the ventricles through the truncus during septum development. The result is the creation of two channels: the pulmonary trunk and the aorta. The bulbus cordis is gradually incorporated into the ventricles.[26,112]

Cardiac Valves. Part of the septation process involves the development of the cardiac valves. This includes the development of the semilunar valves of the aorta and the pulmonary artery and the atrioventricular valves (tricuspid and mitral valves). The cellular and molecular mechanisms that control heart valve cell differentiation are similar to those involved in the formation of cartilage, tendons, and bones.[93]

The semilunar valves develop from a swelling of subendothelial tissue that appears on each side of the ventricular end of the bulbar ridges. These swellings consist of loose connective tissue covered by endothelium. Eventually the swellings become hollowed out and reshaped to form three thin-walled cusps.[26,112] The atrioventricular valves develop from local

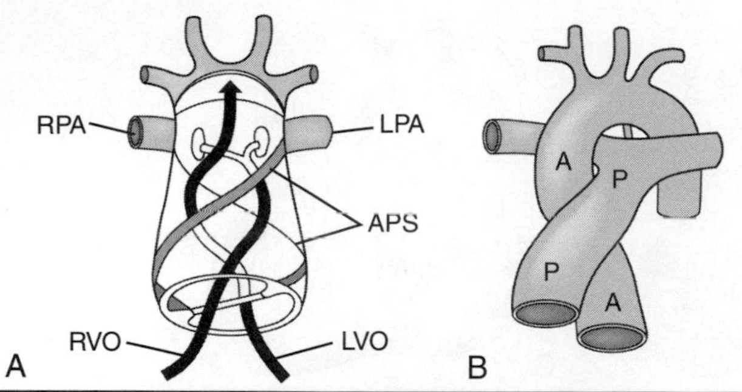

FIGURE 9-10 Septation of the truncus arteriosus. **A,** Diagram showing the aorticopulmonary septum, which separates the systemic arterial flow *(solid dark line)* from the pulmonary arterial flow *(broken line)*; **B,** the mature pulmonary artery and aorta after septation and separation, showing the persistent spiral relationship. *A,* Aorta; *APS,* aorticopulmonary septum; *LPA,* left pulmonary artery; *LVO,* left ventricular outflow pathway; *P,* pulmonary trunk; *RPA,* right pulmonary artery; *RVO,* right ventricular outflow pathway. (From Reller, M.D., et al. [1991]. Cardiac embryology. Basic review and clinical correlations. *J Am Soc Echocardiogr, 4,* 519.)

proliferation of subendocardial tissue as well as from connective tissue under the endocardium of the atrioventricular canals. These, too, become hollowed out, but on the ventricular side. The atrioventricular valves remain connected to the ventricular wall via muscular strands that are both papillary muscles and chordae tendineae. The mitral valve develops two cusps; the tricuspid has three.[26,101,112]

Conducting System

The initial pacemaker of the cardiac muscle is located in the caudal part of the left cardiac tube. Because the muscle layers of the atrium and ventricle are continuous, this temporary pacemaker is effective in controlling contractions throughout the primitive heart. Once the sinus venosus develops, the excitatory center (sinoatrial node) is found in the right wall. This node is incorporated into the right atrium along with the sinus venosus, where it lies near the entrance of the superior vena cava.[26,112]

Once the sinus venosus is incorporated into the atrium, cells from the left wall of the sinus venosus can be found in the base of the interatrial septum. When combined with cells from the atrioventricular canal, the atrioventricular (AV) node and the bundle of His are formed. These structures can be identified in embryos early in the second month of gestation.[26,112]

The Purkinje fibers constitute one of the most unusual features of the heart muscle. These cells are responsible for the initiation and propagation of the cardiac impulse and ensuring a regular contraction sequence within the organ. Although they are cardiac muscle cells, they are specialized through differentiation for conduction rather than contraction. These cells have fewer fibrils and are larger in diameter than the rest of the cardiac muscle cells. Purkinje cells are located external to the endocardium and run without interruption from the atrium to the ventricle as the atrioventricular bundle.[26] A fibrous band of connective tissue eventually separates the muscles of the atria and ventricles. This results in the atrioventricular node and bundle of His being the only conductive pathways between the upper and lower halves of the heart.

Blood Vessels

Blood vessels consist of an endothelial lining stabilized by an outer coat of connective tissue. The formation of blood vessels involves either vasculogenesis or angiogenesis. Vasculogenesis is "process by which endothelial progenitor cells are recruited and differentiate into mature endothelial cells to form new blood vessels."[51, p. 1293] Angiogenesis involves sprouting of new blood vessels from existing ones.[51] In most organ systems, both processes are involved.

The earliest vessels are derived from angioblastic tissue, which differentiates from the mesenchyme that covers the yolk sac, within the connecting stalk and in the wall of the chorionic sac. The impetus for vascular differentiation seems to be the reduction of nutrients within the yolk sac, which leads to an urgent need for a vascular system to supply nutrients to the cells.[26,61,112]

Masses of isolated angioblasts come together and form blood islands. Soon spaces can be seen in these islands, around which the angioblasts will arrange themselves. This results in lumen formation and the development of a primitive endothelial layer. The isolated vessels fuse to form a network of channels and extend to adjacent areas either through growth (endothelial budding) or by fusion with other independently formed vessels. Mesenchymal cells surrounding the primitive endothelial vessels differentiate into the muscle and connective layers of the vessels.[112]

Endothelial tissue first appears in the yolk sac wall as isolated cellular cords that develop a lumen. As these vessels join together, a network of endothelial vitelline vessels is formed. By extension and growth the network progressively reaches the embryonic body.[26] Primitive plasma and blood cells are developed from endothelial cells trapped within the vessels of the yolk sac and allantois. Blood formation in the embryo begins in the liver after 5 to 6 weeks (see Chapter 8).[26,112]

The endothelial lining of vessels develops before circulation begins. However, once circulation begins, the hemodynamics of blood flow influences the growth of the endothelium and the differentiation of the other parts of the vessel wall. The developing organs and the temporal sequence and metabolic demands of those organs may also influence the differentiation of vessels.[26]

The first vessels seen within the embryonic body seem to form from a diffuse network that runs throughout the embryonic mesenchyme. As tissues and organs differentiate, the regional networks elaborate to meet metabolic demands. The earliest vessels are simple endothelial tubes; differentiation of arteries from veins is not possible. As development continues, the tunica media and tunica adventitia of the definitive arteries and veins arise from mesenchymal tissue.[26]

Arteries. The aortic arches are essential in the primitive circulatory system. These vessels arise from the aortic sac and terminate in the dorsal aorta. A total of five pairs develop;

however, the third, fourth, and fifth arches are the only ones to contribute to the great vessels. By the end of the eighth week, the adult pattern has been established.[112]

The right and left dorsal aortae are the primary embryonic arteries. Initially these vessels are continuations of the endocardial tubes and can be divided into three portions: a short, ventral, ascending portion that supplies blood to the forebrain; a primitive first aortic arch that lies in the mesenchyme of the mandibular arch (pharynx); and a relatively long, descending portion that distributes blood to the embryonic body, yolk sac, and chorion via the segmental plexuses, vitelline vessels, and umbilical branches, respectively. The paired dorsal aortae initially run the length of the embryo. As development continues, the two fuse just caudal to the branchial region so that there is only a single midline vessel in the caudal part of the embryo.[26]

There are three major arterial branches that run off the dorsal aorta above the level of right and left aortic fusion. The intersegmental arteries are a group of 30 or more vessels that pass between and carry blood to the somites and their derivatives, which will form the muscular and bony elements of this region. In the cervical region the first seven intersegmental arteries are connected by a longitudinal anastomosis that forms the vertebral artery. The proximal segments of the first six arteries disappear, and the seventh intersegmental artery becomes the subclavian artery.[112]

The somatic arteries also arise from this group of vessels. Eventually the intercostal arteries, lumbar arteries, common iliac arteries, and lateral sacral arteries can be identified.[112] The midline branches of the dorsal aorta run to the yolk sac, allantois, and chorion. There are two main groups: the lateral branches and the ventral branches. The ventral or vitelline arteries supply the yolk sac and the gut. These vessels will eventually be reduced to three persisting vessels: the celiac, superior mesenteric, and inferior mesenteric arteries. These vessels service the foregut, midgut, and hindgut, respectively.[112] The lateral branches supply the nephrogenic ridge and its derivatives. At first there are several branches, but retrogression results in four vessels remaining in the mature organism. These vessels are the phrenic, suprarenal, renal, and gonadal arteries.

Umbilical Arteries. By far the largest of the dorsal aortic vessels are the paired umbilical arteries (UAs). These vessels pass through the connecting stalk (umbilical cord) and become continuous with the chorionic vessels in the developing placenta. After delivery the proximal portions of these arteries become the internal iliac and superior vesical arteries. The distal portions are obliterated and become the medial umbilical ligaments.

Veins. There are three sets of paired veins that drain into the heart of the 4-week-old (6 weeks menstrual age) embryo. These are the vitelline veins, which return blood from the yolk sac; the umbilical veins, which bring oxygenated blood from the chorion; and the cardinal veins, which return blood from the body.[175]

Vitelline Veins. The vitelline veins follow the yolk stalk and ascend on either side of the foregut. They then pass through the septum transversum and enter the sinus venosus of the heart. As the primitive liver grows into the septum transversum, the hepatic sinusoids become linked with the vitelline veins. As the right vitelline vein begins to disintegrate, parts are incorporated into the developing hepatic vessels. The portal vein develops from the vitelline-derived vessels that surround the duodenum.

Umbilical Veins. The umbilical veins originate as a pair of vessels; however, the right vein and part of the left degenerate so that only a single vessel remains to return blood from the placenta to the fetus. As these vessels degenerate, the DV develops in the liver and connects the remaining umbilical vein with the inferior vena cava. At birth the umbilical vein and the DV are obliterated with the cutting of the umbilical cord and the modifications in the circulation. The remnants of the vessels are the ligamentum teres and ligamentum venosum, respectively.

Cardinal Veins. Very early in the embryonic period, the cardinal vessels are the main drainage system. The anterior and posterior cardinal veins bring blood from the cranial and caudal regions and empty into the heart via a common cardinal vein that enters the sinus venosus on each side. By the eighth week the anterior cardinal veins are connected through an anastomosis that allows for shunting of blood from the left vein to the right. This connection becomes the left brachiocephalic vein. The right anterior and right common cardinal veins form the superior vena cava. The posterior cardinal veins are transitional vessels. These vessels service the mesonephric kidneys and disappear when these transient kidneys degenerate. The subcardinal and supracardinal vessels develop gradually and facilitate perfusion of the mesonephric kidneys. These vessels do not degenerate entirely, as do the posterior cardinal veins, but contribute to the development of the inferior vena cava.

The inferior vena cava is the result of a series of changes in the embryonic veins of the trunk. The four main segments of the inferior vena cava are derived from the hepatic vein and hepatic sinusoids (hepatic segment), the right subcardinal vein (prerenal segment), the subcardinal and supracardinal anastomosis (renal segment), and the right supracardinal vein (postrenal segment).[112,175]

Developmental Basis for Common Anomalies

Development of the heart is controlled by a group of cardiac genes and transcription factors that are expressed in a specific sequence. Alterations in these genes or factors or in their sequencing may lead to agenesis or aplasia (failure in development), hypoplasia (incomplete or defective development), dysplasia (abnormal development), malposition, failure of fusion of adjoining parts, abnormal fusion, incomplete reabsorption, persistence of a vessel, or early obliteration of a vessel and thus cardiac defects.[26] Cardiac defects are the most common congenital defect and are seen in 0.8% to 1% of liveborn infants and 10% of spontaneous abortions.[21,163] About one fourth of spontaneous abortions with cardiac defects have other noncardiac problems.[26,174] The most common heart defects arise from alterations in sepatation, valve formation, and patterning of the great vessels.[168]

Currently 57% to 83% of critical cardiac malformations and one-third of all congenital heart defects are detected by prenatal ultrasound.[163] Doppler evaluation of the fetal cardiovascular system includes arterial (evaluation of individual arterial beds such as the uterus, umbilical artery and cerebral circulation), venous (evaluation of the ductus venosus, inferior vena cava, umbilical vein, and hepatic veins), and intracardiac evaluations. Doppler evaluations are used to evaluate fetal growth restriction and to assess potential complications such as preeclampsia, twin to twin transfusion, fetal hydrops and, arrhythmias.[14,15,155,175]

The major structures of the heart are completed by 8 weeks after fertilization (10 weeks postmenstrual age).[168] Timing of development of major anomalies is summarized in Table 9-7. Most major defects arise during weeks 6 to 7 of development. However, lesions may continue to evolve during the remainder of gestation. For example, ventricular inflammation, outflow tract obstruction, arch obstruction, ventricular, aortic or pulmonary artery hypoplasia may develop or progress. Arterioventricular or semilunar valve regurgitation may compromise fetal circulation. Alterations in rhythms may lead to myocardial disease or heart failure may develop. Newer imaging techniques and fetal echocardiography have led to a better diagnosis of congenital heart defects before birth and the potential for the development of earlier therapies.[14,15,104,153,175] These therapies are done to decrease the risk of fetal or early neonatal death or to decrease the risk of a primary anomaly developing into a more severe one.[104] Therapies can be either pharmacologic interventions (see Chapter 7) or procedures such as fetal aortic valvuloplasty done via percutaneous needle insertion in infants with aortic stenosis or hypoplastic left heart syndrome with atrial septum restriction, pulmonary atresia, or pulmonary stenosis.[104]

The brain and heart develop simultaneously and share genes and signaling pathways. Children with alterations in development of the heart have a higher frequency of focal brain injury and white matter injury.[105] This may be due to abnormal cerebral blood flow in early development, especially in infants with hypoplastic left heart syndrome and d-transposition of the great vessels, with increased risk of injury.[105]

The etiology of most congenital heart defects is incompletely understood, but is thought to include both genetic and environmental factors in most nonsyndrome congenital heart defects.[163] In about 8% of children there is a clear genetic cause; most are associated with obvious chromosomal anomalies (e.g., Down, Cri-du chat, trisomy 18, trisomy 13, and Turner syndrome). The incidence of cardiac defects is about 40% in infants with Down syndrome and higher in infants with trisomy 13 and 18.[174] Many of the single-gene and other inherited syndromes, including Marfan, Williams, and DiGeorge syndromes, are associated with heart disease. However, these syndromes account for only about 3% of all congenital heart defects.[21] Environmental factors may also play a role in the etiology of congenital cardiac malformations. Fetal exposure to teratogens through maternal ingestion of drugs such as antiepileptic drugs or warfarin, or alcohol, as well as viral infections (e.g., rubella or cytomegalovirus), can result in alterations in cardiac development. These variables account for about 2% of known congenital heart disease. Maternal disorders such as diabetes mellitus and phenylketonuria also increase the risk of fetal cardiac defects.[21] For example, the frequency of cardiac defects in infants of women with diabetes mellitus is two to four times higher than normal. Systemic lupus erythematosus is associated with fetal heart block (see Chapter 13).

In the remaining 85% of infants with defects, there is no clear cause. Some are due to multifactorial inheritance (see Chapter 1) in which there may be a heritable predisposition for cardiac anomalies. This combined with some type of environmental trigger during a vulnerable period results in abnormal development. Implications of selected congenital heart defects are discussed in "Clinical Implications for Neonatal Care."

Functional Development

Functional development of the heart involves maturation of the fetal myocardium, myocardial performance, fetal circulation, control of fetal circulation, oxygenation, and heart rate. Heart rate, fetal acid-base balance, control of heart rate, and fetal responses to hypoxia and asphyxia are discussed in depth in Chapter 6.

Fetal Myocardium

The fetal myocyte has a small amount of contractile tissue, which is restricted to the subsarcolemmal region. About 60% of the myocardial tissue consists of noncontractile mass in the fetus (versus 30% in adults).[99,142,158,178] The fetal myocardium has fewer myofibrils, which are arranged in a more random fashion rather than in a parallel organization as occurs in adults.[5,47,139] These changes, along with the decreased number of sarcomeres per gram of ventricular muscle and increased water content, limit the amount of force that the fetus can generate per unit of area.[140] The sarcoplasmic reticulum in the fetal myocardium is reduced and less organized, reducing calcium sequestration and altering calcium transport and thus contractility.[177] Therefore the fetal heart is more dependent on trans-sarcolemmal calcium movement with lower intracellular concentrations. As a result, the fetal myocardium develops less contractile force, with a lower velocity of shortening and reextension.

The fetal myocardium is less compliant than that of the adult, although the relationship between muscle length and force is qualitatively similar. The decreased compliance may be due in part to constraint of the pericardium, lungs, and chest.[83] As extrauterine growth occurs, the compliance of both ventricles increases. Right-side pressures are greater than left-side pressures in the fetus, so blood flows from right to left across the foramen ovale from the right atrium to left atrium or across the ductus arteriosus (DA) from the pulmonary artery to aorta.[5,83,140]

Metabolism is also immature in the fetal myocardium. Lactate is the main energy source in the fetal and neonatal myocardium versus long chain fatty acids (LCFAs) in adults due to limitations in fatty acid transport from decreased activity of enzymes needed to transport LCFAs into the mitochondria.[142,177] However, the fetal heart has an increased ability to utilize anaerobic metabolism, which partially compensates for these limitations.

Myocardial Performance

After birth, when circulation flows in series (Figure 9-11, *B*), the stroke volume of the RV equals that of the LV. However, in the fetus, which is not dependent upon the lungs to oxygenate the blood, circulation is arranged in a parallel fashion (see Figure 9-11, *A*). This arrangement allows for mixing of oxygenated blood with deoxygenated blood at the atrial and great vessel levels. Blood from the RV and LV is mixed in the descending aorta below the DA. The modifications in the circulation that allow for this mixing divert blood from the immature lungs to the placenta, where oxygen–carbon dioxide exchange occurs. Stroke volumes of the two fetal ventricles are not equal. The fetus sends 65% of the venous return to the RV and 25% to the LV; therefore RV stroke volume is 28% greater than that in the LV.[47] As a result of these differences, cardiac output in the fetus is defined as the total output of the RV and LV, or the combined cardiac output (CCO).[47] The RV pumps up to two thirds of the combined ventricular output.[125,140] RV stroke volume is greater than that of the LV and plays a major role in maintaining CCO.[118,142] The RV is responsible for delivering blood to the descending aorta, lower body, and placenta; LV output goes primarily to the cerebral and coronary circulations with little going to the lower body.[118,142]

The fetal resting cardiac output is the highest of any time of life with a CCO of 450 to 500 mL/min/kg at term.[85] The high fetal cardiac output may be necessary to meet the high fetal oxygen consumption demands. When compared to that of the adult, fetal oxygen consumption is 1½ to 2 times higher. This may be an adaptive mechanism for the low oxygen tension found in the fetal state.[7] The ability to maintain this high output is due to the elevated heart rate and the cardiac shunts. Changes in fetal cardiac output seem to be directly related to fetal heart rate (FHR) changes, with reduced sensitivity to preload and afterload.[177] A 10% increase in FHR above the resting level is associated with an increase in both right and left ventricular output; a decrease in heart rate results in a decrease in combined ventricular output.

In the fetal heart, the RV and LV have stages of filling that are similar to those in the adult; however, the end-diastolic dimensions of the RV are larger than those of the LV. There also seems to be a difference in the rate of filling between the ventricles. In the fetus, an increase in RV volume or afterload

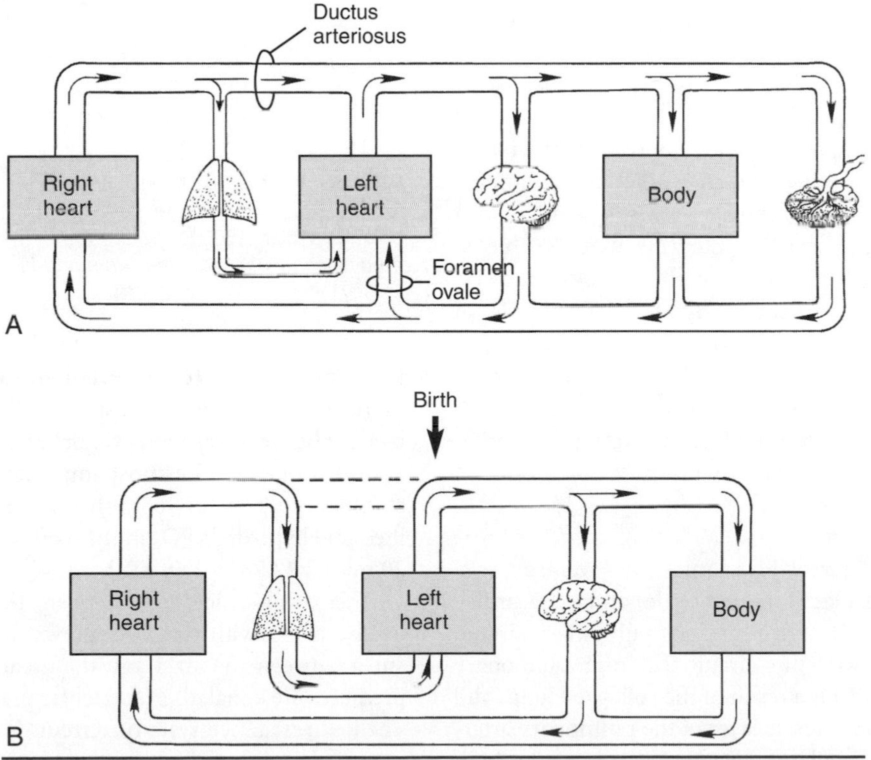

FIGURE 9-11 Comparison of **(A)** fetal (parallel) with **(B)** adult (series) circulatory systems. (Modified from Dawes, G.S. [1968]. *Fetal and neonatal physiology.* Chicago: Year Book, by Bloom, R.S. [2006]. Delivery room resuscitation of the newborn. In R.J. Martin, A.A. Fanaroff, & M.C. Walsh [Eds.]. *Fanaroff and Martin's Neonatal-perinatal medicine: Diseases of the fetus and infant* [8th ed.]. Philadelphia: Mosby.)

interferes with LV filling. The Frank-Starling relationship is present and a primary regulator of fetal cardiac output.[5,47,83] However, fetal cardiac function is less responsive to changes in preload and afterload.[101] There may be less functional reserve because the fetal heart functions at the maximum and interventions such as volume infusion do not significantly increase stroke volume and output.[142] Heart rate is the most effective way for the fetus to increase ventricular function and cardiac output.[83,101,118]

In terms of afterload, the fetal myocardium shortens more slowly when compared with adult tissue. This fetal liability is to be expected given the maturation of the force-generating ability of the myocardium. Arterial pressure is a major component of afterload and has a significant effect on ejection (the higher the pressure, the smaller the stroke volume). This relationship holds throughout development, although the neonate seems to be less tolerant of increases in arterial pressure.[9,102]

Changes in inotropy (the strength of myocardial contractions) reflect a change in the ability of the myocardium to contract, and maturational development affects inotropy in the fetus and neonate. These changes are probably related to the availability of calcium and the control of cytosolic calcium. The development of the sarcomeres and their intracellular control mechanisms is integrally tied to this process. The sarcoplasmic reticulum calcium pump is immature and less able to remove calcium, leading to less relaxation of the fetal heart in response to sympathetic stimulation.[101]

Heart rate also affects the strength of contraction in a positive way in the fetus, neonate, and adult. In fetal lambs, however, as heart rate increases, stroke volume decreases. This is most likely due to a decrease in end-diastolic volume that is a natural consequence of the increased heart rate. Conflicting data have been found in studies of the human fetus, although the majority of studies suggest a positive effect of heart rate on ventricular output. This may be due to additional factors that have inotropic effects.[9] Systemic systolic blood pressure is 15 to 20 mmHg (1.99 to 2.66 kPa) at 16 weeks rising to 30 to 40 mmHg (3.99 to 5.32 kPa) at 28 weeks.[83] Diastolic is $<$5 mmHg ($<$0.67 kPa) at 16 to 18 weeks and 5 to 15 mmHg (0.67 to 1.99 kPa) at 19 to 26 weeks.[83] Umbilical venous pressure increases from 4.5 mmHg (0.60 kPa) at 18 weeks to 6 mmHg (0.80 kPa) at term.[83]

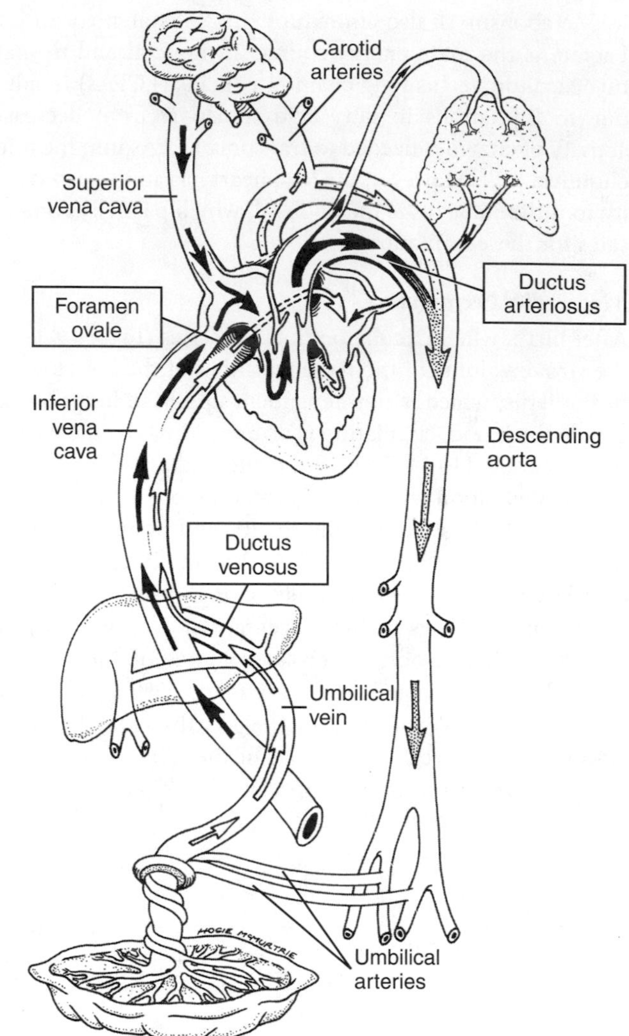

FIGURE 9-12 Fetal circulation. (From Bloom, R.S. [2006]. Delivery room resuscitation of the newborn. In R.J. Martin, A.A. Fanaroff, & M.C. Walsh [Eds.]. *Fanaroff and Martin's Neonatal-perinatal medicine: Diseases of the fetus and infant* [8th ed.]. Philadelphia: Mosby.)

Fetal Circulation

The fetal circulation (Figure 9-12) is unique in several aspects: (1) presence of intracardiac (foramen ovale) and extracardiac (DV and DA) shunts; (2) high-resistance pulmonary circuit; and (3) low-resistance systemic circuit. The high pulmonary vascular resistance (PVR) is a result of the collapsed lungs and the thick medial smooth muscle layer of the pulmonary arteries (see Pulmonary Vasculature).[140] As a result of the high PVR and collapsed lungs, blood flow to the lungs is low in the fetus, although some is retained to support lung growth and development (see Pulmonary Vasculature). The high resting tone and PVR in the fetus are thought to be maintained by mechanical factors (compression of small pulmonary arteries by the fluid-filled alveolar spaces), the low fetal PO_2, and a balance between vasoconstrictors and vasodilators that favors vasoconstriction. The most important pulmonary vasoconstrictors are probably endothelin, arachidonic acid metabolites, and hypoxia.[17] PO_2 in the fetal pulmonary circuit is 17 to 20 mmHg (2.26 to 2.66 kPa).

The communication between the atria (i.e., foramen ovale), along with the DA, allows for equalization of pressures between the atria and the great vessels. Because these pressures are equal, the ventricular pressures are also equal.[180] The low-resistance systemic circuit is also due to the passive nature of umbilical and placental blood flow.[180]

As noted previously, blood flow in the fetus is arranged in a parallel fashion (see Figure 9-11, *A*). This arrangement results in mixing of oxygenated blood at the atrial and great vessel levels. The fetal shunts allow for this mixing, which diverts blood from the immature lungs to the placenta, where oxygen-carbon dioxide exchange takes place. As a result, 40% to 50% of the fetal cardiac output is directed toward the placenta, with 14% to brain and no more than 10% to 12% to lungs.[19] The remainder is divided among the gastrointestinal tract, kidneys, and the rest of body. The fetal liver is the first organ to receive maternal substances, followed by the heart and brain.

As the blood returns from the placenta to the fetus via the umbilical vein (UV), it passes either into the portal system's microcirculation to later run off into the inferior vena cava (IVC) or into the DV. The DV is a narrow trumpet–shaped structure that originates from the UV as it turns below the liver.[14,83] The DV is narrowest at the UV end with a mean diameter of 0.5 mm at midgestation increasing to no more than 2 mm by term.[83] The DV connects, via the umbilical vein–portal sinus, to the IVC just below the diaphragm (see Figure 9-12). The DV is important in nutrient and oxygen partitioning.[14] At 20 weeks, 30% of the blood flow from the UV is shunted across the DV, decreasing to 18% to 20% by 32 weeks.[17,83,98,175] By late pregnancy, 70% to 80% of the oxygenated blood from the placenta goes first to the liver, reflecting an increased priority of the liver needs near term.[83] DV shunting is influenced by its diameter, pressure gradients and blood viscosity.[98] An increase in the diameter of the DV increases the proportion of DV blood reaching the heart and down regulates the volume of blood going to the left lobe of the liver.[14] With hypovolemia or hypoxemia, more blood is shunted across the DV and thus to the heart.[17,83] Shunting across the DV is also increased in fetal growth restriction, even under stable conditions.[83]

The liver blood supply consists of blood from the UV (80%), portal vein (15%), and hepatic artery (5%).[47] UV blood entering the liver flows to both lobes; portal venous blood is directed primarily to the right lobe.[123] Therefore 95% of the blood flow to the left lobe comes from the UV. The right lobe blood supply comes from the UV (40% to 60%), portal vein (30% to 50%), and hepatic artery (10%).[47,63]

The DV is a low-resistance channel that allows a portion of relatively well-oxygenated blood to enter the heart directly. Normal flow is phasic and anterograde. Abnormal flow patterns in the DV may indicate fetal stress.[142] The DV is under tonic adrenergic control and dilates in the presence of nitric oxide, prostaglandins, and hypoxemia.[83,126] The blood entering the IVC from the UV via the DV joins with the blood that returns from the lower half of the fetal body. The blood that reaches the IVC from the umbilical vein has a greater oxygen content and kinetic energy and so stays in a stream that is separate from the blood returning from the lower body.[14,19,83] Because of this preferential streaming, DV blood is found along the left dorsal wall of the IVC.[47,93] Altered DV flow in early pregnancy and low velocity IVC flow are associated with fetal acidemia, aneuploidy, hydrops, arrhythmias, and cardiac defects.[14,98,117,161]

As the IVC blood enters the right atrium, a tissue flap, the eustachian valve, at the junction of the RA and IVC directs blood from the dorsal portion of the IVC (i.e., where the more highly oxygenated blood from the UV streams) toward the crista dividens and foramen ovale; the lower velocity blood is directed toward the tricuspid valve.[47,175] The foramen ovale is formed by the overlap of the atrial septum secundum over the atrial septum primum (see Figure 9-9). Patency of the foramen ovale is maintained by increased blood flow and pressure in the right versus left atrium.[19,83] The crista dividens (the free edge of the atrial septum) separates the flow into two streams, with 50% to 60% being diverted across the foramen ovale into the left atrium.

In the left atrium the blood from the IVC mixes with the (minimal) pulmonary venous return and passes through the mitral valve into the LV. Thus most of the blood in the LA and LV is the more oxygenated umbilical vein blood. Upon contraction of the heart, this blood is ejected into the ascending aorta to feed the coronary, left carotid, and subclavian arteries. Only 10% of fetal CO continues across the aortic isthmus into the descending aorta.[85]

The aortic isthmus (between the left subclavian and ductus arteriosus) is the area between blood ejected from the RV and LV. Normally flow is both systolic and diastolic and anterograde across the isthmus, but with fetal stress diastolic flow may become retrograde as a compensatory response to preserve cerebral perfusion.[142]

The blood flowing along the anterior portion of the IVC consists of hepatic and lower body desaturated blood. This blood mixes with blood from the superior vena cava (SVC) and coronary sinus in the right atrium. This blood flow is directed downward across the tricuspid valve and into the RV. Very little of the SVC blood return crosses the foramen ovale to the left atrium. Venous return to the RA is about two thirds blood from the IVC (about one third of which is blood from the UV and DV), about one third from the SVC, and about 3% from the coronary sinus.[47]

The mixed blood in the right ventricle is then ejected into the pulmonary artery, where increased PVR prevents more than 10% to 12% of the RV blood flow (or about 8% of the CCO) from entering the pulmonary bed. In the second half of pregnancy, less than 40% of the CCO is shunted across the DA to enter the descending aorta and the low-resistance systemic and placental circulations.[83,85] Blood flow to the pulmonary bed increases after 30 weeks to up to 30% of the CCO, perhaps due to growth and thus increased metabolic need of the lungs.[47,83] Decreased diastolic flow and increased pulsations are associated with placental infection and twin-to-twin transfusion.[142]

The DA is similar in size to the descending aorta and pulmonary artery. The medial layer of the DA consists of longitudinal and spiral layers of smooth muscle surrounded by concentric layers of elastic tissue; the intima consists of thick neointimal cushions made up of smooth muscle and endothelial cells.[59] The DA smooth muscle is the site of oxygen sensors; the endothelium releases vasoactive substances such as PGE_2 and PGI_2 to modulate DA tone.[59]

The low fetal PO_2 and high levels of circulating prostaglandins (especially PGE_1, PGE_2, and PGI_2) maintain patency of the DA in utero. Prostaglandins are normally metabolized in the lungs. Because pulmonary blood flow is so low in the fetus, PGs are metabolized more slowly and therefore levels remain high. PGE_2 is the most powerful and interacts with receptors (EP_2, EP_3, EP_4) on the ductal wall. This interaction activates adenylate cyclase, which increases cAMP to decrease sensitivity of the ductus to calcium and help maintain relaxation. Stimulation of EP_3 opens K-ATP channels to hyperpolarize the ductus and reduces tone.[32] Reactivity of the DA increases in the late third trimester increasing its vulnerability to the constricting effects of prostaglandin synthatase inhibitors such as indomethacin.[83] Blood returns to the placenta via the two UAs, which arise from the internal iliac arteries. The UAs spiral around the umbilical vein in the cord, then anastomose near the placental surface to equalize arterial pressures.[2] The UA wall is relatively thick in comparison to its lumen size with several layers of vascular smooth muscle cells but no internal elastic lamina.[2]

Fetal circulation is not significantly altered by increased intrauterine pressure with uterine contractions in the healthy fetal-placental unit. Even with compression of the placental vessels, the vessels are relatively unreactive to short-term changes.[47]

Oxygen Content

The oxygen content of the fetus is lower than that of the neonate, child, or adult. The highest oxygen content is found in the blood returning from the placenta via the umbilical vein, which is 30 to 35 mmHg (3.99 to 4.65 kPav) and 80% to 90% saturated.[47,85] This falls to 26 to 28 mmHg (3.45 to 3.72 kPav) (saturation, 65%) by the time it reaches the left atrium and mixes with blood from the IVC and pulmonary veins and is ejected into the ascending aorta.[85]

The umbilical return that mixes with the superior vena caval blood (PO_2, 12 to 14 mmHg [1.59 to 1.86 kPav]; saturation, 40%) is reduced to a PaO_2 of 15 to 25 mmHg (1.99 to 3.32 kPaa).[47,85,140] This blood is destined for the pulmonary arteries, descending aorta (55% saturated), upper torso, and placenta. Therefore the blood with the highest oxygen content is delivered to the coronary arteries and brain, whereas the blood with the lowest PaO_2 is shunted toward the placenta, where reoxygenation occurs.

Another fetal adaptation to low oxygen tension is the presence of fetal hemoglobin. This specific type of hemoglobin has a high affinity for oxygen even at low oxygen tensions, thereby improving saturation and facilitating transport of oxygen to the tissues. The perfusion rate is greater in the fetus than adult, which helps compensate for the lower oxygen saturations and increased oxygen-hemoglobin affinity.[19] The low oxygen tension in the fetus keeps the pulmonary vasculature constricted and, along with PGE_2, the DA dilated.[19] See Chapters 8 and 10 for a further discussion of fetal hemoglobin and oxygenation.

Control of Fetal Circulation

Fetal circulation is controlled by neural inputs and humoral factors, such as catecholamines, vasopressin, angiotensin II, and prostaglandins. Baroreceptors in the aortic arch and carotid arteries are sensitive to changes in systemic arterial pressure. With development, the sensitivity of the arterial baroreflex changes and is reset as blood pressure increases.[146] The mechanism for this is not well understood but involves both peripheral and central resetting. Endogenous nitric oxide, angiotensin II, serotonin, and changes in basal autonomic nerve sensitivity may all modulate this process.[146] Carotid receptor stimulation leads to a mild tachycardia and marked increase in blood pressure, whereas stimulation of aortic chemoreceptors leads to bradycardia and a slight increase in blood pressure.[47] Natriuretic peptides are functional by midgestation and have a role in volume and blood pressure regulation.[37]

Sympathetic innervation is immature, with parasympathetic (vagal) dominance. Both vagal and sympathetic tone increase with fetal hypoxia. Parasympathetic stimulation has a primary job in maintaining FHR and beat-to-beat variability. The sympathetic nervous system provides a reserve to improve the heart's pumping ability during intermittent stress. Cholinergic fibers develop early in gestation. α-Adrenergic and β-adrenergic fibers also appear early and increase with gestation.[47] If oxygen content of the fetal blood decreases, blood flow to the brain, myocardium, and adrenals increases; pulmonary blood flow and flow to the lower body decreases.[47] Autonomic control of fetal circulation is discussed further in Chapter 6.

NEONATAL PHYSIOLOGY

The cardiovascular system is designed to deliver adequate oxygen and nutrients to the tissues and remove metabolic by-products at all stages of development. The coordinated functioning of respiratory, cardiovascular, and endocrine systems is essential to meet the cellular metabolic needs, especially in times of stress. During fetal, neonatal, and adult life, these processes are quite different, and maturational processes continue after birth. Alterations or a delay in transitional circulation processes in the preterm infant can result in low systemic blood flow and hypotension.[86]

Transitional Events

At birth the cardiac output (CO) is redistributed with increased pulmonary blood flow. Pulmonary and systemic pressure change as pulmonary vascular resistance (PVR) decreases and systemic vascular resistance (SVR) increases. The ventricles begin working in series (see Figure 9-11, *B*), which is the adult configuration, rather than in parallel, and the fetal extracardiac and intracardiac shunts close. With birth, oxygenation is moved from the placenta to the lungs, and air ventilation results in increased oxygen availability, with a concomitant rise in PO_2 levels.

Epinephrine and norepinephrine levels increase during labor and at birth, decreasing to prebirth levels within four hours, although the increase in sympathetic outflow is maintained for at least 6 hours.[5,71,146] This surge may be related to the alterations in blood gases with birth, decreased ambient temperature, cord clamping, increased intracranial pressure, or other events during transition.[146] In addition, control mechanisms may override arterial baroreflexes to maintain high sympathetic tone with transition.[146] Epinephrine mediates increased CO and myocardial contractility, which are important for changes in myocardial function with birth and for enhancing contractility with the stresses of transition.[146] These responses may be attenuated in preterm infants.[146]

The changeover from fetal to neonatal circulation is linked directly with the development and function of the pulmonary vasculature and changes in PVR (see "Pulmonary Vasculature"). At delivery the low-resistance placental circulation is removed, leading to an increase in SVR.[102] The increased SVR is due to the increased volume of blood in the arterial system (i.e., blood that no longer has a placenta to return to), which must be accommodated in the systemic circulation, and to the decreasing PVR. As a result of these changes, systemic blood pressure demonstrates a sustained increase over the first hours to days after birth.[102,109]

The increased SVR may lead to transient myocardial dysfunction in very low birthweight infants due to the limited capacity of their myocardium and decreased systemic perfusion. Immature compensatory mechanisms may reduce cerebral blood flow and brain oxygen delivery increasing the risk of white matter injury or increase the risk of periventricular-intraventricular hemorrhage during the subsequent reperfusion phase.[118]

The initiation of air breathing leads to lung expansion, an increase in alveolar oxygen concentration, and vasodilation of the pulmonary vascular bed. As vasodilation occurs, PVR falls rapidly. At birth the PVR falls by almost 80%, resulting in a dramatic increase in pulmonary blood flow and a fall in ductal shunting. Before birth the high PVR and low SVR result in 90% of the right ventricle (RV) output going through the ductus. After delivery, 90% of this flow goes to the pulmonary arteries.[47] The left ventricle (LV) must now pump the entire CO (approximately 350 mL/kg). This change is mediated by the increase in circulating catecholamines and myocardial β-adrenergic receptors.[85]

Factors decreasing PVR at birth include lung aeration; increasing PO_2; and release of vasodilators such as bradykinin (which increases as PO_2 increases), PGE_1, PGE_2, PGI_2 (prostacyclin), nitric oxide, and endothelial-derived releasing factor (EDRF). Lung aeration and PO_2 are the most critical factors. Lung inflation and increasing PO_2 either alone or together (greatest effect) decrease PVR and increase nitric oxide.[17,140] Lung inflation stimulates pulmonary stretch receptors, leading to a reflexive vasodilation and a 4- to 10-fold increase in pulmonary blood flow.[47,140] Currently the major pulmonary vasodilators at birth are thought to be nitric oxide and prostacyclin, whose release may be mediated by gaseous expansion of the lungs. Adenosine, bradykinin, and possibly adrenomedullin may also have important roles.

Nitric oxide, a main component of endothelial-derived relaxing factor, is released by the endothelium and stimulated by oxygen.[17] Studies in fetal lambs suggest that both increased PO_2 and rapid increase in pulmonary blood flow (creating shear stress) induce endothelial nitric oxide synthetase (NOS) and thus increase nitric oxide levels with birth.[140] Increased NOS expression with oxygen stimulation develops late in gestation as the pulmonary vasculature become more sensitive to nitric oxide. Pulmonary vasoconstriction in utero is thought to be mediated by inhibition of nitric oxide production by substances such as endothelins.[180] Prostacyclin increases late in gestation and in the early postbirth period. Its action is thought to be stimulated by rhythmic lung distention rather than increased oxygenation. Oxygen may also mediate dilation by opening oxygen-sensitive potassium channels in the pulmonary smooth muscle.[140]

Umbilical blood flow is reduced to less than 20% of fetal values within 40 to 60 seconds after birth; diameters of the umbilical vein and arteries decrease significantly within 120 seconds. The exact cause of these changes is not clear, but may be related to exposure of the cord to the cooler, more highly oxygenated room temperature, although these are not the only factors in that contraction precedes the increase in oxygenation and cooling leads to transitional, not sustained, constriction.[2] Local vasoconstrictors such as serotonin may also play a role.[2]

Closure of the Ductus Venosus

The ductus venosus (DV) is functionally closed within minutes of birth due to cessation of blood flow. Cessation of placental blood flow is mediated by mechanical stimulation with stretching of the umbilical cord and its blood vessels. This enhances initial constriction of the umbilical blood vessels. The rapid increase in PO_2 with initiation of breathing maintains constriction of the umbilical vessels.[47] The DV is obliterated by one week in three fourths of term infants and in most by 10 to 14 days.[49] The DV remains open longer in preterm infants and infants with persistent pulmonary hypertension and cardiac malformations.[83] Closure is probably mediated by endothelin-1 and thromboxane A_2.[101]

Closure of the Foramen Ovale

Alterations at birth lead to pressure changes within the cardiac chambers and the movement from parallel circulation to in-series circulation. The pressure changes result from the rapid drop in systemic venous return via the inferior vena cava (IVC) and the increase in pulmonary venous return. The left atrial pressure rises, exceeding the right atrial pressure, and the foramen ovale's flap valve closes, functionally separating the two atria. The foramen ovale usually closes anatomically by 30 months but may remain patent into childhood or longer.[47,101,123] In 15% to 25% of adults the flaps remain open enough for a probe to be easily passed through them. This opening occurs without significant right to left shunting.[44,85,140] A patent foramen ovale in adults is associated with a risk of paradoxical systemic embolism, refractory hypoxemia in individual with myocardial infarction or pulmonary disease, migraine headaches with aura, and neurologic decompression illness in divers, high altitude pilots, and astronauts.[44]

Closure of the Ductus Arteriosus

The ductus arteriosus (DA) begins to close almost immediately after birth but remains patent for several hours to days following delivery. The pulmonary vascular resistance (PVR) may remain higher than the systemic vascular bed for a short time following the first breath. This allows for a small right-to-left shunt to remain and for desaturated blood to mix with oxygenated blood in the descending aorta. If the PVR remains high or is increased during the first hours or days after delivery, the right-to-left shunt may become clinically significant, as is seen in persistent pulmonary hypertension of the newborn.

As the systemic vascular resistance (SVR) continues to increase and stabilize and the PVR continues to fall, the movement of blood across the DA reverses and becomes left to right. For a time, flow is bidirectional, with both right-to-left and left-to-right flow, but then right-to-left flow ceases. Within the first 10 to 15 hours of extrauterine life in most term infants, the DA achieves functional closure through smooth muscle constriction.[101] By 96 hours of age, the DA is functionally closed in nearly all term infants.[32,49,123] The DA remains open for a longer period in preterm infants (see Patent Ductus Arteriosus in the Preterm Infant). In most healthy preterm infants greater than 30 weeks' gestation, the DA has closed functionally by 4 days. Only 11% of these infants have a patent ductus arteriosus (PDA) versus 65% of infants younger than 30 weeks' gestation with severe respiratory distress.[32]

Anatomic closure takes longer and is usually achieved within 2 to 3 months. During this time, the ductus may be reopened if hypoxia or increased PVR is encountered. This may occur with prolonged crying or with pathologic problems. Anatomic closure involves neointimal thickening with endothelial destruction and loss of smooth muscle cells from the inner muscle media, proliferation of subintimal tissue, and formation of connective tissues to form a fibrous strand known as the ligamentum arteriosus.[47,77] By term the DA has a very thick wall and requires an intramural vasa vasorum to provide nutrients to the outer muscle. Constriction of the DA obliterates the vasa vasorum and the muscle becomes avascular and hypoxic. This ischemic hypoxia of the ductal wall inhibits PGE_2 and NO and induces growth factors and apoptosis of smooth muscle in the ductal wall.[77]

Functional closure of the DA at birth is influenced primarily by oxygen and vasoactive substances (particularly prostaglandins) rather than primarily hemodynamic changes, as is seen with closure of the foramen ovale and DV.[47] Factors favoring DA dilation include PGE_1, PGE_2, PGI_2, hypoxia, and acidosis, whereas factors favoring DA constriction include PGF_2, prostaglandin synthetase, increased PO_2 and pH, endotheklin-1, and bradykinin.[19,59,76,123]

Although there is a relative hypoxia present at birth (when compared with adult oxygen levels), within 10 minutes the neonate has a PaO_2 of 50 mmHg (6.65 kPaa). This continues to increase over the first hour to approximately 62 mmHg (8.24 kPaa). Arterial oxygen concentrations stabilize between 75 and 85 mmHg (9.97 to 11.30 kPa) over the first 2 days, with a concomitant fall in PVR and improved ventilation-perfusion ratios. The fall in PVR continues for the next several weeks; however, the adult circulatory pattern is usually achieved within the first 2 days.[7]

The increased PaO_2 alters ductal smooth muscle membrane potential mediated by a cytochrome P450 hemoprotein, which leads to increased calcium influx and contraction or by altering potassium channels. Potassium modulates voltage-gated calcium channels, opening them to increase the influx of calcium.[59] Potassium channels in the ductus change during gestation to ones that can be inhibited by oxygen.[32] Endothelin-1, which may be induced by the increased PaO_2 after birth, increases intracellular calcium via G-protein coupling.[76] The Rho/Rho kinase pathways induce calcium sensitization (via persistent myosin light chain phosphorylation) and vasoconstriction.[59,76] Platelets may also be involved in DA closure by enhancing sealing of the constricted DA; proinflammatory cytokines inhibit this thrombic sealing.[42,59]

PGE_2 is thought to be primarily responsible for maintaining the patency of the DA during fetal life. The DA is extremely sensitive to PGE_2, and it is the loss of this reactivity that keeps the ductus closed after birth. Just before birth there is a decrease in circulating PGE_2 concentrations, possibly due to an increase in pulmonary blood flow that enhances delivery of PGE_2 to the lungs for metabolism. This may prepare for or enhance ductal closure at the time the infant converts to air breathing and active ductal constriction occurs.[7,47] Prostaglandin receptors in the ductal wall also decrease, further reducing PGE_2 efficacy. The continued decrease in PGE_2 with birth is related to increased pulmonary blood flow and increased lung metabolic activity as well as removal of the placenta, the main source of PGE_2 in the fetus.[47,59,108,120]

Neonatal Myocardium

The myocardium undergoes structural and functional changes after birth. The newborn myocardium has less sarcoplasmic reticulum and t-tubule synthesis with shorter, more rounded and disorganized myofibrils.[12] The myocardium also contains more fibrous non-contractile tissue than older individuals and has decreased sympathetic innervation.[12] The myocytes become more cylindrical; myofibrils increase and become more organized.[101,120,178] In the first month, growth occurs due to increases in myocyte numbers; by the second month, increases are due to changes in cell size.[5] The major physiologic change in the myocardium is the improved ability to generate force and of the myofibrils to shorten. The weeks following birth bring about a change in ventricular mass, with the left increasing more than the right.[139,145] However, during this process the RV becomes more compliant. As a result, changes in RV volume have a greater impact on LV filling in the fetus and newborn than in the adult.[7,9]

Myocardial compliance increases rapidly during the first few days of extrauterine life. Changes in connective tissue content can be seen during this time and may explain the change in compliance, although additional explanations may lie in collagen, extracellular matrix, or matrix attachment site differences between the fetus and the adult. In immature infants the myometrium has a higher water content and less contractile mass; therefore the ventricles are less distensible and generate less force per unit weight.[32]

Pulmonary Vasculature

As noted in the previous section, with transition to extrauterine life, blood flow to the lungs increases 8- to 10-fold with the marked decrease in PVR.[69] Failure of PVR to fall at birth can lead to persistent pulmonary hypertension (see Chapter 10). The high PVR in the fetus is due to a thick muscular coat of medial smooth muscle. This muscle involutes rapidly after birth. Toward the periphery the encircling smooth muscle is less complete and is absent in the most peripheral arteries.[17]

Changes in the pulmonary vasculature after birth occur in two phases (Figure 9-13). The first phase is prominent during the first 24 hours after birth, with dilation and recruitment of nonmuscularized and partially muscularized arteries.[130] The second phase involves further involution from 24 hours of age to 6 to 8 weeks. The partially muscularized arteries become nonmuscularized and the completely muscularized vessels become partially muscularized with thinning of the remaining muscle layer.[130] As a result of these changes, the vessel lumen size increases, the ability of the pulmonary arteries to constrict decreases, and PVR continues to fall. By 6 to 8 weeks after birth, PVR reaches adult values and the pulmonary vasculature becomes less sensitive to the effects of PO_2 changes.

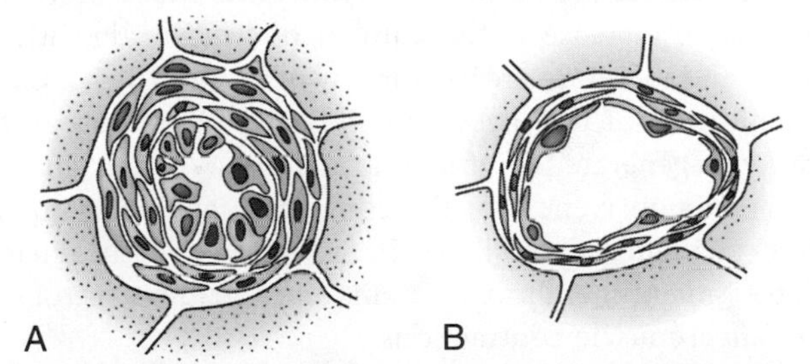

FIGURE 9-13 Changes in the small muscular pulmonary arteries during transition. Muscularized small pulmonary arteries from a near-term gestation fetus **(A)** demonstrate swollen endothelial cells and increased thickness of the muscular layer. Within 24 hours after birth **(B)**, a considerable increase in luminal diameter is noted secondary to flattening of the endothelial cells, spreading of the smooth muscle cell, and an increase in external diameter caused by relaxation of the smooth muscles. These events contribute to the drop in pulmonary vascular resistance after birth. (From Lakshminrushimha, S. & Steinharn, R.H. [1999]. Pulmonary vascular biology during neonatal transition. *Clin Perinatol, 26,* 604.)

Metabolic Rate and Oxygen Transport

Metabolic rate is measured as oxygen consumption and is much higher in the neonate than in the adult. The neonatal metabolic rate is also higher than that of the fetus because of independent extrauterine functioning and growth requirements. The components of oxygen consumption are related to energy expenditure and include basal metabolic rate, growth, heat production, and physical activity. The growth component is approximately 2% to 3% of the total metabolic rate and is higher in preterm infants. Oxygen consumption in the neonate increases exponentially with physical activity, placement in a nonneutral thermal environment, therapeutic and diagnostic procedures, and increased work of breathing.[177]

The oxygen availability, which is the product of the CO and the arterial oxygen content, is also elevated in the neonate. The estimated delivery of oxygen in the neonate at rest is 75% higher than in the adult. Three major processes impair oxygen availability: ventilation-perfusion mismatching from either intrapulmonary or extrapulmonary sources, reduced oxygen-hemoglobin–binding capacity, and reduced CO. In addition to these processes, a cardiovascular system that is unable to respond to an increased metabolic demand can result in decompensation.[177]

Endocrine, respiratory, and cardiovascular responses to altered oxygenation are similar to those found in the adult, the major difference being that the neonate functions close to maximum capacity normally and therefore has little reserve to compensate for further demands. Therefore, when impaired oxygen transport results in increased CO (due primarily to an increased heart rate), the maximum is readily reached. Further oxygen demands are associated with an increase in oxygen extraction and a decrease in oxygen saturation.[75]

Hypoxemia results in a decrease in oxygen consumption, oxygen availability, and SVR and an increase in oxygen extraction by the tissues. Heart rate and CO increase, because the ability to deliver and release oxygen to the myocardium is essential for the myocardium to respond to the hypoxemia and compensate for impaired oxygen transport. Isovolemic anemia results in a significant decrease in arterial and mixed venous oxygen content, mean aortic pressure, and SVR. CO and stroke volume increase regardless of the hemoglobin content; however, heart rate increases are seen only with hemoglobin levels of 6 g/dL (60 g/L) or less. If oxygen affinity is reduced, CO and stroke volume increase to a greater degree. These events, once again, occur only when myocardial function is maintained. Impaired CO results in redistribution of blood flow, with flow directed to the heart and brain preferentially and shunted away from the peripheral organ systems. This is reflected in an increase in vascular resistance in the lower body, with no change in upper body resistance.

Over the first 2 to 4 months of life, there is a fall in hemoglobin concentration, an increase in adult hemoglobin (HbA), and a rightward shift in the oxygen-hemoglobin dissociation curve (see Chapters 8 and 10). This enables more oxygen to be released to the tissues at the same capillary oxygen tension. However, the increased metabolic demands of extrauterine life (including physical activity) must be accompanied by an increase in the P50 to compensate for the total hemoglobin concentration. The pattern of changes during these first 2 to 4 months includes a decline in total hemoglobin (reaching its lowest point at 8 to 12 weeks in term infants); a progressive shift in P50 to the right; and an increase in 2,3-diphosphoglycerate (2,3-DPG) (see Chapter 8). There may also be an increase in CO and an increase in oxygen extraction. The latter is adjusted depending on the oxygen consumption, total hemoglobin, and P50. Once hemoglobin levels fall below a critical point, however, CO is unable to compensate for the reduced oxygen availability, necessitating a redistribution in CO.[75]

Myocardial Performance in the Neonate

Myocardial performance is influenced by ventricular preload, myocardial contractility, heart rate, and ventricular afterload. The adaptation to neonatal life is characterized by an increase in heart rate, end-diastolic volume, and enhanced inotropy due to sympathetic stimulation.[5] Even at rest the neonate is functioning near full capacity with reduced reserve in contractility, preload, and afterload.[12] This functional state is needed to meet the increased vascular loading that occurs with birth. Consequently, the newborn heart has less ability to adapt to additional acute pressure (afterload) or volume (preload) stresses.[5] Since many inotropic agents increase afterload, this may reduce positive inotropic effects.[12] The increased sympathetic stimulation with birth may be one reason that the newborn is less able to significantly increase CO with hypotension.[146]

Preload

Ventricular preload is a measure of end-diastolic volume (EDV). Myocardial fiber length changes with EDV in a predictable manner as described by the Frank-Starling law. According to this law, up to critical length, increased EDV leads to increased fiber length and improved contractility. This leads to increased stroke volume (SV) and CO.

Ventricular preload in the neonate is influenced by the less compliant ventricles. The neonatal heart does function under the Frank-Starling law, but under homeostatic conditions it operates at the upper limit of this law. Compared to the adult heart, the neonatal heart requires a higher filling pressure and this filling pressure is reached at lower volumes. In addition, neonates have a higher CO due to increased metabolism.

The neonatal heart must deal with the increased preload generated by the high volume load at delivery. Moreover, the low compliance of the LV decreases the preload reserve volume. Heart rates in neonates are high, falling during the 6 weeks following delivery. Whether infants can augment CO through further increases in heart rate continues to be debated, as does the effectiveness of inotropic support in the neonate without contractility failure. If increases in afterload or preload are associated with decreased contractility, as with sepsis or asphyxia, inotropic support can rapidly improve CO.[5]

In the fetus and newborn, an increase in RV volume interferes with LV filling.[5] The impact of one chamber on another is also more marked with decreasing compliance. So if there are changes in RV diastolic or loading pressures in the fetus, the LV is compromised and stroke volume is reduced. Once the pulmonary vascular resistance (PVR) drops at delivery and throughout the neonatal period, LV filling is enhanced and stroke volume is improved. Therefore neonates are more compromised than adults are if there is an increase in RV preload (i.e., rapid administration of a large fluid bolus) or afterload with specific pathologic conditions (e.g., pulmonary hypertension).

Contractility

Myocardial contractility relates to the heart's intrinsic pumping ability, which is dependent on calcium influx in myocardium. Acidosis, hypercarbia, and hypoxia alter cell permeability and the NA-K pump and lead to decreased contractility.

Contractile capabilities are dependent upon the force of contraction, shortening velocity (preload), inotropy, and afterload (load carried at the time of contraction). The maximum shortening of muscle is obtained when there is zero load; however, as the afterload increases, the velocity of muscle shortening decreases. If the load is so great that no external shortening is possible, the contraction is considered isometric. Changing the muscle length can alter the force of the contraction; force development is related to the number of cross-bridges (the greater the number, the greater the force).[9]

An increase in contractility and development of force is part of the maturation process of the myocardium. There is no sudden change in force-generating ability with birth, but rather a slow progression over time as the entire cardiac system matures into adulthood. Most of these maturational processes are related to structural changes in the myocardial anatomy. As myofibril content increases, there is an increase in the number of cross-bridge attachments and therefore greater force generation. The increased organization of the myofibrils may also contribute to the ability to generate forceful contractions. Whether changes in the responsiveness of the contractile apparatus to calcium facilitate any of these changes is currently unclear. Maturation of membrane systems and calcium control may also affect muscle contractions.

The maturational increase in the force-generating ability of the myocardium begins to be seen in late gestation and continues until adulthood. Ventricular filling, pressure development, and ejection in the fetus are similar to those in the neonate and the adult, except that at birth there is a marked increase in combined ventricular output.[47] With birth, RV output increases by one third, whereas LV output triples. An increase in pulmonary venous return, improved inotropy (strength of contraction), increased heart rate, and the diastolic and systolic interactions of the right and left ventricles may contribute to the change in combined ventricular output. LV output increases significantly while the DA is still patent. A PDA increases the volume load of the heart, which may initiate a Frank-Starling response. The doubling of the LV stroke volume seen at birth may be related to release of ventricular constraint (from the chest wall, lungs, and pericardium) with lung aeration and clearance of lung fluid (see Chapter 10), thus increasing ventricular preload.

In the weeks after birth, LV output returns to fetal levels or lower, whereas systolic and end-diastolic pressures continue to rise. Other indicators of the increased birth inotropy also return to fetal baselines. A clear explanation for this is not known, although it may have to do with the reaccumulation of reserves after the birth process. Therefore diseases that place an additional demand on the heart to produce more CO in the first days of extrauterine life can result in cardiovascular compromise in the neonate.[9]

Myocardial contractility is altered in the neonate due to the infant's decreased ventricular compliance and reduced contractile mass. As a result, neonates rely more on heart rate than on stroke volume to increase CO. Yet this mechanism is also limited due to parasympathetic domination in the neonate and immaturity of the sympathetic nervous system. In addition the neonate is vulnerable to metabolic and biochemical alterations that can further compromise contractility. Increasing heart rate may only improve CO slightly in the neonate, because CO is near maximum under homeostatic conditions.

Because myocardial contractility in neonates is high during the first week of life, there is little reserve in contractility. This implies that inotropic drugs will do little to improve the contractile state of the normally functioning neonatal heart. One mechanism for this increased inotropic state and the elevated CO is the high level of adrenergic stimulation that occurs around birth. However, the increased CO that remains for several weeks postnatally cannot be explained by continued catecholamine activity.

Heart Rate

The baseline heart rate is determined by the intrinsic depolarization rate of the sinoatrial node, which is actively inhibited by tonic parasympathetic input. Myocardial sympathetic innervation is incomplete at birth, with decreased norepinephrine levels during the first 3 weeks. As a result, vagal effects predominate, with limited response to catecholamine stimulation of β-adrenergic receptors. As the parasympathetic system matures, the resting heart rate decreases.[7] Tachycardia (more than 160 beats per minute) is usually seen with events that lead to catecholamine release, sympathetic stimulation, or parasympathetic withdrawal. A higher heart rate is also seen in the extremely premature infant, in whom control of cardiac function is dominated by the sympathetic nervous system.

Afterload

Ventricular afterload is the resistance against which the heart pumps (i.e., PVR, SVR). Afterload affects contractility. Increased afterload leads to decreased contractility, whereas decreased afterload leads to increased contractility. Even though PVR decreases significantly at birth, PVR remains higher in the neonate than in the adult for 6 to 8 weeks after birth. During this time, PVR gradually decreases to adult values as the medial muscle layer of pulmonary arterioles is restructured (see "Pulmonary Vasculature"). In addition, neonatal pulmonary vasculature is characterized by increased reactivity of pulmonary arterioles, with a tendency toward vasoconstriction and increased PVR.

The LV end-diastolic volume increases with birth. This probably contributes to the neonatal increase in output via the Frank-Starling relationship. These changes may be due to the circulatory transition that occurs at delivery and the fall in PVR and increased pulmonary venous return. LV filling may be augmented by a decrease in RV afterload. Therefore a fall in pulmonary artery pressure would enhance LV output by decreasing RV afterload, which would improve RV ejection and result in a smaller RV end-diastolic volume. The LV is then able to fill to a larger volume at a comparable filling pressure. This interaction is magnified in the fetus and neonate because of the reduced cardiac compliance.[9]

Regulation of Fetal and Neonatal Circulation

As in the adult, medullary, hypothalamic, and cerebral cortical activity presumably influence fetal and neonatal cardiovascular functions. The medullary centers appear to influence cardiovascular responses in a variable fashion in the fetus and the newborn; however, higher cortical or hypothalamic activities are associated with an increase in heart rate and hypertension. This stimulation and response are quite different than the baroreflex, which is a peripheral response by the baroreceptors to hypertension that is itself secondary to increased peripheral resistance. Baroreceptor and chemoreceptor function is reviewed in the box in Chapter 6 on p. 165.

Complex neurohumoral and metabolic responses maintain blood pressure, heart rate, and distribution of blood flow in the fetus and the newborn. These include systemic sensors (stretch receptors and neural and hormonal mediators) as well as local responses that allow an organ to regulate flow. The interaction of the two systems allows the fetus and the newborn to respond to stress events by redistributing blood flow to spare high-priority organs with specific oxygen requirements.

The arterial baroreflex modulates heart rate and peripheral vasodilation by altering autonomic activity and regulating release of substances such as angiotensin II and arginine vasopressin.[146] Baroreceptors that are sensitive to changes in blood pressure are located in the aortic arch and the carotid sinuses (see Figure 6-2). These sensors cause changes in heart rate and, in the fetus, may be responsible for stabilizing fetal blood pressure, with increasing sensitivity as gestational age advances. Baroreceptor activity has been implicated in the decreasing fetal heart rate (FHR) baseline seen in later gestation as blood pressure rises. In late gestation and in the early postbirth period, the baroreflex is reset toward higher pressures paralleling the gradual increase in blood pressure.[96,146] Short-term increases in blood pressure do not cause resetting, although this is seen in adults.[146] Chemoreceptors can be found in both the peripheral and central nervous systems and may alter FHR in response to hypoxemia and acidosis (see Chapter 6). Present in the latter half of gestation, they appear to be responsive to changes in pH and carbon dioxide tension and give rise to bradycardia while CO and umbilical blood flow are preserved. Following birth, hypoxia leads to tachycardia and an increase in CO associated with increased respiratory effort.[7]

Sympathetic intervention is present and functional in the fetus and newborn, increasing responsiveness with increasing gestational age. Stimulation results in tachycardia, augmented myocardial contractility, and increased systemic arterial blood pressure. The newborn has limited α-receptors and myocardial sympathetic innervation.[12] Sympathetic nerves may exhibit "denervating hypersensitivity" (maximal stimulation with small amounts of catecholamines).[12] β-adrenoreceptors are low in extremely low-birth weight infants, but increase to term and are higher in term infants than at older ages. Responses of α- and β-receptors have a more limited effect on cardiac contractility in the newborn with fewer β2-receptors (important for vasodilation and bronchodilation) and many active α-receptors (which increase cardiac inotrophy, vascular tone, and thus blood pressure and afterload).[12]

Parasympathetic input also increases with advancing gestational age. The major effector is the vagus nerve, which provides an inhibitory effect on FHR. Short-term variability of the FHR is modulated primarily by impulses from the vagus nerve (see Chapter 6). With increasing gestational age the parasympathetic system has a greater role in heart rate regulation, especially after 28 to 30 weeks, and increases more rapidly after 37 to 38 weeks, suggesting a marked increase in vagal tone.[146]

Humoral regulation of the cardiovascular system is related to the impact of catecholamines, vasopressin, renin-angiotensin, and prostaglandins on the heart and vascular bed.[146] Catecholamines are secreted by the adrenal medulla and may be involved in fetal cardiovascular system regulation before the development of the sympathetic nervous system. Fetal myocardium appears to have similar responsiveness to catecholamines compared to the adult.[7] As noted earlier, catecholamine levels increase markedly with birth, reaching pharmacologic levels.[96]

Arginine vasopressin is produced by the fetal pituitary gland early in gestation. Although usually undetectable, the concentration of vasopressin increases during hypoxia, hypotension, or hypernatremia. This results in vasoconstriction of the vessels in the musculoskeletal system, skin, and gut while increasing flow to the brain and heart. Prostaglandins may also play a role in augmenting blood flow to the brain during hypoxic episodes. These mechanisms may play a major role in the redistribution of blood flow seen in the fetus during significant hypoxia (see Chapter 6).[7]

Stimulation of the renin-angiotensin system leads to an increase in FHR, blood pressure, and combined ventricular output. Blood flow to the lungs and myocardium increases; flow to the renal system falls off. Angiotensin II seems to exert a vasotonic effect on the peripheral circulation. These effects may support the fetus during episodes of significant blood loss.[7]

CLINICAL IMPLICATIONS FOR NEONATAL CARE

Cardiovascular disturbances in the neonate include congestive heart failure (CHF), cyanosis, murmurs, and arrhythmias. Cardiac malformations occur in 0.8% to 1% of live births and represent about 10% of all congenital malformations. Murmurs that are due to the normal turbulence of transitional circulation (i.e., ductal closure) or physiologic turbulence in the pulmonary artery are considered benign. Gestational age and disease also affect the cardiovascular system and are factors in patent ductus arteriosus (PDA) and bronchopulmonary dysplasia (BPD).

Assessment of Heart Sounds

The newborn's heart rate ranges from 120 to 160 beats per minute, with significant state-related variations. Heart rate increases with birth and remains higher for the first hour, although there is marked variability between individual infants. Because heart rate is the most effective method for the neonate to increase CO, cardiorespiratory illness, sepsis, and metabolic problems are often accompanied by tachycardia.

The neonatal heart accounts for 0.75% of body weight in the neonate (versus 0.35% in adults). On chest roentgenogram the neonatal heart generally occupies about 40% of the field (versus 35% in adults). Because the heart is positioned more transversely, the apical pulse is felt to the left of the sternal border. A visible precordial impulse may be seen along the left sternal border for 4 to 6 hours after birth.[64]

Heart sounds are of higher pitch, shorter duration, and greater intensity; and functional murmurs, hums, and clicks may be heard. Murmurs are heard in about one third of healthy infants in the first 24 hours after birth and in two thirds in the first 48 hours. A systolic DA murmur is heard in about 15% of infants while the ductus is still patent, most often around 5 to 6 hours of age. Sinus arrhythmias are common in infants and children.[153] The most common significant arrhythmias in infants are bradycardia and supraventricular tachycardia.[64] Sinus bradycardia is seen due to the predominant parasympathetic innervation of the sinus node in the neonate. Bradycardia may occur due to vagal stimulation or secondary to hypoxemia or acidosis. Bradycardia may not be well tolerated in infants since heart rate comprises a greater portion of CO than stroke volume. Arrhythmias often do not compromise systemic perfusion or CO as much in neonates as in older individuals. Abnormal sinus rhythms in infancy may indicate underlying cardiac anomalies that alter reflexive mechanisms for heart rate control.[64]

Cardiac Shunts

Right-to-left cardiac shunts involve shunting of blood from systemic venous circulation to the arterial circulations without oxygenation. These shunts are usually characterized by obstruction to flow on the right side of the heart distal to an abnormal communication. Right-to-left shunting is characteristic of fetal circulation; that is, placental blood moves from the venous circulation to the arterial circulation bypassing the lungs via either the foramen ovale or DA. Pathologic examples of right-to-left cardiac shunts include persistent pulmonary hypertension of the newborn (PPHN), in which the foramen ovale or DA or both remain open; pulmonary stenosis or atresia, in which blood is shunted from right to left via a PDA, foramen ovale, or ventricular septal defect (VSD); or transposition of the great vessels.

Left-to-right cardiac shunts are characterized by recirculation of oxygenated blood through the lungs, bypassing the peripheral circulation. Left to right shunting at the atrial level increases the amount of blood pumped by the pulmonary ventricle (normally the RV). Left-to-right shunting at the level of the great vessels or ventricles increases the volume load on the systemic ventricle (usually the LV). With a large VSD, there may also be increased stress on the pulmonary ventricle.[88] Examples of left-to-right shunting include a PDA (shunting of blood from the aorta to the pulmonary artery and thus back to the lungs) or a VSD with shunting of oxygenated blood from the LV to the RV and thus back to the lungs. Common clinical manifestations of left-to-right shunts are tachypnea (due to pulmonary edema), tachycardia (due to catecholamine release), diaphoresis in older infants (due to catecholamine release), poor weight gain (due to increased energy demands of the heart and other systems), and sometimes hepatomegaly (due to altered hemodynamics).[89]

Cyanosis

Cyanosis is a physical sign characterized by blue gray mucous membranes, nail beds, and skin. Central cyanosis occurs after 5 g/dL (50 g/L) of hemoglobin has been desaturated. Hypoxemia is a state of abnormally low arterial blood oxygen concentration. The degree of hypoxemia may or may not correlate with cyanosis, depending on the blood hemoglobin concentration and the ability of the observer to detect cyanosis. The most common causes of cyanosis in the neonate are cardiac disease and pulmonary disease. The ability to be able to distinguish between these two is essential. Therefore when congenital heart disease is suspected, the degree of hypoxemia must be related to the volume of pulmonary blood flow.

Hypoxemia in these infants is due to right-to-left shunting (diversion of blood from the lungs); therefore ventilation and oxygen delivery do not improve oxygenation. This is the basis for the hyperoxia challenge test. With adequate ventilation and 100% oxygen, the PaO_2 should rise above 150 mmHg (19.95 kPaa). If the PaO_2 does not increase above 100 mmHg (13.30 kPaa), cyanotic congenital heart disease is most likely the cause of the cyanosis. Between 100 and 150 mmHg (13.30 to 19.95 kPaa), cardiac disease is possible but further diagnostic testing needs to be conducted (e.g., echocardiography). Selected congenital anomalies are discussed in the next section to demonstrate these principles.

Patent Ductus Arteriosus in the Preterm Infant

There are three general physiologic characteristics of a PDA in the preterm infant: (1) increased flow through the lungs with diastolic volume overload; (2) increased flow through the left atrium, LV, and aorta; and (3) left-to-right shunting to the pulmonary circulation. Blood is shunted from the upper and lower aortic circulations with a large ductus and multiorgan effects.

The DA in the preterm infant is thin walled and less dependent on the vasa vasorum, so it does not develop the ischemia-hypoxia–stimulated remodeling unless there is complete cessation of blood flow.[32] The preterm ductus is also less likely to constrict with birth due to the presence of immature myosin isoforms, potassium channels that are less responsive to oxygen inhibition, altered Rho/Rho kinase pathways, higher circulating PGE_2 levels secondary to decreased clearance by the immature lungs, and especially increased sensitivity to the vasodilating effects of PGE_2 and NO.[32,59,76,108,120] Thus cyclooxygenase inhibitors such as indomethacin and ibuprofen, which inhibit prostaglandin synthetase and thus prostaglandin production, are effective in constricting the ductus.[55,59,108,120]

The preterm infant has less pulmonary arterial muscle (see Closure of the Ductus Arteriosus) and an immature pulmonary parenchyma. The presence of a patent ductus arteriosus (PDA) is associated with interstitial edema and decreased compliance of the lung due to pulmonary edema. Ductal closure results in an increased compliance and a decreased need for ventilatory support (especially end-expiratory pressure). Prolonged ventilatory support due to a PDA increases the risk of bronchopulmonary dysplasia in preterm infants.

Perfusion of peripheral organ systems is dependent upon adequate systolic and diastolic flow. With a PDA, blood flow is redistributed with decreased flow to the skin, bone, and skeletal muscle, followed by the gastrointestinal system and kidneys.[31] The preterm infant even with limitations in myocardial performance is able to increase LV output and maintain effective systemic blood flow with a small to moderate PDA by increasing stroke volume (secondary to a simultaneous decrease in afterload resistance and increase in LV preload).[32] If a large PDA exists, systemic diastolic arterial flow is compromised and may even be reversed in the descending aorta. This can lead to decreased renal perfusion and contribute to the development of volume overload and CHF.

Gastrointestinal effects are also related to a decrease in flow and intestinal ischemia. Preterm infants with intestinal ischemia as a result of a PDA are at risk for developing necrotizing enterocolitis. Cerebral ischemia may also occur as blood is diverted from the upper body. Cerebral blood flow changes can also increase the incidence of intraventricular hemorrhage.

A large left-to-right shunt through the PDA increases the left atrial and ventricular volume, leading to enlargement of these two chambers. The increased LV size also increases the myocardial wall stress, which could lead to myocardial ischemia in the preterm infant. If LV compromise exists, inotropic support may be needed until PDA closure is achieved. Treatments have included supportive management, pharmacologic therapy and surgical intervention.[59,108,120]

Congenital Heart Defects

Most cardiac defects are compatible with intrauterine life and only become significant at birth. Even defects that significantly alter hemodynamics and flow in the fetal heart are often tolerated well since the fetal shunts allow for compensation (see Figures 9-11, *A*, and 9-12). The exceptions to this include defects with atrioventricular valve regurgitation and myocardial dysfunction, which tend to be less well tolerated.[47,123] With any severe defect, birth may result in acute compromise as the fetal shunts close. Closure of the DA can be life-threatening in infants with ductal dependent pulmonary blood flow (PDA allows left to right shunting to send blood to lungs) or ductal dependent systemic blood flow (PDA allows right to left shunting to send blood to body).[143] Thus initial management is often directed at maintaining fetal shunts. Table 9-8 classifies congenital cardiac defects by physiologic consequence. Hemodynamic consequences with transition to extrauterine life of selected disorders are described in the following sections.

Total Anomalous Venous Return

In this condition, the pulmonary veins do not connect with the left atrium; rather, some or all of the pulmonary veins form a confluence or collecting vessel that usually lies posterior to the left atrium. There may be one or more sites of connection between the pulmonary venous collecting vessel or individual pulmonary veins and the systemic venous

Table 9-8 Classification of Congenital Cardiac Disease

CLASSIFICATION	EXAMPLES
Severe cyanosis caused by separate circulation and poor mixing	D-transposition of the great arteries D-transposition of the great arteries and ventricular septal defect Double-outlet right ventricle with subpulmonary ventricular septal defect (Taussig-Bing)
Severe cyanosis caused by restricted pulmonary blood flow	Tetralogy of Fallot Double-outlet right ventricle with subaortic ventricular septal defect and pulmonary stenosis Tricuspid atresia Pulmonary atresia with intact interventricular septum Critical pulmonary stenosis Ebstein anomaly Single ventricle with pulmonary stenosis Persistent pulmonary hypertension
Mild cyanosis caused by complete mixing with normal or increased pulmonary blood flow	Total anomalous pulmonary venous connection Truncus arteriosus Single ventricle without pulmonary stenosis Double-outlet right ventricle with subaortic ventricular septal defect
Systemic hypoperfusion and congestive heart failure with mild or no cyanosis	Aortic stenosis* Coarctation of the aorta and aortic arch interruption Hypoplastic left heart syndrome Multiple left heart defects Single ventricle with subaortic stenosis or coarctation of the aorta Myocardial disease: cardiomyopathy and myocarditis* Cardiac tumor* Arteriovenous malformation* Hypertension*
Acyanosis with no or mild respiratory distress	Normal murmurs Pulmonary stenosis Ventricular septal defect† Atrial septal defect Endocardial cushion defect† Patent ductus arteriosus† Aorticopulmonary window* D-transposition of the great arteries Arteriovenous malformation Hypertension

From Zahka, K.G. & Lane, J.G. (2006). Approach to the neonate with cardiovascular disease. In R.J. Martin, A.A. Fanaroff, & M.C. Walsh. *Neonatal-perinatal medicine: Diseases of the fetus and infant* (8th ed.). St. Louis: Mosby.
*No symptoms with mild forms of disease.
†Congestive heart failure may develop as left-to-right shunt increases with decrease in pulmonary vascular resistance.

circuit. Usually the pulmonary veins drain directly or, more commonly, indirectly into the right atrium via one of the normal embryonic channels. The embryonic defect involves failure of development of the common pulmonary vein normally connecting the developing pulmonary venous plexus with the posterior aspect of the left atrium.[143,179]

The postnatal presentation depends on the degree of obstruction of pulmonary venous drainage. If obstruction is severe, presentation occurs within the first week of life. If obstruction is mild, presentation may not occur until the latter half of the first year. The presence of an intra-atrial communication—either a patent foramen ovale or a true atrial septal defect (ASD)—is necessary to sustain life postnatally. The hemodynamic impact of total anomalous pulmonary venous return does not occur until pulmonary blood flow increases at the time of delivery. Pulmonary edema is the usual result. Oxygenation is interrupted because of edema, right-to-left shunting, and increased pulmonary resistance.

Transposition of the Great Arteries

This defect arises from abnormal septation of the truncus arteriosus so that the aorta arises from the RV and the pulmonary artery from the left. The foramen ovale and DA develop normally and, in a simple transposition, the coronary arteries arise from the aorta. At birth, with closure of the foramen ovale and DA, and in the absence of other defects, two separate circulations exist. In one, desaturated blood returning from the body to the RA flows to the RV and out the aorta to the body without being oxygenated. In the other circulation, oxygenated blood from the lungs returns to the LA, then flows to the LV and back to the lungs via the pulmonary artery. Both RV and LV workload is increased.[143] Survival at birth is dependent on bidirectional flow via the foramen ovale and DA or the presence of other defects such as an atrial septal defect or ventricular septal defect (VSD). Severe cyanosis develops as the fetal shunts (particularly the DA) close. PGE_2 is given to maintain ductal patency until the infants can be taken to surgery.[47,177,179] Infants with transposition tend to be large for gestational age, possibly due to a higher oxygen saturation (~65%) in blood sent to the lungs and lower body (and thus the gastrointestinal tract and pancreas).[105] The decreased saturation of blood going to the brain may increase the risk of ischemia and white matter injury.[105]

Truncus Arteriosus

Truncus arteriosus is a single great artery that arises from the base of the heart that supplies the coronary, pulmonary, and systemic arteries. This defect is thought to result from septation failure. Up to one third of infants with truncus arteriosus have a microdeletion of chromosome 22.[143] In utero, the main consequence of truncus arteriosus is complete mixing of the systemic and pulmonary venous return above the truncal valve. The truncal valve is abnormal (stenotic, thickened, or regurgitant) in 50%.[143] The truncus is usually quite large, and the DA arising from the pulmonary arteries may be smaller than normal. Because blood flow through the heart is normal, the rest of the heart develops normally.

Postnatally the flow of the pulmonary arteries and systemic arteries is a function of the relative resistances in the two circuits. Initially the pulmonary resistance is high and pulmonary flow will equal or slightly exceed systemic flow. Over the first hours or days of life, the pulmonary arteriolar resistance decreases and pulmonary blood flow increases. As the pulmonary venous return increases, the LV must eject an increasing volume load, which eventually leads to CHF. Because there is common mixing of systemic and pulmonary venous blood above the truncal valve, the degree of hypoxemia decreases as the pulmonary flow increases so that these infants are only mildly cyanotic until left heart failure and pulmonary edema interfere with oxygen exchange and pulmonary venous desaturation ensues.[143]

Tricuspid Atresia

In tricuspid atresia there is a failure in the development of the right atrioventricular valve; therefore an intra-atrial communication is necessary for survival. This communication is usually in the form of a patent foramen ovale. Along with this, there is usually a VSD connecting a large LV cavity with a hypoplastic chamber that is the outflow portion of the RV. The great arteries may be either normally related or transposed. There may also be an atresia.

Fetal growth and development are uncompromised, so the alterations in cardiovascular status must be compatible with normal growth and development in utero. All systemic venous return is diverted across the foramen ovale into the left atrium and LV. If there are no further abnormalities, the entire ventricular volume is ejected into the aorta. If the VSD is large, some of the LV output passes through the VSD into the hypoplastic RV, exiting via the pulmonary artery if the vessels are normally related or via the aorta if transposition is present.

After delivery there is little change in the circulation, but the normal postnatal alterations impose significant liabilities. Neonates with pulmonary atresia or severe pulmonary stenosis continue to depend on the DA for pulmonary blood flow. When the DA begins to close, severe hypoxemia, acidosis, and eventually death follow. In infants with a large VSD and no pulmonary stenosis, the pulmonary blood flow increases as the pulmonary arteriolar resistance drops and congestive heart failure (CHF) ensues, usually in the first month of life.

Left-Sided Obstructive Lesions

The major lesions in this group are critical aortic stenosis (i.e., blood flow depends on a PDA), interrupted aortic arch, hypoplastic left heart syndrome (small or absent LV and hypoplastic or atretic mitral and aortic valves), and coarctation of the aorta (see next section). Some infants present soon after birth with CHF with or without circulatory failure and shock. Others do well initially until they present at 1 to 2 weeks with circulatory failure and shock.[143] Obstruction of LV outflow in the fetus leads to hypertrophy and hyperplasia.

LV compliance is decreased with decreased blood flow through the foramen ovale (blood flow may even reverse). RV output is increased as more of the IVC blood flows to the RV and thus across the DA to the lower body. With aortic atresia, all atrial output is via the RV and all systemic blood crosses the DA. Some of this blood follows the normal path via the descending aorta, some via retrograde flow into the ascending aorta to the coronary arteries, upper body, and head.[13,47,105,177,179] These infants have decreased blood flow to the brain which may increase the risk of neurodevelopmental alterations.[105]

Even if the defect is severe, the fetus does well because of the parallel fetal circulation (see Figure 9-11, *A*). At birth the onset of symptoms varies with severity: the more severe the defect, the earlier the onset is. Infants with severe aortic stenosis develop increased left atrial pressure as pulmonary blood flow increases and LV compliance decreases. The foramen ovale closes or remains open with left-to-right shunting of blood from the LA to the RA. Initially, systemic blood flow is also partially maintained via the RV and DA. When the ductus closes, all systemic flow is from the LV via the stenotic aorta. Therefore, in these infants, symptoms of poor perfusion and circulatory failure coincide with closing of the ductus.[13,47,143]

In infants with aortic atresia and hypoplastic left heart syndrome, all systemic blood is routed from the RV to the aorta via the DA. Pulmonary blood flow crosses the foramen ovale left to right (LA to RA). Symptoms arise within the first 24 hours if the ductus is narrow or closes at birth. If the ductus remains open, symptoms may not appear for several weeks.[13,47,143,177]

Coarctation of the Aorta

This defect involves a constriction in the aorta distal to the left subclavian artery, usually at the junction of the DA and the aortic isthmus between the ductus and the left subclavian artery. There may be tubular hypoplasia of the aortic arch and intracardiac anomalies, and these must be ruled out during evaluation. About one third of infants with this defect also have a VSD.[47]

Because there is normally very little flow across the aortic isthmus in utero, the tubular hypoplasia and narrowing of the arch does not affect fetal growth and development, and blood is shunted across the DA. After birth the constriction in the aorta increases the LV afterload. If a VSD exists, this increased systemic resistance leads to a large left-to-right shunt. As the pulmonary vascular resistance (PVR) falls, the left-to-right shunt increases, resulting in a volume as well as a pressure overload of the LV. In addition to CHF, there is failure of the blood to pass from ascending to descending aorta if the coarctation is severe. This results in tissue hypoxia, lactic acidosis, and eventual death after the DA closes.

Those neonates with a juxtaductal coarctation but no other associated anomalies have slightly different hemodynamics. Closure of the DA leads to an acute increase in LV afterload, because blood must be pumped through the narrowed segment; before ductal closure, blood is able to circumvent the coarctation via a shelf of tissue at this insertion point. Since no obstruction was present in utero, no collateral vessels have developed. The neonatal myocardium is unable to respond to the increased workload; consequently CHF with elevation of LV end-diastolic, left atrial, and pulmonary venous pressures develops.[47,177] If the constriction is less severe, the infant may present with decreased femoral pulses and differences between the upper and lower extremity pulses.

Ventricular Septal Defect

Ventricular septal defects (VSDs) are the most common congenital heart defect (1/250 live births). These may be isolated defects or associated with other congenital cardiac defects.[143] The most common site for a VSD is the membranous portion of the septum that lies between the crista supraventricularis and the papillary muscle of the conus when the heart is viewed from the RV side. Less common sites are the area above the crista, the muscular portion of the septum below the tricuspid valve, and the anterior trabecular portion of the ventricular septum near the apex of the RV.

Because the right and left sides of the heart are arranged in a parallel fashion before birth, the presence of a large communication at the ventricular level in addition to the normal ductus connection at the great vessels does not significantly alter the fetal circulation. After birth, however, the hemodynamics depend on the size of the defect and the pulmonary and systemic vascular resistances. If the defect is large, it offers no resistance to flow. The systolic pressure in the ventricles and great vessels is approximately equal and the systemic and PVRs determine the degree of intracardiac shunting. As the PVR gradually falls, the volume of blood in the LV increases. Therefore more blood is ejected through the VSD into the pulmonary artery. When the pulmonary blood flow is about three times greater than the systemic flow, the volume load can no longer be accommodated, and CHF develops. Moderate to large VSDs usually become hemodynamically significant by 4 to 6 weeks of age as the PVR decreases and pulmonary blood flow increases (see "Pulmonary Vasculature").[143] The right atrium and RV are not volume overloaded, but in the presence of a large defect the RV must generate pressures equal to those of the LV, so there is usually RV hypertrophy without significant dilation. Preterm infants often develop symptoms earlier than term infants because PVR is lower in these infants due to decreased muscularization of the pulmonary arteries.[47,143,177]

If the VSD is small, it does offer resistance to flow, and the pressures in the two ventricles may differ. Infants with this type of defect are a heterogeneous group, with the hemodynamics depending on the size of the defect rather than the PVR. If the defect is very small, the RV and pulmonary artery pressures may be normal and the pulmonary blood flow less than twice the systemic flow. These infants are rarely symptomatic but usually exhibit a murmur. Up to half of isolated VSDs close spontaneously in infancy or childhood.[143]

Tetralogy of Fallot

Tetralogy of Fallot involves a combination of VSD, pulmonary valve stenosis, RV hypertrophy, and rightward displacement of the aortic root. If the VSD is large, right and left ventricular pressures are similar, so the amount of shunting is determined primarily by the degree of pulmonary stenosis and SVR.[47] In the fetus the portion of the combined ventricular output from the aorta is increased, as is the diameter of the aorta. Thus blood flow in utero is usually adequate.[6,41,47]

If the infant has mild to moderate pulmonary stenosis, closure of the DA may not alter pulmonary blood flow enough to reduce PO_2. With severe pulmonary stenosis, closure of the ductus significantly reduces pulmonary blood flow and the infant develops progressive severe cyanosis.[47] PGE_2 infusions are used to maintain ductal patency and pulmonary blood flow until the infant can be taken to surgery.

MATURATIONAL CHANGES DURING INFANCY AND CHILDHOOD

The changes in the cardiovascular system at birth include a redistribution of workload between the RV and LV as flow changes from a parallel to an in-series circuit (see Figure 9-11). These changes result in an increase in CO, with the RV ejecting blood against a lower afterload and the LV ejecting against a higher afterload. The ventricular mass changes in response to these new demands, with the LV wall thickness increasing significantly while the right remains unchanged. This change in wall thickness is secondary to an increase in cell number and size, beginning soon after birth. Because of the increased workload of the LV, cell replication occurs more rapidly in the left myocardium. Ventricular size and compliance change gradually during infancy and childhood, so cardiac function is similar to that of adults by adolescence.[97,142]

There is little change in heart size for 4 to 6 weeks after birth; then heart size doubles by 1 year. Heart size increases with somatic growth, with a four-fold increase by 5 years and six-fold increase by 9 years. Changes in heart size are due primarily to fat deposition. Changes in heart size are accompanied by descent of the diaphragm, increasing the room for cardiac movement and expansion of the respiratory system. The heart, which is more transverse in the infant, comes to lie more oblique and lower in relation to the ribs. The position of the heart becomes more vertical by 7 years. As a result, the apical impulse is lower and nearer the midclavicle line.[64,97]

The cross-sectional area of cardiac muscle fibers increases sevenfold to adulthood. Increased numbers of small blood vessels, whose growth parallels changes in weight and height, accompanies this change. The thickness of the great vessel walls doubles between birth and puberty, and their lumens increase 2½-fold. By 2 to 3 years of age, the child's cardiac shadow is similar to that of the adult.[97]

The myocardial cells change in size, shape, and architecture following birth. The LV matures more rapidly after birth, which can be seen in myocyte shape changes. The immature cells are rounder and have a smoother surface. As cells mature, their shape becomes increasingly irregular, with identifiable step changes along their lateral borders. The myocytes become longer and acquire a larger cross-sectional area. Volume of the LV myocytes increases 30- to 40-fold from infancy to adolescence.[142]

Stimulation for these changes may be related to the sympathetic nervous system. During the neonatal period, α-adrenoceptors and circulating norepinephrine levels are higher than at any other stage of development. In tissue cultures, stimulation of α_1-receptors (e.g., with norepinephrine) results in cell growth. Therefore it can be inferred that the presence of increased receptors and stimulant results in induction of myocardial cell growth.

Myofilament and sarcomere changes also occur with maturation. The sarcomere A-I bands are more irregular; the Z band disk is thicker, although more variable; and the M band is absent initially. The myofibrils are more disorganized and often are not oriented in the same direction as the long axis. Instead they are arranged around a large central mass of nuclei and mitochondria, which may persist for weeks following birth. Eventually the myofibrils assume the adult position and are distributed across the cell.

The increase in the proportion of cell volume that contains myofilaments, organizational changes, and modification of the sarcomeres leads to improved contraction ability. Other changes that are indicative of maturation include a postnatal mitochondrial increase, which is most likely in response to metabolic changes in the muscle tissue. Initially there is a dramatic increase in the number of mitochondria; with further maturation the mitochondria become highly ordered in their arrangement. This occurs weeks after delivery. The arrangement facilitates energy transfer to the sarcomere during contraction.

Stroke volume and ventricular EDV increase with age. Stroke volume is 5 to 10 mL (1.5 mL/kg) in the infant versus 70 to 90 mL in the adolescent. EDV is 40 mL/m² body surface area (BSA) in infants, increasing to 70 at 2 years of age. CO per unit of weight falls from 350 mL/kg in the infant to 150 mL/kg at 2 months to 100 mL/kg in the adolescent (versus 75 in the adult); absolute CO increases from 0.6 L/min at birth to 6 L/min in adult.[64,85,97,101] Infants and young children, like neonates, increase CO primarily by increasing heart rate rather than stroke volume.

Sinus arrhythmias are common in infants and children. The most common significant arrhythmia in children is bradycardia; ventricular tachycardia and ventricular fibrillation are more common in the adult.[64] As collagenous material increases among the fibers of the SA node, the frequency of insignificant arrhythmias decreases.

The cardiac index (CO/m² BSA) is 3.5 to 4.5 L/min in the child (slightly higher than in an adult); low CO is less than 2.1 to 2.5 L/min at any age. Right-axis deviation on the electrocardiogram (ECG) is seen for the first few months. LV dominance appears by 3 to 6 months as the LV muscle mass increases, with a net reduction in RV mass. The right and left ventricles are of equal size by 6 to 10 months. By 7 years the LV is larger than the right, with the LV wall twice as thick as the RV wall (i.e., the adult relationship).[64,97] Increased P-wave duration, RR interval, and QRS duration and magnitude are observed on the ECG until about 6 years of age. By this age the ECG is similar to that seen in older adolescents.[70]

PVR decreases to adult values by 6 to 8 weeks, and as soon as 3 weeks in some infants. Myocardial response to volume therapy is similar to the response of the adult by this age. This means that the infant can increase stroke volume and CO with fluid challenges or with a moderate increase in afterload. By one to two years, myocardial function is similar to that of an adult.

The pulse rate decreases from birth to late adolescence, and the range of normal pulse becomes narrower. The heart rate ranges from 90 to 140 beats per minute in the toddler, 80 to 110 beats per minute in the preschool child, and 75 to 100 beats per minute in childhood. After about 10 years, heart rate varies by gender, with higher rates in females than in males. Smaller quantitative changes in vital signs may be qualitatively more significant in infants and children than in adults. Gender differences in pulse rate are evident after 10 years, with rates higher in females than in males.[64,111]

Blood pressure—systolic more than diastolic—rises with increasing age. Systolic blood pressure begins to rise after 4 weeks.[73] Increases in systolic blood pressure after puberty are related to changes in height and weight, with a greater change seen in males. Blood pressure levels plateau in females at 15 to 17 years and in males by 20 years.

The rapid growth in heart size between 9 and 16 years of age is associated with changes in weight and height. The heart reaches adult size by the end of adolescence. A marked increase in heart muscle is also seen with this growth spurt, along with increased length and thickness of blood vessels. These changes—along with the increase in blood pressure and SV and the decrease in HR—may result in the transient sensation of chest fullness or discomfort with palpitations in the adolescent.[97]

SUMMARY

To achieve extrauterine stability, the newborn undergoes significant alterations in cardiovascular status that convert it from a parallel system to an in-series system that must integrate with the respiratory system in order to maintain oxygenation. The complex development of the heart and cardiovascular system places the neonate at greater risk for alterations in normal development that can lead to postnatal compromise affecting multiple systems. Close assessments during the transitional period result in early identification and treatment of cardiovascular disease while promoting normal growth and development. Table 9-9 summarizes recommendations for clinical practice.

Table 9-9 Recommendations for Clinical Practice Related to the Cardiovascular System in Neonates

Monitor cardiovascular adaptation to extrauterine life (pp. 280-283).
Assess and evaluate the neonate for changes in cardiovascular performance related to transitional changes (pp. 284-285).
Conduct a thorough cardiovascular assessment of any infant presenting with a murmur during the transitional period, especially if associated with cyanosis (pp. 286-287).
Develop an understanding of the embryonic mechanisms that may result in cardiac congenital anomalies (pp. 270-276).
Provide continuous physiologic monitoring for infants suspected of cardiac disease (pp. 286-292).
Monitor infants with cardiac defects for signs of congestive heart failure and shock (pp. 286-292).
Evaluate all preterm infants serially for signs of a patent ductus arteriosus (pp. 287-288).
Monitor infants with a patent ductus arteriosus for signs of increasing respiratory distress and congestive heart failure (pp. 287-288).
Monitor and evaluate cardiovascular function in infants at risk for persistent pulmonary hypertension (pp. 282-283, 287, Chapter 10).

References

1. Abbas, A.E., Lester, S.J., & Connolly, H. (2005). Pregnancy and the cardiovascular system. *Int J Cardiol, 98,* 179.
2. Adamson, S.L., et al. (2012). Regulation of umbilical blood flow. In R.A. Polin, W.W. Fox, & S.H. Abman (Eds.). *Fetal and neonatal physiology* (4th ed.). Philadelphia: Saunders.
3. Ahmed, A. (2011). New insights into the etiology of preeclampsia: Identification of key elusive factors for the vascular complications. *Thromb Res, 127,* S72.
4. American College of Obstetricians and Gynecologists. (2002). Exercise during pregnancy and the postpartum period (technical bulletin no. 267). *Obstet Gynecol, 99,* 171.
5. Anderson, P.A.W., et al. (2004). Cardiovascular function during development and the response to hypoxia. In R.A. Polin, W.W. Fox, & S.H. Abman (Eds.). *Fetal and neonatal physiology* (3rd ed.). Philadelphia: Saunders.
6. Apitz,C., Webb, G.D., & Redington, A.N. (2009). Tetralogy of Fallot. *Lancet, 374,* 1462.
7. Arnold-Aldea, S.A. & Parer, J.T. (1990). Fetal cardiovascular physiology. In R.D. Eden & F.H. Boehm (Eds.). *Assessment and care of the fetus: Physiological, clinical, and medicolegal principles.* Norwalk, CT: Appleton & Lange.
8. Artal, R. (2003). Exercise: The alternative therapeutic intervention for gestational diabetes. *Clin Obstet Gynecol, 46,* 479.

9. Artman, M., Mahoney, L. & Teitel, D. (2010). *Neonatal cardiology*. New York: McGraw Hill.
10. Bahado-Singh, R.O. & Jodicke, C. (2010). Uterine artery Doppler in first-trimester pregnancy screening. *Clin Obstet Gynecol, 53,* 879.
11. Bajolle, F., Zaffran, S., & Bonnet, D. (2009). Genetics and embryological mechanisms of congenital heart diseases. *Arch Cardiovasc Dis, 102,* 59.
12. Barrington, K.J. (2008). Hypotension and shock in the preterm infant. *Semin Fetal Neonatal Med, 13,* 16.
13. Barron, D.J., et al. (2009). Hypoplastic left heart syndrome. *Lancet, 374,* 551.
14. Baschat, A.A. (2010). Ductus venosus Doppler for fetal surveillance in high-risk pregnancies. *Clin Obstet Gynecol, 53,* 858.
15. Baschat, A.A. (2011). Examination of the fetal cardiovascular system. *Semin Fetal Neonatal Med, 16,* 2.
16. Bédard, E., Dimopoulos, K., & Gatzoulis, M.A. (2009). Has there been any progress made on pregnancy outcomes among women with pulmonary arterial hypertension? *Eur Heart J, 30,* 256.
17. Bellotti, M., et al. (2000). Role of ductus venosus in distribution of umbilical flow in human fetuses during second half of pregnancy. *Am J Physiol, 279,* H1256.
18. Blanchard, D.G. & Shabetal, R. (2009). Cardiac disease. In R.K. Creasy, et al. (Eds.). *Creasy & Resnik's Maternal-fetal medicine: Principles and practice* (6th ed.). Philadelphia: Saunders Elsevier.
19. Bloom, R.S. (2006). Delivery room resuscitation of the newborn. In R.J. Martin, A.A. Fanaroff, & M.C. Walsh (Eds.). *Fanaroff and Martin's Neonatal-perinatal medicine: Diseases of the fetus and infant* (8th ed.). Philadelphia: Mosby.
20. Brankston, G.N., et al. (2004). Resistance exercise decreases the need for insulin in overweight women with gestational diabetes mellitus. *Am J Obstet Gynecol, 190,* 188.
21. Brennan, P. & Young, I.D. (2001). Congenital heart malformations: Etiology and associations. *Semin Neonatol, 6,* 17.
22. Bridges, E.J., et al. (2003). Hemodynamic monitoring in high-risk obstetrics patients, I. Expected hemodynamic changes in pregnancy. *Crit Care Nurse, 23,* 53.
23. Brooks, V.L., Dampney, R.A., & Heesch, C.M. (2010). Pregnancy and the endocrine regulation of the baroreceptor reflex. *Am J Physiol Regul Integr Comp Physiol, 299,* R439.
24. Carbillon, L., et al. (2000). Pregnancy, vascular tone, and maternal hemodynamics: A crucial adaptation. *Obstet Gynecol Surv, 55,* 574.
25. Carlin, A. & Alfirevic, Z. (2008). Physiological changes of pregnancy and monitoring. *Best Pract Res Clin Obstet Gynaecol, 22,* 801.
26. Carlson, B.M. (2008). *Human embryology and developmental biology* (4th ed.). St. Louis: Mosby Elsevier.
27. Caulin-Glaser, T. & Setaro, J.F. (2004). Pregnancy and cardiovascular disease. In G.N. Burrow, T. Duffy, & J.A. Copel (Eds.). *Medical complications during pregnancy* (6th ed.). Philadelphia: Saunders.
28. Clapp, J.F. (1989). Oxygen consumption during treadmill exercise before, during and after pregnancy. *Am J Obstet Gynecol, 161,* 1458.
29. Clapp, J.F. (1991). Maternal exercise performance and early pregnancy outcome. In R.A. Mittelmark, R.A. Wiswell, & B.L. Drinkwater (Eds.). *Exercise in pregnancy* (2nd ed.). Baltimore: Williams & Wilkins.
30. Clapp, J.F. (2000). Exercise during pregnancy. A clinical update. *Clin Sports Med, 19,* 273.
31. Clapp, J.F. 3rd (2003). The effects of maternal exercise on fetal oxygenation and feto-placental growth. *Eur J Obstet Gynecol Reprod Biol, 110,* S80.
32. Clyman, R.I. (2012). Mechanisms regulating closure of the ductus arteriosus. In R.A. Polin, W.W. Fox, & S.H. Abman (Eds.). *Fetal & neonatal physiology* (4th ed.). Philadelphia: Saunders.
33. Cruz, M.O., Briller, J., & Hibbard, J.U. (2010). Update on peripartum cardiomyopathy. *Obstet Gynecol Clin North Am, 37,* 283.
34. Cunningham, G., et al. (2009). *Williams obstetrics* (23rd ed.). New York: McGraw-Hill.
35. Curry, R., Swan, L., & Steer, P.J. (2009). Cardiac disease in pregnancy. *Curr Opin Obstet Gynecol, 21,* 508.
36. Damm, P., Breitowicz, B., & Hegaard, H. (2007). Exercise, pregnancy, and insulin sensitivity—what is new? *Appl Physiol Nutr Metab, 32,* 537.
37. Das, B.B., Raj, S., & Solinger, R. (2009). Natriuretic peptides in cardiovascular diseases of fetus, infants and children. *Cardiovasc Hematol Agents Med Chem, 7,* 43.
38. Dempsey, F.C., Butler, F.L., & Williams, F.A. (2005). No need for a pregnant pause: Physical activity may reduce the occurrence of gestational diabetes mellitus and preeclampsia. *Exerc Sport Sci Rev, 33,* 141.
39. Dietl, J. (2000). The pathogenesis of preeclampsia: New aspects. *J Perinat Med, 28,* 464.
40. Duffy, T.P. (2004). Hematologic aspects of pregnancy. In G.N. Burrows, T.P. Duffy, & J.A. Copel (Eds.). *Medical complications during pregnancy* (6th ed.). Philadelphia: Saunders.
41. Duro, R.P., Moura, C., & Leite-Moreira, A. (2010). Anatomophysiologic basis of tetralogy of Fallot and its clinical implications. *Rev Port Cardiol, 29,* 591.
42. Echtler, K., et al. (2010). Platelets contribute to postnatal occlusion of the ductus arteriosus. *Nat Med, 16,* 75.
43. Falcao, S., et al. (2010). Exercise training can attenuate preeclampsia-like features in an animal model. *J Hypertens, 28,* 2446.
44. Fazio, G., et al. (2010). Patent foramen ovale and thromboembolic complications. *Curr Pharm Des, 16,* 3497.
45. Ferrero, S., Colombo, B.M., & Ragni, N. (2004). Maternal arrhythmias during pregnancy. *Arch Gynecol Obstet, 269,* 244.
46. Fisher, S.J., McMaster, M., & Roberts, J.M. (2009). The placenta in normal pregnancy and preeclampsia. In M.D. Linhheimer, J.M. Roberts, & G. Cunningham (Eds.). *Chesley's hypertensive disorders in pregnancy* (3rd ed.). New York: Academic Press.
47. Friedman, A.H. & Fahey, J.T. (1993). The transition from fetal to neonatal circulation: Normal responses and implications for infants with heart disease. *Semin Perinatol, 17,* 106.
48. Fu, Q. & Levine, B.D. (2009). Autonomic circulatory control during pregnancy in humans. *Semin Reprod Med, 27,* 330.
49. Fugelseth, D., et al. (1997). Ultrasonographic study of ductus venosus in healthy neonates. *Arch Dis Child Fetal Neonatal Ed, 77,* F131.
50. Ganzevoort, W., et al. (2004). Plasma volume and blood pressure regulation in hypertensive pregnancy. *J Hypertens, 22,* 1235.
51. Gao, Y. & Raj, J.U. (2010). Regulation of the pulmonary circulation in the fetus and newborn. *Physiol Rev, 90,* 1291.
52. Garovic, V.D. (2000). Hypertension in pregnancy: Diagnosis and treatment. *Mayo Clin Proc, 75,* 1071.
53. Gei, A.F. & Hankins, G.D. (2001). Cardiac disease and pregnancy. *Obstet Gynecol Clin North Am, 28,* 465.
54. Gelson, E., et al. (2011). Effect of maternal heart disease on fetal growth. *Obstet Gynecol, 117,* 886.
55. Giliberti, P., et al. (2009). The physiopathology of the patent ductus arteriosus. *J Matern Fetal Neonatal Med, 22,* 6.
56. Gowda, R.M., et al. (2003). Cardiac arrhythmias in pregnancy: Clinical and therapeutic considerations. *Int J Cardiol, 88,* 129.
57. Gregg, A.R. (2004). Hypertension in pregnancy. *Obstet Gynecol Clin North Am, 31,* 223.
58. Hale, R.W. & Milne, L. (1996). The elite athlete and exercise in pregnancy. *Semin Perinatol, 20,* 277.
59. Hamrick, S.E. & Hansmann, G. (2010). Patent ductus arteriosus of the preterm infant. *Pediatrics, 125,* 1020.
60. Harris, I.S. (2011) Management of pregnancy in patients with congenital heart disease. *Prog Cardiovasc Dis, 53,* 305.
61. Harris, I.S. & Black, B.L. (2010). Development of the endocardium. *Pediatr Cardiol, 31,* 391.
62. Hartmann, S. & Bung, P. (1999). Physical exercise during pregnancy—Physiological considerations and recommendations. *J Perinat Med, 27,* 204.
63. Haugen, G., et al. (2004). Portal and umbilical venous blood supply to the liver in the human fetus near term. Ultrasound *Obstet Gynecol, 24,* 599.
64. Hazinski, M.F., & van Stralen, D. (1990). Physiologic and anatomic differences between children and adults. In D.L. Levin & F.C. Morris (Eds.). *Essentials of pediatric intensive care.* St. Louis: Quality Medical Publications.

65. Hegewald, M.J. & Crapo, R.O.(2011). Respiratory physiology in pregnancy. *Clin Chest Med, 32,* 1.
66. Higgins, J.R. & de Swiet, M. (2001). Blood-pressure measurement and classification in pregnancy. *Lancet, 357,* 131.
67. Hilfiker-Kleiner, D., Sliwa, K., & Drexler, H. (2008). Peripartum cardiomyopathy: Recent insights in its pathophysiology. *Trends Cardiovasc Med, 18,* 173.
68. Hill, C.C. & Pickinpaugh, J. (2008). Physiologic changes in pregnancy. *Surg Clin North Am, 88,* 391.
69. Hislop A. (2005). Developmental biology of the pulmonary circulation. *Paediatr Respir Rev, 6,* 35.
70. Hosier, D.M. (1978). Changes in the electrocardiogram with age. In T.R. Johnson, W.M. Moore, & J.E. Jeffries (Eds.). *Children are different.* Columbus, OH: Ross.
71. Iwamoto, H.S. (2004). Endocrine regulation of the fetal circulation. In R.A. Polin, W.W. Fox, & S.H. Abman (Eds.). *Fetal and neonatal physiology* (3rd ed.). Philadelphia: Saunders.
72. Jim, B., et al. (2010). Hypertension in pregnancy: A comprehensive update. *Cardiol Rev, 18,* 178.
73. Johnson, T.R. (1978). Changes in the developing cardiovascular system in relation to age. In T.R. Johnson, W.M. Moore, & J.E. Jeffries (Eds.). *Children are different.* Columbus, OH: Ross.
74. Joles, J.A. & Poston, L. (2010). Can exercise prevent preeclampsia? *J Hypertens, 28,* 2384.
75. Kafer, E.R. (1990). Neonatal gas exchange and oxygen transport. In W.A. Long (Ed.). *Fetal and neonatal cardiology.* Philadelphia: Saunders.
76. Kajimoto, H., et al. (2007). Oxygen activates the Rho/Rho-kinase pathway and induces RhoB and ROCK-1 expression in human and rabbit ductus arteriosus by increasing mitochondria-derived reactive oxygen species: A newly recognized mechanism for sustaining ductal constriction. *Circulation, 115,* 1777.
77. Kajino, H., et al. (2002). Vasa vasorum hypoperfusion is responsible for medial hypoxia and anatomic remodeling in the newborn lamb ductus aeriosus. *Pediatr Res, 51,* 228.
78. Kametas, N.A., et al. (2003). Maternal cardiac function in twin pregnancy. *Obstet Gynecol, 102,* 806.
79. Kametas, N.A., et al. (2004). Maternal cardiac function during pregnancy at high altitude. *BJOG, 111,* 1051.
80. Katz, V.L. (2003). Exercise in water during pregnancy. *Clin Obstet Gynecol, 46,* 432.
81. Kilpatrick, S.J. (2009). Anemia and pregnancy. In R.K. Creasy, et al. (Eds.). *Creasy & Resnik's Maternal-fetal medicine: Principles and practice* (6th ed.). Philadelphia: Saunders Elsevier.
82. Kirkpatrick, C.A.(2010). The HELLP syndrome. *Acta Clin Belg, 65,* 91.
83. Kiserud, T. (2005). Physiology of the fetal circulation. *Semin Fetal Neonatal Med, 10,* 493.
84. Kita, N. & Mitsushita, J. (2008). A possible placental factor for preeclampsia: sFlt-1. *Curr Med Chem, 15,* 711.
85. Kleigman R.M., et al. (2011). *Nelson's textbook of pediatrics* (19th ed). Philadelphia: Saunders Elsevier.
86. Kluckow, M. (2005). Low systemic blood flow and pathophysiology of the preterm transitional circulation. *Early Hum Dev, 81,* 429.
87. Kramer, M.S. (2006). Regular aerobic exercise for women during pregnancy. *Cochrane Database Syst Rev, 3,* CD000180.
88. Kulik, T.J. (2012). Physiology of congenital heart disease in the neonate. In R.A. Polin, W.W. Fox, & S.H. Abman (Eds.). *Fetal & neonatal physiology* (4th ed.). Philadelphia: Saunders.
89. Kung, G.C. & Triedman, J. (2005). *Pathophysiology left to right shunts.* UpToDate online13.2; available at http:www.uptodateonline.com; Accessed July 23, 2011.
90. Lee, W. & Cotton, D.B. (1990). Maternal cardiovascular physiology. In R.D. Eden and F.H. Boehm (Eds.). *Assessment and care of the fetus: Physiological, clinical, and medicolegal principles.* Norwalk, CT: Appleton & Lange.
91. Leet, T. & Flick, L. (2003). Effect of exercise on birthweight. *Clin Obstet Gynecol, 46,* 423.
92. Levine, R.J. & Karumanchi, S.A. (2005). Circulating angiogenic factors in preeclampsia. *Clin Obstet Gynecol, 48,* 372.
93. Lincoln, J., Lange, A.W., & Yutzey, K.E. (2006). Hearts and bones: Shared regulatory mechanisms in heart valve, cartilage, tendon, and bone development. *Dev Biol, 294,* 292.
94. Lindheimer, M.D., Taler, S.J., & Cunningham, F.G. (2009). American Society of Hypertension. ASH position paper: Hypertension in pregnancy. *J Clin Hypertens (Greenwich), 11,* 214.
95. Lindheimer, M.D., Taler, S.J., & Cunningham, F.G. (2010). Hypertension in pregnancy. *J Am Soc Hypertens, 4,* 68.
96. Long, W.A., et al. (2004). Autonomic and central neuroregulation of fetal cardiovascular function. In R.A. Polin, W.W. Fox, & S.H. Abman (Eds.), *Fetal and neonatal physiology* (3rd ed.). Philadelphia: Saunders.
97. Lowrey, G.H. (1986). *Growth and development of children.* Chicago: Year Book Medical Publishers.
98. Maiz, N. & Nicolaides, K.H. (2010). Ductus venosus in the first trimester: Contribution to screening of chromosomal, cardiac defects and monochorionic twin complications. *Fetal Diagn Ther, 28,* 65.
99. Makikallio, K., Jouppila, P., & Rasanen, J. (2005). Human fetal cardiac function during the first trimester of pregnancy. *Heart, 91,* 334.
100. Malone, F.D. & D'Alton, M.D. (2009). Multiple gestation: Clinical characteristics and management . In R.K. Creasy, et al. (Eds.). *Creasy & Resnik's Maternal-fetal medicine: Principles and practice* (6th ed.). Philadelphia: Saunders Elsevier.
101. Mann, D. & Mehta, V. (2004). Cardiovascular embryology. *Int Anesthesiol Clin, 42,* 15.
102. Marsal, K. (2012). Fetal and placental circulation during labor. In R.A. Polin, W.W. Fox, & S.H. Abman (Eds.), *Fetal and neonatal physiology* (4th ed.). Philadelphia: Saunders.
103. Maynard, S.E., et al. (2003). Excess placental soluble fms-like tyrosine kinase 1 (sFlt1) may contribute to endothelial dysfunction, hypertension, and proteinuria in preeclampsia. *J Clin Invest, 111,* 649.
104. McElhinney, D.B., Tworetzky, W., & Lock, J.E. (2010). Current status of fetal cardiac intervention. *Circulation, 121,* 1256.
105. McQuillen, P.S. & Miller, S.P. (2010). Congenital heart disease and brain development. *Ann N Y Acad Sci, 1184,* 68.
106. Mehers, S. & Duley, L. (2006). Exercise or other physical activity for preventing preeclampsia and its complications. *Cochrane Database Syst Rev, 10,* CD005942.
107. Melzer, K., et al. (2010). Physical activity and pregnancy: Cardiovascular adaptations, recommendations and pregnancy outcomes. *Sports Med, 40,* 493.
108. Mercanti, I., Boubred, F., & Simeoni, U. (2009). Therapeutic closure of the ductus arteriosus: Benefits and limitations. *J Matern Fetal Neonatal Med, 22,* 14.
109. Mercanti, I., et al. (2011).Blood pressure in newborns with twin-twin transfusion syndrome. *J Perinatol, 31,*417.
110. Mittelmark, R.A., Wiswell, R.A., & Drinkwater, B.L. (1991). *Fetal responses to maternal exercise. Exercise in pregnancy* (2nd ed.). Baltimore: Williams & Wilkins.
111. Monga, M. (2009). Maternal cardiovascular, respiratory and renal adaptation to pregnancy. In R.K. Creasy, et al. (Eds.). *Creasy & Resnik's Maternal-fetal medicine: Principles and practice* (6th ed.). Philadelphia: Saunders Elsevier.
112. Moore, K.L., & Persaud, T.V.N. & Torchia, M.G. (2011). *The developing human: Clinically oriented embryology* (9th ed.). Philadelphia: Saunders Elsevier.
113. Morris, S.N. & Johnson, N.R. (2005). Exercise during pregnancy: A critical appraisal of the literature. *J Reprod Med, 50,* 181.
114. Muñoz-Chápuli, R. & Pérez-Pomares, J.M. (2010). Cardiogenesis: An embryological perspective. *J Cardiovasc Transl Res, 3,* 37.
115. Myatt, L. & Webster, R.P. (2009). Vascular biology of preeclampsia. *J Thromb Haemost, 7,* 375.
116. Nama, V., et al. (2011). Mid-trimester blood pressure drop in normal pregnancy: Myth or reality? *J Hypertens, 29,* 763.

117. Nicolaides, K.H. & Chitty, L.S. (2011). Fetal therapy: Progress made and lessons learnt. *Prenat Diagn, 31,* 619.
118. Noori, S., Stavroudis, T.A., & Seri, I. (2009). Systemic and cerebral hemodynamics during the transitional period after premature birth. *Clin Perinatol, 36,* 723.
119. Ntusi, N.B. & Mayosi, B.M. (2009). Aetiology and risk factors of peripartum cardiomyopathy: A systematic review. *Int J Cardiol, 131,* 168.
120. Ohlsson, A., Walia, R., & Shah, S.S. (2010). Ibuprofen for the treatment of patent ductus arteriosus in preterm and/or low birth weight infants. *Cochrane Database Syst Rev, 4,* CD003481.
121. O'Toole, M.L. (2003). Physiologic aspects of exercise in pregnancy. *Clin Obstet Gynecol, 46,* 379.
122. Parsons, M. (1988). Effects of twins: Maternal, fetal, and labor. *Clin Perinatol, 15,* 41.
123. Patel, C.R., et al. (2002). Fetal cardiac physiology and fetal cardiovascular assessment. In A.A. Fanaroff & R.J. Martin (Eds.). *Neonatal-perinatal medicine: Diseases of the fetus and infant* (7th ed.). Philadelphia: Mosby.
124. Patterson, A.J. & Zhang, L. (2010). Hypoxia and fetal heart development. *Curr Mol Med, 10,* 653.
125. Pelech, A.N. (2004). The physiology of cardiac auscultation. *Pediatr Clin North Am, 51,* 1515.
126. Perreault, T. & Coceani, F. (2003). Endothelin in the perinatal circulation. *Can J Physiol Pharmacol, 81,* 644.
127. Pivarnik, J.M., Perkins, C.D., & Moyerbrailean, T. (2003). Athletes and pregnancy. *Clin Obstet Gynecol, 46,* 403.
128. Pritchard, J. (1965). Changes in blood volume during pregnancy and delivery. *Anesthesiology, 26,* 393.
129. Pritchard, J.A., et al. (1972). Blood volume changes in pregnancy and the puerperium. II. Red blood cell loss and changes in apparent blood volume during and following vaginal delivery, cesarean section, and cesarean section plus total hysterectomy. *Am J Obstet Gynecol, 84,* 1271.
130. Rabinovitch, M. (2012). Developmental biology of the pulmonary vasculature. In R.A. Polin, W.W. Fox, & S.H. Abman (Eds.). *Fetal and neonatal physiology* (4th ed.). Philadelphia: Saunders.
131. Redman, C.W. & Sargent, I.L. (2005). Latest advances in understanding preeclampsia. *Science, 308,* 1592.
132. Resnik, R. (2004). The puerperium. In R.K. Creasy, R. Resnik, & J.D. Iams (Eds.). *Maternal-fetal medicine: Principles and practice* (5th ed.). Philadelphia: Saunders Elsevier.
133. Riemann, M.K., et al. (2000). Effects on the foetus of exercise in pregnancy. *Scand J Med Sci Sports, 10,* 12.
134. Roberts, J.M. & Cooper, D.W. (2001). Pathogenesis and genetics of pre-eclampsia. *Lancet, 357,* 53.
135. Roberts, J.M., et al. (2003). National Heart Lung and Blood Institute. Summary of the NHLBI Working Group on Research on Hypertension During Pregnancy. *Hypertension, 41,* 437.
136. Roberts, J.M. (2005). Preeclampsia: Recent insights. *Hypertension, 46,* 1243.
137. Roberts, J.M. & Funai, E.F. (2009). Pregnancy-related hypertension. In R.K. Creasy, et al. (Eds.). *Creasy & Resnik's Maternal-fetal medicine: Principles and practice* (6th ed.). Philadelphia: Saunders Elsevier.
138. Romem, A., et al. (2004). Incidence and characteristics of maternal cardiac arrhythmias during labor, *Am J Cardiol, 93,* 931.
139. Rudolph, A.M. (2000). Myocardial growth before and after birth: Clinical implication. *Acta Paediatr, 89,* 129.
140. Rudolph, A.M. (2003). Fetal circulation and cardiovascular adjustments after birth. In A.M. Rudolph & C.D. Rudolph (Eds.). *Rudolph's pediatrics* (21st ed.). New York: McGraw-Hill.
141. Rudolph, A.M. (2010). Congenital cardiovascular malformations and the fetal circulation. *Arch Dis Child Fetal Neonatal Ed, 95,* F132.
142. Rychik, J. (2004). Fetal cardiovascular physiology. *Pediatr Cardiol, 25,* 201.
143. Scholz, T.D. & Reinking, B.E.. (2012). Congenital heart disease. In C.A. Gleason & S. Devaskar (Eds.). *Avery's diseases of the newborn* (9th ed.). Philadelphia: Saunders.
144. Schrier, R.W. (2010). Systemic arterial vasodilation, vasopressin, and vasopressinase in pregnancy. *J Am Soc Nephrol, 21,* 570.
145. Sedmera, D. (2005). Form follows function: Developmental and physiological view on ventricular myocardial architecture. *Eur J Cardiothorac Surg, 28,* 526.
146. Segar, J.L. (2012). Neural regulation of blood pressure during fetal and neonatal life. In R.A. Polin, W.W. Fox, & S.H. Abman (Eds.). *Fetal & neonatal physiology* (4th ed.). Philadelphia: Saunders.
147. Shah, D.M. (2011). Hypertensive disorder of pregnancy. In R.J. Martin, A.A. Fanaroff, & M.C. Walsh (Eds.). *Fanaroff and Martin's neonatal-perinatal medicine: Diseases of the fetus and infant* (9th ed.). Philadelphia: Mosby Elsevier.
148. Shenoy, V., Kanasaki, K., & Kalluri, R. (2010). Pre-eclampsia: Connecting angiogenic and metabolic pathways. *Trends Endocrinol Metab, 21,* 529.
149. Sibai, B., Dekker, G., & Kupferminc, M. (2005). Pre-eclampsia. *Lancet, 365,* 785.
150. Sibai, B.M. (2005). Diagnosis, prevention, and management of eclampsia. *Obstet Gynecol, 105,* 402.
151. Silva, L.M., et al. (2008). No midpregnancy fall in diastolic blood pressure in women with a low educational level: the Generation R Study. *Hypertension, 52,* 645.
152. Siu, S.C., et al. (2002). Adverse neonatal and cardiac outcomes are more common in pregnant women with cardiac disease. *Circulation, 105,* 2179.
153. Sklansky, M. (2003). New dimensions and directions in fetal cardiology. *Curr Opin Pediatr, 15, 463.*
154. Soultanakis-Aligianni, H.N. (2003). Thermoregulation during exercise in pregnancy. *Clin Obstet Gynecol, 46,* 442.
155. Strasburger, J.F. & Wakai, R.T. (2010). Fetal cardiac arrhythmia detection and in utero therapy. *Nat Rev Cardiol, 7,* 277.
156. Streuling, I., Beyerlein, A., & von Kries, R. (2010). Can gestational weight gain be modified by increasing physical activity and diet counseling? A meta-analysis of interventional trials. *Am J Clin Nutr, 92,* 678.
157. Tappero, E.P. & Honeyfield, M.E. (2009). *Physical assessment of the newborn: A comprehensive approach to the art of physical examination* (4th ed). Santa Rosa, CA: NICU Ink.
158. Teitel, D.F. (2004). Physiologic development of the cardiovascular system in the fetus. In R.A. Polin, W.W. Fox, & S.H. Abman (Eds.). *Fetal and neonatal physiology* (3rd ed.). Philadelphia: Saunders.
159. Thornburg, K.L., et al. (2000). Hemodynamic changes in pregnancy. *Semin Perinatol, 24,* 11.
160. Tsen, L.C. (2005). Gerard W. Ostheimer "What's new in obstetric anesthesia" lecture. *Anesthesiology, 102,* 672.
161. Turan, O.M., et al. (2011). The duration of persistent abnormal ductus venosus flow and its impact on perinatal outcome in fetal growth restriction. *Ultrasound Obstet Gynecol.* 2011 Apr 4. [Epub ahead of print.]
162. Ueland, K., & Hansen, J.M. (1969). Maternal cardiovascular dynamics. II. Posture and uterine contractions. *Am J Obstet Gynecol, 103,* 1.
163. van der Bom, T., et al. (2011). The changing epidemiology of congenital heart disease. *Nat Rev Cardiol, 8,* 50.
164. Veille, J.C. (1996). Maternal and fetal cardiovascular response to exercise during pregnancy. *Semin Perinatol, 20,* 250.
165. Volman, M.N., et al. (2007). Haemodynamic changes in the second half of pregnancy: A longitudinal, noninvasive study with thoracic electrical bioimpedance. *BJOG, 114,* 576.
166. Walker, S.P., et al. (1999). The diastolic debate: Is it time to discard Korotkoff phase IV in favor of phase V for blood pressure measurements in pregnancy? *Med J Aust, 169,* 203.
167. Walther, N.K.A. & Peeters, L. (2005). Severe cardiac disease in pregnancy. Part I: Hemodynamic changes and complaints during pregnancy, and general management of cardiac disease in pregnancy. *Curr Opin Crit Care, 11,* 430.

168. Wantanabe, M., et al. (2011). Cardiac embryology. In R.J. Martin, A.A. Fanaroff, & M.C. Walsh (Eds.). *Fanaroff and Martin's Neonatal-perinatal medicine: Diseases of the fetus and infant* (9th ed.). Philadelphia: Mosby Elsevier.
169. Warnes, C.A. (2004). Pregnancy and pulmonary hypertension. *Int J Cardiol, 97,* 11.
170. Weissgerber, T.L., et al. (2006). Exercise in the prevention and treatment of maternal-fetal disease: A review of the literature. *Appl Physiol Nutr Metab, 31,* 661.
171. Weissgerber, T.L., Davies, G.A., & Roberts, J.M. (2010). Modification of angiogenic factors by regular and acute exercise during pregnancy. *J Appl Physiol, 108,* 1217.
172. Williams, D. (2003). Pregnancy: A stress test for life. *Curr Opin Obstet Gynecol, 15,* 465.
173. Williams, R.G., et al. (2006). Report of the National Heart, Lung, and Blood Institute Working Group on research in adult congenital heart disease. *J Am Coll Cardiol, 47,* 701.
174. Wolfe, L.A. & Weissgerber, T.L. (2003). Clinical physiology of exercise in pregnancy: A literature review. *J Obstet Gynaecol Can, 25,* 473.
175. Yagel, S., et al. (2010). The fetal venous system, part I: Normal embryology, anatomy, hemodynamics, ultrasound evaluation and Doppler investigation. *Ultrasound Obstet Gynecol, 35,* 741.
176. Young, B.C., Levine, R.J., & Karumanchi, S.A.(2010). Pathogenesis of preeclampsia. *Annu Rev Pathol, 5,* 173.
177. Zahka, K.G. (2011). Genetic and environmental contributions to congenital heart disease. In R.J. Martin, A.A. Fanaroff, & M.C. Walsh (Eds.). *Fanaroff and Martin's Neonatal-perinatal medicine: Diseases of the fetus and infant* (9th ed.). Philadelphia: Mosby Elsevier.
178. Zahka, K.G. (2011). Principles of neonatal cardiovascular hemodynamics. In R.J. Martin, A.A. Fanaroff, & M.C. Walsh (Eds.). *Fanaroff and Martin's Neonatal-perinatal medicine: Diseases of the fetus and infant* (9th ed.). Philadelphia: Mosby Elsevier.
179. Zahka, K.G. & Erenberg, F. (2011). Congenital defects. In R.J. Martin, A.A. Fanaroff, & M.C. Walsh (Eds.). *Fanaroff and Martin's Neonatal-perinatal medicine: Diseases of the fetus and infant* (9th ed.). Philadelphia: Mosby Elsevier.
180. Zahka, K.G. & Lane, J.R. (2011). Approach to the neonate with cardiovascular disease. In R.J. Martin, A.A. Fanaroff, & M.C. Walsh (Eds.). *Fanaroff and Martin's Neonatal-perinatal medicine: Diseases of the fetus and infant* (9th ed.). Philadelphia: Mosby Elsevier.

CHAPTER 10

Respiratory System

Respiration is the totality of those processes that ultimately result in energy being supplied to the cells. In pregnancy the respiratory system undergoes significant changes. The increased metabolic needs of the pregnant woman, fetus, and placenta require improved maternal respiratory efficiency to ensure adequate oxygenation. The placenta functions as the respiratory system for the fetus, providing nutrients and oxygen and removing carbon dioxide. This makes the relationship between the mother and fetus not only intimate but also interdependent. At birth, tremendous energy is expended by the neonate to generate sufficient negative pressure to convert to an air-liquid interface in the alveoli and maintain functional residual capacity (FRC). Transitional events continue over the first week of life as the neonate adjusts to the new environment, more alveoli are recruited, and the surfactant system stabilizes. This chapter examines alterations in the respiratory system and acid-base homeostasis during the perinatal period and their implications for the mother, fetus, and neonate. Fetal blood gases and responses to hypoxia are discussed in Chapter 6.

MATERNAL PHYSIOLOGIC ADAPTATIONS

Changes in the respiratory system during pregnancy increase the volume of air and gas exchange with each breath enhancing oxygen availability to and carbon dioxide removal from the fetus. These changes are mediated by hormonal and biochemical changes as well as by the enlarging uterus. As the muscles and cartilage in the thoracic region relax, the chest broadens and tidal volume (V_T) is improved with a conversion from abdominal to thoracic breathing. This leads to a 50% increase in air volume per minute. These changes result in a mild respiratory alkalosis. For the fetus, this mild alkalosis enhances gas exchange across the placenta.

Antepartum Period

Pregnancy is associated with major changes in the respiratory system, including changes in lung volumes and ventilation. Both biochemical and mechanical factors interact to increase the delivery of oxygen and the removal of carbon dioxide.[147] Otolaryngeal changes are discussed in Chapter 15.

Factors Influencing Respiratory Function

Mechanical Factors. The gradual enlargement of the uterus leads to changes in abdominal size and shape, shifting the resting position of the diaphragm up to 4 cm above its usual position to accommodate the growing uterus (Figure 10-1).[23,43,96,147,247] The thoracic circumference increases by 5 to 7 cm and the transverse diameter of the chest by about 2 cm in response to the increased intraabdominal pressure with a flaring of the lower ribs.[43,96,247] The subcostal angle progressively increases from 68 to 103 degrees in late gestation.[23,96,247] Not all of these changes can be attributed to intraabdominal pressure, in that the increase in the subcostal angle occurs before the increasing mechanical pressure.[147,247,250] Relaxation of the ligamentous rib attachments increases rib cage elasticity. This change is similar to those seen in the pelvis and mediated by similar factors, such as relaxin (see Chapter 15).

Although the aforementioned changes suggest that diaphragmatic motion decreases, the reverse is actually true. Diaphragmatic movement actually increases about 2 cm during pregnancy, with the major work of breathing being accomplished by the diaphragm rather than by the costal muscles.[23,43,96,147] These changes in thoracic structures modify the abdominal space, perhaps in preparation for the increase in uterine size and peak at 37 weeks.[96] The changes in thoracic configuration have a major impact on lung volumes, however, to which the increasing intra-abdominal pressure contributes.

Biochemical Factors. Hormones and other biochemical factors are important in stimulating changes in the respiratory system in pregnancy. These substances can act centrally via stimulation of the respiratory center or directly on smooth muscle and other tissues of the lung. The most important influences are mediated by progesterone, in combination with estradiol (which increases progesterone receptors in the hypothalamus) and prostaglandins (PGs).[108]

Serum progesterone levels increase progressively throughout pregnancy and are thought to be a major factor in the changes seen in ventilation.[250] Progesterone is a respiratory stimulant. The administration of progesterone to nonpregnant subjects increases minute ventilation and enhances responses to hypercapnia.[96,108,147] This suggests an increased

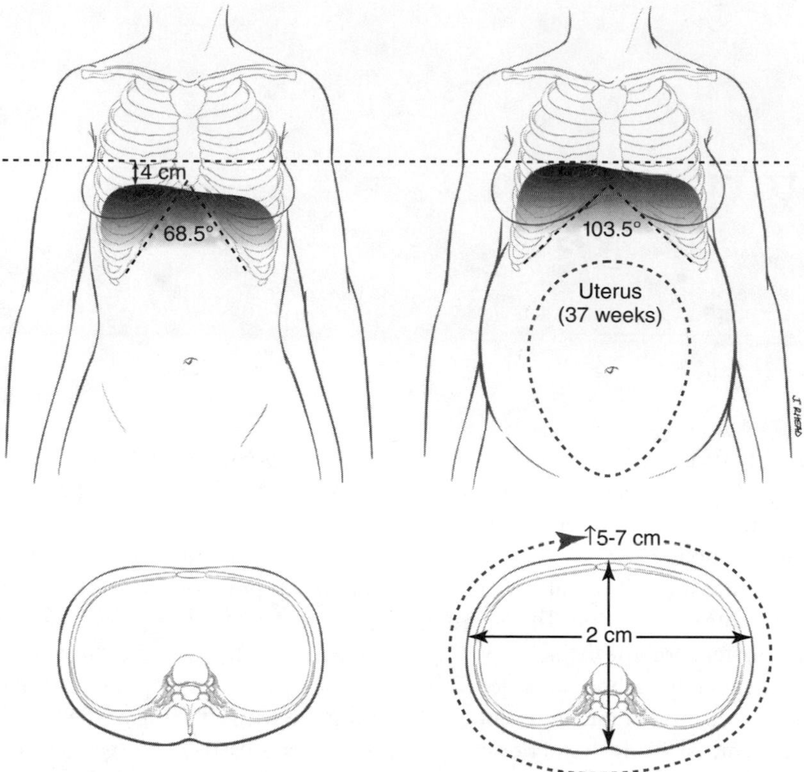

FIGURE 10-1 Chest wall changes that occur during pregnancy. The subcostal angle increases, as does the anterior-posterior and transverse diameters of the chest wall and the chest wall circumference. These changes compensate for the 4-cm elevation of the diaphragm so that the total lung capacity is not significantly reduced. (From Hegewald, M.J. & Crapo, R.O. (2011). Respiratory physiology in pregnancy. *Clin Chest Med*, 32, 1.)

sensitivity to carbon dioxide by the respiratory center and that progesterone lowers the carbon dioxide threshold of the respiratory center.[3,108,250] For example, in the nonpregnant woman, an increase of 1 mmHg (0.13 kPa) in the $PaCO_2$ results in a 1.5 L/min increase in ventilation, whereas during pregnancy the same 1-mmHg increase in $PaCO_2$ leads to a 6-L/min increase in ventilation.[247] More than 60% of the increase in CO_2 sensitivity occurs by 20 weeks' gestation.[213]

This increased sensitivity most likely contributes to the sensation of dyspnea that is experienced by many pregnant women and may also lead to some of the hyperventilation that occurs during the second stage of labor after pushing efforts (as carbon dioxide levels increase during breath holding).[147] Progesterone may also exert a local effect on the lung, causing water retention in the lung that results in decreased diffusion capacity. Therefore hyperventilation is an attempt to maintain normal PO_2 levels.[247]

Progesterone may also play a role in decreasing airway resistance (up to 50%), thereby reducing the work of breathing and facilitating a greater airflow in pregnancy. Relaxation of bronchiole smooth muscle has been attributed to progesterone. This counteracts the expected increase in airway resistance that would be the result of lungs that are less distended.

PGs may also play a role in ventilatory changes by affecting the smooth muscle tissue of the bronchial airways. $PGF_{2\alpha}$ is a bronchial smooth muscle constrictor, whereas PGE_1 and PGE_2 have bronchodilator effects. PGs may balance or counteract the consequences of structural changes in the respiratory system during pregnancy (e.g., decreased lung distention as a result of elevated diaphragm) and modify respiration to meet fetal requirements (maternal respiratory alkalosis promotes carbon dioxide transfer from the fetus).

Lung Volume

Changes in lung volumes begin in the middle of the second trimester and are progressive to term (Figure 10-2). The most significant change is a 30% to 40% (from 500 to 700 mL) increase in V_T, with a progressive 15% to 20% decrease in expiratory reserve volume (ERV), 20% to 25% decrease in residual volume (RV), and 20% to 30% decrease in FRC.[96] The FRC is further decreased in the supine position at term.[96] The decreased FRC may increase uptake and elimination of inhaled anesthetics.[23] Along with the change in V_T, there is a concomitant increase in inspiratory capacity (IC) by 5% to 10%, thereby allowing the total lung capacity (TLC) to remain relatively stable, with a slight decrease of up to 5% by term.[23,96,147] Vital capacity (VC) and inspiratory reserve

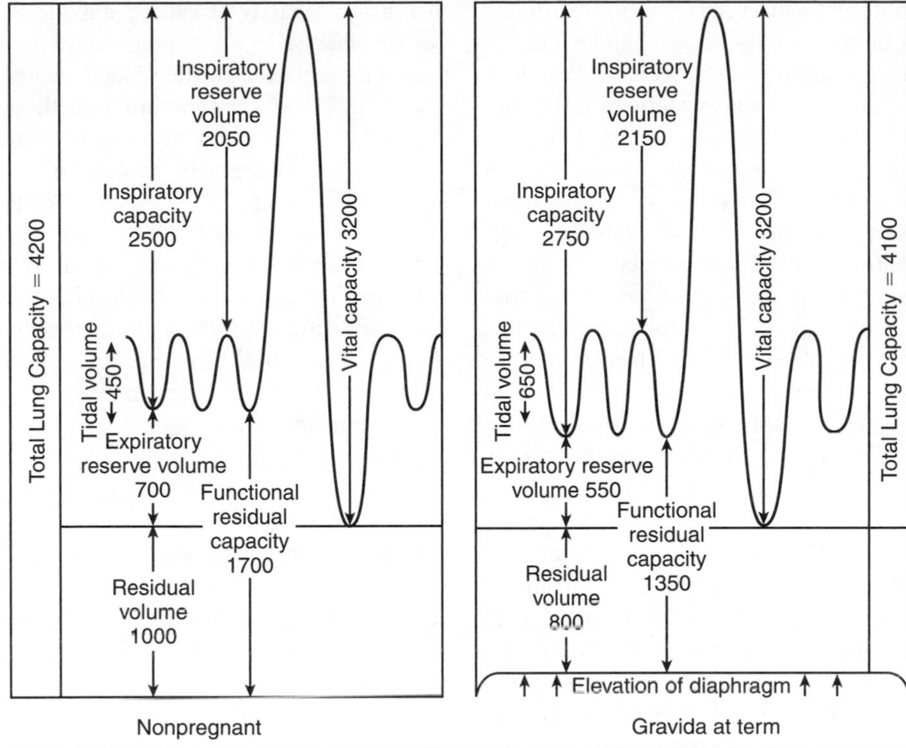

FIGURE 10-2 Lung volume changes in pregnancy (units in mL). (From Gardner, M.O. & Doyle, N.M. [2004]. Asthma in pregnancy. *Obstet Gynecol Clin North Am, 31,* 390.)

volume (IRV) are essentially unaltered, although some literature notes a small change in IRV.[147,247,250] Peak expiratory flow rates tend to decrease during pregnancy, possibly due to mechanical changes in the respiratory system.[95] Physiologic dead space is increased by 60 mL.[247]

The decreased RV, in conjunction with an elevated metabolic rate, increases the risk of hypoxia if respiratory depression occurs.[250] On the other hand, forced expiratory volume in 1 second (FEV_1) does not change nor does the FEV_1/VC ratio.[147,250] These assessments are used in individuals with asthma and are generally thought to be reliable in pregnant women.[43,147,250] However, recent studies suggest that peak inspiratory flow rates are altered by maternal position (lower in supine versus standing or sitting) and may in fact decrease to some extent during pregnancy.[95]

Changes in lung volumes result from the elevation of the diaphragm and the changes in the configuration of the chest. The alteration in RV is also the result of a 35% to 40% decrease in chest wall compliance; lung compliance is unchanged.[43,96,147,247] The decreased chest wall compliance is caused by hormonal influences as well as changes in abdominal pressure. This reduction in compliance allows for more inward movement of the chest wall and reduces the amount of trapped air (residual trapped volume) that contributes to the RV. Therefore the RV decreases 200 to 300 mL. This, along with an approximately 200 mL decrease in ERV, brings the total deficit in the FRC to 500 mL (see Figure 10-2). The FRC falls progressively from 20 weeks' gestation for a change of 10% to 24% by term.[147,250]

Lung Function

Changes in lung function are related to three major factors: ventilation, airflow, and diffusing capacity.[147] Oxygen consumption increases during pregnancy; however, the arterial oxygen pressure (PaO_2), though it increases, does not change significantly, even though the arteriovenous oxygen difference decreases. This indicates that there must be a change in ventilation.[247]

Ventilation. Minute ventilation (V_T x Respiratory rate [RR]) increases up to 30% to 50% during pregnancy.[23,147] Changes begin by 8 weeks' gestation and result in an increase in minute volume, from 6.5 to 7.5 L/min in early pregnancy to 10 to 10.5 L/min at term.[108] The elevated resting ventilation exceeds the demands in oxygen consumption, indicating that women tend to hyperventilate during pregnancy.[147,247,250] The greater increase in resting ventilation is thought to be due to the stimulatory effects of progesterone on the respiratory center.[147] Progesterone may also increase red blood cell levels of carbonic anhydrase B, which facilitates CO_2 transfer and lowering of the PCO_2.[247] The hyperventilation of pregnancy and associated respiratory system alterations are also mediated by the interaction of acid-base balance changes, increased breathing drive, increased central chemoreflex sensitivity, increased metabolism and decreased cerebral blood flow.[109-111]

The increase in minute ventilation is probably due primarily to the 30% to 40% increase in V_T rather than changes in respiratory rate, which usually is unchanged.[23,43,96,247] It is much more efficient to increase alveolar ventilation through an increase in V_T than with a proportionately equal increase in respiratory rate. The increased metabolic rate and carbon dioxide production also influence V_T changes.[250] Maximal inspiratory and expiratory pressures are not altered in pregnancy. The reduced RV further enhances alveolar ventilation. This change in RV decreases the amount of gas mixing that occurs with each tidal exchange in the alveolus, thereby improving gas exchange at the alveolar level. Alveolar ventilation increases by 50% to 70% during pregnancy.[15,147,247]

Airflow. Airflow is dependent upon resistance encountered in the bronchial tree. Two important determining factors for resistance are smooth muscle tone in the bronchi and the degree of congestion encountered in bronchial wall capillaries. Despite the changes in minute ventilation and the concomitant increase in alveolar ventilation, the work of breathing (airway resistance and lung compliance) remains unchanged. In the larger airways, congestion has very little to do with resistance. Airway resistance does not change significantly during pregnancy because of a balance between bronchoconstricting ($PGF_{2\alpha}$, decreased RV, and decreased $PaCO_2$) and bronchodilating (PGE_2 and progesterone) forces.[96,147]

Assessment of small airway function is most often determined by evaluation of closing volume (CV) and closing capacity (CC). CV is the point at which the small airways close (collapse and cease to ventilate) in the lowest part of the lung. Small airway ($<$1 mm) patency is believed to be the result of transpulmonary pressure, compliance of the airway walls, and the presence of sufficient surfactant. Closure in the lung bases normally occurs somewhere between the RV and FRC. CV is usually expressed as a percentage of vital capacity (CV/VC). CC is the term applied to the sum of the CV and RV (CC = CV + RV) and is expressed as a percentage of total lung capacity (CC/TLC).[43,147,250]

Under normal circumstances, airway closure does not occur during tidal breathing. When closure occurs at a higher than normal volume, however, gas exchange may be affected because ventilation to the lung bases is decreased. In pregnancy, airway closure above the FRC has been reported near term and is attributed to the 20% to 30% decrease in ERV.[147] Airway closure is more likely to occur in supine versus sitting.[147] This alteration changes gas distribution and may result in a decrease in oxygen content and PaO_2 in the third trimester.[43,147,247,250] When airway closure is at or above FRC, there is the possibility of altering PaO_2 due to ventilation-perfusion ($\dot{V}/\dot{Q}$) mismatch in the lung bases. If these differences are significant, compensatory maternal physiologic responses such as an increase in respiratory rate may result. However, this is not a usual event in healthy women who compensate by changes in the hemoglobin-oxygen dissociation curve (see "Acid-Base Changes").[26]

Diffusing Capacity. Diffusing capacity refers to the ease with which gas is transferred across the pulmonary membrane. Diffusion capacity of carbon dioxide may show an increase or no change in early pregnancy, followed by a decrease, reaching a plateau in the second half of pregnancy in many women. These changes are not thought to be clinically significant.[23,33,96,147] Carbon dioxide production increases by 30% due to changes in cholesterol and fat metabolism.[250] Oxygen consumption increases by 32 to 58 mL/min.[171] This change is accounted for by the needs of the fetus (average of 12 mL/min) and placenta (4 mL/min), and by increased maternal cardiac output (7 mL/min), ventilation (2 mL/min), renal function (7 mL/min), and extra tissue in the breasts and uterus (5 mL/min). The increase in carbon dioxide production exceeds the changes in oxygen consumption, leading to an increase in the respiratory quotient from 0.70 to 0.83 by term.[247]

Acid-Base Changes

Oxygen consumption, carbon dioxide production, and basal metabolic rate all increase due to the increased metabolic demands from the mother, placenta, and fetus.[96] The normal pregnant woman is in a state of compensated respiratory alkalosis, which is thought to be the result of the effects of progesterone on the respiratory system and lung volume changes, especially the increased minute volume.[247,250] The result is a reduction in arterial and alveolar carbon dioxide and a slight increase in PaO_2. The fall in PCO_2 begins early in pregnancy, paralleling changes in ventilation.[147,247] Definitions of common terms used in acid-base physiology are listed in Table 6-1 on p. 165.

The purpose of the respiratory alkalosis seems to be facilitation of carbon dioxide transfer from the fetus to the mother by increasing the arterial carbon dioxide pressure ($PaCO_2$) gradient. Hyperventilation leads to average $PaCO_2$ values of 27 to 32 mmHg (3.59 to 4.25 kPaa) and a concomitant decrease in serum bicarbonate levels to between 18 and 21 mEq/L (mmol/L) with a base deficit of -3 to -4 mEq/L (mmol/L).[23,147] The latter is a consequence of increased renal excretion of bicarbonate, reflecting a metabolic compensation for the lower $PaCO_2$. The lower $PaCO_2$ produces a gradient within the intervillous space that enhances fetal offloading of carbon dioxide.[23] This may be the primary function of the hyperventilation of pregnancy.[160] $PaCO_2$ values vary with the altitude at which the mother resides; the decrease in $PaCO_2$ is greater at higher altitudes (compensatory hyperventilation to maintain and adequate PaO_2.[23,96,247] The pH increases to the high end of normal (7.40 to 7.45) to maintain homeostasis. These changes are stable throughout pregnancy until the onset of labor.[33,43,147] The reduction in blood buffer reduces the mother's ability to compensate for a metabolic acidosis that could develop during prolonged labor or other states in which tissue perfusion may be reduced.

In contrast, PaO_2 levels increase from those of prepregnancy (95 to 100 mmHg [12.63 to 13.30 kPaa]) because of the increase in alveolar ventilation. During the first trimester, PaO_2 levels range from 106 to 108 mmHg, dropping to 101 to 104 mmHg (13.43 to 13.83 kPaa) by the third trimester.[247]

Even though the PaO_2 level remains elevated, the alveolar-arterial PO_2 gradient ($AaDO_2$) is unchanged throughout most of pregnancy, but may increase near term due to an attempt to offset hyperventilation.[147] Oxygen delivery is maintained within normal limits during pregnancy due to the increased carbon dioxide, which compensates for changes in the respiratory system and the decrease in red blood cells.[247] Supine positioning versus sitting in late pregnancy further decreases PaO_2 levels and increases the $AaDO_2$ gradient.[147,247] However, these changes are thought to have little clinical significance.[147]

Oxygen-Hemoglobin Dissociation Curve. The oxygen-hemoglobin dissociation curve (see Box 10-1 below) demonstrates that once the plateau of the curve is achieved it takes large changes in oxygen concentration in order to make small changes in SaO_2. The P_{50} increases from 26 to 30 mmHg (3.45 to 3.99 kPaa) by term (Figure 10-3), thus decreasing the affinity of hemoglobin and enhancing transfer of oxygen from mother to fetus.[247,250] These changes are mediated by the increase in 2,3-diphosphoglycerate (2,3-DPG), which is stimulated by the increase in maternal pH.[43] The increased 2,3-DPG shifts the oxygen-hemoglobin dissociation curve to the right to enhance oxygen release to the fetus.

It is unclear whether the small changes seen in PaO_2 levels during pregnancy are significant to the maternal-fetal oxygen gradient and therefore to the fetus. Considering that fetal PaO_2 levels are between 25 and 35 mmHg (3.32 and 4.65 kPaa), this seems unlikely. However, this increase may reflect increased maternal pulmonary circulation, with a greater volume of blood contained within the pulmonary vasculature at any given point in time. This may be significant at higher altitudes (see "Effects of Altitude and Air Travel"). SaO_2 does not change significantly during pregnancy, although saturations below 96% may be seen in women who smoke.

Intrapartum Period

The major effect of labor upon the respiratory system is related to the increased muscular work, metabolic rate, and oxygen consumption, which increases 40% to 60% during labor.[23] Consequently, alterations in ventilation and acid-base status can be anticipated. The healthy woman tolerates these changes since oxygen delivery is much greater than needs, but this can become a problem in the compromised woman.[247]

With the onset of labor, there is an increased demand for oxygen; oxygen consumption increases with uterine muscle activity. If there is insufficient time for uterine relaxation and restabilization after a contraction, oxygen content is lower and myometrial hypoxia as well as metabolic acidosis may occur with the next contraction. Over time this can lead to inadequate oxygenation, which increases the severity of the pain experienced. Most studies have evaluated respiratory system changes during active and painful labor. There are few studies evaluating the labor process with the use of sporadic analgesia and psychoprophylaxis. The pain experienced during labor is the result of the interaction of a number of factors (see Chapter 15). The subjective component includes the discomfort that is perceived by the mother. Objective factors are related to changes in the

BOX 10-1 Oxygen-Hemoglobin Dissociation Curve

The oxygen-hemoglobin dissociation curve demonstrates the equilibrium between oxygen and hemoglobin (see Figure 10-3). The curve relates the partial pressure of oxygen to the percentage of hemoglobin that is saturated. There are two aspects of the curve that must be considered: its shape and its position. The shape of the curve is sigmoid, indicating that at higher levels (>50 mmHg [6.65 kPaa]) the curve flattens and an increase in PO_2 produces little increase in saturation. This upper region is the PO_2 range in which oxygen binds to hemoglobin in the lungs. At low PO_2 levels the curve is steep and small changes in PO_2 result in large changes in hemoglobin saturation. In this range, oxygen is released from hemoglobin and cellular activities occur. A small drop in PO_2 here allows a large amount of oxygen to be unloaded to the tissues.

The position of the curve, whether it is shifted to the right or the left, depends on the oxygen affinity for the hemoglobin molecule. The affinity of hemoglobin for oxygen must be sufficient to oxygenate the blood during its movement through the pulmonary circulation. However, it must be weak enough to allow release of oxygen to the tissues. This affinity is expressed as the P_{50}, the oxygen tension at which hemoglobin is half saturated. The higher the affinity the lower the P_{50} and vice versa, indicating an inverse relationship. The P_{50} for adult blood at a pH of 7.40 and a temperature of 37° C (98.6° F) is normally 26 mmHg (3.45 kPa).

Numerous factors, both genetic and environmental, can influence the affinity of hemoglobin and shift the oxygen-hemoglobin dissociation curve.

A shift to the right implies a lowered affinity; a shift to the left indicates that oxygen is more tightly bound to hemoglobin. The structure of the hemoglobin molecule regulates the affinity and can be affected by pH, PCO_2, and temperature. Increasing amounts of carbon dioxide reduce hemoglobin affinity for oxygen. This is termed the *Bohr Effect*. Because of the Bohr Effect, the reciprocal exchange of oxygen for carbon dioxide is facilitated. Elevations in temperature also shift the curve to the right such that saturation is decreased at any given PO_2. The pH increases with release of CO_2, and the curve shifts to the left. The shift indicates an increased affinity for oxygen and favors the uptake of oxygen by hemoglobin.

Because of the sigmoid shape of the curve, a shift in position has little effect on the saturation when the PO_2 is within the normal arterial range (95 to 100 mmHg [12.63 to 13.33 kPaa]). However, in the venous system, in which the PO_2 range is around 40 mmHg (5.32 kPaa), there is a right shift in the curve, leading to an increased unloading of oxygen to the tissues and improving tissue oxygenation. Figures 10-3 and 10-19 illustrate oxygen-hemoglobin dissociation curves for the pregnant woman and the newborn. Changes in oxygen equilibrium after birth in term and preterm infants are illustrated in Figure 10-20.

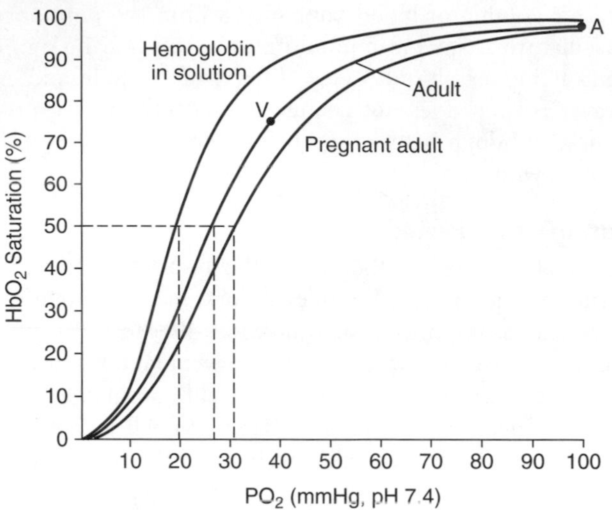

FIGURE 10-3 Oxyhemoglobin dissociation curve under standard conditions for normal blood of pregnant and nonpregnant adults. Also shown is the dissociation curve for hemoglobin in solution. (From Delivoria-Papadopoulos, M. & McGowen, J.E. [1998]. In R.A. Polin & W.W. Fox [Eds.]. *Fetal and neonatal physiology* [2nd ed.]. Philadelphia: Saunders.)

functioning of the cardiorespiratory system, alterations in the autonomic nervous system, and physical changes that occur during labor and delivery.

Ventilatory alterations related to pain vary significantly from patient to patient; therefore, each laboring woman must be evaluated individually. Changes seen during the intrapartum period include an increase in respiratory rate and a change in V_T, with a tendency toward further hyperventilation. Hyperventilation is a natural response to pain and becomes evident as the pain and apprehension of labor increase. Hyperventilation is diminished when pain is alleviated.[21] Maximal inspiratory pressure decreases during strong expulsive efforts, possibly as a result of development of transient diaphragmatic fatigue.

Although pain seems to be the major cause of this hyperventilatory response, anxiety, drugs, and the use of psychoprophylactic breathing exercises can contribute to the elevated respiratory rate. V_T may be further increased during the second stage of labor as hyperventilation following breath holding with expulsive efforts is encountered. Risks of the Valsalva maneuver are discussed in Chapter 4.

Increases in oxygen uptake and minute ventilation are seen during labor, with a significant increase noted between early latent and active phases. Oxygen consumption increases 40% to 60% during labor with further increases (up to twofold) with contractions.[33,247] This is balanced by an increase in cardiac output. Women with low oxygen delivery may become compromised with inadequate oxygen delivery to both the woman and fetus.[247] The increase in ventilation can lead to a progressive and substantial decline in $PaCO_2$. There are wide variations in values between patients; however, a $PaCO_2$ level around 25 mmHg is representative of what might be encountered during the first stage of labor. A transient decline in $PaCO_2$ occurs with each contraction until cervical dilation is complete, at which time the decline in $PaCO_2$ may be seen even between contractions.

The changes in $PaCO_2$ are markedly reduced or eliminated when continuous lumbar epidural anesthesia is used during labor. Variables affecting $PaCO_2$ levels that need to be considered include breath holding (which elevates $PaCO_2$ levels), compensatory hyperventilation following breath holding, length of contractions, and frequency of contractions. The timing of analgesia administration as well as the frequency and efficacy of the analgesia may also alter $PaCO_2$ values.[43] The respiratory alkalosis that ensues from hyperventilation is normally associated with a drop in base excess and possibly a decrease in arterial pH, according to some researchers. Others have documented a rise in pH. In either case, the degree of change indicates that labor and hyperventilation are highly significant events that may lead to alterations in physiologic parameters.[21]

Mild maternal acidosis is not uncommon and can be attributed to isometric muscular contractions that reduce the blood flow to working muscles, leading to tissue hypoxia and anaerobic metabolism in the face of a normal PaO_2. The degree of maternal acidosis is dependent upon the extent of maternal anxiety and tension, intensity of muscular workload, degree of isometric contractions, and duration of labor.

In the first stage of labor, the maternal and fetal $PaCO_2$ levels parallel each other. This may reflect the respiratory nature of these changes. As labor progresses, this paralleling of values is lost. Fetal $PaCO_2$ levels increase when maternal acidosis occurs, reflecting not only fetal base deficit alterations but also the hypoxia within the uterine muscle. Contractions not only decrease the blood flow to the intervillous space but also reduce the oxygen supply to the uterus. The longer and stronger the contractions, the more pronounced the effects are. The local buildup of $PaCO_2$ decreases the fetal elimination of carbon dioxide, which may lead to a drop in fetal pH. During the second stage of labor, maternal $PaCO_2$ levels may rise during pushing efforts. During this stage, a further increase in blood lactate levels due to voluntary muscle activity during bearing down is seen. This is reflected in a substantial decline in blood pH and a fall in blood buffering capability (base deficit).

Significant changes in acid-base status due to hyperventilation and increased oxygen consumption are potentially hazardous to both the mother and fetus.[21] Extremely low $PaCO_2$ levels result in cerebral vasoconstriction and possibly reduce intervillous perfusion and blood flow. The alkalemia that results shifts the oxygen-hemoglobin dissociation curve to the left. This shift impairs the release of oxygen from maternal blood to fetal blood, thereby decreasing the availability of oxygen to the fetus during a time when oxygenation may already be impaired due to uterine contractions.[21] Hyperventilation may lead to dizziness and tingling in the mother due to low $PaCO_2$ levels. Interventions can include counting respirations out loud to help the mother slow her respiratory rate, letting her know when the contraction is ending so that

Table 10-1 **Maternal Blood Gas Alterations During the Intrapartum Period**

STAGE OF LABOR	PARAMETER	RANGE VALUE	ACID-BASE STATUS
Early	$PaCO_2$	21 to 26 mmHg (2.79 to 3.45 kPaa)	Respiratory alkalosis
	Plasma base deficit	−0.9 to 26.9 mEq/L (mmol/L)	
	Blood pH	7.43 to 7.49	
End of first stage	$PaCO_2$	21 to 35 mmHg (2.79 to 4.65 kPaa)	Mild metabolic acidosis compensated by respiratory alkalosis
	Plasma base deficit	−1.2 to 29.2 mEq/L (mmol/L)	Mild respiratory acidosis during bearing down
	Blood pH	7.41 to 7.54	
End of second stage (delivery)	$PaCO_2$	16 to 24 mmHg (2.12 to 3.19 kPaa)	Metabolic acidosis uncompensated by respiratory alkalosis
	Plasma base deficit	−2.3 to −12.3 mEq/L (mmol/L)	
	Blood pH	7.37 to 7.45	

From Burgess, A. (1979). *The nurse's guide to fluid and electrolyte balance.* New York: McGraw-Hill.

she can begin to relax, avoiding the Valsalva maneuver, and promoting deep breathing between contractions to cleanse the system and promote oxygenation and restabilization.

The acid-base changes encountered in the first and second stages of labor quickly reverse in the third stage and postpartum period with compensatory respiratory efforts. These efforts are largely due to a decrease in respiratory rate. Acid-base levels return to pregnancy values within 24 hours of delivery and to nonpregnant levels by several weeks after delivery. Table 10-1 summarizes the changes in arterial blood gases during the intrapartum period.

Research on the effects of labor on acid-base status has been conducted in conjunction with the delivery of epidural analgesia. Psychoprophylaxis (psychoanalgesia) has been shown to reduce the need for medication, reduce tension and pain by self-report, and engender a positive attitude toward the labor and delivery experience. Lamaze psychoprophylaxis is based on the hypothesis that childbirth is a natural physiologic process and that pain can be minimized through education and specified exercises. Education and antenatal preparation are designed to reduce anxiety through knowledge of the processes of labor. Relaxation techniques are designed to reduce skeletal muscle spasm and tension that may contribute to pain. Reduction of pain sensations and perception is achieved through distraction by utilizing conditional responses such as breathing patterns and other nonpharmacologic measures (see Chapter 15).

Postpartum Period

The respiratory tract rapidly returns to its prepregnant state after delivery. This is a direct result of the separation of the placenta and consequential loss of progesterone production, as well as the immediate reduction in intraabdominal pressure with delivery of the infant that allows increased excursion of the diaphragm.

Chest wall compliance changes immediately after delivery due to a decrease in pressure on the diaphragm and reduction in pulmonary blood volume. A 20% to 25% increase in static compliance has been reported following delivery. Changes in rib cage elasticity may persist for months after delivery.[250] V_T and RV return to normal soon after delivery, whereas ERV may remain in an abnormal state for several months. As progesterone levels fall in the first 2 days after delivery, $PaCO_2$ levels rise. Diffusing capacity, which at term is slightly below postpartum levels, increases during the postpartum period. Overall, anatomic changes and ventilation return to prepregnant status by 24 weeks after delivery, although the subcostal angle tends to remain about 20% wider than prepregnancy vaues.[96]

CLINICAL IMPLICATIONS FOR THE PREGNANT WOMAN AND HER FETUS

The respiratory changes that occur with pregnancy can be annoying as well as limiting in some circumstances. Common complaints and experiences include dyspnea, capillary engorgement of the upper respiratory tract, and altered exercise tolerance. As a result, modifications in activity levels as well as in the activities themselves may need to be considered. Discussions with women regarding their usual activities can help provide sufficient information for determining when change is needed. In addition, changes in the maternal respiratory system can influence the course of disease processes (e.g., asthma in some women), affecting not only the mother but also the fetus. Specific areas addressed in this section include dyspnea of pregnancy, upper respiratory capillary engorgement, respiratory infections, asthma, smoking, and anesthesia. Exercise is discussed briefly; further information can be found in Chapter 9.

Dyspnea

The sensation of dyspnea is reported by 60% to 70% of pregnant women, usually beginning during the first or second trimester (Figure 10-4). A maximal incidence is reached between 28 and 31 weeks and remains relatively stable to term.[147,247,250]

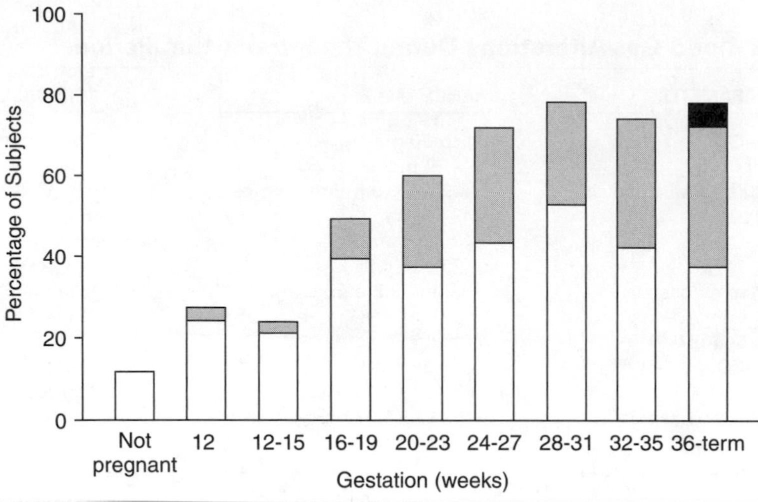

FIGURE 10-4 Incidence, time course, and severity of dyspnea during normal pregnancy. *Solid white areas,* dyspnea present climbing hills or more than one flight of stairs; *solid gray areas,* present on climbing one flight of stairs, walking at an even pace on level ground, during routine performance of housework; *solid black area,* dyspnea present on slightest exertion or at rest. (From Milne, J. [1979]. The respiratory response to pregnancy. *Postgrad Med J, 55,* 318.)

Because abdominal girth has not increased significantly at the time of dyspnea onset, intraabdominal pressure cannot be ascribed as the cause.

Dyspnea during pregnancy is a physiologic dyspnea; that is, it occurs even at rest or with mild exertion.[250] The exact cause remains unclear, but it is thought to be due to the increased respiratory drive and load, changes in oxygenation, or a combination of these events.[250] Increased sensitivity to carbon dioxide and hypoxia may be important contributing factors, especially in early pregnancy. During late pregnancy, mechanical factors may aggravate these changes.[171] The increased V_T and lower $PaCO_2$ have also been implicated. In addition, the heightened maternal awareness of the normal hyperventilation of pregnancy might result in the sensation of dyspnea. An improvement in symptoms in some women with increasing gestation suggests an adjustment to this normal process.

Dyspnea can be quite uncomfortable and anxiety provoking. The hyperventilation and dyspnea may decrease the ability of some pregnant women to maintain their usual activity levels. Pathologic dyspnea—which may occur with disorders such as pulmonary emboli (a complication sometimes seen in pregnancy)—must be differentiated from physiologic dyspnea during pregnancy. Pathologic dyspnea is characterized by respiratory rates greater than 20, PCO_2 below 30 mmHg (3.99 kPaa) or greater than 35 mmHg (4.66 kPaa), or abnormal FEV_1.[250]

Upper Respiratory Tract Capillary Engorgement

Hormonal changes (especially the increase in estrogens) along with the increased blood volume, hyperemia, edema, glandular hypersecretion and increased phagocyte activity alter the mucosa of the oro- and nasopharynx with capillary engorgement throughout the respiratory tract.[96] Progesterone may contribute to engorgement by inducing vascular smooth muscle relaxation and nasal vascular pooling. Increased circulating blood volume may also play a role in this pooling. The results of these changes can be uncomfortable to some women and may be exacerbated in women with preeclampsia.[137] With preeclampsia, the airways may be narrower due to soft tissue edema.[169] In some situations these changes can be hazardous. For example, swelling of the airway along with other physiologic changes in pregnancy (e.g., weight gain, changes in the gastrointestinal system, and increased total body water) increase the risk for the pregnant woman who requires intubation for obstetric or nonobstetric problems.[23,71,169] The rate of failed intubations is seven to eight times higher during pregnancy.[23]

The nasopharynx, larynx, trachea, and bronchi may become swollen and reddened. For some individuals this may be uncomfortable, but it usually does not pose any unusual difficulties. These symptoms can be markedly aggravated with minor upper respiratory infections and preeclampsia. The swelling can lead to inflammation (noninfective in nature) that causes changes in the voice (e.g., hoarseness), make nose breathing difficult, and increase the incidence of nosebleeds. Abrasions and lacerations of the mucosa may occur, and bleeding may ensue.[21,71,169]

Rhinitis (defined as nasal congestion that lasts 6 or more weeks without signs of infection or allergy) is seen in up to 30% of all pregnant women and in approximately two thirds of those who smoke.[62,84,96,137] These symptoms may appear any time but usually begin in the second trimester and parallel increasing estrogen levels.[137] Estrogens and placental growth hormone (a stimulator of nasal mucosal growth) have been implicated in the etiology of pregnancy rhinitis.[62,84,96] Rhinitis usually disappears by 48 hours postpartum, but may take up to 2 weeks in some women.[96] Upper respiratory tract changes may also increase snoring and exacerbate sleep-disordered breathing or increase obstructive sleep apnea.[23,26] These changes are discussed further in Chapter 15.

Exercise

The effect of exercise on the respiratory system is related to alveolar ventilation and is dependent upon the age, body weight, body composition, and physical condition of the individual. Cardiovascular function, uterine blood flow, respiratory function, blood gases, aerobic capacity, metabolism, temperature, and psychologic state are all affected by exercise. Cardiorespiratory changes with exercise during pregnancy are discussed further in Chapter 9.

The usual changes in maternal respiratory function during pregnancy are similar to those with mild to moderate exercise.[111,180] Studies of respiratory rates with exercise in pregnant and nonpregnant women demonstrate that respiratory rates in pregnant women are higher than those in nonpregnant women during mild exercise, but this difference disappears during moderate exercise. V_T and minute volume remain higher in pregnant subjects during all levels of exercise.[180] Ventilation increases 38% and oxygen consumption is 15% greater during exercise in pregnant versus nonpregnant women.[147,180] The efficiency of gas exchange does not seem to be impaired in the pregnant woman during exercise. During prolonged exercise, however, PaO_2 increases and $PaCO_2$ decreases. This decrease in $PaCO_2$ is most likely due to the effects of progesterone on the respiratory center. Oxygen consumption also increases with advancing gestational age. Part of this increase is due to the increased work of carrying the extra weight associated with pregnancy. Exercise-induced changes in acid-base balance are similar in pregnant and nonpregnant women.

Effects of Altitude and Air Travel

With increasing altitude, compensatory decreases in PaO_2 and changes in other parameters can be seen. These are an attempt by the maternal system to maintain higher PaO_2 levels under relatively hypoxic conditions.[147,153] The change in altitude has a significant effect on oxygen saturation and changes the oxygen-hemoglobin dissociation curve. Pregnant women living at high altitude have a higher minute ventilation, FRC, TLC, forced VC, forced expiratory volume, and diffusion capacity than women at sea level.[23,121] The hyperventilation of pregnancy is also accentuated, and maternal dyspnea may be more prominent; therefore patients need to be given assurance that it is normal.[8] The woman increases her ventilation and oxygen saturation during the first trimester, while diffusing capacity decreases to the third trimester, leading to decreased oxygen content by term. These changes are not significant if the woman comes from a family that has lived at altitude for at least 3 generations.[23,121] Pregnancy at high altitude is also associated with morphologic differences in placental villi with increased capillary diameter.[64] Women living at altitude have lower birth weight infants. Birth weight is decreased by an average of 100 g for each 3000 ft (1000 m) increase in altitude.[23]

Commercial aircraft are usually pressurized to 6000 to 8000 feet (1829 to 2434 meters) above sea level, so flying results in a transient exposure to altitude. During ascent, the pregnant woman may experience transient cardiopulmonary adaptations (increased heart rate and blood pressure; decreased aerobic capacity).[4] The fetal heart rate may also increase transiently during both takeoff and landing, but stays within normal limits.[71] Pregnant women who travel by airplane may also experience an increase in dyspnea and respiratory rate as their bodies attempt to compensate for the increased altitude. Fetal hemoglobin (HbF) and the fetal circulation protect the fetus from desaturation during commercial flights.[201] Thus flying in commercial aircraft is generally not a risk in women with uncomplicated pregnancies.[4,35,71,145] The American College of Obstetricians and Gynecologists states that "in the absence of obstetric or medical complications, pregnant women can observe the same general precautions for air travel as the general population and can fly safely."[4] Most airlines allow travel up to 36 weeks of pregnancy, with travel up to 7 days before the woman's expected due date permitted with a certificate from their health care provider.[4] For international travel the cutoff may be earlier.

Pregnant women may be at greater risk of thromboembolism during air travel due to changes in hemostasis (see Chapter 8) and hemoconcentration due to the low cabin humidity (<25%) and should be sure to stretch, perform isometric exercises, and walk around the cabin at regular intervals.[201] However, a retrospective study did not find any increased risk of thromboembolism up to 2 weeks after air travel.[71] Because of the low cabin humidity, the woman should also maintain hydration with frequent intake of nonalcoholic beverages, because hydration is important for placental blood flow.[201]

Pulmonary Disease and Pregnancy

Pulmonary disorders may be aggravated by the changes in the respiratory system during pregnancy. Respiratory infections and asthma are discussed here. Women with pulmonary hypertension (see Chapter 9) and cystic fibrosis (see Chapter 1) are also at increased risk for complications during pregnancy. Outcomes depend on their status at the onset of pregnancy.[28]

Adult respiratory distress syndrome (ARDS) is an acute lung injury involving diffuse interstitial infiltrates, decreased lung compliance, and hypoxia.[33] ARDS is usually triggered by sepsis but may also be triggered by other factors, including disseminated intravascular coagulation (see Chapter 8), preeclampsia, amniotic fluid embolism, abruptio placenta, or fetal demise.[147,247] Physiologic changes during pregnancy, especially changes in colloid osmotic pressure, may increase the risk of ARDS following lung injury.[33]

Respiratory Infection

Changes in the immune (see Chapter 13) and pulmonary systems in the pregnant woman, along with upper airway hyperemia and edema, not only make having an upper respiratory infection more uncomfortable but can also potentiate movement of the infection into the lungs.[197] Infections associated with lung involvement can potentially increase airway resistance, thereby increasing the work of breathing, and lead to decreased V_T and RV. This may lead to decreased maternal and subsequently fetal PaO_2 levels. The increased oxygen requirements of pregnancy, elevated diaphragm, decreased FRC, increased lung water, and changes in closing volume may increase the severity of respiratory problems.[27,43] Avoidance of those situations in which infections might be contracted and avoidance of individuals carrying infections when possible is a good practice. Most upper respiratory infections are only annoyances and do not lead to significant consequences for the mother or fetus.

Pneumonia, although rare, is a common cause of nonobstetric maternal death in North America.[27,84] The prevalence of bacterial pneumonia is similar during pregnancy in nonpregnant, healthy women.[57,84,247] However, pregnant women are more susceptible to viral pneumonia and the pneumonia may progress more rapidly during pregnancy.[33,84,247] The risk of pneumonia increases with each trimester and by the third trimester, the risk of hospitalization from pneumonia is five times higher in pregnant than nonpregnant women.[84,247] The risk of influenza related morbidity is 10.5/10,000 during pregnancy versus 1.91/10,000 in nonpregnant women.[84] As a result, influenza vaccinations are recommended for all pregnant women during flu season, regardless of trimester.[34] Pregnancy may also increase the risk of varicella pneumonia.[84,247] Pneumonia increases the risk of preterm labor, altered fetal growth, and maternal and perinatal mortality.[33,34,84,247] Although chronic infections such as tuberculosis (TB) have often been reported to reactivate and worsen with pregnancy, recent evidence suggests that in women with drug-sensitive TB who have received adequate therapy, fetal and maternal outcomes are generally good.[147,247] Respiratory infections are discussed further in Chapter 13 (see section on Risk of Maternal Infection).

Asthma

Asthma is an obstructive disease characterized by increased airway resistance, decreased expiratory flow rates, hyperinflation with premature airway closure, and some loss of lung compliance. These factors lead to an increase in the work of breathing. Along with this, hyperinflation and exaggerated negative pleural pressures can lead to increased demands on the right ventricle. This can be seen as a rise in pulmonary arterial pressure. These factors decrease left stroke volume, arterial systolic pressure, and pulse pressure.[147]

The restrictive processes in asthma are usually reversible and are due to an increased responsiveness of the airways to a variety of stimuli. When stimulated, the characteristic responses include contraction of the bronchial smooth muscle, mucous hypersecretion, and mucosal edema. The mechanism for this responsiveness is unclear and may be different from patient to patient.[147]

Several mechanisms have been implicated in the etiology of asthma. These include an immunologic response, blocked β-adrenergic function, β-adrenergic amine deficiency, cholinergic dominance, intrinsic smooth muscle defect, or some combination of these. Other possibilities include an imbalance in cyclic nucleotides. Cyclic adenosine monophosphate (cAMP) and cyclic guanosine monophosphate (cGMP) are involved in the modulation of airway tone, with the former contributing to bronchodilation and the latter to bronchoconstriction.[41] A major pathogenic characteristic is airway inflammation with release of inflammatory mediators (e.g., leukotrienes, histamine, eosinophil chemotactic factor of anaphylaxis, platelet-activating factor), and disruption of the mucosal epithelial barrier.[147]

The prevalence of asthma has increased in the general population, leading to an increase in pregnant women with asthma.[171] As a result, asthma is the most common pulmonary problem seen during pregnancy, occurring in approximately 8% of pregnant women.[173] Asthma may improve (about 23%), worsen (about 30%), or remain unchanged (about 47%) during pregnancy.[57] Trying to predict an individual's course during pregnancy is extremely difficult. Women with more severe asthma before pregnancy are more likely to have severe asthma, and require hospitalization, during pregnancy, although this is not always the case.[18,57,147,247] No change in perinatal mortality has been reported in women with mild to moderate asthma when the asthma was medically managed; women with severe asthma are at high risk for exacerbation and pregnancy complications, including preterm delivery, low birth weight, fetal growth restriction, increased perinatal mortality and morbidity, and preeclampsia.[14,57,147,171,203] Worsening of symptoms during the intrapartum period occurs in 10% to 40%; most return to their prepregnancy status by 3 months postpartum.[80,171]

Asthma may lead to maternal hypoxia or hyperventilation with resultant hypocapnia and alkalosis, potentially affecting fetal well-being.[247] Transient hypoxia is not generally as great a concern as chronic hypoxia, which increases the risk of preterm birth, altered fetal growth, and mortality.[247] Acute hypocapnia and alkalosis, however, can contribute to fetal depression by reducing umbilical and uterine blood flow secondary to vasoconstriction. Alkalosis also increases maternal hemoglobin affinity for oxygen, thereby reducing availability to the fetus.

The normal alterations of the respiratory system during pregnancy may influence asthma in both positive and negative ways (Table 10-2). The hyperventilation of pregnancy may be more distressful for the asthmatic woman.[80] The increase in circulating cortisol levels may augment cAMP functioning as well as reduce inflammation through steroid action. Progesterone levels decrease bronchomotor tone—relaxing smooth muscle tissue—and thereby decrease airway resistance. Elevated serum cAMP levels may also promote bronchodilation. Thus improvement of asthma during pregnancy may be

Table 10-2 Factors Affecting Asthma in Pregnancy

IMPROVEMENT
Increased progesterone-mediated bronchodilation
β-Adrenergic-stimulated bronchodilation
Decreased plasma histamine levels
Increased free cortisol levels
Increased glucocorticoid-mediated β-adrenergic responsiveness
Increased PGE-mediated bronchodilation
PGI_2-mediated bronchial stabilization
Increased half-life of bronchodilators
Decreased protein-binding of bronchodilators
WORSENING
Pulmonary refractoriness to cortisol effects
Increased $PGF_{2\alpha}$-mediated bronchoconstriction
Decreased functional residual capacity, causing airway closure and altered ventilation-perfusion ratios
Increased major basic protein in lung
Increased incidence of viral or bacterial respiratory infection
Increased gastroesophageal reflux
Increased stress

Data from Schatz, M. & Hoffman, C. (1987). Interrelationships between asthma and pregnancy: Clinical and mechanistic considerations. *Clin Rev Allergy, 5*, 301.

secondary to increased free cortisol, decreased plasma histamine, decreased bronchial smooth muscle tone due to progesterone, and decreased airway resistance due to decreased tone.[147,171,247] Conversely, worsening may be due to increased progesterone and mineral steroids that compete for glucocorticoid receptors, increased β2-adrenoreceptor responsiveness, increased viral respiratory infections and thus bronchial inflammation, increased $PGF_{2\alpha}$, and hyperventilation.[147] The increased tendency for gastroesophageal reflux (see Chapter 12) during pregnancy may also exacerbate the asthma.[171] Therefore, the effect of pregnancy on the course of asthma in an individual woman depends on the balance of these factors in her system.

Pharmacologic treatment and the selection of an appropriate agent are based on the risk-to-benefit ratio of bronchodilator effect and hypoxia avoidance versus possible adverse consequences.[173] Oral corticosteroids in the first trimester have been linked to an increased risk of cleft lip with or without cleft palate, and increase in preeclampsia, preterm delivery, and low birth weight.[57,183] Thus inhaled corticosteroids are generally advocated as a first line therapy.[57,173,247] Maternal physiologic changes may alter the pharmacokinetics, although most agents seem to be as effective during pregnancy as in nonpregnant women.[247] Women with exacerbations may need stepwise increase in therapies; women who improve may also need changes in treatment.[173] Decreased compliance (up to ⅓) with use of inhaled corticosteroids during pregnancy is associated with an increased frequency of exacerbations.[57] The National Asthma Education and Prevention Program has published guidelines for management of the pregnant asthmatic woman and notes that "it is safer for pregnant women with asthma to be treated with asthma medication than it is for them to have asthma symptoms and exacerbations."[173] General management includes careful history taking and evaluation, patient education, avoidance of known triggers, and medical therapy. Education about the medical regimen and recognition of early symptoms so that treatment may be initiated early and hypoxia prevented are essential. Women need to be counseled to use only those medications prescribed and to avoid over-the-counter medications. Prescribed medications should be taken only as directed; maternal and fetal side effects need to be explained clearly and concisely.[147]

Smoking

"Smoking during pregnancy is among the leading preventable causes of adverse maternal and fetal outcomes."[171] Maternal smoking increases perinatal morbidity and mortality. Smoking may also interfere with a woman's ability to conceive.[170] Risks for the pregnant woman include increased rates of spontaneous abortion, abruptio placenta, placenta previa, early or late bleeding, premature rupture of membranes, and preterm labor.[22,63,147,170,171]

Fetal and neonatal risks of maternal smoking include low birth weight (two- to threefold increase), preterm delivery, and fetal growth restriction.[22,147,170] Infants of women who smoke on average weigh 200 g less at birth than infants of women who do not smoke.[170,233] There is a dose-related effect of the number of cigarettes per day and the decrease in birth weight, especially in women who continue smoking past 32 weeks' gestation.[147,170,190] The degree of risk for low birth weight in women who smoke may be influenced by maternal genotype, especially genetic polymorphisms that affect the activity of specific enzymes needed to metabolize the various chemicals in cigarettes.[238] Paternal smoking is also associated with decreased birth weight although not to the degree seen with maternal smoking.[170]

The exact mechanism for these complications is not completely understood, but include indirect effects on uterine blood flow and direct effects due to transfer of toxins such as nicotine, which appears to be the toxin causing the most maternal and fetal harm, across the placenta (see Chapter 7).[22,170,209] Nicotine and its main metabolite, cotinine, are lipid soluble and readily crosses the placenta.[170,209] Fetal levels are generally 90% of maternal levels and may be higher.[171] Nicotine may also compete with nutrients for placental nutrient carriers, reducing nutrient transfer and thus fetal growth. Many of the risks seen with smokers are related to the placenta or consequences of altered placental function. This supports an etiology mediated by changes in placental structure and alterations in uteroplacental blood flow and oxygenation.[147]

Placentas of smokers are proportionately greater in weight (as related to fetal weight) than placentas of nonsmokers and demonstrate histologic changes, suggesting hypoxia with a compensatory hypertrophy. Women who experience chronic anemia or live at high altitudes have similar compensatory mechanisms because of the chronic intrauterine hypoxia. The placentas of smokers also have more areas of calcification, an increased incidence of fibrin deposits, an increased frequency of necrosis and inflammation in the margin, and evidence of deoxyribonucleic acid (DNA) changes.[147] In addition, an increased risk of placental lesions has also been identified. These findings suggest that smoking causes some direct damage to the blood vessels of the placenta that may lead to placental underperfusion.

If the alterations seen in the placenta are due to a decrease in uterine blood flow, the fetal consequences may be acidosis and hypoxemia. Because diffusion of oxygen to the fetus is dependent on blood flow, a decrease in flow could lead to chronic hypoxia that over time may have a cumulative effect on development. This decrease in uterine blood flow may be mediated by the release of catecholamines from the adrenal glands as a consequence of nicotine exposure. An increased maternal heart rate and an elevation of blood pressure are clinical indications of catecholamine release with smoking. The catecholamines trigger peripheral vasoconstriction, which leads to a decrease in perfusion of the uteroplacental vasculature (underperfusion).

Chronic underperfusion leads to fibrin deposition in arteries, inflammation and necrosis of tissue, and the development of lesions and calcifications. The perimeter of the placenta would be affected first, because perfusion is lower in these regions. The reduction of blood flow brought about by these defects could affect the placenta such that it would not be able to sustain itself, leading to an increased incidence of abruption. The overall impact of these changes would be a reduction in placental blood flow, leading to a decrease in available oxygen to the fetus and hypoxia.

The risk of hypoxia is further increased by carbon monoxide, a by-product of smoking, which equilibrates between maternal and fetal blood.[147] Because carbon monoxide has a higher affinity for hemoglobin than oxygen, the oxygen-carrying capacity of the blood in smokers is reduced. These effects have been demonstrated by highly elevated levels of carboxyhemoglobin in the fetus at birth. Along with this, carbon monoxide greatly increases the affinity of oxygen for hemoglobin. With increased affinity, oxygen is less readily unloaded to the fetal tissues. This, in turn, reduces fetal oxygenation further.

Children of smokers are at risk for later problems as well, including behavioral difficulties; long term learning memory; and mood, conduct, and attention-deficit disorders.[22,56,170,209] Changes in the central nervous system may be due to alterations in expression of neurotransmitters in the fetus, fetal adrenergic activation leading to sympathetic nervous system dysfunction, or alterations in the serotonin system.[111] Alterations in lung function have been reported with in utero exposure to smoking and often persist to late childhood and possibly longer.[56] Sudden infant death syndrome and the incidence of childhood respiratory disorders, including asthma, pneumonia, and bronchitis, are also higher.[56,147,170,171] Offspring of smokers also are reported to have a higher incidence of non-Hodgkin lymphoma, acute lymphoblastic leukemia, and Wilms tumor, with a dose-response relationship.[56,147]

Inhalation Anesthesia

The use of inhalation anesthesia in pregnant women usually occurs only during emergencies. Intubation may be more difficult in the pregnant women (see "Upper Respiratory Tract Capillary Engorgement"). The effect on the maternal respiratory system is related to maternal cardiorespiratory status before induction and the type and adequacy of ventilation following induction. Light to moderate anesthesia with adequate oxygen mixing should provide no difficulties to the well-hydrated, stable, pregnant woman.[21] Because of the reduced functional residual capacity and increased closing volumes during pregnancy, as well as the higher metabolic requirements, the pregnant woman is less tolerant of apnea and is at higher risk for a difficult or failed intubation.[135,136] Oxygen partial pressure levels drop rapidly in these situations, leading to hypoxia, hypoxemia, and acidosis. These events not only place the mother at risk, but also jeopardize the status of the fetus.

Inhalation agents are dose and time-dependent compounds affecting the fetus directly through transplacental movement of drugs or indirectly by altering maternal homeostasis or changing uteroplacental blood flow.[21,193] If fetal depression does occur, it is an indication of impaired placental blood flow, possibly due to decreased maternal cardiac output.[21,43,147] Most of the time, no serious depression occurs. However, uteroplacental blood flow may be altered through several mechanisms: (1) change in perfusion pressure, (2) modification of vascular resistance, (3) alterations in uterine contractions and basal tone, and (4) interference in fetal cardiovascular function (umbilical circulation). Uterine blood flow varies directly with perfusion pressure across the uterine vascular bed (uterine arterial pressure minus uterine venous pressure) and inversely with uterine vascular resistance. The balance between perfusion pressure and vascular resistance is the primary basis for acute changes in uterine blood flow.[21,141]

Adverse responses or heavy anesthesia can precipitate a hazardous sequence of events. Maternal cardiac output may fall, precipitating a fall in blood pressure and an increased likelihood of maternal acidosis and decreased uterine blood flow. The result is a decreased uteroplacental blood flow with decreased nutrient supply to the fetus. Fetal heart rate and blood pressure may fall due to direct fetal cardiovascular depression (drug response) or the indirect effect of decreased uteroplacental perfusion. The decreased cardiac output and low blood pressure culminate in fetal hypoxia and acidosis, as reflected in low oxygen saturations, elevated PCO_2 levels, and falling base excess. Fetal status before induction affects the severity of the response.[21,141] This same sequence of events may occur with severe maternal hyperventilation. Marked reductions in maternal PCO_2 reduce uteroplacental blood flow and maternal cardiac output and can lead to fetal hypoxemia and acidosis.

SUMMARY

The maternal respiratory alterations that occur during pregnancy ensure an adequate supply of oxygen to the developing fetus and its supporting structures. These demands are increased with activity and labor and are usually compensated for without difficulty. However, subjective interpretation of labor and the pain experienced can trigger maternal hyperventilation and alter fetal homeostasis. Adequate education of the mother about the normal physiologic changes and the labor experience is essential to maternal-fetal well-being. Psychoprophylaxis, analgesia, and anesthesia can moderate the experience and can be used safely during the intrapartum period. Careful monitoring with all these methods is important to safeguard the fetus. Clinical implications for the pregnant woman and her fetus are summarized in Table 10-3.

DEVELOPMENT OF THE RESPIRATORY SYSTEM IN THE FETUS

Embryonic development of the lung and the role of lung fluid and fetal breathing movements in development, as well as surfactant synthesis and secretion, set the stage for understanding the changes that occur with transition to extrauterine life. Respiratory system development is stimulated by multiple genes and a complex interplay of regulatory molecules, including growth factors, transcription factors (DNA binding proteins), extracellular matrix molecules, integrins, intracellular adhesion molecules, morphogens, and exogenous factors such as retinoic acid and antioxidants.[40,83,123,163,198,240] Lung development is also stimulated by mechanical forces especially stretch of lung tissue by fetal breathing movements and accumulation of lung fluid.[38] Mechanical forces increase the rate of cell proliferation and differentiation, especially of the alveolar epithelium.[90]

Table 10-3 Clinical Implications for the Respiratory System in the Pregnant Woman and Fetus

- Understand the normal respiratory changes that occur during pregnancy (pp. 297-301, 303-304).
- Explain to the pregnant woman the changes that can occur in the respiratory system early in pregnancy and how they can affect daily activities and exercise tolerance (pp. 298-300, 303-305).
- Encourage prelabor preparation to reduce discomfort, hyperventilation, and anxiety during labor (pp. 301-303).
- Reduce hyperventilation during labor by counting respirations slowly, discouraging breath holding, and encouraging deep breathing between contractions (pp. 301-303).
- Discuss upper airway changes that may lead to nasal congestion and other symptoms (pp. 304-305).
- Counsel women regarding respiratory infections during pregnancy (pp. 305-306).
- Counsel pregnant women to get an influenza vaccine if they are pregnant during flu season (p. 306).
- Discuss usual exercise routines and changes that may be necessary (p. 305 and Chapter 9).
- Counsel pregnant women regarding air travel (p. 305).
- Counsel asthmatic women who are pregnant to follow their medical regimen as directed, to avoid known precipitating factors, and seek medical intervention when symptoms persist (pp. 305-307).
- Encourage and support pregnant women in reducing or eliminating cigarette consumption both during and after pregnancy (pp. 207-308, Chapter 7).

Anatomic Development

Lung growth occurs in five stages: embryonic (3 to 6 weeks' gestation), pseudoglandular (6 to 16 weeks' gestation), canalicular (16 to 26 weeks' gestation), saccular (26 to 36 weeks' gestation), and alveolar (36 weeks' gestation to 2 to 3 years postbirth).[114,129] These stages are summarized in Figure 10-5.

The embryonic stage of lung development lasts from 3 to 6 weeks' gestation. Around day 24, a ventral diverticulum (outpouching) can be seen developing from the foregut. This groove extends downward and is gradually separated from the future esophagus by a septum (see Chapter 12). Two to 4 days later, the first dichotomous branches can be seen (Figure 10-6). By the end of this stage, 3 main divisions are evident on the right and 2 on the left, with 10 rudimentary bronchopulmonary segments on the right and 8 or 9 on the left.[164,230,240] Lung bud branching is mediated by fibroblast growth factors (FGF)-1 and -2 secreted by the heart, transforming growth factor-β (TGF-β), which is controlled by retinoic acid (RA) via RAR-α and RAR-β (deletions of these receptors can lead to pulmonary agenesis, tracheal esophageal fistula, and lobar agenesis) and many other endodermal and mesenchymal factors.[40,163]

Between 6 and 16 weeks' gestation, a tree of narrow tubules forms. New airway branches arise through a combination of cell multiplication and necrosis. These tubules have thick epithelial walls made of columnar or cuboidal cells. This morphologic structure, along with the loose mesenchymal tissue surrounding the tree, gives the lungs a glandular appearance (hence the term pseudoglandular stage).[114,164,240] The principal pulmonary arteries are in place by 14 weeks.[114] By 16 weeks, branching of the conducting portion of the tracheobronchial tree is established. These preacinar airways can from this point forward increase only in length and diameter, not in number. The most peripheral structures at this time are the terminal brochioles.[240] Fifteen to 20 generations of airways develop (all branches to the level of the alveolar ducts).[114,120]

Epithelial-mesenchymal interaction is critical for early lung and pulmonary vasculature development and branching morphogenesis mediated by FGF-10, FGF-7, endothelial GF, and TGF-α.[90,120,198,199] The mesenchymal tissue surrounding the airways has an inductive influence via expression of multiple growth and transcription factors and other signaling molecules. Removal of this tissue interrupts epithelial branching until regeneration occurs. Mesenchyme that surrounds the endodermal tree contributes to the nonepithelial elements of the bronchial tree. Another type of mesenchyme

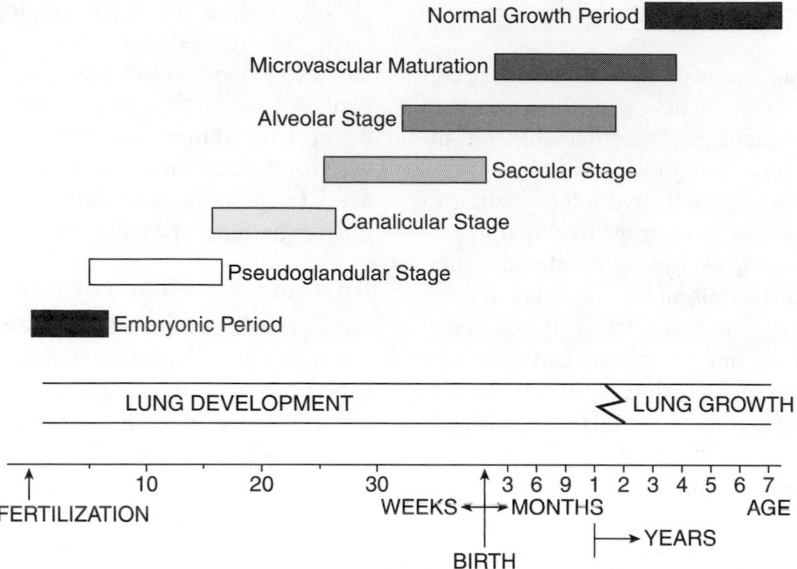

FIGURE 10-5 Timetable for lung development. The period of lung development continues 1 to 2 years, followed by continued lung growth into childhood. The timing of the saccular and alveolar stages and the period of microvascular maturation overlap with indeterminate initiation and end points. (Modified from Zeltner, T.B., et al. [1987]. The postnatal development and growth of the human lung. II: Morphology and end points. *Respir Physiol, 67,* 269.)

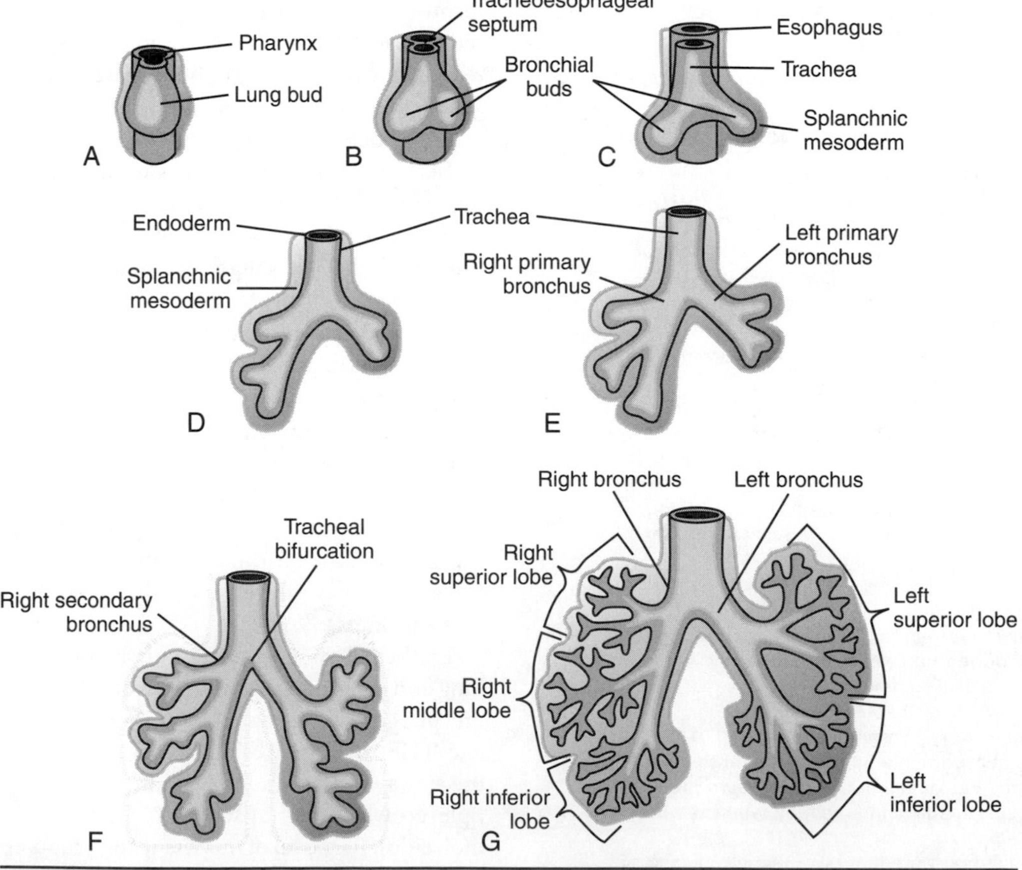

FIGURE 10-6 Successive stages in the development of the bronchi and lungs. **A** through **C,** Four weeks. **D** and **E,** Five weeks. **F,** Six weeks. **G,** Eight weeks. (From Moore, K.L. & Persaud, T.V.N. [1993]. *The developing human: Clinically oriented embryology* [5th ed.]. Philadelphia: Saunders.)

develops into the pleura, subpleural connective tissue, intralobular septa, and cartilage of the bronchi. Toward the end of the pseudoglandular period, rudimentary forms of cartilage, connective tissue, muscle, blood vessels, and lymphatic vessels can be identified.[104] Ciliated cells appear in the upper airway by 7 weeks and in the bronchi by 13 weeks. Mucus-producing glands appear in the bronchi by 13 weeks.[114,240] Mucus production begins by 14 weeks.[114] Primitive arteries appear by 14 weeks.[114]

Around 16 weeks, the epithelial cells of the distal air spaces (future alveolar lining) begin to flatten (becoming more cuboidal) and increase in glycogen (which serves as a substrate for surfactant synthesis), signaling the beginning of the canalicular stage.[192] This stage is called canalicular because of the vascular capillaries that begin to multiply in the interstitial space.[240] A rich vascular supply begins to proliferate in the interstitial space, and with the changes in mesenchymal tissue, the capillaries are brought closer to the airway epithelium to form alveolar-capillary membranes (future gas exchange areas) by 19 weeks.[114,240] Primitive respiratory bronchioles begin to form during this stage, delineating the acinus (gas-exchanging section of the lung) from the conducting portion of the lung (Figure 10-7, *A*). Type II and then type I alveolar epithelial cells begin to differentiate.[240] Between 20 and 24 weeks, the cuboidal type II cells lining the terminal portions of the airway begin to develop lamellar bodies, indicating the beginning of surfactant production.[114,120,192]

The canalicular stage continues until 26 weeks' gestation. By 24 to 26 weeks, terminal air sacs begin to appear as outpouchings of the terminal bronchioles, marking the beginning of the saccular stage (see Figure 10-7, *B*). During the saccular stage the number of terminal sacs increases, forming multiple pouches off a common chamber (the future alveolar duct). Glucocorticoid receptors on these cells increase with increasing gestation.[90] Around 30 weeks' gestation, lung surface area and volume increase sharply.[156,240] As blood vessels develop, they stretch and thin the epithelium that covers them, bringing the double capillary network (see Pulmonary Vasculature) into closer proximity with the developing airways (see Figure 10-7, *B* and *C*).[164,240] The number of air spaces (initially saccules, then later alveoli) increase from 65,000 at 18 weeks to 240,000 by 24 weeks, 4 million by 32 to 36 weeks and 50 to 150 million by term (versus 500 million in adults).[114,115,120]

The alveolar stage begins around 36 weeks' gestation (see Figure 10-7, *C*). Shallow cup-shaped indentations in the saccule walls can be detected. These primitive alveoli consist of smooth-walled transitional ducts and saccules with primitive septa with double capillary loops.[38] These saccules will deepen and multiply via septation postnatally to form true alveoli and markedly increase the gas exchange surface area.[38,240] Only about 20% of the alveoli are formed by term. Alveolarization also involves thinning of the distal airways and alveolar walls and growth of lung capillary network.[6,255] These processes are stimulated by growth and can be disrupted by hypoxia or hyperoxia.[120,255] The alveolar stage is also a time of microvascular maturation with further thinning of the gas exchange membrane and intraalveolar walls and formation of a single capillary network (see Pulmonary Vasculature).[90,198] Disruption of lung development between 32 weeks and term interferes with alveolarization and can have both short- and long-term effects on lung function.[114]

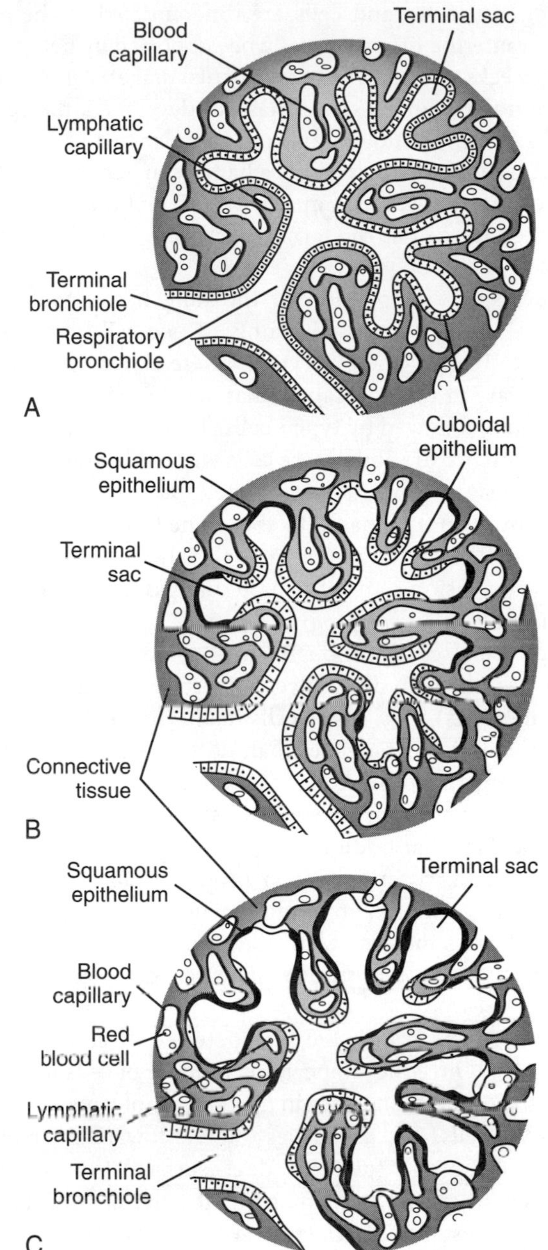

FIGURE 10-7 Diagrammatic sketches of histologic sections illustrating progressive stages of lung development. **A,** Late canalicular stage (approximately 24 weeks' gestation). **B,** Early saccular stage (approximately 26 weeks' gestation). **C,** Newborn infant (early alveolar stage). Note that the alveolar capillary membrane is thin and some of the capillaries have begun to bulge into the terminal air sacs (future alveoli). (From Moore, K.L. & Persaud, T.V.N. [2008]. *The developing human: Clinically oriented embryology* [8th ed.]. Philadelphia: Saunders Elsevier, p. 204.)

Lung structures and cells are differentiated to the point that extrauterine life can usually be supported by between 24 and 26 weeks' gestation (late canalicular stage). Although the normal number of air spaces has not developed, the epithelium has thinned enough and the vascular bed has proliferated to the point that oxygen exchange can occur. The 24- to 26-week lung, however, is markedly different than that of the term neonate, just as the term infant's lung is different from that of the child or adult.

The respiratory portion of the lung has a continuous epithelial lining composed mainly of two cell types: type I and type II cells (pneumocytes). These cell types begin to differentiate in the late canalicular stage.[198,240] Type II cells appear first, followed by type I cells. Type I cells attenuate or flatten with maturation. These cells with their long cytoplasmic extensions cover approximately 93% of the alveolar surface by term (compared to about one third of the surface in adults).[240] The thinnest area of the alveolus is composed of these extensions, and it is here that gas exchange occurs most rapidly.

The type II cells, although more numerous than type I, occupy less than 5% of the alveolar surface (versus about two thirds in adults).[192,240] These cells retain their cuboidal shape and contain more organelles than do type I cells. Mitochondria are larger, and the Golgi apparatus, rough endoplasmic reticulum, ribosomes, and multivesicular bodies are more extensive. Lamellar bodies and glycogen lakes appear within the cytoplasm.[240] Surfactant is produced and secreted by the lamellar bodies. With development, numbers and size of lamellar bodies increase with storage of surfactant lipids. As the density of lamellar bodies increases, cytoplasmic glycogen decreases.[240]

The first type II cells are seen between 20 and 24 weeks' gestation.[114] Once they appear, the number of cells increases, with a concomitant increase in the number of lamellar bodies within the cells. The organelles migrate toward the luminal plasma membrane (alveolar duct surface), which forms prominent microvilli, extending into the alveolar duct toward the end of gestation. Surfactant secretion occurs along this border.

Surfactant secretion from type II cells is detectable between 24 and 25 weeks' gestation.[99] Surfactant proteins (SPs) also begin forming. SP-A expression begins at 75% to 80% of gestation; SP-B and SP-C begin by mid-gestation.[155,240] Along with surfactant production and secretion, type II pneumocytes appear to be the chief cells involved in the repair of the alveolar epithelium. This suggests that type I cells are more susceptible to injury and differentiate from type II pneumocytes.

Pulmonary Vasculature

Vascular development involves two stages: vasculogenesis (development of blood vessels) and angiogenesis ("sprouting" of new blood vessels from existing ones).[6] Development of the pulmonary vasculature and lymphatic system requires continuous coordinated interaction between epithelial and mesenchymal tissue.[74,158,220] The relatively hypoxic uterine environment is essential for development of the lung and pulmonary vasculature. This hypoxic vasoconstriction is mediated by hypoxia inducible factor-1 (HIF-1), which regulated vascular endothelial growth factor (VEGF) and allows the pulmonary circulation to increase 60% by term without a dramatic redistribution of blood to the lungs prior to birth.[74] The lung vasculature development is regulated by multiple transcription factors and other mediators. VEGF is critical both prior to and after birth. Alterations in VEGF also decrease alveolarization.[158] Other factors mediating pulmonary vasculature development include angioproteins, platelet derived GF, bone morphogenetic proteins, WNT, and NOTCH signaling pathways (see Chapter 3).

Pulmonary vessel development occurs in conjunction with the branching of the bronchial tree. The arteries have more branches than the airways; the veins develop more tributaries. The preacinar region has an arterial branch (referred to as a conventional artery) that runs along each conducting airway; supernumerary arteries feed the adjacent alveoli. All the preacinar bronchi along with the pulmonary arteries are present by 16 to 17 weeks' gestation (end of the pseudoglandular period).[6,74,220] If for any reason there is a decrease in the number of airways, there is a concomitant decrease in conventional and supernumerary arteries. From 16 weeks on, the preacinar vessels increase in length and wall structure only.[74,104,192,240]

With movement into the canalicular and saccular stages, intraacinar arteries appear and continue their development into the postnatal period. The conventional arteries continue their development for the first 18 months of life, and the supernumerary arteries continue to be laid down for the first 8 years. These latter vessels are smaller and more numerous, servicing the alveoli directly.[104] If blood flow through the conventional arteries is reduced or blocked, the supernumerary arteries may serve as collateral circulation, thereby maintaining lung function during periods of ischemia or increased pulmonary vascular resistance. Postnatally, the intraacinar vessels multiply rapidly as alveoli appear.

The pulmonary veins develop more slowly. By 20 weeks, however, preacinar veins are present. The development of the veins parallels that of the arteries and conducting airways, although supernumerary veins outnumber supernumerary arteries. Both types of veins (supernumerary and conventional) appear simultaneously.[104] Formation of additional veins as well as lengthening of existing veins continues postnatally.

Further development of the pulmonary circulation is related to the changes in muscle wall thickness and extension of muscle into arterial walls. Because of the low intrauterine oxygen tension, the pulmonary artery wall is very thick. The wall thins as oxygen tension rises after birth. With thinning, the medial layer elastic fibrils become less organized. The pulmonary vein, in contrast, is found to be deficient in elastic fibers at birth and progressively incorporates muscle and elastic tissue over the first 2 years of life.[99]

The intrapulmonary arteries have thick walls as well. The smaller arteries have increased muscularity and dilate actively with the postnatal increase in oxygen tension. There is a concomitant fall in pulmonary vascular resistance.[104] Between 3 and 28 days postnatally, these vessels achieve their adult wall thickness–to–external diameter ratio; the larger arteries take longer to achieve adult levels (4 to 18 months).[99]

The arteries of the fetus are more muscular than those of the adult or child. Muscle thickness–to–external diameter ratio decreases postnatally based on postnatal age and the size of the vessel.[104] After delivery, muscle distribution changes, and this process continues over the first 19 to 20 years of life. Antenatally, muscle development can be seen in the arteries of the terminal bronchioles; by 4 months' postnatal age, the arteries of the respiratory bronchioles have incorporated muscle tissue.

The pulmonary capillary network develops along with the terminal air sacs and alveoli. During the canalicular stage there is a marked increase in lung capillaries around the developing air spaces. In areas where the capillaries come into close approximation with the cuboidal epithelium, the epithelium begins to thin as initial air-blood barriers develop.[38,74,99,220] During the saccular stage, capillaries form a double layer between thick intrasaccular septa, with a capillary network on either side of a central connective tissue core.[99,114,220,240] During the early alveolar stage, the intraalveolar septa attenuates and the capillary bilayer fuses into a single layer accompanied by further microvascular growth and development. This is mediated by many stimuli including VEGF, transcription factors, crosstalk between the epithelium and mesenchyme, and the low intrauterine oxygen tensions.[220,237] VEGF is important in maintaining alveolar structure and development of the alveolar-epithelial capillary interface. Platelet derived GF, FGF family, collagenases, and proteoglycans are also important in alveolar development at this stage.[40]

Congenital Anomalies of the Lungs

Most lung abnormalities arise during the embryonic and pseudoglandular stages.[240] Pulmonary agenesis in the embryonic period probably occurs secondary to failure of initial (lung agenesis) or later (lobar-bronchial agenesis) branching. Primary pulmonary hypoplasia is related to abnormalities in the transcription factors or GF critical for early lung development.[120] Agenesis is rare, but when it occurs is often associated with tracheal stenosis or esophageal atresia.[240] Lack of adequate amniotic fluid during the canalicular or saccular periods can lead to pulmonary hypoplasia.[40] Pulmonary hypoplasia may arise due to intrinsic abnormalities in lung development, and is most damaging during the canalicular stage when the conducting airways are developing.[114] Hypoplasia may occur secondary to external compression, as with congenital diaphragmatic hernia (CDH), or from oligohydramnios, as occurs with renal agenesis (and thus inadequate amniotic fluid production in Potter syndrome.[74,120] The mechanisms for pulmonary hypoplasia with oligohydramnios (see Chapter 3) is not well understood but may be due to mechanical restriction of the chest wall (lack of space to grow due to lack of amniotic fluid in the amniotic sac), interference with fetal breathing movements, or failure to produce adequate fetal lung fluid.[240] Pulmonary hypoplasia with decreased alveoli and a reduced pulmonary vascular bed can result in abnormal muscularization of preacinar and intracinar arterioles and lead to persistent pulmonary hypertension.[74]

CDH occurs in 1/2200 to 1/4000 live births and is due to malformations in the diaphragm with alterations in lung development.[3,74] The cause of the malformation is unknown and the defect in the diaphragm may be secondary to altered lung development.[3,74] Hypotheses include that the diaphragmatic defect is due to (1) abnormal development of the adjacent lung, (2) abnormal muscle innervation by the phrenic nerve, (3) improper myotubule formation, (4) failure of closure of the pleuroperitoneal canal, or (5) defective pleuroperitoneal fold development.[83] CDH results in lung compression by the herniated portions of the gastrointestinal system. The lung on the side of the herniation is most severely affected, but the lung on the contralateral side is also affected. The lung hypoplasia in CDH involves a developmental as well as a compression defect, possibly due to down regulation of signaling molecules, with delayed lung maturation, altered pulmonary vasculature development and defects in surfactant maturation.[6,83,90,114,138,232]

Bronchiogenic cysts—usually single lesions ranging in size from small cysts to those covering an entire lobe—develop early in gestation. These cysts arise from abnormal budding of the foregut diverticulum with cystic duplication of the tracheobronchial tree.[40] Congenital cystic adenomatoid malformations arise from alterations in the development of the terminal respiratory bronchioles.[40,229] These defects are characterized lung tissue with a discordant spacial arrangement due to abnormal airway patterning and abnormal branching of immature bronchioles accompanied by overgrowth of terminal bronchioles and a decreased number of alveoli.[40] Other events that can alter fetal and postnatal lung development include fetal growth restriction, altered fetal breathing movements, decreased nutrient supply, nicotine exposure, and preterm birth.[150]

Functional Development

The functional development of the lung includes development of the surfactant system, defenses against inflammation and oxidative stress, lung fluid, and fetal breathing movements. The lung secretes various substances and has its own macrophage function. Macrophages are found in groups of three or four cells lying free within the alveolar space. Ingested foreign bodies are seen as osmiophilic inclusions within the cell. These cells are spherical in shape and are derived from hematopoietic tissue.[157] Larger particles (e.g., bacteria) not swept away by ciliary action are removed and destroyed by pulmonary macrophages. Foreign material, once identified, is engulfed and destroyed by the macrophage. These cells are critical for protection of the lung environment and removing surfactant from the alveolar surface.

Surfactant

Surfactant is of major importance to the adequate functioning of the lung and has many roles (Table 10-4), including reduction of surface tension at the air-liquid interface within alveoli (Figure 10-8) , altering lung mechanics, and is lung innate host defenses.[244] Pulmonary surfactant is a lipoprotein, composed of 70% to 80% phospholipids (Figure 10-9).[120,246] The majority (80%) of the lipid is saturated phosphatidylcholine (PC), of which dipalmitoyl phosphatidylcholine (DPPC) is the most abundant. The latter is the component responsible for decreasing the surface tension to almost zero when compressed at the surface during inspiration. Phosphatidylglycerol (PG) accounts for another 5% to 10% of the phospholipids present in surfactant. PG is unique to lung cells, bronchoalveolar fluid, and amniotic fluid. This makes PG a good marker for surfactant. Immature lungs contain large amounts of phosphatidylinositol PI. Levels of PI decrease as PG increases with lung maturity.[114,120] Neutral lipids include primarily cholesterol along with esters and acylglycerol fatty acids.[246] The other components are involved in intracellular transport, storage, exocytosis, adsorption, spreading of the monolayer, clearance at the alveolar lining, and immunoprotection (see Box 10-2 on page 315).[246]

Table 10-4 Classic and "Nonsurfactant" Functions of Pulmonary Surfactant

CLASSIC FUNCTIONS	"NONSURFACTANT" FUNCTIONS
Lung mechanics	Nonspecific host defenses
Reduction of surface tension in relation to surface area	Maintaining the surfactant film stability as a pathogen barrier
Stabilizing lung volume at low transpulmonary pressures	Facilitating microciliary transport
Prevention of lung collapse and atelectasis	Antioxidant activity
Gas exchange:	Antibacterial-antiviral activity
Maintaining the gas exchange area of the lung	Specific host defenses role:
Reduction of pulmonary shunt flow	SP-A and SP-D are "collectins" with a pathogen-recognizing function
	SP-A and SP-D serve as opsonins, modulating chemotaxis, and phagocytosis
	SP-A interacts with alveolar macrophages through a specific receptor
	Alteration of cytokine/ inflammatory mediator release

From Frerking, I., et al. (2001). Pulmonary surfactant: Functions, abnormalities and therapeutic options. *Intensive Care Med, 27,* 1700.
SP, Surfactant protein.

The four surfactant proteins (SPs) are SP-A, SP-B, SP-C, and SP-D. These make up 10% of the surfactant.[114] SPs are involved in surfactant function, modulate alveolar macrophages, and influence innate immunity and surfactant catabolism.[244] SP-A, SP-B, and SP-C are produced by Clara cells (conducting airway epithelial cells). SP-A and SP-D are hydrophilic collectins (innate host defense proteins). SP-B and SP-C are hydrophobic.[143] SP-A is the most abundant SP and is needed for surfactant turnover, formation of tubular myelin (Figure 10-10 and Box 10-2 on p. 315), and nonimmune host defenses within the lungs.

SP-A maintains the surfactant monolayer at the air-liquid interface.[44] The major function of SP-A is in innate host defenses in the alveoli and airways. SP-A acts as an opsonin in modifying inflammatory responses and promotes phagocytosis and clearance of pathogens by alveolar marcophages.[114,120] Deficiency

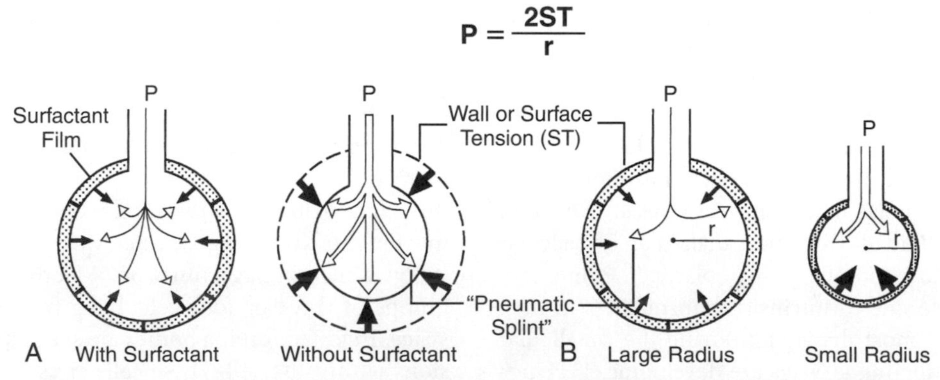

FIGURE 10-8 Illustration of the LaPlace relationship and the effects of surfactant film **(A)** and alveolar radius **(B)** on wall or surface tension. The degree (reflected in the size of the *open arrows*) of airway or intraalveolar pressure (P) needed to counteract the tendency of alveoli to collapse (represented by the *solid arrows*) is directly proportional to double the surface tension (ST) and inversely proportional to the size of the radius (r). Distending airway pressure applied during assisted ventilation can be likened to a "pneumatic splint." (From Keszler, M., Abubakar, M.K., & Wood, B.R. [2011]. Physiologic principles. In J.P. Goldsmith & E.H. Karotkin [Eds.]. *Assisted ventilation of the neonate* [5th ed.]. Philadelphia: Saunders, p. 23.)

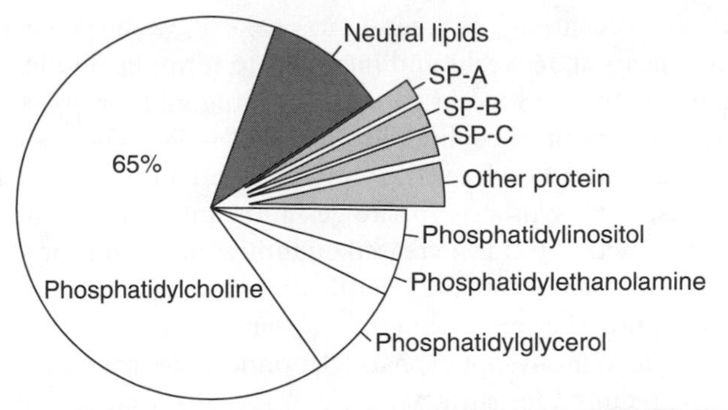

FIGURE 10-9 Composition of pulmonary surfactant. (From Jobe, A.H. [1999]. Fetal lung development, tests for maturation, induction of maturation, and treatment. In R.K. Creasy & R. Resnik [Eds.]. *Maternal-fetal medicine* [4th ed.]. Philadelphia: Saunders.)

of SP-A increases the risk of pulmonary infection. SP-B acts with SP-A to form tubular myelin (see Figure 10-10).[24,46,156,243,246] SP-A may also act to make surfactant less vulnerable to inactivation by edema and inflammatory byproducts after lung injury, in binding exotoxins and in gram negative and gram positive organism opsonization.[114] SP-A levels are low in preterm infants with respiratory distress syndrome (RDS).[120] Decreased SP-A to phospholipid ratios increase the risk of RDS, bronchopulmonary dysplasia (BPD), and death.[114]

SP-B maintains the surface tension–lowering effects of surfactant, enhances spreading of the monolayer, and stimulates lipid adhesion and surface film formation.[157] SP-B is essential for production of lamellar bodies and reprocessing of surfactant.[44,114,120] SP-C working with SP-B facilitates spreading,

BOX 10-2 Surfactant Biosynthesis

Surfactant is synthesized in the type II alveolar cells mediated by multiple enzymes. Phospholipids are synthesized in the endoplasmic reticulum from glucose, phosphate, and fatty acids. The surfactant components then move from the endoplasmic reticulum to the Golgi apparatus and lamellar bodies (see Figure 10-10). The lamellar bodies, which are large lipid rich intracellular organelles, are formed by fusion of multivesicular bodies forming lipid bilayers. Lamellar body formation is enhanced by ATP-binding cassette (ABC) transporter A3, a transmembrane protein involved in lipid transport.[246] The lamellar bodies contain surfactant lipids (PC, PG), SP-B, and SP-C.[245] The lamellar bodies are secreted by exocytosis into the alveolar space in response to mechanical stimuli (lung distention, hyperventilation), beta-agonists, and purines such as adenosine triphosphate.[114,120,246] Here the lamellar body unravels to form tubular myelin. This process requires the interaction of SP-A, SP-B, and calcium. Tubular myelin is a long, rectangular tubule that forms a lattice-like structure with SP-A at the corners. This structural change enhances spreadability and adsorption. Tubular myelin spreads over the alveolar surface in a monolayer (and likely in multilayers in some areas).[114,119,191,246]

Surfactant reduces surface tension within the alveoli. Surface tension is the attraction between molecules at the gas liquid interface within the alveoli. Surface tension is constricting force causing alveoli to constrict and collapse. Surfactant acts to prevent this attractive force. Phospholipids contain hydrophilic (polar) and hydrophobic (nonpolar) groups. The surface film is oriented so that the polar groups interact with the moist alveolar lining and the nonpolar with the air molecules. During expiration the molecules of this surface film are compressed preventing interaction of gas and liquid molecules in the alveoli and thus reducing surface tension (see Figure 10-8).[114,246]

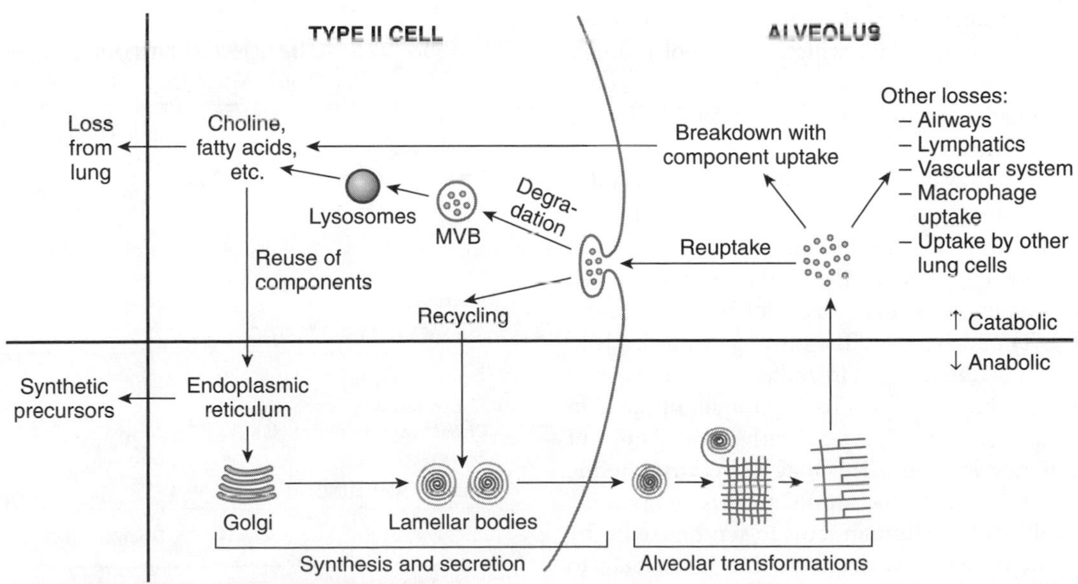

FIGURE 10-10 Metabolic pathways of surfactant phosphatidylcholine from synthesis to secretion by type II cells to alveolar transformation and reuptake by the type II cell. *MVB,* Multivesicular body. (From Jobe, A.H. [1999]. Fetal lung development, tests for maturation, induction of maturation, and treatment. In R.K. Creasy & R. Resnik [Eds.]. *Maternal-fetal medicine* [4th ed.]. Philadelphia: Saunders.)

surface absorption, and lipid uptake.[24,114,156,243] SP-D has a similar function to SP-A in innate host defenses and is increased with acute lung injury.[24,114,156,243] SP-D is also important in surfactant structure and regulating the alveolar surfactant pool and reuptake. SP-D binds bacteria, fungi, viruses, and promotes macrophage opsonization and Phagocytosis.[245]

Mutations in genes for SP-A, SP-B, and SP-C and transporter proteins such as ABCA3 can lead to inborn errors in surfactant production and acute or chronic respiratory problems after birth.[243,245] Mutations in the SP-B gene on the short arm of chromosome 2 result in a recessive disorder that has a neonatal onset with surfactant deficiency, respiratory failure, and increased risk of air leak and pulmonary hypertension. Complete lack of SP-B results in severe RDS that does not respond to surfactant replacement therapy. These infants need a lung transplant to survive. These infants are usually term and die within 3 to 6 months. Infants with partial or transient SP-B defects have a better outcome.[41,156] SP-C mutations had a variable onset of symptoms such as tachypnea, cyanosis, and failure to thrive. ABCA3 (transport protein located in the lining of lamellar bodies) deficiency can also result in severe surfactant deficiency and a lethal form of RDS in term infants.[114,245] Alterations in SP-C can lead to interstitial lung disease.[114,120]

Surfactant Biosynthesis. The biosynthesis of surfactant entails a series of events including glycerophospholipid production, apoprotein synthesis, glycosylation and surfactant apoprotein processing, integration of surfactant component parts, transport of components from synthesis sites to integration sites (lamellar bodies), and finally breakdown and recycling of components. This process is summarized in Box 10-2 on page 315 and in Figure 10-10.

PC and PG are composed of a three-carbon glycerol backbone with fatty acids esterified to the hydroxyl groups. The asymmetric arrangement of these molecules results in a hydrocarbon-rich fatty acid tail, which is nonpolar, and a phosphodiester region, which is polar. This allows for a monolayer film (and sometimes multilayers) to be established at the air-liquid interface within the alveoli.[114,191,196,246]

There are two pathways for phosphatidylcholine (also called lecithin) synthesis. Key precursors for PC synthesis include glycerol, fatty acids, choline, glucose, and ethanolamine. The major pathway is the cytidine diphosphate (CDP) choline system, which is critical for mature alveolar structural integrity and stability. The other pathway leads to phosphatidylethanolamine (PE) formation and is termed the *methyltransferase system.* This has minor significance in the adult lung and seems to play a relatively insignificant role in fetal lung development. This may be because choline is incorporated more effectively into PC than is methionine. However, the ability of the human fetus to synthesize PC by N-methylation of PE early in gestation may contribute to survival with premature delivery.

The increasing biosynthesis of phosphatidylcholine (PC), phosphatidylinositol (PI), and phosphatidylglycerol (PG) in late gestation depends on the biosynthesis of phosphatidic acid. PI appears by 28 weeks and peaks at 32 to 35 weeks; PG appears at 36 weeks and increases to term; PC gradually increases from 28 weeks to term, peaking after 36 weeks.[88] The majority of phospholipid produced is PC. The choline pathway and the diglyceride synthesis mechanisms that yield increased PC synthesis in late gestation interact. Although this interaction yields increased quantities of PC, it is not the highly saturated version identified in the final surfactant compound. The remodeling of PC that occurs in the phosphatidylcholine-lysophosphatidylcholine cycle provides the DPPC required for surfactant.[156,196]

As gestation advances, phospholipid content and saturation increase. This is accompanied by an increase in lamellar bodies within the type II cells. Choline incorporation, which is low in early gestation, increases abruptly in late gestation. This suggests that pathway regulatory mechanisms are enhanced in order to meet postnatal needs. Increases in surfactant before birth are due to increased synthesis; increases during and immediately after birth are due to increased secretion.[196] In late gestation in term infants, the surfactant pool increases to levels similar to those in adults. Table 10-5 summarizes differences in surfactant components in mature versus immature lungs. Markers of lung maturation include loss of glycogen lakes in type II cells, increased fatty acid synthesis, increased β-receptors, and increased production of PC via the choline incorporation pathway.[156]

Enzymatic changes in the phospholipid synthesis pathway correlate to the surge in saturated PC and increase in PG with concomitant decrease in PI.[156,196] Whether this surge is due to a change in enzyme or substrate concentration, an adjustment in catalytic efficiency, a change in substrate affinity, or the activation of latent enzymes is not clear.

Table 10-5 Changes in Surfactant with Development

VARIABLES	IMMATURE LUNG	MATURE LUNG
TYPE II CELLS		
Glycogen lakes	High	None
Lamellar bodies	Few	Many
Microvilli	Few	Many
SURFACTANT COMPOSITION		
Sat PC/Total PC	0.6	0.7
Phosphatidylglycerol (%)	<1	10
Phosphatidylinositol (%)	10	2
SP-A (%)	Low	5
SURFACTANT FUNCTION		
	Decreased	Normal

From Jobe, A.H. (2006). Lung development and maturation. In R.J. Martin, A.A. Fanaroff, & M.C. Walsh (Eds.). *Neonatal-perinatal medicine: Diseases of the fetus and infant* (8th ed.). Philadelphia: Mosby, p. 1076.
Sat PC, Saturated phosphatidylcholine; *SP-A,* surfactant protein A.

Influences on Fetal Lung Maturation

A complex interaction of hormones, growth factors, and other substances controls surfactant synthesis. Normal lung function is dependent upon the presence of surfactant, which permits a decrease in surface tension at end-expiration (to prevent atelectasis) and an increase in surface tension during lung expansion (to facilitate elastic recoil on inspiration). Surfactant provides the lung with the stability required for maintenance of homeostatic blood gas pressures while decreasing the work of breathing.[82] Surfactant may play a role in the cascade of events that leads to the initiation of labor and parturition. Secretion of surfactant phospholipids into amniotic fluid with fetal breathing during the third trimester may stimulate PGE synthesis in the amnion by serving as a source of arachadonic acid. SP-A, which is secreted after 80% of gestation and reaches maximal levels right before term, may serve as a stimulus for activation of inflammatory signals that eventually lead to labor onset.[116,120]

Hormones that stimulate or accelerate lung maturity include glucocorticoids , thyroid hormones, estradiol, vascular epithelial growth factor, fibroblast growth factor, prolactin, thyrotropin-releasing hormone, catecholamines, TGF-α, and epidermal growth factor.[143,196] Estradiol stimulates phospholipid synthesis and helps prepare the pulmonary circuit for the decreased pulmonary vascular resistance after birth.[213] Thyroxine (T_4) and triiodothyronine (T_3) have also been shown to increase the rate of phospholipid synthesis.[196] Thyroid hormones, like glucocorticoids, enhance production of PC through choline incorporation. They do not, however, increase PG synthesis or stimulate the production of surfactant-specific proteins. Whereas glucocorticoids increase fatty acid synthetase activity, thyroid hormone seems to decrease its activity. These differences suggest different sites of action for these hormones as well as the need for action in conjunction with other hormones. However, trials of thyrotropin releasing hormone either alone or in combination with glucocorticoids have demonstrated a lack of efficacy and an increase in complications.[41]

Glucocorticoids and thyroid hormones play a role in enhancing the synthesis of phospholipids; catecholamines stimulate the secretion of surfactant into the alveolar space. This appears to be a direct action of adrenergic compounds on type II cells. The increase in surfactant and saturated phosphatidylcholine in lung fluid improve lung stability. An added benefit is the inhibition of fetal lung fluid secretion and possible reabsorption of the fluid within the alveoli at the time of delivery. These two effects (the increase in surfactant and decrease in lung fluid) work together in preparing for respiratory conversion at birth.[71] Other factors influencing type II cell maturation and surfactant biosynthesis are summarized in Table 10-6.

Table 10-6 Regulators of Alveolar Type II Cell Differentiation

AGENT	PROPOSED PHYSIOLOGIC ROLE
INDUCERS	
Glucocorticoid (cortisol)	Major endogenous modulator of alveolar development and surfactant production
β-Adrenergic agonists (especially epinephrine, cyclic AMP)	Increase surfactant production and secretion, especially during labor and delivery
Thyroid hormones (T_3, T_4)	Enhance glucocorticoid effects on lipid synthesis
Retinoic acid	May interact with glucocorticoids to regulate lipid and SP-B production
Bombesin-related peptides	May contribute to surfactant lipid synthesis
Parathyroid hormone-related protein	?
INHIBITORS	
Protein kinase C activators (proinflammatory cytokines)	Inhibit surfactant protein gene transcription during infections, inflammation
Transforming growth factor-β family	Inhibit type II maturation during early gestation and with inflammation
Tumor necrosis factor-α	Inhibit SP-B and SP-C gene transcription during infection
Insulin	Inhibit surfactant protein gene transcription in infants of diabetic mothers with poorly controlled disease
Dihydrotestosterone	Delayed type II cell maturation in males

From Guttentag, S. & Ballard, P.L. (2004). Lung development: Embryo growth, maturation and developmental biology. In H.W. Tausch, R.A. Ballard, & C.A. Gleason (Eds.). *Avery's diseases of the newborn* (8th ed.). Philadelphia: Saunders, p. 610.

Glucocorticoids. Glucocorticoids are critical for the normal pattern of surfactant synthesis and fetal lung maturation.[91,196] Glucocorticoids bind to gene promoter regions and induce lipogenic enzymes needed for phospholipid production and desaturation of PC, an induce enzymes for Na and K flux.[156] Glucocorticoids increase the rate of glycogen depletion and glycerophospholipid biosynthesis. The depletion in glycogen leads to direct anatomic changes in alveolar structures by thinning the interalveolar septa and increasing the size of the alveoli. Morphologic changes include an increase in the number of type II cells and an increase in the number of lamellar bodies within those cells. These changes occur in conjunction with functional maturation, leading to an accelerated synthesis of surfactant phospholipid.[24,91,156] Glucocorticoids may also play a role in early lung development.[24] Glucocorticoids act directly on lung tissue, increasing the number of β-adrenergic receptors and enhancing elastin and collagen production, thus improving lung compliance.[156,196] Glucocorticoids also increase antioxidant enzymes to assist in protecting cells during the transition from the low oxygen intrauterine to high oxygen extrauterine environment, enhance lung fluid clearance and lung parenchyma maturation.[89,156] Levels of glucocorticoids increase near term enhancing lung maturation by increasing fatty acids needed for phospholipid synthesis, and increasing expression of SP-B, SP-C, and SP-D (primarily by increasing transcription of genes that code for these proteins).[89,143] The actions of glucocorticoids may be mediated by the expression of 11β-hydroxysteroid dehydrogenase (see Chapter 19).[75]

Antenatal Corticosteroids. Administration of antenatal corticosteroids (ACS) can accelerate normal lung maturation both morphologically and functionally as described above, inducing structural maturation, and increasing lung volume, compliance, and responses to exogenous surfactant therapy.[94] Current ACOG recommendations are: "A single course of corticosteroids is recommended for pregnant women between 24 weeks' and 34 weeks' gestation who are at risk of preterm delivery within 7 days. A single course of antenatal corticosteroids should be administered to women with premature rupture of membranes before 32 weeks' gestation to reduce the risks of respiratory distress syndrome, perinatal mortality, and other morbidities. The efficacy of corticosteroid use at 32 to 33 completed weeks' gestation for preterm premature rupture of membranes is unclear, but treatment may be beneficial, particularly if pulmonary immaturity is documented."[5,p.422] Either betamethasone or dexamethasone may be used, with no clear proof of efficacy of one drug over the other. Some studies suggest that betamethasone may be safer and more protective, but this has not been found in others.[174,242] ACS treatment reduces the incidence of RDS by about 50% in infants younger than 31 weeks' gestational age, decreases neonatal mortality by 30%, and decreases the incidence of intraventricular hemorrhage, necrotizing enterocolitis and the severity of disease in infants with RDS.[20,91,93,120,143,186] Concerns have been raised about the effects of corticosteroids on the developing brain and fetal growth with repeated courses of ACS.[5,13,20,127,175,186,242] Multiple courses may decrease the risk of RDS, but they also increase the risk of fetal growth alterations.[13,20,42,93,178,186,235] However, a recent study reported that a single repeat dose (>7 days) was not associated with differences in physical growth or neurodevelopment at 2 years.[185] Another recent study found that multiple courses (2 to 9) were associated with a dose-dependent decline in fetal growth.[178] ACOG recommends that a "single rescue course of antenatal corticosteroids may be considered if the antecedent treatment was given more than 2 weeks prior, the gestational age is less than 32 6/7 weeks, and the women are judged by the clinician to be likely to give birth within the next week. However, regularly scheduled repeat courses or multiple courses (more than two) are not recommended. Further research regarding the risks and benefits, optimal dose, and timing of a single rescue course of steroid treatment is needed."[5,p.422]

Factors Enhancing and Delaying Lung Maturation. In addition to the use of antenatal steroids, other factors may also influence fetal lung maturation. Maternal-fetal events that lead to stress, and increased fetal catecholamine and corticosteroid levels have been associated with accelerated lung maturity and a decreased risk of RDS.[156] However, stressed infants do not consistently have a lower incidence of RDS. Maturation of lung function is variable. Although lung maturation usually occurs after 35 to 36 weeks, lung maturation may occur earlier or later. Some infants seem to have spontaneous early lung maturation. Lung maturation can be induced as early as 24 weeks by antenatal corticosteroids or exposure to inflammation.[116,120] About 20% of infants born <28 weeks have low oxygen needs with no or minimal RDS.[140] Some infants born at 24-25 weeks can be transitioned to air breathing with continuous positive airway pressure (CPAP) or maintained on CPAP from birth.[10,165]

Lung maturation is delayed in infants of diabetic mothers (IDMs) and infants with RH isoimmunization with hydrops. The major causative factor influencing pulmonary maturation in IDMs seems to be adequacy of blood glucose control.[156] Hyperglycemia and hyperinsulinemia decrease choline incorporation into PC; hyperinsulinemia delays PC production by the type II cell and delays morphologic maturation of the lung.[156] Maturation of surfactant synthesis occurs at the same time that glycogen is depleted from the lungs and liver. Insulin inhibits glycogen breakdown, thereby decreasing the substrate available for PC synthesis as well as altering the natural anatomic changes that occur with glycogen depletion. The effect of cortisol on choline incorporation may be altered by insulin, although some have found either no effect or a synergistic effect. Insulin may inhibit surfactant protein gene transcription in women with poorly controlled diabetes.[69] However, in vivo studies suggest that hyperglycemia rather than hyperinsulinemia may be a more important cause of altered lung maturation in an IDM.[196]

Androgens also delay type II cell maturation.[69] At any stage of gestation, the female fetal lung is about 1 week more mature. This may be why male preterm infants are more prone to RDS than female infants of similar gestations.[196]

Assessment of Fetal Lung Maturity

Accurate assessment of fetal lung maturity is important in the management of preterm labor and birth. This is especially true when the date of the last menstrual period is not known or if preeclampsia, placenta previa, multiple pregnancy, Rh isoimmunization, diabetes, or fetal growth restriction is present. The presence of surfactant phospholipids in the amniotic fluid allows determination of lung maturity because their concentrations change as the surfactant system matures. Gluck and colleagues initially demonstrated that the ratio of lecithin (L) to sphingomyelin (S) (the L/S ratio) is a reliable index and a good predictor of whether RDS will develop if the infant is born within the 48 hours following amniocentesis.[156] Sphingomyelin is a membrane lipid not related to lung maturation that remains relatively stable. Lecithin levels rise sharply at around 34 to 35 weeks' gestation, thereby providing the basis for achieving a ratio between the two. An L/S ratio greater than 2:1 indicates lung maturity and a negligible risk for RDS. Values less than 1.5:1 to 2:1 indicate lung immaturity, with a high incidence of RDS if the ratio is <1:1.[120] A higher incidence of inaccurate readings is found in complicated pregnancies.

Factors that influence phospholipid concentrations in the amniotic fluid include volume of amniotic fluid (varies inversely) and contamination of the sample with blood, meconium, or antiseptics. PC levels are falsely high with blood contamination (fetal or maternal). PG is only slightly affected, however, because blood does not contain PG in significant amounts. The presence of PG is an indication that the major synthesis pathway for surfactant is present and functioning. Therefore, when PG is present in the amniotic fluid, there is little risk for RDS regardless of the L/S ratio value.[156] Other techniques for assessing fetal lung maturity include the complete lung profile, a modified profile (L/S ratio and PG only), and techniques such as the fluorescent polarization (FP) assay, lamellar body count, surfactant to albumin ratio, and foam stability.[88,156]

Antioxidant Defenses

Another biochemical system that develops antenatally and is needed for successful adaptation to extrauterine life is the antioxidant system (AOS). The AOS is designed to scavenge or detoxify the highly reactive oxygen metabolites produced during aerobic respiration. The potentially cytotoxic oxygen metabolites (e.g., superoxide radical, hydrogen peroxide, hydroxyl radical, singlet oxygen, peroxide radical) are produced intracellularly in excess amounts under hyperoxic conditions. The detoxifying antioxidant enzymes include superoxide dismutase, catalase, and glutathione peroxidase.

The placenta contains all major antioxidant systems.[29,49,172] Oxidative stress is a part of the normal process of early development of the fetus and placenta (see Chapter 3). For example, low levels of oxidative stress are needed for placental angiogenesis and to establish blood flow in the intervillous space. Initial embryologic development occurs in a low oxygen environment. The onset of full intervillous space blood flow (and thus increased exposure to reactive oxygen species) occurs at the same time that maternal, placental, and fetal AO systems increase. Production of reactive oxygen species may be important in signaling during pregnancy, stimulating labor onset and enhancing myometrial contractility. Excess oxidative stress, however, can increase the risk of miscarriage. In addition, oxidative stress is increased with preeclampsia, diabetes, and fetal growth restriction.[29,172]

The transition to the extrauterine environment is a move from a relatively hypoxic state to a more hyperoxic one. In utero, the fetal lung is exposed to low PaO_2 levels, with even lower oxygen tensions existing in the fetal lung fluid that fills the alveolar spaces and bronchiole tubes. At delivery the alveolar and airway cells are abruptly exposed to hyperoxic tensions. Therefore it is important to have an AOS in place that can reduce damage by oxygen radicals. Concerns about oxidative stress is one of the bases for studies of the use of room air or low oxygen levels rather than 100% oxygen for delivery room resuscitation.[39,124,184,187,226,235]

The development of the antioxidant enzymes occurs in the second half of gestation. For example, activity of superoxide dismutase, the major antioxidant enzyme, appears around the time that surfactant synthesis begins in the type II cells and continues to mature to term.[132] Thus the preterm infant is particularly vulnerable to lung injury from oxidative stress.[255] Antioxidant levels appear to be strongly correlated to the degree of protection that can be expected from oxygen radical–induced lung injury.[11] When enzyme levels are increased (as with exogenous treatment), there is increased tolerance to hyperoxia. Although there are other protective mechanisms in place, it does not appear that increased amounts of these will result in an increased level of protection. However, deficiencies within these other pathways will result in an increased susceptibility to cellular damage. This suggests that the other antioxidants play a secondary role in providing protection. Antioxidant enzymes provide primary protection by direct detoxification of reactive oxygen radicals. This prevents damage to cell proteins and DNA structure. The other systems terminate reactions already initiated by oxygen radical attack.

Lung Fluid

Fluid is present in the lung lumen as early as 6 weeks' gestation and is actively secreted beginning in the canalicular stage.[74,181] This fluid is derived from alveolar epithelium secretions and is not an ultrafiltrate or mixture of plasma or amniotic fluid.[30] Lung fluid is thought to be secreted primarily by type I and II alveolar cells.[126]Active transport is required to attain the final ion concentrations found in the fluid; this is achieved by the active transport of chloride, with sodium following passively.[74,126] The water flux can be attributed to the osmotic force of sodium chloride (NaCl).[30] Osmolarity and sodium and chloride levels are higher in lung fluid than in amniotic fluid, whereas pH, bicarbonate, potassium, and protein levels are lower.[74,114,126]

Estimated lung fluid production in term infants is 4 to 5 mL/kg/hr or about 300 to 400 mL per day for the average infant and is slightly greater than the functional residual capacity (FRC) after birth.[74,114,120] Of the fluid produced, some is swallowed and a small amount moves into the amniotic fluid via periodic opening of the larynx. Most remains in the lungs due to the higher pressure within the fetal thoracic cavity compared to amniotic fluid.[114] Movement of lung fluid into amniotic fluid increases with fetal breathing movements, but these movements do not alter lung fluid production rate.[120,240] The amount of lung fluid contributed to the amniotic pool is relatively insignificant when compared to that contributed by micturition (see Chapter 3).

Lung fluid plays an important part in cell maturation and development as well as in determining formation, size, and shape of the developing air space. Alterations in fluid dynamics affect pulmonary cell proliferation and differentiation. If production of lung fluid is decreased or if significant chronic leakage of amniotic fluid is experienced (both of which lead to oligohydramnios), there is risk of lung hypoplasia.[74,126,181] In comparison, excessive lung fluid or tracheal obstruction of a chronic nature leads to hyperplasia, with an increase in the number of alveoli, although these alveoli are functionally immature.[126,240]

Lung fluid production slows in late pregnancy, with a decrease in volume to 65% of previous values. Absorption of lung fluid begins in early labor so that after birth only about 35% of the original lung fluid volume needs to be cleared (see Transitional Events).[114,156,192] Infants born by cesarean delivery prior to labor onset will have a greater volume of lung fluid to clear at birth, increasing the risk of transient tachypnea of the newborn. Preterm infants also have more lung fluid at birth (up to 25% greater than term infants).[126]

Fetal Blood Gases

Usual fetal blood gases are listed in Table 10-7. Factors that affect maternal-to-fetal diffusion of oxygen include maternal and fetal PO_2 relationships, maternal and fetal oxygen-hemoglobin dissociation curves (see Box 10-1 on page 301), HbF concentrations, and the Bohr effect.[159] Fetal PO_2 is lower (20 to 30 mm Hg) than after birth, but the oxygen content is only slightly below that of adults due to the increased affinity of fetal hemoglobin for oxygen (see Chapter 8) and lower oxygen demands due to decreased metabolic needs.[81] Carbon dioxide transfer is affected by hydrogen ion concentration and the Haldane effect. Fetal blood gases and evaluation of fetal acid-base status are described in Chapter 6.

Fetal Breathing Movements

Fetal breathing movement (FBM) are rhythmic diaphragmatic, laryngeal, and intercostal muscle contractions.[47] FBM can be seen on ultrasound as early as 10 weeks' gestation, and they occur 6% of the time by 19 weeks.[38,90,194] FBM are rapid and irregular, occurring intermittently early in gestation. These early movements probably originate in the spinal cord.[1] Later movements require differentiation of the respiratory motor neurons and functional innervation of these neurons.[87] As gestation progresses, the strength and frequency of FBM increase, and they occur approximately 30% to 40% of the time in the last 10 weeks, with a rate of 30 to 70 breaths per minute.[9,48,162,194] FBM are associated with fetal state and tend to occur in rapid eye movement-like sleep. Large movements (gasping) occur 5% of the total breathing time, one to four times per minute. FBM decrease in frequency immediately before term labor onset.[194]

The rapid and irregular respiratory activity contributes to lung fluid regulation and stretches the lung tissues, thereby influencing lung growth.[1,74,90] The diaphragm seems to be the major structure involved, with minimal chest wall excursion encountered (4- to 8-mm change in transverse diameter). Movement of the diaphragm is necessary for chest wall muscle and diaphragm training and development, building adequate strength for the initial breath.[48] The movement of the diaphragm also influences the course of lung cell differentiation and proliferation. Bilateral phrenectomy in animal models results in altered lung morphology with an increase in type II over type I cells. Presumably the innervated diaphragm increases the size of the thorax and thereby increases tissue stress, affecting morphology.

With increasing gestational age, FBM become more organized and vigorous.[162] Even with these gestational changes, tracheal fluid shifts are negligible—the pressure generated being no more than 25 mmHg (3.32 kPaa). Fetal maturation leads to the appearance of FBM cycles, with an increase in breathing movements during daytime hours. Although the patterns of FBM vary according to rate, amplitude, and character, they seem to be correlated mostly with fetal behavioral states and occur most often during rapid eye movement sleep.[1,9,48,194]

The mechanism for the initiation of FBM is unknown, although they can be stimulated by maternal inhalation of carbon dioxide, adrenergic and cholinergic compounds, and PG synthesis inhibitors. Other factors affecting FBM, including maternal glycemia, nicotine use, alcohol ingestion, and labor, are summarized in Table 10-8.[47,157,194] These Altered breathing patterns can be seen during periods of

Table 10-7 Normal Fetal pH and Blood Gas Data

	UMBILICAL VEIN	DESCENDING AORTA	ASCENDING AORTA
pH	7.40-7.43	7.36-7.39	7.37-7.40
PO_2 (torr)	28-32	20-23	21-25
[kPa]	[3.72-4.25]	[2.66-3.05]	[2.79-3.32]
PCO_2 (torr)	38-42	43-48	41-45
[kPa]	[5.05-5.58]	[5.71-6.38]	[5.45-5.98]

From Fineman, J.R., Clyman, R., & Heymann, M.A. (2004). Fetal cardiovascular physiology. In R.K. Creasy, R. Resnik, & J.D. Iams (Eds.). *Maternal-fetal medicine: Principles and practice* (5th ed.). Philadelphia: Saunders, p. 172.

Table 10-8 Factors Affecting Fetal Breathing Movements

FACTOR	EFFECT
Glucose concentrations; glucose infusions	Increased FBM in patients who have fasted
Cigarette smoking	Increased frequency of FBM, although incidence remains unchanged
Caffeine	Increased FBM with chronic exposure; no effect with acute exposure
Ethanol	Dramatic decrease in FBM
Methadone	Decreased FBM with chronic exposure
Tocolytics	Dramatic increase in FBM

Adapted from Richardson, B.S. & Gagnon, R. (2004). Fetal breathing and body movements. In R.K. Creasy, R. Resnik, & J.D. Iams (Eds.). *Maternal-fetal medicine: Principles and practice* (5th ed.). Philadelphia: Saunders, p. 184.

FBM, Fetal breathing movements.

fetal hypoxia. Mild hypoxemia decreases the incidence of FBM, while severe hypoxemia may lead to cessation of FBM for several hours. The onset of asphyxia leads to gasping.[9] The onset of mild hypoxemia (as with umbilical artery occlusion of short duration) may lead to quiet sleep, which decreases activity expenditure and oxygen consumption in the fetus. Although paradoxic in nature, this conservation mechanism may protect the fetus while cardiac output is redistributed toward the placenta.

NEONATAL PHYSIOLOGY

The neonatal respiratory system is still immature at birth and undergoes significant changes during transition to extrauterine life and in early postnatal life. As described in "Development of the Respiratory System in the Fetus," the final stage of lung development begins in late gestation and continues well into the postnatal period. Changes in the lungs with growth are summarized in Table 10-9.

Transitional Events

Transitional events are those activities that must occur within organ systems to achieve appropriate functioning in the extrauterine environment. The most critical of these is the establishment of an air-liquid interface at the alveolar level and the acquisition of sustained rhythmic respirations by the neonate. This must occur within seconds of placental separation, or pulmonary and cardiovascular changes will not occur and resuscitation will be necessary. Respiratory changes at birth are linked with the cardiovascular changes discussed in Chapter 9.

In most instances, transition to extrauterine life is smooth. Approximately 10% of newborns will require some assistance at birth; <1% require extensive resuscitation.[92] When intervention is needed, evidence-based guidelines are available from the International Liaison Committee on Resuscitation (ILCOR), which are incorporated into the Neonatal Resuscitation Program (NRP).[124,125,206,253]

Establishment of Extrauterine Respiration

At term, the acinar portion of the lung is well established, although "true" alveoli have only begun to develop. The pulmonary blood vessels are narrow; less than 10% to 12% of the cardiac output perfuses the lungs to meet cellular nutrition needs. This low-volume circulation is in part due to the high pulmonary vascular resistance created by constricted arterioles.

Lung aeration is complete when lung fluid is replaced with an equal volume of air and the functional residual capacity (FRC) is established. A substantial amount of air is retained from the early breaths, and within an hour of birth 80% to 90% of the FRC is created. The retention of air is due to surfactant and a decrease in surface tension. Surfactant decreases the tendency toward atelectasis; promotes capillary circulation by increasing alveolar size, which indirectly dilates precapillary vessels; improves alveolar fluid clearance; and protects the airway.[19,72] The blood gas levels that are encountered in the fetal state would result in significant hyperventilation if encountered postnatally. This indicates a diminished responsiveness of the respiratory centers to chemical stimuli in the blood in the prenatal period. Postnatal breathing is responsive to stimuli from arterial and central chemoreceptors (via oxygen and carbon dioxide tension in the blood); stimuli from the chest wall and lungs, musculoskeletal system, and skin; and environmental and behavioral stimuli. The changes that take place at birth and the increase in aerobic metabolism are not only rapid but irreversible. Within a few hours of birth, the full-term neonate is responsive to hypoxia and hypercapnea in much the same manner as an adult.[83]

During the course of labor, progressive changes are seen in fetal blood gases. The PO_2 slowly decrease, PCO_2 increases, pH decreases, and a base deficit is seen; these usual changes are not significant enough to cause depression at birth.[81] Changes in blood gases with transition are summarized in Figure 10-11. Delivery is an oxidative stress and associated with up-regulation of antioxidant defenses.[40] Antioxidant

Table 10-9 Changes in Lung Size with Growth

PARAMETER	30 WEEKS' GESTATION	FULL TERM	ADULT	FOLD INCREASE AFTER BIRTH
Lung volume	25 mL	150-200 mL	5 L	23
Lung weight	20-25 g	50 g	800 g	16
Alveolar number		50 m	300 m	8
Surface area	0.3 m^2	3-4 m^2	75-100 m^2	23
Surface area/kg		0.4 m^2	1 m^2	2.5
Alveolar diameter	32 mm	150 μm	300 μm	22
Number of airways	24	23-24	22-24	0
Tracheal length		26 mm	184 m	7
Main bronchi length		26 mm	254 m	10

From Hodson, W.A. (1998). Normal and abnormal structural development of the lung. In R.A. Polin & W.W. Fox (Eds.). *Fetal and neonatal physiology* (2nd ed.). Philadelphia: Saunders.

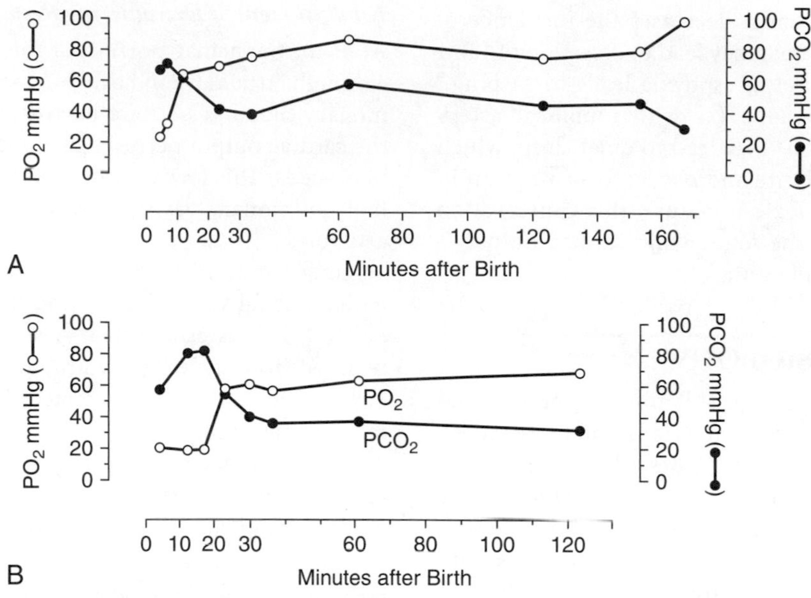

FIGURE 10-11 Changes in PO_2 and PCO_2 during the first minutes after birth in normal infants **(A)** and in asphyxiated infants **(B)** with delayed onset of respiration. (Courtesy of R. Turnell, M.D. From Carlo, W.A. & DiFiore, J.M. [2002]. Assessment of pulmonary function. In A.A. Fanaroff & R.J. Martin [Eds.]. *Neonatal-perinatal medicine: Diseases of the fetus and infant* [7th ed.]. St. Louis: Mosby.)

potential (antioxidant enzymes and nonenzymatic antioxidants) is reduced in infants born by cesarean delivery and in preterm infants increasing the risk of injury from reactive oxygen species.[49] Use of room air or low oxygen levels for resuscitation reduces oxidative stress at birth.[39,124,187,226,235] Resuscitation with low oxygen levels has been associated with less oxidative stress, inflammation, and chronic lung disease in preterm infants.[234] Oxygenation changes gradually with birth and may take a healthy term newborn 5 to 15 (median 7.9) minutes to achieve a percutaneous oxygen saturation (SpO_2) >90%.[51,235] Infants born by cesarean delivery and preterm infants take longer.[235] Preductal values are higher than postductal and are representative of brain values.[52,149,235] A predictive nomogram is available for preductal SpO_2 changes in the first 10 minutes after birth in term and preterm infants (data from infants who did not require medical intervention in the delivery room).[51]

Many factors have been suggested to stimulate the first breath including stimulation of chemoreceptors, changes in PaO_2, hypercapnea, cord clamping, cold, touch, and other sensory stimuli. Establishment of continuous respirations after birth requires resetting of thresholds of both peripheral and central chemoreceptors.[76] Hormonal or chemical mediators may also be critical and perhaps as important as low oxygen or sensory input. Occlusion of the umbilical cord stimulates peripheral and central chemoreceptors, perhaps mediated by adenosine, prostaglandins, and endorphins.[9,76,81]

The actual mechanics of respiratory conversion begins with the passage of the fetus through the birth canal. The thorax is markedly depressed during this passage, and external pressures of 160 to 200 cmH_2O (15.68 to 19.61 kPa) and intrathoracic pressures of 89 cmH_2O (8.72 kPa) or greater are generated.[176] As the face or nares are exposed to atmospheric pressure, a small amount of lung fluid is expelled.[81] Recoil of the chest to predelivery proportions allows for passive inspiration of air. This initial step helps reduce forces that must be overcome in order to establish an air-liquid interface in the alveoli.[171]

The forces that must be overcome in the first breaths include the viscosity of the lung fluid column, tissue resistive forces (compliance), and surface tension forces at the air-liquid interfaces. The viscosity of lung fluid provides resistance to movement of fluid in the airways. The maximal resistance takes place at the beginning of the first breath, and the greatest displacement occurs in the trachea.[176] The dissipation of tracheal fluid during the vaginal squeeze reduces the amount of pressure that must be generated to move the liquid column down the conducting airways.

As the column progresses down the conducting branches, the total surface area of the air-liquid interface increases as the bronchiole number increases and diameter is reduced. The surface tension, however, increases.[162] The surface tension forces are the most difficult forces to overcome during the first breath events. Maximal forces are encountered where the radial curvature of the airways is smallest (terminal bronchioles); here the viscous forces are at their nadir.[162,176,241] In this locality, the intraluminal pressure must be at its peak in order to prevent closure by tension in the intraluminal walls (Laplace relationship).[241] If these smaller airways were fluid-filled only (no air-liquid interface), the pressures needed would be considerably less; however, this would make alveolar expansion more difficult. Surface tension forces drop again once air enters the terminal air sacs.[162,241] As the air-liquid interface is established, tubular myelin is formed and spreads over the lining layer.[192] During labor and immediately after birth, alveolar surfactant production increases with secretion of lamellar bodies and formation of tubular myelin.[119] Surfactant biosynthesis and function is described in Box 10-2 on page 315 and in Table 10-4.

Tissue resistive forces at birth are unknown. However, the fluid within the terminal air sacs enhances air introduction, possibly by modifying the configuration of the smaller units of the lung. The fluid enlarges the radius of the alveolar ducts and terminal air sacs, thereby facilitating expansion (Laplace relationship). The lung fluid also reduces the possibility of obstruction of the small ducts by cellular debris.

Pulmonary vascular resistance (PVR) falls with lung expansion, endothelial changes, vasodilation, and mediators such as endothelial derived nitric oxide (NO), prostacyclin (PGI_2), and bradykinin (see Chapter 9). The low PO_2 and pulmonary blood flow in utero suppress NO and PGI_2. The increasing PaO_2 and sheer stress (rapid increase in blood flow to the lungs) with birth increases levels of these vasodilators facilitating maintenance of pulmonary vasodilation and further enhancing pulmonary blood flow.[45,74,236] Endogenous nitric oxide increases soluble guanylate cyclase, which increases cyclic guanosine monophosphate (cGMP); cGMP causes intracellular calcium to decrease and the pulmonary vascular smooth muscle to relax.[236] Prostaglandins increase cyclic adenosine monophosphate (cAMP), which enhances vasodilation by increasing endogenous nitric oxide.[236]

With birth, the lungs must move from secretion to absorption of lung fluid. Because lung fluid production slows in late pregnancy and absorption of lung fluid begins in early labor, after birth only about 35% of the original lung fluid volume needs to be cleared.[114,156,181,192] Ventilation leads to liquid dispersion across the pulmonary epithelium into the pulmonary microcirculation (Figure 10-12). The pulmonary epithelium undergoes a reversible increase in solute permeability, leading to a rapid transfer of lung fluid solutes, the interstitial spaces and lymphatic vessels become distended during the first 4 to 6 hours of life, and an increase in pulmonary lymph flow can be seen.[16,181]

Epithelial sodium channels (ENaC) and Na^+-K^+-ATPase play key roles in lung fluid removal. Increased catecholamines during labor and the catecholamine surge at birth trigger the switch from lung fluid secretion to reabsorption by activating β-adrenergic receptors, including those in type II alveolar cells, and increasing sodium conductance via ENaC and Na^+ pump activity via increases in Na^+-K^+-ATPase and ENaC expression.[16,30,74,120,126,181] Glucocorticoids, acting in conjunction with thyroid hormones, also help regulate sodium transport by increasing ENaC.[75,120] This process is accelerated by the rise in oxygenation with birth.[181] Removal of lung fluid is also mediated by differences in protein in the interstitial space and blood versus lung fluid. This creates an osmotic gradient that pulls liquid from the lungs into the interstitial space and then into the capillaries.[30,157] Approximately 10% to 20% of lung fluid is reabsorbed by the lymphatics.[30]

The drop in PVR with lung aeration and the rise in oxygen tension increase the number of alveolar capillaries perfused, resulting in an increase in blood flow and fluid removal capacity. With the increased lymphatic flow and the dramatic change in the pulmonary blood flow, lung fluid is dispersed within the first few hours after delivery.[30] Loss of lung fluid distention of the lung, along with elastic recoil, results in movement of the lung away from the chest wall. This generates a negative intrapleural pressure. Initially this pressure is about 2 cmH_2O (0.19 kPa), increasing to −5 cmH_2O (−0.48 kPa) as the chest wall becomes less compliant and opposes the lung recoil.

During the interval between recoil and the generation of first breath pressures, the infant may generate a positive pressure within the mouth by glossopharyngeal breathing. This "frog breathing" may facilitate lung expansion and

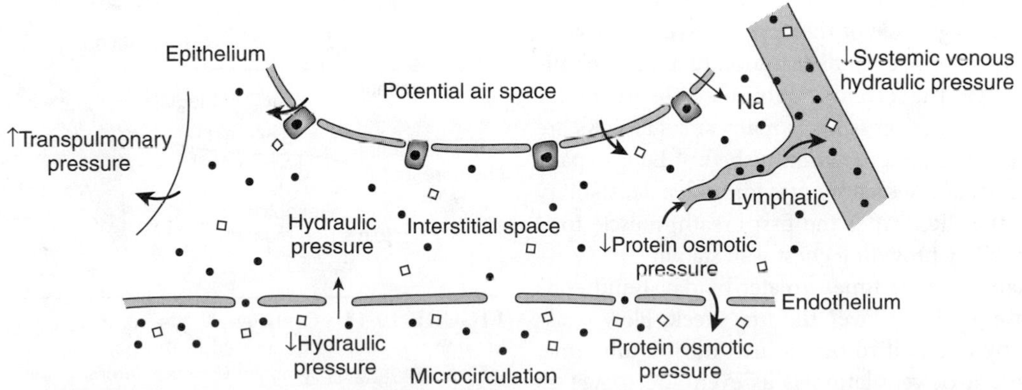

FIGURE 10-12 Schematic diagram of the fluid compartments in the fetal lung showing the forces that affect fluid clearance near birth. *Circles,* Albumin molecules; *squares,* globulin. (From Bland, R.D. [1987]. Pathogenesis of pulmonary edema after preterm birth. *Adv Pediatr, 34,* 175.)

reduce the pressure needed during the first inspiration. However, this is probably not a significant source of pressure in most infants.[162]

Another contributor to lung expansion is the increase in pulmonary blood flow with birth. The increased flow is due to compression of the placenta during labor and delivery with transfer of blood to the fetus and neonate.[157] Jaykka proposed that this flow leads to capillary erection (expansion) as pulmonary capillaries uncoil and may increase transpulmonary pressure and lung stability.[106,107] Because alveoli are attached to their surrounding capillary network by elastic fibers in the extracellular matrix, expansion of the capillaries would pull open the alveoli to allow air entry.[157] Mercer and Skovgaard proposed that neonatal transition was dependent on the presence of adequate blood volume (to mediate capillary erection and alveolar opening in the lungs) and red blood cell volume for oxygen delivery to stimulate respiration and maintenance of oxygenation.[157] Thus placental transfusion may have an important role in respiratory transition (see Chapter 8).[157]

The first diaphragmatic inspiration has been noted to begin within 9 seconds of delivery and generates large positive intrathoracic pressures (mean, 70 cmH_2O [6.85 kPa]). Air enters as soon as the intrathoracic pressure begins to drop, with mean inspiratory pressures of 30 to 35 cmH_2O (2.93 to 3.42 kPa) pressure.[162] The large transpulmonary pressure generated by the diaphragm lasts only 0.5 to 1 second, pulling in 10 to 70 mL of air to establish the functional residual capacity (FRC). The alveolar surfactant lining layer becomes established after the first breath. This layer prevents interaction of air and liquid molecules, reducing surface tension and collapsing forces and preventing alveolar collapse at end expiration as the film is compressed.[191] Surfactant secretion is stimulated by lung distention (stretch) and hyperventilation with the initial breaths as well as the increase in catecholami nes.[81,114,120] Term infants have an estimated surfactant pool of about 100 mg/kg, whereas infants with respiratory distress syndrome have pools of 2 to 10 mg/kg.[114] Pool size increases significantly over the first 3 to 5 days, which helps to "explain why the uncomplicated clinical course of respiratory distress syndrome (RDS) lasts from 3 to 5 days."[57]

The first expiration is also active, establishing a residual volume of air. The magnitude of the expiratory pressure contributes to FRC formation, even distribution of air, and elimination of lung fluid.[162] The second and third breaths are similar to the first but require less pressure as many small airways are open and surface active forces are diminished.[176] Lung expansion augments surfactant secretion, providing alveolar stability and establishing the FRC. After the first breath, muscle tone helps maintain FRC by providing chest wall stability.[162]

Lung compliance is four times greater by day 1 and continues to increase gradually over the first week. Flow resistance decreases by one half to one fourth during this time, and the distribution of ventilation is as even after day 1 as it is on day 3.[162]

Structural and functional changes in the pulmonary circulation occur after birth, with extensive remodeling of the pulmonary arteries during the first weeks after birth. The fall in PVR with birth described above and changes in PVR after birth are transitional events mediated by vasoactive agents and their signaling pathways including endothelial derived NO, PGI2, endothelin-1, platelet activating factor-1, and postnatal remodeling of the pulmonary vasculature.[74] Changes in the pulmonary vasculature and pulmonary vascular resistance after birth are discussed further in Chapter 9. In conjunction with the local vascular changes in the pulmonary bed, there are major organizational changes within the cardiovascular system. The first breath events and cardiovascular events (see Chapter 9) are interdependent and must occur together for transition to be successful.

Control of Respiration

Breathing is controlled by discharge of inspiratory and expiratory neurons in the medulla. Inspiration is active and controlled by an "off switch;" expiration is passive. The inspiratory "off switch" is controlled by pulmonary volume sensors and the pontine pneumotaxic center (for changes in both rate and depth of respiration) and is modulated by peripheral and central chemoreceptors, chest wall proprioceptors, and the cerebral cortex.[248] An overview of the ventilatory control system is in Figure 10-13. The goal of respiration is to meet oxygen and carbon dioxide metabolic demands through extraction of oxygen from the atmosphere and removal of carbon dioxide produced by the individual. The brain respiratory center is responsible for matching the level of ventilation to the metabolic demand. The assessment of metabolic needs and alteration of ventilation is accomplished by the chemoreceptors.

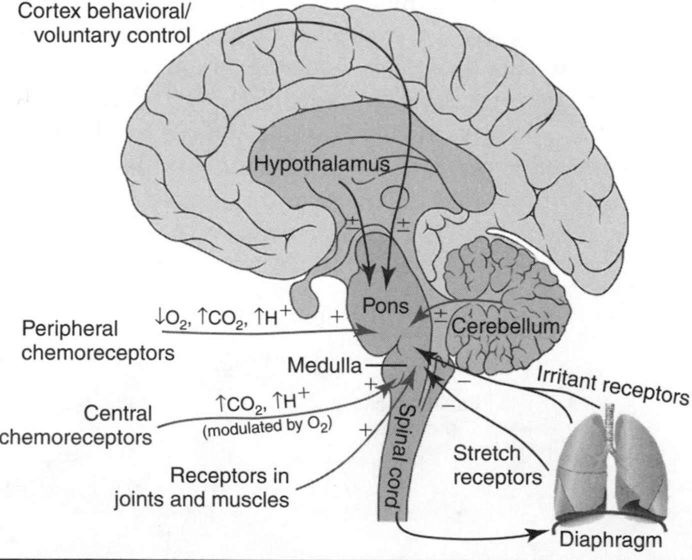

FIGURE 10-13 Overview of the ventilatory control system. Central breathing rhythm is generated in the pons and medulla and modulated by multiple inputs. Symbols: (+) stimulatory, (−) inhibitory, (±) excitatory or inhibitory. Motor output drives diaphragm, upper airway, and other respiratory muscle activity (not shown). (Modified, from original drawing by P.J. Lynch and C.C. Jaffe. From Carroll, J.L. & Agarwal, A. [2010]. Development of ventilatory control in infants. *Paediatr Respir Rev, 11,* 199.)

Ventilator control is immature and unstable in newborns. This physiologic immaturity can be seen in periodic breathing, apnea of prematurity, and probably plays a role in sudden infant death syndrome.[2,32] Factors affecting ventilatory control in newborns are summarized in Table 10-10.

Chemoreceptors

Chemoreceptors provide information about the metabolic needs of the infant, and the mechanoreceptors provide information about the status of the respiratory pump. The central respiratory center integrates this information and establishes a ventilatory pattern that efficiently meets the infant's needs. Each respiratory cycle during a stable state (e.g., quiet sleep) is uniform for amplitude, duration, and waveform. Behavioral influences as well as active sleep states (REM sleep) alter the regularity of breathing. The information received from the various receptors helps to determine the inspiratory time, the expiratory time, the lung volume at which the breath should occur (FRC), the rate of inspiration, and the braking of the expiration. The recruitment and adjustment of the various respiratory muscle groups result in the predetermined lung volume being achieved.[48,241]

The information just described is received by the respiratory controller in the brainstem, which is responsible for initiating automatic respiration and adjustments.[241] The respiratory control center is divided into three areas: the

Table 10-10 Factors Affecting Control of Ventilation in the Spontaneously Breathing Neonate

NEUROLOGIC FACTORS

Maturity of the CNS

Degree of myelinization, which largely determines speed of impulse transmission and response time to stimuli affecting ventilation.

Degree of arborization or dendritic interconnections (synapses) between neurons, allowing summation of excitatory potentials coming in from other parts of the CNS and largely setting the neuronal depolarization and response level of the respiratory center.

Sleep State (i.e., REM sleep vs. quiet or non-REM sleep)

REM sleep is generally associated with irregular respirations (both in depth and in frequency), distortion, and paradoxic motion of the rib cage during inspiration, inhibition of Hering-Breuer and glottic closure reflexes and blunted responses to CO_2 changes.

Quiet sleep is generally associated with regular respirations, a more stable rib cage, and a directly proportional relationship between PCO_2 and degree of ventilation.

Reflex Responses

Hering-Breuer reflex, whereby inspiratory duration is limited in response to lung inflation senses by stretch receptors located in major airways. Not present in adult humans, this reflex is active during quiet sleep of newborns, but absent or weak during REM sleep.

Head's reflex, whereby inspiratory effort is further increased in response to rapid lung inflation. Thought to produce the frequently observed biphasic signs of newborns that may be crucial for promoting and maintaining lung inflation (and thereby breathing regularity) after birth.

Intercostal-phrenic reflex, whereby inspiration is inhibited by proprioception (position-sensing) receptors in intercostal muscles responding to distortion of the lower rib cage during REM sleep.

Trigeminal-cutaneous reflex, whereby tidal volume increases and respiratory rate decreases in response to facial stimulation.

Glottic closure reflex, whereby the glottis is narrowed through reflex constriction of the laryngeal adductor muscles during respiration, thereby breaking exhalation and increasing subglottic pressure (as with expiratory grunting).

CHEMICAL DRIVE FACTORS (CHEMORECEPTORS)

Response to hypoxemia (falling PaO_2) or to decreases in O_2 concentration breathed (mediated by peripheral chemoreceptors in carotid and aortic bodies).

Initially there is increase in depth of breathing (tidal volume), but subsequently if hypoxia persists or worsens, there is depression of reparatory drive, reduction in depth and rate of respiration, and eventual failure of arousal.

For the first week of life at least, these responses are dependent on environmental temperature, i.e., keeping the baby warm.

Hypoxia is associated with an increase in periodic breathing and apnea.

Response to hyperoxia (increase in FIO_2 concentration breathed): enriched O_2 breathing causes a transient respiratory depression, stronger in term than in preterm infants.

Response to hypercapnia (rising $PaCO_2$ or $[H^+]$) or to increase in CO_2 concentration breathed (mediated by central chemoreceptors in the medulla).

Increase in ventilation is directly proportional to inspired CO_2 concentration (or more accurately stated, to alveolar CO_2 tension), as is the case in adults.

Response to CO_2 is in large part dependent on sleep state; in quiet sleep, a rising $PaCO_2$ causes an increase in depth and rate of breathing, whereas during REM sleep, the response is irregular and reduced in depth and rate. The degree of reduction closely parallels the amount of rib cage deformity occurring during REM sleep.

Ventilatory response to CO_2 in newborns is markedly depressed during behavioral activity such as feeding and easily depressed by sedatives and anesthesia.

From Greenspan J.S., et al. (2004). Assisted ventilation: Implications and complications. In R.A. Polin, W.W. Fox, & S.H. Abman (Eds.). *Fetal and neonatal physiology* (3rd ed.). Philadelphia: Saunders, p. 963.

CNS, Central nervous system; *REM,* rapid eye movement.

apneustic center, the pneumotaxic center, and the medullary center. The pneumotaxic center may be responsible for switching inspiration to expiration. The apneustic center seems to be responsible for cutting off inspiration. Both centers are located in the pons and neither seems to be necessary for rhythmic expiration. The medullary center is thought to be responsible for respiratory rhythm. These centers are connected to the cerebral cortex, thereby allowing voluntary control of respiration. The spinal cord is responsible for the integration and relay of commands to the muscles of the respiratory pump via the phrenic and intercostal nerves.

The peripheral chemoreceptors (carotid and aortic bodies) sense PaO_2 and $PaCO_2$, and the central chemoreceptors (medullary) are sensitive to PCO_2^- $[H^+]$ in the extracellular fluid of the brain. When the PaO_2 falls below the acceptable range, the chemoreceptors increase efferent neural activity to the brain respiratory center, resulting in an increase in ventilation. At birth, the fetal PaO_2 of approximately 25 mmHg (3.32 kPaa) (sufficient for intrauterine growth) increases to 50 to 70 mmHg (6.65 to 9.31 kPaa) within the first few breaths and then to 70 mmHg (9.31 kPaa) in the first hours.[76] This increase in oxygen tension exceeds the demands for oxygen, yielding a relative neonatal hyperoxia at birth. The change in oxygen tension causes the chemoreceptors to become less responsive to stimuli ("silenced") during the first few days of life.[2,31] As a result, fluctuations in oxygen tension levels may not lead to an immediate chemoreceptor response during this period with a gradual increase in the slope of the hypoxic stimulus curve.[48,77,119,139] After this lag time, however, the chemoreceptors reset and become increasingly oxygen-sensitive and a major controller of respiration.[2,9,31,48,77,78] This change is due to increases in the density of K^+ channels, greater increases in intracellular calcium in response to hypoxia, and changes in neurotransmitters.[77] The carotid bodies are the main arterial oxygen sensors. Carotid body oxygen response is low at birth, increasing with increasing postnatal age with further maturation taking to 10 weeks.[32] By 2 weeks of age, peripheral chemoreceptor activity is similar to that of adults.[2] Term infants have adult-like central chemoreceptor activity at birth, whereas preterm infants take 4 or more weeks to achieve this level of response.[76,77]

Sustained hyperventilatory efforts during hypoxia cannot be maintained by the neonate. Newborns have a biphasic response with an initial hyperventilatory response (due to stimulation of peripheral chemoreceptors, especially those in the carotid body) followed by a subsequent fall in ventilation (primarily due to a decrease in frequency), to levels below baseline in some preterm infants, and oxygen tension.[1-3,32,47,78] This biphasic response persists for several days in term infants and up to 4 to 6 weeks in preterm infants.[3,76,151] Preterm infants may not have the initial hyperventilation, only the sustained decrease in ventilation.[76] The reason for this lack of sustained response is unknown but may be due to a weak chemoreceptor output, a central inhibitory effect of hypoxia on ventilation mediated by the interaction of neurotransmitters or via descending inhibitory pontine tracts, or changes in pulmonary mechanics.[1,3,48]

The neonate's response to carbon dioxide is also limited in the early neonatal period. Although this is more mature than the response to hypoxia, the neonate can only increase ventilation by three to four times baseline ventilation in comparison to the 10-fold to 20-fold increase that can be achieved by adults. Furthermore, the threshold of tolerance is initially higher, progressively declining over the first month of life.[47,250] This too may be due to the increased $PaCO_2$ levels found in the fetal state (45 to 50 mmHg [5.98 to 6.65 kPaa]) and the need to reset chemoreceptors.[9,48] Hypercapnic ventilatory responses are weaker in preterm infants. Although with hypercapnia, preterm infants develop a sustained increase in tidal volume (V_T), they also have an increase in the expiratory phase that may lead to a net decrease in their respiratory rate.[2,254]

Modification of ventilatory patterns is dependent upon inspiratory muscle strength, rib cage rigidity and compliance, airway resistance, and lung compliance. The status of these parameters at any given time, as well as their integrative functioning, affects the performance of the respiratory pump and is mediated by specific reflex arcs.

Chest Wall Reflexes

Most of the reflexes for the respiratory pump arise from the chest wall via the muscle spindles through local spinal reflex arcs and centrally mediated reflexes. The diaphragm is scantily innervated; however, the intercostal muscles have abundant fibers from which this information is obtained. These stretch-sensitive mechanoreceptors detect chest wall and workload forces.[152]

Excessive stretch is modulated by alpha motor neuron activity altering respiratory muscle activity or recruiting more muscles. Further sensory information is obtained by proprioceptors that sense changes in rib position and tension applied across the joint space. Cutaneous stimulation of the thoracic wall causes a generalized increase in sensory and motor neuron stimulation of the respiratory muscles, augmenting muscle contractions and ventilation.

Chest wall distortion during inspiration stimulates muscle spindles that trigger central reflex arcs, leading to reflex inhibition of intercostal, phrenic, and laryngeal neurons. This is possibly a protective mechanism in the neonate. Termination of distorted inefficient breathing may lead to energy conservation and reduce the possibility of muscle fatigue.

Laryngeal and Pulmonary Reflexes

The mechanoreceptors of the large lung airways include stretch receptors, irritant receptors, and C receptors. The sensory feedback mechanisms for these receptors are along the vagus nerve to the central respiratory center.

The stretch receptors sense lung inflation and deflation, with neural output proportional to lung volume or tension.[9,48] Lung inflation initiates inhibitory impulses that terminate inspiration and prolong expiratory time. This is termed the Hering-Breuer reflex. Once triggered, respiratory frequency slows and may lead to apnea. Although not found in adults, this reflex is active in the neonate for reasons that are not well understood. It may be a protective mechanism for the neonate, because inspiratory occlusion results in an increase in inspiratory effort and inspiratory time. Responses vary in individual infants and may play a role in apnea of prematurity.[1,3,9,227]

The irritant receptors of the mucosal lining in the airways are extremely sensitive to mechanical stimulation and are responsible for the cough reflex seen clinically. In infants over 35 weeks' gestation, there is the typical adult response to stimulation: increased breathing, coughing, arousal, and gross body movement. For infants less than 35 weeks, however, these responses are not usually elicited. These infants may have either no response or a brief cough followed by apnea, slowing of respiration, or immediate respiration.[9] The reason for this difference is unknown but may be due to a functional immaturity or the possibility that unmyelinated irritant receptors may be inhibitory in nature.[227]

The reflex of Head (seen as a sigh) is more prevalent in infants than children or adults. This may be due to a need to recruit more alveoli to maintain adequate gas exchange. Sighs are also more frequent during rapid eye movement (REM) sleep and with periodic breathing.[9]

The laryngeal chemoreflex (LCR) leads to inhibition of breathing in the neonate when the laryngeal mucosa is stimulated chemically (water or acidic solutions) or mechanically.[105] The LCR is associated with glottis closure, swallowing, bradycardia and a decrease in blood pressure. The LCR may be exaggerated in preterm infants.[3]

Upper Airway

The nares are oriented more vertically in infants with a shorter anteroposterior diameter. Nasal resistance is about one third the total pulmonary resistance (versus 45% in adults).[206] Neonates tend to be nasal breathers, although most term infants will breathe orally with nasal occlusion.[19] The nasal route is the primary route of air entry due to the high position of the epiglottis and the position of the soft palate.[206]

The epiglottis and hyoid, thyroid, and cricoid cartilage are stabilized in the term infant by fatty superficial fascia. This fascia is absent in preterm infants, leading to flexibility and increasing the risk of airway obstruction.[206] The pharyngeal airway is shorter and wider in neonates, with the cricoid cartilage at the level of the fourth cervical vertebrae (versus the seventh in adults). The pharyngeal airway is also prone to collapse in preterm infants, leading to obstruction and apnea.[206]

Newborns are able to adduct their vocal cords during expiration to increase their FRC. This can lead to grunting as expired air is released across the partially closed glottis. This mechanism is often seen in more mature preterm infants or term infants with respiratory distress, but it is also noted in healthy infants during the first few days after birth. In these infants, use of this mechanism is thought to assist in maintaining lung volumes during transition.[206]

Respiratory Pump

The movement of gas in and out of the lungs is based on the functioning of the respiratory pump, which is composed of the rib cage and respiratory muscles. The pump must move sufficient oxygen and carbon dioxide into and out of the lungs to replace the oxygen consumed and wash out the carbon dioxide that accumulates in the alveoli. Ventilatory efforts in the neonate are dependent upon the strength and endurance of the diaphragm. When the diaphragm is unable to generate the necessary energy to sustain ventilatory efforts, ventilatory assistance is required.[48]

Diaphragm

The diaphragm inserts on the lower six ribs, the sternum, and first three lumbar vertebrae. It is innervated bilaterally by the phrenic nerves and expends its work on the lung, the rib cage, and the abdomen. To maximize diaphragmatic work, the intercostal muscles must stabilize the rib cage and the abdominal muscles should stabilize the abdomen.[48,148] In the term infant, the coordination of these efforts is reduced; the preterm infant is even less effective at coordinating these events. During REM sleep (the most predominant sleep state in the neonate), the intercostal and abdominal muscles are less efficient, contributing to respiratory instability.

The diaphragm works most efficiently when the dome is high in the thorax (relaxed position, optimal fiber length), increasing the thoracic volume while compressing the abdominal contents and moving the abdominal wall.[148] The neonatal diaphragm is situated differently than that of the adult. In its relaxed state, it is located higher in the thorax, favoring more efficient generation of inspiratory pressures. In the adult, the diaphragm is flatter and generally lower, making it more inefficient mechanically. This difference is made up for by the stability of the chest wall in the adult.

The composition of the muscle fibers in the neonate is also different. In adults, 60% of the fibers are fast-oxidative, fatigue-resistant type I fibers; 30% are type IIa fast-oxidative fatigue-sensitive fibers; and the rest are type IIb slow-oxidative, fatigue-resistant fibers.[128] In contrast, the neonatal diaphragm and intercostal muscles have a lower proportion of fatigue-resistant muscle fibers (20% type I fibers) and more type IIa fibers.[48,128] Type I fibers increase in number from 24 weeks' gestation on. At 24 weeks, they comprise 10% of the total fiber content.[48,86,128]

Contraction and relaxation times, as well as the latent period, are longer in premature babies than in adults. A lack of sarcoplasmic reticulum in the diaphragmatic muscle may result in a slower initiation as well as termination of contractions. Therefore when high respiratory rates occur, there may be ischemia of the muscle with fatigue related to inadequate substrate availability.[152] Because of these developmental patterns and other limitations (Table 10-11), the infant is particularly vulnerable to diaphragmatic muscle fatigue, especially when the work of breathing is increased. This vulnerability increases with lower gestational age.

The neonate's diaphragm is attached to a chest wall that is more pliable than that of the adult. This can lead to distortion

Table 10-11 Potentially Important Predisposing Factors for Diaphragmatic Fatigue in Newborns

PROBLEM	PREDISPOSING FACTOR
Decreased efficiency	Thoracic shape/rib orientation Soft rib cage (magnified by prematurity) REM sleep-induced intercostal muscle activity depression Normally flat diaphragm with decreased zone of apposition
Decreased oxygen and/or substrate supply	Hypoxemia acidosis and/or hypotension Poor compensatory increase in diaphragmatic blood flow Insufficient nutritional intake and/or decreased substrate stores
Decreased maximal force potential	Small muscle fiber diameter Increased lung volume at end expiration

From Murphy, T. & Woodrum, D. (1998). Functional development of respiratory muscles. In R.A. Polin & W.W. Fox (Eds.). *Fetal and neonatal physiology* (2nd ed.). Philadelphia: Saunders.
REM, Rapid eye movement.

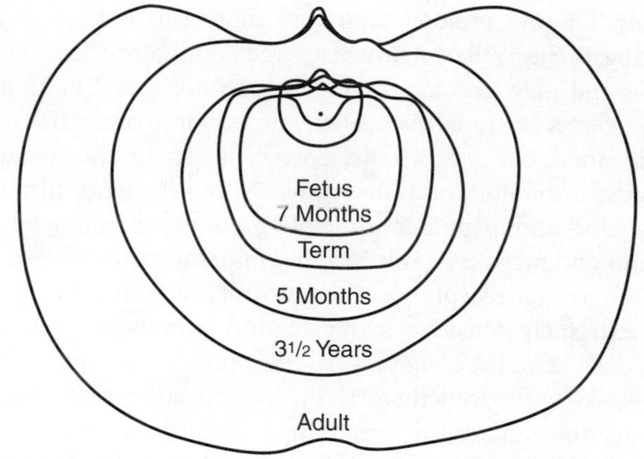

FIGURE 10-14 Superimposed outlines of thoracic skeletal contours at various ages. Outlines are aligned relative to the vertebral body. (From Fenn, W.O. & Rahn, H. [1964]. *Handbook of physiology.* Bethesda, MD: American Physiological Society.)

of the lower portion of the chest wall during contraction, especially with a forceful contraction. The decreased efficiency of the contraction and reduced tidal volume (V_T) can make ventilation less effective, requiring adjustments in the respiratory pattern.[48]

Rib Cage and Chest Wall Muscles

The muscles of the rib cage include the external intercostal muscles (inspiration); the internal intercostal muscles (expiration); and the accessory muscles, including the sternocleidomastoid, pectoral, and scalene muscles. The major role of these muscles is to fixate the chest wall by tonic contraction during diaphragmatic excursion. If they are unable to accomplish this goal, collapse and distortion of the chest wall is likely to occur during inspiratory efforts. If the needed stability is provided, the contraction of the inspiratory muscles of the rib cage can contribute to the thoracic volume by elevating the anterior end of each rib. During sighing, the increase in V_T is largely due to this increased chest wall excursion.

The rib cage of the newborn is more boxlike, with nearly equal anteroposterior and transverse diameters (versus the elliptical shape of the adult) (Figure 10-14). The ribs are articulated to the rib cage more horizontally, in a position similar to that of the adult at full inspiration. This reduces the mechanical efficiency of chest wall excursions in the newborn since most of the V_T must be generated by the diaphragm.[86,142]

Chest Wall Compliance

The chest wall in the infant is cartilaginous, soft, and pliable. This structure allows for compression during passage through the birth canal without rib fractures and for further growth and development. Nelson described the rib cage as a loosely fitting glove surrounding the neonatal lung.[176] The high compliance dictates that for any given change in volume there is minimal change in pressure.[177] The increased compliance is highest in the preterm infant but is significant in the full-term infant as well. As a result, there is a tendency of the chest wall to collapse and the infant to retract as he or she tries to generate the negative pressures needed for lung expansion.

Elastic recoil is that property of a body structure that causes it to return to its resting position after having been stretched or deformed.[177] In the older child and adult, once the chest wall has reached the FRC it tends to recoil outward; however, the tendency of the lung to collapse toward the RV provides a counterbalance.[55,177,241] In other words, at resting lung volumes (FRC) the elastic recoil of the chest wall is equal and opposite to that of the lungs.

At V_T, the chest wall of the neonate has similar compliance to the lungs.[70] The lack of opposition by the thorax to the recoil of the lung causes the newborn's respiratory system to come to equilibrium at a resting volume very close to the collapse volume (Figure 10-15).[70,176] The activity of the intercostal muscles during normal breathing is a major determinant of the elastic characteristics of the chest wall and thus FRC. Therefore during tidal breathing, some of the dependent airways fall into their closing volume range and the bronchioles collapse and are not in communication with the main stem bronchus. Bronchiole compliance contributes to these dynamics.

Elastic recoil of the chest wall increases during the first two weeks after birth, although it remains considerably less than that of the adult for a longer period of time. The continued change in recoil pressures is presumed to be the result of progressive ossification, improvement in intercostal muscle tone, and development of a negative pressure on the abdominal side of the diaphragm.[177]

For the infant (with a small abdomen) lying in a supine position, the outward recoil of the chest is presumably

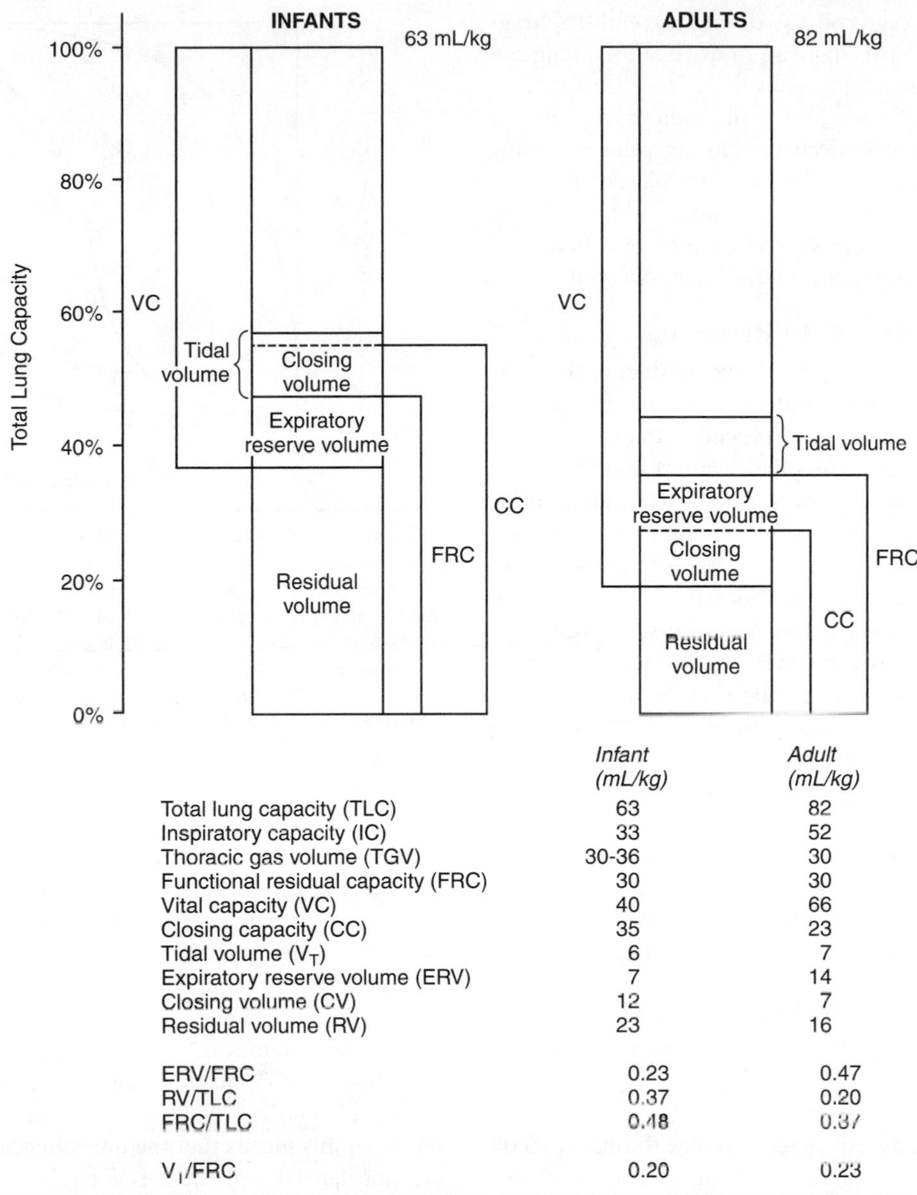

	Infant (mL/kg)	*Adult (mL/kg)*
Total lung capacity (TLC)	63	82
Inspiratory capacity (IC)	33	52
Thoracic gas volume (TGV)	30-36	30
Functional residual capacity (FRC)	30	30
Vital capacity (VC)	40	66
Closing capacity (CC)	35	23
Tidal volume (V_T)	6	7
Expiratory reserve volume (ERV)	7	14
Closing volume (CV)	12	7
Residual volume (RV)	23	16
ERV/FRC	0.23	0.47
RV/TLC	0.37	0.20
FRC/TLC	0.48	0.37
V_I/FRC	0.20	0.23

FIGURE 10-15 Lung volumes in the infant and adult. (From Nelson, N. M. [1976]. Respiration and circulation after birth. In C.A. Smith & N.M. Nelson [Eds.]. *The physiology of the newborn infant.* Springfield, IL: Charles C. Thomas.)

inhibited. Once the infant learns to stand and the abdomen has grown, the contents of the abdominal cavity shift away from the upper abdomen, thereby creating an increase in negative subdiaphragmatic pressure. This change in pressure favors outward recoil of the chest wall.[177]

The clinical implications of a highly compliant chest are related to the ease at which lung collapse is possible in the neonate. The low elastic recoil pressure of the neonatal lung and the high compliance of the thorax result in the majority of tidal breathing in the infant occurring near the closing capacity of the lung. This contributes to the possibility of alveolar collapse and affects gas distribution. These characteristics can also alter breathing patterns with the risk of paradoxical or asynchronous patterns.[86]

The mechanical liabilities of a highly compliant chest wall after delivery include a compromised ability to produce a large V_T, requiring the generation of greater pressures. As a result the infant must perform more work to move the same amount of V_T.[177] This is especially true in preterm infants with lung diseases associated with decreased lung compliance (e.g., RDS). Lung disease causes the respiratory drive (response to stimulus) to increase in an attempt to generate stronger contractions with high inspiratory pressures in order to expand their stiffer, less compliant lungs.

Increased diaphragmatic force and the pliable chest wall lead to chest distortion.[48,176] Therefore a portion of the energy and force of the contraction is wasted. Retractions are the clinical signs of these distortions and are indications of the degree of inward rib cage collapse during forceful diaphragmatic contractions.[177] This increase in work of breathing can lead to fatigue and eventually apnea.

The compliance of the chest wall—combined with the compliance of the lungs—affects the closing volume, closing capacity, expiratory reserve volume, and FRC. For the neonate, this means that a high closing volume and high closing capacity combine with a low expiratory reserve volume and FRC, culminating in a propensity toward alveolar collapse.[176]

Mechanical Properties of the Respiratory System

The work of breathing is the cumulative product of the pressure and volume of air moved at each instant. The work is done by the muscles as energy is expended to overcome the elastic and resistive forces (compliance and resistance) of the lung and thorax as well as the frictional resistance to air movement. The respiratory muscles expend about half their energy on inspiration. The rest is stored within the tissues (which have been stretched) as potential energy. As the potential energy is released, expiration occurs passively.

There are two major sources of resistance that the respiratory muscles must overcome during each breath: (1) tissue elastic resistance that is created by displacement of the lung and chest wall from their resting positions (compliance) and (2) resistance presented by gas molecules flowing through the airways.

The system is most efficient when the respiratory rate and V_T are set to require the minimum expenditure of work. This can be assessed by evaluating the amount of oxygen used in performing the work. Under normal circumstances the oxygen consumed is only a small fraction of the total metabolic requirement. The newborn infant expends the least amount of energy when breathing 30 to 40 breaths per minute.

Lung Compliance

The pressure gradient necessary to overcome the elastic recoil force encountered in the lung depends on V_T and lung compliance. Compliance is the measurement of the elastic properties opposing a change in volume (mL) per unit of change in pressure (cmH_2O) (Hooke law). Static compliance reflects the elastic properties of the lung; dynamic compliance reflects both elastic and resistive forces.[240] Compliance can be demonstrated in a pressure-volume curve (Figure 10-16) that relates a change in lung volume to the change in the alveolar-to-intrapleural pressure gradient (i.e., transpulmonary pressure). The slope of the curve indicates the compliance. The flatter the curve, the stiffer the lung.[166,176]

Lung compliance depends on the tissue elastic characteristics of the parenchyma, connective tissue, and blood vessels, as well as the surface tension in the alveoli and the initial lung volume before inflation. When the lung must be inflated from a very low lung volume, the required pressure gradient is greater.

Changes in lung compliance are sensed by lung stretch receptors. These receptors, along with muscle spindle fibers from the respiratory muscles, transmit information to the respiratory center in order to modify the drive necessary to maintain ventilation. For the healthy, more mature preterm infant, lung compliance is similar to that of the full-term infant. Lung compliance decreases (lungs become less elastic) with decreasing gestational age. Lung disease usually leads to a decrease in lung compliance, which translates to a smaller volume change for pressure change.

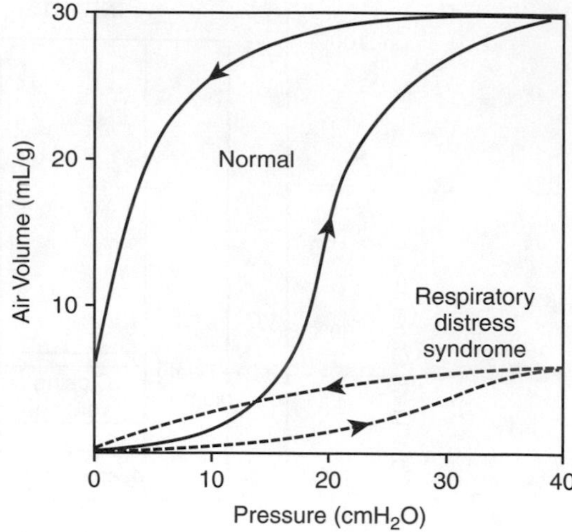

FIGURE 10-16 Air-pressure–volume curves of neonatal and abnormal lung. Volume is expressed as milliliters of air per gram of lung. The lung of an infant with respiratory distress syndrome accepts a smaller volume at all pressures. Note also that the deflation pressure-volume curve follows very closely the inflation curve for the affected lung. (From Keszler, M., Abubakar, M.K., & Wood, B.R. [2011]. Physiologic principles. In J.P. Goldsmith & E.H. Karotkin [Eds.]. *Assisted ventilation of the neonate* [5th ed.]. Philadelphia: Saunders, p. 23.)

The most significant determinant of elastic properties is the alveolar air-liquid interface. When molecules are aligned at an air-liquid interface, they lack opposing molecules on one side; this means that the intermolecular attractive forces are unbalanced and there is a tendency for the molecules to move away from the interface. This reduces the internal surface area of the lung and therefore augments elastic recoil.

Surfactant varies surface tension, allowing for high surface tensions at large lung volumes and low tensions at low volumes. Surfactant forms an insoluble surface film upon compression and thereby lowers surface tension. This tends to stabilize air spaces of unequal size and prevents their collapse. Without surfactant, smaller alveoli tend to empty into larger ones, resulting in microatelectasis alternating with hyperaeration (see Figure 10-8).

Alveolar collapse occurs in a number of diseases; probably the most notable is RDS (see "Respiratory Distress Syndrome"). In RDS, surfactant deficiency is directly related to gestational age and developmental immaturity of the lungs. Surfactant synthesis, however, is also dependent on normal pH and pulmonary perfusion. Therefore any disease or event that interferes with these processes (e.g., asphyxia, hemorrhagic shock, pulmonary edema) may lead to surfactant deficiencies.[166]

Airway Resistance

Lung resistance is dependent upon the size and geometric arrangements of the airways, viscous resistance of the lung tissue, and the proportion of laminar to turbulent airflow. Resistance varies inversely with lung volume—meaning that the greater the lung volume, the less resistance is encountered, and vice versa. This is because the diameter of the airways increases with the expansion of the parenchyma.

Gas flows through a tube from a point of higher pressure to a point of lower pressure. Two patterns of flow have been identified based on the magnitude of the pressure drop and its relationship to the rate of gas flow. These patterns are termed *laminar* and *turbulent*. In laminar flow, resistance is determined by the radius and length of the tube during the flow. Laminar flow can become turbulent if the flow rate rises excessively or when the angle or diameter of the tube changes abruptly (e.g., at branch points).

Airway resistance in the term infant is 20 to 40 $cmH_2O/L/sec$, which is 16-fold greater than in adults (1 to 2 $cmH_2O/L/sec$).[154] Even mild edema will significantly increase the resistance. In adults, the upper airways (especially the nose) account for the major portion of total airway resistance.[176] In neonates and children younger than 5 years of age, the peripheral airways contribute the most to airway resistance.[162] For example, in infants, 50% of the total airway resistance is due to the small airways versus less than 20% in adults.[154] The decreased diameter of airways (especially in the periphery) is the reason for this increased resistance. The distal airway growth in diameter and length lags behind proximal growth during the first 5 years of life. Therefore a small decrement in the caliber of airways can lead to a very large increase in peripheral airway resistance.[129,177]

Cartilage provides the support for stability of the conducting airways. With ongoing development, there is an increase in the number of cartilage rings during the first 2 months of life and an increase in total area of support over the remainder of childhood. The lack of support in the neonate can lead to dynamic compression of the trachea during situations associated with high expiratory flow rates and increased airway resistance (e.g., crying).

In disease states, resistance is increased either by a decrease in the intraluminal size of the airway or through compression or contraction of the walls of the airway.[129,177] Peripheral airways are tethered open by the elastic mesh of the pulmonary parenchyma and the transmural pressure gradient (intraluminal airway pressure greater than the intrapleural pressure). During forced expiration, intrapleural pressure rises significantly; this is transmitted to the alveoli and increased even further by the pulmonary parenchyma elastic recoil pressure. Initially this maintains a favorable pressure gradient. However, a pressure drop must occur from alveolus to mouth during active expiration, and there is a point in the airway at which intraluminal pressure will equal intrapleural pressure (equal pressure point). As the gas continues to move toward the mouth, the forces maintaining airway patency are overwhelmed and the airway collapses.[177] If the elastic parenchyma meshwork is destroyed, as with bronchopulmonary dysplasia (BPD), airway collapse is even more likely.

Resistance increases with decreasing gestational age and with specific lung diseases (e.g., RDS, BPD) that are prominent in preterm infants. The increased resistance is sensed by respiratory muscles, leading to an increase in ventilatory drive. Changes in the radius of the larynx or trachea because of edema (e.g., with repeated intubation) or as a result of intubation also increase resistance. This effect may be quite pronounced because the resistance is generated in the large airways, where resistance should be at its lowest.

Time Constants

Time constants reflect the combined effect of resistance and compliance on the lung. The time needed for a given lung unit to fill to 63% of its final capacity is the product of resistance and compliance. If the resistance and compliance are equal in two adjacent lung units (alveoli), the time constant will be the same and there will be no redistribution of gases between the alveoli.[177] If the time constant of one unit is longer but the compliances remain equal, the two alveoli will eventually reach the same volume. However, the longer the time constant, the slower the filling will be due to the increased resistance. In this instance, the intraluminal pressure in the alveolus with the least resistance will be higher and lead to redistribution of its gases into the adjacent, slower-filling alveolus.[129]

The time constant can also be lengthened when compliance is increased, but resistance remains the same. In this circumstance, the less compliant alveolus will fill faster than its adjacent, more compliant neighbor. This is due to the decreased volume that the less compliant alveolus can hold. Redistribution of gases will occur if inflation is interrupted prematurely due to the increased pressure in the less compliant alveolus as compared to the adjacent lung unit.[177] This redistribution of gases in the lung is not a major factor in the normal lung, in that the alveoli are relatively stable and do not change much in size.[177] This is a result of the effect of surfactant upon the lung.

Ventilation

Once air enters the lungs, it must come in contact with the blood in order to effect gas exchange. The drop in negative pressure causes air to move by bulk flow down the air passages to the level of the bronchioles. From this point forward, the movement of air into the acinar portion of the lungs is due to the random movement of the molecules from a higher area of concentration to a lower area of concentration (diffusion). Any factor that impedes the flow of gas to the acinus reduces gas exchange and influences the partial pressure of gas within the blood. Therefore the effective interface of ventilation with blood flow is responsible for the adequacy of oxygen uptake and carbon dioxide removal. In this section, the factors that affect ventilation at the alveolar level are discussed.

Collateral ventilation between alveoli and bronchioles is decreased in the newborn and young infant. Collateral ventilation between alveoli occurs via the 3- to 13-mm pores of Kohn in the alveolar walls. These pores allow air to move between contiguous alveoli. Lambert's canals allow air to flow from bronchioles into bronchiolar channels. Both structures are poorly developed at birth and "consequently limit the homogenous distribution of ventilation at the alveolar level and prevent ventilation distal to obstructed airways through collateral ventilation."[154]

Dead Space Ventilation

A variable portion of each breath is not involved in gas exchange and is therefore wasted; this is considered dead space ventilation. There are two types of dead space: anatomic dead space and alveolar dead space. Anatomic dead space is that volume of gas within the conducting airways that cannot engage in gas exchange. Alveolar dead space is the volume of inspired gas that reaches the alveolus but does not participate in gas exchange because of inadequate perfusion of that alveolus. The total dead space (anatomic and alveolar) is termed *physiologic dead space.* Physiologic dead space is usually expressed as a fraction of the V_T and is approximately 0.3 in infants and adults.[177] Patients experiencing respiratory failure have elevated dead space–to–V_T ratios, which results in hypoxia and hypercarbia unless counteracted by an increase in the amount of air expired per minute.[177]

Pleural Pressure

The differences in pleural pressure within the lung play a significant role in determining the distribution of gases. During spontaneous breathing, a greater proportion of gas is distributed to the dependent regions of the lung. It is assumed that the difference in subatmospheric (negative) intrapleural pressure at the base and at the apex is the reason for this distribution pattern. Interestingly, alveolar pressure remains constant in all regions of the lung. Subsequently, the transpulmonary distending pressure in the dependent regions is decreased, leading to a reduced lung volume in these areas. The smaller alveoli in the dependent lung regions lie on the steeper slope of the transpulmonary pressure–to–lung volume curve, resulting in a greater portion of the V_T being directed to the dependent alveoli during normal breathing.[177] A greater portion of the pulmonary perfusion goes to the dependent regions as well, thereby matching ventilation and perfusion more closely.

Lung Volumes

Lung volumes in the newborn are illustrated in Figure 10-15.

Functional Residual Capacity

The FRC is established during the first breaths, forming an alveolar reservoir at end-expiration, allowing for continuous gas exchange between respiratory efforts, stabilizing PaO_2. Normally the FRC comprises 30% to 40% of the total capacity of the lung and may change volume from breath to breath. Immediately following birth, the FRC is low, increasing rapidly with successive breaths. In preterm infants with lung disease, the FRC stays low until the lung disease resolves. The goal is to keep the FRC above the passive resting volume of the lung, which may be difficult for neonates due to their pliable, more compliant chest wall. The role of the FRC is crucial in the energy expenditure of the respiratory musculature. FRC minimizes the work of breathing while optimizing the compliance of the system and maintaining a gas reservoir during expiration.[48] In the neonate, the FRC is about 20-30 mL/kg.[119]

Closing Capacity

As noted earlier, in the neonate (especially the preterm infant) it is possible for lung volumes to be reduced below the FRC during quiet breathing in dependent regions of the lung.[154] Closing volume is the lung volume above which airway closure occurs. When the closing capacity exceeds the FRC, the ventilation-perfusion ratio drops and hypoxia and hypercarbia occur. If total atelectasis exists, then the closing capacity exceeds not only the FRC but also the V_T, and these portions of the lung are closed during both expiration and inspiration. The use of end-expiratory pressure is designed to raise the FRC above closing capacity.[177] Continuous distending pressure is used in the neonatal population when chest wall compliance leads to marked distortion and altered lung volumes, as well as during disease states associated with alveolar collapse (e.g., RDS).

The greater closing capacity seen in children younger than 6 years of age and in adults older than 40 years of age is probably due to decreased elastic recoil in the lung.[168] Elastic recoil is that property of the lung that allows it to retract away from the chest wall, creating a subatmospheric pressure in the intrapleural space. The decrease in elastic recoil results in the subatmospheric pressure in the intrapleural space being raised, leading to increased airway closure in dependent regions.[177]

Perfusion

Alveolar ventilation is dependent not only on the functioning of the airways, but also on the functioning of the pulmonary vasculature. Pulmonary vascular muscle thickness is a function of gestational age, with the preterm infant having less well-developed smooth muscle. This incomplete development results in a drop in pulmonary vascular resistance much sooner after delivery, predisposing the infant to a faster onset of congestive heart failure and left-to-right shunting (see Chapter 9).[177]

Normal Pulmonary Blood Flow

The majority of pulmonary blood flow is distributed to the dependent regions of the lungs due to gravitational forces. In zone 1 (apex of the lung), the alveolar pressure is greater than the pulmonary artery and venous pressures. As a result, the pulmonary vessels collapse, with concomitant loss of gas exchange and wasted ventilation.[129] In zone 2, pulmonary artery pressure exceeds alveolar pressure, and blood flow increases. The perfusion pressure increases as blood flows downward; this results in a linear increase in blood flow. Slowing of blood occurs when the pulmonary venous pressure and alveolar pressure are equal.[177] Pulmonary venous pressure and pulmonary artery pressure increase, exceeding alveolar pressure in zone 3, the base of the lungs. In the more dependent regions of this zone, the transmural pressure increases, with resultant dilation of the vessels, and blood flow increases.[129,177]

Posture differences between the upright adult and supine-lying infant probably also affect pulmonary blood distribution. The general principles still apply, but may be to a lesser extent. Wasted ventilation in the apices due to lack of perfusion is probably much less likely in the supine position, helping to balance some of the limitations encountered in the neonatal lung.

Ventilation-Perfusion Relationships

Mismatching of ventilation and perfusion is the most common reason for hypoxia and is a frequent result of the neonatal respiratory system's liabilities. Efficient gas exchange in the lungs requires matching of pulmonary ventilation and perfusion. The relationship between ventilation and perfusion is expressed as a ratio and reflects the correlation between alveolar ventilation and capillary perfusion for the lung as a whole. $\dot{V}/\dot{Q}$ relationships are summarized in Box 10-3 below.

The ventilation of the air space should be adequate to remove the carbon dioxide delivered to it from the blood, and the perfusion of the air space should be no greater than that which allows oxygenation and complete saturation of the blood during its brief passage through the alveolar capillaries. Ideal efficiency would occur if ventilation were perfectly matched to perfusion, yielding a ratio of 1 (Figure 10-17).

In healthy adults, capillary blood spends 0.75 second in the alveolus, and the oxygen–carbon dioxide exchange occurs across the alveolar-capillary membrane. As the blood leaves the alveolus, the blood gas tensions are identical with those of the alveolar gas. The gas tensions achieved at equilibrium are dependent upon rate of ventilation, membrane thickness, membrane area, capillary blood flow, venous gas tensions, and inspired gas tensions.[228] In order for equilibrium to be achieved rapidly, the area for exchange must be large enough to allow the blood to be spread thinly over the vessel wall and blood and gas must actively mix together.[129,241]

Matching of ventilation to perfusion is dependent upon gravity to a large extent. Both ventilation and perfusion increase as air and blood move down the lung, with perfusion increasing more than ventilation. Right ventricular pressure is inadequate to fully perfuse the apices of the lung. On the other hand, lung weight leads to a relatively greater negative intrapleural pressure at the apex than at the base, resulting in the apical alveoli being better expanded but receiving a smaller portion of each V_T than the bases. Along with this, there is reduced perfusion in the apices, creating a high ($\dot{V}/\dot{Q}$) ratio (Figure 10-18, *A*).[176,228,241]

$\dot{V}/\dot{Q}$ ratios of zero are characteristic of shunts (see Figure 10-18, *C*). In this situation, no ventilation takes place during the passage of blood through the lungs. The pulmonary capillary blood arrives in the left atrium with the same gas tensions it had when it was mixed venous blood. Examples of shunts include the normal bronchial and thebesian circulations, perfusion of an atelectatic area, venoarterial shunts, and cyanotic congenital heart disease with blood flowing directly from the right to the left side of the heart.

BOX 10-3 Ventilation-Perfusion Ratios

Ventilation-perfusion ($\dot{V}/\dot{Q}$) ratios are based on the distribution of gases, the distribution of the pulmonary circulation, and the interrelationship between these two factors. This interrelationship is affected by the rate of airflow into the lungs (which is a function of depth of inspiration, rate of inspiration, airway resistance, and lung compliance) and pulmonary circulation (which is influenced by cardiac output and pulmonary vascular resistance). The ideal ratio occurs when ventilation and perfusion are matched such that the sites available on the hemoglobin molecules are equal to the concentration of oxygen molecules in the alveoli and there is sufficient time for the diffusion of oxygen across the membranes and attachment of hemoglobin. The "ideal" lung is depicted in Figure 10-17. In this instance, neither ventilation (oxygen) nor blood flow is wasted. Interestingly, the usual distribution of gases and blood is neither equal nor ideal.

Maldistribution of pulmonary blood flow is the most frequent cause of reduced oxygenation of arterial blood. The degree of nonuniformity of distribution is probably greater for pulmonary circulation than it is for gas distribution. The uneven distribution not only occurs between the two sides of the lungs but also between lobes and alveolar segments. This is usually manifested by a reduction in PaO_2.

Distribution can range from unventilated to unperfused alveoli, with all degrees of variation in between. Ventilated alveoli that are not perfused comprise the alveolar dead space and have PaO_2 and $PaCO_2$ values that are essentially equivalent to those of inspired air. This is because there is no alveolar gas exchange with the blood to modify the gas concentrations in the alveoli. On the other hand, alveoli that are perfused but not ventilated result in intrapulmonary shunts in which PaO_2 and $PaCO_2$ values are the same as those in mixed venous blood. In this situation, the air trapped within the alveoli equilibrates with the venous blood traversing the capillaries of the alveoli (see Figure 10-18). Some degree of gas exchange occurs in all other situations.

When there is a low ventilation-perfusion ratio (<1) the alveoli are under ventilated with respect to perfusion or overperfused with respect to ventilation. In circumstances in which the alveoli are overventilated for the perfusion available, there is a high ventilation-perfusion ratio (>1). In these abnormal or disease states, the ventilation-perfusion inequalities may increase in magnitude, involving greater and greater numbers of alveoli. The net result is a significant impact on gas exchange and blood gases.

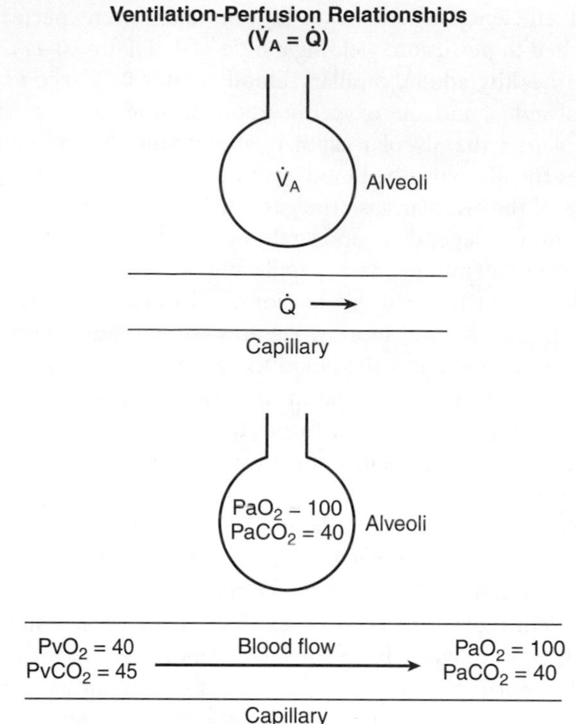

FIGURE 10-17 Ideal lung ventilation-perfusion.

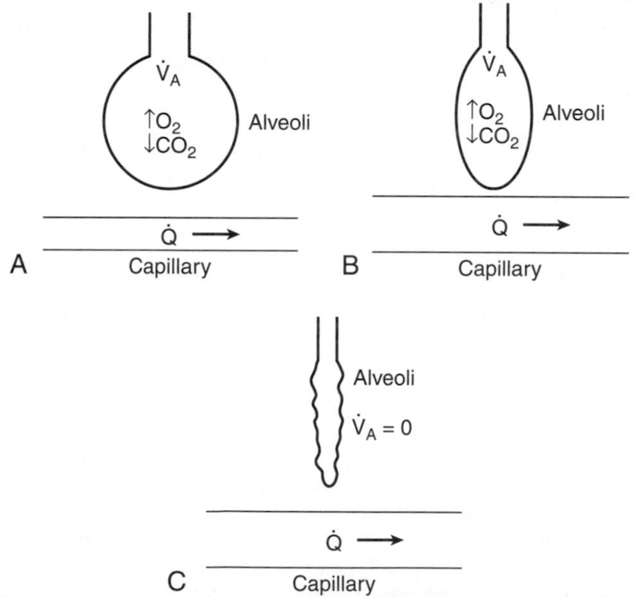

FIGURE 10-18 Ventilation-perfusion mismatching. **A,** High ventilation-perfusion. **B,** Low ventilation-perfusion. **C,** Intrapulmonary shunt.

High ($\dot{V}/\dot{Q}$) ratios (Figure 10-18, *A*) are the result of increased dead space and may also occur if the blood flow is reduced. Rapid equilibration occurs, but a large amount of ventilation is required.[241] Ventilation is wasted, either in anatomic conducting airways or in poorly perfused alveoli (alveolar dead space). Thus a large amount of ventilation is wasted on a relatively small amount of blood without significantly changing the oxygen content. This inefficient gas exchange will eventually result in carbon dioxide retention.[177]

On the other hand, alveolar underventilation results in low ($\dot{V}/\dot{Q}$) ratios (see Figure 10-18, *B*). In this situation, ventilation is low in relation to perfusion but not entirely absent. This is the normal state for the lung bases in an erect position. It is also found in disease in which airway obstruction reduces ventilation to alveolar units (e.g., asthma, cystic fibrosis).

The blood perfusing the underventilated alveoli is incompletely oxygenated and a lower amount of carbon dioxide is removed. Partial venoarterial shunts contribute incomplete arterialized blood to the arterial stream; this is termed venous admixture. This is reflected in an elevated partial pressure of carbon dioxide upon blood gas evaluation.

Abnormalities of ($\dot{V}/\dot{Q}$) ratios may be secondary to either too much or too little ventilation to an area with normal blood flow, too much or too little blood flow with normal ventilation, or some combination of the two. Whichever occurs, the lung's regulatory mechanisms work to achieve and maintain the ideal relationship. In areas where the ($\dot{V}/\dot{Q}$) ratio is high and carbon dioxide levels are low, local airway constriction occurs in order to reduce the amount of ventilation going to the area. When the opposite occurs, the airways dilate in an attempt to increase ventilation to the area and improve the carbon dioxide exchange. When oxygenation is also affected and low alveolar oxygen concentrations are found, the lung reduces blood flow to the region. These mechanisms are finite, however.

In newborns, most of the ventilated areas are well perfused and there is little dead space. However, in newborn infants, significant amounts of perfusion are wasted on unexpanded air spaces (intrapulmonary shunts) as transitional events progress. The lower PaO_2 in the newborn demonstrates the widened alveolar-to-arterial PO_2 gradient, reflecting the increased venous admixture. Although perfusion of unexpanded air spaces may play a significant role in this, the continued right-to-left shunting through transitional circulatory circuits is another contributory factor. The premature infant is at even greater risk for shunting and venous admixture due to developmental immaturity.

Intrapulmonary shunting (see Figure 10-18, *C*) and wasted ventilation are normal features of the newborn lung. The latter results from transition from fluid-filled to air-filled lungs, in which alveoli are underventilated but normally perfused. These effects begin to dissipate after 1 to 2 hours of air breathing. During the first few days of life, the neonatal lung—compared to that of the adult—has a greater shunt component and a larger proportion of low $\dot{V}/\dot{Q}$ areas. However, V_T, alveolar volume, and dead space volume per breath are similar (when expressed in mL/kg). The arterial-alveolar differences in both oxygen and carbon dioxide persist in the full-term infant for about a week due to the venoarterial shunting. These gradually dissipate as adult values are achieved.[176,228]

Effect of $\dot{V}/\dot{Q}$ Mismatching on Oxygen

As inspired gas moves to the level of the arterial circulation, there is a stepwise decrease in oxygen tension. This results in reduced oxygen content in the alveoli; however, alveolar oxygen levels remain higher than those in the arterial blood. This maintains a concentration gradient that supports oxygen diffusion. If the ideal were maintained, at the end of equilibration the alveolar and arterial oxygen concentrations would be the same. This, however, is not the case. There remains a difference between the two ($AaDO_2$), which is reflective of the imperfect matching of ventilation to perfusion (see Figure 10-18).

Under normal circumstances, this difference is relatively small and is secondary to the anatomic shunts through the thebesian and bronchial circulations. The hypoxemic patient, however, may have additional shunts (congenital heart disease) or increased $\dot{V}/\dot{Q}$ mismatching. Both situations result in an increased venous admixture.

$\dot{V}/\dot{Q}$ mismatching affects oxygenation by lowering the arterial PO_2 and widening the $AaDO_2$. This occurs for two reasons, the first being an increased blood flow through low $\dot{V}/\dot{Q}$ segments rather than high $\dot{V}/\dot{Q}$ segments. This results in an increased volume of desaturated blood. The second reason is the sigmoid shape of the oxygen-hemoglobin dissociation curve. This implies that the alveolar PO_2 is not proportional to oxygen content or saturation.

On the oxygen-hemoglobin dissociation curve (Figure 10-19 and Box 10-1 on p. 301), low $\dot{V}/\dot{Q}$ segments, with lower alveolar PO_2 values, will have a proportionately greater drop in oxygen content. This is because of their position on the steep portion of the curve. The high $\dot{V}/\dot{Q}$ segments will have higher alveolar PO_2 values but will not exhibit the expected increase in oxygen content because they lie on the flat portion of the curve. In this area of the curve, changes in PO_2 have very little effect on oxygen content or saturation. The net effect is one of low $\dot{V}/\dot{Q}$ segments negating high ones. Although the oxygen content is higher in the latter, it is not high enough to compensate for the markedly lower oxygen content found in the low $\dot{V}/\dot{Q}$ segments. Therefore arterial desaturation occurs.

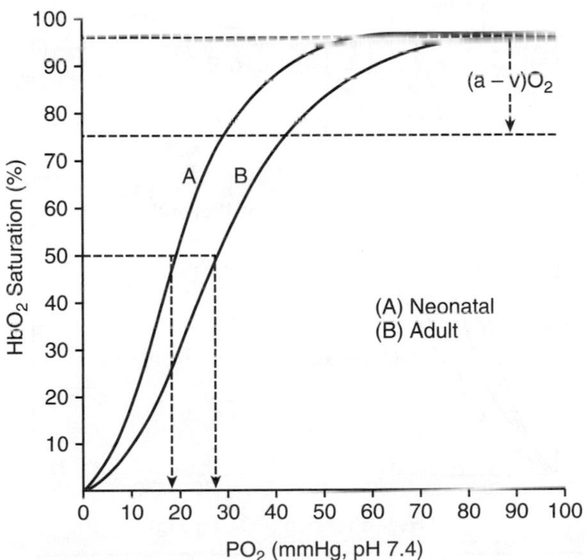

FIGURE 10-19 Oxyhemoglobin curves of blood from term infants at birth and from adults. (From Delivoria-Papadopoulos, M. & McGowen, J.E. [1998]. In R.A. Polin & W.W. Fox [Eds.]. *Fetal and neonatal physiology* [2nd ed.]. Philadelphia: Saunders.)

Measurement of $\dot{V}/\dot{Q}$ mismatching as it relates to desaturation is difficult. Venous admixture is a convenient way to describe the amount of mixed venous blood it would take to obtain the observed arterial oxygen content. Venous admixture can be expressed as the ratio of shunted blood to total pulmonary blood flow, reflecting the efficiency of the lung in oxygenating the blood. The magnitude of this ratio determines in part what effect an increase in fractional inspired oxygen (FIO_2) will have on PaO_2. If the ratio is equal to zero, there will be a linear increase in PaO_2 with increasing inspired oxygen. Once the ratio is 0.5 or greater, increasing the FIO_2 will have little effect on PaO_2.[177]

Effect of $\dot{V}/\dot{Q}$ Mismatch on Carbon Dioxide

$PaCO_2$ is determined mainly by the degree of alveolar ventilation in relation to the carbon dioxide produced by the cells. When alveolar ventilation is reduced secondary to an increase in alveolar dead space (alveoli are ventilated but not perfused or are underperfused), carbon dioxide levels in the blood begin to rise. This is reflected in the widened gradient between end-expiratory PCO_2 and alveolar PCO_2, with end-expiratory PCO_2 being lower due to the addition of alveolar dead space gas, which does not contain carbon dioxide.[177]

The difference between alveolar and capillary PCO_2 is usually low due to the diffusibility of carbon dioxide. This means that even with a large venous admixture load, there would be only a slight increase in arterial PCO_2. The small change occurs because the carbon dioxide dissociation curve is linear and relatively steep (within the normal range), meaning that large changes in carbon dioxide content produce small changes in carbon dioxide tension.

Developmental Differences in $\dot{V}/\dot{Q}$ Matching

In term infants, markedly lower PaO_2 levels are found. This is indicative of a widened alveolar-to-arterial PO_2 gradient and an increase in venous admixture being added to the arterial blood. Persistent right-to-left shunting through fetal vascular channels—along with atelectatic areas of the lung being perfused—is the source of the admixture. In adults the major component of venous admixture is the maldistribution of ventilation.[177]

These differences stabilize as transition progresses, lasting a week or so in the full-term infant. The preterm infant, however, is at greater risk for desaturation because of increased chest wall deformation and increased ductal shunting. For the preterm infant it may be several weeks before complete transition and stabilization occur.[176]

Hypoxemia and thermal stress may result in ductal opening and shunting during the early transitional period for both term and preterm infants. Venous admixture does not fall to adult levels until late infancy and early childhood. Beyond 7 years of age, the PaO_2 does not vary much, stabilizing between 95 and 100 mmHg (12.63 to 13.3 kPaa).[177]

Alveolar-Capillary Membrane

The alveolar-capillary membrane is the physical barrier separating the alveolar gases from the pulmonary capillary blood. The barrier also helps prevent liquid movement from the circulation into the alveolus, thereby preventing alveolar flooding and collapse. Transudation of fluid resulting in pulmonary edema is a major cause of respiratory failure in all age groups.

Diffusion is the movement of gases from an area of high concentration to an area of lower concentration until equilibrium is achieved. This is the mechanism by which gas exchange occurs at the alveolar-capillary membrane. The rate of diffusion is directly proportional to both the surface area available and the solubility of the gases, and it is inversely proportional to the diffusion distance. The diffusion capacity for oxygen is greatly affected by the time it takes for the oxygen to combine with hemoglobin. The surface area in the normal lung is determined by the amount of ventilated and perfused tissue available, increasing with age, height, and body surface area.

Oxygen-Hemoglobin Dissociation Curve

Because of the low-oxygen environment in which the fetus lives, the need for an increased affinity for oxygen is essential to survival. Fetal hemoglobin (HbF) (see Chapter 8) alters this affinity, and 2,3-diphosphoglycerate (2,3-DPG) regulates it.[54] When 2,3-DPG binds with fetal gamma chains, it does not lower oxygen affinity as it does with binding to adult hemoglobin beta chains. The fetal oxygen-hemoglobin dissociation curve therefore lies to the left of the adult curve (see Figure 10-19). This means that in the fetus and neonate the affinity of oxygen for hemoglobin is greater and the release of oxygen to the tissues is somewhat less than in the adult at any given PO_2. The left shift in the very-low-birth-weight infant who has greater HbF may influence SpO_2 measurements.[210]

The "30-60-90" rule can be used to remember general relationships between PaO_2 and saturation: at a PaO_2 of 30 mmHg (3.99 kPaa), the saturation is about 60%; at a PaO_2 of 60 mmHg (7.98 kPaa), saturation is about 90%, and at a PaO_2 of 90 mmHg (11.97 kPaa), saturation is about 95%. Changes in the oxygen-hemoglobin dissociation curve in term and preterm infants at different postbirth ages are illustrated in Figure 10-20. The oxygen-hemoglobin dissociation curve is reviewed in Box 10-1 on page 301.

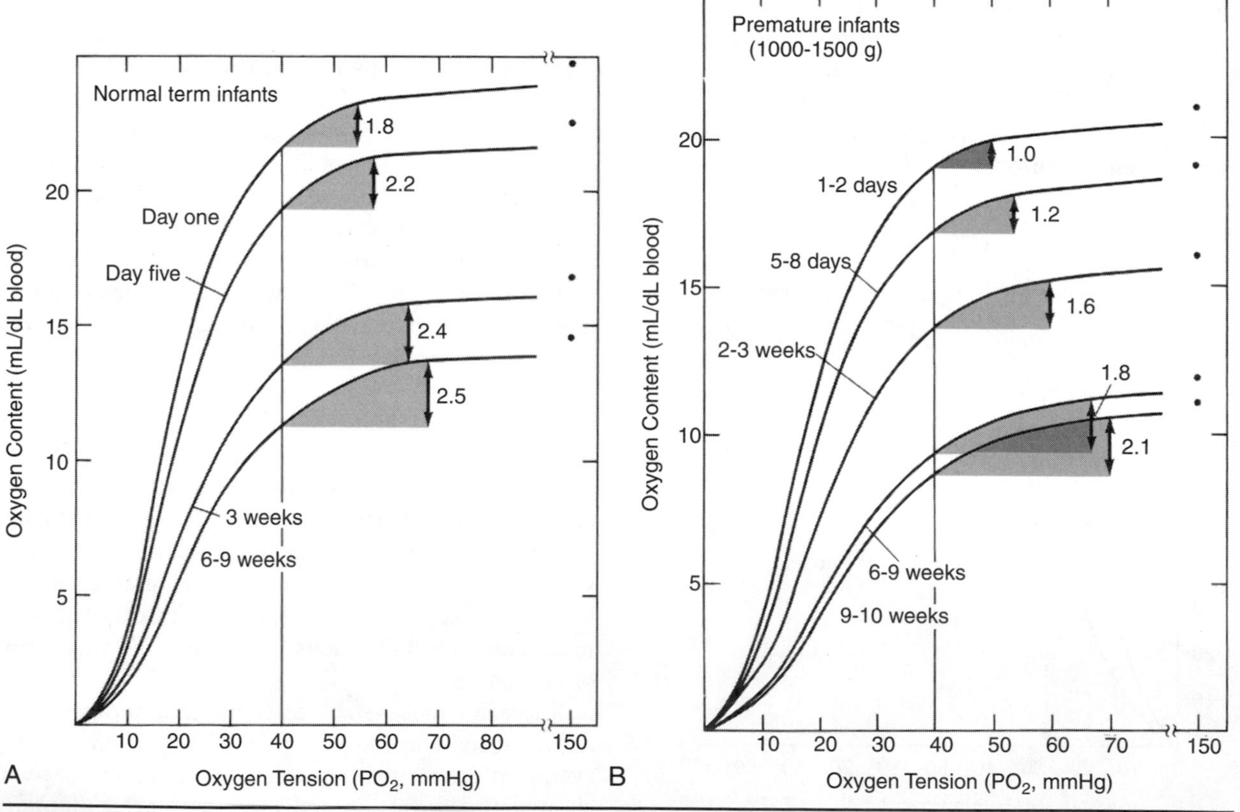

FIGURE 10-20 Oxygen equilibrium curves of blood in term infants **(A)** and preterm infants with birth weight 1000 to 1500 g **(B)** at different postnatal ages. *Double arrows* represent the oxygen unloading capacity between a given "arterial" and "venous" PO_2. Points corresponding to 150 mmHg (14.7 kPa) on the abscissa are the O_2 capacities; each curve represents the mean value of the infant studied in each age group. (From Delivoria-Papadopoulos, M. & McGowen, J.E. [2004]. Oxygen transport and delivery. In R.A. Polin, W.W. Fox, & S.H. Abman (Eds.). *Fetal and neonatal physiology* [3rd ed.]. Philadelphia: Saunders, p. 887.)

Oxygen Consumption

Oxygen consumption in the newborn infant is twice that of the adult in relation to weight. One of the major factors affecting oxygen consumption in the neonate is temperature (see Chapter 20). The neutral thermal environment is that environmental temperature at which oxygen consumption is minimal. Small changes in environmental temperature can result in dramatic increases in oxygen consumption. Decreases of 2° C (3.33° F) in environmental temperature can double oxygen requirements. If the infant is unable to increase oxygen delivery to meet these needs, tissue oxygenation falls and may become insufficient. When oxygen availability is compromised, the cell switches to anaerobic metabolism to meet energy and work needs.

Tissue Respiration

The ultimate purpose of oxygenation of arterial blood is for consumption by the cells during aerobic metabolism. Aerobic metabolism is desirable because 20 times more energy is made available when substrates are metabolized aerobically versus anaerobically.[177] Molecular oxygen is used in oxidation-reduction reactions in cells, in which oxidation is the loss of electrons from an atom or molecule and reduction is the gain of electrons.[168]

When one substance is oxidized, another is reduced. Reducing agents give up electrons; electron acceptors are oxidizing agents. Oxygen is an oxidizing agent. Food molecules (substrate), such as glucose, are reducing agents. Within the cell mitochondria, oxygen serves as final acceptor in the process of cell respiration. Energy is derived from this process and is used to form adenosine triphosphate (ATP) from adenosine diphosphate (ADP) and inorganic phosphate. When energy is later released, ATP is hydrolyzed to ADP. The hydrolysis reaction and cellular work activities allow ATP to provide the energy to accomplish cellular functions. Hypoxia and hyperoxia are discussed in "Clinical Implications for Neonatal Care."

CLINICAL IMPLICATIONS FOR NEONATAL CARE

Although there are many liabilities within the neonatal respiratory system, the healthy term infant achieves transition to the extrauterine environment without any difficulties. However, the developmental stage of the system increases the possibility of respiratory distress and failure above that seen in older individuals. Maturation of both anatomic and functional development are required to achieve adult functioning; therefore both contribute to respiratory vulnerability and the risk of distress. Implications of neonatal respiratory system characteristics are summarized in Table 10-12.

Anatomic risk factors include the incomplete development of the bone and cartilage that make up the thoracic cavity and are a part of the respiratory pump. The increased compliance of the thorax makes it extremely important that the intercostal muscles be able to contract and fixate the chest so that adequate pressure can be generated and inspiration occurs. Although full-term infants appear to compensate well, the intercostal muscles and accessory muscles are still not completely developed. This contributes to diaphragmatic breathing and chest wall instability, which can lead to higher closing volumes and a decreased FRC. In disease states in which increased resistance occurs, the high inspiratory pressures necessary to fill the lungs may result in retractions of the chest wall.

The ability to stabilize the chest wall is directly related to increasing gestational age. Therefore, preterm infants are highly susceptible to chest wall deformation and atelectasis during tidal breathing. This may result in hypoxemia, hypercarbia, and apnea, necessitating supplemental oxygen or ventilatory support.

Airway resistance is increased due to the smaller nares, shorter airways with multiple bifurcations, and peripheral airway diameter. Therefore upper airway congestion and minor small airway infections may lead to increased resistance and place the infant at risk for respiratory distress, muscle fatigue, and respiratory failure. Edema secondary to trauma or infection of upper airway passages can easily result in obstruction with a marked increase in resistance to airflow. This distress can be seen in nasal flaring, retractions, and tachypnea.

Until the age of 5 years, the small peripheral airways contribute 50% of the airway resistance that must be overcome. This is compared with 20% in the adult, who has a much larger cross-sectional area for flow. Bronchi constrict in response to numerous factors, including inhaled irritants, hypoxemia, hypercarbia, and cold. This constriction significantly increases airway resistance and the work of breathing.

The surface area of the lung is also decreased because of the characteristic structure of the chest. The ribs are rounder, giving the typical barrel chest configuration seen in the term infant after birth. However, this results in thoracic crowding due to the relative size of the abdominal organs. The surface area of the lung is consequently decreased and lung expansion is reduced.

The lung compliance is decreased. If compounded by disease states that reduce elasticity (e.g., pulmonary congestion, pulmonary fibrosis), the compliance drops even further and the work of breathing must increase in order to compensate.

Cartilaginous support is essential for the stability of the conducting airways. This too is a function of gestational age and development. Cartilage rings continue to increase in number for up to 2 months in age. Weakness secondary to lack of support can result in dynamic compression of the trachea in situations associated with high expiratory flow rates and increased airway resistance. Although bronchiolitis and asthma are common disease entities that cause this, it can also occur during episodes of crying, resulting in reduced saturations.

The gas-exchange portion of the lung in the term infant is made up of terminal air sacs and alveoli. Terminal air sacs

Table 10-12 **Implications of Alterations in Respiratory Function in Neonates**

ALTERATION	IMPLICATION
Immature alveoli; decreased size and number of alveoli	Risk of respiratory insufficiency and pulmonary problems
Thicker alveolar wall; decreased alveolar surface area	Less efficient gas transport and exchange
Continued development of alveoli until childhood	Possible opportunity to reduce effects of discrete lung injury
Decreased lung elastic tissue and recoil	Decreased lung compliance requiring higher pressures and more work to expand increased risk of atelectasis
Fewer pores and channels for collateral ventilation	Greater distress with airway obstruction Increased risk of air leak and pulmonary edema Increased risk of atelectasis
Compliant boxlike rib cage with almost horizontal insertion of ribs and immature musculature	Difficulty in taking deep breaths Less effective movement of thoracic cage Less effective in generating intrathoracic pressures needed for lung expansion Greater reliance on diaphragmatic and abdominal musculature for respiration Retractions Difficulty maintaining functional residual capacity and increasing tidal volume Risk of atelectasis Increased work of breathing
Reduced diaphragm movement and maximal force potential, with more horizontal position and smaller muscle fiber diameter	Less effective respiratory movement Difficulty generating negative intrathoracic pressures Risk of atelectasis Possible increased risk of muscle fatigue with respiratory insufficiency and failure
Tendency to nose breathe; altered position of larynx and epiglottis	Enhanced ability to synchronize swallowing and breathing Risk of airway obstruction Possibly more difficult to intubate
Small compliant airway passages with higher airway resistance and immature reflexes	Risk of airway obstruction and apnea
Increased pulmonary vascular resistance with sensitive pulmonary arterioles	Risk of ductal shunting and hypoxemia with events such as hypoxia, acidosis, hypothermia, hypoglycemia, and hypercarbia Possible protection against the development of congestive heart failure in first few weeks in infants with defects (e.g., a large ventricular septal defect)
Increased oxygen consumption	Increased respiratory rate and work of breathing Risk of hypoxia
Increased intrapulmonary right-left shunting	Increased risk of atelectasis with wasted ventilation Lower $PaCO_2$
Immature development of lung capillary basement membrane	More vulnerable to collapse of terminal bronchioles and alveoli
Decreased functional residual capacity	Less oxygen reserves with increased risk of atelectasis and hypoxia Increased work of breathing
Closing volume nearer tidal volume	Areas of airway collapse and atelectasis Risk of hypoxia and hypercarbia Increased work of breathing
Immaturity of pulmonary surfactant system in immature infants	Increased risk of atelectasis and respiratory distress syndrome Increased work of breathing
Immature respiratory control	Irregular respiration with periodic breathing Altered respiratory threshold Instability of respiratory drive Risk of apnea Inability to rapidly alter depth of respiration Difficulty in compensating for hypoxemia and hypercarbia

Adapted from Blackburn, S. (1992). Alterations in the respiratory system in the neonate: Implications for practice. *J Perinat Neonatal Nurs 6,* 46.

lack the cupped shape of alveoli and are longer and narrower. They require higher pressures in order to maintain expansion, and once collapsed, increased pressures must be generated in order to reopen them. The alveoli that are present are smaller and predisposed to collapse. Preterm infants have only terminal air sacs because true alveoli have not yet developed.

The surface area available for diffusion is reduced in the neonate. During disease states, this may be reduced even further, requiring an increase in minute ventilation. Much of neonatal disease may be related to an alteration in FRC, closing capacity, or both. When the closing capacity is high, the pleural pressure exceeds the intraluminal pressure, resulting in early closure of bronchi, making them unavailable for gas exchange. A reduction in FRC can lead to unstable blood gases between respiratory efforts.

Without collateral ventilation, the neonate cannot divert ventilation to distal airways when obstruction occurs. Although anatomic pathways have not been found on histologic sectioning of neonatal lungs, radiologic evidence suggests that alternative pathways may exist. Without channels for collateral ventilation, there is an increased risk for atelectasis or emphysematous change and ventilation-perfusion mismatching.[177]

Biochemical immaturity of the surfactant system can result in progressive atelectasis. Primary surfactant deficiency is found in premature infants, resulting in RDS. However, surfactant production may be interrupted by numerous events, including cytogenic oxygen toxicity, ischemia of the pulmonary bed, pulmonary edema, and hemorrhagic shock. Synthesis of surfactant is dependent upon a normal pH and adequate pulmonary perfusion.

Prematurity may also result in increased susceptibility to oxygen-induced cytotoxicity. The development and maturation of the antioxidant system parallels the maturation of the surfactant system, both occurring late in gestation. Without the ability to detoxify reactive oxygen metabolites, these metabolites are released into the immediate environment, where they can injure normal cells.[43] This may lead to cell death or cause pulmonary edema, surfactant synthesis disruption, and scarring of lung tissues.

Physiologic Basis for Clinical Findings

The presence of increased work of breathing indicates a primary pulmonary disorder. The signs of increased work of breathing are chest wall retractions (subcostal, intercostal, suprasternal) and the use of accessory muscles (alar flare). Patients with respiratory failure have elevated ratios of dead space volume to V_T; such a condition results in hypoxia and hypercarbia unless counteracted by an increase in expired minute ventilation.[171]

Respiratory patterns change with increased respiratory work. Tachypnea may be the only sign of abnormalities in lung functioning. Tachypnea is the most efficient way for neonates to increase ventilation and compensate for hypoxia and hypercarbia. Respiratory rates fall as fatigue sets in.

In mild to moderate disease there is tachypnea, slight substernal and intercostal retractions, slight increase in anterior-to-posterior diameter, and intermittent expiratory grunting without cyanosis. Retractions occur because of the increased compliance of the chest wall, the immaturity of the intercostal muscles, and the increased inspiratory pressure generated. As the severity of the disease increases, the retractions become more marked. Deformation of the chest leads to paradoxic breathing (asynchrony of chest and abdominal movements), which is the result of diaphragm fatigue, inability of the intercostal muscles to fixate the chest wall, and increased inspiratory pressures.

Expiratory grunting elevates the end-expiratory pressure and slows the expiratory flow rate. This is accomplished by laryngeal braking through partial closure of the glottis. These maneuvers help maintain expansion and preserve oxygenation between respirations. Grunting is usually not seen in very low birth weight infants. Nasal flaring results from increased inspiratory pressure.

Periodic Breathing and Apnea of Prematurity

Breathing in newborns, especially in preterm infants, tends to be irregular, with marked breath-to-breath variability and episodes of periodic breathing.[9,47] Periodic breathing is defined as "pauses in respiratory movements that last for up to 20 seconds alternating with breathing."[9] Periodic breathing is common in preterm infants and is also seen in term infants, and even adults, at altitude. Periodic breathing is thought to be benign.[9] Periodic breathing can also be induced by hypoxemia and respiratory depression; respiratory stimulants such as caffeine alleviate periodic breathing.[47] Mechanisms for periodic breathing and apnea are unclear but they are probably due to alterations in or instability of the respiratory control center. These patterns are more common during REM sleep, possibly due to decreased intercostal muscle tone, diaphragmatic activity, and upper airway adductor muscle tone during REM sleep.[3,9]

Apnea involves longer pauses and changes in heart rate, often to less than 80 beats per minute. Three types of apnea have been described in preterm infants: central (10% to 25% of the episodes), obstructive (10% to 20%), and mixed (50% to 75%).[9,161] Central apnea is characterized by no airflow or breathing effort and obstructive apnea by no airflow with breathing efforts. Mixed apnea begins as central apnea and ends as obstructive.[3,9,200] These patterns are illustrated in Figure 10-21.

Apnea is common in preterm infants, and more frequent in infants with chronic lung disease or other respiratory problems. The incidence of central apnea decreases with increasing gestational age, is seen in most infants born at less than 1000 g, and may last until these infants reach 43 to 44 weeks postmenstrual age.[3] Factors involved in the pathogenesis of apnea of prematurity include central mechanisms (decreased central chemosensitivity, ventilatory depression, up regulation of inhibitory neurotransmitters such as γ-aminobutyric acid [GABA] and adenosine), altered peripheral reflex pathways (altered carotid body activity, laryngeal chemoreflex, increased bradycardic response to hypoxia) and genetic predisposition.[2,3] Physiologic immaturity and depression of the respiratory drive, sleep state, less well-developed ventilatory responses to carbon dioxide, paradoxic responses to hypoxia (that increase baseline chemoreceptor activity and may destabilize breathing), exaggerated inhibitory reflexes, altered responses to sensory input by the upper airway, and a predisposition to pharyngeal collapse may all contribute to apnea of prematurity.[1,3,9,77] Neonatal sepsis with release of proinflammatory cytokines may alter respiratory control via PG-mediated pathways.[2,3] Methylxanthines (e.g., caffeine, theophylline) are used in management of the preterm infant with apnea. These agents have a central stimulatory effect on brainstem respiratory structures.[2,3,200] Caffeine is the preferred agent due to its efficacy and fewer side effects and potential for improvement in long

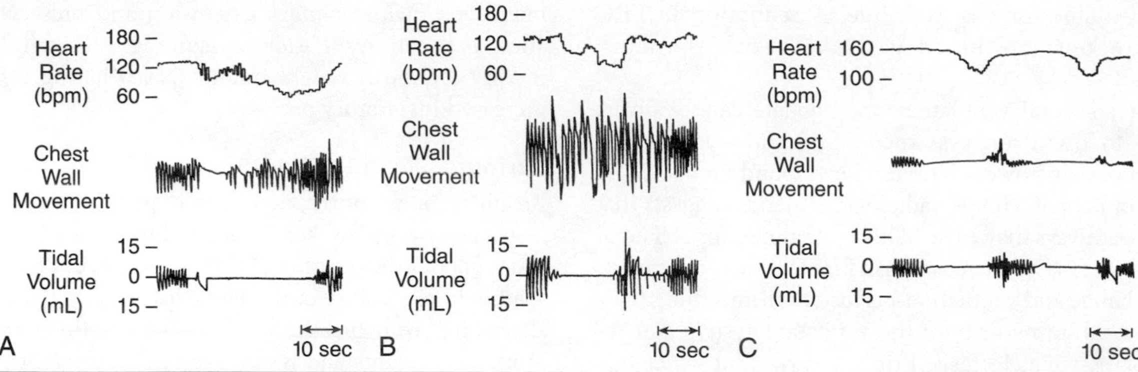

FIGURE 10-21 Illustration of types of apnea. **A,** Mixed apnea. Obstructed breaths precede and follow a central respiratory pause. **B,** Obstructive apnea. Breathing efforts continue, although no nasal airflow occurs. **C,** Central apnea. Both nasal airflow and breathing effort cease simultaneously. (From Miller, M. [1986]. Diagnostic methods and clinical disorders in children. In N. Edelman & T. Santiago [Eds.]. *Breathing disorders of sleep.* New York: Churchill Livingstone.)

term developmental outcomes.[50,97,98,204,205,222] Caffeine may improve neurodevelopmental outcome by altering neurotransmitters (GABA, adenosine) and providing protection against hypoxia-induced periventricular leukomalacia (PVL) by inhibiting adenosine receptors.[2]

Hypoxia and Hyperoxia

Hypoxia

Hypoxia involves a decreased oxygen level of the tissues, whereas hypoxemia involves a decreased oxygen content of the blood. When hypoxia occurs, aerobic metabolism is impaired and there is a subsequent depletion in the supply of ATP. Therefore those processes that require energy will not occur and free radicals will accumulate damaging the cell (Figure 10-22 and Chapter 6). If the hypoxic event is not too severe or too long, cellular activities may be disrupted only for a short period of time, and damage may be reversible. Fetal hypoxia and its consequences are discussed in Chapter 6. Definitions of common terms used are in Table 6-1.

Cell death occurs when the loss of ATP leads to failure of the sodium pump. Once pump failure develops, sodium is free to flow into the cell, bringing water with it. The cell and intracellular structures swell with this increased fluid volume. Along with this, anaerobic metabolism is activated, leading to a fall in cellular pH. The lowered pH interferes with enzyme activities and alters the permeability of the cell membrane. Increased permeability allows calcium to diffuse into the cell, resulting in oxidative phosphorylation uncoupling and a further reduction in ATP formation. As the fluid influx increases, the ribosomes located on the endoplasmic reticulum are shed, and protein synthesis is disrupted.[168,177]

Cell rupture and death may occur if enzymes leak from the intracellular lysosomes. Once released into the intracellular fluid, the enzymes are activated by the low pH, and cell disintegration is inevitable. Enzyme levels (e.g., creatinine phosphokinase) can be measured once cellular disintegration occurs and the enzymes are released into the extracellular fluid.

Abnormal functioning of organ systems is due to the energy-dependent cellular activities. In the brain, aerobic metabolism is necessary for maintaining the sodium-potassium pump, which allows for nerve impulse transmission and synthesis of the synaptic chemicals. Decreased mental activity, impaired judgment, and neuromuscular incoordination may occur when cellular hypoxia is present.

Muscle weakness and fatigue are signs of muscle cell hypoxia. Skeletal muscles have increased compensatory mechanisms and are therefore less susceptible to hypoxic damage than other organ systems.

Respiratory responses include an increase in frequency and depth of respiration. This is an attempt to provide an increased oxygen supply to the blood. Acidosis may occur, contributing to the respiratory compensation. Heart rate and cardiac output also increase as the cardiovascular system attempts to deliver more oxygenated blood to the tissues.

Hematologic responses include stimulation of erythropoietin by low circulating oxygen levels through the kidneys. This results in stimulation of the bone marrow with formation and maturation of red blood cells, which are then released into vascular circulation. In acute hypoxia, immature red blood cells are released. If a chronic hypoxic state exists, the marrow produces more cells and the volume of mature cells increases. This response is an attempt to increase the oxygen-carrying capacity of the blood, thereby improving the oxygen availability to the tissues.

Multiple factors affect the availability of oxygen to the cells. Hypoxia can be categorized—depending on which of these factors is responsible for the alterations in tissue oxygenation—into hypoxic, anemic, circulatory, and histologic hypoxia.

Hypoxic hypoxia occurs when tissue oxygenation is inadequate because the PaO_2 is reduced and hemoglobin is only partially saturated. This situation may be the result of decreased inspired oxygen (altitude), impaired pulmonary diffusion (pulmonary edema), altered perfusion of the lung (persistent pulmonary hypertension), or some combination of these events.[168]

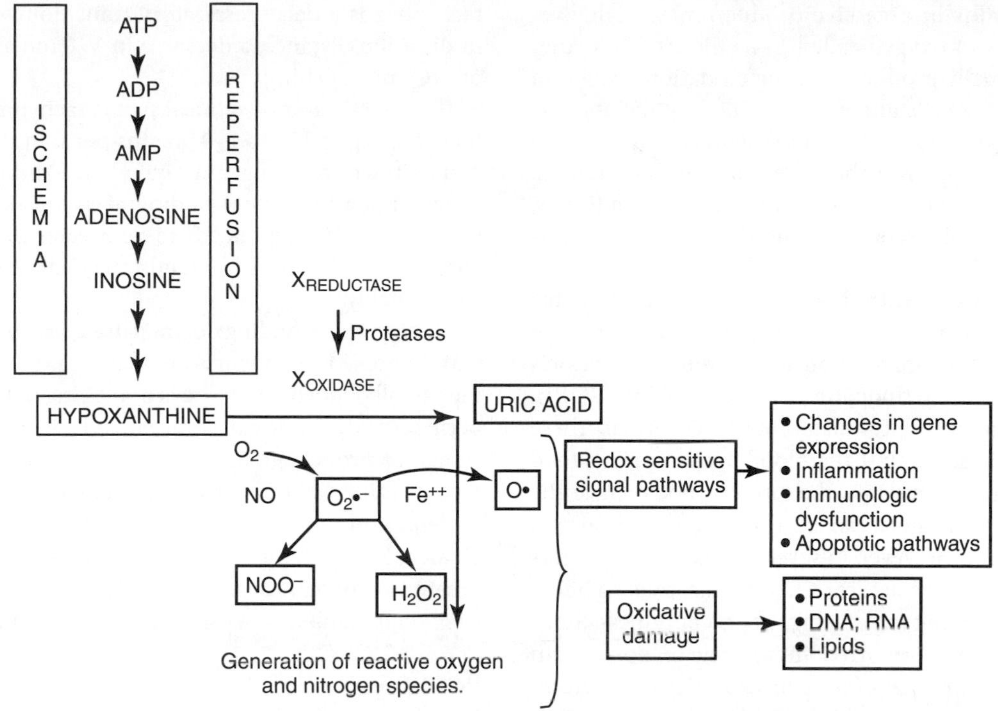

FIGURE 10-22 Events during hypoxia. During hypoxia, adenosine triphosphate (ATP) is exhausted, and complete rebuilding is not achieved. Purine derivatives (e.g., hypoxanthine) accumulate. During reoxygenation, specific proteases transform xanthine reductase ($X_{REDUCTASE}$), which uses oxygen as a substrate generating a burst of reactive oxygen species such as superoxide anion ($O_2^{\bullet -}$), hydrogen peroxide (H_2O_2), and hydroxyl radical ($O^\bullet$) In the presence of ferrous iron (Fe^{++}), large amounts of superoxide anion are generated. Superoxide anion easily combines with abundant nitric oxide (NO) generating peroxynitite ($NOO^\bullet$), an aggressive nitrogen free radical. Free radicals are capable of damaging nearby molecules and organelles, but also act as signalling molecules, causing changes in gene expression, promoting inflammation, altering immune responses, and inducing apoptosis. (From Goldsmith, J.P. [2011]. Delivery room resuscitation of the newborn: Overview and initial management. In R.J. Martin, A.A. Fanaroff, & M.C. Walsh [Eds.]. *Fanaroff and Martin's Neonatal-perinatal medicine: Diseases of the fetus and infant* [9th ed.]. Philadelphia: Mosby Elsevier, p. 469.)

Anemic hypoxia indicates that the hemoglobin available to transport oxygen is reduced although hemoglobin is completely saturated. PaO_2 levels are usually normal in this situation. Anemia may be the result of excessive loss or destruction of red blood cells or impaired production of hemoglobin or red blood cells. Physiologic compensation for anemia includes an increased heart rate and cardiac output. Hypoxia results in vasodilation and decreased blood viscosity, thereby increasing blood flow in an attempt to maintain normal tissue oxygenation.[168,177]

When tissue oxygenation is decreased due to inadequate blood flow (as with hyperviscosity syndrome), the infant is at risk for circulatory hypoxia. The oxygen content of the blood may be normal, but the blood flow to the tissues is reduced; consequently oxygen availability is also reduced.

Histologic hypoxia is reduced oxygen uptake capacity of cells or the reduced oxygen utilization of the cells. Blood flow and oxygen tensions are usually not disturbed. Some toxins (e.g., cyanide, arsenic, and some barbiturates) may interfere with oxidative phosphorylation. Deficiencies in thyroid hormone or niacin also can impair cellular energy production and oxygen use, thereby potentiating cellular hypoxia and altered cellular activity levels.[168]

Hyperoxia

Oxygen can be a toxic agent when too much is available. Prolonged exposure to high concentrations (as in ventilatory support) or increased oxygen pressure (e.g., deep sea diving) can lead to oxygen toxicity. In either situation, time is a critical factor. If the hyperoxia is not reversed, tissue injury may result.

For the premature infant, hyperoxia is a relative term and must be evaluated in light of the PaO_2 levels that are normally encountered in utero. Therefore, small increases in PO_2 may represent a hyperoxic state and place the infant at risk for oxygen injury. The pulmonary system, central nervous system, and retina have been identified as being particularly susceptible to oxygen injury. These systems and organs recognize different levels of oxygen as damaging.[146]

Hyperoxia results in excessive production of highly reactive metabolites of oxygen called *free radicals*. These metabolites are normally produced during oxidation-reduction reactions within the cells and are detoxified by the antioxidant system. In hyperoxic states, this system is overwhelmed and unable to keep up with the generation of free radicals. This can result in cellular damage through irritation (lungs, see section on Chronic Neonatal Lung Disease) or vasoconstriction (retina).

In the eye, high concentrations of PaO_2 cause reversible vasoconstriction. In premature infants, this constriction of blood vessels leads to obliteration of the immature vessels and retinal hypoxia (retinopathy of prematurity [ROP]). Capillary development is stimulated but is abnormal. There is a lack of organization, and the blood vessels may extend beyond the retinal surface into the vitreous body. Once the hyperoxia is resolved, there can be resolution with normal retinal development. However, in severe cases, retinal hemorrhages can occur and fibrous scar tissue forms, causing buckling of the retina, leading to detachment and blindness. Similar changes have been reported in severely hypoxic term infants. Lower target ranges of oxygen saturation for preterm infants have been recommended in recent years to decrease the risk of ROP. A recent randomized clinical trial found that lower (85% to 89%) versus higher (91% to 95%) saturations did not significantly decrease the composite outcome of severe ROP or death, but did increase mortality and decrease severe ROP among survivors.[223] Transfusion of preterm infants with large aliquots of adult blood rapidly increases the amount of adult hemoglobin, altering the oxygen-carrying capacity, and may transiently increase the risk of retinopathy of prematurity.

Transient Tachypnea of the Newborn

Transient tachypnea of the newborn (TTNB) is a disorder characterized by inadequate or delayed clearance of lung fluid leading to a transient pulmonary edema.[3] The population most likely to experience TTNB are full-term infants born by cesarean section prior to labor onset (since these infants will have a greater volume of lung fluid at birth) or who have experienced a perinatal hypoxic stress event.[126] The incidence of TTNB is 5.7/1000 live births in term infants.[3] Possible bases for TTNB include alteration in permeability of the pulmonary capillary vessels, aspiration of amniotic fluid during gasping efforts in utero, and lack of or decreased vaginal thoracic squeeze. The first two explanations would result in an increased protein concentration in the lung fluid, preventing transfer of fluid into the pulmonary circulation (see Figure 10-12). The vaginal thoracic squeeze during a vertex delivery was once thought to be an important mechanism of lung fluid removal. However, because much of the lung fluid is removed before birth, this mechanism probably has only a minor effect on fluid clearance.[81] Immaturity or decreased expression of ENaC slows lung fluid removal.[126] Genetic variations in β-adrenergic receptor expression in the alveoli may also alter lung fluid clearance.[12,126] The net result of transient tachypnea is a delay respiratory transition, with an increase in diffusion distance, a decrease in V_T, and an increased risk of $\dot{V}/\dot{Q}$ mismatching.

The most common clinical sign is tachypnea with respiratory rates up to 120 to 140 breaths per minute. Mild to moderate retractions and grunting may be exhibited. Cyanosis is usually not a prominent finding; if oxygen supplementation is necessary, it rarely needs to be greater than 40%. Air exchange is good; breath sounds may initially be moist but clear quickly.

Radiographic findings demonstrate vascular engorgement with increased pulmonary vascular markings. Central markings are ill defined, but there is branching outward toward the periphery. Moderate cardiomegaly may be evident, and occasional air bronchograms can be identified. The overall lung volume is increased, indicating hyperaeration. The diaphragm is depressed, and the anterior-to-posterior diameter is increased. Symptoms and findings clear within 48 to 72 hours.[3] Treatment modalities are supportive in nature and based on symptoms exhibited. Sepsis must be ruled out.

Respiratory Distress Syndrome

RDS is a developmental deficiency in surfactant synthesis accompanied by lung immaturity and hypoperfusion. The incidence of RDS is inversely related to gestational age. RDS is the most common cause of respiratory failure in the preterm infant and is exacerbated by asphyxia. The pathophysiology of RDS is summarized in Figure 10-23.

RDS is characterized by alterations in surface tension, in which increased pressure is required to keep the alveoli open. Pressures in adjacent alveoli are unequal, therefore time constants are changed, with some alveoli taking longer to fill and others filling normally. This leads to overdistention of the normal alveoli. As the alveoli reach their elastic limit, the infant must generate greater transpulmonary pressure in order to inspire the same amount of volume. The loss of elasticity and the progressive collapse of smaller alveoli reduce lung compliance. This results in uneven $\dot{V}/\dot{Q}$ ratios, with concomitant hypoventilation, decreased FRC, and increased closing capacity.

When the closing volume exceeds the FRC, some segments of the lung are closed during a portion of tidal breathing. As a result, the $\dot{V}/\dot{Q}$ ratio falls and hypoxemia and hypercarbia ensue. The hypoxemia and carbon dioxide retention are usually progressive, culminating in metabolic and respiratory acidosis, which further affect the ability of the type II cells to produce surfactant.[94,119,147]

If the closing volume exceeds both the FRC and V_T, lung segments are closed during inspiration and expiration. This represents complete atelectasis and is characterized as a "white-out" on chest roentgenogram. The use of continuous positive airway pressure (CPAP) and positive end-expiratory pressure (PEEP) prevents alveolar collapse during expiration and increases FRC above closing capacity.

Atelectatic areas of the lung contribute to the dead space within the entire lung. This changes the dead space–to–V_T

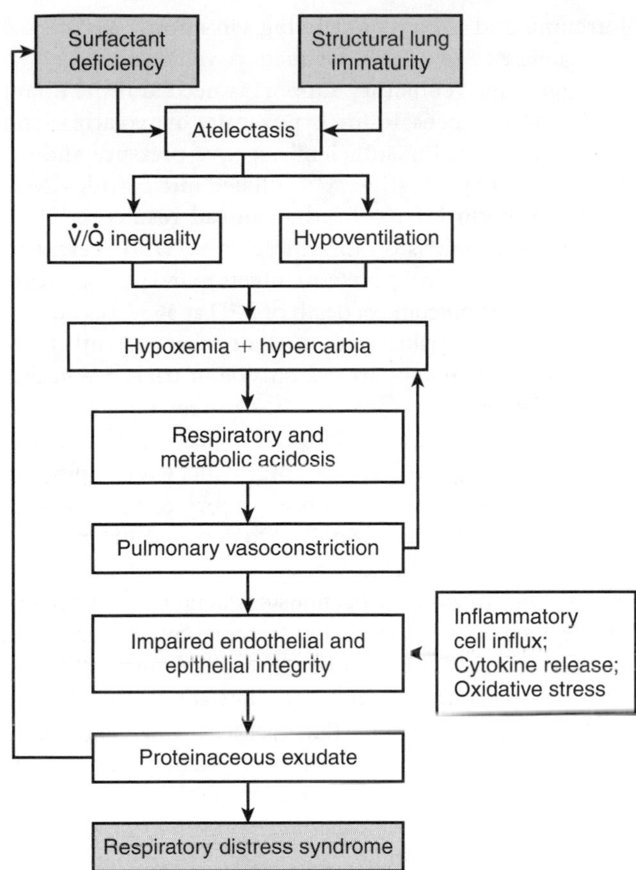

FIGURE 10-23 Schematic representation of the complex series of acute and chronic events that lead to neonatal respiratory distress syndrome. (From Rodriguez, R.J., et al. [2002]. Respiratory distress syndrome and its management. In A.A. Fanaroff & R.J. Martin [Eds.], *Neonatal-perinatal medicine: Diseases of the fetus and infant* [7th ed.]. St. Louis: Mosby.)

ratio and leads to hypoxia and hypercarbia unless there is a concomitant increase in expired minute ventilation. An increase in respiratory rate reflects the infant's attempt to compensate. If dead space has increased to the point that alveolar ventilation is compromised, respiratory failure may be the result. Dead space may increase up to 70% in severe RDS.[177]

As hypoxemia and hypercarbia become more severe, pulmonary artery vasoconstriction occurs. Pulmonary perfusion is compromised, and right-to-left shunting occurs through the foramen ovale and ductus arteriosus. Hypoperfusion and hypoxemia compound local ischemia, leading to continued alveolar and capillary epithelial damage.[94]

The increased subatmospheric intrapleural pressure created by the infant in an attempt to maintain adequate airflow, along with the low serum protein that is common in preterm infants, causes the shift of alveolar and interstitial fluid toward the alveolar space. Combined with the increased alveolar surface tension, pulmonary edema and alveolar flooding ensue. Fibrinogen in the exudate is converted to fibrin. Fibrin lines the alveoli; it binds blood products and cellular debris found in the alveoli, resulting in formation of hyaline membranes.

The excess alveolar fluid and membrane formation result in an increased diffusing distance and reduced lung surface area. Gas exchange is hampered, and ventilation-perfusion mismatching is compounded. Further hypoxemia and hypercarbia are the end result. This becomes a vicious circle that may increase in severity over the first days of life. Recovery is characterized by regeneration of alveolar tissue and concomitant increase in surfactant activity.

RDS is characterized by impaired or delayed surfactant synthesis (see Box 10-2 on page 315 and Figure 10-23). The surfactant synthesis rate and surfactant pool size are lower in infants with RDS. The preterm infant has a decreased number of type II pneumocytes secondary to lung immaturity. Surfactant must not only be present at the time of delivery, but also must be regenerated at a rate consonant with its use. This implies that type II cells must be present, viable, and intact in order to maintain normal surface tension. Inadequate amounts of surfactant at birth may be due to a variety of problems. These include extreme immaturity of the alveolar lining cells, diminished or impaired production rates resulting from transient fetal or neonatal stress, impaired release mechanisms from within the cell, and damage to type II cells. Extreme immaturity and impaired release mechanisms probably explain the inability of the very early fetus to survive.

The surfactant pool is lower in preterm infants and increases more slowly after birth with slower clearance.[120] The half-life of surfactant is 3 to 5 days in preterm infants versus 12 hours in adults.[120] Surfactant components are also altered in immature infants. Surfactant produced by these infants has a decreased surfactant protein-to-lipid ratio, is more rapidly converted to immature forms, is less effective in improving lung compliance, and is more susceptible to inactivation by proteinaceous pulmonary edema.[119]

Lung hypoperfusion with extrapulmonary and intrapulmonary shunting is another component of RDS pathogenesis. An ischemic injury that occurs either in utero or at the time of delivery results in hypoperfusion of the lung. The more immature the lung and smaller the capillary bed, the greater the ease with which the nutritional blood supply to the developing lung can be compromised. At 35 weeks, the type II cells are presumably differentiated to the point that the pathway for PC synthesis is more resistant to fetal stress and the nutritional blood supply is more abundant and therefore more difficult to compromise.

Oxidative stress may also have a role. Preterm infants are more vulnerable to this stress as a result of decreased levels of antioxidant enzymes (e.g., catalase, glutathione peroxidase) and endogenous free-radical scavengers (e.g., α-tocopherol) and decreased binding proteins (e.g., transferrin, ceruloplasmin).[76]

Clinical Manifestations

Clinically the infant attempts to compensate for the progressive respiratory and metabolic acidosis by increasing both inspiratory pressures and respiratory rate. Grunting may occur in term or more mature preterm infants in an attempt to slow expiratory flow rates and maintain a higher FRC. All of the clinical signs appear early and usually increase in severity over the first 72 hours. The infant may also present with pitting edema, cyanosis, and diminished breath sounds.

Cyanosis is a result of an excessive concentration of deoxygenated hemoglobin in the capillaries, although hypoxia can occur without cyanosis. Factors contributing to cyanosis include alveolar hypoventilation, impaired diffusion across the alveolar-capillary membrane, and right-to-left shunting through fetal channels or through completely atelectatic lungs. Hypoxia and cyanosis are usually progressive, requiring increasing concentrations of oxygen.

Grunting is forced expiration against a partially closed glottis so that end-expiratory pressure is increased and expiratory flow is retarded. This maintains the lung at a slightly higher volume for a longer period of time, thereby increasing gas exchange time. There is usually a very short expiratory phase; this reduces the time in which the lung can become airless before the next inspiratory effort. The tachypnea and grunting help maintain a more normal FRC. Grunting is uncommon in very low-birth weight infants.

Retractions are indicative of the increased inspiratory pressure, decreased lung compliance, and increased chest wall compliance. They can be quite marked in RDS, with substernal retractions pulling to the backbone. This dysfunctional respiratory effort results in cephalocaudal expansion only (paradoxic breathing), with increased negative pressures being generated in the bases. Therefore hyperinflation occurs in the bases and atelectasis in the apices. Marked abnormalities in $\dot{V}/\dot{Q}$ ratios are the result.

Treatment

Interventions are supportive as well as active in nature. Adequate, effective resuscitation with maintenance of body temperature is essential for reducing the incidence and severity of the disease. Therapy is aimed at maintaining oxygenation, adequate ventilation, normal pH, and adequate perfusion and tissue oxygenation. Hydration is important, but overhydration increases the risk of congestive heart failure. A systolic murmur, bounding pulses, active precordium, tachycardia, tachypnea, apnea, and carbon dioxide retention, as well as worsening ventilatory requirements, are indications of patent ductus arteriosus (see Chapter 9) and congestive heart failure. Active interventions include administration of exogenous surfactant and the use of continuous distending pressure or continuous negative pressure in an attempt to keep FRC above closing capacity. Many of the effects of surfactant therapy can be achieved by using CPAP to prevent end alveolar collapse, decrease work of breathing, and decrease ventilation-perfusion mismatch.[101,225] Infants can be stabilized with CPAP at delivery and treated with surfactant as needed to avoid mechanical ventilation and decrease their risk for bronchopulmonary dysplasia (BPD).[67,94,117,134,195,202,221] Bubble CPAP and flow driven CPAP are both effective.[92] Bubble CPAP may reduce volutrauma and the accompanying vibrations may mimic those generated by high frequency ventilation.[25,82,92,234] More aggressive ventilatory support is needed if the infant is unable to compensate for hypoxemia, hypercarbia, and acidosis by generating sufficient negative pressure and increasing minute ventilation.[94,101] Inhaled nitric oxide (iNO) use with preterm infants has had mixed results.[17,58,102,130] A recent meta-analysis on the efficacy of iNO to prevent or treat respiratory failure in preterm infants found a 7% decrease in the composite outcome of death of BPD at 36 weeks but not in the individual variables and concluded that currently there was no evidence to support use outside of trials.[58] A recent Cochrane review concluded that "iNO as rescue therapy for the very ill preterm infant does not appear to be effective. Early routine use of iNO in preterm infants with respiratory disease does not affect serious brain injury or improve survival without BPD. Later use of iNO to prevent BPD might be effective, but requires further study."[17]

Surfactant Therapy. Exogenous surfactant therapy stabilizes the lung until postnatal surfactant synthesis matures. Surfactant therapy became generally available in 1990 after a series of successful clinical trials. "Surfactant therapy has been the single most important factor in reducing overall neonatal mortality rates."[44] Surfactant therapy reduces the risk of RDS and the severity of RDS in those with established disease.[114] Surfactant therapy has been associated with a 30% reduction in mortality and a decrease in pneumothorax, oxygen requirements, and ventilator requirements.[118,224] Effects on bronchopulmonary dysplasia, intraventricular hemorrhage and patent ductus arteriosus have been inconsistent.[224] The combined use of antenatal corticosteroids and surfactant therapy has additional beneficial effects.[94,114] Long-term outcome studies have not demonstrated adverse effects related to surfactant therapy.[224] What is currently known and still unknown regarding surfactant therapy is summarized in Box 10-4 on p. 345.

Both synthetic and natural animal-derived surfactant preparations are used. Surfactant phospholipids and proteins are recycled with little catabolism; lipids in surfactant have a slow catabolic rate so are not rapidly degraded.[120] Surfactant therapy does not inhibit endogenous surfactant production. Surfactant therapy increases the infant's alveolar and tissue pools of surfactant as it is taken up into the type II alveolar cell and recycled. As part of the recycling the surfactant is transformed into a better form of surfactant.[120] Exogenous surfactant mixes with the infant's own surfactant. This mixture appears to enhance the function of endogenous surfactant, making it less sensitive to inactivation.[119]

Three types of surfactant are available: animal-derived (natural), synthetic without protein components, and synthetic with protein components. Both animal-derived and synthetic surfactants are effective in reducing RDS.[94,215-218,] Animal-derived surfactant has a more rapid physiologic response, greater reduction in air leak and possibly an improved survival rate than the original synthetic surfactants (no longer used in most countries), possibly due to the presence of SPs in

BOX 10-4 Surfactant Therapy for Respiratory Distress Syndrome

RESOLVED

Improved mortality from respiratory distress syndrome (RDS)
Greatest benefit when antenatal corticosteroids are also employed
Exogenous surfactant does not inhibit endogenous surfactant synthesis
Retreatment may be required in severe RDS
Major component for lowering surface tension: phosphatidylcholine
Endotracheal intubation required for administration of fluid suspension
Improvement in oxygenation, functional residual capacity, and lung compliance
Protein-containing preparations show a faster therapeutic response
Decrease incidence of air leaks
Prophylactic or early use beneficial in infants with extremely low birth weight (<29 weeks' gestation)
Efficacy of surfactant therapy, early extubation, nasal continuous positive airway pressure (CPAP) strategy

UNRESOLVED

Factors predicting likelihood of success of an initial CPAP-based strategy
Optimal ventilator strategy to maximize surfactant response
Effect on incidence and severity of bronchopulmonary dysplasia
Role of surfactant as modulator of the immune system and inflammatory response
Role for recombinant surfactant protein-based preparations

From Hamvas, A (2011). Pathophysiology and management of respiratory distress syndrome and its management. In R.J. Martin, A.A. Fanaroff, & M.C. Walsh (Eds.). *Fanaroff and Martin's Neonatal-perinatal medicine: Diseases of the fetus and infant* (9th ed.). Philadelphia: Mosby Elsevier, p. 1111.

the animal derived preparations.[44,188,218,224,225] Newer synthetic surfactant preparations composed of synthetic phospholipids and hydrophobic surfactant protein analogues (including SP-B and/or SP-C) have been developed and tested.[188,225] Studies to date indicate that these preparations appear to work as well as animal-derived preparations.[167,189,211] Long-term studies are not yet available.

Exogenous surfactant can be given shortly after birth in at-risk infants (prophylactic) or once the infant begins to show signs of RDS (treatment). Both approaches reduce the severity of RDs and mortality.[114] Prophylactic therapy (generally within 15 minutes of birth) has usually been used in infants weighing less than 1000 g. A meta-analysis of early (within the first 30 to 120 minutes) versus later treatment demonstrated decreased mortality, pulmonary interstitial emphysema, and pneumothorax.[251] It is unclear which babies benefit most from prophylactic use, although general practice is to reserve prophylactic use for the most immature babies (<28 to 30 weeks' gestation).[44,94,114,224] Currently surfactant therapy requires that the infant be intubated, although nasopharyngeal instillation and other modes of delivery have been investigated in the past and are currently being re-evaluated.[66,123] Early use of surfactant followed by extubation to nasal CPAP had been associated with a decreased need for later mechanical ventilation, air leak, and BPD.[221,224] Multiple doses are often needed to overcome inactivation of surfactant by soluble proteins in the small airways and alveoli.[214] Multiple doses have been associated with a further decrease in the risk of air leak.[224] Surfactant therapy has also been used for other disorders, including adult RDS (ARDS), bronchiolitis, pneumonia, pulmonary hemorrhage, and meconium aspiration.[44,65,224,225]

Bronchopulmonary Dysplasia

In 1967, Northway and colleagues originally described a sequence of radiographic changes in infants with RDS that came to be known as bronchopulmonary dysplasia (BPD).[179] This sequence of events is rarely seen in current clinical practice. Although the incidence of BPD has not changed significantly in the past decade, the pattern of the disorder has changed since the introduction of surfactant therapy (Table 10-13).[173] There is a slower, subtler onset, with the gradual development of lung abnormalities that persist after 20 to 30 days of life.[15,24] Birth weight and gestational age are the best predictors of BPD.[117]BPD is seen primarily in infants weighing less than 1000 g at birth or who are younger than 30 weeks' gestation.[113,117] Chronic lung disease (CLD) or the "new" BPD, is characterized by oxygen requirements after 28 days of age or at 36 weeks' postconceptional age, but without the characteristic sequence of BPD radiographic changes.[24] Infants with this disorder have decreased

Table 10-13 Differences in Pathologic Features of "New" and "Old" Bronchopulmonary Dysplasia

PRE-SURFACTANT ("OLD")	POST-SURFACTANT ("NEW")
Alternating atelectasis with hyperinflation	Less regional heterogeneity of lung disease
Severe airway epithelial lesions (e.g., hyperplasia, squamous metaplasia)	Rare airway epithelial lesions
Marked airway smooth muscle hyperplasia	Mild airway smooth muscle thickening
Extensive, diffuse fibroproliferation	Rare fibroproliferative changes
Hypertensive remodeling of pulmonary arteries	Fewer arteries, but "dysmorphic"
Decreased alveolarization and surface area	Fewer, larger, and simplified alveoli

From Kinsella, J.P., Greenough, A., & Abman, S.H. (2006). Bronchopulmonary dysplasia. *Lancet, 367,* 1422.

alveolarization, including alveolar hypoplasia and variable saccule wall fibrosis but with minimal airway disease.[122] Most preterm infants who develop BPD require mechanical ventilation and oxygen therapy; very immature infants without significant lung disease are also at risk.[131]

Participants in a workshop organized by the National Institute of Child Health and Human Development; the National Heart, Lung, and Blood Institute; and the Office of Rare Diseases reviewed the definition of BPD and CLD.[112,113] This group recommended that the name **BPD** be retained rather than CLD as the term for chronic neonatal lung disease. They proposed a revised definition with new diagnostic criteria based on gestational age and severity as evidenced by need for oxygen and/or positive pressure ventilation.[113] These criteria, which do not include specific radiographic criteria due to inconsistent interpretation of findings, have been validated in several studies to reflect the severity of lung injury and outcome risks.[61,100]

BPD is due to lung injury, probably mediated by an inflammatory reaction with cytokine release and oxidative damage (Figure 10-24).[219] These responses can be caused by many factors, including structural lung immaturity, oxidative stress and oxidant injury, pulmonary vascular damage, chorioamnionitis, nosocomial infection, inflammation, volutrauma/barotrauma, edema, and undernutrition.[15,122,133,219] "BPD represents the response of the lung during a critical period of lung growth, usually during the canalicular period (17 to 26 weeks), which is a time during which airspace septation and vascular development increases dramatically."[220] BPD involves disruption of vasculogenesis as well as alterations in alveolar structure.[158] Characteristics include alveolar fibroproliferation, vascular smooth muscle hypertrophy, narrowing of the vascular lumens, increased pulmonary vascular resistance, decreased compliance, and inhibition of distal lung formation with decreased alveolarization.[6,220] Alterations in the pulmonary vasculature seen include a decreased number of arteries, medial hypertrophy, abnormal vasoreactivity, and altered muscularization in distal arteries leading to pulmonary hypertension.[74]

Treatment for BPD has been multifaceted. Some modalities are centered on primary prevention; others are employed

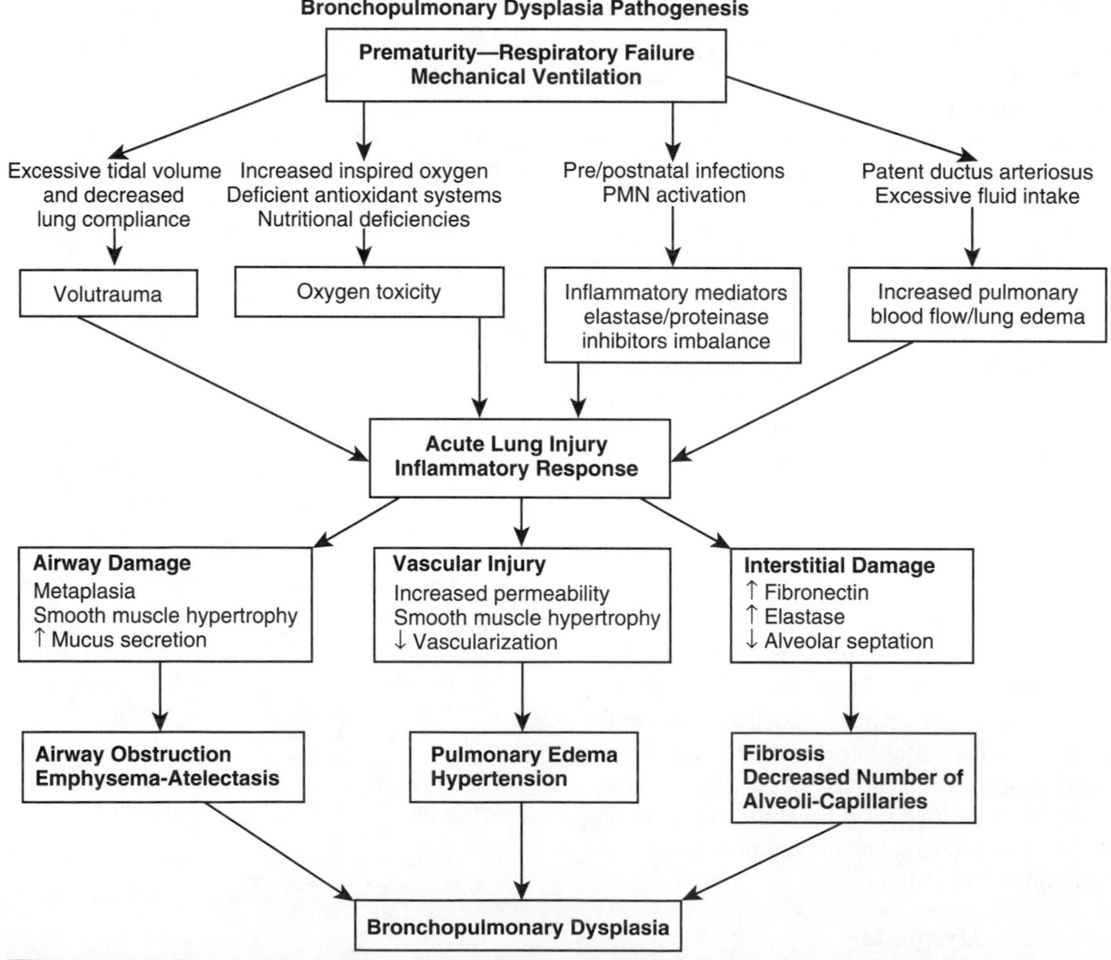

FIGURE 10-24 Pathogenesis of Bronchopulmonary Dysplasia. *PMN,* Polymorphonucleocytes. (From Bancalari, E. & Walsh, M. [2011]. Bronchopulmonary dysplasia. In R.J. Martin, A.A. Fanaroff, & M.C. Walsh (Eds.). *Fanaroff and Martin's Neonatal-perinatal medicine: Diseases of the fetus and infant* (9th ed.). Philadelphia: Mosby Elsevier, p. 1185.)

after the disease process is diagnosed. Primary prevention includes the following: (1) reducing the incidence of premature births through patient education and recognition of early labor, (2) using drugs to delay preterm birth and using antenatal steroids to mature surfactant synthesis pathways and enhance lung development, (3) identifying and treating chorioamnionitis, (4) providing effective resuscitation, (5) avoiding hyperventilation and hyperoxia, (6) using permissive hypercapnia, and (7) providing exogenous surfactant.[15,53,207] Secondary treatment modalities include the following: (1) providing ventilatory support using various techniques and modalities including reducing volutrauma via use of targeted ventilatory strategies such as volume generated ventilation and bubble CPAP, (2) supplying adequate nutrition for growth and healing, (3) facilitating closure of the ductus arteriosus through pharmacologic or surgical treatment, and (4) using bronchodilators and anti-inflammatory agents to decrease resistance to airflow and improve distribution of ventilation.[15,37,53,60,82,131,207] Corticosteroid therapy has been used to reduce inflammation and facilitate weaning from the ventilator. Postnatal steroid use, especially early administration, is controversial because adverse neurologic and other outcomes have been reported in infants on prolonged therapy.[15,36,59,60,208,239] Several studies reported that use of postnatal corticosteroids in infants at high risk to develop BPD reduced the composite outcome of death or altered neurodevelopment.[59,249] The American Academy of Pediatrics statement on postnatal corticosteroids has recently been updated.[239] Research has also focused on enhancing or modifying lung maturation through the use of antioxidants, epithelial growth–promoting enzymes, and iNO (see previous section) to improve adaptation to extrauterine life.[131,207]

Meconium Aspiration Syndrome

Meconium aspiration syndrome (MAS) is a cause of respiratory failure in term and postterm infants. Elimination of meconium into amniotic fluid is often associated with some degree of fetal distress, but it may occur in normal or breech delivery without evidence of asphyxia. Approximately 4% to 14% of all babies delivered release meconium into the amniotic fluid.[7] These infants are usually small for gestational age, postterm, or with cord compression or alterations in uteroplacental circulation. Of infants with meconium-stained fluid, approximately 3% to 12% develop MAS.[7]

Meconium may be passed in utero due to hypoxic stress. Fetal hypoxia or stress increases intestinal peristalsis. The hypoxia and acidosis are probably responsible for the gasping activity that leads to aspiration of meconium before delivery. In about one fourth of infants with meconium-stained amniotic fluid, there is no demonstrable evidence of fetal hypoxia and severe MAS only occurs in about 11% (range, 2% to 36%) of infants with meconium staining.[8,79] Amnioinfusion is not useful in settings with adequate obstetrical care and its use may increase the risk of cord prolapse, placental abruption, hypertonia and uterine rupture.[103] Suctioning of the nasopharynx or oropharynx before the shoulders are delivered does not decrease the risk of MAS or its complications.[231] Routine suctioning of meconium stained infants who are vigorous at birth is also not useful.[7,92] ILCOR states that the "available evidence does not support or refute the routine endotracheal suctioning of depressed infants born through meconium stained amniotic fluid"[124] and due to lack of randomized controlled studies does not currently recommend a change in the current practice of endotracheal suctioning of nonvigorous infants with meconium stained ammonic fluid.[124,187]

Whether MAS is actually due to aspiration of meconium or meconium in the lungs is an incidental finding is unclear.[79] Ghidini and Spong suggest three pathologic factors (chronic hypoxia, acute hypoxia, and infection) may alone or in combination lead to meconium passage in utero, direct damage of the lung, and interference with the ability of the lungs to remove aspirated meconium.[79] The lower airways become partially obstructed, resulting in air trapping and overinflation distal to the obstruction. Small airway obstruction produces an alteration in $\dot{V}/\dot{Q}$ ratios and reduced lung compliance. The alveolar hypoventilation leads to carbon dioxide retention, hypoxemia, and acidosis. When the obstruction is complete, the distal alveoli collapse, increasing the intrapulmonary shunt and compounding arterial hypoxemia. Meconium induces inflammation and cytokine activation.[3] Obstruction may also be potentiated by epithelial inflammation in the bronchi and alveoli. This results in a chemical pneumonitis with increased airway resistance and decreased diffusing capacity. Each of these events contributes to the hypoxemia seen clinically. The pneumonitis may also explain the decreased lung compliance, because elasticity is lost with inflammation. The pathophysiology of meconium aspiration syndrome is illustrated in Figure 10-25.

Meconium damages type II alveolar cells and alters surfactant synthesis and activity.[3,24,85] Meconium decreases SP-A and SP-B, decreases surfactant synthesis, and may form aggregates with surfactant proteins interfering with monolayer formation.[65] Free fatty acids in meconium inactivate surfactant; the cholesterol and other lipids in meconium tend to fluidize the surface film and interfere with the ability of surfactant to lower surface tension during compression.[46,85] Surfactant inactivation, along with the chemical pneumonitis, leads to atelectasis and intrapulmonary shunting (see Figure 10-25). Surfactant therapy has been used for infants with MAS.[85] These infants develop hypoxemia and acidosis and are at risk for persistent pulmonary hypertension.[65]

Minute ventilation is increased in order to compensate for the $\dot{V}/\dot{Q}$ alterations. The increase is usually due to an increase in respiratory rate; however, carbon dioxide retention continues because the V_T is reduced, thereby increasing dead space and reducing alveolar ventilation. The chest roentgenogram demonstrates patchy areas that have reduced aeration. There are sometimes confluent areas alternating with hyperlucent ones. The diaphragm may be depressed. Blood gas levels show a metabolic acidosis and hypoxemia that are reflective

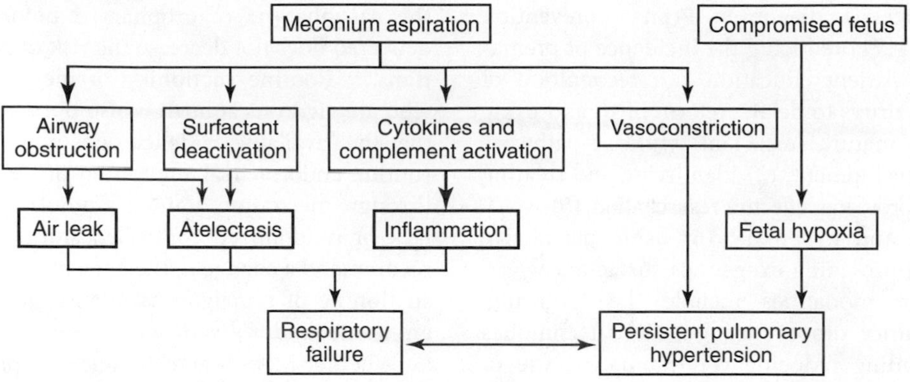

FIGURE 10-25 Pathophysiology of meconium aspiration syndrome. (From Abu-Shaweesh, J.M. [2011]. Respiratory disorders in preterm and term infants. In R.J. Martin, A.A. Fanaroff, & M.C. Walsh (Eds.). *Fanaroff and Martin's Neonatal-perinatal medicine: Diseases of the fetus and infant* (9th ed.). Philadelphia: Mosby Elsevier, p. 1158.)

of upon the degree of pulmonary bed involved. These findings are more pronounced if persistent pulmonary hypertension is present. The infant may be able to compensate initially; therefore $PaCO_2$ levels may be normal. However, this usually does not last.

If the process continues, respiratory failure is likely. Pneumothorax or pneumomediastinum may also occur because of the alveolar distention that occurs with air trapping. Right-to-left shunting is common, especially if persistent pulmonary hypertension is present. Secondary bacterial infections frequently occur but may be difficult to diagnose by chest roentgenogram, especially during the acute phase of the syndrome.

Persistent Pulmonary Hypertension of the Newborn

Persistent pulmonary hypertension of the newborn (PPHN) is a syndrome of acute respiratory distress with hypoxemia and acidemia caused by decreased pulmonary blood flow due to elevated pulmonary vascular resistance (PVR). PVR is high in utero and normally decreases markedly at birth to accommodate the increased blood flow with the switch from placental to pulmonary gas exchange with birth. The decrease in PVR is mediated by lung expansion, endocrine changes, and increases in vasodilators such as endogenous nitric oxide, PGI_2, and bradykinin.[45,236]

Infants with PPHN have central cyanosis associated with right-to-left shunting across the fetal shunts (foramen ovale and ductus arteriosus). This syndrome may represent failure to achieve transition to air breathing or may be secondary to cardiomyopathies, meconium aspiration, alveolar hypoventilation, pulmonary hypoplasia, polycythemia, hypoglycemia, or other lung injury which impedes the normal decreases in PVR.[45,252]

Vascular injury results from endothelial dysfunction secondary to inflammation, hypoxia, and mechanical forces. Hypoxia impairs NO synthetase activity so that cGMP is decreased and intracellular calcium is unregulated. Treatment with inhaled NO can reverse these changes. Increased vasoconstricting prostaglandins mobilize calcium and thus vascular smooth muscle contraction (leading to vasoconstriction). Hypoxia also leads to increases in hypoxia inducible factor (HIF-1) and vascular endothelial growth factors (VEGFs). The increased calcium HIF-1 and VEGF activate vascular smooth muscle proliferation.[45,212] Smooth muscle dysfunction is also seen in PPNH which may be one reason why about one fourth to one third of infants do not respond to inhaled NO therapy.[45] With sepsis or MAS, the increased inflammatory cytokines increase vasodilating prostaglandins and calcium mobilization, and lead to further endothelial and smooth muscle dysfunction. In addition, failure of the pulmonary vasculature to dilate at birth reduces the capacity of these vessels and may result in injury from large volumes of blood under pressure trying to flow through these constricted vessels.[45]

Thus PPHN is a transitional event with failure of pulmonary vessels to dilate adequately so that the PVR remains high.[252] This results in inadequate oxygenation secondary to ventilation-perfusion abnormalities. The continued elevated PVR and increased right heart pressure, combined with the resulting hypoxemia and acidosis, lead to maintenance of fetal circulatory channels. Blood flow tends to bypass the lungs and follow the fetal pathways; therefore the pulmonary hypoperfusion, hypoxia, and acidosis continue. This sets up a cyclic, downward spiral, with a negative feedback loop that escalates these problems. Unless aggressive intervention occurs, death due to inadequate oxygenation is the result. The goals of management are to "lower the pulmonary vascular resistance (PVR:SVR) ratio, reduce intracardiac shunting and right ventricular afterload, improve postductal oxygen saturation without systemic hypotension, as well as correct the underlying cause of the PPHN."[236]

This cycle is aggravated by the increased musculature of the pulmonary blood vessels and heightened reactivity of these vessels.[182] The low fetal PO_2 within these vessels results in constriction and augments the increased PVR created by the increased muscle tissue. As gestational age advances, the constrictor response becomes stronger. The neonatal pulmonary bed is also highly reactive to hypoxic episodes. This may be due to the increased medial wall thickness or the lower density of arteries encountered in the newborn versus the adult. At birth, constriction of the vessels continues if oxygen levels do not rise, so that systemic and pulmonary vascular pressures change. This constriction results in the persistence of fetal circulatory patterns without the benefit of the placenta, the result being hypoxia secondary to transition failure and altered ventilation and perfusion.[212]

Additional hypoxia for any reason (hypoventilation, upper airway obstruction, or interstitial disease) contributes to these mechanisms. If acidosis or hypercarbia exists, they may react synergistically to further increase the PVR. A vicious circle may be set up in which hypoxia leads to reactive vasoconstriction, which in turn leads to increased right-to-left shunting, thereby increasing the degree of hypoxemia and decreasing the normal postnatal transition events that result in pulmonary artery vasodilation. This results in continued pulmonary vasoconstriction and shunting.

MATURATIONAL CHANGES DURING INFANCY AND CHILDHOOD

The functional and anatomic maturation of the respiratory system continues through childhood until the bony thorax stops growing. Functional development is essentially secondary to anatomic development and is tied to the continued growth of the airways and multiplication of the alveoli (see Table 10-9). Preterm infants as a group are more likely to have reduced lung function in the first months after birth and are at risk for later alterations in growth and function.[73]

At the time of term birth, there are 50 to 150 million air spaces—a combination of terminal air sacs and alveoli.[114] From then on, alveoli beget alveoli, gradually replacing all of the terminal air sacs. The greatest change is in the first 2 years.[120] By 6 months, 85% to 90% of all alveoli are formed, although additional alveoli continue to develop until 1.5 to 2 years of age. After 2 to 3 years, lung growth is proportional to body growth.[99,240] By 8 years of age (range, 5 to 13 years), the alveolar number approximates 300 million (versus 500 million in adults).[114,240] The gas exchange surface area of the lungs increases 20-fold from birth to adulthood.[32]

Alveolar diameter doubles in size during maturation. At 2 months of age, alveoli measure 150 to 180 mm; by adulthood, they are 250 to 300 mm.[240] This indicates that there is a steady increase in surface area during childhood. Alveolar surface area increases from 3 to 4 m^2 at birth to 32 m^2 at 8 years, reaching 75 to 100 m^2 by adulthood.[240] This improves the oxygen-diffusing capacity of the organ systems.

Lung compliance increases rapidly during the first year and then more slowly.[141] Lung elastic tissue continues to develop until early adulthood. Collateral ventilation also develops during childhood, thereby providing protection against obstruction of small airways and atelectasis. The pores of Kohn appear sometime between the first and second years of life. Lambert channels begin to be evident by 6 years of age. Interbronchiolar channels are not found in normal lungs but may develop in disease situations.[144]

By 2 years, the type 1 muscle fibers account for 58% of all muscle fibers in the diaphragm.[86] Rib cage compliance remains altered during infancy. The peripheral airways contribute the most to airway resistance until 5 years, when the upper airways predominate (as in adults).[142] Cartilage support for the conducting airways increases rapidly in the first 2 months and then more slowly throughout childhood. Closing capacity decreases after 6 years.[168]

Changes in the shape of the thorax to adulthood are illustrated in Figure 10-14. Infants are predominately nose breathers for the first 3 to 4 months. Until 8 years the cricoid cartilage is the narrowest portion of the larynx (versus the vocal cords in older individuals). Density of mucus glands decreases until adulthood, from 10 to 20 per mm^2 to 1 per mm^2. Venous admixture does not reach adult values until early childhood.[177]

Respiratory rates fall from birth to early adolescence. The greatest change is from birth to 2 years of age (median of 44 breaths/min at birth verus 26 by 2 years of age).[68]

Oxygen affinity continues to increase over the first 6 months of life with conversion from fetal to adult hemoglobin (see Chapter 8). At that time, over 90% of the hemoglobin is the adult type. This improves the diffusion of oxygen to the tissues, meeting the increased metabolic needs of the cells.

From 10 months to 11 years, the pulmonary arteries grow and enlarge; the small arteries are mostly nonmuscular or minimally muscular during this time. At the end of this growth period, the muscular arteries have reached the level of the alveolar duct where the vessels are 130 mm in diameter. Between 11 years and maturation, which occurs around 19 years of age, muscle extension continues, reaching the alveolus where vessels are 75 mm in diameter. Intrapulmonary veins, on the other hand, are thinner than their counterparts, and muscle extension does not spread as far peripherally. Once this is achieved, the system is considered mature.

SUMMARY

Although the respiratory system is not fully developed at birth, the infant demonstrates capabilities and strategies necessary to achieve sustained respirations, blood gas tension, and acid-base homeostasis and compensatory mechanisms to maintain that balance even in disease states. The transition to extrauterine life is a process that takes several days. Knowledge of these differences and the progression toward extrauterine stability can guide therapeutic interventions and determine clinical assessment.

The infant has prepared throughout gestation for this transition. The respiratory muscles have exercised and trained to take over the function of the respiratory pump itself, although fatigue may be encountered quickly. Intercostal muscles can stabilize the chest wall, so that effective ventilation

Table 10-14 Clinical Implications for the Respiratory System in Neonates

Understand the normal anatomic and functional development of the respiratory system in the fetus and neonate (pp. 309-337 and Tables 10-9 and 10-12).
Know what factors stimulate fetal lung development, what factors inhibit functional development, and what therapies are utilized with potential preterm delivery (pp. 317-318, Table 10-6).
Identify the various tests utilized to assess fetal lung maturity (pp. 318-319).
Describe the expected changes in blood gases during the intrapartum and transitional periods (pp. 320-322, 324-326, Chapter 6).
Identify various steps in respiratory transition at birth (pp. 321-324).
Identify infants at risk for hypoxia and asphyxia (pp. 340-342, Chapter 6).
Understand the consequences of hypoxia and hyperoxia (pp. 340-342 and Figure 10-22).
Acquire and maintain neonatal resuscitation skills (pp. 340-342, Chapter 6).
Monitor head and neck positioning in preterm infants to maintain airway patency (p. 327).
Assess respiratory function on a regular basis (pp. 337-339, Table 10-12).
Evaluate preterm infants for periodic breathing and apnea (pp. 339-340).
Identify and evaluate infants at risk for transient tachypnea (p. 342).
Identify and evaluate risk factors and clinical symptomatology associated with respiratory distress syndrome (pp. 342-345).
Monitor infants with respiratory distress syndrome (pp. 343-345).
Identify and evaluate infants at risk for developing bronchopulmonary dysplasia (pp. 345-347).
Identify and monitor infants who either are at risk for or who have meconium aspiration (pp. 347-348).
Identify and monitor infants who either are at risk for or who have persistent pulmonary hypertension (pp. 348-349).

can be achieved. The difficulties come when disease or immaturity are encountered. There is little reserve to increase ventilatory efforts or sustain increased respiratory activity. The ability to recruit accessory muscles, the use of laryngeal braking (grunting), and the recruitment of new alveoli help improve gas exchange and increase the pulmonary surface area. Each infant responds uniquely to the process of transition and to pathology. The development of refined clinical skills and further research may give additional clues as to when and how the respiratory system prepares and achieves its sustained activity. Clinical implications for the neonate are summarized in Table 10-14.

References

1. Abu-Shaweesh, J.M. (2004). Maturation of respiratory reflex responses in the fetus and neonate. *Semin Neonatol, 9,* 169.
2. Abu-Shaweesh, J.M. & Martin, R.J. (2008). Neonatal apnea: What's new? *Pediatr Pulmonol, 43,* 937.
3. Abu-Shaweesh, J.M. (2011). Respiratory disorders in preterm and term infants. In R.J. Martin, A.A. Fanaroff, & M.C. Walsh (Eds.). *Fanaroff and Martin's Neonatal-perinatal medicine: Diseases of the fetus and infant* (9th ed.). Philadelphia: Mosby Elsevier.
4. ACOG (American College of Obstetricians and Gynecologists) Committee on Obstetric Practice. (2009). Committee opinion: Number 443, October 2009. Air travel during pregnancy. *Obstet Gynecol, 114,* 954
5. ACOG (American College of Obstetricians and Gynecologists) Committee on Obstetric Practice. (2011). ACOG Committee Opinion: Number 475. Antenatal corticosteroid therapy for fetal lung maturation. *Obstet Gynecol, 117,* 422.
6. Ad Hoc Statement Committee, American Thoracic Society. (2004). Mechanisms and limits of induced postnatal lung growth. *Am J Respir Crit Care Med, 170,* 319.
7. Aguilar, A.M. & Vain, N.E. (2011). The suctioning in the delivery room debate. *Early Hum Dev, 87,* S13.
8. Ahanya, S.N., et al. (2005). Meconium passage in utero: Mechanisms, consequences, and management. *Obstet Gynecol Surv, 60,* 45.
9. Alvaro, R.E. & Rigatto, H. (2012). Control of breathing in fetal life and onset and control of breathing in the newborn In R.A. Polin, W.W. Fox, & S.H. Abman (Eds.). *Fetal and neonatal physiology* (4th ed.). Philadelphia: Saunders.
10. Ammari, A., et al. (2005). Variables associated with the early failure of nasal CPAP in very low birth weight infants. *J Pediatr, 147,* 341.
11. Asikainen, T.M. & White, C.W.C. (2005). Antioxidant defenses in the preterm lung: Role for hypoxia-inducible factors in BPD? *Toxicol Appl Pharmacol, 203,* 177.
12. Aslan, E., et al. (2008). Transient tachypnea of the newborn (TTN): A role for polymorphisms in the beta-adrenergic receptor (ADRB) encoding genes? *Paediatr, 97,* 1346.
13. Asztalos, E.V., et al. (2010). Multiple courses of antenatal corticosteroids for preterm birth study: 2-year outcomes. *Pediatrics, 126,* e1045.
14. Bakhireva, L.N., et al. (2008). Asthma control during pregnancy and the risk of preterm delivery or impaired fetal growth. *Ann Allergy Asthma Immunol, 101,* 137.
15. Bancalari, E. & Walsh, M. (2011). Bronchopulmonary dysplasia. In R.J. Martin, A.A. Fanaroff, & M.C. Walsh (Eds.). *Fanaroff and Martin's Neonatal-perinatal medicine: Diseases of the fetus and infant* (9th ed.). Philadelphia: Mosby Elsevier.
16. Barker, P.M. & Olver, R.E. (2002). Invited review: Clearance of lung liquid during the perinatal period. *J Appl Physiol, 93,* 1542.
17. Barrington, K.J. & Finer, N. (2010). Inhaled nitric oxide for respiratory failure in preterm infants. *Cochrane Database Syst Rev, 12,* CD000509.
18. Belanger, K., et al. (2010). Effect of pregnancy on maternal asthma symptoms and medication use. *Obstet Gynecol, 115,* 559.
19. Bergeson, P.S. & Shaw, J.C. (2001). Are infants really obligatory nasal breathers? *Clin Pediatr (Phila), 40,* 567.
20. Bevilacqua, E., Brunelli R., & Anceschi, M.M. (2010). Review and meta-analysis: Benefits and risks of multiple courses of antenatal corticosteroids. *J Matern Fetal Neonatal Med, 23,* 244.
21. Birnbach, D.J., et al. (2000). *Textbook of obstetric anesthesia.* New York: Churchill Livingstone.
22. Blood-Siegfried, J. & Rende, E.K. (2010). The long-term effects of prenatal nicotine exposure on neurologic development. *J Midwifery Womens Health, 55,* 143.
23. Bobrowski, R.A. (2010). Pulmonary physiology in pregnancy. *Clin Obstet Gynecol, 53,* 285.
24. Bolt, R.J., et al. (2001). Glucocorticoids and lung development in the fetus and preterm infant. *Pediatr Pulmonol, 32,* 76.

25. Bonner, K.M. & Mainous, R.O. (2008). The nursing care of the infant receiving bubble CPAP therapy. *Adv Neonatal Care, 8,* 78.
26. Bourjeily, G., Ankner, G., & Mohsenin, V. (2011). Sleep-disordered breathing in pregnancy. *Clin Chest Med, 32,* 175.
27. Brito, V. & Niederman, M.S. (2011). Pneumonia complicating pregnancy. *Clin Chest Med, 32,* 121.
28. Budev, M.M., Arroliga, A.C., & Emery, S. (2005). Exacerbation of underlying pulmonary disease in pregnancy. *Crit Care Med, 33,* S313.
29. Burton, G.J. & Jauniaux, E. (2004). Placental oxidative stress: From miscarriage to preeclampsia. *J Soc Gynecol Investig, 11,* 342.
30. Carlton, D.P. (2012). Regulation of liquid secretion and absorption by the fetal and neonatal lung. In R.A. Polin, W.W. Fox, & S.H. Abman (Eds.). *Fetal and neonatal physiology* (4th ed.). Philadelphia: Saunders.
31. Carroll, J.L. (2003). Developmental plasticity in respiratory control. *J Appl Physiol, 94,* 375.
32. Carroll, J.L. & Agarwal, A. (2010). Development of ventilatory control in infants. *Paediatr Respir Rev, 11,* 199.
33. Catanzarite, V. & Cousins, L. (2000). Respiratory failure in pregnancy. *Immunol Allergy Clin North Am, 20,* 775.
34. Centers for Disease Control and Prevention. (2010). Prevention and control of influenza with vaccines: Recommendations of the Advisory Committee on Immunization Practices (ACIP). *MMWR, 59,* 1.
35. Chibber, R., Al-Sibai, M.H., & Qahtani, N. (2006). Adverse outcome of pregnancy following air travel: A myth or a concern? *Aust N Z J Obstet Gynaecol, 46,* 24.
36. Committee on Fetus and Newborn. (2002). Postnatal corticosteroids to treat or prevent chronic lung disease in premature infants. *Pediatrics, 109,* 330.
37. Cools, F., et al. (2010). Elective high-frequency oscillatory versus conventional ventilation in preterm infants: A systematic review and meta-analysis of individual patients' data. *Lancet, 375,* 2082.
38. Copland, I. & Post, M. (2004). Lung development and fetal lung growth. *Paediatr Respir Rev, 5,* S259.
39. Corff, K.E. & McCann, D.L. (2005). Room air resuscitation versus oxygen resuscitation in the delivery room. *J Perinat Neonatal Nurs, 19,* 379.
40. Correia-Pinto, J., et al. (2010). Congenital lung lesions—underlying molecular mechanisms. *Semin Pediatr Surg, 19,* 171.
41. Crowther, C.A., et al. (2004). Thyrotropin-releasing hormone added to corticosteroids for women at risk for preterm birth for preventing neonatal respiratory disease. *Cochrane Database Syst Rev, 2,* CD000019.
42. Crowther, C.A. & Harding, J.E. (2007). Repeat doses of prenatal corticosteroids for women at risk of preterm birth for preventing neonatal respiratory disease. *Cochrane Database of Systematic Reviews, 3,* CD003935.
43. Cunningham, G., et al. (2009). *Williams obstetrics* (23rd ed.). New York: McGraw-Hill.
44. Curley, A.E. & Halliday, H.L. (2001). The present status of exogenous surfactant for the newborn. *Early Hum Dev, 61,* 67.
45. Dakshinamurti, S. (2005). Pathophysiologic mechanisms of persistent pulmonary hypertension of the newborn. *Pediatr Pulmonol, 39,* 492.
46. Dargaville, P.A., et al. (2001). Surfactant and surfactant inhibitors in meconium aspiration syndrome. *J Pediatr, 128,* 113.
47. Darnall, R.A. (2010). The role of CO(2) and central chemoreception in the control of breathing in the fetus and the neonate. *Respir Physiol Neurobiol, 173,* 201.
48. Davis, G.M. & Bureau, M.A. (1987). Pulmonary and chest wall mechanics in the control of respiration in the newborn. *Clin Perinatol, 14,* 551.
49. Davis, J.M. & Auten, R.L. (2010). Maturation of the antioxidant system and the effects on preterm birth. *Semin Fetal Neonatal Med, 15,* 191.
50. Davis, P.G., et al. (2010). Caffeine for Apnea of Prematurity trial: Benefits may vary in subgroups. *J Pediatr, 156,* 382.
51. Dawson, J.A., et al. (2010). Defining the reference range for oxygen saturation for infants after birth. *Pediatrics, 125,* e1340.
52. Dawson, J.A. & Morley, C.J. (2010). Monitoring oxygen saturation and heart rate in the early neonatal period. *Semin Fetal Neonatal Med, 15,* 203.
53. Deakins, K.M. (2009). Bronchopulmonary dysplasia. *Respir Care, 54,* 1252.
54. Delivoria-Papadopoulos, M. & McGowen, J.E. (2012). In R.A. Polin, W.W. Fox, & S.H. Abman (Eds.). *Fetal and neonatal physiology* (4th ed.). Philadelphia: Saunders.
55. DiBlasi, R.M. Richardson, C.P., & Hansen, T.N. (2012). Pulmonary physiology of the newborn. In C.A. Gleason & S. Devaskar (Eds.). *Avery's diseases of the newborn* (9th ed.). Philadelphia: Saunders.
56. DiFranza, J.R., Aligne, C.A., & Weitzman, M. (2004). Prenatal and postnatal environmental tobacco smoke exposure and children's health. *Pediatrics, 113,* 1007.
57. Dombrowski, M.P. & Schatz, M. (2010). Asthma in pregnancy. *Clin Obstet Gynecol, 53,* 301.
58. Donohue, P.K., et al. (2011). Inhaled nitric oxide in preterm infants: A systematic review. *Pediatrics, 127,* e414.
59. Doyle, L.W., et al. (2005). Impact of postnatal systemic corticosteroids on mortality and cerebral palsy in preterm infants: Effect modification by risk for chronic lung disease. *Pediatrics, 115,* 655.
60. Doyle, L.W., et al. (2006). Low-dose dexamethasone facilitates extubation among chronically ventilator-dependent infants: A multicenter, international, randomized, controlled trial. *Pediatrics, 117,* 75.
61. Ehrenkranz, R.A., et al. (2005). Validation of the National Institutes of Health consensus definition of bronchopulmonary dysplasia. *Pediatrics, 116,* 1353.
62. Ellegard, E.K. (2006). Pregnancy rhinitis. *Immunol Allergy Clin North Am, 26,* 119.
63. Enriquez, R., et al. (2006). Cessation of asthma medication in early pregnancy. *Am J Obstet Gynecol, 195,* 149.
64. Espinoza, J., et al. (2001). Placental villus morphology in relation to maternal hypoxia at high altitude. *Placenta, 22,* 606.
65. Finer, N.N. (2004). Surfactant use for neonatal lung injury: Beyond respiratory distress syndrome. *Paediatr Respir Rev, 5,* S289.
66. Finer, N.N., et al. (2010). An open label, pilot study of Aerosurf(R) combined with nCPAP to prevent RDS in preterm neonates. *J Aerosol Med Pulm Drug Deliv, 23,* 303.
67. Finer, N.N., et al. (2010). Early CPAP versus surfactant in extremely preterm infants. *N Engl J Med, 362,* 1970. Erratum in: N Engl J Med. 2010 Jun 10;362(23):2235.
68. Fleming, S., et al. (2011). Normal ranges of heart rate and respiratory rate in children from birth to 18 years of age: A systematic review of observational studies. *Lancet, 377,* 1011.
69. Fraga, M.V. & Guttentag, S. (2012). Lung development: Embryology, growth, maturation, and developmental biology. In C.A. Gleason & S. Devaskar (Eds.). *Avery's diseases of the newborn* (9th ed.). Philadelphia: Saunders.
70. Frappell, P.B. & MacFarlane, P.M. (2005) Development of mechanics and pulmonary reflexes. *Respir Physiol Neurobiol, 149,* 143.
71. Freeman, M., et al. (2004). Does air travel affect pregnancy outcome? *Arch Gynecol Obstet, 269,* 274.
72. Frerking, I., et al. (2001). Pulmonary surfactant: Functions, abnormalities and therapeutic options. *Intensive Care Med, 27,* 1699.
73. Friedrich, L., et al. (2006). Reduced lung function in healthy preterm infants in the first months of life. *Am J Respir Crit Care Med, 173,* 442.
74. Gao, Y. & Raj, J.U. (2010). Regulation of the pulmonary circulation in the fetus and newborn. *Physiol Rev, 90,* 1291.
75. Garbrecht, M.R., et al. (2006). Glucocorticoid metabolism in the human fetal lung: Implications for lung development and the pulmonary surfactant system. *Biol Neonate, 89,* 109.
76. Gauda, E.B. & Martin, R.J. (2002). Control of breathing. In C.A. Gleason & S. Devaskar (Eds.). *Avery's diseases of the newborn* (9th ed.). Philadelphia: Saunders.
77. Gauda, E.B., et al. (2004). Maturation of peripheral arterial chemoreceptors in relation to neonatal apnoea. *Semin Neonatol, 9,* 181.
78. Gaultier, C. & Gallego, J. (2005). Development of respiratory control: Evolving concepts and perspectives. *Respir Physiol Neurobiol, 149,* 3.
79. Ghidini, A. & Spong, C.Y. (2001). Severe meconium aspiration syndrome is not caused by aspiration of meconium. *Am J Obstet Gynecol, 185,* 931.

80. Gluck, J.C. (2004). The change of asthma course during pregnancy. *Clin Rev Allergy Immunol, 26*, 171.
81. Goldsmith, J.P. (2011). Delivery room resuscitation of the newborn: Overview and initial management. In R.J. Martin, A.A. Fanaroff, & M.C. Walsh (Eds.). *Fanaroff and Martin's Neonatal-perinatal medicine: Diseases of the fetus and infant* (9th ed.). Philadelphia: Mosby Elsevier.
82. Goldsmith, J.P. & Karotkin, E.H. (2011). *Assisted ventilation of the neonate* (5th ed.). Philadelphia: Saunders.
83. Gosche, J.R., Islam, S., & Boulanger, S.C. (2005). Congenital diaphragmatic hernia: Searching for answers. *Am J Surg, 190*, 324.
84. Graves, C.R. (2010). Pneumonia in pregnancy. *Clin Obstet Gynecol, 53*, 329.
85. Greenough, A. (2000). Expanded use of surfactant replacement therapy. *Eur J Pediatr, 159*, 635.
86. Greenspan, J.S., Miller, T.L., & Shaffer, T.H. (2005). The neonatal respiratory pump: A developmental challenge with physiologic limitations. *Neonatal Netw, 24*, 15.
87. Greer, J.J. & Funk, G.D. (2005). Perinatal development of respiratory motoneurons. *Respir Physiol Neurobiol, 149*, 43.
88. Grenache, D.G. & Gronowski, A.M. (2006). Fetal lung maturity. *Clin Biochem, 39*, 1.
89. Grier, D.G. & Halliday, H.L. (2004). Effects of glucocorticoids on fetal and neonatal lung development. *Treat Respir Med, 3*, 295.
90. Groenman, F., Unger, S., & Post, M. (2005). The molecular basis for abnormal human lung development. *Biol Neonate, 87*, 164.
91. Gross, I. & Ballard, P.L. (2012). Hormonal therapy for prevention of respiratory distress syndrome. In R.A. Polin, W.W. Fox, & S.H. Abman (Eds.). *Fetal and neonatal physiology* (4th ed.). Philadelphia: Saunders.
92. Gupta, S., et al. (2009). A randomized controlled trial of post-extubation bubble continuous positive airway pressure versus Infant Flow Driver continuous positive airway pressure in preterm infants with respiratory distress syndrome. *J Pediatr, 154*, 645.
93. Halliday, H.L. (2004). Use of steroids in the perinatal period. *Paediatr Respir Rev, 5* S321.
94. Hamvas, A. (2011). Pathophysiology and management of respiratory distress syndrome and its management. In R.J. Martin, A.A. Fanaroff, & M.C. Walsh (Eds.). *Fanaroff and Martin's Neonatal-perinatal medicine: Diseases of the fetus and infant* (9th ed.). Philadelphia: Mosby Elsevier.
95. Harirah, H.M., et al. (2005). Effect of gestational age and position on peak expiratory flow rate: A longitudinal study. *Obstet Gynecol, 105*, 372.
96. Hegewald, M.J. & Crapo, R.O. (2011). Respiratory physiology in pregnancy. *Clin Chest Med, 32*, 1.
97. Henderson-Smart, D.J. & De Paoli, A.G. (2010). Methylxanthine treatment for apnoea in preterm infants. *Cochrane Database Syst Rev, 12*, CD000140.
98. Henderson-Smart, D.J. & Steer, P.A. (2010). Caffeine versus theophylline for apnea in preterm infants. *Cochrane Database Syst Rev, 1*, CD000273.
99. Hislop, A.A. (2002). Airway and blood vessel interaction during lung development. *J Anat, 201*, 325.
100. Hjalmarson, O. & Sandberg, K.L. (2005). Lung function at term reflects severity of bronchopulmonary dysplasia. *J Pediatr, 146*, 86.
101. Ho, J.J., et al. (2002). Continuous distending pressure for respiratory distress syndrome in preterm infants. *Cochrane Database Syst Rev, 4*, CD002271.
102. Hoehn, T., Krause, M.F., & Buhrer, C. (2006). Meta-analysis of inhaled nitric oxide in premature infants: An update. *Klin Padiatr, 218*, 57.
103. Hofmeyr, G.J. & Xu, H. (2010). Amnioinfusion for meconium-stained liquor in labour. *Cochrane Database Syst Rev, 1*, CD000014.
104. Inselman, L.S. & Mellins, R.B. (1981). Growth and development of the lung. *J Pediatr, 98*, 1.
105. Jadcherla, S.R., Hogan, W.J., & Shaker, R. (2010). Physiology and pathophysiology of glottic reflexes and pulmonary aspiration: From neonates to adults. *Semin Respir Crit Care Med, 31*, 554.
106. Jaykka, S. (1954). A new theory concerning the mechanism of the initiation of respiration in the newborn. *Acta Paediatr Scand, 43*, 399.
107. Jaykka, S. (1958). Capillary erection and the structural appearance of fetal and neonatal lungs. *Acta Paediatr Scand, 47*, 484.
108. Jensen, D., et al. (2005). Effects of human pregnancy on the ventilatory chemoreflex response to carbon dioxide. *Am J Physiol Regul Integr Comp Physiol, 288*, R1369.
109. Jensen, D., Webb, K.A., & O'Donnell, D.E. (2007). Chemical and mechanical adaptations of the respiratory system at rest and during exercise in human pregnancy. *Appl Physiol Nutr Metab, 32*, 1239.
110. Jensen, D., et al. (2008). Physiological mechanisms of hyperventilation during human pregnancy. *Respir Physiol Neurobiol, 161*, 76.
111. Jensen, D. & O'Donnell, D.E. (2011). The impact of human pregnancy on perceptual responses to chemoreflex vs. exercise stimulation of ventilation: A retrospective analysis. *Respir Physiol Neurobiol, 175*, 55.
112. Jobe, A.H. & Bancalari, E. (2001). NICHD/NHLBI/ORD workshop summary: Bronchopulmonary dysplasia. *Am J Respir Crit Care Med, 163*, 1723.
113. Jobe, A.H. & Ikegami, M. (2001). Prevention of bronchopulmonary dysplasia. *Curr Opin Pediatr, 13*, 124.
114. Jobe, A.H. (2009). Fetal lung development and surfactant. In R.K. Creasy, et al. (Eds.). *Creasy & Resnik's Maternal-fetal medicine: Principles and practice* (6th ed.). Philadelphia: Saunders Elsevier.
115. Jobe, A.H. (2010). Lung maturation: the survival miracle of very low birth weight infants. *Pediatr Neonatol, 51*, 7.
116. Jobe, A.H. (2010). "Miracle" extremely low birth weight neonates: Examples of developmental plasticity. *Obstet Gynecol, 116*, 1184.
117. Jobe, A.H. (2011). The new bronchopulmonary dysplasia. *Curr Opin Pediatr, 23*, 167.
118. Jobe, A.H. (2012). Surfactant treatment. In R.A. Polin, W.W. Fox, & S.H. Abman (Eds.). *Fetal and neonatal physiology* (4th ed.). Philadelphia: Saunders.
119. Jobe, A.H. & Ikegami, M. (2012). Pathophysiology of respiratory distress syndrome and surfactant metabolism. In R.A. Polin, W.W. Fox, & S.H. Abman (Eds.). *Fetal and neonatal physiology* (4th ed.). Philadelphia: Saunders.
120. Jobe, A.J. (2011). Lung development and maturation. In R.J. Martin, A.A. Fanaroff, & M.C. Walsh (Eds.). *Fanaroff and Martin's Neonatal-perinatal medicine: Diseases of the fetus and infant* (9th ed.). Philadelphia: Mosby Elsevier.
121. Julian, C.G. (2011). High altitude during pregnancy. *Clin Chest Med, 32*, 21.
122. Kallapur, S.G. & Jobe, A.H. (2006). Contribution of inflammation to lung injury and development. *Arch Dis Child Fetal Neonatal Ed, 91*, F132.
123. Kattwinkel, J. (2005). Synthetic surfactants: the search goes on [commentary]. *Pediatrics, 115*, 1075.
124. Kattwinkel, J., et al. (2010). Part 15: Neonatal resuscitation: 2010 American Heart Association Guidelines for Cardiopulmonary Resuscitation and Emergency Cardiovascular Care. *Circulation, 122*, S909.
125. Kattwinkel, J. (2011). *Textbook of neonatal resuscitation* (6th ed.). ELK Grove, IL: American Academy of Pediatrics, American Heart Association.
126. Katz, C., Bentur, L., & Elias, N. (2011). Clinical implication of lung fluid balance in the perinatal period. *J Perinatol, 31*, 230.
127. Kay, H.H., et al. (2000). Antenatal steroid treatment and adverse fetal effects: What is the evidence? *J Soc Gynecol Investig, 7*, 269.
128. Keens, D.H. & Ianuzzo, C.D. (1979). Development of fatigue-resistant muscle fibers in human ventilatory musculature. *Am Rev Respir Dis, 119*, 139.
129. Keszler, M., Abubakar, M.K., & Wood, B.R. (2011). Physiologic principles. In J.P. Goldsmith & E.H. Karotkin (Eds.). *Assisted ventilation of the neonate* (5th ed.). Philadelphia: Saunders.
130. Kinsella, J.P., et al. (2006). Early inhaled nitric oxide in premature newborns with respiratory failure. *N Engl J Med, 355*, 354.
131. Kinsella, J.P., Greenough, A., & Abman, S.H. (2006). Bronchopulmonary dysplasia. *Lancet, 367*, 1421.
132. Kotecha, S. (2000). Lung growth: Implications for the newborn infant. *Arch Dis Child Fetal Neonatal Ed, 82*, F69.

133. Kramer, B.W., et al. (2009). Prenatal inflammation and lung development. *Semin Fetal Neonatal Med, 14,* 2.
134. Kribs, A., et al. (2010). Surfactant without intubation in preterm infants with respiratory distress: First multicenter data. *Klin Padiatr, 222,* 13.
135. Kuczkowski, K.M., Reisner, L.S., & Benumof, J.L. (2003). Airway problems and new solutions for the obstetric patient. *J Clin Anesth, 15,* 552.
136. Kuczkowski, K.M. (2005). Anesthetic management of labor pain: What does an obstetrician need to know? *Arch Gynecol Obstet, 271,* 97.
137. Kumar, R., Hayhurst, K.L., & Robson, A.K. (2011). Ear, nose, and throat manifestations during pregnancy. *Otolaryngol Head Neck Surg, 145,* 188.
138. Lally, K.P., et al. (2004). Surfactant does not improve survival rate in preterm infants with congenital diaphragmatic hernia. *J Pediatr Surg, 39,* 829.
139. Land, S.C. (2004). Hochachka's "Hypoxia Defense Strategies" and the development of the pathway for oxygen. *Comp Biochem Physiol B Biochem Mol Biol, 139,* 415.
140. Laughon, M., et al. (2009). Patterns of respiratory disease during the first 2 postnatal weeks in extremely premature infants. *Pediatrics, 123,* 1124.
141. Littleford, J. (2004). Effects on the fetus and newborn of maternal analgesia and anesthesia: A review. *Can J Anaesth, 51,* 586.
142. Lowrey, G.H. (1986). *Growth and development of children.* Chicago: Year Book.
143. Lyons, C.A. & Garite, T.J. (2002). Corticosteroids and fetal pulmonary maturity. *Clin Obstet Gynecol, 45,* 35.
144. Macklem, P.T. (1971). Airway obstruction and collateral ventilation. *Physiol Rev, 51,* 368.
145. Magann, E.F., et al. (2010). Air travel and pregnancy outcomes: A review of pregnancy regulations and outcomes for passengers, flight attendants, and aviators. *Obstet Gynecol Surv, 65,* 396.
146. Maltepe, E. & Saugstad, O.D. (2009). Oxygen in health and disease: Regulation of oxygen homeostasis—clinical implications. *Pediatr Res, 65,* 261.
147. Mandel, J. & Weinberger, S.E. (2004). Pulmonary diseases. In G.N. Burrow, T.P. Duffy, & J.A. Copel (Eds.). *Medical complications during pregnancy* (6th ed.). Philadelphia: Saunders.
148. Mantilla, C.B., Fahim, M.A., & Sieck, G. (2012). Functional development of respiratory muscles. In R.A. Polin, W.W. Fox, & S.H. Abman (Eds.). *Fetal and neonatal physiology* (4th ed.). Philadelphia: Saunders.
149. Mariani, G., et al. (2007). Pre-ductal and post-ductal O_2 saturation in healthy term neonates after birth. *J Pediatr, 150,* 418.
150. Maritz, G.S., Morley, C.J., & Harding, R. (2005). Early developmental origins of impaired lung structure and function. *Early Hum Dev, 81,* 763.
151. Martin, R.J. & Abu-Shaweesh, J.M. (2005). Control of breathing and neonatal apnea. *Biol Neonate, 87,* 288.
152. Martin, R.J. & Haxhiu, M.A. (2012). Regulation of lower airway function. In R.A. Polin, W.W. Fox, & S.H. Abman (Eds.). *Fetal and neonatal physiology* (4th ed.). Philadelphia: Saunders.
153. McAuliffe, F., et al. (2004). Respiratory function in pregnancy at sea level and at high altitude. *BJOG, 111,* 311.
154. Melo, M.F. (2004). Clinical respiratory physiology of the neonate and infant with congenital heart disease. *Int Anesthesiol Clin, 42,* 29.
155. Mendelson, C.R. (2009). Minireview: Fetal-maternal hormonal signaling in pregnancy and labor. *Mol Endocrinol, 23,* 947.
156. Mercer, B.D. (2009). Assessment and induction of fetal pulmonary maturity. In R.K. Creasy, et al. (Eds.). *Creasy & Resnik's Maternal-fetal medicine: Principles and practice* (6th ed.). Philadelphia: Saunders Elsevier.
157. Mercer, J. & Skovgaard., R. L. (2002). Neonatal transitional physiology: A new paradigm. *J Perinat Neonat Nurs, 15,* 56.
158. Merritt, T.A., Deming, D.D., & Boynton, B.R. (2009). The 'new' bronchopulmonary dysplasia: Challenges and commentary. *Semin Fetal Neonatal Med, 14,* 345.
159. Meschia, G. (2009). Placental respiratory gas exchange and fetal oxygenation. In R.K. Creasy, et al. (Eds.). *Creasy & Resnik's Maternal-fetal medicine: Principles and practice* (6th ed.). Philadelphia: Saunders Elsevier.
160. Meschia, G. (2011). Fetal oxygenation and maternal ventilation. *Clin Chest Med, 32,* 15.
161. Miller, M.J. & Martin, R.J. (2012). Pathophysiology of apnea of prematurity. In R.A. Polin, W.W. Fox, & S.H. Abman (Eds.). *Fetal and neonatal physiology* (4th ed.). Philadelphia: Saunders.
162. Milner, A.D. & Vyas, H. (1982). Lung expansion at birth. *J Pediatr, 101,* 879.
163. Miura, T. (2008). Modeling lung branching morphogenesis. *Curr Top Dev Biol, 81,* 291.
164. Moore, K.L., & Persaud, T.V.N. & Torchia, M.G. (2011). *The developing human: Clinically oriented embryology* (9th ed.). Philadelphia: Saunders Elsevier.
165. Morley, C.J., et al. (2008). Nasal CPAP or intubation at birth for very preterm infants. *N Engl J Med, 358,* 700.
166. Mortola, J.P. (2012). Mechanics of breathing. In R.A. Polin, W.W. Fox, & S.H. Abman (Eds.). *Fetal and neonatal physiology* (4th ed.). Philadelphia: Saunders.
167. Moya, F.R., et al. (2005). A multicenter, randomized, masked, comparison trial of lucinactant, colfosceril palmitate, and beractant for the prevention of respiratory distress syndrome among very preterm infants. *Pediatrics, 115,* 1018.
168. Muir, B.L. (1988). *Pathophysiology* (2nd ed.). New York: John Wiley.
169. Munnur, U., de Boisblanc, B., & Suresh, M.S. (2005). Airway problems in pregnancy. *Crit Care Med, 33,* S259.
170. Murin, S., Rafii, R., & Bilello, K. (2011). Smoking and smoking cessation in pregnancy. *Clin Chest Med, 32,* 75.
171. Murphy, V.E. & Gibson, P.G. (2011). Asthma in pregnancy. *Clin Chest Med, 32,* 93.
172. Myatt, L. & Cui, X. (2004). Oxidative stress in the placenta. *Histochem Cell Biol, 122,* 369.
173. National Asthma Education and Prevention Program (NAEPP). (2005). Managing asthma during pregnancy: Recommendations for pharmacological treatment. *J Allergy Clin Immunol, 115,* 34.
174. National Institutes of Health Consensus. (1995). Consensus Developmental Conference on the Effects of Corticosteroids for Fetal Maturation on Perinatal Outcomes. *JAMA, 273,* 413.
175. National Institutes of Health. (2000). Antenatal corticosteroids revisited: Repeated courses. *NIH Consensus Statement, 17,* 1.
176. Nelson, N.M. (1976). Respiration and circulation after birth. In C.A. Smith & N.M. Nelson (Eds.). *The physiology of the newborn infant.* Springfield, IL: Charles C Thomas.
177. Nichols, D.G. & Rogers, M.C. (1987). Developmental physiology of the respiratory system. In M.C. Rogers (Ed.). *Textbook of pediatric intensive care* (vol. 1). Baltimore: Williams & Wilkins.
178. Norberg, H., et al. (2011). Antenatal corticosteroids for preterm birth: Dose-dependent reduction in birthweight, length and head circumference. *Acta Paediatr, 100,* 364.
179. Northway, W.H., et al. (1967). Pulmonary disease following respiratory therapy of hyaline membrane disease: Bronchopulmonary dysplasia. *N Engl J Med, 276,* 357.
180. O'Tolle, M.L. (2003). Physiologic aspects of exercise in pregnancy. *Clin Obstet Gynecol, 46,* 379.
181. Olver, R.E., Walters, D.V.M., & Wilson, S. (2004). Developmental regulation of lung liquid transport. *Annu Rev Physiol, 66,* 77.
182. Parker T.A. & Kinsella, J.P. (2012). Respiratory failure in the term infant. In C.A. Gleason & S. Devaskar (Eds.). *Avery's diseases of the newborn* (9th ed.). Philadelphia: Saunders.
183. Park-Wyllie, L., et al. (2000). Birth defects after maternal exposure to corticosteroids: Prospective cohort study and meta-analysis of epidemiological studies. *Teratology, 62,* 385.
184. Patel, A., et al. (2009). Exposure to supplemental oxygen downregulates antioxidant enzymes and increases pulmonary arterial contractility in premature lambs. *Neonatology, 96,* 182.
185. Peltoniemi, O.M., et al. (2009). Two-year follow-up of a randomized trial with repeated antenatal betamethasone. *Arch Dis Child Fetal Neonatal Ed, 94,* F402.

186. Peltoniemi, O.M., Kari, M.A., & Hallman, M. (2011). Repeated antenatal corticosteroid treatment: A systematic review and meta-analysis. *Acta Obstet Gynecol Scand, 90,* 719.
187. Perlman, M., et al. (2010). Part 11: Neonatal resuscitation: 2010 international consensus on cardiopulmonary resuscitation and emergency cardiovascular care science with treatment recommendations. *Circulation, 122,* S516.
188. Pfister, R.H. & Soll, R.F., (2005). New synthetic surfactants: the next generation? *Biol Neonate, 87,* 338.
189. Pfister, R.H., Soll, R.F., & Wiswell, T. (2007). Protein containing synthetic surfactant versus animal derived surfactant extract for the prevention and treatment of respiratory distress syndrome. *Cochrane Database Syst Rev, 3,* CD006069.
190. Polakowski, L.L., Akinbami, L.J., & Mendola, P. (2009). Prenatal smoking cessation and the risk of delivering preterm and small-for-gestational-age newborns. *Obstet Gynecol, 114,* 318.
191. Possemayer, F. (2012). Physiochemical aspects of pulmonary surfactant. In R.A. Polin, W.W. Fox, & S.H. Abman (Eds.). *Fetal and neonatal physiology* (4th ed.). Philadelphia: Saunders.
192. Randell, S.H. & Young, S.L. (2012). Structure of alveolar epithelial cells and the surface layer during development. In R.A. Polin, W.W. Fox, & S.H. Abman (Eds.). *Fetal and neonatal physiology* (4th ed.). Philadelphia: Saunders.
193. Reynolds, F. & Seed, P.T. (2005). Anaesthesia for caesarean section and neonatal acid-base status: A meta-analysis. *Anaesthesia, 60,* 636.
194. Richardson, B.S. & Gagnon, R. (2004). Fetal breathing and body movements. In R.K. Creasy, R. Resnik, & J.D. Iams (Eds.). *Maternal-fetal medicine: Principles and practice* (5th ed.). Philadelphia: Saunders
195. Rojas, M.A., et al. (2009). Very early surfactant without mandatory ventilation in premature infants treated with early continuous positive airway pressure: A randomized, controlled trial. *Pediatrics, 123,* 137.
196. Rooney, S.A. (2012). Regulation of surfactant-associated phospholipid synthesis and secretion. In R.A. Polin, W.W. Fox, & S.H. Abman (Eds.). *Fetal and neonatal physiology* (4th ed.). Philadelphia: Saunders.
197. Rosene-Montela, K. & Bourjeily, G. (2009). *Pulmonary problems in pregnancy.* NY: Humana Press.
198. Roth-Kleiner, M. & Post, M. (2003). Genetic control of lung development. *Biol Neonate, 84,* 83.
199. Roth-Kleiner, M. & Post, M. (2005). Similarities and dissimilarities of branching and septation during lung development. *Pediatr Pulmonol, 40,* 113.
200. Sale, S.M. (2010). Neonatal apnoea. *Best Pract Res Clin Anaesthesiol, 24,* 323.
201. Samuel, B.U. & Barry, M. (1998). The pregnant traveler. *Infect Dis Clin North Am, 12,* 325.
202. Sandri, F., et al. (2010). Prophylactic or early selective surfactant combined with nCPAP in very preterm infants. *Pediatrics, 125,* e1402.
203. Schatz, M. & Dombrowski, M.P. (2009). Clinical practice. Asthma in pregnancy. *N Engl J Med, 360,* 1862.
204. Schmidt, B., et al. (2006). Caffeine therapy for apnea of prematurity. *N Engl J Med, 354,* 2112.
205. Schmidt, B., et al. (2007). Long-term effects of caffeine therapy for apnea of prematurity. *N Engl J Med, 357,* 1893.
206. Shaffer, T.H. & Wolfson, M.R. (2012). Upper airway: Structure, function, regulation and development. In R.A. Polin, W.W. Fox, & S.H. Abman (Eds.). *Fetal and neonatal physiology* (4th ed.). Philadelphia: Saunders.
207. Shah, P.S. (2003). Current perspectives on the prevention and management of chronic lung disease in preterm infants. *Paediatr Drugs, 5,* 463.
208. Shah, V., et al. (2007). Early administration of inhaled corticosteroids for preventing chronic lung disease in ventilated very low birth weight preterm neonates. *Cochrane Database Syst Rev, 4,* CD001969.
209. Shea, A.K. & Steiner, M. (2008). Cigarette smoking during pregnancy. *Nicotine Tob Res, 10,* 267.
210. Shiao, S.Y. (2005). Effects of fetal hemoglobin on accurate measurements of oxygen saturation in neonates. *J Perinat Neonatal Nurs, 19,* 348.
211. Sinha, S.K., et al. (2005). A randomized, controlled trial of lucinactant versus poractant alfa among very premature infants at high risk for respiratory distress syndrome. *Pediatrics, 115,* 1030.
212. Sluiter, I., et al. (2011). Vascular abnormalities in human newborns with pulmonary hypertension. *Expert Rev Respir Med, 5,* 245.
213. Soliz, J. & Joseph, V. (2005). Perinatal steroid exposure and respiratory control during early postnatal life. *Respir Physiol Neurobiol, 149,* 111.
214. Soll, R.F. (2000). Multiple versus single dose natural surfactant extract for severe neonatal respiratory distress syndrome. *Cochrane Database Syst Rev, 2,* CD000141.
215. Soll, R.F. & Morley, C.J. (2000). Prophylactic versus selective use of surfactant for preventing morbidity and mortality in preterm infants. *Cochrane Database Syst Rev, 2,* CD000510.
216. Soll, R.F. (2003). Prophylactic natural surfactant extract for preventing morbidity and mortality in preterm infants. *Cochrane Database Syst Rev, 2,* CD000511.
217. Soll, R.F. (2003). Prophylactic synthetic surfactant for preventing morbidity and mortality in preterm infants. *Cochrane Database Syst Rev, 2,* CD001079.
218. Soll, R.F. (2003). Synthetic surfactant for respiratory distress syndrome in preterm infants. *Cochrane Database Syst Rev, 2,* CD001149.
219. Speer, C.P. (2006). Inflammation and BPD: A continuing story. *Semin Fetal Neonatal Med, 11,* 354.
220. Stenmark, K.R. & Abman, S.H. (2005). Lung vascular development: Implications for the pathogenesis of bronchopulmonary dysplasia. *Annu Rev Physiol, 67,* 623.
221. Stevens, T.P., et al. (2007). Early surfactant administration with brief ventilation vs. selective surfactant and continued mechanical ventilation for preterm infants with or at risk for respiratory distress syndrome. *Cochrane Database Syst Rev, 4,* CD003063.
222. Supcun, S., et al. (2010). Caffeine increases cerebral cortical activity in preterm infants. *J Pediatr, 156,* 490.
223. SUPPORT Study Group of the Eunice Kennedy Shriver NICHD Neonatal Research Network & Carlo, W.A., et al. (2010). Target ranges of oxygen saturation in extremely preterm infants. *N Engl J Med, 362,* 1959.
224. Suresh, G.K. (2011). Pharmacological adjuncts II: Exogenous surfactants. In J.P. Goldsmith & E.H. Karotkin (Eds). *Assisted ventilation of the newborn* (5th ed.). Philadelphia: Saunders Elsevier.
225. Sweet, D.G. & Halliday, H.L. (2009). The use of surfactants in 2009. *Arch Dis Child Educ Pract Ed, 94,* 78.
226. Tan, A., et al. (2005). Air versus oxygen for resuscitation of infants at birth. *Cochrane Database Syst Rev, 2,* CD002273.
227. Thach, B.T. (2001). Maturation and transformation of reflexes that protect the laryngeal airway from liquid aspiration from fetal to adult life. *Am J Med, 111,* 69S.
228. Truog, W.E. (2012). Pulmonary gas exchange in the developing lung. In R.A. Polin, W.W. Fox, & S.H. Abman (Eds.). *Fetal and neonatal physiology* (4th ed.). Philadelphia: Saunders.
229. Tsao, K., Albanese, C.T., & Harrison, M.R. (2003). Prenatal therapy for thoracic and mediastinal lesions. *World J Surg, 27,* 77.
230. Turner, B.S., Bradshaw, W., & Brandon, D. (2005). Neonatal lung remodeling: Structural, inflammatory, and ventilator-induced injury. *J Perinat Neonatal Nurs, 19,* 362.
231. Vain, N.E., et al. (2004). Oropharyngeal and nasopharyngeal suctioning of meconium-stained neonates before delivery of their shoulders: Multicentre, randomized controlled trial. *Lancet, 364,* 597.
232. Van Meurs, K. & Congenital Diaphragmatic Hernia Study Group. (2004). Is surfactant therapy beneficial in the treatment of the term newborn infant with congenital diaphragmatic hernia? *J Pediatr, 145,* 312.
233. Vardavas, C.I., et al. (2010). Smoking and smoking cessation during early pregnancy and its effect on adverse pregnancy outcomes and fetal growth. *Eur J Pediatr, 169,* 741.

234. Vento, M., et al. (2009). Preterm resuscitation with low oxygen causes less oxidative stress, inflammation, and chronic lung disease. *Pediatrics, 124,* 439.
235. Vento, M. & Saugstad, O.D. (2011). Oxygen supplementation in the delivery room: Updated information. *J Pediatr, 158,* e5.
236. Verklan, M.T. (2006). Persistent pulmonary hypertension of the newborn: Not a honeymoon anymore. *J Perinat Neonatal Nurs, 20,* 108.
237. Voelkel, N.F., Vandivier, R.W., & Tuder, R.M. (2006). Vascular endothelial growth factor in the lung. *Am J Physiol Lung Cell Mol Physiol, 290,* L209.
238. Wang, X., et al. (2002). Maternal cigarette smoking, metabolic gene polymorphism, and infant birth weight. *JAMA, 287,* 195.
239. Watterberg, K.L. & American Academy of Pediatrics Committee on Fetus and Newborn. (2010). Policy Statement: Postnatal corticosteroids to prevent or treat bronchopulmonary dysplasia. *Pediatrics, 126,* 800.
240. Wert, S.E. (2012). Normal and abnormal structural development of the lung. In R.A. Polin, W.W. Fox, & S.H. Abman (Eds.). *Fetal and neonatal physiology* (4th ed.). Philadelphia: Saunders.
241. West, J.B. (2012). *Pulmonary pathophysiology: the essentials* (8th ed.). Philadelphia: Lippincott.
242. Whitelaw, A. & Thoresen, M. (2000). Antenatal steroids and the developing brain. *Arch Dis Child Fetal Neonatal Ed, 83,* F154.
243. Whitsett, J.A., Wert, S.E., & Xu, Y. (2005). Genetic disorders of surfactant homeostasis. *Biol Neonate, 87,* 283.
244. Whitsett, J.A. (2010). Review: the intersection of surfactant homeostasis and innate host defense of the lung: Lessons from newborn infants. *Innate Immun, 16,* 138.
245. Whitsett, J.A., Wert, S.E., & Weaver, T.E. (2010). Alveolar surfactant homeostasis and the pathogenesis of pulmonary disease. *Annu Rev Med, 61,* 105.
246. Whitsett, J.A. (2012). Composition of pulmonary surfactant lipids and proteins. In R.A. Polin, W.W. Fox, & S.H. Abman (Eds.). *Fetal and neonatal physiology* (4th ed.). Philadelphia: Saunders.
247. Whitty, J.E. & Dombrowski, M.P. (2009). Respiratory diseases in pregnancy. In R.K. Creasy, et al. (Eds.). *Creasy & Resnik's Maternal-fetal medicine: Principles and practice* (6th ed.). Philadelphia: Saunders Elsevier.
248. Widmaier, E., Raff, H., & Strang, K.T. (2005). *Vander's Human physiology: the mechanism of body function* (10th ed.). New York: McGraw-Hill. Williams & Wilkins.
249. Wilson-Costello, D., et al. (2009). Impact of postnatal corticosteroid use on neurodevelopment at 18 to 22 months' adjusted age: Effects of dose, timing, and risk of bronchopulmonary dysplasia in extremely low birth weight infants. *Pediatrics, 123,* e430.
250. Wise, R.A., Polito, A.J., & Krishnan, V. (2006). Respiratory physiologic changes in pregnancy. *Immunol Allergy Clin North Am, 26,* 1.
251. Yost, C.C. & Soll, R.F. (2000). Early versus delayed selective surfactant treatment for neonatal respiratory distress syndrome. *Cochrane Database Syst Rev 2,* CD001456.
252. Zahka, K.G. (2011). Cardiovascular problems of the neonate. In R.J. Martin, A.A. Fanaroff, & M.C. Walsh (Eds.). *Fanaroff and Martin's Neonatal-perinatal medicine: Diseases of the fetus and infant* (9th ed.). Philadelphia: Mosby Elsevier.
253. Zaichkin, J. & Weiner, G.M. (2011). Neonatal Resuscitation Program (NRP) 2011: New science, new strategies. *Adv Neonatal Care, 11,* 43. Erratum in: Adv Neonatal Care. 2011 Jun;11(3):221.
254. Zhang, L., et al. (2003). Hypercapnia-induced activation of brainstem GABAergic neurons during early development. *Resptr Physiol Neurobiol, 136,* 25.
255. Zoban, P. & Czerny, M. (2003). Immature lung and acute lung injury. *Physiol Res, 52,* 507.

Renal System and Fluid and Electrolyte Homeostasis

CHAPTER 11

The kidneys are critical organs in maintaining body homeostasis by regulation of water and electrolyte balance, excretion of metabolic waste products and foreign substances, regulation of vitamin D activity and erythrocyte production (via erythropoietin), and gluconeogenesis.[161] The kidneys also have an important role in control of arterial blood pressure through the renin-angiotensin system and regulation of sodium balance. This chapter examines the alterations in basic renal processes and regulation of fluids and electrolytes observed in the pregnant woman, fetus, and neonate, and discusses the implications of these changes for clinical practice. Basic renal processes are summarized in Figure 11-1 and Box 11-1 on page 358.

MATERNAL PHYSIOLOGIC ADAPTATIONS

The renal system undergoes a variety of structural and functional changes during pregnancy, with many of the structural changes persisting well into the postpartum period. Pregnancy is characterized by sodium retention and increased extracellular volume, which are mediated by alterations in renal function. Many parameters normally used to evaluate renal function and fluid and electrolyte homeostasis are altered in pregnancy, and subclinical renal problems may not be easily recognized.

Antepartum Period

The renal system must handle the effects of increased maternal intravascular and extracellular volume and metabolic waste products as well as serve as the primary excretory organ for fetal wastes. Changes in the renal system are related to hormonal effects (particularly the influence of progesterone on smooth muscle), pressure from the enlarging uterus, effects of position and activity, and alterations in the cardiovascular system and vasoactive substances. Cardiovascular system changes that interact with alterations in renal hemodynamics include increased cardiac output, increased blood and plasma volume, and alterations in the venous system and plasma proteins (see Chapters 8 and 9). The predominant structural change in the renal system during pregnancy is dilation of the renal pelvis and ureters; functional changes include alterations in hemodynamics, glomerular filtration, and tubular handling of certain substances. Changes in fluid and electrolyte homeostasis result from changes in renal handling of water and sodium and alterations in the renin-angiotensin system. Table 11-1 summarizes changes in the renal system during pregnancy and their clinical implications. Even with these changes, renal reserve is maintained during pregnancy, so that the pregnant woman has the capacity for further vasodilation and filtration above baseline if needed.

Structural Changes

Pregnancy is characterized by physiologic hydroureter and hydronephrosis. Significant dilation of the renal calyces, pelvis, and ureters beginning as early as the seventh week, is seen in up to 80% of women.[21,53,78,113,125] The mean kidney length increases by approximately 1 cm due to the increased renal blood flow (RBF), renal vascular and volume, and renal hypertrophy.[66,113] Renal volume increases by 30%.[78,113] The diameter of the ureteral lumen increases with hypertonicity and hypomotility of the ureteral musculature. Hypomotility and reduced peristaltic movements of the ureters may be mediated by prostaglandin E_2 (PGE_2).[21,54]

The ureters elongate and become more tortuous, especially during the last half of pregnancy as they are laterally displaced by the growing uterus.[21] These changes are seen within the renal pelvis and the upper portion of the ureters to the pelvic brim. The portion of the ureters below the pelvic brim (linea terminalis) is usually not enlarged. The ureters may contain as much as 300 mL of urine by the third trimester.[54] This reservoir of urine leads to stasis and can interfere with evaluation of glomerular filtration rate (GFR), tubular function, and influence the accuracy of 24-hour urine collections.[113,125] The stasis increases the risk of ascending urinary tract infection (UTI), nephrolithiasis, and pyelonephrosis.[53,68,70,113,125]

The etiology of physiologic hydroureter is unclear. Dilation begins before the uterus reaches the pelvic brim, so initial changes are probably hormonally mediated. Hormonal influences, particularly progesterone, may induce hypertrophy of the longitudinal smooth muscles surrounding distal portions of the ureters and hyperplasia of periurethral connective tissue.[21,54,113] This may lead to a temporary stenosis and mild dilation of the upper portion of the ureters. These findings are similar to those seen in women on

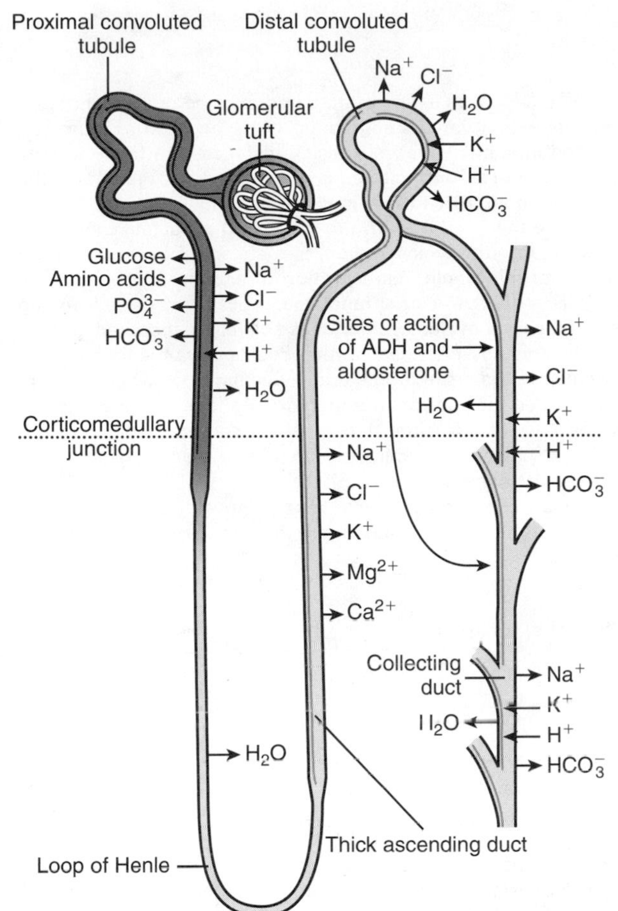

FIGURE 11-1 The nephron. Substances enter the tubule from the blood via glomerular filtration or tubular secretion and are reabsorbed back into the blood by tubular reabsorption (see Box 11-1 on page 358. Any substances that are not reabsorbed are lost in the urine. Water is reabsorbed in the proximal tubule together with glucose, amino acids, phosphate, sodium, and bicarbonate, and from the distal tubule under the influence of arginine vasopressin and the hypertonic medulla. In the distal tubule, sodium is reabsorbed under the influence of aldosterone with associated tubular secretion of potassium and hydrogen ions. (From Modi, N. [2005]. Fluid and electrolyte balance. In J.M. Rennie [Ed.], *Roberton's textbook of neonatology* [4th ed.]. Edinburgh: Churchill Livingstone, p. 335 [as adapted from Cumming, A.D. & Swanson, C.P. [1995]. Disturbances in water, electrolyte and acid-base balance. In C.R.W. Edwards, et al. [Eds.], *Davidson's principles and practices of medicine*. Edinburgh: Churchill Livingstone, p. 587.)

oral contraceptives and in postmenopausal women given estrogen and progesterone.[54]

The major contributing factor to hydronephrosis in later pregnancy is probably external compression of the ureters at the pelvic brim. As pregnancy progresses, the ureters are compressed at the pelvic brim by the iliac arteries, enlarging ovarian vein complexes, and the growing uterus, leading to further marked dilation and urinary stasis.[51] Dilation is more prominent in the primipara, whose firmer abdominal wall may increase resistance and pressure on the ureters.[21]

In most women, the right ureter is dilated to a greater extent than the left.[51,78,113] These differences become more prominent after midgestation.[51] The right ureter makes a right-angle turn as it crosses the iliac and ovarian veins at the pelvic brim; the turn of the left ureter is less acute, and it parallels rather than crosses the left ovarian vein. The iliac vessels are more rigid on the right than on the left, thus further compressing the ureters. Compression is maximal by around 30 weeks' gestation, with no further significant changes to term. The sigmoid colon contributes to dextroversion of the uterus and may increase ureteral compression on the contralateral side during the last trimester.[21,54,78,113] The position of the fetus does not seem to influence ureteral dilation. The site of placental attachment may increase venous flow on that side with subsequent compression of the ureters by the dilated vessels.[54]

Bladder tone decreases as a result of the effects of progesterone on smooth muscle. Bladder capacity doubles by term. The bladder becomes displaced anteriorly and superiorly by the end of the second trimester. Under the influence of estrogen, the trigone undergoes hyperplasia with hypertrophy of the bladder musculature. The bladder mucosa becomes hyperemic with increased size and tortuosity of the blood vessels. The mucosa becomes more edematous and vulnerable to trauma or infection after engagement of the presenting part.[54]

The baseline intravesical pressure doubles due to the enlarged uterus.[106] The decreased bladder tone and flaccidity may lead to incompetence of the vesicoureteral valve and reflux of urine. Vesicoureteral reflux is seen in up to 3.5% of pregnant women, especially in the third trimester.[106] Predisposing factors for this reflux include hypertrophy and hyperplasia of the ureteral wall, increased elasticity of the ureters, increased bladder pressure, and decreased peristalsis in the distal ureter.[106] Alterations in bladder placement by the growing uterus stretch the trigone and displace the intravesical portion of the ureters laterally. This shortens the terminal ureter, decreasing intravesical pressure. If intravesical pressure subsequently increases with micturition, urine regurgitates into the ureters.[54]

Urodynamic Changes

Urine output increases from a mean of 1475 to 1919 mL per 24 hours primarily because of changes in sodium excretion.[106] Mean flow rate decreases in the second and third trimesters with an increase in flow time and time to maximal flow throughout pregnancy.[106] The number of voids per day and mean daily urine output increase throughout gestation.[152] Studies of changes in bladder capacity during pregnancy have reported variable findings. Increased bladder capacity due to the decreased tone has been reported by some investigators, especially in primiparas.[10] Others have found a mean bladder capacity similar to that of the nonpregnant state in the first two trimesters, but decreased capacity in the third trimester due to elevation of the trigone and the size of the presenting part.[142] Another study reported that the pregnant woman's bladder has a larger capacity with a lower pressure

BOX 11-1 Basic Renal Processes

Glomerular filtration—Plasma is filtered from blood moving through the glomerulus into the Bowman capsule. The glomerulus is freely permeable to water and small molecules but impermeable to colloids and larger molecules, including most protein-bound substances. Filtration is influenced by hydrostatic and colloid osmotic pressure.

Tubular reabsorption—Water and other substances appear in the urine in smaller quantities than were originally filtered due to reabsorption in the tubules. Tubular reabsorption of substances from the tubular lumen back into the blood in the peritubular capillaries occurs through simple diffusion, facilitated diffusion, and active transport. These mechanisms can only transport limited amounts (transport maximum [Tm]) of certain substances, such as glucose, due to saturation of the carriers. Any amount filtered in excess of this quantity cannot be reabsorbed and appears in the urine. The proximal tubule is the major site for reabsorption of glucose, amino acids, sodium, protein, and other organic nutrients. The movement of water, sodium, and chloride through the kidneys is interrelated and affected by concentration gradients within various segments of the nephron and the surrounding interstitial spaces. These substances are freely filtered and 99% of the amount filtered is reabsorbed: 65% to 80% in the proximal tubule, 20% to 25% in the ascending limb of the loop of Henle, and the remainder in the distal and collecting tubes. The processes through which sodium is reabsorbed vary in different portions of the tubule. Reabsorption of sodium in the proximal tubule is an active, carrier-mediated process. In the ascending limb of the loop of Henle, chloride is actively reabsorbed and sodium follows passively. Sodium reabsorption is mediated by aldosterone in the distal tubule and collecting duct, where sodium is exchanged for potassium and hydrogen ions. Water reabsorption by passive diffusion or osmosis is sodium dependent but also depends on permeability of the tubular membrane (which is altered by arginine vasopressin).

Tubular secretion—This involves the movement of substances from the peritubular capillaries into the lumen of the tubules.

Adapted from Widemaier, E., Raff, H., & Strang, K. (2010). *Vander, Sherman & Luciano's human physiology: The mechanism of body function* (12th ed.). New York: McGraw-Hill.

Table 11-1 Changes in the Renal System During Pregnancy

PARAMETER	ALTERATION	SIGNIFICANCE
Renal calyces, pelvis, and ureters	Dilation (more prominent on right)	Increased risk of urinary tract infection in pregnancy and postpartum
	Elongation, decreased motility, and hypertonicity of ureter	Altered accuracy of 24-hour urine collections Increased risk of urinary tract infection in pregnancy
	May last up to 3 months postpartum	Increased risk of urinary tract infection postpartum
Bladder	Decreased tone, increased capacity	Increased risk of urinary tract infection Urinary frequency and incontinence Alteration in accuracy of 24-hour urine collections
	Displaced in late pregnancy	Urinary frequency
	Mucosa edematous and hyperemic	Risk of trauma and infection
	Incompetence of vesicoureteral valve	Risk of reflux and infection Alteration in accuracy of 24-hour urine collections
Renal blood flow	Increases 50%-80% by mid-second trimester, then decreases to term	Increased glomerular filtration rate Increased solutes delivered to kidney
Glomerular filtration rate	Increases 40%-60%	Increased filtration and excretion of water and solutes Increased urine flow and volume Decreased serum blood urea nitrogen, creatinine, uric acid Altered renal excretion of drugs with risk of subtherapeutic blood and tissue levels
Renal tubular function	Increased reabsorption of solutes (may not always match increase in filtered load)	Maintenance of homeostasis Avoid pathologic solute or fluid loss
	Increased renal excretion of glucose, protein, amino acids, urea, uric acid, water-soluble vitamins, calcium, hydrogen ions, phosphorus, bicarbonate	Tendency for glycosuria, proteinuria Compensation for respiratory alkalosis Increased nutritional needs (i.e., calcium, water-soluble) vitamins Decreased serum bicarbonate levels
	Net retention of sodium and water	Accumulation of sodium and water to meet maternal and fetal needs
Renin-angiotensin-aldosterone system	Increase in all components	Maintain homeostasis with expanded extracellular volume
	Resistance to pressor effects of angiotensin II	Retention of water and sodium Balance forces favoring sodium excretion Maintain normal blood pressure
Arginine vasopressin and regulation of osmolarity	Osmostat reset at lower baseline osmolarity	Expansion of plasma volume and other extracellular volume Maintenance of volume homeostasis despite reduction in plasma osmolarity

per volume.[134] In nonpregnant women the first urge to void was at a bladder capacity of 150 to 200 mL and maximum at 450 to 550 mL with an intravesicular pressure of 20 cmH_2O (1.96 kPa); in pregnant women the first urge to void was at a bladder capacity of 250 to 400 mL (intravesical pressure of 4 to 8 cmH_2O [0.39 to 0.78 kPa]) and often did not reach maximum until 1000 to 1200 mL (intravesicular pressure of 12 to 15 cmH_2O [1.17 to 1.47 kPa]).[134]

Changes in Renal Hemodynamics

Significant hemodynamic changes occur within the kidneys beginning early in pregnancy in conjunction with systemic vasodilation (see Chapter 9). RBF and GFR increase. Increases in these parameters, although not to the degree seen in pregnancy, also occur during the luteal phase of the menstrual cycle.[78]

RBF increases up to 50% to 80% by the mid–second trimester and then slowly decreases to term.[91,113] The higher values are seen in the left lateral recumbent position.[33] This change is accompanied by increased glomerular filtration rate (GFR), decreased renal vascular resistance (RVR), and activation of the renin-angiotensin-aldosterone system. Renal hemodynamic changes begin before significant expansion of plasma volume and are thought to be primarily related to the decrease in systemic vascular resistance (SVR), which may stimulate decreased RVR leading to increased RBF and GFR, and by sodium retention. These changes may be mediated by nitric oxide (NO), prostacyclin (PGI_2), atrial natriuretic factor (ANF), progesterone, endothelin B, and relaxin, possibly via their effects on GFR. Increased flow is enhanced by vasodilation of preglomerular and postglomerular capillaries.[33,78,113,125] Another measure of renal hemodynamics is the effective renal plasma flow (ERPF), which increases 80% by midpregnancy.[40,113,153] ERPF then gradually decreases during the third trimester to values 50% greater than nonpregnant values.[66,113]

Changes in Glomerular Filtration

The GFR increases 40% to 60% during pregnancy.[29,34,66,91,113] The rise begins as early as 6 weeks and precedes plasma volume expansion and cardiac output (see Chapter 9).[29,91] Changes in GFR are detectable 3 to 4 weeks after conception, with 25% of the increase occurring by 2 weeks postconception, peak at 9 to 16 weeks, then remain relatively stable to near term.[113] Values for GFR in pregnancy, as measured by creatinine clearance, average 110 to 150 mL/min.[113] Differences in reported values for RBF and GFR during pregnancy vary with the method of measurement. The increased GFR is related to the increased glomerular blood flow (and glomerular capillary hydrostatic pressure) and decreased colloid osmotic (plasma oncotic) pressure due to a reduction in the concentration of plasma proteins.[71,91] Failure of the GFR to increase early in pregnancy has been associated with pregnancy loss.[163]

The increases in renal plasma flow (RPF) and GFR parallel each other, although RPF changes are slightly greater than GFR changes. This alters the filtration fraction (GFR/RPF), the portion of the RBF that is filtered.[70,78,113] The filtration fraction is decreased in the first half of gestation and increased in late gestation as ERPF decreases.[78,91] As a result, renal excretion of amino acids, glucose, protein, electrolytes, and vitamins increases, whereas serum urea, creatinine, blood urea nitrogen (BUN), and uric acid levels decrease (Table 11-2).

The causes of the increased GFR during pregnancy are still not completely clear, but the primary factor is the increased RPF and decreased renal vascular resistance.[32,91,144] These changes are stimulated by relaxin (which up-regulates vascular gelatinase activity and leads to activation of endothelin receptors causing vasodilation), increased GFR, and relaxation of the small renal arteries. This process is mediated by NO, which is a potent renal vasodilator.[41,91] Other factors that may play a role are prostacyclin, ANF, human placental lactogen, and human chorionic gonadotropin, which stimulates relaxin secretion.[32,33,41]

During pregnancy, 24-hour urine volumes are higher due to the increased GFR. The degree to which renal handling of substances is altered during pregnancy depends on the renal process involved (see Figure 11-1). For example, because urea and creatinine are processed only by glomerular filtration, the increased GFR leads to a significant decrease in serum urea and creatinine levels.[91,113] The increased GFR also alters renal excretion of drugs (see Chapter 7).[9]

Table 11-2 Changes in Laboratory Values Associated with Renal Function during Pregnancy

VARIABLE	NONPREGNANT VALUES	VALUES DURING PREGNANCY	VALUES REQUIRING FURTHER INVESTIGATION
Creatinine clearance	85-120 mL/min	110-150 mL/min	
Plasma creatinine	0.65 ± 0.14 mg/dL	0.46 ± 0.13 mg/dL	>0.80 mg/dL
Blood urea nitrogen	13 ± 3 mg/dL	8.7 ± 1.5 mg/dL	>14 mg/dL
Urinary protein	<100-150 mg/24 hours	<250-300 mg/24 hours	>300 mg/24 hours
Urinary glucose	20-100 mg/24 hours	>100 mg/24 hours (up to 10 g/24 hours)	
Plasma urate	4-6 mg/dL	2.5-4 mg/dL	>5.8 mg/dL
Urinary amino acids		Up to 2 g/24 hours	>2 g/24 hours

Alterations in Tubular Function

The elevated GFR increases the concentration of solutes and volume of fluid within the tubular lumen by 50% to 100%. Tubular reabsorption increases in order to prevent rapid depletion from the body of sodium, chloride, glucose, potassium, and water. There is actually a net retention of most of these substances during pregnancy. Conversely, tubular reabsorption rates cannot always accommodate the increased filtered load. This results in increased excretion of substances such as glucose and amino acids. Alterations in GFR and tubular function result in altered plasma values of many substances during pregnancy.

Renal glucose excretion increases soon after conception and remains high to term. Urinary glucose values may be 10- to 100-fold greater than the nonpregnant values of 20 to 100 mg per 24 hours due to alterations in reabsorption of glucose in the loop of Henle and collecting ducts.[40,113] Glycosuria is more common during pregnancy and can vary from day to day and within any 24-hour period. Glycosuria is discussed in Evaluation of Renal Function during Pregnancy.

Excretion of amino acids, urea, and protein increases in pregnancy. Protein excretion rises from less than 100 mg per 24 hours to up to 250 to 300 mg per 24 hours, with marked day-to-day variation.[40,66] The primary amino acids whose excretion is markedly increased throughout pregnancy are alanine, glycine, histidine, serine, and threonine; excretion of cysteine, leucine, lysine, phenylalanine, taurine, and tyrosine increases in early pregnancy, but decreases later.[113] Increased urea clearance leads to decreased plasma urea nitrogen levels by 8 to 10 weeks.[40] Plasma urea levels may be only 63% of nonpregnant values by the third trimester.

Proteinuria occurs more frequently during pregnancy with increases in both total protein and urinary albumin.[78] The filtered load of amino acids during pregnancy may exceed tubular reabsorptive capacity with small amounts of protein lost in the urine. Values of 1+ protein on dipsticks are common and do not necessarily indicate the presence of glomerular pathology or preeclampsia.[5,160] Urinary protein excretion during pregnancy is not considered abnormal until values exceed 300 mg per 24 hours.[68,78,113,125] Protein excretion does not correlate with the severity of renal disease, and increased protein excretion in a pregnant woman with known renal disease does not necessarily indicate progression of the disease.[40] However, proteinuria associated with hypertension in the pregnant woman is associated with a greater risk of an adverse pregnancy outcome.[68,162]

Uric acid is normally handled by filtration, secretion, and reabsorption (see Box 11-1 on 358), so less than 10% of the filtered load appears in urine. During pregnancy, filtration of uric acid increases up to 30% in the first 16 weeks, and net reabsorption is decreased and secretion enhanced.[163] As a result, serum uric acid levels decrease up to 25% to 35%, beginning as early as 8 weeks, to a nadir of 2 to 3 mg/dL by 24 weeks.[78,113] Levels gradually increase toward nonpregnant values after that point as tubular reabsorption of uric acid increases. This increase may also be a result of the rise in RPF that alters the filtration fraction at this stage of gestation.[40,113] In women with preeclampsia, uric acid clearance is reduced with higher serum levels.[78]

Potassium excretion is decreased, with retention of an additional 300 to 350 mEq that is thought to be due to increased proximal tubular reabsorption.[91,113] Serum potassium levels do not rise, because the additional potassium is used for maternal tissues and by the fetus. The mechanisms for increased potassium reabsorption in pregnancy are not well documented. These changes occur despite the increase in aldosterone that normally would increase urinary potassium loss. Therefore the altered potassium excretion may be due to antagonistic action of progesterone on renal tubular actions of aldosterone.[91]

Renal acid-base balance is altered to compensate for the respiratory alkalosis that develops secondary to an increased loss of carbon dioxide from changes in ventilation during pregnancy (see Chapter 10). The respiratory alkalosis is compensated for by increased renal loss of bicarbonate. This is accomplished by renal retention of H^+ ions and a decrease in serum bicarbonate. As a result, serum bicarbonate levels fall 4 to 5 mEq/L (mmol/L) during the first trimester to 20 to 22 mEq/L (mmol/L).[66,125] This change may limit buffering capacity in the pregnant woman.[78]

Urinary calcium excretion is increased, possibly due to the increased GFR, and serum calcium and phosphorus levels decrease. This is balanced by increased intestinal absorption of calcium, so serum ionic calcium levels remain stable (see Chapter 17).[113] To maintain homeostasis and meet fetal demands, women need 1200 mg of calcium per day in their diet. Excretion of water-soluble vitamins also increases, so maternal diet must be evaluated to ensure adequate supplies of vitamins B_1, B_2, B_6, and C; folate; and niacin (see Chapter 12).

Fluid and Electrolyte Homeostasis

The pregnant woman must retain additional fluid and electrolytes to meet her needs and those of her growing fetus. In order to do this, renal excretory responses are modified and a new balance achieved. Because fluid and electrolyte balance is mediated predominantly by sodium and water homeostasis, pregnancy changes primarily involve alterations in these substances. The hormonal systems involved in regulation of sodium and water homeostasis, e.g. arginine vasopressin (AVP) and the renin-angiotensin-aldosterone system, must also be altered in order to react appropriately to the new equilibrium.

Sodium Homeostasis. The filtered load of sodium increases up to 50% as a result of the increased GFR. The nonpregnant woman filters approximately 20,000 mEq of sodium per day; the pregnant woman filters 30,000.[41,113] To prevent excessive urinary sodium loss, tubular reabsorption of sodium also increases so that 99% of the filtered sodium is reabsorbed. As a result, there is a net retention of 900 to 950 mg (2 to 6 mEq/day) of sodium during pregnancy.[40,41,78,113] Sodium retention occurs gradually with an increase in late pregnancy.[41]

Much of the sodium is used by the fetus and placenta; the rest is distributed in maternal blood and extracellular fluid (ECF) (Table 11-3).[163]

Despite these alterations, the pregnant woman remains in sodium balance and responds normally to changes in both sodium and water balance. The specific mechanisms for sodium retention during pregnancy are unclear. The maintenance of sodium balance during pregnancy is multifactorial and related to a balance (Figure 11-2) between natriuretic factors favoring sodium excretion (increased GFR, decreased RVR, decreased plasma oncotic pressure, decreased serum albumin, vasodilating prostaglandins, increased ANF, and the diuretic-like and aldosterone-antagonistic actions of progesterone) and antinatriuretic factors favoring sodium conservation (increased renin, aldosterone, deoxycorticosterone, human chorionic somatomammotropin [human placental lactogen], and estrogen).[113,161,163] ANF is released by the atrial endothelial lining and increases early in pregnancy. ANF opposes the action of progesterone and inhibits the renin-angiotensin-aldosterone system, thus stimulating sodium loss. Relaxin also mediates sodium balance during pregnancy. Relaxin is associated with osmoregulatory changes, vasodilation, and increased GFR.[29,33,125] As a result of these changes, sodium retention in pregnancy is proportional to water accumulation and the woman remains in homeostatic balance.

Renin-Angiotensin-Aldosterone System

The renin-angiotensin-aldosterone system is important in fluid and electrolyte homeostasis and maintaining arterial blood pressure (Figure 11-3 and Box 11-2 on page 362). Pregnancy is characterized by increases in components of the renin-angiotensin-aldosterone system and decreased sensitivity to the pressor effects of angiotensin II (ANTII).[11] Changes in most of these components peak at 30 to 32 weeks. The changes are mediated by estrogens, progesterone, prostaglandins, and alterations in renal processing of sodium.[64] Although the renin-angiotensin-aldosterone system is altered during pregnancy, this system responds normally, but at a new set point, to interventions that alter volume such as salt restriction, diuretics, and positional changes.[92]

During pregnancy, major sites for renin production include the uterus, placenta, and fetus as well as the kidneys.[26,75] Renin peaks at levels two to three times higher than normal during the first trimester and remains elevated, with a tendency to reach a plateau by about 32 weeks. The increase in renin is due primarily to increased inactive renin; however, both active renin and plasma renin activity (PRA) (a measure of the capacity of plasma to generate angiotensin I) also increase.[64,148] PRA increases 4 to 10 fold during the first trimester, peaking at 12 weeks, and then remaining high to term with a possible decrease in the third trimester noted by some investigators.[139,148]

Table 11-3 Storage of Sodium during Pregnancy

STORAGE SITE	SODIUM (MEQ [MMOL/L])
Fetus	290
Edema fluid	240
Plasma	140
Amniotic fluid	100
Uterus	80
Placenta	57
Breasts	35
Red cells	5
Total	947

From Sullivan, C.A. & Martin, J.N. (1994). Sodium and pregnancy. *Clin Obstet Gynecol* 37, 558.

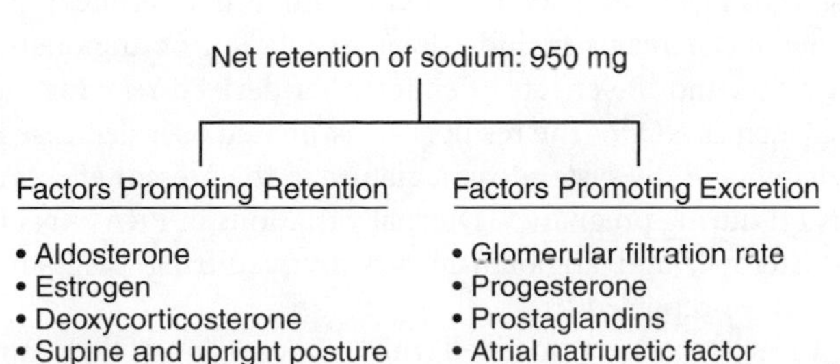

FIGURE 11-2 Factors influencing the regulation of sodium excretion in pregnancy. (From Monga, M. [1999]. Maternal cardiovascular and renal adaptation to pregnancy. In R.K. Creasy & R. Resnik [Eds.], *Maternal-fetal medicine* [4th ed.]. Philadelphia: Saunders.)

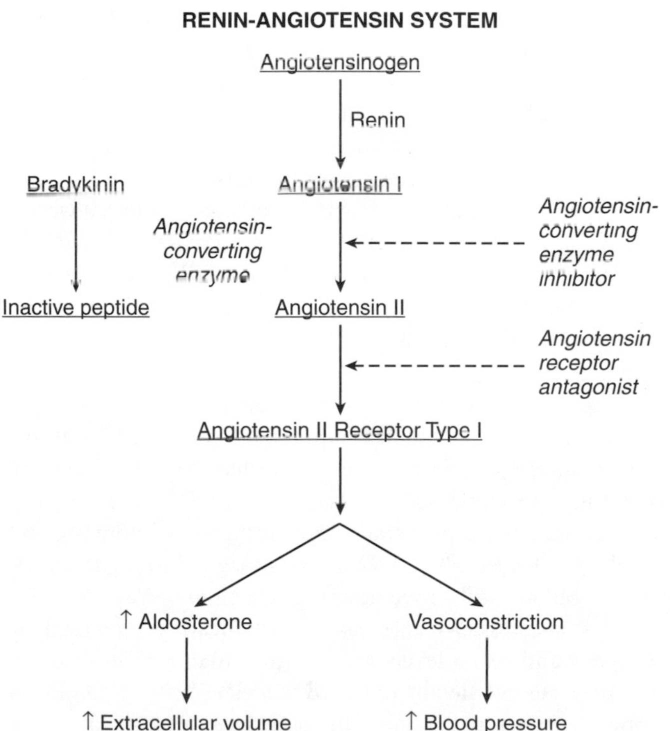

FIGURE 11-3 Renin-angiotensin-aldosterone system. (From Quan, A. [2006]. Fetopathy associated with exposure to angiotensin-converting enzyme inhibitors and angiotensin receptor antagonists. *Early Hum Dev, 82,* 23.)

BOX 11-2 Renin-Angiotensin-Aldosterone System

The renin-angiotensin-aldosterone system has key roles in blood pressure regulation and fluid and electrolyte homeostasis. Angiotensinogen (plasma renin substrate) is produced in the liver and is always present in the blood. Renin is a proteolytic enzyme found in blood in active and inactive forms. Renin is secreted and stored primarily in the juxtaglomerular cells surrounding afferent arterioles of cortical nephron glomeruli. Renin is also synthesized in extrarenal sites such as the brain, vascular smooth muscle, the genital tract, and the fetoplacental unit. Stretch receptors in the juxtaglomerular cells sense changes in renal perfusion and afferent arteriole pressures and increase renin release.

Renin release is also influenced by the sympathetic nervous system and concentrations of circulating potassium, angiotensin II (ANTII), and possibly sodium. Renin acts on angiotensinogen to form angiotensin I, whose actions include stimulating catecholamine release, facilitating norepinephrine release from peripheral sympathetic veins, and reducing renal blood flow in the cortex and the medulla. A measure of the capacity of plasma renin to generate angiotensin I (ANTI) is plasma renin activity (PRA). ANTI is broken down by angiotensin-converting enzyme (ACE) to ANTII in the pulmonary circulation. ANTII is a potent vasoconstrictor that stimulates adrenal production and release of aldosterone and constriction of the renal vasculature to reduce glomerular filtration rate (GFR) and the effective renal plasma flow (ERPF). ANTII helps to maintain the arterial blood pressure and peripheral perfusion. Atrial natriuretic factor (ANF) also influences blood pressure and stimulates urinary sodium excretion.

Angiotensin$_1$ (AT_1) receptors are found on vascular smooth muscle, adrenal gland, and other tissues. Simulation of AT_1 receptors by ANTII increases intracellular calcium leading to increased vasoconstriction, sympathetic activity, and aldosterone release.[76] AT_2 receptors are found in the fetal kidney. Stimulation of these receptors enhances fetal renal development. Expression of these receptors decreases after birth.[76]

Aldosterone is a mineralocorticoid secreted by the outer zona glomerulosa cells of the adrenal cortex. The two major activities of aldosterone are regulation of extracellular fluid (ECF) balance by altering sodium retention and excretion and regulation of potassium. Aldosterone regulates fluid volume via a direct effect on renal distal tubular transport of sodium to increase sodium reabsorption and decrease potassium reabsorption. As sodium is reabsorbed, potassium and hydrogen ions are secreted into the tubular lumen. Increased reabsorption of sodium results in increased water retention, since water is passively reabsorbed along with the sodium, thus increasing body ECF volume. Aldosterone is regulated via feedback mechanisms involving potassium and ECF volume.[60,76,148,161]

Renin release is stimulated by estrogens (which also increase concentrations of angiotensinogen), decreased blood pressure, increased levels of plasma and urinary PGE, and the aldosterone-antagonizing effects of progesterone.[11,139,148] Increases in plasma renin are also seen during the later part of the secretory phase of the menstrual cycle, peaking at twice normal levels with the luteinizing hormone surge and persisting until midway into the luteal phase. These changes coincide with progesterone release.

Angiotensinogen (plasma renin substrate) levels double by 8 to 10 weeks, increase twofold to threefold by 20 weeks, and peak at 30 to 32 weeks.[11,26] This increase is due to the effects of estrogen on the liver, which synthesizes this substrate.[139] Low angiotensinogen levels are associated with spontaneous abortion and may reflect reduced placental estrogen production.

Angiotensin-converting enzyme (ACE) levels may be similar or slightly lower than nonpregnant values, although increases after 30 weeks have been reported.[26,139] ACE levels are also high in the uterus and placenta.[11] ANTII increases early in pregnancy and peaks at two to three times nonpregnant levels by 30 weeks.[26,139] ANTII levels may fall in the third trimester but are still above nonpregnant values.

Plasma aldosterone levels are significantly increased by 8 weeks and reach levels 4 to 6 times higher than those in nonpregnant women by the third trimester.[41,66,102,148] Aldosterone increases again later in gestation, peaking at about 36 weeks at levels 8 to 10 times higher than nonpregnant values. The increased aldosterone opposes the sodium-losing effects of progesterone and allows a progressive accumulation of sodium in maternal and fetal tissues.

Despite these changes, the pregnant woman remains responsive to both sodium depletion and loading, suggesting that a new equilibrium has been established.[41,148] The expanded intravascular and ECF compartments are sensed as "normal" by the woman's vascular and renal volume-regulating mechanisms. The elevated levels of aldosterone may be necessary to maintain the expanded extracellular volume. This new equilibrium is protected against further increases or depletion in a manner similar to that in nonpregnant individuals.[66]

ANTII is a potent vasopressor. Yet despite markedly elevated levels during pregnancy, the blood pressure does not rise and in fact actually decreases along with the peripheral vascular resistance (see Chapter 9).[11] The basis for resistance of the pregnant woman to the pressor effects of ANTII and other vasoactive substances is unclear. This refractoriness may be due to decreased vascular smooth muscle responsiveness to ANTII, perhaps mediated by local action of vasodilating prostaglandins, such as PGI_2, and progesterone.[75,77,151] Other mechanisms include down-regulation of angiotensin receptors and the effects of endothelial-derived relaxing factors such as NO.[151] The result is an estimated 60% decrease in sensitivity of the systemic vasculature to the pressor effects of ANTII during pregnancy. Diurnal variations in PRA, ANTII, aldosterone, and angiotensin sensitivity during pregnancy have been reported.[42]

Preeclampsia is associated with a suppression of the renin-angiotensin-aldosterone system.[26,76,77] The increases in renin, aldosterone, and ANTII are smaller in women with preeclampsia than in normotensive women. The preeclamptic woman is highly sensitive to the vasopressor effects of ANTII.

The angiotensin II type I receptor agonistic autoantibodies seen in preeclamptic women may play a role in the pathogenesis of preeclampsia (see Chapter 9).[76,77]

Volume Homeostasis and Regulation of Osmolarity

Because ECF volume is determined by sodium, the accumulation of sodium in pregnancy is accompanied by accumulation of water. Both extracellular and intravascular volumes expand during pregnancy. The largest portion of this expansion is in the vascular component, favoring placental perfusion. The amount of water filtered by the kidneys increases 50% or more during pregnancy due to the increased GFR. Pregnant women accumulate 6 to 7 L of water (Table 11-4) to meet their needs and those of the fetoplacental unit.[92,113] About 70% to 75% of maternal weight gain is due to increased body water in the extracellular spaces. Interstitial fluid volume increases 2 to 3 L beginning at 6 weeks and peaks at 24 to 30 weeks, with the greatest accumulation during the second half of pregnancy.[41,163] Accumulation of greater than 1.5 L of interstitial fluid is associated with edema. Alterations in blood volume are discussed in Chapters 8 and 9.

The exact mechanisms for water retention in pregnancy are still unclear with disagreement regarding the significance of these volume changes during pregnancy and how pregnant women "sense" these changes.[91,92,99] Lindheimer noted: "All agree that normal pregnancy is characterized by an absolute increment in both extracellular and intravascular volume (by some 6–7 L, at that), but investigators disagree on the meaning of these changes. For some ('under-fill' theory) it is an incomplete response to both the systemic vasodilation and markedly increased arterial global compliance characteristic of normal pregnancy, and indeed, the lower blood pressure and markedly stimulated renin-angiotensin system and aldosterone levels that persist during normal pregnancy are consistent with this paradigm. For others, this is an absolute hypervolemia perhaps due to the higher levels of salt-retaining steroids that accompany gestation ('over-fill' theory), and to still others, there is a constant resetting of the 'volumestat' as pregnancy progresses ('normal-fill' theory), the gravida always acting as if her current volume status were 'normal.'"[92, p. 1712]

The increase in plasma volume occurs despite decreases in plasma osmolarity and colloid osmotic pressure, changes that would normally stimulate decreases in intravascular volume. Estrogen and progesterone may play a role through dilation of the venous capacitance vessels so that they can accommodate additional volume without stimulation of atrial baroreceptors to alter AVP and aldosterone release.[40]

Plasma osmolarity decreases from conception, reaching 8 to 10 mOsm/kg below nonpregnant values of 290 mOsm/kg by 10 weeks' gestation and remaining low to term.[41,66,78,113,125,137,151] This change is associated with changes in sodium, urea, and other ions and may arise from the decrease in PCO_2 and subsequent compensatory adjustments in renal ion excretion. A decrease in plasma osmolarity of this magnitude in a nonpregnant person would significantly reduce the osmotic threshold for thirst, suppress AVP release, and lead to a massive water diuresis (as occurs in diabetes insipidus). However, the pregnant woman senses this change in osmolarity as normal. At this new baseline, she responds to water loading and deprivation and concentrates and dilutes urine in a manner similar to that in nonpregnant individuals.[113] Because of these changes, the urine of pregnant women is concentrated at levels below nonpregnant values.

Arginine Vasopressin. AVP (also known as antidiuretic hormone) secretion and its effect on renal reabsorption of water are similar in pregnant and nonpregnant women, as is AVP secretion in response to changes in baseline plasma osmolarity.[163] During pregnancy, the osmostat for AVP is reset, so the threshold at which the osmoreceptors signal the need for increased release is reduced from 280 to 270 mOsm/kg.[27,41,66,125] The thirst threshold (usually 10 mOsm/L [mmol/L] above the osmostat) is also reset during pregnancy, falling from 290 to 280 mOsm/L (mmol/L).[66,137]

AVP metabolites increase in pregnancy, probably due to placental metabolism, but maternal circulating AVP levels do not change significantly. The threefold to fourfold increase in plasma AVP clearance, which peaks at 22 to 24 weeks, is secondary to placental vasopressinases.[66,151] The posterior pituitary responds to this increased clearance by releasing more AVP to maintain normal plasma levels.[66] These changes in osmoregulation parallel the progressive increase in vasopressin metabolism and placental vasopressinases. The increased plasma vasopressinase in multiple pregnancies may be a basis for polyuria in these women.[137]

Nonosmotic factors regulating AVP secretion in pregnancy are poorly understood. In nonpregnant individuals a decrease in arterial blood pressure stimulates AVP secretion. In pregnancy the fall in plasma osmolarity occurs weeks

Table 11-4 Estimates (In mL) of Average Accumulated Extracellular and Intracellular Water at the End of Pregnancy

	TOTAL WATER	EXTRACELLULAR	INTRACELLULAR
Fetus[a]	2414	1400	1014
Placenta[b]	540	260	280
Amniotic fluid[c]	792	792	0
Uterus[d]	800	528	272
Mammary gland	304	148	156
Plasma	920	920	0
Red cells	163	0	163
Total	5933	4048	1885

From Davison, J.M. (1997). Edema in pregnancy. *Kidney Int Suppl*, 59, S90.
For the purposes of the above estimates, the following assumptions have been made:
[a]Extracellular space = 41.2% of body weight.
[b]48% is extracellular water.
[c]99% is water.
[d]66% of water is extracellular.

before the decline in blood pressure, and the lowered osmolarity is still sensed as normal at term when the blood pressure has returned to nonpregnant values. AVP release is also influenced by plasma volume (decreased plasma volume increases AVP release and increased plasma volume decreases AVP release). During pregnancy the threshold for the release of AVP is reset to accommodate the increase in extracellular volume at a lower baseline plasma osmolarity.[40,66] Human chorionic gonadotropin may also have a role in resetting the thirst and osmostat receptors during pregnancy.[66] The lowering of the osmotic threshold is probably due to the systemic arterial vasodilation leading to vasopressin simulation and up-regulation of aquaporin 2 water channels in the collecting ducts.[137]

Intrapartum Period

The renin-angiotensin systems of both the fetus and the mother are further altered during labor and delivery. At delivery, maternal renin, PRA, and angiotensinogen, as well as fetal renin and angiotensinogen levels, are elevated. These changes may be important in control of uteroplacental blood flow during the intrapartum and immediate postbirth periods.

Because the changes in renal function may also affect handling and excretion of drugs, drug doses and responses must be carefully monitored (see Chapter 7). General anesthesia decreases GFR, RPF, and sodium excretion and is associated with renal vasoconstriction, which may be magnified by the effects of stress with catecholamine release.[127] Thus monitoring of fluid and electrolyte status is especially important following use of general anesthesia for cesarean birth or with nonobstetric surgery during pregnancy.

Some pregnant women are also at risk for iatrogenic water intoxication during late pregnancy and the intrapartum period. This risk may result from the loss of electrolytes by use of saluretics; forcing fluids in a woman with preeclampsia and compromised renal function; or oxytocin infusion during labor, because the antidiuretic action of oxytocin reduces water excretion.

Some bladder and urethral trauma probably occurs in most women during the intrapartum period.[106] With contractions, intravesicular pressure increases by about 5 cmH_2O (0.49 kPa); however, bearing down increases pressure by up to 50 cmH_2O (4.90 kPa). Therefore prolonged straining during the second stage of labor may be more important in causing injury to the bladder than are contractions.[106]

Postpartum Period

RPF decreases markedly in the first 5 days after delivery.[129] GFR remains elevated (by about 40%) during the first day postpartum and then decreases over the next 2 weeks but remains about 20% elevated.[71] RPF, GFR, plasma creatinine, creatinine clearance, and BUN return to nonpregnant levels by 2 to 3 months postpartum.[10,129] Urinary excretion of calcium, phosphate, vitamins, and other solutes generally returns to normal by the end of the first week, but hyperfiltration may be maintained for up to 4 weeks due to decreased glomerular oncotic pressure.[148] Immediately after delivery, the creatinine clearance increases, but by 6 days is similar to nonpregnant levels.[40] PRA and ANTII concentrations fall to nonpregnant values immediately after delivery and then rise again and remain elevated for up to 14 days.[148] These changes may reflect the loss of renin from the fetoplacental unit, with subsequent "overshooting" by the maternal system.[148] Urinary glucose excretion returns to nonpregnant patterns by 1 week postpartum, and pregnancy-associated proteinuria is resolved by 6 weeks.[21,40] Plasma osmolality returns to nonpregnant levels by 2 weeks.[151]

The postpartum period is characterized by rapid and sustained natriuresis and diuresis, especially prominent on days 2 to 5, as the sodium and water retention of pregnancy is reversed.[40] Fluid and electrolyte balance is generally restored to nonpregnant homeostasis by 21 days postpartum and often earlier. Persistence of more than a trace of edema after this time is indicative of sodium retention or a protein-losing state.

The decrease in oxytocin contributes to diuresis because oxytocin acts similarly to AVP in promoting reabsorption of free water. As oxytocin levels decrease, the diuresis becomes more pronounced, with up to 3000 mL of urine excreted per 24 hours on the second through fifth days after delivery.[38,66,101] A normal voiding for the postpartum woman may be 500 to 1000 mL, several times greater than a nonpostpartum individual. Water may also be lost via night sweats.

Women with preeclampsia may become hypervolemic during the postpartum period as water accumulated in the interstitial space returns to the vascular compartment. If the woman's renal function remains impaired, the normal diuresis may be delayed. She may be unable to rapidly excrete this increased fluid volume and in rare cases may develop congestive heart failure or pulmonary edema.

The alterations in tone of the ureters and bladder during pregnancy do not permanently impair function of these structures in most women unless damage from infection has incurred.[21,102,113] Morphologic changes in the urinary tract may last 3 to 4 months.[66,113] In many women the dilation of the bladder, ureters, and renal pelvis has decreased significantly by the end of the first week, although the potential for distensibility of these structures may persist for several months. In most women these structures return to their nonpregnant state by 6 to 8 weeks; in some women these changes may persist for 12 to 16 weeks or longer.[40,66] In up to 10% of women, the anatomic changes in the ureters and bladder persist.[129]

The decreased tone, edema, and mucosal hyperemia of the bladder can be aggravated immediately postpartum by prolonged labor, forceps delivery, analgesia, or anesthesia.[21] These events may also lead to submucosal hemorrhages. Pressure of the fetal head on the bladder during labor can result in trauma and transient loss of bladder sensation in the first few days or weeks postpartum. This can lead to overdistention of the bladder, with incomplete emptying (in about 20%) and an inability to void.[129] Stress incontinence is also seen postpartum, although it usually develops before delivery.[152] Altered sphincter tone may increase the frequency of incontinence with events such as coughing.

Decreased urine flow rates are seen after vaginal delivery, with an increased voided volume, total flow time, and time to peak flow on the first day postpartum returning to non-pregnant levels by 2 to 3 days.[128] Urinary retention is reported in 1.7% to 17.9% of women and is more common after the first vaginal delivery, epidural anesthesia, and catheterization before delivery.[134] Retention is a result of the continuing bladder hypotonia after delivery without the weight of the pregnant uterus to limit its capacity.[134]

CLINICAL IMPLICATIONS FOR THE PREGNANT WOMAN AND HER FETUS

Changes in the renal system and fluid and electrolyte homeostasis during pregnancy are associated with events such as urinary frequency, nocturia, dependent edema, and an inability to void postpartum that are experienced by many pregnant women. These events are usually not pathologic but can be annoying and are often amenable to nursing interventions. However, renal changes are also associated with an increased risk of pathologic events such as UTI and pyelonephritis and can interfere with the recognition and evaluation of renal disease during pregnancy. In addition, renal system changes interact with or are aggravated by preeclampsia and other renal and hypertensive disorders.

Urinary Frequency, Incontinence, and Nocturia

Urinary frequency (more than 7 daytime voidings) occurs in about 60% of women.[106] Urinary frequency is progressive and maximum at term.[152] Frequency begins in the first trimester before the uterus is large enough to put significant pressure on the bladder.[152] Throughout most of pregnancy, urinary frequency is primarily due to the effects of hormonal changes, hypervolemia, and the increased RBF and GFR.[53,152] Pressure of the pregnant uterus probably influences urinary frequency during the third trimester. Alterations in bladder sensation postpartum can lead to overdistention with incomplete emptying and overflow incontinence.[21]

During pregnancy, 30% to 50% of women (versus about 8% of nonpregnant women) experience incontinence.[106] Urinary incontinence can begin in any trimester, but once it begins, an increase in severity until delivery is noted.[106,142,152] An increase is seen in both stress incontinence and urge incontinence.[53] Stress incontinence is reported in up to 41% of pregnant women, urge incontinence in 3% to 15%.[53,55] Urinary incontinence regresses after delivery in the majority of women, but often returns in subsequent pregnancies.[106] Onset of stress incontinence after delivery is associated with continued symptoms at 1 year postpartum in 24% of women.[55]

Nocturia results from increased sodium excretion, with an obligatory, concomitant loss of water. During the day, water and sodium are trapped in the lower extremities because of venous stasis and pressure of the uterus on the iliac vein and inferior vena cava. At night, when the pregnant woman lies down, pressure on the iliac vein and inferior vena cava is reduced, promoting increased venous return, cardiac output, RBF, and glomerular filtration with subsequent increase in urine output. However, since pregnant women excrete large amounts of sodium at night, diurnal differences in sodium, and therefore water, excretion may be the primary cause of nocturia.[53,106] Nursing interventions for women experiencing urinary frequency and nocturia are summarized in Table 11-5.

Dependent Edema

Dependent edema is seen in up to 70% of pregnant women and is more common as pregnancy progresses.[41] Edema is more common in obese women and is associated with larger babies.[41] The forces resulting in the movement of fluid out of the vascular space include capillary hydrostatic pressure and colloid osmotic (plasma oncotic) pressure, which is generated primarily by albumin.[41] Compression of the iliac vein and inferior vena cava by the growing uterus increases capillary hydrostatic pressure below the uterus, with filtration of fluid into the interstitial spaces of the lower extremities. The net reduction in plasma albumin during pregnancy reduces plasma colloid osmotic pressure, interfering with return of fluid to the vascular compartment. However, Theunissen and colleagues suggest that the increased interstitial fluid is not due to the decreased plasma oncotic pressure, because interstitial oncotic pressure is reduced to an even greater degree by increased flow of protein into the lymphatic system to maintain the transcapillary osmotic gradient.[151] They suggest the basis of the edema is alterations in capillary permeability and changes in interstitial ground substance. These changes reduce the margin of safety against edema, but increase the margin of safety for vascular engorgement and provide a transcapillary pool of fluid that can be mobilized with delivery.[151]

Dependent edema is more likely to develop in women who are in supine or upright positions for prolonged periods. The development of edema in pregnancy is associated with the amount of water accumulation in maternal tissues. Women with no visible edema have an accumulation of approximately 1.5 L. Pedal edema is associated with an accumulation of 2 L or more; women with generalized edema have accumulated 4 to 5 L or more of water. Edema in the lower legs increases the risk of varicosities and thromboembolic complications (see Chapter 8). Nursing interventions are summarized in Table 11-5 and include leg elevation, increased fluids, activity changes, and water immersion.[41] Leg elevation uses gravity to decrease capillary hydrostatic pressure and thus reabsorption of interstitial fluid into the vascular space.[41] Water immersion also changes hydrostatic pressure to help move water back into the vascular space. Increased urine flow and diuresis are noted after immersion.

Effects of Position on Renal Function

Position can markedly alter renal function during pregnancy, especially during the third trimester. These postural effects are magnified in women with preeclampsia and hypertension. As pregnancy progresses, there is pooling of blood in

Table 11-5 Nursing Interventions for Common Problems during Pregnancy Related to the Renal System

PROBLEM	NURSING INTERVENTIONS
Urinary frequency	Restrict fluids in evening. Ensure adequate intake over 24-hour period. Encourage to void when there is sensation to reduce accumulation of urine. Limit intake of natural diuretics (e.g., coffee, tea, cola with caffeine). Teach the mother signs of urinary tract infection.
Nocturia	Use the left lateral recumbent position in the evening to promote diuresis. Reduce fluid intake in evening. Ensure adequate fluid intake over 24-hour period. Avoid coffee, tea, and cola with caffeine in the evening.
Dependent edema	Avoid the supine position. Avoid the upright position for extended periods. Rest in the left lateral recumbent position with legs slightly elevated. Elevate the legs and feet at regular intervals and when sitting. Use water immersion. Use support hose or elastic stockings. Avoid tight clothing on lower extremities (e.g., tight pants, socks, girdles, garter belts, knee-high stockings). Engage in regular exercise. Restrict intake of high-salt foods and beverages. Assess for signs of preeclampsia (e.g., increased blood pressure, proteinuria, generalized edema).
Inability to void postpartum	Assess for bladder distention and urine retention. Promote adequate hydration. Promote early ambulation. Provide privacy. Administer analgesic before voiding attempt. Place ice on perineum to reduce swelling and pain. Pour warm water over perineum. Turn on the water in the bathroom. Provide fluid during the voiding attempt.
Risk of urinary tract infection	Screen urine culture on initial prenatal visit. Encourage use of the left lateral position to maximize renal output and urine flow. Teach perineal hygiene. Encourage adequate fluid intake.

the pelvis and lower extremities while sitting, lying supine, or standing. The pooling of blood leads to a relative hypovolemia and decreased cardiac output. In order to compensate and maintain adequate perfusion of vital organs such as the heart and brain, blood vessels supplying less vital organs such as the kidneys are constricted.[22] Renal plasma flow is maximal in the left lateral position.[113]

During the second half of pregnancy, the supine and upright positions are associated with a reduction in GFR and in urine output.[113] As a result, pregnant women excrete water poorly and have a reduced urine volume when lying supine and, to a lesser extent, when upright.[113] For example, renal excretion of a water load while in the supine position may be decreased by 40% in late pregnancy. Water excretion is enhanced by the lateral recumbent position. However, this position interferes with the ability of the woman to concentrate urine, possibly because of mobilization of fluid from the lower extremities with increased intravascular volume and subsequent suppression of AVP.

Renal handling of sodium is also affected by postural changes. Moving from a lateral recumbent to a supine or sitting position is associated with sodium retention and, in some cases, with an increase in plasma renin and aldosterone levels.[163] Sodium excretion may be decreased in the supine and upright positions. This sodium retention is associated with weight gain and occasional ankle swelling that comes and goes rapidly depending on the woman's activity patterns and position and does not necessarily indicate pathology. Therefore in evaluating sudden weight gain and edema in the extremities during pregnancy, data regarding recent activity patterns are essential.

Inability to Void Postpartum

Postpartum urinary retention is defined as the "lack of spontaneous micturition 6 hours after a vaginal delivery or removal of an indwelling catheter."[53] Urinary retention is reported in 0.45% to 17.9% of postpartum women, with an increased risk after first labors, instrument delivery, cesarean birth, epidurals, labor longer than 13 to 14 hours, and perineal lacerations.[53] Immediately after delivery, the woman has a hypertonic bladder with an increased capacity and decreased sensation, leading to incomplete emptying. Women should void within 6 to 8 hours of delivery. Some women experience an inability to void after delivery, which is related to the following factors: (1) trauma to the bladder from pressure of the presenting part during labor, with transient loss of bladder sensation; (2) edema of the urethra, vulva, and meatus and spasm of the sphincter from the forces of delivery; (3) decreased intraabdominal pressure immediately postpartum due to continuing distention of the abdominal wall; (4) decreased sensation of the bladder due to regional anesthesia and catheter use; and (5) hematomas of the genital tract.[101] Nursing interventions are summarized in Table 11-5.

Risk of Urinary Tract Infection

UTI occurs with increased frequency during pregnancy and is related to anatomic changes in the renal system. Asymptomatic bacteriuria (ASB) occurs in 2% to 10% of pregnant women, which is similar to rates in sexually active nonpregnant women.[106,162] However, during pregnancy, 12.5% to 30% of women with untreated ASB develop pyelonephritis.[162]

Dilation of the urinary tract, along with partial obstruction of the ureters from ureteral compression at the pelvic brim, results in urinary stasis. Large volumes of urine may be sequestered in the ureters and hypotonic bladder during pregnancy. These static pools increase the risk of ASB, especially because the urine may contain glucose, protein, and amino acids, which provide additional substrates for bacterial growth. Edema and hyperemia of the bladder mucosa also increase susceptibility to infection. The static column of urine in the hypoactive ureters also facilitates ascending bacterial migration, increasing the risk of pyelonephritis.[106] Women with sickle cell anemia and trait are at higher risk for UTI. UTI has been associated with preterm labor (see Chapters 4 and 13).[162]

UTIs are also more common during the postpartum period. Factors that increase the risk of UTIs postpartum include pregnancy-induced changes in the bladder (hypotonia, edema, and mucosal hyperemia) that may be aggravated by the trauma of labor and delivery. Decreased bladder sensation from pressure of the fetal head during labor leads to incomplete emptying and urinary stasis, further predisposing to UTI for the first few postpartum weeks. Recommendations to reduce the risk of UTI during pregnancy and the postpartum period are summarized in Table 11-5.

Fluid Needs in Labor

Fluid needs of women in labor are controversial; the routine use of intravenous (IV) infusions has been questioned and even discontinued in some practices.[82,98,119,155] Before use of general anesthesia for delivery, food and fluid intake was maintained during labor. With introduction of general anesthesia, food and fluid were prohibited and IV administration of fluids and glucose became routine to provide fluid and calories to prevent dehydration and ketosis.[98,100,155] Routine IV use has continued in many settings even with the decline in use of general anesthesia. There is little documentation supporting either the benefits of this therapy or the risk of oral intake for most women.[87,122,143,155] A recent Cochrane review of 5 studies (n=3130) found no benefit or harm of oral fluids in labor and concluded that "there is no justification for the restriction of fluids and food in labor for women at low risk for complications."[14] Current guidelines from professional groups support oral intake during labor in low-risk women.[7,8,84]

IV infusions may be needed for anesthesia or medication administration and must be carefully monitored. However, there is little evidence to support routine use of IV infusions in otherwise healthy women not receiving these agents. O'Sullivan notes the following: "Intravenous therapy is seldom necessary during the first 12 hours of labor, irrespective of the finding of ketonuria; when it is prescribed, the indication for its use should be clearly documented and fluid balance charts should be meticulously maintained. In fact, the judicious use of oral fluids should mitigate the need for intravenous fluids in many patients."[124,p.39] In addition, it may be harder for the woman to change her position during IV therapy, leading to increased use of the supine position. IV therapy is also linked to increased use of medications because there is an accessible line.[82] Volume loading with colloids prior to or during can blunt the hemodynamic alterations with spinal anesthesia in pregnant women.[37,140] Crystalloids administered 20 to 30 minutes before spinal anesthesia have been found to have no advantage over administration during the preocedure.[150] Complications such as infection, phlebitis, hyponatremia, and fluid overload can occur with IV therapy.[87,119]

Acute hydration can lead to hypervolemia, with a greater risk in pregnant women who already have expanded body water and plasma volume. The use of hypertonic glucose infusions can lead to elevations in maternal blood glucose, which can in turn result in fetal hyperglycemia and hyperinsulinemia and eventually neonatal hypoglycemia.[19,82,98,112,119,121,155] Lower cord blood sodium values and increased neonatal weight loss in the first 48 hours have been reported following the administration of 5% dextrose solutions to laboring women.[38]

Although rare, the pregnant woman is at increased risk for water intoxication.[111] Oxytocin infusions have been associated with water intoxication and maternal and fetal hyponatremia.[87,111] The risk of water intoxication is increased when oxytocin is administered with large volumes of hypertonic dextrose solution.[87,111] The hypertonic solution pulls fluid into the vascular compartment from the interstitial space, resulting in hemodilution. However, the additional fluid cannot be readily excreted due to the antidiuretic effects of oxytocin. Water intoxication results in electrolyte imbalances such as hyponatremia, which can affect both mother and fetus and in severe cases can lead to seizures and hypoxia.[19,87,121] Thus not only must oxytocin infusions be carefully monitored, but maternal electrolyte and fluid status and urine output must also be carefully evaluated for any woman receiving this type of infusion.

Maternal-Fetal Fluid and Electrolyte Homeostasis

Fetal fluid and electrolyte balance is dependent on maternal homeostasis and placental function. Because serum osmolarity is similar in the fetus and the mother, changes in maternal or fetal osmolarity will lead to transfer of water from the opposite compartment to achieve homeostasis. Water is continuously exchanged between mother and fetus, with a net flux in favor of the fetus, placenta, and amniotic fluid. Factors that influence the rate and direction of water exchange between the mother and the fetus include maternal and fetal blood flow to and from the placenta, osmotic and hydrostatic pressure gradients across the placenta, and availability of cellular transport mechanisms.[91]

Fetal balance is affected by any maternal or fetal conditions that alter the supply, demand, and transfer of water. Maternal events such as altered nutrition, electrolyte imbalance, diabetes, hypertension, or the excessive use of diuretics are associated with alterations in fetal fluid and electrolyte status, amniotic fluid volume, and fetal growth.[24] For example, fetal urine flow can be increased by volume loading of maternal blood or administration of diuretics, because acute changes in maternal plasma osmolarity induce parallel changes in the fetus due to transplacental movement of fluid, with decreased urine flow and increased AVP.[24] In addition, because fetal free water is derived from the mother, net movement of water to the fetus is decreased when maternal osmolarity increases; this leads to decreased fetal urine flow and increased tubular reabsorption of water. The fluid and electrolyte status of the infant reflects maternal balance during labor.[151] A reduction in fetal plasma volume with increased fetal osmolarity occurs in most infants during labor. These changes are more pronounced following prolonged labor, with administration of hyperosmolar glucose solutions to the mother, or during fetal hypoxia because fluid is redistributed from the extracellular fluid (ECF) to intracellular fluid (ICF) compartments. Maternal electrolyte imbalances result in similar alterations in the fetus. Administration of hypotonic fluid to the mother can, by increasing the maternal ECF volume, lead to decreases in fetal osmotic pressure and serum sodium and has resulted in maternal and neonatal hyponatremia and an increased risk of neonatal complications.[49] If this therapy is used, the fluid and electrolyte status of both mother and newborn infant must be carefully monitored.

Evaluation of Renal Function During Pregnancy

The marked increase in GFR during pregnancy significantly reduces serum blood urea nitrogen (BUN), plasma urea, uric acid, and creatinine by the end of the first trimester. As a result, values that are normal for nonpregnant individuals may actually be elevations for the pregnant woman and reflect pathologic alterations in renal function. Thus it is critical for health care providers to know the normal values for these parameters during pregnancy (see Table 11-2) so that early signs of renal impairment are not missed. In a pregnant woman, serum creatinine decreases in each trimester an average 0.5 mg/dL versus nonpregnant values of 0.80 mg/dL.[78] Serum creatinine levels greater than 0.80 mg per 100 mL, plasma urea nitrogen levels greater than 14 mg per 100 mL (6 mmol/L), or plasma BUN and creatinine levels that do not decrease to expected values by mid-gestation may indicate a significant reduction in renal function and require further investigation.[40,66,162,163]

GFR is best measured by endogenous creatinine clearance (C_{cr}) during pregnancy as other measures have been demonstrated to underestimate GFR.[68,145] The 24-hour C_{cr} is generally a good index of GFR in both pregnant and nonpregnant women but is less valid in women with severe renal impairment or diminished urine production.[91] In the latter case, the amount of creatinine secreted by the proximal tubule can markedly alter urinary creatinine values.[40] The C_{cr} rises approximately 45% by 4 weeks postconception and remains elevated to or near term, when it may begin to fall.[40,91]

Dilation of the urinary tract with stasis and retention of large volumes of urine can lead to collection errors. Accuracy of clearance measures in pregnancy can be improved by using 24-hour collections to avoid "washout" from diurnal changes in urine flow, ensuring that the woman is well hydrated to ensure a high urine flow rate, discarding the first morning specimen, and having the woman assume a lateral recumbent position for 1 hour before the start and 1 hour before the end of the collection. Dietary intake has to be evaluated in the timing of blood samples during a clearance period in that recent ingestion of cooked meat can increase plasma creatinine levels up to 0.18 mg per 100 mL (1.59 μmol/L). Plasma creatinine levels, used to estimate GFR, are influenced by age, height, weight, and gender. In the pregnant woman, body size and weight may not accurately reflect kidney size.[40]

Interpretation of diagnostic studies such as ultrasound or IV pyelography in the pregnant woman must be done in light of the normal structural changes.[162] Because structural changes in the urinary system may persist for several months after delivery, these alterations also need to be considered when evaluating postpartum renal function. Evaluation of renal function is considered if the GFR during the postpartum period decreases more than 25% to 30% from predelivery values or if the serum creatinine rises above nonpregnant levels.[18]

Glycosuria

Chemically detectable glycosuria is found in more than 50% of pregnant women.[5,28,163] Glucose excretion may be 10 to 100 times greater than the nonpregnant levels of 20 to 100 mg per 24 hours.[113] About 70% of pregnant women excrete more than 100 mg of glucose per 24 hours; in up to 50%, glucose excretion is greater than 150 mg per 24 hours.[18,40,163] Large day-to-day variation in glucose excretion is reported, with little correlation between excretion rate, plasma glucose levels, and the stage of pregnancy.[40,163] Few women with glycosuria have abnormal glucose tolerance test results. Thus glycosuria in pregnancy does not reflect alterations in carbohydrate metabolism but rather alterations in renal function.[113,163]

The basis for glycosuria in pregnancy is secondary to the increases in GFR and tubular flow rate that exceeds the maximal tubular reabsorptive capacity for glucose (200 to 240 mg/dL).[5,78,113] As the GFR increases during pregnancy, renal reabsorptive capacity for glucose also increases but not to the same extent. Thus as the filtered load of glucose increases, more glucose is excreted, leading to glycosuria at normal plasma glucose levels.[163] When glucose excretion increases, alterations in reabsorption seem to occur primarily in that portion of the glucose load that escapes reabsorption in the proximal tubules (usually 5% of the filtered glucose) and is normally reabsorbed in the loops of Henle and collecting duct.[40,78,113]

Glycosuria during pregnancy has not been associated with alterations in perinatal mortality or morbidity or with subsequent development of diabetes or renal disorders.[5,28] However, Davison suggests that women with greater than the usual degree of glycosuria during pregnancy may have sustained renal tubular damage from earlier untreated UTIs.[40] How this alters renal handling of glucose is unclear. Infection is known to cause a temporary impairment of distal tubular function. In some women, sites for glucose reabsorption may not be completely healed and thus are unable to deal with the stresses imposed by the increased filtered load of glucose during pregnancy.

Because of the high incidence of glycosuria in normal pregnant women, glycosuria is not useful in screening for pregnancy-related glucose intolerance.[78] In addition, urinary glucose may not be a reliable indicator of plasma glucose control in pregnant diabetics, thus decreasing the usefulness of urinary glucose concentrations for monitoring these women.[40] In the pregnant diabetic, any elevation of blood glucose results in a greater urinary loss of glucose than in the nonpregnant state. Because water and electrolytes are normally lost along with glucose, volume depletion and polydipsia occur sooner in the pregnant than in the nonpregnant diabetic woman (see Chapter 16).

Hypertension and the Renal System

The kidneys play a critical role in the regulation of blood pressure; therefore alterations in renal function often lead to hypertension. During the perinatal period, renal disorders associated with hypertension often have a poorer outcome for both mother and infant. Preeclampsia involves specific lesions and functional alterations in the renal system (see Table 9-5). The renal lesion usually seen in preeclampsia is glomerular capillary endotheliosis, which decreases the diameter of the glomerular capillary lumina, resulting in decreased GFR and RPF.[68,86] In women with preeclampsia, GFR and RPF are decreased from values seen in healthy pregnant women.[86] The renin-angiotensin-aldosterone system is altered in preeclampsia (see p. 362). An exaggerated response to ANTII, which antedates the onset of clinically detectable hypertension, has also been noted in women with preeclampsia.[148] Sodium excretion is reduced in these women due to the decreased GFR, increased vascular resistance, decreased RPF (with decreased perfusion of the peritubular capillaries), alterations in plasma and blood volume, and possibly inadequate tubular reabsorptive mechanisms.[68,76,77] Further discussion of vascular changes associated with pregnancy, preeclampsia, and the impact of preeclampsia and chronic hypertension can be found in Chapter 9.

Renal Disease and Pregnancy

Regardless of the specific disorder, as the severity of renal disease and reduction in renal function increase, the ability to conceive and sustain a pregnancy also decreases.[39,40,125,162] In general, normotensive women with mild renal disease before pregnancy do well during pregnancy, although the risk of preeclampsia, preterm birth and fetal growth restriction increases, and their renal prognosis is not significantly altered by pregnancy.[125,145] Women with moderate to severe disease have a greater risk of worsening renal function, hypertension, preeclampsia, preterm birth, or other pregnancy complications.[125,145,162] A normal pregnancy is rare if, before conception, the woman has a plasma creatinine greater than 2.5 mg/dL (220 μmol/L) or a urea nitrogen above 30 mg/dL (10.72 mmol/L).[125] Table 11-6 summarizes the effects of pregnancy on chronic renal problems. Management of women with chronic renal problems includes careful monitoring of maternal functional status and signs of increasing severity of the disease and fetal assessment.

Pregnancy Following Renal Transplantation

Having a transplant improves fertility within 1 to 12 months in women who have been on dialysis.[80,125,162] Many women have conceived following renal transplantation. Overall 71% to 76% of pregnancies result in a live birth.[35] Of those women who carried the pregnancy beyond the first trimester, more than 90% have had a successful pregnancy outcome, although pregnancy complications such as hypertension, preterm birth, preeclampsia, and fetal growth restriction were increased.[35,46,79,80,89,125,162] The transplanted kidney undergoes the usual renal changes seen in pregnancy. Renal hemodynamics often improve with pregnancy, but some women have impairment of renal function during pregnancy that may persist.[33,66] However, a recent review did not find any negative effects of pregnancy on either maternal survival or the transplanted kidney.[79] Pregnancy is generally not recommended for at least 1 year following transplantation in stable women to ensure that the transplant is successful and able to function under the increased demands of pregnancy.[80,104] Optimal immunosuppressant therapy during pregnancy is unknown but the woman may need to be switched to safer drugs as a few agents have been found to be associated with an increased risk of fetal anomalies.[79,125] Long-term follow-up data are still sparse, especially for the newer drugs.[162]

SUMMARY

The renal system is critical to maintenance of fluid and electrolyte homeostasis within the body. Relatively small changes in renal function can significantly alter this homeostasis, leading to a variety of volume and electrolyte disorders. Renal function and many related laboratory parameters are altered significantly during pregnancy to levels that would be of concern in a nonpregnant individual. In most cases the pregnant woman readily adapts to these changes and establishes a new equilibrium for volume and electrolyte homeostasis. At this new equilibrium, she responds to alterations in fluid and electrolyte intake in a manner similar to that of a nonpregnant individual. Pathophysiologic conditions that alter renal function or volume homeostasis affect the health of both the pregnant woman and her infant. Monitoring and health counseling related to fluid and electrolyte status are essential during pregnancy. Clinical recommendations for nurses working with pregnant women based on alterations in the renal system and fluid and electrolyte balance are summarized in Table 11-7.

Table 11-6 **Chronic Renal Disease and Pregnancy**

RENAL DISEASE	EFFECTS
Chronic glomerulonephritis and focal glomerular sclerosis (FGS)	Incidence of high blood pressure late in gestation is increased, but there is usually no adverse effect if renal function is preserved and hypertension is absent before gestation. Some disagree, believing coagulation changes in pregnancy exacerbate disease, especially immunoglobulin A (IgA) nephropathy, membranoproliferative glomerulonephritis, and FGS.
IgA nephropathy	Some cite risks of sudden escalating or uncontrolled hypertension and renal deterioration. Most note good outcome when renal function is preserved.
Chronic pyelonephritis (infectious tubular disease)	Bacteriuria occurs in pregnancy and may lead to exacerbation.
Reflux nephropathy	In the past, some emphasized risks of sudden escalating hypertension and worsening of renal function. Consensus now is that results are satisfactory when preconception function is only mildly affected and hypertension is absent. Vigilant screening for urinary tract infection is necessary.
Urolithiasis	Ureteral dilation and stasis do not seem to affect natural history, but infections can be more frequent. Stents have been successfully placed, and sonographically controlled ureterostomy has been performed during gestation.
Polycystic kidney disease	Functional impairment and hypertension usually minimal in childbearing years.
Diabetic nephropathy	There are no adverse effects of the renal lesion. Frequencies of infection, edema, and preeclampsia increase.
Systemic lupus erythematosus	Prognosis is most favorable if disease is in remission 6 or more months prior to conception. Some authorities increase steroid dosage in immediate postpartum period.
Periarteritis nodosa	Fetal prognosis is poor. Associated with maternal death. Therapeutic abortion should be considered.
Scleroderma	For onset during pregnancy, there can be rapid overall deterioration. Reactivation of quiescent scleroderma can occur during pregnancy and after delivery.
Previous urologic surgery	Depending on original reason for surgery, there may be other malformations of urogenital tract. Urinary tract infection is common during pregnancy, and renal function may undergo reversible decrease. No significant obstructive problem but cesarean section may be necessary in case of abnormal presentation or to avoid disruption of the continence mechanisms if artificial sphincters or neourethras are present.
After nephrectomy, solitary and pelvic kidneys	Pregnancy is well tolerated. Condition may be associated with other malformations of the urogenital tract. Dystocia rarely occurs with a pelvic kidney.

From Williams, D.J. & Davison, J.M. (2009). Renal disorders. In R.K. Creasy, et al. (Eds.), *Creasy & Resnik's Maternal-fetal medicine: Principles and practice* (6th ed.). Philadelphia: Saunders, p. 916.

DEVELOPMENT OF THE RENAL SYSTEM IN THE FETUS

Although functionally different, the renal and genital systems (see Chapter 1) are closely linked embryonically and anatomically. Both develop from a common ridge of mesodermal tissue and end in the cloaca. Anatomic development of the kidneys begins early in gestation, with formation of the adult number of nephrons by around 34 to 36 weeks. Urine formation begins by 9 to 10 weeks; during the second half of gestation, urine production by the fetus is a major component of amniotic fluid. Renal function does not reach levels comparable to adults until about 2 years of age.

Renal development is under the control of many genes, including *PAX-2* and *WTI*, and their protein products. These genes are differentially expressed to form transcription factors and other proteins that encode for extracellular matrix, cell adhesion, and growth factors, and cell receptor proteins (e.g., angiotensin II receptors).[30] Factors influencing nephrogenesis include glial-derived neurotrophic factor, bone morphogenetic proteins, FOXcl, Cxal, roundabout-2, fibroblast growth factors, transforming growth factor-β, insulin-like growth factors, platelet-derived growth factor, protein phosphatases, and the renin-angiotensin system.[30,102]

Anatomic Development

Development of the Kidneys

The kidneys arise from a ridge of mesodermal tissue (called the *nephrogenic cord*) that runs along the posterior wall of the abdominal cavity on either side of the primitive aorta. The kidney develops through three successive, overlapping stages. The initial steps involve formation of transient nonfunctional structures (called the *pronephros* and *mesonephros*) on either side of midline, from which the metanephros, or permanent kidney, develops. The pronephros arises in the cervical region in the third week, extends in a cranial-to-caudal direction, and then degenerates beginning in the fourth week. Each pronephros consists of 7 to 10 solid cell groups. The pronephric ducts are incorporated into the mesonephric kidneys.

The mesonephros appears late in the fourth week, forming a large ovoid organ on either side of midline next to the developing gonads in the thoracic and lumbar regions (Figure 11-4). The mesonephros and gonad form the urogenital ridge. The mesonephros consists of S-shaped tubules with glomeruli and collecting ducts that enter a common large duct. This mesonephric duct persists in the male as the wolffian duct and gives rise to the male genital ducts

Table 11-7 Recommendations for Clinical Practice Related to Changes in the Renal System and Fluid and Electrolyte Homeostasis in Pregnant Women

Recognize the usual changes in the renal system during pregnancy and postpartum (pp. 356-365 and Table 11-1).
Recognize the usual values for renal function tests and patterns of change during pregnancy and postpartum (pp. 359-360, 368 and Table 11-2).
Recognize that individual laboratory values must be evaluated in light of clinical findings and previous values (pp. 359-360, 368).
Teach women to recognize and reduce the risk of urinary tract infection during pregnancy and postpartum (pp. 366-367).
Recognize the effects of altered renal function on pharmacokinetics of drug elimination by glomerular filtration (pp. 359-360, 364 and Chapter 7).
Monitor and evaluate maternal responses to drugs for evidence of subtherapeutic doses (pp. 359-360, 364 and Chapter 7).
Assess maternal nutritional status in relation to calcium and water-soluble vitamins and provide nutritional counseling (p. 360 and Chapters 12 and 17).
Know the influences of position on renal function (pp. 365-366).
Counsel women regarding appropriate positions and activity patterns (pp. 365-366).
Assess activity patterns and position in evaluating changes in weight gain and edema (p. 365).
Monitor fluid and electrolyte status and renal function following use of general anesthetics (pp. 364, 367).
Monitor oxytocin and intravenous infusions during labor and delivery to avoid overload (pp. 364-367).
Use fluids, ice chips, and other alternatives to use of intravenous infusions with women with uncomplicated labors (p. 367).
Know the benefits and risks for the mother, fetus, and neonate of different types of intravenous fluids (pp. 367-368).
Avoid use of hypertonic solutions during labor (pp. 367-368).
Know indications for intrapartum intravenous therapy (pp. 367-368).
Monitor maternal fluid and electrolyte status and urine output (especially in women receiving an oxytocin infusion or with preeclampsia or compromised renal function) during labor for development of water intoxication (pp. 364, 367-368).
Teach women the common experiences associated with changes in the renal system (urinary frequency, dependent edema, nocturia) and implement appropriate interventions (pp. 365-367 and Table 11-5).
Monitor women with dependent edema for varicosities and thromboembolism (p. 365 and Chapter 8).
Know usual values and monitor for glycosuria and proteinuria in the pregnant woman (pp. 360, 368-369).
Monitor fluid and electrolyte status of women with preeclampsia, chronic hypertension, and diabetes, recognizing that alterations may occur more rapidly than in other pregnant women (pp. 368-369).
Monitor fluid and electrolyte status, renal function, amniotic fluid volume, and fetal growth in women on diuretics (pp. 367-368).
Counsel women with renal disorders regarding the impact of their disorder on pregnancy and of pregnancy on their disorder (p. 369 and Table 11-6).
Monitor women with chronic renal problems for signs of initiation of preterm labor, fetal growth restriction, hypertension, and alterations in maternal renal function (p. 369 and Table 11-6).
Evaluate bladder function and voiding postpartum (pp. 366, 364-365).
Implement interventions to encourage postpartum voiding (p. 366, Table 11-5).
Observe for signs of pulmonary edema and congestive heart failure post birth in women with preeclampsia and impaired renal function (p. 364).
Recognize that structural changes in the urinary system may persist for 6 months or more following birth (pp. 364-365).

(see Chapter 1). The rest of the mesonephros regresses by 8 to 10 weeks as the metanephros begins to function.[114,164]

The permanent kidneys (metanephros) arise during the fifth week from the ureteric bud at the caudal end of the mesonephric duct. Formation of the permanent kidney involves two separate, interrelated processes. The ureteric bud grows out into the surrounding mesoderm (metanephric blastema), dilates, and branches to form the ureters, renal pelvis, and collecting ducts (see Figure 11-4). Failure of this bud to arise results in renal agenesis. The number of ureteric bud branches determines the eventual number of nephrons. Usually 15 branch generations are formed, the first 9 by 15 weeks' gestational age and the reminder by 20 to 22 weeks.[102,132] These branches induce formation of the nephrons, with formation of 4 to 7 nephrons around each terminal collecting duct branch. The growth of the ureteric bud into the surrounding mesoderm induces formation of small vesicles that elongate to form primitive renal tubules (nephrons). The proximal ends of these tubules form the Bowman capsule. The distal end comes into contact with the blind ends of the collecting ducts and fuses.[114,133,164]

Nephron formation begins at about 8 weeks in the juxtamedullary area and progresses toward the cortex. Induction of nephron formation involves the release of a cascade of gene transcription factors and signaling molecules.[102] Nephron formation is illustrated in Figure 11-5.

By 20 to 22 weeks, branching of the collecting ducts is complete and one third of the nephrons have been formed. Nephrons continue to develop until 34 to 35 weeks, when adult numbers of nephrons are reached.[132,159] Nephron development continues in the preterm infant born before 35 weeks' gestation until the infant reaches 34 to 35 weeks' postconceptional age. Maturation and hypertrophy of the nephrons continue into infancy with growth of glomeruli and tubules.[83,114] Renal vascularization parallels nephrogenesis.[60]

Initially the kidneys are in the pelvic area. With straightening of the embryo and growth of the sacral and lumbar areas, the kidneys undergo a series of positional changes and migrate upward. During this process, the kidneys rotate 90 degrees so that the renal pelvises face midline.[164] Failure of the kidneys to ascend leads to pelvic kidneys. Abnormal ascent and rotation can result in configurations such as

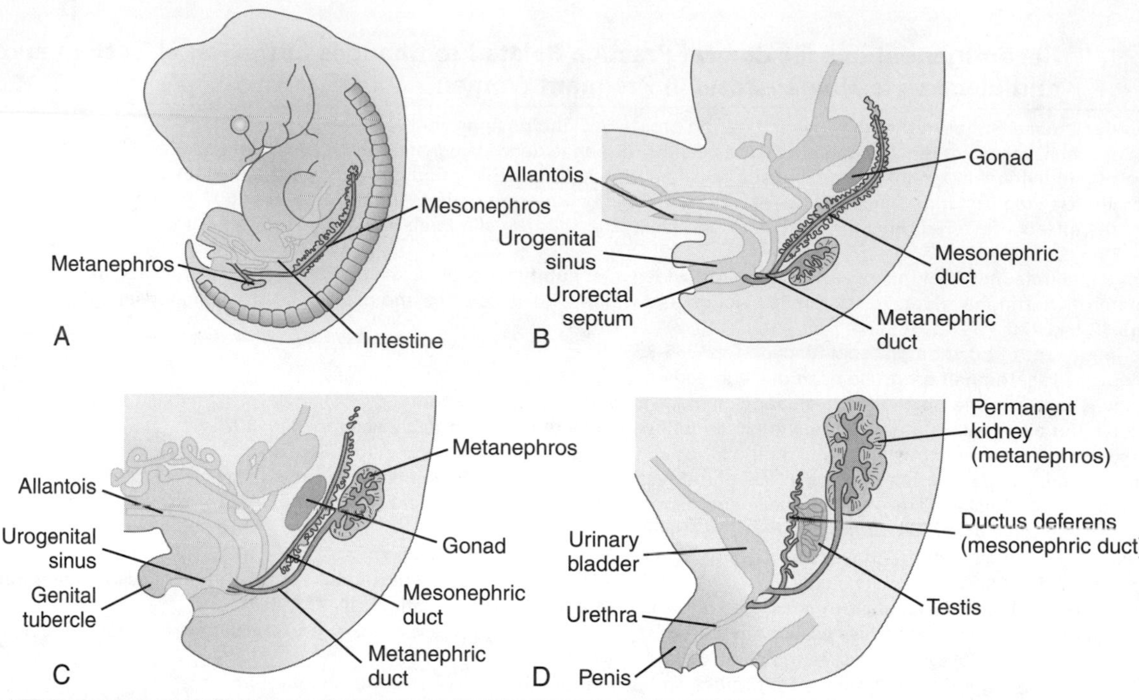

FIGURE 11-4 Formation of the kidneys. **A**, At 6 weeks; **B**, at 7 weeks; **C**, at 8 weeks; **D**, at 3 months (male). (From Carlson, B.M. [2004]. *Human embryology and developmental biology* [3rd ed.]. St. Louis: Mosby, p. 395.)

horseshoe-shaped kidneys (in which the caudal ends of the kidneys are pushed together and fuse).

Development of the Urinary System

The urinary system develops following division of the cloaca. The cloaca is the dilated end of the hindgut and is involved in the development of the terminal portions of the genital (see Chapter 1), urinary, and gastrointestinal (see Chapter 12) systems. Downward growth of the urorectal septum at 5 to 6 weeks divides the cloaca into the posterior anorectal canal and anterior primitive urogenital sinus (see Figure 11-4, *C*). The upper and largest part of the urogenital sinus becomes the bladder and is initially continuous with the allantois. The allantois eventually becomes a thick fibrous cord (the urachus, or median umbilical ligament). The ureters are incorporated into the bladder wall. The urethra develops from the lower urogenital sinus along with portions of the external genitalia.[114,164] Bladder capacity increases from 10 mL at 32 weeks to 40 mL by term.[59]

Developmental Basis for Common Anomalies

Alterations in renal function in adults may be due to altered programming during renal development by poor maternal nutrition, decreased placental blood flow, and epigenetic changes.[103] Fetal or neonatal insults can also alter nephrogenesis and programming of the kidney.[83,131] Preterm infants and infants with fetal growth restriction have fewer glomeruli and smaller kidneys at birth with impaired growth into early childhood and an increased risk of later hypertension and renal disease.[15,83,131,136] These changes may be due to poor maternal nutrition, chronic fetal hypoxemia, or increased maternal glucocorticoids and altered intrauterine nutrient availability (which suppresses the renin-angiotensin-aldosterone system and alters sodium transport), and endothelial dysfunction.[13] Other factors that may alter renal development include maternal hyperglycemia, alterations in the renin-angiotensin system, decreased vitamin A availability, and pharmacologic agents.[88,105]

Major malformations of the renal system and urinary tract can be divided into three broad categories: agenesis-dysplasia of the renal system, polycystic kidneys, and malformations of the lower urinary tract. Several events are critical for the normal development of the kidneys. If the ureteric bud does not arise from the end of the mesonephric duct or if the ureteric bud does not induce formation of the renal cortex and nephrons, unilateral or bilateral renal agenesis, aplasia, or hypoplasia results. If the ureteric bud splits early or if two buds arise on one side, there may be duplication of the kidneys or ureters. Renal agenesis and hypoplasia are often associated with oligohydramnios. The marked decrease in amniotic fluid with bilateral renal agenesis, as occurs in Potter sequence, is thought to result in adverse effects on extrarenal fetal development (see Chapter 3).[49]

Increased use of routine fetal ultrasound has resulted in more fetuses being identified with hydronephrosis with an incidence of 1:100 to 1:500.[17] The significance of this finding is controversial.[17] Mild unilateral dilation of the renal pelvis, without any renal or urinary tract abnormalities, is usually

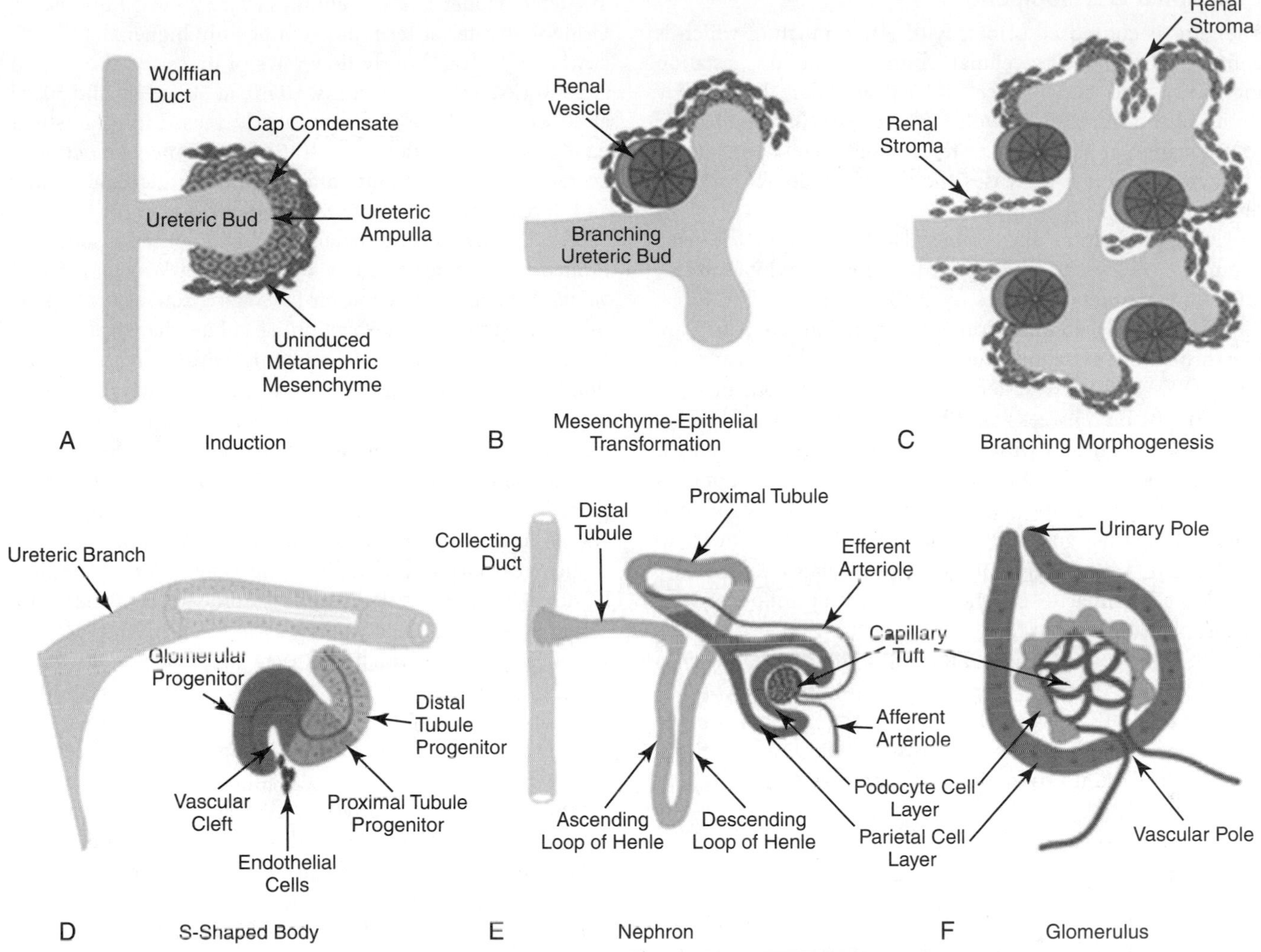

FIGURE 11-5 Stages of kidney formation. (**a**) Induction of the metanephric mesenchyme by the ureteric bud promotes aggregation of mesonephric cells around the tip of the ureteric bud. (**b**) Polarized renal vesicles are formed next. (**c**) Stromal cells secrete factors that influence nephrogenesis and branching morphogenesis. (**d**) Formation of S-shaped body involves the formation of a proximal cleft that is invaded by angioblasts. (**e**) Complete nephron joined to collecting duct. (**f**) Glomerulus demonstrating organization of the capillary tuft, podocytes, and parietal cells. (From Rosenblum, N.D. [2008]. Developmental biology of the human kidney. *Semin Fetal Neonatal Med, 13*, 125.)

transient and secondary to a larger renal pelvic area and an increased urine flow rate.[17,45] Thirty percent to 80% of these infants have a normal postnatal renal appearance.

Polycystic kidneys are a heterogeneous group of disorders that arise from environmental and genetic causes. The specific embryologic basis for these defects is unknown. Theories that have been proposed include (1) failure of the collecting ducts to develop, with subsequent cystic degeneration; (2) failure of the developing nephrons to unite with the collecting tubules; (3) persistence of remnants of early rudimentary nephrons, which normally degenerate but instead remain and form cysts; and (4) secondary to a concomitant urinary tract obstruction with urine retention leading to cyst formation in the nephrogenic area.[114] The latter theory has been proposed as a possible cause of adult-onset polycystic kidneys.

Malformations of the lower urinary tract include obstructive uropathy and exstrophy. Obstructive uropathy arises from obstructions at the ureteropelvic junction due to adhesions, aberrant blood vessels, or strictures, or in the urethra from posterior urethral valves. Severe forms result in fetal renal damage from hydronephrosis. Anomalies of other systems may occur secondary to oligohydramnios (see Chapter 3). Percutaneous placement of a diverting shunt into the fetal bladder to drain urine into amniotic fluid has been used to promote drainage of the urinary tract and prevent irreversible renal damage before birth.[102] The effectiveness of this therapy is currently being evaluated in a multicenter randomized controlled trial.[116] Exstrophy of the bladder arises from incomplete midline closure of the inferior part of the anterior abdominal wall, with concurrent abnormalities in the mesoderm of the bladder wall.[114]

Functional Development

The fetus is composed primarily of water, much of which is contained in the extracellular compartment. As gestation increases, total body water and extracellular fluid slowly decrease and intracellular volume increases (Figure 11-6).[126] Maintenance of this high water content may be mediated by prolactin, which increases the water binding capacity of fetal cells.

Urine production and glomerular filtration in the fetus begin at 9 to 10 weeks; the loop of Henle functions by 14 weeks, and tubular function begins by 9 to 12 weeks.[30,56,130] Renal blood flow (RBF) and the glomerular filtration rate (GFR) are low throughout gestation, due to the high renal vascular resistance (RVR) and low systemic blood pressure, but increase between 20 and 35 weeks and then level off to birth.[30,56] This increase is concurrent with increases in numbers and growth of nephrons. In adults, 20% to 25% of the cardiac output goes to the kidneys. In the fetus, 40% to 50% of the combined ventricular output goes to the placenta and only 2% to 7% to the kidneys.[48] Fetal fluid and electrolyte balance is therefore maintained primarily by the placenta and influenced by maternal balance.

Although fetal RBF and GFR are low, this does not lead to low fetal urine output.[49] Fetal urine is an important component for amniotic fluid production, and the primary component of amniotic fluid after 18 weeks.[130,159] Fetal urine output and amniotic fluid production both increase with gestation.

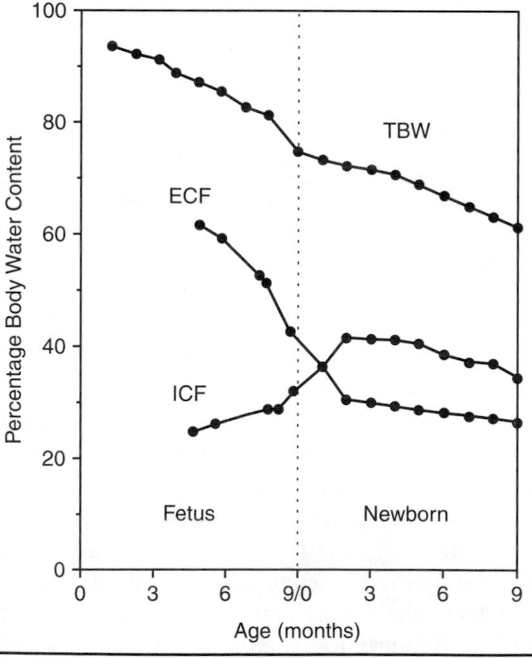

FIGURE 11-6 Total body water (TBW) content and fluid distribution between intracellular fluid (ICF) and extracellular fluid (ECF) compartments in humans during the fetal and neonatal periods and during the first 9 months after birth. (From Brace, R.A. [1998]. Fluid distribution in the fetus and neonate. In R.A. Polin, W.W. Fox, & S.H. Abman [Eds.], *Fetal and neonatal physiology* [3rd ed.]. Philadelphia: Saunders, p. 1342.)

The fetal bladder fills and empties every 20 to 30 minutes.[130] Urine flow rates at term are significantly higher than in the newborn.[17] Mean hourly flow rates of urine are about 2 mL at 20 weeks, 5 mL at 10 weeks, 10 mL at 30 weeks, and 30 mL at 40 weeks.[59] Urine flow rates are decreased in infants with fetal growth restriction.[18] Alterations in urine production or excretion can significantly alter both amniotic fluid volume and development of other systems (see Chapter 3).

Fetal ability to concentrate urine and conserve sodium is limited, with a concentrating ability about 20% to 30% of adult values. Fetal urine is hypotonic (averaging 200 mOsm/kg) due to greater tubular reabsorption of solute than water.[30,59,117] Fetal urine becomes less hypotonic with increasing gestation.[159] The major solute in fetal urine is sodium, decreasing from 120 mEq/L (mmol/L) at 16 weeks to 50 mEq/L (mmol/L) from 24 to 40 weeks. The fetus is not dependent on the kidneys for sodium conservation in that sodium is readily trans ported across the placenta. The expanded extracellular fluid (ECF) compartment of the fetus may stimulate decreased tubular reabsorption of sodium and water. During the third trimester, fetal urine may become isotonic with plasma during severe stress.[24] The fetal kidney is less sensitive to arginine vasopressin (AVP), which is present by 12 weeks, possibly as a result of immaturity of AVP receptors or presence of antagonists such as prostaglandins.[93,159,164] Osmoreceptors and volume receptors in the fetus stimulate prolonged secretion of AVP from about 26 weeks' gestation.

The renin-angiotensin system (see Figure 11-3 and Box 11-2 on 362) is active in the fetus, with increased renal and extrarenal production of all components. An intact renin-angiotensin system is necessary for normal development and fetoplacental circulation.[6,57,60,69,76] Angiotensin II (ANTII) acts as a growth modulator and renal growth factor.[4,30,76] Angiotensin type 2 (AT_2) receptors are denser early in development; later in gestation, both AT_2 and angiotensin type 1 (AT_1) receptors increase in the fetus. Both types of receptors are also found in the placenta. After birth the density of AT_2 (but not AT_1) receptors decreases.[4,6,69,76] Therefore it is thought that AT_2 receptors regulate morphogenesis, whereas AT_1 may be important in later neurovascular development.[4,69,76,94,154] Blocking of AT receptors in developing animals leads to congenital anomalies of the kidneys and urinary tract.[146] Exposure to angiotensin-converting enzyme (ACE) inhibitors is associated with altered renal hemodynamics and development.[60]

Angiotensinogen is produced in the yolk sac and found in the immature renal tubule by 30 days. Renin is found by 4 to 6 weeks in the mesonephros and by 8 weeks in the metanephros.[69] Renin concentration and activity are both elevated in the fetus, decreasing to term but still higher than adult levels. The juxtamedullary cells produce increasing amounts of renin from the third month of gestation. Renal responsiveness to aldosterone is decreased in the fetus, which may lead to increased sodium loss. Endothelial cells lining the villous capillaries and the cells of the trophoblast are rich in ACE; the fetal membranes and amniotic fluid contain large amounts of renin. ACE is found by 30 days, primarily in the proximal tubules. The chorion also produces renin and angiotensinogen.[148] Placental circulation is a major site for conversion of angiotensin I to ANTII (similar to processes in the pulmonary circulation after birth), which is involved in control of placental blood flow in the fetus. The increased ANTII appears important in modulating fetal blood pressure and renal hemodynamics, especially at birth.[146]

During the last 20 weeks of gestation, the weight of the kidney increases in a linear relationship to gestational age, body weight, and body surface area. Before 5 months, renal growth occurs primarily in the inner medullary area, which contains mostly collecting ducts. From 5 to 9 months, major growth is in the cortex and outer medullary areas. After birth, nephron growth occurs primarily in the tubules and the loop of Henle. At birth, approximately 20% of the infant's loops of Henle are too short to reach into the medulla, which can lead to problems in concentrating urine. The rate of tubular growth after birth is reflected in changes in glomerular-to-tubular surface area. This ratio is 27:1 at birth, 8:1 by 6 months, and 3:1 in adults.

NEONATAL PHYSIOLOGY

The newborn's kidney differs from that of the older child and adult in glomerular and tubular function. The adult number of nephrons is achieved by 34 to 35 weeks, but the nephrons are shorter and less functionally mature. Alterations in renal function and fluid and electrolyte balance are heightened in preterm infants who have not yet achieved their full complement of nephrons. When evaluating postnatal renal function, both gestational age and postbirth age must be considered, because postnatal renal maturation is more a function of postbirth than gestational age; that is, a preterm infant who is several weeks old may have more mature renal function than a newborn term infant. Basic renal processes are summarized in Box 11-1 on page 358. Alterations in neonatal renal function and their implications are summarized in Table 11-8.

Table 11-8 Implications of Alterations in Renal Function in Neonates

ALTERATION	IMPLICATIONS
Decreased glomerular filtration rate	Difficulty excreting water loads with risk of overhydration and water intoxication Narrow margin of safety for fluid management Tendency for water retention and edema (especially pulmonary edema) Increased half-lives of drugs such as antibiotics, barbiturates, and diuretics Altered drug doses and dosing intervals Risk of hyperglycemia in very low–birth weight (VLBW) infants
Altered tubular function: sodium	Increased sodium loss in urine, especially in VLBW infants Alterations in other electrolytes with risk of acidosis, hyperkalemia, hypocalcemia, and hypoglycemia Limited ability to excrete excess sodium
Altered tubular function: glucose	Unable to handle exogenous glucose Risk of glycosuria Load with risk of hyperglycemia Risk of hyponatremia and dehydration Less able to compensate for acid-base abnormalities with risk of acidosis, especially in VLBW infants
Decreased concentrating ability	Risk of dehydration

From Blackburn, S. (1994). Renal function in the neonate. *J Perinat Neonatal Nurs, 8,* 37.

Transitional Events

During intrauterine life, the placenta is the major organ of excretion, handling many functions that are normally performed by the lungs and kidney. With birth, the kidneys must rapidly take over control of fluid and electrolyte balance, excretion of metabolic wastes, and other renal functions. Activity of arginine vasopressin (AVP) and the renin-angiotensin system increases with birth, perhaps stimulated by catecholamines, prostaglandins, hypercarbia, and the renin-angiotensin, kinin-kallikrein, and other systems. As a result, blood pressure increases, with peripheral vasoconstriction and redistribution of blood flow to the vital organs (see Chapter 9). Tubular sodium reabsorption decreases during the intrapartum period, so the first urine has a higher fractional sodium excretion.[159] Renal blood flow (RBF) may not increase immediately at birth, but does increase significantly by 24 hours as renal vascular resistance (RVR) falls.[58] Activity of the renin-angiotensin system increases further during the first few days after birth. Transient increases in glomerular filtration rate (GFR) may occur during the first 2 hours after birth. These changes are variable, decreasing to previous levels by 4 hours.[18]

Body Composition

Body composition changes with gestational age and is influenced by maternal fluid and electrolyte balance. Newborns have higher total body and extracellular water and less intracellular water than older individuals. With advancing gestation, total body water content and extracellular water decrease, whereas intracellular water increases as cells proliferate and organs mature.[24] The fetus is 83% water at 32 weeks' gestation and 78% at term.[18] Extracellular fluid (ECF) decreases from 59% at 24 weeks' gestation, to 53% at 32 weeks' gestation, and 44% at term; intracellular water increases from 27% to 34% (see Figure 11-6).[18,26,44,76,109] The relative interstitial volume of the newborn is three times greater than that of the adult.[118,122] This increases the risk of periorbital, peripheral, and pulmonary edema.[118] Pulmonary edema can interfere with gas exchange; in the brain germinal matrix edema may increase the risk of germinal matrix and intraventricular hemorrhage (see Chapter 15).[118]

Electrolyte composition also changes with gestational age. Because the electrolyte composition of extracellular water is primarily Na^+ and Cl^-, the preterm infant (with more extracellular water) has more Na^+ and Cl^- and fewer intracellular ions (K^+, Mg^{2+}, PO_4) per unit weight. Protein, fat, and carbohydrate composition of the body also increases with age. Infants that are small for gestational age (SGA) have more water and less fat, whereas infants that are large for gestational age (LGA) have more fat and less water.

Before onset of labor, the infant's arterial blood pressure rises due to increases in catecholamines, atrial natriuretic factor (ANF) or peptide, cortisol, and movement of additional blood from the placenta into the fetus.[126] These changes plus alterations in the acid-base status of the fetus during labor lead to increased capillary permeability with a shift in fluid from the intravascular to the interstitial space. This results in up to a 25% decrease in fetal plasma volume and 14% decrease in fetal blood volume during the intrapartum period.[24,108] With birth, ECF volume increases further, primarily due to placental transfusion (see Chapter 8). With increased oxygenation and changes in vasoactive hormones after birth, capillary integrity is gradually restored and fluid begins to move from the interstitial space back into the vascular space.[126]

The increase in ECF volume is followed by a diuresis as fluid in the interstitial space is mobilized and eliminated and the extracellular space contracts.[44,65,96] The postbirth fluid decrease in ECF volume is thought to be related to increases in GFR, increased levels of epithelial transport proteins, which enhance tubular function, and primarily to decreases in ANF, which is elevated in the fetus and for the first week after birth.[107,110,126] These changes are primarily due to decreased pulmonary vascular resistance and not renal maturation.[108] The decreased pulmonary vascular resistance after birth increases pulmonary blood flow and left atrial return. This stretches the atrial wall with release of ANF.[107] The fluid shifts are greater in the extremely low–birth weight (ELBW) infant.[16] In the first 72 hours, the ELBW infant may have a water loss of up to 10 mL/kg or more due to immature renal function, high transepidermal insensible water loss (IWL), and changes in the extracellular space.[16] Loss of fluid from the interstitial space may lead to hypernatremia, hyperglycemia, and hyperkalemia.[16]

Loss of 5% to 10% (usually less than 7%) of birth weight (up to 10% to 15% in many preterm infants) is usually seen during the first week following birth due to these changes in body water compartments.[18,24,44,96,126,149] Contraction of the extracellular space increases with decreasing gestational age at birth.[95] Losses are also higher in preterm infants because they produce a more dilute urine and have greater urine sodium (and therefore additional obligatory water) loss. Fluid therapy during the first week must account for these changes; otherwise fluid overload, which is associated with increased morbidity including a risk of congestive heart failure, necrotizing enterocolitis (NEC), and symptomatic patent ductus arteriosus (PDA), may occur.[44,96]

Urine Output

Urine output varies with fluid and solute intake, renal concentrating ability, perinatal events, and gestational age. Generally, term infants excrete 15 to 60 mL/kg of urine per day and preterm infants 1 to 3 mL/kg/hour (24 to 48 mL/kg/day) during the first few days. Urine output less than 0.5 mL/kg/hour after 24 hours is considered oliguria. Output increases over the first month to 250 to 400 mL/day. In the first 2 days after birth, frequency of micturition is two to six times per hour; subsequently, micturition occurs one or more times with each feeding.[159] Preterm infants less than 32 weeks' gestational age tend to void once per hour, have more interrupted voids (two to three small voids within 10 minutes), and have smaller voids with residuals.[141] These differences may be due to immaturity of the detrusor sphincter complex. Bladder capacity is about 13 mL at 32 weeks, 20 mL by 36 weeks, and 40 mL by term.[59,141]

The initial voiding after birth usually occurs within 24 hours but may be delayed. Approximately 13% to 21% of newborns void in the delivery room, over 95% by 24 hours, and all (unless there are problems) by 48 hours.[31] If infants urinate for the first time in the delivery room, this event may be missed or not recorded. The force and direction of the urine stream are as important in assessing the urinary system as is the time of first voiding. A delay in spontaneous voiding, in the absence of renal anomalies, is usually due to inadequate perfusion with contraction of the intravascular compartment and temporary expansion of interstitial fluid volume. Delayed voiding may occur in infants whose mothers received magnesium sulfate before delivery. Side effects of magnesium sulfate in the newborn include neuromuscular blockade with hypotonia and urine retention.

Renal Blood Flow and Glomerular Filtration

RBF in both term and preterm infants at birth is lower than in adults, primarily because the RVR is high in infants. RVR is inverse to gestational age and falls after birth, but it is still higher than in adults.[58] RVR is high in the fetus because renal function is primarily needed in utero only for amniotic fluid production. Therefore only a small percentage of the fetal cardiac output perfuses the kidney. During the first 12 hours after birth, 4% to 6% of the cardiac output perfuses the kidneys, increasing to 8% to 10% (versus 25% in adults) over the next few days.[18] RVR falls as RBF and GFR increase.[59,60] A similar pattern is seen in preterm infants greater than 34 to 35 weeks' gestational age, but the decrease in RVR is more gradual, with a slower increase in GFR. The higher RVR and low blood flow to the outer cortex of the kidney in preterm infants may be due to the predominance of sympathetic tone in these infants.

Effective renal blood flow (ERBF) increases with postconceptional age. ERBF is 20 mL/min per 1.73 m^2 at 30 weeks, increasing to 45 at 35 weeks and 83 at term, versus about 300 mL/min per 1.73 m^2 at 3 months and 650 by 12 to 24 months (1.73 m^2 is a correction factor for differences in surface area that allows comparison of values between persons of different sizes).[146] Changes in RBF after birth are due to formation of new glomeruli; vascular remodeling; decreased RVR; and vasoactive substances such as adenosine, endothelin, angiotensin II, prostaglandins (especially PGE_2 and PGI_2), ANF, nitric oxide (NO), and the renin-angiotensin and kinin-kallikrein systems.[58,59,146] Because the newborn has a higher RVR and sensitivity to vasoconstrictors than older individuals, the increase in RBF in early infancy is related to decreases in vasoconstrictor influences (Figure 11-7).[146] In newborns, the juxtamedullary nephrons are more mature than the outer cortical nephrons and a greater proportion of the blood perfuses the inner cortical and medullary nephrons versus the outer cortical nephrons. After birth, perfusion of the outer cortex increases rapidly, perhaps in response to catecholamines and redistribution of placental blood flow.

A major difference in renal function between the newborn and the adult is the lower GFR in the newborn, which is even lower when the infant's smaller size and surface area are considered. The GFR is approximately 20 to 25 mL/min per 1.73 m^2 at term or after 35 weeks, 10 to 13 mL/min per 1.73 m^2 in infants less than 28 weeks' gestational age, and as low as 2 mL/min per 1.73 m^2 at 25 weeks.[65,117] The GFR (Figure 11-8) and RBF increase rapidly after birth, doubling by 2 weeks of age.[56] The pattern of maturation is similar in preterm infants over 34 to 35 weeks' gestation and term infants, although preterm infants may exhibit a slower increase, especially during the first week. The GFR is lower in preterm infants less than 34 to 35 weeks' gestational age and remains low until their full complement of nephrons has developed at about 34 to 35 weeks' gestational age. After this point, maturation of RBF and GFR increases rapidly (up to fivefold) and is similar to that of term infants.[117] The decreased GFR in very low–birth weight (VLBW) infants may limit their ability to respond to physiologic stress such as hypoxia and apnea, or to nephrotoxic drugs, such as indomethacin, that impair renal perfusion.[47]

Although the preterm infant continues to develop nephrons until 34 to 35 weeks, nephrogenesis may be altered with decreased numbers of glomeruli, smaller kidneys, and altered distal tubular function.[120,135] This alteration in development is particularly apparent in infants born at less than 1000-g birth weight.[56,73,120] This can lead to long-term impairment in renal function in some infants.[56,81,83,103,115,120] Factors that may alter renal development in preterm infants include fetal and extrauterine growth restriction, maternal glucocorticoids and medications such as aminoglycosides, indomethacin, ibuprofen, and hyperoxia (compared to what the infant experiences in utero).[56] These infants are at increased risk for hypertension in adulthood.[15,50,56,115,135]

The increase in GFR after birth (see Figure 11-8) is due to redistribution of placental blood flow with increased RBF and perfusion pressure, decreased RVR, and increased systemic blood pressure, which increases glomerular capillary hydrostatic pressure, along with increasing glomerular surface area (initially glomerular surface area is about 10% that of an adult) and increased permeability of the glomerular membrane.[58] Increased angiotensin II (ANTII) may help maintain the GFR in the face of a low mean arterial pressure. GFR correlates with gestational age in infants prior to 35 weeks, so that after the postbirth increase in GFR, GFR increases with postmenstrual age.[58,61] After 35 weeks, GFR is more closely related to weight, length, and postbirth age. Maturation of GFR and other aspects of renal function may occur at varying rates in preterm infants, so infants must be evaluated individually in determining dosages of many pharmacologic agents (see Chapter 7).[137]

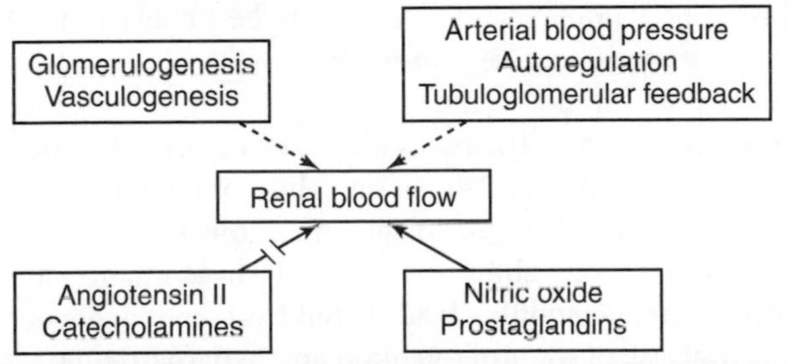

FIGURE 11-7 Factors that influence the development of renal blood flow include anatomic factors (glomerulogenesis and vasculogenesis), physical factors (arterial blood pressure, myogenic autoregulatory response), and vasoactive factors (autoregulation, tubuloglomerular feedback, nitric oxide, and prostaglandins). Other vasoactive agents can regulate renal blood flow, although renal vascular resistance regulation in the newborn is probably the result of a balance between the vasoconstrictor influences of angiotensin II and catecholamines or renal nerves and the vasodilatory influences of nitric oxide and prostaglandins. (From Solhaug, M.J. & Jose, P.A. [2012]. Postnatal maturation of renal blood flow. In R.A. Polin, W.W. Fox, & S.H. Abman [Eds.], *Fetal and neonatal physiology* [4th ed.]. Philadelphia: Saunders, p. 1243.)

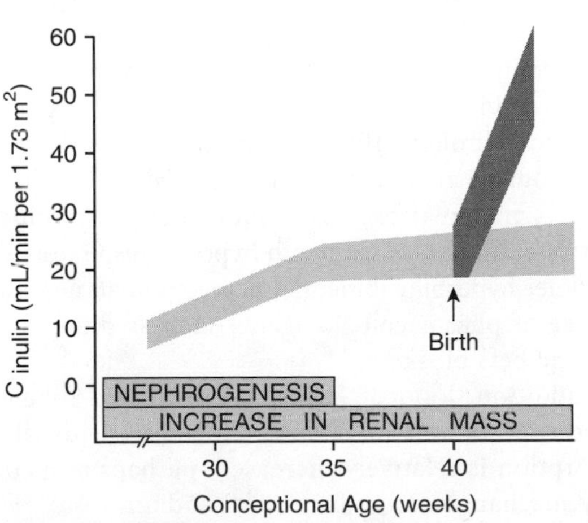

FIGURE 11-8 Maturation of glomerular filtration rate in relation to conceptional age. (From Guignard, J.P. [1981]. The neonatal stressed kidney. In A.B. Gruskin & M.E. Norman [Eds.], *Pediatric nephrology*. The Hague: Martinus Nijhoff.)

Tubular Function

Tubular function is also altered in the neonate. The decreased RBF and GFR reduce the volume of solutes per unit time that the tubules must handle. However, the neonate has a smaller tubular reabsorptive surface area, fewer solute transporters, decreased Na^+-K^+-ATPase activity, and altered control of H^+ transport.[72] Tubular thresholds for reabsorption of many solutes are also reduced and neonates are more likely to lose sodium, glucose, and other solutes in urine. Although tubular function is quite adequate for the healthy infant, immature infants or compromised infants are at risk for fluid and electrolyte problems. Infants treated with antenatal steroids, which increases Na^+-K^+-ATPase mRNA, have more mature renal function at birth.[109]

Sodium

Immediately after birth, both term and preterm infants are in negative sodium balance due to the physiologic natriuresis stimulated by ANF changes with birth.[47,61] This rapidly changes to a positive sodium balance in term infants. Rapidly growing infants are in positive sodium balance (sodium intake greater than output). Excretion of sodium in neonates is reduced in comparison to adults, possibly because of increased plasma renin activity (PRA) and aldosterone levels, decreased Na^+-K^+-ATPase activity (especially in infants less than 34 weeks' gestation), as well as incorporation of sodium into the new tissue.[49,61] Renal tubular handling of sodium undergoes rapid changes after birth as the reabsorptive capacity for sodium and other solutes increases.

Term newborns readily conserve sodium with increased responsiveness of the distal tubule to aldosterone and a rapid increase in Na^+-K^+-ATPase activity after birth.[61,109,159] The pattern for renal reabsorption of sodium is different in the infant than in an older child or adult, primarily because of the altered distribution of blood flow and changes in reabsorption in the proximal versus distal tubules. In infants, a greater portion of RBF is to juxtamedullary nephrons, whereas in the adult the majority of RBF is to the cortical area and only about 10% goes to the medullary area. Because the juxtamedullary nephrons tend to be more involved in conservation than excretion of sodium, an infant's ability to excrete a sodium load is limited. This limitation increases the tendency toward sodium retention, with increased ECF volume and edema formation if excess sodium is given.[18,117] Increased urinary sodium loss is seen with hypoxia, respiratory distress syndrome, hyperbilirubinemia, acute tubular necrosis, and with use of pharmacologic agents such as diuretics, dopamine, and beta blockers.[44]

In addition, loop of Henle and proximal tubule reabsorption of sodium in infants is decreased; distal tubule reabsorption is relatively increased, perhaps as a compensatory mechanism to reduce renal sodium loss.[59,61,159] The increased distal tubule reabsorption is enhanced by elevated levels of aldosterone. Tubular reabsorption of sodium is greater in term infants than in preterm infants, who have increased urinary sodium losses and lower plasma sodium levels. Factors that influence natriuresis are summarized in Table 11-9.

Sodium Balance in Preterm Infants. Preterm infants are more likely to be in negative sodium balance (sodium intake less than output) and have difficulty conserving sodium during the first few weeks after birth.[43,44,52] Negative sodium balance has been observed in 100% of infants less than 30 weeks' gestation, 70% at 30 to 32 weeks, and 40% between 33 and 35 weeks.[4] Factors leading to the negative sodium balance in these infants include decreased Na^+-K^+-ATPase, high ECF volume, reduced tubular aldosterone sensitivity (with a lack of epithelial sodium channels in the distal tubule that normally increase in response to aldosterone), and other factors listed in Table 11-9.[52,117,159] Even though the GFR is lower in the preterm infant (so the kidneys have less sodium to handle at any given time), the altered tubular reabsorption with decreased proximal tubular reabsorption (where 80% to 90% of sodium is reabsorbed in adults), decreased loop of Henle reabsorption (only 20% of adult capacity), and increased distal tubule load results in increased fractional sodium excretion.[52,109] Antenatal steroids may decrease the alterations in sodium and water balance in preterm infants by decreasing insensible water loss and hypernatremia.[44] These infants tend to have an earlier diuresis and natriuresis after birth, possibly due to earlier maturation of epithelial transport systems in the kidney.[44]

Decreased proximal tubule reabsorption of sodium in preterm infants may be due to the shorter length of the tubules and immature transport mechanisms. As a result, greater amounts of fluid and electrolytes such as Na^+ remain in the lumen and are sent to the distal tubule. The distal tubule is unable to increase its reabsorptive capacity to handle the additional sodium load despite elevated PRA and aldosterone levels, so more sodium is lost in the urine. The ability of the distal tubule to respond to aldosterone may be reduced or the distal tubule may already be under maximal aldosterone stimulation and thus may be unable to further increase its reabsorptive capacity.[159]

Thus preterm infants have a limited ability to both excrete and retain sodium.[61] The result is a narrow margin for sodium homeostasis in the VLBW infant. These infants lose excess sodium in their urine due to the limitations in sodium conservation described above. In addition, these infants cannot readily excrete a sodium load. If fluid intake is inadequate, they are at risk of sodium retention and hypernatremia, especially in the first week after birth.[107]

The fractional sodium excretion (FE_{Na}) is the amount of urinary sodium excretion as a percent of the filtered sodium.[52] FE_{Na} is highest in the first 10 days after birth and by 1 month is less than 0.4% to 1%. There is an inverse relationship between (FE_{Na}) and gestational age.[56] For example, there is a greater than 10-fold increase in FE_{Na} between 23 and 31 weeks' gestation.[43] In the larger preterm infant, FE_{Na} is 1% to 5% versus 5% to 15% in VLBW infants and 0.5% to 1% in term infants.[44] Adult values of less than 0.5% are reached by 2 weeks' postbirth age.[118] FE_{Na} is a measure of

Table 11-9 Factors Affecting Natriuresis and Urine Output in Fetuses and Newborn Infants

FACTOR	EFFECT ON NATRIURESIS	EFFECT ON URINE OUTPUT
Low renal blood flow (e.g., PDA)	↓	↓
Indomethacin for PDA	Variable	↓
Limited GFR:		
prerenal failure	↓	↓
Intrinsic or postrenal failure	↑	↑ or ↓
Tubular function: low tubular Na^+-K^+-ATPase	↑	
Prenatal glucocorticoid administration (up-regulates transcription)	↓	
High cord levels of DLIF (inhibit Na^+-K^+-ATPase)	↑	
Dysfunction: aminoglycosides, amphotericin	↑	↑
Dopamine (note that receptor is probably not present in ELBW infants)	↑	↑
Renin-angiotensin-aldosterone system/ high PRA and angiotensin activity:*		
Aldosterone (low level at birth later stimulated by sodium depletion)	↓	
Progesterone (limits tubule sensitivity to aldosterone)	↑	
High circulating level of atrial natriuretic factors	↑	
High concentration of AVP	May↑	↓
Prostaglandins (limit effect of AVP)		↑
Osmotic diuresis caused by hyperglycemia	↑	↑
Diuretics	↑	↑

From Brion, L.P., Bernstein, J., & Spitzer, A. (1997). Kidney and urinary tract. In A.A. Fanaroff & R.J. Martin (Eds.), *Fanaroff & Martin's Neonatal-perinatal medicine: Diseases of the fetus and infant* (6th ed.). St. Louis: Mosby.

AVP, Arginine vasopressin; *DLIF,* circulating endogenous digoxin-like immunoreactive factors; *ELBW,* extremely low birth weight; *GFR,* glomerular filtration rate; *Na^+-K^+-ATPase,* sodium potassium adenosine triphosphatase; *PDA,* patent ductus arteriosus; *PRA,* plasma renin activity.

*Increased natriuresis caused by extracellular fluid expansion mediated by ADH; decreased natriuresis if sodium depletion.

From Ramanathan, S. & Turndorf, H. (1988). Renal disease. In F.M. James, A.S. Wheeler, & D.M. Dewan (Eds.), *Obstetric anesthesia: The complicated patient* (2nd ed.). Philadelphia: F.A. Davis.

tubular function (as GFR is a measure of glomerular function) and is calculated as follows:

$$FE_{Na} = \frac{\text{Urine sodium}}{\text{Serum sodium}} \times \frac{\text{Serum creatinine}}{\text{Urine creatinine}} \times 100$$

Tubular reabsorption of sodium (T_{Na}) can be estimated by the formula $T_{Na} = 100\% - FE_{Na}$. The greater the FE_{Na}, the more sodium is lost in the urine. To determine whether FE_{Na} is excessive, sodium and fluid intake must be considered.[49,52] By several weeks of age, most preterm infants are in positive sodium balance as tubular function matures. Maturation takes longer in VLBW infants, who are at risk for fluid and electrolyte disturbances for a longer period.[22,159]

Glucose

The ability of the tubules to reabsorb glucose and the transport maximum (T_m) for glucose are decreased in the preterm infant but similar to or exceed those of adults in term infants.[65,159] The lower T_m in the preterm is due to low levels of sodium-glucose transporters in the proximal tubule.[159] Even at term, the renal threshold for glucose (corrected for surface area) is lower in the infant. Even with this lower threshold, most normoglycemic infants (unless very immature) are not glycosuric. This is probably because the glucose T_m-to-GFR ratio is high.[159] Although the glomerulotubular balance for glucose filtration and reabsorption can be demonstrated as early as 25 weeks' gestation, low renal thresholds for glucose (less than 100 to 150 mg/dL [less than 5.55 to 8.32 mmol/L]) and increased fractional excretion of glucose are seen in some VLBW infants less than 28 weeks' gestation.[72,117] Urinary glucose levels are increased in preterm infants, with higher fractional glucose excretion, less reabsorption of glucose, and a tendency toward glycosuria.[18] VLBW infants are also at risk for hyperglycemia, because they are unable to readily excrete a glucose load. Because renal handling of glucose is interrelated with that of water, Na^+, K^+, and other solutes, attempts to excrete a glucose load may lead to hyponatremia, dehydration, and other abnormalities. Therefore VLBW infants with glucose IV must be monitored for hyperglycemia, glycosuria, and fluid and electrolyte status. Glucose metabolism is discussed in Chapter 16.

Renal Handling of Other Solutes

In general, renal excretion of solutes increases with both gestational and postnatal age. Potassium excretion is low during gestation, and the newborn is less able to excrete a potassium load. With the lower GFR, less sodium is delivered to and reabsorbed by the tubules. Because K^+ is exchanged for Na^+ in the distal tubule, less K^+ is secreted and subsequently excreted.[18] Healthy term and growing preterm infants are in positive potassium balance; stressed or ill infants may have a negative balance. Transient hyperkalemia (up to 5.5 to 6 mEq/L [mmol/L]) occurs in some VLBW infants (especially those less than 27 to 28 weeks' gestational age), probably due to their low GFR, decreased tubular response to aldosterone, and decreased Na^+-K^+-ATPase activity.[51,95] The turnover of potassium is related to that of energy needs and nitrogen. Stressed infants have greater energy needs. After other energy sources (i.e., carbohydrate and fat stores) have been used, protein will be catabolized for energy, with release of nitrogen. This leads to a negative nitrogen balance and increase in K^+ secretion and excretion. A negative potassium balance is also associated with the use of diuretics and parenteral fluid therapy.

Uric acid levels are higher in preterm than term infants (averaging 7.7 versus 5.2 mL/dL [457.99 versus 309.20 μmol/L]) and decrease with gestation. Serum levels are higher in infants due to increased production of uric acid as a by-product of nucleotide breakdown.[164] Serum uric acid levels may also be elevated in hypoxic infants or following asphyxia. Uric acid crystals may occasionally be seen as reddish staining of the diaper in normal newborns and can be misinterpreted as blood. Urea excretion is usually decreased in the neonate in that they are using nitrogen for growth. Urinary protein excretion is greater at birth, gradually decreasing over the first few weeks. Transient proteinuria may occur during the first 5 days.[159]

The fractional renal reabsorption of amino acids is greater than 98% for all but histidine. Newborns may have a mild but not usually clinically significant aminoacidemia due to immaturity of proximal tubule transporters for glycine, taurine, and proline.[65] Amino acid excretion is increased in preterm infants, especially for taurine, which may be 38% to 68%.[65]

Renal excretion of phosphorus, calcium, and magnesium is interrelated with sodium reabsorption and excretion. During the first week, calcium excretion varies inversely with gestational age and directly with urine flow and sodium excretion, thus increasing the risk for hypocalcemia in the VLBW infant.[18] Alterations in sodium intake and excretion alter renal handling of these solutes in ill infants, so liberal sodium supplementation may lead to development or exacerbation of hypocalcemia.[20] Phosphorus excretion is higher during the first weeks after birth and is related to gestational age and type of oral feeding. Calcium and phosphorus metabolism are discussed in Chapter 17.

VLBW infants are at higher risk for nephrocalcinosis with an incidence of 16% to 64%.[3,67,158] Contributory factors are the high urinary calcium excretion, low serum phosphorus, metabolic acidosis, and elevated urinary oxalate and urate excretion.[67,158] Urinary calcium and phosphorus excretion are increased with use of furosemide.[3] Nephrocalcinosis increases the risk of osteopenia and rickets.

Acid-Base Homeostasis

Serum bicarbonate levels and plasma pH are lower in neonates due to a lower renal threshold for and reduced capacity to reabsorb bicarbonate. The lower threshold (serum level at which bicarbonaturia occurs) might be the result of altered transport capacity for bicarbonate (due to weak expression of enzymes and transporters needed for bicarbonate reabsorption) or may be related to expansion of ECF volume.[18,59,164] The more immature the infant, the lower the bicarbonate levels. Initially, serum bicarbonate levels may be as low as 12 to 16 mEq/L (mmol/L) in VLBW, 16 to 20 mEq/L (mmol/L) in LBW, and 19 to 22 mEq/L (mmol/L) in term infants (versus 24 to 28 mEq/L in adults).[25,59] Serum bicarbonate levels in preterm infants increase to values greater than 20 mEq/L within the first 1 to 2 weeks. Urinary pH is 6 to 7 initially, with minimum values (4.5 to 5.3) reached by 1 to 2 weeks. The occurrence of alkaline urine along with a metabolic acidosis suggests renal tubular acidosis.

Term and preterm infants are able to excrete an acid load, although the ability of the kidneys to respond to an acid load increases with gestational and postnatal age.[25,59,159] The decreased response to an acid load in the VLBW infant may result from immaturity of the hydrogen ion–secreting mechanism, decreased excretion of urinary buffers, or unresponsiveness of the distal tubule to aldosterone, as well as the lower GFR.[65,117] Normally most newborns are probably secreting near to their maximal ability, with little reserve to cope with any disorders that produce acidosis. Thus any event that increases the potential for acidosis, such as cold stress, hypoxemia, or malnutrition, is more likely to produce alterations in acid-base status in the newborn.

Water Balance

Regulation of water balance by the newborn is similar to that of the adult but it occurs within a narrower range. The ability of newborns to dilute urine is similar to that of adults, whereas their ability to concentrate urine is limited. The ability to dilute is defined as the minimum amount of solute (electrolytes, protein) that can be excreted in a volume of urine; that is, there is an obligatory amount of solute that the body must lose in order to excrete water in urine. Since diluting segments of the distal tubule and ascending loop of Henle develop early, term newborns and preterm infants of more than 35 weeks' gestation can dilute their urine to an osmolarity of 50 mOsm/L (mmol/L) (similar to adult values) or lower; preterm infants of less than 35 weeks' gestation can dilute to 70 mOsm/L (mmol/L).[44,93] However, neither term nor preterm infants can handle large or rapidly administered water loads due to their low GFR.[93,117] Therefore the neonate is at risk for overhydration, water retention, and fluid overload. The decreased ability to excrete a water load is related primarily to a lower GFR and perhaps decreased sensitivity of the tubules to AVP. The ability to excrete a water load increases after 3 to 4 days in term infants and preterm infants born at 35 weeks' gestation or more.[164]

The ability to concentrate urine relates to the maximum amount of solute that can be excreted within a volume of urine (i.e., the ability to excrete a solute load without becoming dehydrated). To excrete more solute, the body would have to increase the amount of water in the urine. The ability to concentrate urine is mediated by vasopressin and occurs via aquaporins (water channel proteins).[93] The concentration of solutes in urine depends on a complex interaction of events called the *countercurrent multiplier system* (see Box 11-3 on page 381). The newborn can maximally concentrate urine to

BOX 11-3 Countercurrent Multiplier System

The ability to concentrate urine is the maximum amount of solute that can be excreted within a volume of urine. Adults concentrate to a maximum of 1200 to 1400 mOsm/L (mmol/L); term newborns to 600 to 700 mOsm/L (mmol/L). To excrete more solute, the amount of urine water would have to be increased. Concentration of solutes in urine depends on the countercurrent system, which involves movement of Na^+, water, and other solutes between the tubular lumen, collecting ducts, and surrounding interstitial fluid.

This system can be summarized as follows: Fluid entering the descending limb of the loop of Henle is hypoosmotic due to movement of solutes out of the proximal tubule (see Figure 11-1). Because water but not Na^+ is reabsorbed in the descending limb, the fluid in the loop of Henle becomes hyperosmotic. As the filtrate moves through the ascending limb, Na^+ and Cl^- (but not water) move out of the lumen, so that the filtrate again becomes hypoosmotic and the surrounding interstitial fluid becomes hyperosmotic. The longer the loops of Henle, the more concentrated the urine. As the filtrate passes through the distal tubule and collecting duct, Na^+ reabsorption is mediated by aldosterone and Na^+ is exchanged for secreted H^+ and K^+. There is little water movement in the distal tubule. In the collecting duct, arginine vasopressin (AVP) controls water reabsorption. When AVP is present, water reabsorption increases, resulting in a hypertonic urine.

Adapted from Ramanathan, S. & Turndorf, H. (1988). Renal disease. In F.M. James, A.S. Wheeler, & D.M. Dewan (Eds.), *Obstetric anesthesia: The complicated patient.* Philadelphia: F.A. Davis.

approximately half of adult levels (600 to 800 mOsm/L [mmol/L] versus 1200 to 1400 mOsm/L [mmol/L]). This ability is further decreased in preterm infants, with maximum urinary concentration of 245 to 450 mOsm/kg/L in 1300- to 1500-g infants at 1 to 3 weeks of age and even lower levels in more immature infants. By 4 to 6 weeks after birth, preterm infants can concentrate similarly to term infants.[159] The limitation in concentrating ability is due to several factors:

1. Decreased medullary osmotic gradient related to decreased accumulation of urea and other solutes and increased medullary blood flow.
2. Lower concentrations of blood urea. Urea is a solute that sets up the concentration gradient. Because urea is an end product of nitrogen metabolism, growing infants—who use nitrogen to make protein and new tissue—metabolize less nitrogen and produce less urea.
3. Decreased solute levels for the concentration gradients in the interstitial space due to decreased reabsorption and increased excretion of Na^+, Cl^-, glucose, and urea, possibly mediated by increased prostaglandin production.
4. Decreased length of loops of Henle and collecting ducts and immature tubular function.
5. Decreased response to circulating AVP and immaturity of AVP-signal transducer pathways; decreased transcription of aquaporin 2 (AQP2) water channels in the collecting ducts.
6. Interference of prostaglandins with the hypoosmotic action of AVP.
7. Reduced expression of AQP2 water channels.[23,44,93,108,117,159,164]

Hormonal Regulation

Renin-Angiotensin-Aldosterone System

Renin-angiotensin-aldosterone system activity (see Figure 11-3 and Box 11-2 on page 381) is inversely related to gestational age.[141,146] Values in the newborn are higher than in adults and decrease gradually over the first months.[94,117,141,146] Angiotensinogen and PRA are particularly high (Figure 11-9).[52,94,117,] PRA is inversely related to gestational age and 3 to 5 times higher in infants than adults.[117] PRA remains high for the first 2 to 3 weeks in all newborns and then begins to slowly decrease. Circulating ANTII is also high at birth, and the decrease parallels the decrease in PRA.[94] The high ANTII levels may be mediated by decreased end organ responsiveness in the newborn.[94,117] Hyperfunction of this system may be due to the low systemic blood pressure and RBF, sodium wasting, and normal decrease in ECF volume after birth.[164] The increased renin and aldosterone concentrations may be also mediated by prostaglandins, which are elevated at birth.[18] By increasing sodium reabsorption by the distal tubules, or by influencing vasoconstriction, aldosterone modulates changes in GFR to protect the renal tubules from overload with loss of electrolytes and other solutes in the urine.

In the VLBW infant, adrenal production of aldosterone is decreased compared to that in the term infant, and the distal tubule is less responsive to aldosterone.[18,159] These changes increase the risk of hyponatremia and dehydration. Hypertension in the newborn is usually related to factors that activate the renin-angiotensin system to stimulate ANTII production (e.g., renal vein thrombosis, coarctation of the aorta, bronchopulmonary dysplasia, and glucocorticoid administration).[94] The basis for the decreased response to aldosterone is uncertain but may relate to lack of receptors, the presence of an undetermined antagonist, or the deficiency of intracellular transport system enzymes. At the same time, inhibition of aldosterone release is decreased, which increases the risk of sodium overload if too much supplemental sodium is given.[61]

Arginine Vasopressin

Although the distal tubule and the collecting ducts of the infant respond to AVP, the responses of the collecting ducts to AVP are immature at birth possibly due to low expression of AQP2.[90] Aquaporins are vasopressin-sensitive water channels that are needed for water reabsorption.[90] AVP works by inserting aquaporins (water channels) into the apical membranes of collecting duct cells. These proteins are decreased in immature infants.[108] AQP2 is the main target of AVP in regulating collecting duct permeability and the ability to concentrate urine.[74] AVP binds to arginine-vasopressin V2 receptors that stimulate signaling pathways to promote movement of preformed vesicles containing AQP2 channels to the

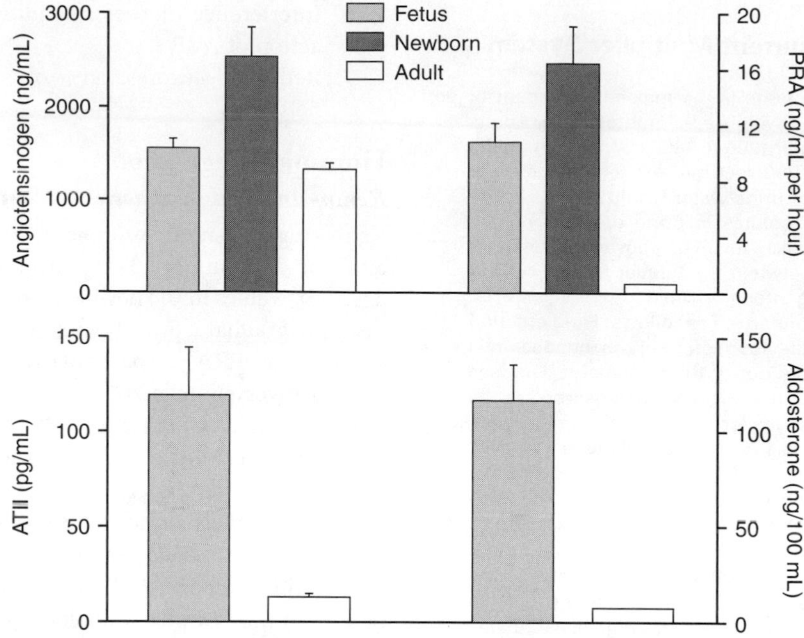

FIGURE 11-9 Circulating levels of angiotensinogen, plasma renin activity (PRA), angiotensin II (ATII), and plasma aldosterone in fetal cord blood, newborn infants, and normal adults. (From Tufro-McReddie, A. & Gomez, R.A. [1993]. Ontogeny of the renin-angiotensin-aldosterone system. *Semin Nephrol, 13,* 519.)

membrane surface, making the collecting duct membrane more permeable to water.[44]

AVP increases at birth, especially in infants born vaginally (possibly stimulated by head compression).[23,117,126] Sensitivity of volume receptors and osmoreceptors in neonates is similar to that in adults. However, tubular response to circulating AVP is decreased in preterm infants with resistance of the immature kidney to AVP, due to immature transcription of AQP2.[23,74,90,117,126,159] Plasma and urinary AVP are increased following hypoxic-ischemic events (possibly mediated by catecholamines) and in infants with intracranial hemorrhage, respiratory distress syndrome (RDS), meconium aspiration syndrome, and pneumothorax. These findings may be due to decreased osmolarity in the medullary interstitium (from decreased tubular function and decreased reabsorption of solutes) or inhibition of AVP by increased levels of prostaglandin E_2 (PGE_2).[49,93,126] The increase in AVP at birth may enhance extrauterine adaptation by increasing blood pressure and peripheral vasoconstriction and enhancing postnatal fluid homeostasis.

Factors regulating AVP secretion in neonates are not fully understood. Increased AVP and water retention may be important in the etiology of later hyponatremia in VLBW infants.[159] Chronically increased sodium excretion with contraction of the ECF compartment may stimulate the renin-angiotensin-aldosterone system and AVP secretion. AVP increases renal water reabsorption to restore ECF volume but may also decrease plasma sodium. As noted above, AVP is increased with stressful events such as birth, surgery, intraventricular hemorrhage, and other complications.[61] The result is increased water and subsequently sodium loss with a risk of water retention and hyponatremia.[61,107]

Other Regulating Factors

Renal function and hemodynamics are influenced by other substances in addition to the renin-angiotensin-aldosterone system and AVP. The kallikrein-kinin system is activated at birth and modulates RBF and handling of sodium and water by stimulating formation of bradykinins and prostaglandins and by acting as an antagonist to the renin-angiotensin-aldosterone (RAA) system and AVP.[146] The kidneys produce dopamine (precursor to norepinephrine and epinephrine) in the proximal tubules of superficial nephrons.[126] Dopamine inhibits renal sodium absorption (thus increasing sodium excretion), increases water excretion by inhibiting AVP release from the pituitary, and alters water transport in the collecting ducts.[126] Prostaglandins also mediate RBF and may be important in regulating RBF during stress; they may also balance the increased renin-angiotensin-aldosterone activity.[94,146]

ANF is released by the atrial myocardium in response to atrial stretch. ANF has natriuretic and diuretic actions. ANF increases at birth, peaking at 48 to 72 hours, the time of maximal postbirth diuresis.[18] Birth results in decreased pulmonary vascular resistance, increased pulmonary blood flow, and thus increased blood return to the left atrium. This stretches the left atrium and stimulates ANF release. The ANF response is blunted in preterm infants, perhaps due to decreased cyclic guanosine monophosphate, more rapid clearance of ANF, and altered renal hemodynamics.[117]

Bladder

The neonate's bladder is almost entirely in the abdominal cavity and is cigar shaped (as opposed to the pyramidal shape in adults); therefore the ureters are short. As a result, distention of the bladder compresses the abdomen and increases pressure on the diaphragm. As the pelvic cavity increases in size during infancy and early childhood, the bladder gradually sinks into the pelvis and the ureters lengthen.[97]

CLINICAL IMPLICATIONS FOR NEONATAL CARE

The newborn infant is able to regulate sodium and water balance, but within a much narrower range than in the older child or adult. As a result, the neonate is much more likely to develop fluid and electrolyte disturbances within a shorter period of time, with a small margin between homeostasis and overload or underload. Careful calculation and monitoring of needs are essential to maintain homeostasis. Immaturity of renal function limits the ability of the infant, especially if preterm or ill, to cope with additional stress and increases the risk of renal dysfunction following pathophysiologic events such as hypoxia, ischemia, or RDS. In addition, alterations in renal function affect excretion of drugs and influence serum levels and drug half-life values, increasing the risks of side effects and toxicity.

Management of Fluid and Electrolyte Balance

Birth represents a major change in the infant's fluid and electrolyte status, which in fetal life is maintained by the placenta and mother. During the transitional period, infants undergo a physiologic diuresis and natriuresis (see Transitional Events) resulting in an isotonic contraction of the extracellular space and a transient negative sodium and water balance. If caregivers do not allow this normal transition, the infant is at risk of fluid retention, including accumulations of pulmonary interstitial fluid.[107] Lorenz notes that, in light of these changes after birth, "the goal is not to maintain fluid and electrolyte status after birth but rather to allow these changes to occur appropriately."[95,p.205] Early volume expansion of VLBW infants without cardiovascular compromise has not been documented to improve outcomes.[123]

Calculation of fluid needs for any infant involves consideration of maintenance needs, replacement of losses, and provision of allowances for growth. Maintenance needs include consideration of endogenous water produced by oxidative metabolism plus insensible water loss (IWL) and loss of water in urine and stool. Usual values for these parameters are known and can be used to calculate fluid needs. In healthy term or large preterm infants, individual variations from these values, unless major, are probably not crucial, in that the infant's kidneys will adjust to ensure fluid and electrolyte homeostasis.[44] However, ill or VLBW infants may not be able to adjust, because their renal function is inefficient or compromised by illness. In addition, these infants are more likely to be in environments (e.g., incubator, radiant warmer, or phototherapy) that can markedly alter IWL.[44]

Stool water loss is estimated at 5 to 10 mL/kg/day under basal conditions but can increase markedly with diarrhea. Stool water losses are considered to be minimal during the first few days after birth and thus are not included in calculation of initial fluid needs. Approximately 5 to 10 mL/kg/day of endogenous water is produced by oxidation. This water is often ignored in calculation of fluid requirements, because it offsets fecal losses.[18] Water for growth varies with body water composition. For example, if an infant is assumed to have water content of 70%, water needed for growth would be 0.70 mL per gram of weight gain. Because body water composition is not static, water for growth is generally estimated at 10 to 20 mL/kg/day, with the higher values used for more immature infants who have a larger proportion of body water.[44] In the first week after birth, during the period of physiologic weight loss, calculation of maintenance fluid needs does not include replacement of water for growth but is based primarily on calculation of IWL and urine water loss.

Insensible Water Loss

IWL is water loss from the skin (70%) and respiratory tract (30%). IWL generally consists of about 32% of the total water requirement, unless IWL is markedly increased.[18] Basal levels of IWL in the neonate are 20 mL/kg/day or 0.7 to 1.6 mL/kg/hour.[18] IWL is markedly increased in the preterm infant. In ELBW infants with thin, gelatinous skin, these losses are particularly high (see Chapter 14).[16] Skin water loss is proportional to surface area, and these infants have greater ratios of surface area to weight. Preterm infants also have greater IWL because of increased permeability of their epidermis to water, greater percentage of body water, and increased skin blood flow in relation to metabolic rate.[18,44,126] IWL can be significantly altered by conditions that increase the basal metabolic rate and by therapeutic modalities such as phototherapy, radiant warmers, heat shields, humidity, and incubators.[16,18] Lower ambient humidity or higher ambient temperature increase IWL; higher ambient humidity or humidified oxygen lower IWL.[44] For example, water loss increases 100% in infants older than 26 weeks' gestational age if the ambient humidity is decreased from 60% to 20%.[2] Factors that increase or decrease IWL in neonates are summarized in Table 11-10.

Urine Water Loss

Urine water loss generally accounts for about 56% of total body water requirements (generally about 50 to 100 mL/kg/day).[18] The amount of water the infant must excrete in urine, the maximum urine concentrating ability (urine osmolarity), and the renal solute load are all interrelated and can be calculated using the following formula:

$$\text{Urine volume (mL/kg)} = \frac{\text{Solute load (mOsm/kg)}}{\text{Urine osmolarity (mOsm/L[mmol/L])}} \times 1000$$

Table 11-10 Factors Influencing Insensible Water Loss in Neonates

INCREASE INSENSIBLE WATER LOSS	DECREASE INSENSIBLE WATER LOSS
Immaturity (50%-300%)	Plastic heat shields (30%-50%)
Radiant warmer (50%-200%)	Double-wall incubator or heat shield (30%-50%)
Forced convection incubator (30%-50%)	Plastic blanket under radiant warmer (30%-50%)
Phototherapy (40%-100%)	High humidity (50%-100%)
Respiratory distress	Transport thermal blanket (70%)
Elevated body or ambient temperature*	Assisted ventilation with warmed and humidified air (20%-30%)
Skin breakdown or injury	Increasing postnatal age
Congenital defects (omphalocele, gastroschisis, neural tube defect)	Semipermeable dressing or topical agents (50%)
Motor activity, crying (up to 70%)	
Other factors that increase metabolic rate	

Compiled from references 16, 18, 44, 95, 109, 136, 159.

*A 1-degree increase in body temperature is equal to a 30% increase in insensible water loss.

Variations in renal solute load can markedly alter obligatory urinary water losses. For example, a nongrowing infant who could concentrate to a maximum of 300 mOsm/L would have to excrete about 25 mL/urine/kg to get rid of a solute load of 7.5 mOsm/kg; the same infant would be obligated to lose 50 mL/urine/kg if receiving a solute load of 15 mOsm/kg ($7.5/300 \times 1000 = 25$ mL/kg urine versus $15/300 \times 1000 =$ 50 mL/kg urine) and would be at greater risk for dehydration. The renal solute load is the amount of solutes from metabolic end products (especially nitrogenous compounds and electrolytes) and exogenous sources that must be excreted by the kidneys. Endogenous solutes are produced from catabolism of tissues when caloric and protein intake is inadequate. Exogenous solutes are derived from parenteral solutions and enteral intake. The solute load from exogenous sources can be calculated from the following formula:

$$\text{Solute load (mOsm/L [mmol/L])} = 4\text{ (g protein per dL)} + 1\,(Na^+ + K^+ + Cl^-)$$

Renal solute load varies with the type of oral intake and whether or not the infant is receiving an intravenous solution with additional electrolytes and other solutes.

Renal solute load is lowest for growing infants fed human milk and highest for infants who are starved or receiving high osmolar parenteral fluids or a high-protein formula. Renal solute loads for commercial formulas can be found in the manufacturer's formula handbook. Renal solute loads for parenteral fluids average 10 to 20 mOsm of solute per 100 kcal expended (in infants less than 10 kg, mL/kcal = mL/kg). For example, an intravenous line with a 10% glucose solution would average 10 mOsm/kg/day, and a maintenance IV with 3 mEq NaCl and 2 mEq KCl would yield an additional 10 mOsm/L (mmol/L) of solute from these electrolytes (i.e., 3 from Na, plus 3 from Cl, plus 2 from K, plus 2 from Cl).[18]

Various factors can modify renal solute load and urine water excretion. In the growing preterm infant who is incorporating protein and other solutes into new tissue, each gram of weight gain decreases the renal solute load by about 1 mOsm. The decrease in solute load is reflected in decreased obligatory urine water loss. Urine water volume and thus fluid needs may be increased with glycosuria or furosemide therapy and decreased in infants on positive-pressure ventilation or with the syndrome of inappropriate secretion of antidiuretic hormone (SIADH [ADH is the former term for AVP]) or acute renal tubular necrosis.[18]

Estimating Fluid and Electrolyte Needs

During the first few days following birth, maintenance fluid requirements are based on IWL and urine water loss. With increasing postbirth age, fluid requirements increase due to increased stool water losses and growth. There are many variations in specific recommendations for fluid and electrolyte needs. Fluid needs for the first few days are generally calculated to account for the normal physiologic weight loss of birth weight. If IWL is increased (see Table 11-10), fluid needs are also increased. On the other hand, fluid needs are reduced in infants with acute renal failure or congestive heart failure. Fluid needs are higher in infants weighing less than 1000 g due to markedly increased IWL and decreased renal concentrating ability (which increases obligatory urine water loss). Current recommendations for fluid and electrolyte management are available.[44,85,149,156]

Sodium Requirements of Preterm Infants

There are differing viewpoints on the management of fluid and electrolyte status in preterm infants. Sodium intake is usually calculated at 1 to 3 mEq/kg/day. Sodium supplementation is usually lower for the first few days due to the relatively volume-expanded state of most infants.[44] Preterm infants, particularly those less than 30 to 32 weeks' gestation, may be unable to maintain sodium balance on the standard sodium intake due to increased urinary Na loss, and may require higher sodium intakes.[44,47,52] Dell recommends 1 to 2 mEq/kg/day for the first 3 to 7 days, then 2 to 3 after that, perhaps increasing to 4 to 5 in VLBW infants due to increased urinary sodium losses in the first few weeks.[44]

Early administration of sodium can also increase the risk of hypernatremia and respiratory problems by interfering with the normal extracellular water loss after birth.[49,62,63,108] Hartnoll and colleagues studied early (day of life 1) versus late (one infant had lost 6% of birth weight) administration of 4 mEq/kg of supplemental sodium.[62,63] Infants with early sodium intake had less of a decrease in extracellular water and increase in respiratory problems both at 1 week and 28 days. The investigators thought that the increased respiratory problems were due to persistent extracellular volume expansion with increased pulmonary interstitial fluid.[62] Restriction of sodium intake in the first 5 days decreased the incidence of hypernatremia, whereas fluid restriction led to hyponatremia.[36] Modi notes that, if given liberal fluid intake with sodium supplementation, infants will not have the usual initial postbirth weight loss. However, eventually most infants will experience the typical postbirth changes in fluid compartments.[109] "The well recognized diuresis that accompanies improving respiratory function in babies with RDS is in fact a natriuresis and is an example of delayed postnatal maturation."[109]

All infants have a reduction in ECF volume in the first few days, which is associated with increased excretion of fluid and sodium. This in part accounts for the increased sodium losses in the first week. Thus correcting the high sodium excretion by increasing sodium intake in the first week may impede the normal postbirth adjustments in body fluid compartment values.[109,159] However, after these adjustments have occurred, sodium balance in the VLBW infant must be carefully evaluated and monitored. Most clinicians agree that sodium supplementation is necessary in VLBW infants after the initial decrease in extracellular volume.[18,159] The more immature the infants, the less able they are to adapt to a low sodium intake.[159] Various protocols have been recommended for management of fluids and electrolytes in VLBW infants. Sodium acetate or sodium bicarbonate may be used to help compensate for the respiratory acidosis from respiratory immaturity and problems and from metabolic acidosis due to renal tubular immaturity.[18] Some formulas as well as human milk may not contain adequate sodium for the VLBW infant with immature renal function. These infants may require sodium supplementation until sodium balance is positive.

Risk of Overhydration and Dehydration

Although the infant can dilute urine to osmolarities of 50 to 70 mOsm/L (mmol/L), the usual diuretic response to a water load often diminishes before the entire load can be excreted.[96] This decreased ability to excrete a water load makes the infant more susceptible to fluid overload. Term and larger preterm infants are more vulnerable to overhydration in the first 5 days following birth, in that maximal dilution is not achieved until after that time.[44] GFR remains low in preterm infants until a gestational age greater than 34 to 35 weeks is reached; thus these infants are at risk for volume overload for a longer period. Fluid overload in preterm infants has been associated with an increased risk of PDA.[147] The expanded extracellular volume secondary to fluid overload may stimulate production of PGE_2, which maintains a patent ductus. In infants with PDA and a large shunt, blood flow to the intestines is reduced, which may result in hypoperfusion, ischemia, and increased risk of necrotizing enterocolitis.

Because of decreased concentrating ability, neonates (especially preterm infants) are at risk for dehydration, particularly if fluid intake is inadequate or extrarenal losses are elevated, as with transepidermal loss in VLBW infants. In evaluating dehydration in the first week, the usual postbirth weight loss must be considered so that infants do not become overhydrated.[44]

Electrolyte Imbalances

Limitations in renal function in preterm and ill neonates increase the risk of electrolyte disturbances from iatrogenic causes. Electrolyte imbalances can also arise from pathophysiologic problems, but these are not considered here.

Hyponatremia

Hyponatremia in preterm or sick infants can occur secondary to alterations in fluid (dilutional hyponatremia) or in sodium balance. Dilutional hyponatremia can arise from excess transfer of free water across the placenta because of rapid or excessive administration of fluids to the woman in labor. Excessive administration of a hypotonic solution overwhelms the limited fetal or neonatal renal capacity to deal with a water overload. This may occur if maintenance fluid requirements for the first week after birth do not allow for the physiologic weight loss, especially in VLBW infants. These events lead to rapid expansion of extracellular volume and reduced serum sodium and are associated with an increased incidence of PDA, congestive heart failure, NEC, intracranial hemorrhage, and bronchopulmonary dysplasia.

Dilutional hyponatremia can also occur subsequent to water retention associated with SIADH. This syndrome is seen with a variety of pathophysiologic problems such as asphyxia, respiratory distress, sepsis, and central nervous system problems and following PDA ligation and other stressful situations. SIADH involves excessive secretion of AVP with normal fluid intake, serum hyponatremia and hypoosmolality, increased urine osmolality and renal sodium excretion, absence of volume depletion and dehydration, and normal renal and adrenal function.[126]

Hyponatremia can also arise from negative sodium balance and excessive loss of sodium by immature kidneys of VLBW infants. In these infants the greater sodium loss increases water loss (renal excretion of sodium must be accompanied by excretion of water), leading to decreased ECF volume and hyponatremia.[126] Urinary sodium loss and subsequent hyponatremia in VLBW infants interfere with renal concentrating ability by changing the osmotic gradient and impairing AVP response. This further reduces water reabsorption and increases sodium loss and risk of hyponatremia.[52] Dilutional hyponatremia is an ever-present risk for VLBW infants in the early postnatal period. This risk may be reduced by increasing sodium intake in VLBW infants during the first few weeks and careful monitoring of intake, output, electrolytes, weight, and fluid status.[18] A late hyponatremia may be seen at 4 to 6 weeks of age in rapidly growing VLBW infants.[47]

Hypernatremia

Hypernatremia related to immaturity of renal function may arise from dehydration caused by excessive sodium intake or increased IWL. The dehydration may be aggravated by limited concentrating ability of the immature kidney.[93] Hypernatremia can also follow intravenous administration of sodium bicarbonate, in that the infant may not be able to rapidly excrete this sodium load. Hypernatremia in VLBW infants is usually secondary to high transepidermal water losses in the first week.[51] Hypernatremia is associated with an increased risk of intracranial bleeding in both term and preterm infants.[14]

Hyperkalemia in Preterm Infants

VLBW infants are also at risk for both oliguric and nonoliguric hyperkalemia because of alterations in renal function and changes in fluid dynamics after birth. The reported incidence of hyperkalemia is up to 53% of infants weighing less than 1000 g at birth.[126] Nonoliguric hyperkalemia may result from shifts in potassium from the intracellular to extracellular space or immaturity of renal tubular K^+ secretion mechanisms. As a result, potassium needs must be carefully monitored and routine replacement may need to be decreased in the first few days.[16,95] Some infants less than 26 to 27 weeks of age have signs of dehydration at 24 to 48 hours, with elevated sodium, potassium, and glucose without oliguria, acidosis, or shock. This may result from excessive evaporative losses (up to 100 to 200 mL/kg/day) due to the immature skin and greater surface area–to–body mass ratio, aldosterone insensitivity, and immaturity of renal Na^+-K^+-ATPase activity or a shift in potassium from the intracellular to extracellular space.[1,95] This is rare today with current management strategies and the use of humidity.

Measurement of Renal Function and Hydration Status

Parameters used to assess hydration status in the neonate include weight, fluid intake, urine specific gravity (1.002 to 1.010) and osmolarity (60 to 300 mOsm), urine output (minimum 1 to 3 mL/kg/hour) and electrolytes, and serum electrolytes and osmolarity. Findings indicative of adequate renal function in the newborn include urine volume greater than 1 to 3 mL/hour, FE_{Na} less than 3%, and urine specific gravity of 1.008 to 1.012.[44] Changes in urine specific gravity are often an early response to alterations in hydration. Urine for this measurement can be obtained reliably from either collecting bags or aspirating several drops from the diaper. Urine output can be assessed by weighing the diaper before and after use and noting the difference (1 g = 1 mL urine). Because urine rapidly evaporates from diapers of infants under radiant warmers, this assessment must be done soon after the infant voids.

Serum osmolarity can be estimated by doubling the serum sodium value (because sodium and its anions are the major components of ECF), or more precisely by the following formula:

$$\text{Serum osmolality (mOSm/L [mmol/L])} = \frac{\text{BUN (mg/dL)}}{2.8} + \frac{\text{Blood glucose (mg/dL)}}{18}$$

2.8 and 18 represent molecular weights divided by 10. Measurement of renal function also involves assessment of GFR.

Plasma creatinine levels at birth reflect maternal values and increase shortly after birth (possibly because of a shift in ECF), followed by a decrease and stabilization at about 0.35 to 0.40 mg/dL (30.94 to 35.96 μmol/L) (range, 0.14 to 0.70 mg/dL [12.37 to 61.88 μmol/L]) by 1 to 2 weeks in term infants and up to 3 weeks in most preterm infants.[47,138] The elevated creatinine levels may be due to immature tubular function with "leaky" tubular membranes. Plasma creatinine levels are higher at birth in ELBW infants and inversely related to gestational age. In VLBW infants, there is a transient increase at birth, peaking at 3 to 4 days followed by a decrease that stabilizes at 3 to 4 weeks.[47,58] Because GFR increases more slowly after birth in these infants, the decrease in plasma creatinine is slower. Therefore, plasma creatinine levels are a poorer predictor of renal function in ELBW infants.[47,95] This measure is also limited in infants and children in general due to the progressive changes in GFR and muscle mass.[138]

Creatinine clearance generally approximates GFR in term infants (as in adults) but is considerably more variable in preterm infants. At lower GFR values, creatinine clearance tends to overestimate GFR.[58,138] Creatinine clearance correlates with birth weight, length, and gestational age. Plasma creatinine and creatinine clearance are useful measurements in stable infants but are less accurate in infants with renal failure or preterm infants whose renal function is rapidly changing with maturation.[138] The formula GFR (mL/min per 1.73 m^2) = KL/P_{cr} (L = length in cm; P_{cr} = plasma creatinine; K = estimate of muscle mass) is a better estimate of GFR than plasma creatinine alone, in that it accounts for percentage of muscle mass. In this formula, K = 0.27 for VLBW, 0.33 for preterm infants with weight appropriate for gestational age (AGA), 0.31 for SGA preterm infants, 0.45 for AGA term infants, and 0.33 for SGA term infants younger than 1 year.[138] This formula can be used after the first week in term infants and until 1 year of age for preterm infants after 34 to 35 weeks' gestational age. The accuracy of this formula has been questioned, however, especially because variations in hydration status and various pathophysiologic states can alter the results.[52,58]

Renal Function during Neonatal Illness

Immaturity in renal function in infants, especially preterm infants, limits their ability to cope with additional stresses and can lead to significant alterations of renal function in association with specific pathologic problems such as RDS, perinatal asphyxia, congestive heart failure, bronchopulmonary dysplasia, and PDA. These disorders can also interfere with maturation of renal hemodynamics and tubular function (Figure 11-10).[159]

During hypoxic-ischemic events, severe RDS, or other hypoxemic events, vascular resistance is increased, GFR decreased, and the renin-angiotensin-aldosterone system activated, further magnifying alterations that normally occur in normal newborns. In addition, cardiac output is redistributed, with increased blood flow to vital organs (heart, brain, and adrenal glands) and reduced flow to less essential areas such as the renal and gastrointestinal systems. The percentage of decrease in flow to these nonessential systems is greater

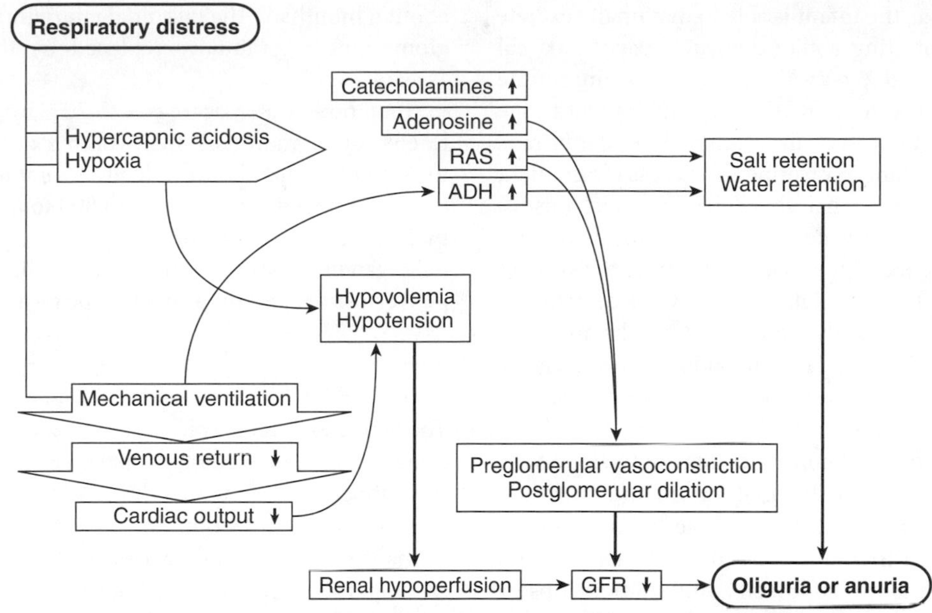

FIGURE 11-10 The main pathways of renal dysfunction in respiratory distress. Mechanical ventilation as well as the hypoxemia-induced activation of vasoactive factors contributes to the development of systemic hypotension and hypovolemia. (From Tóth-Heyn, P., et al. (2000). The stressed neonatal kidney. From pathophysiology to clinical management of neonatal vasomotor neuropathy. *Pediatr Nephrol, 14,* 230.)

in immature animals and perhaps in human preterm infants as well.[44] The decreased blood flow increases the risk of renal and intestinal ischemia and disorders such as acute tubular necrosis and NEC. Following hypoxic-ischemic events, infants are at risk for SIADH, reduced urine output, impaired electrolyte reabsorption, hyperkalemia, and hyponatremia.[12,159] These infants require careful calculation and titration of fluid intake. Oliguria or anuria is most likely to develop within the first 24 hours. Initial fluid intake is limited to replacement of insensible and urinary water losses.

Infants with RDS and hypoxemia have marked changes in renal function with impairment of renal perfusion and reduced urine output by hypoxemia. Oliguria is associated with renal tubular necrosis, decreased renal perfusion, and impaired diluting ability. These impairments can lead to a decreased ability to excrete water, water retention, and edema. The reduction in perfusion is due to vasoconstriction with increased RVR possibly mediated by elevated activity of the renin-angiotensin system. The decreased urine output is due to increased AVP and altered renal hemodynamics with a decreased GFR. In hypoxemic infants, an increase in urine output may occur before improvement in the alveolar-arterial oxygen gradient, suggesting that the improvement in respiratory function may be secondary to renal excretion of fluid sequestered in the lungs. Renal tubular function is also altered in these infants, with increased renal loss of protein, glucose, and sodium, decreased concentrating ability, and impairment of the ability to excrete acid (increasing the risk of renal tubular acidosis).

Positive-pressure ventilation further alters renal function by decreasing cardiac output and renal perfusion, redistributing blood flow, and increasing intrathoracic and inferior vena caval pressure. Positive-pressure ventilation and constant positive airway pressure alter renal function by decreasing GFR. Adequate hydration and careful monitoring of fluid and electrolyte status are especially critical for infants with respiratory problems and those on assisted ventilation.

MATURATIONAL CHANGES DURING INFANCY AND CHILDHOOD

Renal function undergoes rapid maturation during the first 2 years. Thus the first 1 to 2 years are a time of increased risk of fluid and electrolyte problems in infants. Function comparable to that of adults is achieved by around 2 years. Effective renal plasma flow increases rapidly from birth to 3 months and then more slowly reaches adult values by 12 to 24 months.[146] GFR also increases rapidly during the first 3 months, reaching 60 mL/min/1.73 m^2 by 3 months, 80 mL/min/1.73 m^2 by 6 months, 100 mL/min/1.73 m^2 by 12 months, and adult values (120 mL/min/1.73 m^2) by 2 years.[65,159] Values may remain lower in preterm infants, with a lag in reaching values seen in term infants. Creatinine output per unit of body weight increases throughout childhood as muscle mass increases.[69] Plasma creatinine values are stable at values averaging 0.35 to 0.40 mg/dL (30.94 to 35.36 μmol/L) until 2 years of age, when they increase further until adolescence.[138]

By 2 months of age, the infant is able to maximally excrete a water loss; concentrating ability does not reach maximal adult levels until around 2 years.[93] The ability to concentrate urine is probably related to increasing protein content in the diet, which increases urea levels in serum and tubular filtrate. This increase is important in creating the necessary gradient essential for maximizing renal concentrating mechanisms. Maturation of sodium and water reabsorption in the tubules can take up to 18 months of age; prior to this time the kidneys have a limited capacity to regulate salt and water excretion.[83]

PRA decreases significantly from 1 to 6 weeks and then more slowly. Adult values for PRA and aldosterone levels are reached by 6 to 9 years, possibly earlier.[94] The decrease in ANTII parallels the decrease in PRA.[94]

Glomerular development continues after birth, involving primarily hypertrophy.[102] Further maturation and growth of nephrons continues to about 2 years of age.[94] Anatomically the lobulation seen in the newborn kidney disappears and the glomerulus and tubules approach adult relationships by about 6 months.[18] The cuboidal epithelium of the newborn's glomerulus is gradually replaced by thin epithelium by 1 year of age.

Total body water decreases to 70% by 3 months and 60% to 65% by 12 months.[97] ECF volume decreases to 30% by 3 to 6 months and then gradually to adult values by adolescence. Urine output increases to 500 to 600 mL per 24 hours by 1 year of age. The bladder remains a cigar-shaped abdominal organ until early childhood, with achievement of the adult pelvic position and pyramidal shape by about 6 years of age.[97]

SUMMARY

The neonate is vulnerable to significant alterations in volume homeostasis and electrolyte balance due to immaturity of renal function. This vulnerability is especially marked in the preterm infant, in whom there is very little margin for errors in management of fluid and electrolyte status. These infants can rapidly become overhydrated or dehydrated or develop

Table 11-11 Recommendations for Clinical Practice Related to Changes in the Renal System and Fluid and Electrolyte Homeostasis in Neonates

Recognize the usual changes in the renal system in the fetus and neonate (pp. 374-383 and Table 11-8).
Monitor fluid and electrolyte status of infants of mothers who received large volumes or rapidly administered intravenous fluids during labor or hypertonic intravenous solutions (pp. 367-368).
Know normal values for parameters used to assess renal function and fluid and electrolyte status and recognize abnormalities (pp. 376-380, 383-386).
Know expected patterns of weight loss following birth and monitor status (p. 367).
Carefully calculate fluid and electrolyte requirements (pp. 383-385).
Record fluid intake and output and maintain within calculated limits (pp. 383-385).
Use infusion device to administer intravenous fluids, calculate intake hourly, and adjust as needed (pp. 380-381, 383-385).
Assess hydration status of infants using weight, intake and output, urine specific gravity and osmolality, serum osmolality, and electrolytes (pp. 383-386).
Observe for signs of overhydration, water retention, vascular overload, and dehydration (pp. 385, 386).
Know and monitor complications associated with excess fluid (pp. 385-386).
Record time and character of first voiding (p. 376).
Monitor voiding and fluid and electrolyte status in infants with hypoxic-ischemic events and after maternal magnesium sulfate administration (pp. 376, 386-387).
Monitor infants on glucose IVs for glycosuria, hyperglycemia, and fluid and electrolyte status (p. 379 and Chapter 16).
Monitor potassium levels in very low–birth weight (VLBW) infants and in infants with increased energy needs, in infants who are stressed, or in infants on diuretics or volume expanders (pp. 379-380, 386).
Monitor calcium and magnesium levels in VLBW infants or those on sodium supplementation or with increased sodium excretion (pp. 378-380, 384-385).
Monitor blood and urine pH values in low–birth weight (LBW) or ill infants (p. 380).
Know the risk factors for acidosis and observe for acid-base alterations in infants with cold stress, altered nutrition, and fluid and electrolyte alterations (p. 380).
Observe for renal sodium loss and hyponatremia especially in VLBW infants (pp. 376-379, 384-385).
Know effects of illness on renal function and monitor ill or stressed infants for problems such as hyponatremia and dehydration (pp. 386-387 and Figure 11-10).
Recognize and monitor for drug side effects related to immature renal function (pp. 376-377, 383 and Chapter 7).
Know components (e.g., maintenance, replacement of loss, provision for growth) of usual fluid and electrolyte needs for infants and how these needs vary at different gestational ages (pp. 383-385).
Calculate infant fluid and electrolyte needs and renal solute load (pp. 383-385).
Avoid use of high solute load formulas, especially in LBW infants (pp. 380-381, 384).
Recognize factors influencing insensible water loss and act to minimize the effects of these losses (p. 383 and Table 11-10).
Recognize and monitor for effects of neonatal pathophysiologic problems on renal function (pp. 386-387).
Recognize factors placing the infant at risk for overhydration, dehydration, and electrolyte imbalances, and monitor infants for these problems (pp. 385-386).
Recognize parameters associated with the syndrome of inappropriate secretion of antidiuretic hormone (SIADH) and late metabolic acidosis (pp. 384-385).

hyponatremia, hypernatremia, and other electrolyte disorders. By careful assessment and observation, the nurse can prevent or minimize the effects of many of these disorders. Recommendations for clinical practices related to alterations in the renal system and fluid and electrolyte balance are summarized in Table 11-11. By providing care to minimize these alterations, neonatal health can be enhanced, with a reduction in the risks associated with pathophysiologic complications.

References

1. Adamkin, D.H. (1998). Issues in the nutritional support of the ventilated baby. *Clin Perinatol, 25,* 79.
2. Agren, J., Sjörs, G., & Sedin, G. (1998). Transepidermal water loss in infants born at 24 and 25 weeks of gestation. *Acta Paediatr, 87,* 1185.
3. Aladangady, N. (2004). Urinary excretion of calcium and phosphate in preterm infants. *Pediatr Nephrol, 19,* 1225.
4. Alcorn, D., et al. (1996). Angiotensin receptors and development: The kidney. *Clin Exp Pharmacol Physiol Suppl, 3,* S88.
5. Alto, W.A. (2005). No need for glycosuria/proteinuria screen in pregnant women. *J Fam Pract, 54,* 978.
6. Alwan, S., Polifka, J.E., & Friedman, J.M. (2005). Angiotensin II receptor antagonist treatment during pregnancy. *Birth Defects Res A Clin Mol Teratol, 73,* 123.
7. American College of Nurse-Midwives. (2008). Providing oral nutrition to women in labor. *J Midwifery Womens Health, 53,* 276.
8. American Society of Anesthesiologists Task Force on Obstetric Anesthesia. (2007). Practice guidelines for obstetric anesthesia: An updated report by the American Society of Anesthesiologists Task Force on Obstetric Anesthesia. *Anesthesiology, 106,* 843.
9. Anderson, G.D. (2005). Pregnancy-induced changes in pharmacokinetics: A mechanistic-based approach. *Clin Pharmacokinet, 44,* 989.
10. Andriole, V.T. & Patterson, T.F. (1991). Epidemiology, natural history, and management of urinary tract infections in pregnancy. *Med Clin North Am, 75,* 359.
11. Anton, L. & Brosnihan, K.B. (2008). Systemic and uteroplacental renin angiotensin system in normal and pre-eclamptic pregnancies. *Ther Adv Cardiovasc Dis, 2,* 349.
12. Askenazi, D.J., Ambalavanan, N., & Goldstein, S.L. (2009). Acute kidney injury in critically ill newborns: What do we know? What do we need to learn? *Pediatr Nephrol, 24,* 265.
13. Ballermann, B.J. (2005). Glomerular endothelial cell differentiation. *Kidney Int, 67,* 1668.
14. Barnette, A.R., et al. (2010). Sodium intake and intraventricular hemorrhage in the preterm infant. *Ann Neurol, 67,* 817.
15. Baum, M. (2010). Role of the kidney in the prenatal and early postnatal programming of hypertension, *Am J Physiol Renal Physiol, 298,* F235.
16. Baumgardt, S. & Costarino, A.T. (2000). Water and electrolyte metabolism of the micropremie. *Clin Perinatol, 27,* 131.
17. Becker, A. & Baum, M. (2006). Obstructive uropathy. *Early Hum Dev, 82,* 15.
18. Bell, E.F. & Oh, W. (2005). Fluid and electrolyte management. In M.G. MacDonald, M.M.K. Seshia, & M.D. Mullett (Eds.), *Avery's neonatology: Pathophysiology and management of the newborn* (6th ed.). Philadelphia: Lippincott Williams & Wilkins.
19. Bergum, D., Lonnée, H., & Hakli, T.F. (2009). Oxytocin infusion: Acute hyponatraemia, seizures and coma. *Acta Anaesthesiol Scand, 53,* 826.
20. Bert, S., Gouyon, J.B., & Semama, D.S. (2004). Calcium, sodium and potassium urinary excretion during the first five days of life in very preterm infants. *Biol Neonate, 85,* 37.
21. Beydoun, S.N. (1985). Morphologic changes in the renal tract in pregnancy. *Clin Obstet Gynecol, 28,* 249.
22. Bhatia, J. (2006). Fluid and electrolyte management in the very low birth weight neonate. *J Perinatol, 26,* S19.
23. Bonilla-Felix, M. (2004). Development of water transport in the collecting duct, *Am J Physiol Renal Physiol, 287,* F1093.
24. Brauer, K., Brace, R.A., & Stonestreet, B.S. (2012). Fluid distribution in the fetus and neonate. In R.A. Polin, W.W. Fox, & S.H. Abman (Eds.), *Fetal and neonatal physiology* (4th ed.). Philadelphia: Saunders.
25. Brewer, E.D. (2012). Urinary acidification. In R.A. Polin, W.W. Fox & S.H. Abman (Eds.), *Fetal and neonatal physiology* (4th ed.). Philadelphia: Saunders.
26. Brown, M.A., et al. (1997). The renin-angiotensin-aldosterone system in pre eclampsia. *Clin Exp Hypertens, 19,* 713.
27. Brunton, P.J., Arunachalam, S., & Russel, J.A. (2008). Control of neurohypophysial hormone secretion, blood osmolality and volume in pregnancy. *J Physiol Pharmacol, 59,* 27.
28. Buhling, K.J., et al. (2004). The usefulness of glycosuria and the influence of maternal blood pressure in screening for gestational diabetes. *Eur J Obstet Gynecol Reprod Biol, 113,* 145.
29. Carlin, A. & Alfirevic, Z. (2008). Physiological changes of pregnancy and monitoring. *Best Pract Res Clin Obstet Gynaecol, 22,* 801.
30. Chevalier, R.L. & Norwood, V.F. (2012). Functional development of the kidney in utero. In R.A. Polin, W.W. Fox, & S.H. Abman (Eds.), *Fetal and neonatal physiology* (4th ed.). Philadelphia: Saunders.
31. Clark, D.A. (1977). Time of first void and first stool in 500 newborns. *Pediatrics, 60,* 457.
32. Conrad, K.P., et al. (2005). Role of relaxin in maternal renal vasodilation of pregnancy. *Ann N Y Acad Sci, 1041,* 147.
33. Conrad, K.P. (2011). Emerging role of relaxin in the maternal adaptations to normal pregnancy: Implications for preeclampsia. *Semin Nephrol, 31,* 15.
34. Cornelis, T., et al. (2011). The kidney in normal pregnancy and preeclampsia. *Semin Nephrol, 31,* 4.
35. Coscia, L.A., et al. (2010). Report from the National Transplantation Pregnancy Registry (NTPR): Outcomes of pregnancy after transplantation. *Clin Transpl, 24,* 65.
36. Costarino, A.T., et al. (1992). Sodium restriction versus daily maintenance replacement in low birth weight premature neonates: A randomized, blind therapeutic trial. *J Pediatr, 120,* 999.
37. Cyna, A.M., et al. (2006). Techniques for preventing hypotension during spinal anaesthesia for caesarean section. *Cochrane Database Syst Rev 4,* CD002251.
38. Dahlenburg, G.W., Burnell, R.H., & Braybrook, R. (1980). The relation between cord serum sodium levels in newborn infants and maternal intravenous therapy during labour. *Br J Obstet Gynaecol, 87,* 519.
39. Davison, J.M. & Lindheimer, M.D. (2011). Pregnancy and chronic kidney disease. *Semin Nephrol, 31,* 86.
40. Davison, J.M. (1987). Overview: Kidney function in pregnant women. *Am J Kidney Dis, 9,* 248.
41. Davison, J.M. (1997). Edema in pregnancy, *Kidney Int Suppl, 59,* S90.
42. Delemarre, F., et al. (1996). Diurnal variation in angiotensin sensitivity in pregnancy. *Am J Obstet Gynecol, 174,* 259.
43. Delgado, M.M., et al. (2003). Sodium and potassium clearances by the maturing kidney: Clinical-molecular correlates. *Pediatr Nephrol, 18,* 759.
44. Dell, K.M. (2011). Fluids, electrolytes and acid-base homeostasis. In R.J. Martin, A.A. Fanaroff & M.C. Walsh (Eds.), *Fanaroff & Martin's Neonatal-perinatal medicine: Diseases of the fetus and infant* (9th ed.). St. Louis: Mosby Elsevier.
45. Dighe, M., et al. (2011). Fetal genitourinary anomalies—a pictorial review with postnatal correlation. *Ultrasound Q, 27,* 7.
46. Dötsch, J., et al. (2009). The implications of fetal programming of glomerular number and renal function. *J Mol Med, 87,* 841.
47. Drukker, A. & Guignard, J.P. (2002). Renal aspects of the term and preterm infant: A selective update. *Curr Opin Pediatr, 14,* 175.
48. Ellis, D. (2011). Regulation of fluids and electrolytes in infants and children. In P.J. Davis, F.P. Cladis, & E.K. Motoyama (Eds.),

Smith's anesthesia for infants and children (8th ed.), Philadelphia: Mosby Elsevier.

49. Engle, W.D. (1986). Development of fetal and neonatal renal function, *Semin Perinatol, 10,* 113.
50. Fanos, V., et al. (2010). Perinatal nutrient restriction reduces nephron endowment increasing renal morbidity in adulthood: A review. *Early Hum Dev, 86,* 37.
51. Faúndes, A., et al. (1998). Dilatation of the urinary tract during pregnancy: Proposal of a curve of maximal caliceal diameter by gestational age. *Am J Obstet Gynecol, 178,* 1082.
52. Feld, L.G. & Corey, H.E. (2012). Renal transport of sodium during early development. In R.A. Polin, W.W. Fox, & S.H. Abman (Eds.), *Fetal and neonatal physiology* (4th ed.). Philadelphia: Saunders.
53. Fiadjoe, P., Kannan, K., & Rane, A. (2010). Maternal urological problems in pregnancy. *Eur J Obstet Gynecol Reprod Biol, 152,* 13.
54. Freed, S.Z. (1981). Hydronephrosis of pregnancy. In S.Z. Freed & N. Herzig (Eds.), *Urology in pregnancy*. Baltimore: Williams & Wilkins.
55. Granese, R. & Adile, B. (2008). Urinary incontinence in pregnancy and in puerperium: 3 months follow-up after delivery, *Minerva Ginecol, 60,* 15 (in Italian).
56. Gubhaju, L., Sutherland, M.R., & Black, M.J. (2011). Preterm birth and the kidney: Implications for long-term renal health. *Reprod Sci, 18,* 322.
57. Gubler, M.C. & Antignac, C. (2010). Renin-angiotensin system in kidney development: Renal tubular dysgenesis. *Kidney Int, 77,* 400.
58. Guignard, J.P. (2012). Postnatal development of glomerular filtration rate in neonates. In R.A. Polin, W.W. Fox, & S.H. Abman (Eds.), *Fetal and neonatal physiology* (4th ed.). Philadelphia: Saunders.
59. Guignard, J.P. & Sulyok, E. (2012). Renal morphogenesis and development of renal function. In C.A. Gleason & S. Devaskar (Eds.). *Avery's diseases of the newborn* (9th ed.). Philadelphia: Saunders.
60. Guron, G. & Friberg, P. (2000). An intact renin-angiotensin system is a prerequisite for normal renal development. *J Hypertens, 18,* 123.
61. Hartnoll, G. (2003). Basic principles and practical steps in the management of fluid balance in the newborn. *Semin Neonatol, 8,* 307.
62. Hartnoll, G., Bétrémieux, P., & Modi, N. (2000). Randomised controlled trial of postnatal sodium supplementation on body composition in 25 to 30 week gestational age infants. *Arch Dis Child Fetal Neonatal Ed, 82,* F24.
63. Hartnoll, G., Bétrémieux, P., & Modi, N. (2001). Randomised controlled trial of postnatal sodium supplementation in infants of 25-30 weeks gestational age: effects on cardiopulmonary adaptation. *Arch Dis Child Fetal Neonatal Ed, 85,* F29.
64. Hassan, E., et al. (2000). Clinical implications of the ovarian/endometrial renin-angiotensin-aldosterone system. *Ann N Y Acad Sci, 900,* 107.
65. Haycock, G. (2005). Renal function and renal disease in the newborn. In J.M. Rennie (Ed.), *Roberton's textbook of neonatology* (4th ed.). Edinburgh: Churchill Livingstone.
66. Hayslett, J.P. (2004). Renal disease in pregnancy. In G.N. Burrow, T.P. Duffy, & J.A. Copel (Eds.), *Medical complications during pregnancy* (6th ed.). Philadelphia: Saunders.
67. Hein, G., et al. (2004). Development of nephrocalcinosis in very low birth weight infants. *Pediatr Nephrol, 19,* 616.
68. Hennessy, A. & Makris, A. (2011). Pre-eclamptic nephropathy. *Nephrology, 16,* 134.
69. Hilgers, K.F., et al. (1997). Angiotensin's role in renal development, *Semin Nephrol, 17,* 492.
70. Hill, C.C. & Pickinpaugh, J. (2008). Physiologic changes in pregnancy. *Surg Clin North Am, 88,* 391.
71. Hladunewich, M.A., et al. (2004). The dynamics of glomerular filtration in the puerperium, *Am J Physiol Renal Physiol, 286,* F496.
72. Holtbäck, U. & Aperia, A.C. (2003). Molecular determinants of sodium and water balance during early human development. *Semin Neonatol, 8,* 291.
73. Huang, H.P., et al. (2007). Early postnatal renal growth in premature infants. *Nephrology, 12,* 572.
74. Iacobelli, S., et al. (2010). Aquaporin-2 urinary excretion in preterm infants: Relationship to diuresis and vasopressin. *Acta Physiol (Oxf), 200,* 339.
75. Irani, R.A. & Xia, Y. (2008). The functional role of the renin-angiotensin system in pregnancy and preeclampsia. *Placenta, 29,* 763.
76. Irani, R.A., et al. (2010). Autoantibody mediated angiotensin receptor activation contributes to preeclampsia through tumor necrosis factor-alpha signaling. *Hypertension, 55,* 1246.
77. Irani, R.A. & Xia, Y. (2011). Renin angiotensin signaling in normal pregnancy and preeclampsia. *Semin Nephrol, 31,* 47.
78. Jeyabalan, A. & Lain, K.Y. (2007). Anatomic and functional changes of the upper urinary tract during pregnancy. *Urol Clin North Am, 34,* 1.
79. Josephson, M.A. & McKay, D.B. (2010). Pregnancy in the renal transplant recipient. *Obstet Gynecol Clin North Am, 37,* 211.
80. Josephson, M.A. & McKay, D.B. (2011). Pregnancy and kidney transplantation. *Semin Nephrol, 31,* 100.
81. Keijzer-Veen, M.G., et al. (2010). Reduced renal length and volume 20 years after very preterm birth. *Pediatr Nephrol, 25,* 499.
82. Keppler, A.B. (1988). The use of intravenous fluids during labor. *Birth, 15,* 75.
83. Kett, M.M. & Denton, K.M. (2011). Renal programming: Cause for concern? *Am J Physiol Regul Integr Comp Physiol, 300,* R791.
84. King, R., et al. (2011). Oral nutrition in labour: "Whose choice is it anyway?" A review of the literature. *Midwifery, 27,* 674.
85. Kleinman, R.E. (2009). *Pediatric nutrition handbook* (6th ed.). Elk Grove Village, IL: American Academy of Pediatrics.
86. Lafayette, R. (2005). The kidney in preeclampsia. *Kidney Int, 67,* 1194.
87. Lamp, J.M. & Macke, J.K. (2010). Relationships among intrapartum maternal fluid intake, birth type, neonatal output, and neonatal weight loss during the first 48 hours after birth. *J Obstet Gynecol Neonatal Nurs, 39,* 169.
88. Lelièvre-Pégorier, M. & Merlet-Bénichou, C. (2000). The number of nephrons in the mammalian kidney: Environmental influences play a determining role. *Exp Nephrol, 8,* 63.
89. Levidiotis, V., Chang, S., & McDonald, S. (2009). Pregnancy and maternal outcomes among kidney transplant recipients. *J Am Soc Nephrol, 20,* 2433.
90. Li, Y., et al. (2011). Urinary aquaporin-2 excretion during ibuprofen or indomethacin treatment in preterm infants with patent ductus arteriosus. *Acta Paediatr, 100,* 59.
91. Lindheimer, M.D., Conrad, K.P., & Karumanchi, S.A. (2008). Renal physiology and disease in pregnancy. In R.J. Alpern & S.C. Hebert (Eds.), *Seldin and Giebisch's The kidney: Physiology and pathophysiology* (4th ed.). San Diego: Academic Press.
92. Lindheimer, M.D. & August, P. (2009). Aldosterone, maternal volume status and healthy pregnancies: A cycle of differing views. *Nephrol Dial Transplant, 24,* 1712.
93. Linshaw, M.A. (2012). Concentration and dilution of the urine. In R.A. Polin, W.W. Fox, & S.H. Abman (Eds.), *Fetal and neonatal physiology* (4th ed.). Philadelphia: Saunders.
94. Lopez, M.L.S. & Gomez, R.A., et al. (2012). Development of the renin-angiotensin system. In R.A. Polin, W.W. Fox, & S.H. Abman (Eds.), *Fetal and neonatal physiology* (4th ed.). Philadelphia: Saunders.
95. Lorenz, J.M. (1997). Assessing fluid and electrolyte status in the newborn. National Academy of Clinical Biochemistry. *Clin Chem, 43,* 205.
96. Lorenz, J.M. (2012). Fetal and neonatal body water compartment values with reference to growth and development. In R.A. Polin, W.W. Fox, & S.H. Abman (Eds.), *Fetal and neonatal physiology* (4th ed.). Philadelphia: Saunders.
97. Lowrey, G.H. (1986). *Growth and development of children.* Chicago: YearBook Medical.
98. Ludka, L.M. & Roberts, C.C. (1993). Eating and drinking in labor. A literature review. *J Nurse Midwifery, 38,* 199.
99. Luft, F.C., Gallery, E.D.M., & Lindheimer, M.D. (2009). Normal and abnormal volume homeostasis. In M.D. Lindheimer, J.M. Roberts, & F.G. Cunningham (Eds.), *Chesley's Hypertensive disorders in pregnancy* (3rd ed.). San Diego: Elsevier.

100. Maharaj, D. (2009). Eating and drinking in labor: Should it be allowed? *Eur J Obstet Gynecol Reprod Biol, 146,* 3.
101. Malinowski, J. (1978). Bladder assessment in the postpartum patient. *J Obstet Gynecol Neonatal Nurs, 7,* 14.
102. Mann, S., Johnson, M.P., & Wilson, R.D. (2010). Fetal thoracic and bladder shunts. *Semin Fetal Neonatal Med, 15,* 28.
103. Maringhini, S., et al. (2010). Early origin of adult renal disease. *J Matern Fetal Neonatal Med, 23,* 84.
104. McKay, D.B., et al. (2005). Reproduction and transplantation: Report on the AST Consensus Conference on Reproductive Issues and Transplantation. *Am J Transplant, 5,* 1592.
105. Merlet-Bénichou, C. (1999). Influence of fetal environment on kidney development. *Int J Dev Biol, 43,* 453.
106. Mikhail, M.S. & Anyaegbunam, A. (1995). Lower urinary tract dysfunction in pregnancy: A review. *Obstet Gynecol Surv, 50,* 675.
107. Modi, N. (2003). Clinical implications of postnatal alterations in body water distribution. *Semin Neonatol, 8,* 301.
108. Modi, N. (2004). Management of fluid balance in the very immature neonate, *Arch Dis Child Fetal Neonatal Ed, 89,* F108.
109. Modi, N. (2005). Fluid and electrolyte balance. In J.M. Rennie (Ed.), *Roberton's textbook of neonatology* (4th ed.). Edinburgh: Churchill Livingstone.
110. Modi, N., et al. (2000). Postnatal weight loss and contraction of the extracellular compartment is triggered by atrial natriuretic peptide. *Early Hum Dev, 59,* 201.
111. Moen, V. & Irestedt, L. (2009). Water intoxication following labour and surgery: Blaming oxytocin—the easy way out? *Acta Anaesthesiol Scand, 53,* 1226.
112. Moen, V., et al. (2009). Hyponatremia complicating labour: Rare or unrecognised? A prospective observational study. *Br J Obstet Gynaecol, 116,* 552.
113. Monga, M. (2009). Maternal cardiovascular, respiratory, and renal adaptation to pregnancy. In R.K. Creasy et al. (Eds.), *Creasy & Resnik's Maternal-fetal medicine: Principles and practice* (6th ed.). Philadelphia: Saunders Elsevier.
114. Moore, K.L., Persaud, T.V.N., & Torchia, M.G. (2011). *The developing human: Clinically oriented embryology* (9th ed.). Philadelphia: Saunders.
115. Moritz, K.M., et al. (2008). Factors influencing mammalian kidney development: Implications for health in adult life. *Adv Anat Embryol Cell Biol, 196,* 1.
116. Morris, R.K. & Kilby, M.D. (2009). An overview of the literature on congenital lower urinary tract obstruction and introduction to the PLUTO trial: Percutaneous shunting in lower urinary tract obstruction. *Aust N Z J Obstet Gynaecol, 49,* 6.
117. Nafday, S.M. (2005). Renal disease. In M.G. MacDonald, M.M.K. Seshia, & M.D. Mullett (Eds.), *Avery's neonatology, pathophysiology and management of the newborn* (6th ed.). Philadelphia: Lippincott Williams & Wilkins.
118. Nakayama, D.K. (2010). Management of the surgical newborn: Physiological foundations and practical considerations. *J Pediatr Urol, 6,* 232.
119. Newton, N., Newton, M., & Broach, J. (1988). Psychologic, physical, nutritional and technologic aspects of intravenous infusion during labor. *Birth, 15,* 67.
120. Nuyt, A.M. & Alexander, B.T. (2009). Developmental programming and hypertension. *Curr Opin Nephrol Hypertens, 18,* 144.
121. Ophir, E., et al. (2007). Water intoxication—a dangerous condition in labor and delivery rooms. *Obstet Gynecol Surv, 62,* 731.
122. O'Reilly, S.A., et al. (1993). Low risk mothers: Oral intake and emesis in labor. *J Nurse Midwifery, 38,* 228.
123. Osborn, D.A. & Evans, N. (2004). Early volume expansion for prevention of morbidity and mortality in very preterm infants. *Cochrane Database Syst Rev 2,* CD002055.
124. O'Sullivan, G. (1994). The stomach—fact and fantasy: eating and drinking during labor. *Int Anesthesiol Clin, 32,* 31.
125. Podymow, T., August, P., & Akbari, A. (2010). Management of renal disease in pregnancy. *Obstet Gynecol Clin North Am, 37,* 195.
126. Posencheg, M.A. & Evans, J.R. (2012). Acid-base, fluid and electrolyte management. In C.A. Gleason & S. Devaskar (Eds.). *Avery's diseases of the newborn* (9th ed.). Philadelphia: Saunders.
127. Ramanathan, S. & Turndorf, H. (1988). Renal disease. In F.M. James, A.S. Wheeler, & D.M. Dewan (Eds.), *Obstetric anesthesia: The complicated patient*. Philadelphia: F.A. Davis.
128. Ramsay, I.N., et al. (1993). Uroflowmetry in the puerperium. *Neurourol Urodyn, 12,* 33.
129. Resnik, R. (2004). The puerperium. In R.K. Creasy, R. Resnik, & J.D. Iams (Eds.), *Creasy & Resnik's Maternal-fetal medicine: principles and practice* (5th ed.). Philadelphia: Saunders.
130. Reznik, V.M. & Budorick, N.E. (1995). Prenatal detection of congenital renal disease. *Urol Clin North Am, 22,* 21.
131. Ritz, E., et al. (2011). Prenatal programming—effects on blood pressure and renal function. *Nat Rev Nephrol, 7,* 137.
132. Rosenblum, N.D. (2008). Developmental biology of the human kidney. *Semin Fetal Neonatal Med, 13,* 125.
133. Sadler, T.W. (2012). *Langman's medical embryology* (12th ed.). Philadelphia: Lippincott, Williams & Wilkins.
134. Saultz, J.W., et al. (1991). Postpartum urinary retention. *J Am Board Fam Pract, 4,* 341.
135. Schell-Feith, E.A., Kist-van Holthe, J.E., & van der Heijden, A.J. (2010). Nephrocalcinosis in preterm neonates. *Pediatr Nephrol, 25,* 221.
136. Schmidt, I.M., et al. (2005). Impaired kidney growth in low-birth-weight children: Distinct effects of maturity and weight for gestational age. *Kidney Int, 68,* 731.
137. Schrier, R.W. (2010). Systemic arterial vasodilation, vasopressin, and vasopressinase in pregnancy. *J Am Soc Nephrol, 21,* 570.
138. Schwartz, G.J., Brion, L.P., & Spitzer, A. (1987). The use of plasma creatinine for estimating glomerular filtration rate in infants, children, and adolescents. *Pediatr Clin North Am, 34,* 571.
139. Seely, E.W. & Moore, T.J. (1994). The renin-angiotensin-aldosterone system and vasopressin. In D. Tulchinsky & A.B. Little (Eds.), *Maternal-fetal endocrinology* (2nd ed.). Philadelphia: Saunders.
140. Siddik-Sayyid, S.M., et al. (2009). A randomized trial comparing colloid preload to coload during spinal anesthesia for elective cesarean delivery. *Anesth Analg, 109,* 1219.
141. Sillén, U., et al. (2000). The voiding patterns of healthy preterm neonates. *J Urol, 163,* 278.
142. Simeonova, A. & Bengtsson, C. (1990). Prevalence of urinary incontinence among women in a Swedish primary health care centre. *Scan J Prim Health Care, 8,* 203.
143. Singata, M., Tranmer, J., & Gyte, G.M. (2010). Restricting oral fluid and food intake during labour. *Cochrane Database Syst Rev 1,* CD003930.
144. Smith, M., et al. (2005). Renal hemodynamic effects of relaxin in humans. *Ann N Y Acad Sci, 1041,* 163.
145. Smith, M.C., et al. (2008). Assessment of glomerular filtration rate during pregnancy using the MDRD formula. *BJOG, 115,* 109.
146. Solhaug, M.J. & Jose, P.A. (2012). Postnatal maturation of renal blood flow. In R.A. Polin, W.W. Fox, & S.H. Abman (Eds.), *Fetal and neonatal physiology* (4th ed.). Philadelphia: Saunders.
147. Stephens, B.E., et al. (2008). Fluid regimens in the first week of life may increase risk of patent ductus arteriosus in extremely low birth weight infants. *J Perinatol, 28,* 123.
148. Symonds, E.M. (1988). Renin and reproduction. *Am J Obstet Gynecol, 158,* 754.
149. Taylor, S.N., et al. (2010). Fluid, electrolytes, and nutrition: minutes matter. *Adv Neonatal Care, 10,* 248.
150. Teoh, W.H. & Sia, A.T. (2009). Colloid preload versus coload for spinal anesthesia for cesarean delivery: The effects on maternal cardiac output. *Anesth Analg, 108,* 1592.
151. Theunissen, I.M. & Parer, J.T. (1994). Fluid and electrolytes in pregnancy. *Clin Obstet Gynecol, 37,* 3.
152. Thorp, J.M., et al. (1999). Urinary incontinence in pregnancy and the puerperium: A prospective study. *Am J Obstet Gynecol, 181,* 266.

153. Thornburg, K.L., et al. (2000). Hemodynamic changes in pregnancy. *Semin Perinatol, 24,* 11.
154. Tiniakos, D., et al. (2004). Ontogeny of intrinsic innervation in the human kidney. *Anat Embryol (Berl), 209,* 41.
155. Tourangeau, A., et al. (1999). Intravenous therapy for women in labor: Implementation of a practice change. *Birth, 26,* 31.
156. Tsang, R.C. (2005). *Nutrition of the preterm infant: Scientific basis and practical guidelines* (2nd ed.). Cincinnati, OH: Digital Educational Pub.
157. van den Anker, J. (2005). Renal function and excretion of drugs in the newborn. In S.J. Yaffee & J.V. Aranda (Eds.), *Neonatal and pediatric pharmacology: Therapeutic principles in practice* (3rd ed.). Philadelphia: Lippincott Williams & Wilkins.
158. Verhulst, A., et al. (2005). Preconditioning of the distal tubular epithelium of the human kidney precedes nephrocalcinosis. *Kidney Int, 68,* 1643.
159. Vogt, B.A. & Dell, K.M. (2011). The kidney and urinary tract. In R.J. Martin, A.A. Fanaroff, & M.C. Walsh (Eds.), *Fanaroff & Martin's Neonatal-perinatal medicine: Diseases of the fetus and infant* (9th ed.). St. Louis: Mosby Elsevier.
160. Waugh, J.J., et al. (2004). Accuracy of urinalysis dipstick techniques in predicting significant proteinuria in pregnancy. *Obstet Gynecol, 103,* 769.
161. Widemaier, E., Raff, H., & Strang, K. (2010). *Vander's Human physiology: The mechanisms of body function* (12th ed.). New York: McGraw-Hill.
162. Williams, D.J. & Davison, J.M. (2009). Renal disorders. In R.K. Creasy et al (Eds.), *Creasy & Resnik's Maternal-fetal medicine: Principles and practice* (6th ed.). Philadelphia: Saunders Elsevier.
163. Winston, J. & Levitt, M.F. (1985). Renal function, renal disease and pregnancy. In S.H. Cherry, R.L. Berkowitz, & N.G. Kase (Eds.), *Rovinsky and Guttmacher's Medical, surgical and gynecologic complications of pregnancy.* Baltimore: Williams & Wilkins.
164. Yared, A., Barakat, A.Y., & Ichikawa, I. (1990). Fetal nephrology. In R.D. Eden & F.H. Boehm (Eds.), *Assessment and care of the fetus.* Norwalk, CT: Appleton & Lange.

CHAPTER 12

Gastrointestinal and Hepatic Systems and Perinatal Nutrition

The gastrointestinal (GI) system consists of processes involved in intake, digestion, and absorption of nutrients and elimination of by-products in bile and stool.[249] Utilization of nutrients for production of energy and other vital functions is discussed in Chapters 16 and 17. This chapter focuses on the processes involved in preparing nutrients for absorption across the intestinal villi.

Maternal nutrition is one of the most important factors affecting pregnancy outcome. The maternal GI tract must digest and absorb nutrients needed for fetal and placental growth and development and to meet the altered demands of maternal metabolism as well as eliminate unneeded by-products and waste materials from both the woman and the fetus. Structural and physiologic immaturity of the neonate's GI tract can result in alterations in neonatal nutritional status and increase the risk of malabsorption and dehydration. This chapter reviews GI and hepatic function in the pregnant woman, fetus, and neonate and implications for clinical practice. Hepatic function related to drug metabolism is discussed in Chapter 7.

MATERNAL PHYSIOLOGIC ADAPTATIONS

The gastrointestinal (GI) and hepatic systems during pregnancy are characterized by marked anatomic and physiologic alterations that are essential in supporting maternal and fetal nutrition. These changes are related to mechanical forces such as the pressure of the growing uterus and hormonal influences such as effects of progesterone on GI smooth muscle and effects of estrogen on liver metabolism.

Antepartum Period

The antepartum period is characterized by anatomic and physiologic changes in all the organs of the GI system. These changes and their implications are summarized in Table 12-1. Pregnancy is associated with increased appetite; increased consumption of food; and alterations in the types of food desired, including cravings, avoidance of certain foods, and, rarely, pica (craving for nonnutrient substances). Specific changes in food consumption and the types of foods craved or avoided are strongly influenced by cultural and economic factors. Food consumption has been reported to increase 15% to 20% beginning in early pregnancy, peaking at midgestation and decreasing near term.[207] Alterations in food intake and appetite create a positive energy balance during pregnancy to meet the needs of the pregnant woman and fetus and to prepare for lactation (see Chapter 16).[128] Changes in maternal caloric intake do not parallel changes in basal metabolism or fetal growth.

The basis for changes in patterns of food intake is unclear but may be a response to the movement of glucose and other nutrients to the fetus, alterations in taste threshold and acuity, and hormonal changes. Estrogen acts as an appetite suppressant and progesterone as an appetite stimulant. Influences of estrogen and progesterone on patterns of food intake are supported by similar changes during the menstrual cycle. Decreased appetite and food intake have been reported during the follicular phase of the menstrual cycle (when estrogen peaks), and with increased appetite during the luteal phase (when progesterone peaks).[249] During pregnancy, alterations in insulin and glucagon combine with estrogen and progesterone to influence food intake.[249] Leptin serum levels parallel changes in body mass index (BMI) during pregnancy and may also mediate maternal appetite changes. The increased food intake with increased leptin levels suggests the development of leptin insensitivity or resistance, which is mediated by human placental lactogen.[128]

Mouth and Pharynx

Contrary to the old wives' tale regarding the loss of a tooth per baby, pregnancy does not result in demineralization of the woman's teeth. Fetal calcium needs are drawn from maternal body stores, not from the teeth (see Chapter 17). The major component of tooth enamel (hydroxyapatite crystals) is not reduced by the biochemical or hormonal changes of pregnancy.[156,167,214] As a result of gingival alterations, however, the pregnant woman may become more aware of preexisting or newly developed dental caries. Changes in saliva and the nausea and vomiting of pregnancy may increase the risk of caries during pregnancy although this has not been well studied.[167] Dental plaque, calculus, and debris deposits increase during pregnancy and are associated with gingivitis.[21,214] In addition, there may be a transient increase in tooth mobility.[214]

Table 12-1 Alterations in the Gastrointestinal System during Pregnancy

ORGAN	ALTERATION	SIGNIFICANCE
Mouth and pharynx	Gingivitis	Friable gum tissue with bleeding and discomfort with chewing Increased periodontal disease
	Epulis formation	Bleeding and interference with chewing
	Increased saliva production	Annoyance
Esophagus	Decreased lower esophageal sphincter pressure and tone	Increased risk of heartburn
	Widening of hiatus with decreased tone	Increased risk of hiatal hernia
Stomach	Decreased tone and motility with delayed gastric emptying time	Increased risk of gastroesophageal reflux and vomiting Increased risk of vomiting and aspiration with use of sedatives or anesthetics
	Incompetence of pyloric sphincter	Reflux of alkaline biliary material into stomach
	Decreased gastric acidity and histamine output	Improvement of peptic ulcer symptoms
Small and large intestines	Decreased intestinal tone and motility with increased transit time	Facilitated absorption of nutrients such as iron and calcium Increased water absorption in large intestine with tendency toward constipation Increased flatulence
	Increased height of duodenal villi	Increased absorption of calcium, amino acids, other substances
	Altered enzymatic transport across villi; increased activity of brush border enzymes	Increased absorption of specific vitamins and other nutrients; increased sodium and water absorption
	Displacement of cecum and appendix by uterus	Complicates diagnosis of appendicitis
Gallbladder	Decreased tone and motility	Alteration in measures of gallbladder function Increased risk of gallstones
Liver	Altered position	May mask mild to moderate hepatomegaly
	Altered production of liver enzymes, plasma proteins, bilirubin, and serum lipids	Some liver function tests less useful in evaluating liver disorders Early signs of liver dysfunction may be missed Altered early recognition of liver dysfunction
	Presence of spider angiomata and palmar erythema	Discomfort because of itching

Pregnancy may exacerbate existing periodontal disease with an increase in periodontal pocket depth during gestation.[165] Periodontal disease has also been associated with intrauterine infection and an increased risk of preterm birth and low–birth weight risk in some but not all studies.[2,82,150,191,248,261] The mechanism is unclear but may be due to either alterations in maternal and fetal immune responses or translocation of oral bacteria into the uterus with colonization and inflammation of the placenta.[95] Increased prostaglandin (PG) synthesis mediated by proinflammatory cytokines from inflamed gingival tissues or via release of bacterial endotoxins could then initiate labor onset (see Chapter 4).[150,261] These studies lack consistent definitions of periodontal disease with lack of control for confounding variables such as socioeconomic status and smoking in some studies.[261] Several recent meta-analyses concluded that oral prophylaxis and treatment of periodontal disease may reduce preterm and low–birth weight rates and that further evaluation is needed; another analysis did not find an association.[82,191,248]

Gingivitis occurs in 30% to 80% of pregnant women, generally beginning around the second month and peaking in the middle of the third trimester.[156,167,214] The anterior region of the mouth is usually the most affected site.[21] Gingival tissue contains both estrogen and progesterone receptors.[21] Estrogen increases blood flow to the oral cavity and accelerates turnover of gum epithelial lining cells. The gums become highly vascularized (with proliferation of small blood vessels and connective tissue), hyperplastic, and edematous.[21,62,156] Progesterone and estradiol may stimulate located inflammation via production of PGs and decreased levels of inflammatory inhibitors.[21] Development of gingivitis may be related to these alterations in the inflammatory process during pregnancy (see Chapter 13), with increased intensity of localized irritation, or to changes in connective tissue metabolism.[21,143] These changes, along with the decreased thickness of the gingival epithelial surface, result in friable gum tissues that may bleed easily or cause discomfort with chewing. Bleeding with brushing occurs more frequently during pregnancy. The incidence of gingivitis is higher with increasing maternal age and parity, preexisting periodontal disease, and poor dentition.[156,208]

In up to 5% of pregnant women, a specific angiogranuloma known as an *epulis* or *pregnancy tumor* develops.[214,249] Epulis formation generally occurs between the second and third month, but can occur later.[21,167] Epulis may gradually increase in size, but rarely is larger than 2 cm in diameter. The etiology is unknown but is thought to relate to hormonal changes (epulis tissue has estrogen and progesterone receptors) and inflammation.[21] Epulis formation is characterized by gingivitis that is advanced and severe. There is a hyperplastic outgrowth that is generally found along the maxillary gingiva and often appears between the upper anterior maxillary teeth.[21] This mass is purplish red to dark purple, very friable, bleeds easily, and often interferes with chewing.[21] Epulis is usually painless, but may ulcerate and become painful in some women.[21,167] Epulis usually regresses spontaneously after delivery, but may recur in the same locations with subsequent pregnancies. Occasionally these growths may need excising during pregnancy due to bleeding, interference with chewing, or increasing periodontal disease.[156,214]

Saliva becomes more acidic during pregnancy, with alterations in electrolyte content and microorganism load, but it usually does not increase in volume.[167] Some women may experience a sense of increased saliva production due to difficulty in swallowing saliva during the period of nausea and vomiting in early pregnancy.[156] A few women do experience excessive salivation (ptyalism). This uncommon disorder begins as early as 2 to 3 weeks and ceases with delivery. The excessive salivation seems to occur primarily during the day.[62] The pathogenesis of ptyalism is unknown, but it is thought to be due to increased saliva, the inability to swallow due to nausea, or activation of the esophagosalivary reflex during gastroesophageal reflux (GER).[214]

Esophagus

Lower esophageal sphincter (LES) tone decreases. This decrease is thought to be primarily due to the smooth muscle relaxant activity of progesterone.[61,117] The LES is a pressure barrier between the stomach and the esophagus, acting as a protective mechanism to prevent or minimize GER. Resting LES pressure decreases during pregnancy with decreased responsiveness to hormonal and physiological stimuli.[61,62,117] At the beginning of the second trimester, basal LES tone is unchanged, although a marked decrease in the normal rise in LES pressure in response to stimulation with a protein meal has been reported.[62,203] This suggests an inhibitory effect and may signal the loss of an important protective response—that is, the ability to modify LES pressure in response to increased intragastric pressure so that reflux is prevented.[62] LES pressure gradually falls by 33% to 50%, with most of the decrease occurring in the third trimester and reaching a nadir at about 36 weeks.[203]

Changes in the LES in pregnancy are similar to changes seen during the ovarian cycle and in women on oral contraceptives, supporting the theory of a hormonal cause for this alteration. An increased incidence of acid reflux with heartburn, which is associated with decreased LES pressure, is seen in nonpregnant women during the luteal phase of the ovarian cycle, when progesterone levels are highest.[203,249] After delivery or discontinuance of oral contraceptives, LES function returns to normal.[62,76,249] Alterations in LES tone and pressure are etiologic factors in the development of heartburn during pregnancy.

Other changes in the esophagus during pregnancy include an increase in secondary peristalsis and nonpropulsive peristalsis and increased incidence of hiatal hernia. Flattening of the hemidiaphragm causes a loss of the normal acute esophageal-gastric angle, which may also lead to reflux.[62]

Stomach

The stomach of the pregnant woman tends to be hypotonic with decreased motility due to actions of progesterone. GI motility is decreased, with prolonged small intestinal transit time. Incompetence of the pyloric sphincter may result in alkaline reflux of duodenal contents into the stomach.[62,117] Gastric emptying time is thought to be unchanged.[61,76,204,214,228,242,259]

The effect of pregnancy on gastric acid secretion is unclear. In several studies, gastric volume was not increased nor was gastric pH decreased during early pregnancy.[117,242] Others have reported a decrease in acidity during the first and second trimesters along with normal gastrin levels, with an increase in acidity to greater than nonpregnant values during the third trimester, accompanied by an increase in gastrin.[214] In general there seems to be a tendency for decreased gastric acidity in pregnancy, especially during the first and second trimesters, with an increase in the third along with small but statistically significant decreases in both basal and histamine-stimulated acid output.[62] Women with peptic ulcers tend to have fewer symptoms during pregnancy, partly because of these changes (see Pregnancy in Women with Peptic Ulcer Disease).[117]

Secretion of pepsin parallels changes in gastric acid output.[61] Decreased gastric acidity is thought to result from hormonal influences (particularly estrogen) and increased levels of placental histaminase.[62,208] Placental histaminase is thought to mediate acid and pepsin secretion by reducing parietal cell responsiveness to endogenous histamine.[62] Gastrin levels are normal during most of pregnancy, with marked increases late in the third trimester, at delivery, and immediately after delivery. The additional gastrin is probably of placental origin.

Small and Large Intestines

The action of progesterone on smooth muscles decreases intestinal tone and motility. The decreased motility observed in pregnancy may not necessarily be a direct effect of progesterone however, but rather due to inhibition by plasma motilin.[228] Decreased GI tone leads to prolonged intestinal transit time, especially during the second and third trimesters. Alterations in transit time increase with advancing gestation, paralleling the increase in progesterone.

Intestinal transit times during stages of pregnancy have been compared with phases of the ovarian cycle in nonpregnant women. Intestinal motility is altered and transit time prolonged during late pregnancy and the luteal phase of the ovarian cycle when progesterone secretion is elevated. The prolonged transit time in late pregnancy is due to an increase in small bowel transit secondary to inhibition of smooth muscle contraction and not to delayed gastric emptying time. The woman may experience a sense of "bloating" and abdominal distention secondary to the delay in intestinal transit times.[214]

The height of the duodenal villi increases (hypertrophies) during pregnancy, which in turn increases absorptive capacity.[117] This change, along with the influences of progesteronc on intestinal transit time and increased activity of brush border enzymes, increases the absorptive capacity for substances such as calcium, lysine, valine, glycine, proline, glucose, sodium, chloride, and water.[117,249] Progesterone also increases lactase and maltase activity. Absorption of other nutrients (including niacin, riboflavin, and vitamin B_6) is reduced, perhaps due to the influence of progesterone on enzymatic transport mechanisms.[117,214,249] Duodenal absorption of iron increases nearly twofold by late pregnancy, probably in response to a reduction of maternal circulating iron stores due to uptake by the placenta and fetus.[214] As a result of the decreased intestinal motility, nutrients and fluids tend to remain in the intestinal lumen for longer periods of time. This may facilitate absorption of nutrients such as iron and calcium. The amount and efficiency of intestinal calcium absorption increase, mediated primarily by increased 1,25-dihydroxyvitamin D (see Chapter 17).

Progesterone may also enhance absorption of calcium, sodium, and water and increase net secretion of potassium.[214,249] The reduced motility and increased transit time in the large intestine increase water and sodium absorption in the colon.[117] Stools are smaller with lower water content, which contributes to development of constipation during pregnancy. Increased flatulence may also occur due to decreased motility along with compression of the bowel by the growing uterus. The appendix and cecum are displaced superiorly by the growing uterus, so that by term the appendix tends to be located along the right costal margin.

Pancreas

The pancreas contains estrogen receptors, which in the rich estrogen environment of pregnancy may increase the risk of pancreatitis.[249] Serum amylase and lipase decrease during the first trimester. The significance of this change is unclear. Changes in the islet cells and the increased production and secretion of insulin are discussed in Chapter 16.

Gallbladder

Muscle tone and motility of the gallbladder decrease during pregnancy, probably due to the effects of progesterone on smooth muscle. As a result, gallbladder volume is increased and emptying rate decreased, especially in the second and third timesters.[61,214] Most measures of gallbladder function are altered during pregnancy, especially after 14 weeks. Some studies have reported that fasting and residual volumes increase to about 20 weeks' gestation, then remain high to term, paralleling the increase in progesterone.[76] The residual gallbladder volume after fasting and emptying is nearly twice as large in the pregnant woman as in nonpregnant women who are not taking oral contraceptives. The increased fasting volume may also be due to decreased water absorption by the mucosa of the gallbladder. This change results from reduced activity of the sodium pump in the mucosal epithelium secondary to estrogens. As a result, bile is more dilute, with a decreased ability to solubilize cholesterol. The sequestered cholesterol may precipitate to form crystals and stones, increasing the tendency to form cholesterol-based gallstones in the second and third trimesters.[61,76,142] In the third trimester, bile is supersaturated with lithogenic cholesterol, which, in conjunction with biliary stasis and sludging, increases the risk of gallstones (see Cholelithiasis and Pregnancy).[76,142] Alterations in gallbladder tone also lead to a tendency to retain bile salts, which can lead to pruritus.

Liver

During pregnancy the enlarging uterus displaces the liver superiorly, posteriorly, and anteriorly. Hepatic blood flow per se is not significantly altered despite marked changes in total blood volume and cardiac output. This is because much of the increased cardiac output is sent to the uteroplacental circulation. As a result, the proportion of cardiac output delivered to the liver remains constant at 25% to 35%.[121] Histologically, only minor nonspecific changes in the liver such as increased fat and glycogen storage and variations in cell size have been reported. The size of the liver does not increase.[258]

Liver production of plasma proteins, bilirubin, serum enzymes, and serum lipids is altered. These changes arise primarily from estrogen, which increases the rough endoplasmic reticulum and liver protein synthesis, and in some cases from hemodilution.[258] Progesterone increases proliferation of the smooth endoplasmic reticulum and cytochrome P450 isoenzymes.[258] Changes in liver products during pregnancy and their significance are summarized in Table 12-2.

Although liver function is not impaired during pregnancy, most of the changes in liver function tests are in the same direction as seen in individuals with liver disorders. Some liver function tests are less useful in evaluating liver disorders during pregnancy; other tests such as aspartate aminotransferase (AST, or serum glutamic-oxaloacetic transaminase [SGOT]), alanine aminotransferase (ALT, or serum glutamic-pyruvic transaminase [SGPT]), and bilirubin are only slightly lower than nonpregnant values.[61,110,209] Changes in hepatic metabolism of drugs during pregnancy are discussed in Chapter 7.

Spider angiomas (also called *spider nevi*) and palmar erythema (common findings in many liver disorders) are thought to be caused by estrogens and are seen in many pregnant women (see Chapter 14). These findings tend to develop between the second and fifth months and disappear or diminish following delivery. Increases in the size of previously existing spider angiomas may also be noted.

Weight Gain during Pregnancy

Weight gain during pregnancy reflects increased maternal stores as well as those of the developing fetus and placenta (Figure 12-1). Approximately 62% of the gain is water, 30% fat, and 8% protein. About 25% of the total gain is attributable

Table 12-2 Liver Function Tests in Normal Pregnancy and Postpartum

SUBSTANCE	PREGNANCY EFFECT	TRIMESTER OF MAXIMUM CHANGE	RETURN TO NONPREGNANT LEVEL	BASIS AND IMPLICATION
Albumin	↓ 20%-40%	2	?	Result of hemodilution and increased catabolism; leads to decreased protein for binding and increased concentrations of free substances
γ-Globulin	N to sl ↓	3	?	Transfer of immunoglobulin G to fetus in third trimester for protection of fetus from infection
α-Globulin	sl ↑	3	3 weeks	Facilitation of transport of lipids and carbohydrates to the placenta, as well as transport of increased maternal thyroid hormones
β-Globulin	sl ↑	3	3 weeks	Facilitation of transport of lipids, carbohydrates, and iron to placenta, as well as transport of hormones
Total protein	↓ 20%	2	?	Primarily related to a fall in albumin; decreases protein-bound substances and increases concentrations of free protein for transport across the placenta
TBG	↑ 2- to 3-fold	1-3	Decreases with removal of placenta and decreased estrogen	Increases beginning within a few weeks after fertilization and plateaus from midgestation to delivery; alters concentration of free versus bound thyroid hormone
CBG	↑ 2- to 3-fold		Decreases with removal of placenta and decreased estrogen	Alters concentration of free versus bound cortisol
Fibrinogen	↑ 50%	2	2-3 weeks	Protection against excessive blood loss at delivery by facilitating clotting
Ceruloplasmin	↑	3	3 weeks	Involved in the transport of most of the body copper needed by mother, fetus, and placenta
Transferrin	↑	3	?	Involved in the binding and transport of iron to meet increased maternal and fetal needs
Bilirubin	N	—	—	May be a slight increase in bilirubin clearance due to maternal clearance of bilirubin from fetus
BSP	N to sl ↑	3	Soon after delivery	Increased removal associated with decreased albumin; alterations may reflect the mild cholestasis seen in pregnancy
AST (SGOT) and ALT (SGPT) in pregnancy	sl ↓ in upper limit	—	—*	Do not change significantly during pregnancy, so these enzymes can be used as indicators of liver or other organ damage during pregnancy
AST (SGOT) and ALT (SGPT) in labor	↑	In labor	By 2-3 weeks*	Increase during labor and delivery, perhaps reflecting the effects of the mechanical forces of labor
GGT	sl ↓ in upper limit	3	?*	Important in synthesis of amino acids for maternal and fetal use

Continued

Table 12-2 **Liver Function Tests in Normal Pregnancy and Postpartum—cont'd**

SUBSTANCE	PREGNANCY EFFECT	TRIMESTER OF MAXIMUM CHANGE	RETURN TO NONPREGNANT LEVEL	BASIS AND IMPLICATION
Alkaline phosphatase	2- to 4 fold ↑	3	Usually by 3 weeks	Much of increase is probably a result of increased production by the fetus and placenta rather than the maternal liver
Lactic dehydrogenase in pregnancy	sl ↑	3	?	Enzyme associated with tissue injury that catalyzes lactic acid to pyruvic acid
Lactic dehydrogenase in labor	↑	In labor	By 2-3 weeks	Increases further during labor, perhaps reflecting the effects of the mechanical forces of labor
Cholesterol	1½- to 2-fold ↑	2-3	By 10 days with significant decrease within 24 hours	Essential precursor for many lipid substances; needed for alterations in lipid metabolism and increased demands for lipids during pregnancy including production of estrogens and progesterone by the placenta

Modified from Monheit, A.G., Cousins, L., & Resnik, R. (1980). The puerperium: Anatomic and physiologic adjustments. *Clin Obstet Gynecol,* 23, 973.
ALT (SGPT), Serum alanine aminotransferase; *AST (SGOT),* serum aspartate aminotransferase; *BSP,* sulfobromophthalein; *CBG,* cortisol binding globulin; *GGT,* serum γ-glutamyl transferase; *N,* no change; *sl,* slight; *TBG,* thyroid binding globulin.
*May rise for up to 10 days postpartum, especially after cesarean delivery.

to the fetus, 11% to the placenta and amniotic fluid, and the remainder to the mother.[101] Optimal weight gain during pregnancy varies with maternal prepregnancy weight; greater weight gain is generally recommended in women who are underweight, and a lower total weight gain is preferable for women who are obese. Maternal weight gain per se lacks sensitivity and specificity as a predictor of pregnancy outcome, in that many women with good pregnancy outcomes have weight gains outside the recommended range.[37,115] However, higher or lower than usual weight gains do increase the risk of maternal and fetal complications and perinatal mortality rates (Figure 12-2).[1,93,215]

Body mass index (BMI) and energy expenditure (see Chapter 16) must also be considered. Prepregnancy BMI and adiposity also affect perinatal outcome. Underweight women have an increased risk of preterm and small-for-gestational-age

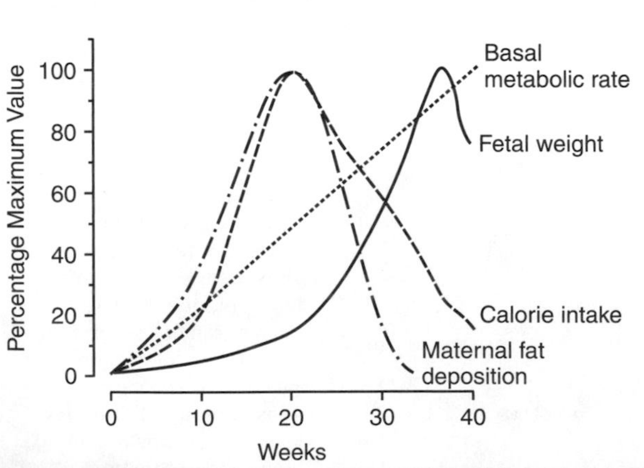

FIGURE 12-1 Changes in maternal caloric intake, maternal fat deposition, fetal weight, and basal metabolic rate during pregnancy. (Values are expressed as a percentage of marginal change.) (From Rosso, P. [1987]. Regulation of food intake during pregnancy and lactation. *Ann N Y Acad Sci,* 499, 191.)

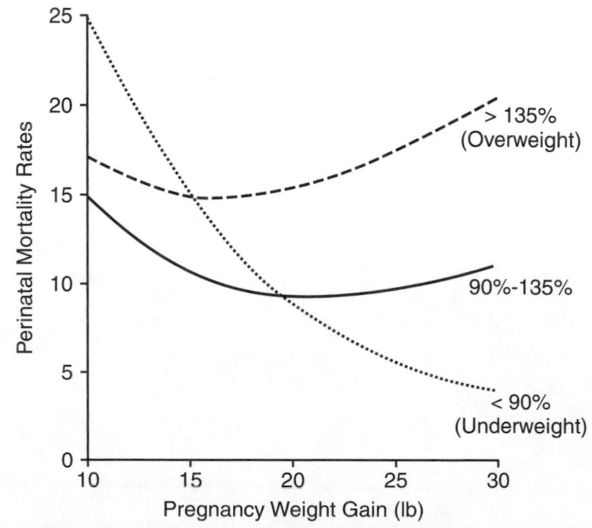

FIGURE 12-2 The relationship between weight gain in pregnancy and perinatal mortality. (From Naeye, R.L. [1979]. Weight gain and the outcome in pregnancy. *Am J Obstet Gynecol,* 135, 3.)

(SGA) infants with decreased macrosomia, preeclampsia and cesarean birth; overweight women have an increase in spontaneous abortion, congenital anomalies, intrauterine death, gestational diabetes, hypertensive disorders, preeclampsia, thromboembolic complications and cesarean birth, and decreased risk of SGA and growth-restricted infants.[215]

The Institute of Medicine (IOM) guidelines for weight gain and the pattern of gain based on prepregnancy weight for height were published in 1990.[103] These guidelines generated controversy, particularly in relation to the weight gain range for obese women, and concern that using them would increase the number of large-for-gestational-age (LGA) infants and maternal and fetal complications.[37,115,202,215] Abrams and colleagues reviewed pregnancy outcomes from studies using the IOM guidelines and found that weight gain within these recommendations was associated with the best maternal and fetal outcome.[1] However, they noted that in most women, weight gain was not within the IOM guidelines.[1] In other studies, only about one third of pregnant women gained weight within the recommended limits, with most gaining more than recommended.[37,38] Chu et al. found that using the 1990 IOM guidelines 30% of normal weight women and 60% of overweight women gained more than recommended; excessive gestational weight gain was correlated with weight retention postpartum and later obesity.[52] Others have found similar outcomes.[178]

In response to concerns of excessive weight gain and later development of obesity, the IOM recently revised these guidelines (see Table 12-3). The revised guidelines also added recommended gain for three subcategories of obesity (class I, II, and III). The current IOM guidelines assume a 1.1- to 4-lb weight gain during the first trimester, followed by a recommended 0.8 to 1 lb (0.36 to 0.45 kg) per week for the second and third trimesters in normal BMI women, with higher gains of 1 to 1.3 lb (0.45 to 0.59 kg) per week in underweight and less per week in overweight women (0.6 to 0.7 lb or 0.23 to 0.32 kg). Obese women are recommended to restrict weight gain during the first trimester to 0.4 to 0.6 lb (0.18 to 0.27 kg).[181,198,199]

Weight gain during the first trimester goes primarily toward maternal fat stores (see Figure 12-1). Weight gained during the second half of pregnancy goes toward growth of the fetus and maternal supportive tissues. Marked or persistent deviations from these patterns should be evaluated.[198,199] Women whose weight gain significantly exceeds these limits or deviates from the expected pattern require similar evaluation. For example, if a woman gains 30 lb in the first 20 weeks of pregnancy, she has added approximately 25 lb (11.33 kg) of fat to her stores (and additional fat is often difficult to lose postpartum). This woman will still need to gain approximately 20 lb (9.07 kg) during the second half of pregnancy to ensure adequate growth of the fetus and her own tissues.[208] Greater gains are needed in women with multifetal pregnancies.[109,181] These women also have increased nutritional needs, including higher energy, vitamin D, linolenic and linoleic acids, calcium, and other minerals.[44]

Intrapartum Period

Gastric motility is further decreased during labor. This decrease is probably influenced by anxiety and pain as well as the effects of opioid administration. The reduced competency of the LES, along with decreased gastric motility and increased gastric acidity, delays gastric emptying time and increases the risk of aspiration with sedatives or anesthesia.

Labor is accompanied by delays in gastric emptying times that differ from both third-trimester and nonpregnant values.[61,259] Opioids may be the main factor in delayed gastric emptying during labor. Opioids also delay gastric emptying and increase the risk of aspiration if used in conjunction with general anesthesia. Reduced use of general anesthesia for delivery has reduced the numbers of women at risk for intrapartum aspiration. However, any use of general anesthesia with a pregnant woman, whether for delivery or nonobstetric surgery, requires careful monitoring and use of interventions to prevent vomiting and aspiration.

During labor, alkaline phosphatase levels, which double during pregnancy, increase further. Serum aminotransferases (AST and ALT), which only change slightly during pregnancy, and lactic dehydrogenase increase up to twice normal values.[185] These enzymes are associated with tissue

Table 12-3 New Recommendations for Total and Rate of Weight Gain during Pregnancy by Prepregnancy Body Mass Index

PREPREGNANCY BMI	BMI* (kg/m²)	TOTAL WEIGHT GAIN (lb)⁺	2nd AND 3rd TRIMESTER MEANS (RANGE) GAIN (lb)/WEEK
Underweight	<18.5	28-40	1 (1-1.3)
Normal weight	18.5-24.9	25-35	1 (0.8-1)
Overweight	25.0-29.9	15-25	0.6 (0.5-0.7)
Obese (includes all categories)	>30.0	11-20	0.5 (0.4-0.6)

From Rasmussen, K.M. & Yaktine, A.L. (2009). *Weight gain during pregnancy: reexamining the guidelines.* Institute of Medicine (US) and National Research Council (US) Committee to Reexamine IOM pregnancy weight guidelines. Washington, DC: National Academies Press.
*BMI is calculated using metric units (BMI = kg/m² × 100).
⁺Calculations assume a 0.5-2 kg (1.1-4.4 lb) weight gain in the first trimester.
BMI, body mass index.

injury and may reflect the stresses of labor on the mother and placenta.

Postpartum Period

During the postpartum period, the anatomic and physiologic changes within the GI and hepatic systems gradually return to their prepregnant state. Delivery results in an average weight loss of 4.5 to 5.8 kg (10 to 13 lb).[60] Findings regarding postpartum weight loss are inconsistent. Some women have further weight loss during the first week; others have no change or gain weight. The increased adrenocortical hormone and arginine vasopressin activity associated with the stress of labor tends to lead to water and sodium retention that may prevent weight loss or lead to a gain. In general, after 4 days, most women begin to show some additional loss, averaging another 2.3 to 3.6 kg (5 to 8 lb) due to diuresis and 0.9 to 1.4 kg (2 to 3 lb) from involution and lochia by the end of the first week.[58] Alterations in energy utilization may alter losses in nonlactating women.[60]

Most women lose weight steadily over the first 3 to 6 months postpartum, with the greatest loss in the first 3 months. Weight loss occurs sooner and to a greater degree in women of lower parity, age, and prepregnant weight.[60] Lactation may facilitate postpartum weight and body fat loss as maternal tissue stores are catabolized to use as energy for milk production.[60] Most women do not lose all of the pregnancy weight gain, with an average retention of 1 kg (2.2 lb) with each pregnancy; 10% retain more than 15 lb (6.8 kg).[60] Women who are overweight or normal weight before pregnancy are more likely to retain weight following pregnancy than women who were underweight.[60] Abrams and colleagues found no evidence that weight gain during pregnancy within the IOM recommendations increased the risk of weight retention following birth.[1] However, weight gain above these recommendations was common and associated with an increased risk of further weight gain during the first postpartum year and perhaps later development of obesity.[180,221] Most studies have small sample sizes and often do not control for activity, diet, and psychosocial factors.

Gingivitis often disappears after delivery but may last for up to 6 months postpartum.[214] Epulis regresses and also usually disappears postpartum, but a scarred area may remain.[214] LES pressure and tone return to normal levels by 4 to 8 weeks postpartum.[203,214] Gallbladder volume returns to normal by 2 weeks postpartum.[76] Gallbladder contractility is enhanced postpartum, enabling the previously atonic gallbladder to empty a larger proportion of its volume and expel microgallstones that developed during pregnancy.[249] Expulsion of these stones can lead to a gallstone pancreatitis.

Most of the liver enzymes return to nonpregnant levels within 3 weeks of delivery.[201] Fatty acids, cholesterol, triglycerides, and lipoproteins tend to reach normal levels by about 10 days.[201] AST, ALT, and serum γ-glutamyl transferase (GGT) (see Table 12-2), which rose during the intrapartum period, may continue to rise for up to 10 days postpartum, especially following cesarean birth.[201] These parameters generally reach nonpregnant levels by 2 to 3 weeks. Alkaline phosphatase decreases after delivery and usually returns to nonpregnant levels by 20 days, but may remain elevated for up to 6 weeks.[185,201]

The appendix returns to its usual position by 10 days postpartum.[228] GI muscle tone and motility are decreased during the intrapartum and early postpartum periods. Decreased gastric motility along with relaxation of the abdominal musculature can result in gaseous distention 2 to 3 days postpartum. Decreased intestinal motility can lead to postpartum ileus and constipation. Bowel movements usually resume 2 to 3 days after birth, with resumption of normal bowel patterns by 8 to 14 days.

CLINICAL IMPLICATIONS FOR THE PREGNANT WOMAN AND HER FETUS

The normal alterations in GI function and structure in the pregnant woman are responsible for some of the more common discomforts of pregnancy, including heartburn and constipation. Alterations in the anatomic position of structures such as the appendix and liver and in concentrations of liver enzymes and other substances, as well as concerns about potential hazards with the use of radiographic contrast studies on the fetus, can lead to difficulty in assessing and diagnosing pathologic processes that arise. This section examines the basis for development of these problems and reviews the effect of pregnancy on selected disorders such as peptic ulcer disease (PUD) and cholelithiasis.

Nutritional Requirements of Pregnancy

The physical and physiologic demands of pregnancy on the mother, along with fetal needs for nutrients, significantly increase nutritional requirements during pregnancy (Table 12-4). Nutrient needs are also altered postpartum and during lactation (see Chapter 5). During pregnancy an additional 300 to 340 kcal per day are needed in the second trimester and up to 450 kcal per day are needed in the third trimester to meet energy and growth demands of the mother and fetus and to conserve protein for cell growth.[181] Energy needs vary considerably from woman to woman with adaptations in individual metabolism to spare energy for fetal growth. Thus the diet should be individualized based on maternal age, trimester, BMI and activity.[116] The woman meets the energy demands of pregnancy by increasing intake, decreasing activity, or limiting maternal fat storage (see Chapter 16).[120] The total minimum energy costs of pregnancy average 80,000 kcal, although some women may need up to 120,000 kcal.[215] Protein requirements increase to 60 g or slightly more to provide nitrogen for maternal, fetal, and placental tissue synthesis and growth.[108,188] Sources of protein should contain all the essential amino acids. Adequate maternal intake of the essential fatty acids, linoleic acid, and α-linolenic acid (an omega-3 fatty acid) is important for fetal growth and development, especially brain and vision development.[215]

Maternal plasma levels of water-soluble vitamins and many minerals gradually decline during gestation. This

Table 12-4 Basis for Increased Nutrient Needs in Pregnancy

NUTRIENT	REASON FOR INCREASED NEED IN PREGNANCY
Protein	Rapid fetal tissue growth Placental growth and development Maternal tissue growth (e.g., uterus, breasts) Increased blood volume (increased hemoglobin, plasma proteins) Maternal storage reserves (for labor, delivery, and lactation)
Calories	Increased basal metabolic rate (BMR), energy needs, and protein sparing
Calcium	Fetal skeleton and tooth bud formation Increased maternal calcium metabolism
Phosphorus	Fetal skeleton and tooth bud formation Increased maternal phosphorus metabolism
Iron	Increased maternal circulating blood volume and increased hemoglobin Fetal liver iron storage; iron cost of pregnancy
Iodine	Increased BMR and thyroxine production
Magnesium	Coenzyme in energy and protein metabolism; enzyme activator Tissue growth; cell metabolism; muscle action
Vitamin A	Essential for cell development and thus for tissue growth Fetal tooth bud formation (development of enamel-forming cells in gum tissue) Bone growth
Vitamin D	Absorption of calcium and phosphorus Mineralization of fetal bone tissue and tooth buds
Vitamin E	Tissue growth Cell wall integrity and red blood cell integrity
Vitamin C	Tissue formation and integrity Increased iron absorption Integrity of connective and vascular tissues
Folic acid	Increased metabolic demands of pregnancy and increased heme production Production of cell nucleus materials
Niacin	Coenzyme in energy and protein metabolism
Riboflavin	Coenzyme in energy and protein metabolism
Thiamin	Coenzyme in energy metabolism
Vitamin B_6	Coenzyme in protein metabolism Increased fetal growth requirement
Vitamin B_{12}	Coenzyme in protein metabolism, especially proteins in nucleic acid Formation of red blood cells

Adapted from Worthington-Roberts, B.S. & Williams, S.R. (1996). *Nutrition in pregnancy and lactation*. New York: McGraw-Hill.

decline is probably primarily due to the effects of hemodilution rather than to greater fetal and maternal demands.[207] With the exception of vitamin D (see Chapter 17) and iron (see Chapter 8), little is known about the effects of pregnancy on metabolism of most vitamins and minerals. Recommended dietary reference intakes (DRIs) for childbearing-age, pregnant, and lactating women are available from the Food and Nutrition Board of the National Academy of Science's Institute of Medicine.[104-108]

During pregnancy, recommended dietary reference intakes for many vitamins are increased by 20% to 100%, including vitamin E, vitamin C, thiamin, riboflavin, niacin, vitamin B_6, and vitamin B_{12}.[2,105,106,188,215] Vitamin E is essential during pregnancy for tissue growth and integrity of cell and red blood cell membranes. Vitamin C increases iron absorption and is needed for collagen formation and tissue formation and integrity. Thiamin, niacin, riboflavin, and vitamins B_6 and B_{12} serve as coenzymes for protein and energy metabolism, which are increased in the pregnant woman.[233] Zinc supplementation has been reported to increase birth weight in undernourished women with low serum zinc levels and decrease the risk of fetal growth restriction.[8] Requirements for minerals and other vitamins are discussed in Chapter 8 (iron and folate), Chapter 17 (calcium, phosphorus, magnesium, and vitamin D), and Chapter 19 (iodine). Absorption of some minerals, including calcium, iron, zinc, and selenium, increases during pregnancy.[8,121] Excessive intake or marked deficiency of specific vitamins and minerals has been reported to be associated with adverse pregnancy outcome, although the number of observations is limited. Excessive vitamin A (retinol) is associated with an increase in birth defects.[8,159,188] The reader is referred to texts on nutrition during pregnancy for further discussion of nutritional assessment and requirements.[103,207,233]

The benefits of routine multivitamin supplementation other than for specific supplements such as folic acid and iron have not been clearly documented.[215,217,223] The IOM recommendations indicate that pregnant women with balanced diets do not need routine multivitamin and mineral supplementation, except iron, and even routine iron supplementation is not without controversy (see Chapter 8).[55,103] Folic acid supplementation is recommended for all women of childbearing age to reduce the incidence of neural tube defects (see Chapter 15).[67] Additional multivitamin and mineral supplementation or supplementation of specific nutrients may be needed by women whose diet is inadequate (which may apply to women both below and above the poverty level) or who have a multiple pregnancy, smoke, or are alcohol or drug abusers. Micronutrient supplementation during pregnancy has been reported to decrease low birth weight but not to affect preterm birth rates or perinatal or neonatal mortality.[51]

Fetal Nutritional Needs

The fetus is dependent on the mother and placenta for transfer of nutrients essential for normal fetal growth and development. (Fetal growth and alterations are discussed in Development of the Gastrointestinal and Hepatic Systems in the Fetus.) Maternal nutrition during pregnancy, whether adequate, inadequate, or excessive, leads to "programming" of fetal tissues and may have long-term consequences for neurobehavioral outcomes and later health of offspring, including risks of hypertension, obesity, and cardiovascular disease.[144]

Nutritional needs of the fetus are met by three mechanisms depending on the stage of development. Before implantation, the blastocyst absorbs nutrients from its surrounding tissues and from fluids within the fallopian tube and uterus. Between implantation and placental development, nutrients are absorbed via a sinusoidal space between maternal and fetal tissues. With formation of the placenta, nutrients are transferred across this structure from mother to fetus via a variety of mechanisms (see Chapter 3). The energy needs of the fetus near term are met through carbohydrates (80%) and amino acids (20%).[207] Fats are not used as a primary energy source by the fetus due to immaturity of fat metabolism. The major fetal energy source is glucose from the mother; free fatty acids are used as an alternative energy source and a substrate for lipid formation (see Chapter 16). Amino acids are actively transported from mother to fetus, and imbalances in maternal plasma amino acid concentrations can result in excessive fetal concentrations and subsequent damage as can occur in women with phenylketonuria (see Chapter 1).

Fetal needs for most vitamins and minerals can be met if maternal intake follows recommended DRIs.[103] Lipid-soluble vitamins (A, D, E, and K) cross the placenta more readily than water-soluble vitamins and with increasing ease with advancing gestation. The vitamins most likely to be associated with deficiencies during pregnancy are folate and B_6 (see Chapter 8).

Calcium and phosphorus are actively transported across the placenta, which allows accumulation of calcium and calcification of the fetal skeleton (see Chapter 17). The fetus needs micronutrients such as zinc, copper, chromium, iodine, magnesium, and manganese. Maternal dietary intake of these elements is usually sufficient. Iron supplementation is recommended to enhance maternal iron stores (see Chapter 8).

Heartburn and Gastroesophageal Reflux

Heartburn (reflux esophagitis with retrosternal burning) arises from reflux of gastric acids into the lower esophagus. Heartburn has been reported in up to 80% of women at some point during pregnancy, with an increased frequency seen in the third trimester.[21,203,214,117,228] Heartburn usually begins during the second trimester, although about 25% experience heartburn in the first trimester. Heartburn intensifies with advancing gestation and disappears following delivery.[203] Interventions are summarized in Table 12-5.

The pathogenesis of heartburn during pregnancy is multifactorial. The major etiologic factor is relaxation of the LES along with alterations in pressure gradients across the sphincter. In nonpregnant women, LES tone increases in response to elevations in intragastric pressure as a protective mechanism to prevent or minimize reflux. Alterations in LES tone during pregnancy eliminate or significantly reduce this protective mechanism.[61,117,228] Pregnant women without heartburn tend to have LES pressures sufficient to maintain the normal pressure gradient across the gastroesophageal junction, whereas women with heartburn do not demonstrate this compensatory mechanism.[208,228] Pregnant women (regardless of whether or not they experience heartburn) have increased nonpropulsive esophageal motor activity with decreased wave amplitude and slower spread of peristaltic waves, with a reduction in secondary peristalsis.[208] These findings are suggestive of reflux and are more prominent in women who experience symptoms of heartburn during pregnancy.

Pressure from the growing uterus increases intragastric pressure and, along with flattening of the hemidiaphragm, causes anatomic distortion of the stomach and decreases the acuteness of the angle at the gastroesophageal junction.[62,117] Elevations in intragastric and intraabdominal pressure are intensified by multiple pregnancy, hydramnios, obesity, lithotomy position, bending over, or application of fundal pressure.[228] The tendency toward reflux is increased by the decreased GI tone and relaxation of the cardiac sphincter.[62,246] As a result of gastric stasis and pyloric incompetence, the refluxed material may be alkaline or acidic. Prolonged reflux of normal pH or alkaline duodenal material can lead to esophagitis.[62] If pharmacologic therapy is needed, histamine$_2$-receptor antagonists, which are Food and Drug Administration (FDA) class B agents, are usually recommended, with cimetidine and ranitidine having the greatest use.[203,228] For more severe GER, proton pump inhibitors, which are FDA class C agents, may sometimes be used. Data on use of these agents during pregnancy are limited, but several studies have reported that use of omeprazole was not associated with major teratogenic risks, especially with use after the first trimester.[177]

The frequency of hiatal hernia is also increased, occurring in 15% to 20% of pregnant women primarily after 7 to 8 months' gestation. This disorder arises from alterations in muscle tone and pressure with widening of the hiatus. Interventions are similar to those for heartburn (see Table 12-5).

Constipation

Constipation occurs in 10% to 30% of women and tends to be worse in the first and third trimesters.[214,228,246] Constipation probably arises primarily from alterations in water transport and reabsorption in the large intestine. The smooth muscle relaxant effects of progesterone decrease intestinal motility and prolong transit time, which increases electrolyte and subsequently water absorption in the large intestine. Progesterone may also inhibit motilin (a stimulating GI hormone) release.[228] Other predisposing factors are compression of the rectosigmoid area by the enlarging uterus and changes in dietary habits and activity

Table 12-5 Recommendations for Common Problems during Pregnancy Related to the Gastrointestinal System

PROBLEM	NURSING RECOMMENDATIONS
Heartburn	Eat small, frequent meals
	Eat bland foods
	Avoid fatty or spicy foods, tomatoes, and highly acidic citrus products
	Avoid late night or large meals
	Avoid foods that reduce lower esophageal sphincter pressure (e.g., alcohol, chocolate, caffeine)
	Avoid lying down for 1-3 hours following meals
	Chew gum
	Sleep with torso elevated
	Avoid lying flat or bending
	Use antacids (calcium-magnesium based) after meals and at bedtime
	Avoid the use of antacids containing phosphorus (alters calcium-phosphorus balance, leading to leg cramps), sodium (increases water retention), or high-dose aluminum (accumulates in woman and fetus; causes constipation)
	Monitor for side effects of chronic antacid use (alteration in muscle tone and deep tendon reflexes, electrolyte imbalance)
	Recognize potential effects of chronic antacid use on malabsorption of K, P, Ca, and drugs such as anticoagulants, salicylates, vitamin E
Constipation	Drink fluids
	Drink hot or cold liquids (especially on an empty stomach)
	Eat high-fiber/bulk laxative foods such as fruits and raw vegetables
	Eat high-fiber bran and wheat foods
	Encourage regular light exercise during pregnancy
	Ambulate early postpartum
	Use stool softeners
	Use bulk-forming fiber-containing agents (which are not absorbed and are therefore safest)
	Use stimulant laxatives with caution and avoid long-term use
	Avoid use of mineral oil in pregnancy (absorbs fat-soluble vitamins including vitamin K)
	Monitor for side effects if laxatives are prescribed (fluid accumulation, sodium retention and edema, cramping)
	Monitor for drug interactions if laxatives are prescribed (decreased serum K with diuretics, decreased effectiveness of anticoagulants and salicylates)
Hemorrhoids	Use sitz bath
	Use astringents such as witch hazel (Tucks), lemon juice, or vinegar
	Eat bulk foods
	Prevent constipation and straining (see above)
Nausea and vomiting	Eat small, frequent, high-carbohydrate, low-fat meals and snacks
	Avoid strong odors, fatty or spicy foods, and cold liquids
	Consume dry crackers or toast before arising
	Consume ginger (e.g., soda, tea, cookies, supplement)
	Suck on hard candy
	Try elastic wrist bands (SeaBands)
	Lie down when first experiencing symptoms
	Practice relaxation techniques
	Avoid factors and situations that precipitate symptoms
	Monitor for side effects of pharmacologic agents (see pp. 404)

and exercise patterns. Interventions for women with constipation are summarized in Table 12-5.

Hemorrhoids

Hemorrhoids arise more frequently during pregnancy and are aggravated by constipation. Factors that contribute to hemorrhoid formation during pregnancy include poor support for hemorrhoidal veins in the anorectal area; lack of valves in these vessels, leading to reversal in the direction of blood flow and stasis; gravity; pressure of the expanding uterus; increased venous pressure in the pelvic veins; venous congestion and engorgement; and enlargement of the hemorrhoidal veins.[18] Interventions for women with hemorrhoids are summarized in Table 12-5.

Nausea and Vomiting

Nausea with or without vomiting is a self-limiting event experienced by up to 70% to 90% of pregnant women in Western cultures.[35,64,138,204] Vomiting occurs in 30% to 45% of these women, but is uncommon in many other cultures.[138,214] Nausea and vomiting in pregnancy (NVP) generally begins between 4 and 6 weeks, but may occur as early as 2 to 3 weeks after the last menstrual period, and peaks at 8 to 12 weeks.[228] NVP usually resolves by 10 to 12 weeks, although a few women (less than 10%) may experience symptoms to term.[228,252] NVP incidence and severity are often linked to dietary cravings and aversions.[54] The most frequent food aversions are to meat, fish, poultry, and eggs.[79] NVP is often thought to occur most prominently before rising in the morning and ingestion of food (hence the term *morning sickness*), but many women experience symptoms in the afternoon, evening, or throughout the day.[64,117] Although NVP usually disappears by 10 to 12 weeks it persists to 14 weeks in 40% of women, 16 weeks in less than 20%, and 20 weeks in less than 10%.[208,214]

The exact cause and function of nausea and vomiting is unknown. Many theories have been proposed, focusing on mechanical, endocrinologic, allergic, metabolic, genetic, and psychosomatic etiologies, but none has substantial research support.[90,100,129,138,208,214,228] An adaptive and protective mechanism for NVP has also been postulated.[79,100] NVP likely results from a combination of metabolic and endocrine factors, many of them placental in origin, mediated by other factors.[138]

The most common hormonal theories are related to rapidly increasing and high levels of estrogen, human chorionic gonadotropin (hCG), and possibly thyroxine. Support for a hormonal basis comes from studies documenting nausea in women on estrogen medications or combined oral contraceptive pills, the high correlation between women who experience nausea with both oral contraceptive use and pregnancy, and parallels between hCG patterns and the timing of symptom appearance and disappearance in NVP.[100,138] However, studies examining the correlation of hCG levels with symptom appearance and intensity in individual women have produced inconsistent results.[90] Increased NVP is seen in women with multiple and molar pregnancies, both of which are characterized by increased hCG.[138] Perhaps a combination of endocrine factors leads to NVP, and individual women may have different sensitivities to these substances. The prevalence of specific hCG isoforms or alterations in hCG receptors may account for differences in NVP prevalence among various populations.[138] NVP has been associated with favorable pregnancy outcomes such as decreased miscarriage rates, low birth weight, and perinatal mortality, although some researchers have found no differences in perinatal mortality and low birth weight.[13,54,79,100,117,231,256] Few studies have been done to document a psychogenic basis to NVP, and many available reports are case studies of women in psychotherapy. Studies that have been done on more representative populations present conflicting findings.

Another hypothesis is that NVP may have an adaptive function to protect the embryo from potentially toxic substances in foods, such as animal products that might contain parasites and other pathogens if not handled correctly, caffeinated beverages, and alcohol.[100] A study of 20 societies in which women experience NVP and 7 in which NVP is rare found that the societies in which NVP was rare were more likely to have plants (corn) as the primary staple rather than animal products.[79]

Decreased energy intake in early pregnancy is correlated with increased placental weight in animal and human studies.[79] Huxley suggests that hCG activates the thyroid, thus increasing thyroxine secretion, which stimulates placental growth. As noted above, hCG (and thyroxine) levels correlate with severity and onset of NVP in some but not all studies. Huxley postulates that NVP reduces maternal energy intake. Maternal levels of anabolic hormones, insulin, and insulin-like growth factor I (IGF-I) are lowered as is maternal tissue synthesis, favoring early placental growth and development, and later fetal growth.[100] Underweight women tend to experience less severe NVP than women with normal preconceptional BMI.[100]

Interventions for women experiencing NVP are summarized in Table 12-5. Pharmacologic treatment may occasionally be required due to severity of symptoms or interference with the woman's responsibilities. Use of pharmacologic agents is fraught with potential problems, in that NVP and thus the administration of any drugs occur during the period of embryonic organogenesis. Until the early 1980s, Bendectin (which combined an antihistamine and pyridoxine) was commonly used to treat NVP. Litigation over the relationship of Bendectin and congenital defects resulted in removal of this drug from the market, although a causal relationship has never been documented.[253] Alternative therapies have been investigated.[114,151,253] Ginger has been reported to be effective in reducing nausea in most studies, although there continue to be concerns about high doses.[35,36,192,252,253] Ginger may work by increasing gastric tone and peristalsis via anticholinergic and antiserotonin actions.[252] Vitamin B_1 has also been shown to reduce NVP.[176] However, studies on the use of acupuncture for NVP have had equivocal findings.[114,151]

Hyperemesis gravidarum, an uncommon disorder seen in 0.3% to 1% of pregnant women, is intractable vomiting associated with alterations in nutritional status, dehydration, electrolyte imbalance, significant weight loss (greater than 5%), ketosis, and acetonuria.[13,61,117,228,252] These women often require hospitalization. Risk factors include primiparas, multiple gestation, family history or hyperemesis in previous pregnancies.[117,138] Hyperemesis has been linked to alterations in thyroid hormones (see Chapter 19) and endocrine changes (especially progesterone and human chorionic gonadotropin), immunologic changes, and metabolic alterations, and is associated with *Helicobacter pylori*.[61,138,228,252] Hyperemesis usually begins by 4 to 10 weeks and resolves by 20 weeks, but persists to delivery in about 10%.[252]

Food and Fluid Intake in Labor

For many years most hospitals in the United States did not allow women in active labor to eat or consume beverages other than ice chips or clear liquids. These prohibitions developed during the period when general anesthesia was commonly used during the second stage of labor; accordingly, there were concerns regarding the risk of aspiration should the anesthetized woman vomit. These constraints have been questioned, with many practitioners advocating more liberal food and fluid policies during labor.[122] Potential benefits include meeting maternal energy needs and reducing maternal stress and the risks of ketosis, hyponatremia, and vomiting.[218] There is little documentation supporting either the benefits of this therapy or the risk of oral intake for most women (see Chapter 11).[145] Most studies have not reported adverse effects of oral intake during labor in low-risk women (studies of high-risk women are lacking).[148,183,218,243] O'Sullivan and associates compared a light diet versus water during labor and found no differences in labor duration, cesarean section rate, incidence of vomiting, or outcomes.[183] A Cochrane review examined oral fluid or food intake during labor and concluded that there was no evidence to support restrictions for low-risk women.[224] Current guidelines from professional groups also support oral intake during labor in low-risk women.[12,122,260]

Individuals opposed to a more liberal food and fluid policy in labor argue that, although rare, aspiration has devastating consequences and can still occur with an endotracheal tube in place or use of regional anesthesia. Pregnant women are at particular risk for pulmonary aspiration because of delayed gastric emptying time in late pregnancy, increased levels of gastrin (resulting in increased gastric volume), and decreased LES tone (which allows stomach contents in an unconscious woman to passively move into the pharynx and into the lungs). Those advocating relaxation of restrictions note that (1) general anesthesia has been replaced by regional anesthesia; (2) the incidence of maternal mortality from aspiration of stomach contents in normal labor is rare; (3) gastric emptying may not be significantly altered in normal women who have not received narcotics; (4) use of intravenous fluid administration is increased; and (5) prolonged fasting during labor has physiologic and psychologic effects.[40,41,145] Sharts-Hopko noted that maternal aspiration "is so rare that a randomized control trial to see if oral intake related to maternal mortality is not even feasible."[218,p.198] General anesthesia, if used, is safer than in the past as the result of changes in anesthetic agents and administrative techniques, such as the use of endotracheal tubes, which prevent aspiration of vomitus. Potential physiologic effects of fasting include increased ketones and fatty acids with decreased alanine, glucose, and insulin. Psychologic effects include increased anxiety and stress.[41] Use of intravenous fluids has been associated with maternal and infant fluid and electrolyte problems (see Chapter 11). Low-risk women who deliver at home or in alternative settings and women in other cultures often consume food and beverages during labor with few complications.

Effects of Altered Maternal Nutrition

Adequate nutrition during pregnancy is essential for optimal fetal growth and development. Most studies demonstrate a correlation between maternal weight gain and birth weight even when other variables that influence birth weight (gestational age, maternal height, and birth order) are held constant. The relationship between weight gain during pregnancy and perinatal mortality varies with maternal prepregnancy weight and pregnancy weight gain (see Figure 12-2). Alterations in maternal nutrition can influence both fetal growth and later outcomes of offspring. For example, undernourished women, especially those with low prepregnancy BMI and low weight gain during pregnancy, have an increased risk of SGA and fetal growth restricted infants. These infants are at risk for later developing obesity and type 2 diabetes.[128,140,215] Infants born to obese women are at later risk of developing obesity and type I diabetes.[140] Specific effects of altered maternal nutrition are listed in Table 12-6. Effects of maternal nutrition on the fetus are discussed further in Fetal Growth.

Undernutrition and Pregnancy

Women who are underweight have a higher incidence of pregnancy loss and SGA infants. These women may fail to gain adequate weight during pregnancy, further increasing the risk of fetal growth restriction and maternal nutritional anemia and malnutrition. Maternal undernutrition can also alter fetal metabolic programming, increasing the risk of later disorders (see "Fetal Growth").[47,78]

Kristal and Rush and others have reviewed studies examining the effects of maternal undernutrition on fetal growth and concluded the following: (1) limitations in the overall amount of maternal food intake from either starvation or iatrogenic limitations lead to a consistent depression in birth weight (up to 550 g); (2) relief of acute undernutrition up to the beginning of the third trimester is associated with return of birth weight to previous levels; (3) results of supplementation studies with pregnant women at risk nutritionally (in developed and developing countries) are consistent, with increases in birth weight of 40 to 60 g; (4) there seems to be a limit in the amount of supplementation a given individual can tolerate and to the effect of these supplements; and (5) a consistent depression in birth weight is seen with use of high-density protein supplements in which more than 20% of calories supplied are protein.[125,126] High-density protein diets have also been associated with an increased incidence of SGA infants and possibly increased neonatal morbidity in some populations.[125] Both caloric and protein deprivation affect the fetus, although it is controversial as to which is most detrimental to fetal growth and development. Human and animal studies suggest that restrictions in caloric intake have the most marked effects on fetal growth, whereas protein deprivation leads to alterations in later development.[93] Providing undernourished women with balanced protein energy supplementation reduces the risk of fetal growth restriction.[102] Studies of supplementation with micronutrients of undernourished women have been sparse (and tend to focus on a single nutrient), although some have reported improvements in maternal and fetal weight.[51]

Maternal Obesity and Pregnancy

Maternal obesity is one of the most common risk factors in pregnant women.[128] Maternal obesity is associated with an increased incidence of macrosomia, LGA infants, delivery

Table 12-6 **Expected Consequences of Inadequate Nutrition in Women during a Reproductive Cycle**

PREPREGNANCY	PREGNANCY	POSTPREGNANCY
	Deficient Nutrition	
Short stature Low body weight Low adiposity Low lean body mass Delayed menarche Low nutrient reserves (including Ca, Fe, I, Zn, vitamin A) Low discretionary activity	Small placenta Reduced duration of pregnancy Risk of low birth weight and fetal growth restriction Inadequate weight gain Low deposition of fat Inadequate volume expansion Inadequate hormonal response Nutrient deficiencies (including Fe, I, Zn, vitamin A, folate, vitamin D) Perinatal complications Lower discretionary activity	Body weight deficient Poor lactation performance Prolonged amenorrhea Longer birth interval Nutrient deficiencies (Fe, Ca, Zn, vitamin A, and so on) Low discretionary activity Poorer prepregnancy nutrition
	Relative Excess of Energy (Obesity)	
Poor health (higher prevalence of hypertension, diabetes) Low discretionary activity	Increased adiposity Risk of macrosomic baby Perinatal complications Risk of preeclampsia and diabetes	Worsening of diabetes and health consequences Low discretionary activity

Adapted from Viteri, F.E., Schumacher, L., & Silliman, K. (1989). Maternal malnutrition and the fetus. *Semin Perinatol*, 13, 236.
IUGR, Intrauterine growth restriction.

complications, and perinatal mortality.[28,128,168] These LGA infants are usually larger than expected in weight but not length due to increased deposition of adipose tissue.[93] The woman's excess adipose tissue reserves may be supplying some of the fuel needed for fetal growth. Cord blood triglyceride levels are elevated, reflecting enhanced fat synthesis by the fetal liver and adipose tissue.[93] Because obese women tend to have LGA infants even when pregnancy weight gain is inadequate, may be difficult to determine whether their infants are growth restricted.

Many of the metabolic changes seen in pregnancy (e.g., increased circulating insulin, insulin resistance) are similar to those seen in obese women.[93] Obese women tend to have more problems during delivery due to increased fetal growth and macrosomia. The incidence of preeclampsia and chronic hypertension, thrombophlebitis, varicose veins, and diabetes mellitus is increased in obese women.[28,93,140,181] These women may gain excess weight during pregnancy, which can be difficult to lose later.[52,178,181] Maternal obesity also has been reported to be a risk factor for neural tube defects.[181]

Caloric restriction during pregnancy is generally not recommended because of potential adverse effects on the fetus. Severe caloric restriction can significantly reduce the availability of glucose (the major fetal energy substrate) and increase maternal serum amino acid and ketone levels. Maternal ketosis has been associated with poor neurologic development in offspring, although some studies have not confirmed this finding.[93] However, caloric restriction may be indicated in the obese pregnant woman to maintain a weight gain that has been associated with an improved pregnancy outcome.

Pregnancy and Gastrointestinal Disorders

The physiologic and anatomic changes of the GI tract during pregnancy have varying effects on disorders of this system. The course of some disorders is minimally affected by pregnancy. Approximately 1/500 to 1/735 pregnant women require nonobstetric surgery.[206] Appendicitis and cholelithiasis are the most common reasons for nonobstetric surgery during pregnancy.[226]

Pregnancy and Acute Appendicitis

Appendicitis is not more common during pregnancy, but may be more severe due to delayed diagnosis.[117] Diagnosis of appendicitis during pregnancy is complicated by anatomic and physiologic changes of pregnancy. Because the appendix is displaced upward and laterally to the right, the point of maximal tenderness may be as high as the right costal margin. By the second trimester, the appendix lies above the iliac crest. As a result, radiated pain associated with suppuration or perforation tends to be felt at the point where the appendix abuts the peritoneum, which becomes higher and more lateral as gestation progresses.[14,226,231]

Guarding and rebound tenderness are often milder and less well localized, in that the uterus is between the appendix and the parietal peritoneum.[228] Nausea is common in the first trimester, and changes in white blood cell counts associated with appendicitis are similar to changes in pregnancy. Suidan and Young suggest that one way to differentiate uterine from appendiceal pain is to turn the woman onto her left side while pressing the point of maximal tenderness. If the pain decreases or ceases, the pain is probably uterine in origin; if not, appendicitis should be suspected.[231] Appendicitis increases the risk of spontaneous abortion and preterm labor, especially if accompanied by perforation and peritonitis.[117,228] The risk of perforation is greatest in the third trimester.[228]

Pregnancy in Women with Inflammatory Bowel Disease

One of the more common GI disorders occurring in the childbearing population is inflammatory bowel disease (IBD), which includes ulcerative colitis and Crohn's disease. Most recent studies report that fertility rates in women with IBD are similar to the general population; however, fertility is reduced after surgical intervention.[27] If these disorders are quiescent at the time of pregnancy the outcome for both mother and fetus is usually good, although these women have an increased risk of preterm delivery (most ≥35 weeks), low birth weight, cesarean delivery, and spontaneous abortion.[27,59,117,147,164,228] If the disorder is active at the time of conception, there is a greater risk of these complications.[27,117,147,164,228] The risk of exacerbation during pregnancy is similar to the risk in nonpregnant women.[27] Risk of exacerbation is highest during the first trimester and postpartum. Long-term detrimental effects of pregnancy on the course of IBD have not been reported.[27]

Pregnancy in Women with Peptic Ulcer Disease

PUD in women is seen more often after menopause and is uncommon during the childbearing years. The risk of PUD is greatest with use of nonsteroidal anti-inflammatory agents in combination with colonization with *Helicobacter pylori.*[228] In women of childbearing age, estrogen may protect the gastric lining from ulcer formation, perhaps by increasing gastric and duodenal mucous secretion.[249] Pregnancy has a further protective effect on the development and progression of PUD.[117,208] Up to 80% of women with PUD im prove during pregnancy, although 50% experience recurrence of symptoms by 3 months postpartum and almost all by 2 years after delivery.[62,208] Women with persistent symptoms during pregnancy usually have other problems such as hyperemesis gravidarum and albuminuria.[208]

The basis for improvement during pregnancy may be due to the normal GI changes that accompany pregnancy, including decreased gastric acidity and motility and increased mucous secretion.[61] Production of hydrochloric acid (both basal and in response to histamine) decreases in pregnancy, with a tendency to return to normal or increased levels of acidity in the third trimester.[228] Decreased gastric acidity, increased plasma histaminase (thought to mediate acid and pepsin secretion by reducing parietal cell responsiveness to endogenous histamine), increased prostaglandins (protective of gastric mucosa), and increased mucous secretion (which protects the gastric mucosa from the effects of acid) may all contribute to improvement in peptic ulcer symptoms.[25,62,214] Gastrin levels are normal during most of pregnancy, with marked increases late in the third trimester, at delivery, and immediately after delivery. Thus, by late pregnancy, gastric pH and pepsin output have returned to nonpregnant levels. It is at this time that peptic ulcer symptoms tend to recur.[62,208]

Cholelithiasis and Pregnancy

The incidence of cholelithiasis, which is more common in women, is increased further during pregnancy and in women taking oral contraceptive agents.[76,142,258] Cholelithiasis is the second most common nonobstetric surgical problem (acute appendicitis being the most common) during pregnancy. A hormonal basis for the risk of gallstones in women has been suggested, in that the increased risk is seen primarily between menarche and menopause. Elevated estrogen and progesterone levels during pregnancy may further aggravate the tendency toward cholelithiasis, as does the increased bile stasis and sludging during pregnancy.[142,258]

There are three forms of gallstones: cholesterol, pigment, and mixed (composed primarily of calcium bilirubinate). The increased incidence of gallstones associated with females and pregnancy is seen primarily with cholesterol gallstones. The process of gallstone development involves (1) production of bile supersaturated with cholesterol; (2) nucleation and crystallization of cholesterol, which initiates stone formation; and (3) growth of the stone.[204] Supersaturation of bile with cholesterol occurs when cholesterol secretion is high or bile acid secretion is low (concentrated bile is more likely to hold cholesterol in solution). Cholesterol production increases during pregnancy. In addition, estrogens and progesterone increase biliary cholesterol saturation and estrogen decreases the proportion of chenodeoxycholic acid. This acid is a component of the bile acid pool that dissolves gallstones by decreasing biliary cholesterol secretion. Altered gallbladder tone during pregnancy, with incomplete emptying and increased fasting and residual volumes, may also increase the risk of gallstone formation by sequestering cholesterol crystals.[76,142,204] Cholelithiasis during pregnancy may increase the risk of chronic gallbladder disease.[142]

Pregnancy and Liver Disease

Liver disease in pregnancy can be divided into two categories: (1) disorders seen only in pregnancy and associated with jaundice and abnormal liver tests (intrahepatic cholestasis, preeclampsia, and fatty liver of pregnancy); and (2) liver diseases that may occur during and are affected by pregnancy.[185] Fetal fatty acid oxidation defects may increase the risk of maternal liver disease, especially acute fatty liver of pregnancy and HELLP syndrome, which includes hemolysis (H); elevated serum levels of liver enzymes, especially AST and ALT (EL); and low platelets (LP).[38,43] The reason for this risk is postulated to be due to accumulation and deposition of fetal 3-hydroxy fatty acid acylcarnitine intermediary metabolites.[43]

The most common liver disease seen in pregnant women is viral hepatitis.[185] Major effects of pregnancy on liver disorders are potential difficulties with diagnosis, increased fetal risk and, especially with hepatitis B, transmission to the fetus. Alterations in some liver function tests during pregnancy can make diagnosis of liver disorders more difficult, although jaundice is always abnormal. Jaundice and liver disorders during pregnancy are discussed in Chapter 18.

Table 12-7 Recommendations for Clinical Practice Related to Changes in the Gastrointestinal System in Pregnant Women

Counsel women regarding changes in appetite, food preferences, and intake during pregnancy (p. 392).
Counsel women regarding gingival changes during pregnancy and the need for dental hygiene (pp. 393-395).
Counsel women regarding common problems (heartburn, nausea and vomiting, constipation, hemorrhoids) associated with the gastrointestinal (GI) system (pp. 395, 402-404 and Table 12-1).
Implement interventions to reduce or relieve heartburn, nausea and vomiting, constipation, and hemorrhoids (pp. 395, 402-404 and Table 12-5).
Counsel women regarding the presence of spider angiomas and palmar erythema (p. 396 and Chapter 14).
Recognize the usual parameters for liver function tests and patterns of change during pregnancy and the postpartum period (pp. 396, 407-408 and Table 12-2).
Know the expected parameters for weight gain during pregnancy and monitor maternal patterns (pp. 396, 398-399 and Table 12-3).
Know the recommended nutritional requirements during pregnancy (pp. 400-401 and Table 12-4).
Assess maternal nutritional status and provide nutritional counseling (pp. 400-402 and Table 12-4).
Recognize potential maternal and fetal/neonatal complications associated with undernutrition and obesity during pregnancy (pp. 405-406 and Table 12-6).
Monitor fluid, food, and caloric intake during labor and the early postpartum period (pp. 404-406).
Counsel women regarding weight loss patterns following delivery (p. 400).
Recommend postpartum exercises to enhance weight loss and return of abdominal and perineal tone (p. 400).
Evaluate GI function postpartum (p. 400).
Recognize factors that increase the risk of gallstone formation and recognize signs of cholelithiasis (pp. 396, 407).
Counsel women with GI and liver problems regarding the effect of their disorder on pregnancy and of pregnancy on the disorder (pp. 406-407).
Recognize signs of appendicitis during pregnancy (pp. 406-407).
Recognize signs of liver disorders that are unique to pregnancy (p. 407 and Chapter 18).
Counsel women with phenylketonuria and other metabolic disorders regarding risks to their infant and need for dietary restrictions (p. 407, Chapter 1).
Know fetal nutritional requirements and counsel women regarding fetal needs and growth patterns (pp. 401-402, 416-417).
Know factors that can alter fetal growth and monitor fetal growth patterns (pp. 401-402, 416-417 and Table 12-6).
Counsel women regarding changes in GI function with use of oral contraceptive agents (pp. 395, 402, 407).

Severe pruritus and jaundice characterize intrahepatic cholestasis (see Table 14-2). The risk of postpartum hemorrhage, gallstones, fetal distress, stillbirth, and prematurity is increased.[175] The basis for this disorder is unclear, although it may have a genetic basis or hormonal cause, in that a similar syndrome occurs with oral contraceptive use.[204] Fatty liver of pregnancy is a rare disorder of unknown cause that usually appears during the third trimester, often in association with preeclampsia, with high fetal and maternal mortality rates. Delivery of the infant results in rapid improvement.[204]

Liver function and histologic changes are associated with preeclampsia (see Table 9-5), with alterations in liver function tests (AST, ALT, GGTP, and bilirubin) reported in some women. The degree of liver abnormality tends to parallel the severity of preeclampsia. The most significant involvement is in women who develop HELLP syndrome (see Chapter 9).[204,258]

SUMMARY

The pregnant woman experiences changes in GI and hepatic function that enhance absorption of nutrients for herself and her fetus. These changes are associated with common experiences and discomforts of pregnancy such as heartburn, constipation, nausea, and vomiting. A major component of interconceptional and prenatal care is nutritional assessment and counseling. Maternal nutrition before and during pregnancy is critical for optimal growth and development of the fetus and prevention of maternal, fetal, and neonatal disorders. Table 12-7 summarizes recommendations for clinical practice related to the GI system and perinatal nutrition.

DEVELOPMENT OF THE GASTROINTESTINAL AND HEPATIC SYSTEMS IN THE FETUS

The development of the gastrointestinal (GI) system can be divided into three phases. During early gestation, anatomic development gives rise to the organs and other structures of this system. During middle to late gestation, functional components such as hormones, enzymes, and reflexes develop (Figure 12-3). Finally, after birth, coordinated function develops with interaction of hormones and enzymes in the digestion of food substances along with maturation of suck-swallow coordination.

The enteric nervous system (ENS) consists of neurons in the wall of the GI tract that modulate motility, microcirculation, secretion, and immune responses. The ENS develops from neural crest cells that colonize the gut by 13 weeks. Failure of migration and colonization can lead to disorders such as Hirschsprung disease.[43] Characteristics and timing of other common GI anomalies are described in the next section and are summarized in Table 12-8. GI anomalies may occur as

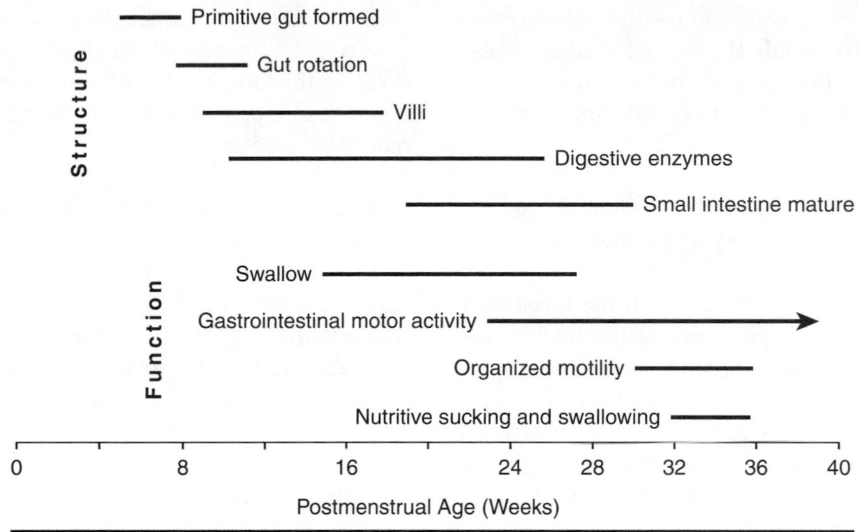

FIGURE 12-3 Timetable of gastrointestinal structural and functional development. (From Newell, S.J. [1996]. Gastrointestinal function and its ontogeny: How should we feed the preterm infants? *Semin Neonatol*, 1, 60.)

Table 12-8 Incidence, Time of Occurrence, and Associated Defects of Various Gastrointestinal Anomalies

ANOMALY	INCIDENCE (PER LIVE BIRTHS)	FETAL AGE AT WHICH DEFECT OCCURS	PRESENCE OF HYDRAMNIOS	OTHER CONCURRENT DEFECTS
Diaphragmatic hernia	1:4000	8th-10th week of fetal life	>75%	Lung hypoplasia, malrotation of bowel, PDA, coarctation of aorta, and neurologic malformations
Tracheoesophageal fistula and esophageal atresias	1:3000 1:4000	4th-5th week of fetal life	>60%	Seen in more than 50% of patients and include GI, skeletal, and cardiac defects
Duodenal atresia	1:10,000 1:40,000	8th-10th week of fetal life	~50%	Down syndrome, GI malformations, and congenital heart disease
Jejunoileal atresia	1:330-1:1500	During fetal life after embryogenesis (after 12 weeks' gestation)	35% jejunal 10%-15% ileal	Infrequent, but volvulus, malrotation, and meconium peritonitis may occur
Colonic atresia	1:5000-1:20,000	Vascular accidents in gestation	Rare	Other defects occur in 30%-40%, and these tend to be associated with abdominal wall defects, vesicointestinal fistulas, and jejunal atresias
Anorectal anomalies	1:5000-1:15,000	5th-8th week of fetal life	Rare	May be familial-associated anomalies in 30%-70%; these anomalies include cardiac, GI, and vertebral anomalies
Omphalocele	1:3000-1:10,000	8th-11th week of fetal life	Common, but incidence unknown	Other defects occur in 60%; cardiac defects 15%-20%; tetralogy of Fallot, and specific syndromes; Beckwith and trisomy D, E, and 21 are also seen
Gastroschisis	1:6000	9th-11th week of fetal life	Incidence unknown	Foreshortened gut and intestinal atresias (15%); cardiac defects (<10%)
Duplications of GI tract	1:1000-1:4000	4th-6th week of fetal life	Unknown	Most common in ileum and esophagus
Meckel's diverticulum	1:50-1:100	5th-7th week of fetal life	Rare	Usually occurs as isolated defect

From Sunshine, P. (1990). Fetal gastrointestinal physiology. In R.D. Eden & F.H. Boehm (Eds.), *Assessment and care of the fetus.* Norwalk, CT: Appleton & Lange.
GI, Gastrointestinal; *PDA*, patent ductus arteriosus.

isolated malformations or in association with malformations of other systems, most frequently the skeletal, cardiovascular, or urogenital systems.[235] Fetal growth restriction is seen in approximately one third of infants with GI malformations.[235]

Anatomic Development

Anatomic development of the GI system begins during the fourth week with partitioning of the yolk sac into intraembryonic and extraembryonic portions. Initially the cranial portion of the GI system develops concurrently with the respiratory system (see Chapter 10). The epithelium of the trachea, the bronchi, and the lungs and digestive tract arise from the primitive gut, a derivation of the yolk sac. The GI system develops in a cranial-to-caudal direction. The yolk sac arises at 8 days and by the fourth week has divided into two parts. The extraembryonic or secondary yolk sac provides for nutrition of the embryo, before development of the mature placenta, and then is assimilated into the umbilical cord by 3 to 4 months. The intraembryonic portion is incorporated into the embryo as the primitive gut (Figure 12-4).

The primitive gut is initially closed at both ends by membranes. The cranial (buccopharyngeal) membrane is reabsorbed during the third week, forming the stomodeum (future site of the mouth); the caudal (cloacal) membrane is absorbed during the ninth week. The midgut remains temporarily connected to the yolk sac by the vitelline duct. Development of the primitive gut and its derivatives can be divided into four sections: pharyngeal gut, foregut, midgut, and hindgut.[159]

Development of the Pharyngeal Gut

The pharyngeal gut extends from the buccopharyngeal membrane (which becomes the stomodeum) to the tracheobronchial diverticulum, forming the pharynx and its derivative, lower respiratory tract, and upper esophagus (Figure 12-5). The pharyngeal area develops from bands of mesenchymal tissue (branchial or pharyngeal arches) separated by deep clefts (branchial or pharyngeal clefts) on the exterior of the embryo. A series of indentations (pharyngeal pouches) appear on the lateral walls of the pharyngeal gut and penetrate into the surrounding mesenchyme but do not communicate with the external clefts.[210] The pharyngeal arches form the muscular and skeletal components of the pharyngeal area, aortic arch, and nerve networks; the mandible; the dorsal portion of the maxillary process; the hyoid bone; the thyroid bone; the laryngeal cartilage; and associated vascular and nerve supplies. The pharyngeal pouches form the eustachian tubes, tonsils, thymus, parathyroid, and part of the thyroid.[159,210]

Development of the Foregut and Common Anomalies

The foregut extends from the tracheobronchial diverticulum to the upper part of the duodenum. Structures formed from the foregut (lower esophagus, stomach, liver, upper portion of the duodenum to the entry of the common bile duct, liver, biliary tree, and pancreas) are all supplied by the celiac artery.[159]

Esophagus. During the fourth week the tracheobronchial diverticulum appears along the ventral wall of the foregut, dividing the foregut into the ventral respiratory primordium and dorsal esophagus. The esophagus is initially short, but quickly elongates with ascent of the pharynx and cranial growth. The rapidly growing endothelium temporarily obliterates the esophageal lumen, with recanalization of the lumen by 8 weeks.

Incomplete division of the foregut into respiratory and digestive portions at 4 to 5 weeks leads to tracheoesophageal fistula with or without esophageal atresia (Figure 12-6; also see Table 12-8). This malformation probably arises from posterior deviation or unequal development of the septum developing between the primitive trachea and esophagus due to genetic and environmental factors.[65,77] Failure of the lumen to recanalize during the eighth week leads to esophageal stenosis or atresia.

Stomach, Duodenum, and Pancreas. The stomach arises during the fourth week as a spindle-shaped dilation in the caudal area of the foregut (see Figure 12-5), and its structure is well established by 6 weeks. The stomach dilates and enlarges, rotating around a longitudinal and an anteroposterior axis. During the longitudinal rotation, the stomach rotates 90 degrees clockwise, ending with the left side facing anteriorly and the right posteriorly. The subsequent greater growth of the posterior wall in comparison with the anterior wall leads to the lesser and greater curvatures of the stomach. Initially the cephalic and caudal ends of the stomach are in midline. During the anteroposterior rotation of the stomach, the caudal (pyloric) portion moves right and upward, and the cephalic (cardiac) portion moves left and slightly downward.[159,210] Embryonic anomalies of the stomach are rare, probably because stomach development is relatively simple. The most common stomach anomaly is pyloric stenosis, which is thought to be genetic in origin.

The duodenum arises from both the foregut and midgut. As the stomach rotates, the duodenum takes on a C-shaped form and rotates to the right. The lumen of the duodenum becomes obliterated by rapidly growing epithelium, with later recanalization beginning at 6 or 7 weeks. Failure to recanalize leads to duodenal atresia or stenosis.

The pancreas appears at about 5 weeks as dorsal and ventral buds in the duodenal area. As the duodenum rotates to the right and becomes C-shaped, the ventral pancreatic bud migrates toward the lower end of the common bile duct. The two pancreatic buds meet and fuse to form the final pancreas by 7 weeks. In individuals with an annular pancreas, the ventral bud encircles the duodenum and may cause obstruction.[210] All pancreatic cell types are seen by 9 to 10 weeks.

Liver and Gallbladder. The liver appears during the third week as a ventral thickening (liver bud or hepatic diverticulum) consisting of rapidly proliferating strands of cells at the distal end of the foregut (see Figure 12-5). The hepatic diverticulum divides into a large cranial portion, which forms the hepatic parenchyma and main bile duct, and a smaller caudal portion, from which the gallbladder arises.[210] The liver initially

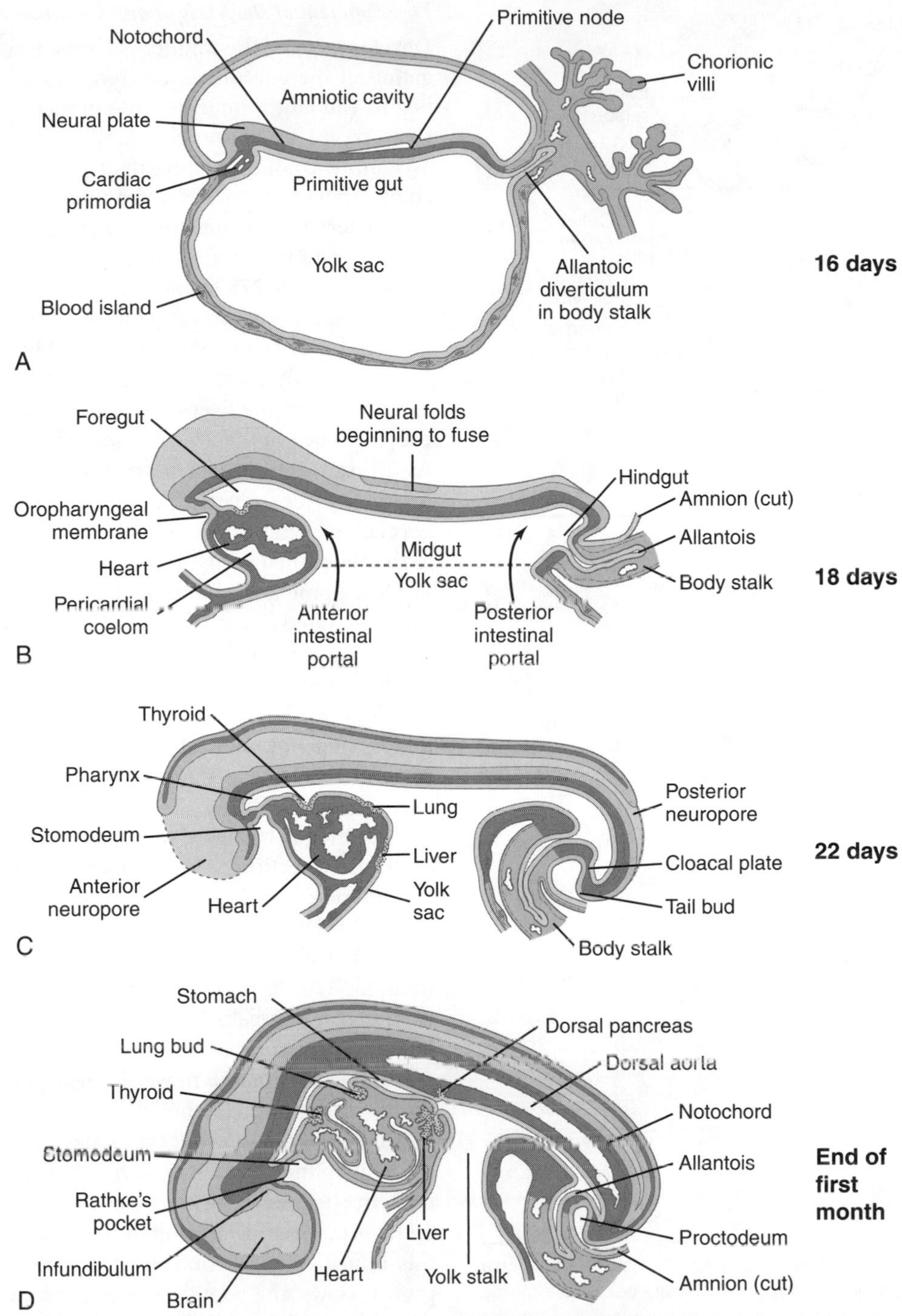

FIGURE 12-4 Sagittal section through human embryos showing the early establishment of the digestive system. **A,** At 16 days. **B,** At 18 days. **C,** At 22 days. **D,** At the end of the first month. (From Carlson, B.M. [2004]. *Human embryology and developmental biology* (3rd ed.). St. Louis: Mosby, p. 121.)

grows into the septum transversum, a thick mesodermal plate separating the yolk sac and the thoracic cavity. The liver grows rapidly, eventually bulging into the caudal part of the abdominal cavity and stretching the mesoderm of the septum transversum until it becomes a thin membrane. The ventral portion of this membrane forms the falciform ligament; the dorsal portion forms the lesser omentum. The cranial portion of the septum transversum forms part of the diaphragm. Further growth of the liver promotes closure of the pleuroperitoneal canals (two large openings on either side of the foregut). Hepatocytes develop as long cords, 3 to 5 cells thick, that insert into the liver stroma.[26]

The lumina of the gallbladder and the intrahepatic and extrahepatic bile ducts are initially open, becoming

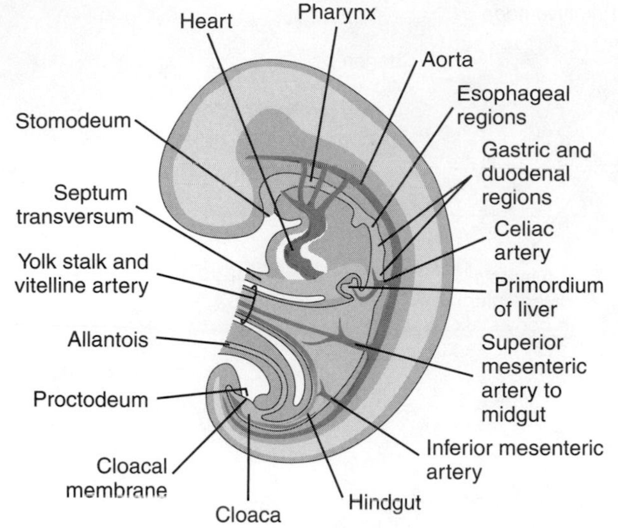

FIGURE 12-5 Early development of the digestive system and its blood supply. (From Moore, K.L. & Persaud, T.V.N. [2003]. *The developing human: Clinically oriented embryology* [7th ed.]. Philadelphia: Saunders.)

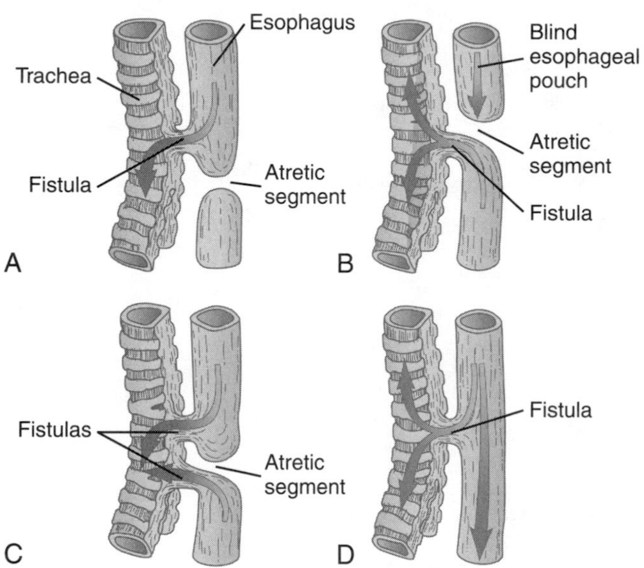

FIGURE 12-6 Varieties of tracheoesophageal fistulas. **A,** Fistula above the atretic esophageal segment. **B,** Fistula below the atretic esophageal segment. **C,** Fistulas above and below the atretic esophageal segment. **D,** Fistulas between the patent esophagus and the trachea. (From Carlson, B.M. [2004]. *Human embryology and developmental biology* (3rd ed.). St. Louis: Mosby.)

temporarily obliterated by proliferating epithelium and later recanalizing. Biliary atresia can arise from failure of recanalization. With complete failure, the ducts are narrow nonfunctional fibrous cords. Failure of part of a bile duct to recanalize results in partial obstruction or atresia of that duct, with distention of the gallbladder and hepatic duct proximal to the atretic area.[159,210]

Development of the Midgut and Common Anomalies

Development of the midgut is characterized by rapid elongation of the gut and associated mesentery.[159] The midgut begins caudal to the liver and gives rise to the small intestine (except for the upper duodenum), cecum, appendix, ascending colon, and proximal portion of the transverse colon. These structures are supplied by the superior mesenteric artery.[159] The intestines increase in length 1000-fold during gestation, doubling in length in the last 15 weeks (mean length is 275 cm at term).[171]

Initially midgut growth parallels the neural tube; however, the rapid growth of the midgut quickly exceeds that of the rest of the body, including the abdominal cavity. This occurs at a time when the liver and kidneys are relatively large, occupying much of the available space in the abdominal cavity. As a result, the midgut herniates into the extraembryonic coelom of the proximal umbilical cord. This physiologic herniation begins in the sixth week, with return of the midgut to the abdominal cavity during the tenth week.

Development of the midgut involves four steps: herniation, rotation, retraction, and fixation (Figure 12-7).[159,210] The midgut initially elongates and forms a U-shaped loop, which projects (herniates) into the proximal umbilical cord (see Figure 12-7, *A*). The cranial limb of this loop grows rapidly, forming coils characteristic of the small intestine with little change in the caudal portion except for appearance of the cecal bud (see Figure 12-7, *B*).

The midgut rotates a total of 270 degrees in a counterclockwise direction around an axis formed by the superior mesenteric artery. Midgut rotation occurs in two stages. The initial 90-degree rotation occurs while the midgut is in the umbilical cord (see Figure 12-7, *A* and *B*); the second rotation (180 degrees) takes place as the gut returns to the abdomen at 10 weeks (see Figure 12-7, *B* and *C*). The initial 90-degree rotation is in a counterclockwise direction. As a result, the cranial limb moves to the right and down and the caudal limb moves to the left and up (see Figure 12-7, *B*). The lumen of the intestines becomes temporarily obliterated by rapid epithelial growth, with later recanalization.

Retraction or return of the midgut to the abdominal cavity occurs rapidly during the tenth week. The stimulus for this return is unknown, but it occurs as the rate of liver growth slows, the relative size of the kidney decreases, and the abdominal cavity enlarges. As the midgut reenters the abdominal cavity, the gut rotates 180 degrees counterclockwise. The jejunum returns first and the area of the cecal bud last; the cecum and appendix end up near the liver in the right upper quadrant (see Figure 12-7, *D*).[210]

The final step in development of the midgut is fixation (see Figure 12-7, *E*). The cecum and appendix descend into the lower right quadrant. The proximal colon lengthens, becoming the ascending colon. The mesenteries are pressed against the posterior abdominal wall and fuse with the wall. In some regions of the midgut, the mesenteries also fuse with the parietal peritoneum so that the ascending colon is rectoperitoneal.

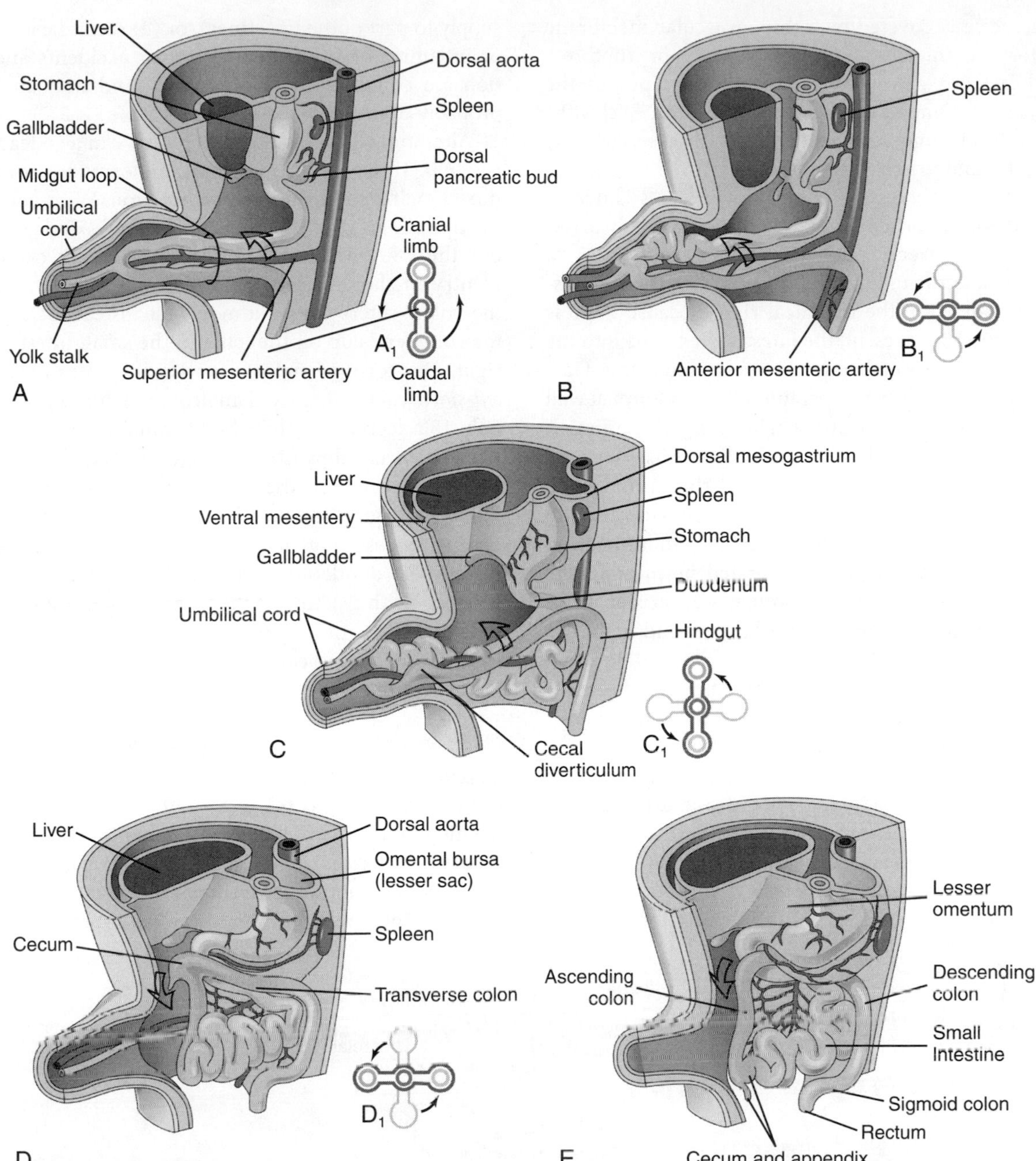

FIGURE 12-7 Development of the midgut (see p. 412). **A,** Midgut loop in proximal umbilical cord at 6 weeks. **A_1,** Transverse section through midgut, showing initial relationships of limbs of midgut loop to artery. **B,** Beginning midgut rotation. **B_1,** 90-degree counterclockwise rotation. **C,** Return of intestines to abdomen at 10 weeks. **C_1,** Additional 90-degree rotation. **D,** After return to abdomen. **D_1,** Final 90-degree rotation (for a total of 270 degrees). **E,** Late fetal period, with cecum rotated to normal position. (From Moore, K.L. & Persaud, T.V.N. [1998]. *Before we are born: Essentials of human embryology and birth defects* [5th ed.]. Philadelphia: Saunders.)

Common Anomalies of the Midgut. Congenital anomalies of the midgut include omphalocele, gastroschisis, umbilical hernia, intestinal stenosis and atresia, and malrotation (see Table 12-8). Omphalocele arises at 8 to 11 weeks' gestation from a developmental arrest at the stage of herniation of the midgut into the umbilical cord with failure of all or part of the gut to return to the abdominal cavity (results in bowel-containing omphalocele). There is often an associated defect in development of the abdominal musculature at the junction of the umbilical cord (results in liver-containing omphalocele). This defect results from a primary failure in the formation of the lateral folds, which along with the cephalic and caudal folds form the abdominal wall.[159] The size of the defect influences the size of the omphalocele, which can range from a single loop of intestine to a mass containing most of the intestines and parts of the liver, bladder, and other organs.

The omphalocele is covered by a thin, avascular membrane (derived from amnion) that may be intact or ruptured. The umbilical cord generally inserts into the apex of the omphalocele sac. Omphalocele is associated with Beckwith-Wiedemann syndrome, congenital heart disease, trisomy 13, trisomy 18, and urinary tract problems.[123]

In gastroschisis, the extrusion of the intestines is due to a defect in the anterior abdominal wall that probably arises between 9 and 11 weeks but may occur as early as 5 to 6 weeks. This defect is usually to the right of, and not necessarily continuous with, the umbilical ring. Because there is usually no hernial sac present, the intestines extrude into the amniotic cavity and are embedded in a gelatinous mass. Gastroschisis arises secondary to a paraumbilical abdominal wall defect that may be a result of (1) failure of differentiation of the lateral fold somatopleure after the bowel has returned to the peritoneal cavity and the umbilical ring has formed; (2) failure in formation of the umbilical coelom with rupture of the amniotic membrane at the base of the umbilical cord; (3) intrauterine rupture of an incarcerated hernia into the cord; or (4) weakness in the abdominal wall arising from alterations in the normal involution of the second umbilical vein or ischemic damage.[94]

An umbilical hernia is associated with an enlarged umbilical ring and failure of the rectus muscles to come together in midline. The protruding viscera are covered with normal skin.

Intestinal stenoses and atresias can arise as primary or secondary defects. Primary stenosis or atresia arises at 8 to 10 weeks, and perhaps as early as 6 to 7 weeks, as a result of partial or complete failure of the intestinal lumen to recanalize. Secondary stenosis or atresia is a result of (1) fetal vascular accidents or infarction (with interruption of blood supply to part of the intestines), or (2) secondary to twisting or inflammatory changes.[91] Vascular accidents and infarction are common causes of jejunal and ileal atresias and probably occur after 12 weeks (see Table 12-8).

Alterations in midgut development can also lead to malrotation. Three of the more common forms are nonrotation, mixed malrotation, and reverse rotation. With nonrotation, the midgut rotates 90 degrees instead of 270 degrees, without the 180-degree rotation that normally occurs upon reentry of the gut into the abdominal cavity. As a result, the colon enters the abdomen first instead of last so that the colon ends up on the left and the small intestine on the right. This form of malrotation is sometimes referred to as *left-sided colon.* In mixed malrotation, the midgut rotates only 180 degrees, so that the terminal ileum reenters first. The cecum is subpyloric and fixed to the abdominal wall, which may compress the duodenum. In reverse rotation, the initial 90-degree rotation is clockwise instead of counterclockwise, resulting in placement of the transverse colon behind the duodenum. Malrotation increases the risk of volvulus, with twisting of the intestinal loops and abnormal fixation of the mesenteries, resulting in excessive mobility of the bowel. This can lead to kinking of the bowel and blood vessels and necrosis.[159,210]

Development of the Hindgut and Common Anomalies

Development of the hindgut and urogenital systems is interrelated. The cloaca is the expanded terminal end of the gut; the hindgut ends at the cloacal membrane (Figure 12-8). The hindgut gives rise to the distal transverse colon, descending and sigmoid colons, rectum, upper anal canal, bladder, and urethra, which are supplied by the inferior mesenteric artery.[159]

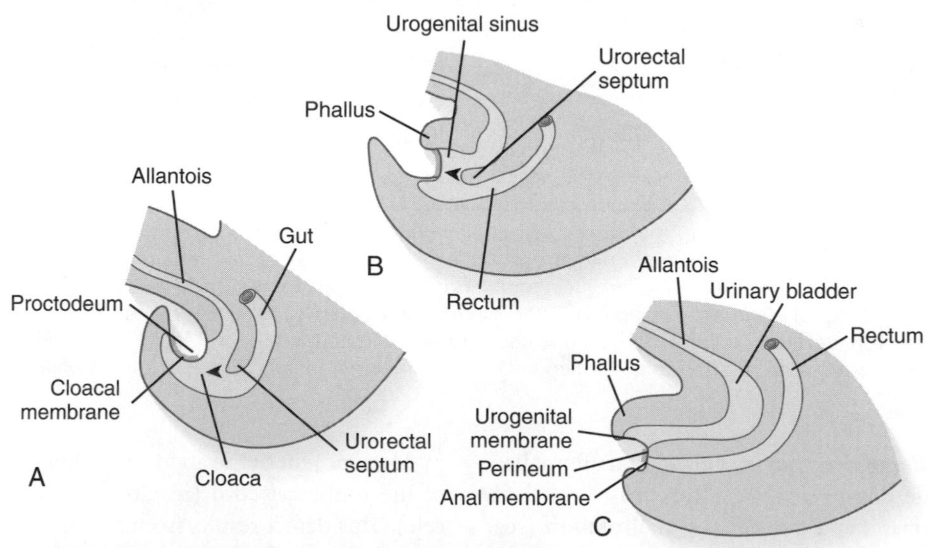

FIGURE 12-8 Stages in the subdivision of the common cloaca by the urogenital septum. **A,** In the fifth week. **B,** In the sixth week. **C,** In the eighth week. The arrowheads indicate the direction of growth of the urorectal septum. (From Carlson, B.M. [2004]. *Human embryology and developmental biology* [3rd ed.]. St. Louis: Mosby, p. 364.)

At 5 to 7 weeks, the cloaca is divided into two parts by the urorectal septum, a wedge of downward-growing mesenchymal tissue. During weeks 6 to 7, the urorectal septum reaches and fuses with the cloacal membrane, forming the perineum. The area of fusion is the perineal body. This fusion divides the cloacal membrane into two parts. The ventral urogenital membrane is incorporated in the terminal portion of the urogenital system (see Chapters 1 and 11); the dorsal part becomes the anal membrane. A pit that develops in the anal membrane ruptures at 8 to 9 weeks, resulting in an open communication between the rectum and the body exterior. The lower portion of the anal canal develops from ectodermal tissue around the site of the anal pit.[210]

Imperforate anus and associated malformations arise from abnormal development of the urorectal septum. In the simplest form of imperforate anus, the anal membrane fails to rupture and the anal canal ends at the membrane. In more complex forms, there may be a layer of connective tissue between the end of the rectum and the body surface. Failure of the anal pit to develop or atresia of the end of the rectum can result in these forms. If the descent of the urorectal septum is arrested, the cloaca may remain, with abnormalities of the urogenital and lower GI systems.

Functional Development

Anatomically the fetal GI tract develops to the stage seen in the newborn by about 20 weeks.[136,124] Functional development begins during fetal life with development of digestive and liver enzyme systems and the absorptive surfaces of the intestine (Table 12-9; see Figure 12-3) and continues into the postbirth period. Most of the processes needed for adequate enteral nutrition are in place by 33 to 34 weeks' gestation.[124] Although the placenta takes care of the nutrient needs of the fetus, function of the fetal GI tract is important in amniotic fluid homeostasis (see Chapter 3). Amniotic fluid in turn contains nutrients, hormones, and growth factors that stimulate secretion of hormones and regulatory peptides and enhance growth and maturation of the gut.[71,124,250]

The major gut-regulating polypeptides, including gastrin, motilin, and somatostatin, are all present by the end of the first trimester and act as local inducing agents regulating growth and development of the gut.[19,174,250] Initially, cells that produce these substances are more widely distributed than in the adult, but they reach adult distribution by 24 weeks. Gastric epidermal growth factor (EGF) receptors appear by 18 weeks. EGF enhances growth and development of the gut and may protect the stomach from hydrochloric acid. Transport of amino acids begins by 14 weeks, glucose transport by 18 weeks, and fatty acids by 24 weeks (see Table 12-9).[134]

The intestinal villi begin to develop around 7 weeks and are present throughout the small intestine by 14 to 16 weeks, with well-developed villi and crypts seen by 19 weeks.[25,171] Intestinal motility and peristalsis develop gradually and mature during the third trimester.[25] Meconium is first found at 10 to 12 weeks and moves into the colon by 16 weeks.[6] Small

Table 12-9 Development of the Gastrointestinal Tract in the Fetus

DEVELOPMENT	GESTATION (WEEKS)
ANATOMIC DEVELOPMENT	
Esophagus	
Superficial glands develop	20
Squamous cells appear	28
Stomach	
Gastric glands form	14
Pylorus and fundus defined	14
Pancreas	
Differentiation of endocrine and exocrine tissue	14
Liver	
Lobules form	11
Small Intestine	
Crypt-villi develop	14
Lymph nodes appear	14
Colon	
Diameter increases	20
FUNCTIONAL DEVELOPMENT	
Sucking and Swallowing	
Swallowing begins	10-14
Only mouthing	28
Immature suck-swallow	33-36
Stomach	
Gastric motility and secretion	20
Pancreas	
Zymogen granules	20
Liver	
Bile metabolism	11
Bile secretion	22
Small Intestine	
Active transport of amino acids	14
Glucose transport	18
Fatty acid absorption	24
Enzymes	
α-Glucosidase	10
Dipeptidases	10
Lactase	10
Enterokinase	26

From Lebenthal, A. & Lebenthal, E. (1999). The ontology of the small intestinal epithelium. *J Parenter Enteral Nutr, 23,* S5.

amounts of meconium may enter the amniotic fluid in the second trimester before development of anal sphincter function at 20 to 22 weeks' gestation.[6]

Fetuses by 13 to 15 weeks respond to oral stimulation with tongue protrusion, rooting, and sucking.[98] Older fetuses have been noted on ultrasound to suck reflexively on their fingers.[14] Nonnutritive sucking begins by 20 weeks.[71] Swallowing begins at 10 to 14 weeks, and by 16 weeks the fetus swallows 2 to 6 mL of amniotic fluid per day, increasing to 200 to 600 mL/day (average, 450 mL/day) by term. About 20% of the fluid swallowed by the fetus is lung fluid not amniotic fluid.[75] Swallowing is important for amniotic fluid homeostasis, regulation of amniotic fluid volume, GI development, and somatic growth.[75] Swallowing may also be important in fetal thirst and appetite programming. About 10% of fetal protein intake comes from swallowed amniotic fluid.[75] Failure of the fetus to swallow amniotic fluid is associated with GI obstruction and polyhydramnios (see Chapter 3).

Most of the metabolic functions of the fetal liver are handled by the maternal liver. The fetal liver is primarily a hematopoietic organ until the latter part of gestation, when bone marrow erythropoiesis and liver metabolic activity increase. Many liver enzyme systems are still immature at birth. Fetal hepatic metabolism of drugs is discussed in Chapter 7.

GI enzymes involved in protein digestion and absorption develop early in gestation and may be important in fetal life to prevent bowel obstruction by cellular debris.[83] Glucose from the mother is the major source of fetal energy (see Chapter 16). Disaccharidase enzymes are present by 9 to 10 weeks, increase rapidly after 20 weeks, and become very active after 27 to 28 weeks (except for lactase, which does not reach mature levels until 36 to 40 weeks).[123,135] Pancreatic amylase activity is minimal in the fetus.[73] Salivary amylase is present by 16 to 18 weeks in amniotic fluid and by 20 weeks in the fetus, but remains low.[73,174] Pancreatic lipase develops by 32 weeks, but remains low; lingual and gastric lipase are present by 26 weeks and increase to term.[73] Proteolytic enzymes are found by 20 to 25 weeks.[73] Trypsin achieves 90% of childhood values by term.[73] Enterokinase activity appears at 26 weeks. Bile acids can be detected in the liver and gallbladder by 14 to 16 weeks and in the intestines by 22 weeks; however, the bile acid pool remains low even at term. The fetal jejunum and liver have decreased capacity for reabsorbing bile acids and poorer enterohepatic recirculation of taurine-conjugated bile acids, the major bile acid at birth.[94,124] Lipase is present by 10 to 12 weeks.[174]

Fetal Growth

Fetal growth is dependent on factors such as genetic determinants, general maternal health and nutrition, availability of growth substrates, presence of fetal growth–promoting hormones, and vascular support via changes in plasma volume during pregnancy and the maternal blood supply to the placenta.[49,86] Availability of growth substrates depends on perfusion of the intervillous spaces and availability of glucose, amino acids, and fats in maternal blood (see Chapter 16). Fetal growth does not seem to be greatly dependent on hormones such as growth hormone, thyroid hormones, glucocorticoids, and sex steroids that are critical for postnatal growth. Hormones and peptide growth factors believed to be necessary for fetal growth include insulin, human placental lactogen (hPL), insulin-like growth factors I and II (IGF-I and IGF-II), epidermal growth factor, platelet-derived growth factor, leptin, and transforming growth factor–α.[188] Insulin and the IGFs (especially IGF-I and IGF-II) are critical in regulating fetal growth, although insulin probably has a permissive rather than a direct effect on fetal growth by stimulating nutrient uptake and utilization.[85] Growth factors appear early in gestation, beginning at the four- to eight-cell stage. "Disruption of the *IGF1, IGF2,* or *IGF1R* [receptor] gene retards fetal growth, whereas disruption of *IGF2R* or overexpressing *IGF2* [genes] enhances fetal growth."[85]

Many of the genes involved in growth regulation are imprinted (see Box 1-2 on p. 9) including IGF-II (paternally imprinted) and its receptor (maternally imprinted).[86,157] Loss of paternal imprinting with reactivation of the maternal allele (gene form) is seen in infants with Beckwith-Wiedemann syndrome, which is characterized by abnormal fetal and postnatal growth.[157]

Early in gestation, placental and embryonic growth are regulated primarily by IGF-II. IGF-II is unaffected by nutrient availability and enhances placental growth and nutrient transfer.[85] Thus embryo and placental growth are maintained even if maternal energy intake is decreased, as often occurs with NVP.[100] During the second and third trimesters, fetal growth becomes dependent on IGF-I, which is sensitive to nutrient status.[86,100] Another factor that is thought to have a role in fetal growth is placental leptin, which is secreted into both maternal and fetal circulations. Leptin (see Chapter 16) is thought to act on the hypothalamus to regulate food intake and satiety. During pregnancy, placental leptin may signal satiety to the maternal hypothalamus, thus resulting in reduced food intake and energy intake, which stimulates placental growth.[20,100] Dysregulation of leptin is seen with fetal growth restriction.[130] Leptin can be found in cord blood by 18 weeks' gestation.[184]

Growth is slow during the first 2 months (period of organ formation), and then accelerates rapidly. Maximum growth rate is achieved from the fourth to eighth months, when the fetus grows at the rate of 5% to 9% per week. Most of the fetal weight is gained from 20 weeks to term, increasing from about 5 g/day at 15 weeks, to 15 to 20 g/day at 20 weeks, and 30 to 35 g/day after 32 to 34 weeks.[157,202] At the cellular level, growth occurs through hypertrophy (increased cell size) or hyperplasia (increased cell numbers). The human fetus undergoes primarily hyperplastic growth from conception to 20 weeks (similar increases in deoxyribonucleic acid [DNA] and organ protein content), followed by a period of simultaneous hyperplasia and hypertrophy from 20 to 28 weeks. From 28 weeks on, growth is predominantly hypertrophic with rapid increases in cell size and accumulation of fat, muscle, and connective tissue.[157,265]

Fetal growth is altered in approximately 15% of pregnancies, with either fetal under- or overgrowth. Fetal overgrowth and macrosomia are discussed in Chapter 16; fetal undergrowth is discussed in the next section. The effects of maternal nutrient restriction or excess depend on the stage of pregnancy, length of restriction, and type of restriction. For example, if maternal nutrients are restricted throughout pregnancy, fetal growth restriction develops. If the restriction is only during the first trimester, infant birth weights tend to be within normal limits, with increased placental weight. Increased food intake in early gestation tends to be associated with infants with lower birth and placental weights. High carbohydrate intake in early pregnancy is associated with lower placental and birth weights. Restricted protein intake (and thus restricted intake of essential amino acids) in early pregnancy has a detrimental effect on both fetal and placental development.[100]

The "developmental origins of health and disease" hypothesis proposes an association between an abnormal fetal environment and later disorders.[22,23,39,47,87] Developmental programming in utero is mediated by nutrients and hormones. Fetal or developmental programming refers to effects of the fetal environment on susceptibility to later disorders. The nutritional and hormonal status during fetal and early post birth life can alter organ development including the hypothalamus and other endocrine structures (see Chapter 19). The mechanisms by which the fetal environment influence later status are not well understood, but are thought to be related to placental adaptive responses to the intrauterine environment. After birth these adaptations may no longer be appropriate for the extrauterine environment and increase the risk for adult onset disorders such as insulin resistance and type 2 diabetes (due to altered endocrine programming or changes in glucose-insulin metabolism); obesity (due to altered leptin and endocrine programming), hypertensive disorders, coronary artery disease (due to alterations in vascular development and lipid metabolism), and osteoporosis (due to alterations in leptin and bone development).[22,23,47,68,74,78,87,88]

In infants with fetal growth restriction and "placental insufficiency," nutritional delivery is decreased due to both decreased blood flow and a smaller placental size, but also down-regulation of nutrient transporters.[111] Conversely with fetal overgrowth, as occurs with maternal diabetes, placental nutritional transporters are up-regulated.[111] Altered programming can influence later metabolic control and these changes may be mediated in part by adipocytokines (hormones secreted by white adipose tissue that modulate metabolism, energy homeostasis, and growth).[39,74,78,119] Adipocytokines are secreted by placental and fetal tissues and include dentin, adiponectin, resistin, vistatin, and apelin, all of which exert effects on fat, muscle, and liver cells in early life.[39] Under- or over-provision of nutrients in utero can program adipose tissue function and amount.[39,87] As noted above, adverse in utero nutrition may have long-term effects on the infants, with an increased risk of altered neurologic development, increased childhood mortality rates, and a predisposition to chronic disease such as hypertension, coronary artery disease, and type 1 (with excess growth) or 2 (with fetal undernutrition) diabetes in adult life.[74,78,86,88,128,140,157,233]

Fetal Growth Restriction

Fetal growth restriction is the failure of a fetus to achieve its genetic growth potential in utero.[157] In practice this is stated as measures of absolute (i.e., low birth weight [LBW]) and relative (i.e., small-for-gestational-age) size. Factors that cause alterations in growth, such as malnutrition during the period of hyperplasia, can decrease the rate of cell division and result in organs or a fetus that is smaller in size with fewer cells. This symmetric form of growth alteration is not reversible after the time when hyperplastic cell growth would normally have ceased. Malnutrition during the period of hypertrophy results in organs or a fetus that are smaller in size (due to reduction in cell size) but has a normal number of cells. This is asymmetric growth restriction, which is seen in about 75% of infants with fetal growth restriction.[157] Hypertrophic growth alterations may be reversible with adequate nutrition. Because fetal tissues are undergoing hyperplastic growth throughout gestation, the fetus is especially vulnerable to irreversible changes at the cellular level.[249]

Factors altering fetal growth can be intrinsic or extrinsic.[157,205,262] Intrinsic factors are those within the fetus arising from chromosomal or genetic abnormalities, infectious agents, or other teratogens that alter the normal process of cell division and usually result in symmetric growth restriction. Extrinsic factors include maternal preeclampsia, placental alterations or insufficiency, and fetal malnutrition. Pathologic changes characteristic of reduction in placental blood flow are seen in placentas of growth-restricted infants.[251] Placental insufficiency due to maternal, fetal, or placental factors often results in caloric restriction to the fetus (inadequate glucose transported to meet fetal growth needs) and tends to occur later in gestation. Caloric restriction usually leads to an asymmetric growth failure in which brain growth is spared. Fetal malnutrition due to maternal protein restriction (arising from maternal malnutrition or significantly protein-reduced diets) generally results in symmetric fetal growth failure in which brain growth is not necessarily spared.[249] Management of fetal growth restriction varies with the underlying cause. Strategies range from fetal therapies to prepregnancy counseling and preventive interventions such as cessation of smoking and alcohol use, promotion of adequate nutrition, and early identification of and interventions for pathologic problems such as preeclampsia. The growth-restricted fetus and neonate are at risk for hypoxic-ischemic events, meconium aspiration, hypoglycemia, and other problems (Table 12-10) and later development of type 2 diabetes, obesity and cardiovascular disease (see previous section).[15,22,23,47,68,111,112,158,220,227,238,257]

Table 12-10 Perinatal Adaptive Problems of Small-for-Gestational-Age Infants

PROBLEM	PATHOGENESIS	PREVENTION
Hypoxic-ischemic events	↓ Placental reserve (insufficiency) ↓ Cardiac glycogen stores	Antepartum and intrapartum fetal heart rate monitoring
Meconium aspiration	Hypoxia/stress phenomenon	Oral-pharyngeal-tracheal suction
Fasting hypoglycemia	↓ Hepatic glycogen ↓ Gluconeogenesis	Early alimentation
Alimented hyperglycemia	"Starvation diabetes"	Avoid excessive carbohydrate loads
Polycythemia-hyperviscosity	Fetal hypoxia, ↑ erythropoietin Placental transfusion	Neonatal partial exchange transfusion
Temperature instability	↓ Adipose tissue ↑ Heat loss	Ensure neutral thermal environment
Pulmonary hemorrhage (rare)	Hypothermia, ↓ oxygen, DIC	Avoid cold stress and hypoxia
Immunodeficiency	"Malnutrition" effect	Unknown

Adapted from Kliegman, R.M. (2006). Intrauterine growth restriction. In R.J. Martin, A.A. Fanaroff, & M.C. Walsh (Eds.), *Fanaroff and Martin's neonatal-perinatal medicine: Diseases of the fetus and infant* (8th ed.). Philadelphia: Mosby.
DIC, Disseminated intravascular coagulation.

NEONATAL PHYSIOLOGY

GI function in the neonate is characterized by functional, anatomic, and physiologic limitations, which are increased in the preterm infant. Provision of adequate nutritional support for growth and development is an ongoing challenge for nurses and other health care providers. As a result of the limitations in GI function, infants are at risk for dehydration, reflux, malabsorption, and electrolyte imbalance.

Transitional Events

Although the fetal GI system is involved with removal of amniotic fluid, digestive and absorptive functions are performed primarily by the placenta. With birth, the infant's GI system, although still functionally immature, must assume responsibility for supplying the infant's energy, nutrient, and fluid needs. The intestinal mucosal barrier (glycocalyx) remains immature for 4 to 6 months. During this period, antigens and other macromolecules can be transported across the intestinal epithelium into the systemic circulation, increasing the risk for both infection and the development of allergies. With maturation of the epithelium (gut closure), uptake of macromolecules decreases. The intestines are sterile at birth, but become rapidly colonized, with colonization influenced by whether the infant is breastfed or formula fed. Intestinal bacteria are an important source of vitamin K. It takes about 6 weeks for adequate amounts to be produced (see Chapter 8).[26] Gut closure and the development of intestinal flora are discussed in Chapter 13.

Maturation of Gastrointestinal Function

Postnatal development of GI function is influenced by the infant's genetic endowment, intrinsic timing mechanisms, initiation of feeding, type of feeding, composition of the diet, hormonal regulatory mechanisms, and gut trophic factors.[19,25,45,134,139,157] Gut trophic factors include nutrients (e.g., iron, zinc, vitamin B_{12}, vitamin A, and folate), hormones (e.g., insulin and growth factor), and peptides (e.g., epidermal growth factor, transforming growth factor, insulin-like growth factors, and somatostatin). Hormonal regulatory mechanisms have a critical role in mediating development of the gut after birth. Postnatal gut maturation is also stimulated by increases in specific GI hormones and enteric neuropeptides, including enteroglucagon (growth of the intestinal mucosa), gastrin (growth of gastric mucosa and exocrine pancreas), motilin and neurotensin (development of gut motor activity), and gastric inhibitory peptide (initiation of enteroinsular axis and subsequent glucose tolerance).[42,45,134,205,250]

A major stimulus for increases in these hormones is initiation of enteral feeding, which induces surges in plasma concentrations of the hormones listed earlier in both term and preterm infants. The response is delayed in preterm infants and in infants on parenteral-only nutrition. Human milk is rich in many GI trophic factors and thus enhances postbirth GI adaptation and maturation and pancreatic function, which in turn enhances absorptive capacities, gut closure, and mucosal defenses (see Chapter 13) and decreases the risk of infection and necrotizing enterocolitis (NEC).[63,73,139] Term infants with fetal distress have increased concentration of GI hormones, especially motilin, which may account for meconium passage. Increases in other hormones may cause redistribution of visceral blood flow in these infants.[19]

Infants demonstrate marked changes in intermediary metabolites and secretions from the gut, pancreas, and pituitary within hours after birth (Table 12-11). Marked differences are seen in hormonal secretion with human milk versus formula by 6 days, with a greater insulin response in formula-fed infants that lasts to at least 9 months. This suggests that early feeding practices may have prolonged and subtle effects on programming hormonal responses to feeding.[73,162,250] Similar changes in intermediary metabolites and secretions are not seen in infants who are being given nothing by mouth (NPO) or are on only parenteral or intravenous feedings.[19,250] These responses are

Table 12-11 Changes in Gastrointestinal Hormones and Enteric Neuropeptides in Neonates

SUBSTANCE	SITE: ROLE	POSTNATAL CHANGES*	IMPLICATIONS
Gastrin	Stomach: Regulates gastric secretions; trophic effect on gastric mucosa	Cord blood levels 4- to 5-fold higher than adult and remain higher for several weeks. Increase further with first feeding. Basal levels decline after 3-4 weeks and surge with feeding	Gastric acid low in spite of high gastrin levels; may be a result of a lack of receptors or inhibitory effects of peptide YY and neurotensin, which allow gastrin to stimulate gastric mucosal maturation without excess acid secretion
Secretin	Duodenum: Neutralizes acidic chyme entering duodenum	Higher basal levels with a more marked increase with feeding in first 3 weeks	May protect mucosa during maturation. Occurs even in absence of feeding
Cholecystokinin (CCK)	Upper small intestine: Stimulates pancreatic enzyme secretion and gallbladder contraction	Postnatal surge	May enhance pancreatic growth
Motilin	Small intestine: Increases gastric emptying and stimulates intestinal motility (interdigestive myoelectric complexes) between feedings	Cord blood levels are low with marked postnatal surge peaking at 2 weeks. Peak is enhanced but delayed in preterm infants	Increased motor activity in the neonatal gut
Glucose-dependent insulinotropic peptide (GIP)	Jejunum: Increases insulin after meals	Low at birth, increasing gradually in first month	Increases associated with development of glucose responses
Neurotensin	Ileum: Inhibits gastric secretion and motility	Increases after feeding. Response develops in first month	Decreases entry of chyme, enhancing early nutrient absorption
Peptide YY	Distal intestine: Inhibits gastric emptying and slows small bowel transit	Elevated in cord blood, increasing further to 2 weeks at 50 times higher than adult levels	Prevents hyperacidity with increased gastrin in neonate
Enteroglucagon and glucagon-like peptides I and II	Small and large intestine: Secreted in parallel; enhance insulin secretion after feeding	Marked postnatal surge peaking in first week	Enhance gut maturation

Based on material from Vanderhoof, J.A., et al. (2005). Gastrointestinal disease. In M.G. MacDonald, M.M.K. Seshia, & M.D. Mullett (Eds.), *Avery's neonatology: Pathophysiology and management of the newborn* (6th ed.). Philadelphia: Lippincott Williams & Wilkins.
*Surges seen only in infants who are fed enterally with milk feedings. All except secretin are low in infants on parenteral-only feedings.

delayed for several days in preterm infants started on enteral feedings, reflecting immaturity of gut responses.[19]

These surges seem to be triggered by small amounts of enteral feeding and are absent in unfed neonates.[19] This finding has implications for gut maturation in infants fed from birth by parenteral nutrition and has led to the use of minimal enteral feeding. Small amounts of enteral feeding may be important to induce surges in gut hormones and maturation of the gut (see Minimal Enteral Feedings). Maturation of gut functions and enzymes is described in the next section.

Initiation of Enteral Feeding

At birth the GI system must adapt to enteral nutrition. This process begins in fetal life and is still immature in the preterm infant. In addition to stimulating release of hormones critical for maturation of gut function, enteral feedings are also important as a source of energy and fluid for the infant. Human milk is the preferred feeding for both term and preterm infants and has benefits for both mother and infants (see section on "Human Milk" and Chapter 5). A healthy infant can be breastfed immediately after delivery. Colostrum is rich in antibodies, nonirritating, easily swallowed, and enhances meconium passage. Bottle-fed infants are usually fed within 4 to 6 hours, but can certainly be fed sooner, especially if at risk for hypoglycemia. Formula is usually preferred. Animal studies suggest that 5% dextrose water (D_5W) is as damaging to the lungs as formula if aspirated. More damaging still may be 10% dextrose water ($D_{10}W$) because of its lower pH and higher glucose content. Aspiration of regurgitated sterile water mixed with gastric acid can also be irritating to lung tissue. Early feeding and adequate fluid intake are associated with decreased bilirubin levels (see Chapter 18). Initiation of feeding in ill or preterm infants depends on infant health status, maturity, and ability to tolerate feeding.

Minimal Enteral Feedings

Lack of early enteral feeding has detrimental effects that can lead to intestinal inflammation, mucosal atrophy, and infection.[171] Minimal enteral feeding, also called gut or GI priming, is early (within the first week after birth) introduction of small amounts of enteral feeding to induce surges in gut hormones and maturation of the gut rather than to meet the infant's nutritional needs, which are supplied by parenteral nutrition.[211] As noted, providing even small amounts of enteral feeding in the first weeks following birth is important to stimulate gut hormones and subsequent maturation of the intestine.[211] There is no postbirth rise in gut hormones in preterm infants on parenteral nutrition, whereas infants fed orally demonstrate a marked increase in these hormones over the first week.[25]

As little as 0.5 to 1.0 mL/kg/hour of enteral feeding appears to be beneficial. These small volumes help build up mucosal bulk and stimulate development of brush border enzymes and pancreatic function; enhance maturation of GI hormones; and reduce the distention, vomiting, and malabsorption that often occur with resumption of enteral feeding. Early minimal feedings have also been reported to improve maturation of gut motor patterns, decrease feeding intolerance; increase lactase activity; improve weight gain; enhance transition to oral feedings; reduce the risk of NEC; and decrease physiologic jaundice, cholestasis, osteopenia, glucose intolerance, and sepsis.[31,34,123,184,211,171] Human milk is the preferred substance for minimal enteral feeding.[31,123] Use of sterile water does not provide the same enhancement of gut maturation and motility as provision of feeding with nutrients.[31] Advantages of minimal enteral feeding are summarized in Table 12-12.

Passage of Meconium

Passage of meconium is an essential step in initiation of intestinal function. Meconium consists of vernix caseosa, lanugo, squamous epithelial cells, occult blood, and bile and other intestinal secretions. Initially meconium is sterile, with bacteria appearing by 24 hours of age. Most term infants pass meconium by 12 (69%) to 24 (94%) hours and almost all (99.8%) by 48 hours of age. Meconium passage is delayed in preterm infants, probably due to immaturity of gut motility patterns. Only 37% of preterm infants pass meconium by 24 hours, 69% by 48 hours, and 99% by 9 days.[255] Although failure to pass meconium is a frequent sign of intestinal obstruction, infants with a high-level complete obstruction such as a duodenal atresia may occasionally pass meconium stool. Delayed passage of meconium is associated with elevated bilirubin levels, probably due to continued action of the intestinal deconjugating enzyme, β-glucuronidase, with reabsorption of the unconjugated bilirubin and recirculation to the liver via the enterohepatic circulation (see Chapter 18).

Table 12-12 Advantages of Gastrointestinal Priming (Minimal Enteral Feedings) With Human Milk

Shortens time to regain birth weight
Improves feeding tolerance
Reduces duration of parenteral nutrition
Enhances enzyme maturation
Reduces intestinal permeability
Improves gastrointestinal motility
Matures hormone responses
Improves mineral absorption, mineralization
Lowers incidence of cholestasis
Reduces duration of phototherapy
Earlier use of mother's milk
Mother begins milk expression earlier
Infant receives more mother's milk
Psychological advantage for mother
Safety

From Schanler, R.J. (2005). Enteral nutrition for the high-risk neonate. In H.W. Taeusch, R.A. Ballard, & C.A. Gleason (Eds.), *Avery's diseases of the newborn* (8th ed.). Philadelphia: Saunders, p. 1044.

Functional and Anatomic Maturation

GI function is still maturing at birth, especially in preterm infants, which increases the risk of malabsorption and malnutrition. Functional and anatomic maturation includes suck-swallow reflexes, esophageal motility, function of the lower esophageal sphincter (LES), gastric emptying, intestinal motility, and development of absorptive surface area.

Sucking and Swallowing

Reflexes needed for food intake mature in the fetus during the third trimester (see Figure 12-3). Sucking and swallowing mature at different rates.[9] The swallow reflex is well developed by 28 to 30 weeks but easily exhausted. Frequency of swallowing is decreased in infants of 30 to 35 weeks' gestation compared to infants older than 35 weeks.[71] This reflex is complete by about 34 weeks. In newborns, air enters the stomach via the nasal passages with swallowing. Because air can compete with milk for space in the infant's stomach and lead to regurgitation, burping is used to release this air. The gag reflex may be present by 18 weeks but is not complete until around 34 weeks.

Maturation of sucking is related to gestational not postnatal age.[84] Infants demonstrate nutritive sucking (NS) and nonnutritive sucking (NNS). NS brings milk into the oral cavity by compression of the nipple and generation of negative pressure. NNS is more rapid than nutritive sucking, and has a regular burst-pause pattern.[24,136] NNS rates are 2 sucks/sec with a 7:1 suck-swallow pattern versus 1 suck/sec with a 1:1 suck-swallow ratio seen with NS. NNS is present in preterm infants, but does not develop a rhythmic pattern until about 32 to 33 weeks and is not mature until 37 weeks.[71,195] Coordination of sucking movements is seen by 28 weeks; however, the intraoral pressure generation is up to 40% lower than in term infants.[182] The sucking reflex usually is not developed enough for consistent nutritive sucking until 32 to 34 weeks.[182] Sucking is thought to stimulate secretion of GI regulatory peptides and thus enhance gastric emptying.

Although all components of sucking and swallowing are present by 28 weeks, the infant is often unable to coordinate these activities with respiration and has a different suck-swallow pattern than seen in term infants.[24,171] Some suck-swallow synchrony is seen at 32 to 34 weeks; synchrony is complete by 36 to 38 weeks. Suck-swallow coordination has been demonstrated earlier in breastfeeding than in bottle-feeding infants.[154] Both term and preterm infants have 1 to 4 sucks/swallow, versus 1 to 2 sucks/swallow in older infants.[182] Maturation of suck-swallow coordination seems to be related to postmenstrual age.[84]

Three stages in the development of suck-swallow patterns have been described: (1) mouthing with no effective sucking (seen before 32 weeks' gestation); (2) an immature sucking pattern with short bursts of sucking not synchronized with swallowing (seen between 32 and 36 weeks' gestation); and (3) a mature pattern with long bursts of sucking accompanied by swallowing and associated with propulsive peristaltic waves in the esophagus emerging around 35 to 36 weeks.[94,182] Sucking is observed in term infants from birth; however, the mature suck-swallow pattern does not appear for several days. A transient immature suck-swallow pattern seen with the first few feedings is characterized by short bursts of 3 to 5 sucks followed by swallowing.[94] Within 24 to 48 hours, a mature pattern emerges, characterized by a prolonged burst of 30 or more sucks, with approximately 1 to 2 sucks per second, swallowing every 5 to 6 sucks, and a 1:1 suck-swallow-breath rate.[98,136,137,182]

In contrast, preterm infants tend to have short bursts of sucking (6- to 9-second bursts of 8 to 10 sucks per burst), usually accompanied by a rest period (for breathing) before sucking resumes.[133,182] Preterm infants are limited in their ability to suck by their weaker flexor control (important for firm lip and jaw closure) and immature musculature. Organization of sucking into a burst-pause pattern seems to occur earlier with breastfeeding than with bottle feeding. Assessment of an infant's suck, swallow, and gag capabilities is important before initiation of enteral feeding.[98]

Infants must also be able to coordinate breathing with sucking and swallowing. "Coordination of suck-swallow-breathing is a function of the infant's ability to suck effectively and swallow rapidly as boluses are formed."[133] As the liquid is propelled toward the pharynx, pharyngeal swallowing reflexes are triggered; before swallowing, an airway inhibitory reflex is triggered.[182] Increased swallowing frequency is seen in preterm infants. Lau and colleagues proposed that feeding difficulties in preterm infants are more likely related to inappropriate swallow-breathe than suck-swallow interactions.[133] Stages in the development of NS and the maturation of suck-swallow-respiration have been characterized.[9,131,132] Oral stimulation has been reported to enhance the expression (stripping/compression of the nipple for milk ejection) component of sucking.[81]

From 38 weeks' gestation to 6 months postbirth, infants can easily coordinate these activities with a 1:1 swallow-to-breathing ratio (less synchronized in preterm infants).[182] The larynx is positioned high in the pharynx in young infants so that the epiglottis overlaps the soft palate, diverting fluid around the laryngeal opening into the espohagus.[182] After 6 months of age, this ability is gradually lost. Until about 3 months of age, solids placed in the infant's mouth will be forced up against the palate by the tongue and then are either swallowed or flow out of the mouth. By 3 to 4 months of age, the infant begins to be able to selectively transfer semisolid food to the back of the mouth for swallowing.

Esophageal Motility and Lower Esophageal Sphincter Function

Esophageal motility is decreased in the newborn, especially during the first 12 hours after birth. Esophageal peristalsis is increased and accompanied by simultaneous nonperistaltic contractions, with poor coordination of esophageal motility and swallowing. (Motility refers to oscillating contractions in small segments that mix food versus the large peristaltic waves that propel food along the GI tract.) The length of the LES is reduced in infants. The LES, which forms a pressure barrier between the esophagus and stomach, is divided into three sections. In children and adults, the upper section is above the diaphragm (under the influence of intrathoracic pressure), the middle section is at the level of the LES, and the lower is below the diaphragm (under the influence of abdominal pressure). This anatomy protects against reflux. In the neonate, the LES is primarily above the diaphragm and reflux is more likely.[00] LES pressures are lower in preterm than in term infants and increase with gestation from a resting pressure of 4 mm Hg at 28 weeks to the adult value of 18 mm Hg by term; however, even the very-low-birth-weight (VLBW) infant is able to generate effective LES pressures.[109,124,171,182]

The infant has transient periods of LES relaxation that increase the risk of reflux.[182] The LES may also relax transiently from pressure on the fundus of the stomach from overdistention, as may occur with delayed gastric emptying.[80] In addition, infants have a shorter esophagus and the angle formed by the fundus of the stomach and esophagus is less acute, also increasing the risk of reflux.[80] Alterations in the LES are related to incomplete development and possibly decreased responsiveness to gastrin (which enhances LES pressure) due to delayed maturation of hormonal receptors. LES tone develops rapidly during the first week; however, the sphincter may remain immature for up to 6 to 12 months.

Gastric Emptying

Gastric motility and muscle tone are decreased and emptying time is delayed in the newborn, especially during the first 3 postnatal days.[182] The delay in gastric emptying may have a hormonal basis with delayed maturation of feedback control mechanisms. The elevated gastrin level in the newborn also delays emptying.[137] Antroduodenal activity (coordination of contractions between the antral portion of stomach and the duodenum) is up to five times lower in preterm infants than in term infants, markedly delaying gastric emptying, especially with formula feeding.[83,182]

Gastric emptying is influenced by other factors such as muscle tone, mucus, pyloric sphincter tone, presence of amniotic fluid, hormones, and type of food. Carbohydrate increases emptying time, and fat decreases emptying time. Medium-chain triglycerides empty faster than long-chain ones.[71,182] Human milk empties up to twice as fast as formula or dextrose water, and D_5W empties faster than $D_{10}W$.[182,212]

Formulas with higher caloric density are retained in the stomach for longer periods (although these formulas are associated with emptying of more calories over comparative periods). Mucus delays gastric emptying, especially during the first 24 hours after birth. Upright or semi-upright positions decrease the likelihood of air passing from the stomach to the duodenum. The gastric capacity of an infant is approximately 6 mL per kilogram of body weight. In preterm infants, large residual gastric volumes may sometimes develop, leading to gastric distention, compromised respiratory function, and interference with delivery of adequate nutrients.

Intestinal Motility

Mature intestinal interdigestive motility patterns involve three phases, which recycle over a 60- to 90-minute period. Phase I is quiescence, phase II is characterized by irregular contractions, and phase III is characterized by regular phasic contractions. Contractions during phase II and III migrate down the intestine and are called *migratory motor complexes* (MMCs).[42,71,182] Intestinal motility patterns and gastric emptying begin to mature after 30 to 32 weeks' gestation but are still somewhat disorganized until near term age. Between 29 and 32 weeks' gestation, infants begin to develop periods of gut quiescence interspersed with short bursts of activity called *clusters*. Between 32 and 36 weeks' gestation, motor activity becomes more organized, with cycling between quiescence and activity clusters.[71] Frequency of clusters decreases with increasing gestational age (from 12 to 14 per minute at 27 to 28 weeks to 6 to 8 per minute by term). As cluster frequency decreases, MMCs appear. MMCs are first seen by 32 to 34 weeks' gestation and are mediated by motilin. Motilin receptors are not functional until 32 weeks' gestation, with an absence of cyclic motilin release in the preterm infant. MMCs are rare during fasting in infants who instead have periods of quiescence alternating with nonmigratory phasic activity. With increasing gestational age, the length of the activity clusters increases and their frequency decreases.

In adults given milk, motor activity increases (mature fed response). Most (85%) term infants have a mature gut fed response. Preterm infants may have a mature fed response but they are more likely to have an immature response (motor activity decreases with feeding) or indeterminate response (motor activity does not change with feeding), especially infants younger than 35 weeks' gestation.[71] Thus most term infants have increased intestinal motility with feeding, whereas in most preterm infants contractions cease, possibly due to vagal immaturity. The cessation of contractions with feeding in preterm infants lasts for 15 to 20 minutes and then gradually resumes. Alterations in motility in preterm infants may limit the ability of these infants to tolerate enteral feedings due to less efficient propulsion of food, delayed gastric emptying, and slower intestinal transit time. Antenatal corticosteroids may enhance maturation of GI motor activity.

Intestinal movement tends to be more disorganized and slower in newborns due to immaturity of the intestinal musculature, poor coordination of peristaltic waves, and a tendency for segmentation of peristalsis.[83] Disorganized motility results in a decreased ability to clear the upper gut, with impaired absorptive function, prolonged transit time in the upper intestine, and more rapid emptying of the ileum and colon. Intestinal transit time averages 4 to 12 hours in adults versus 8 to 96 hours in the preterm infant. Prolonged transit time in the small intestine may also be an advantage by increasing chances for absorption of specific nutrients. However, faster emptying of the colon reduces the time for water and electrolyte absorption, increasing stool water content and the risk of dehydration and electrolyte imbalance. The gastrocolonic reflex is active in the neonate: entry of food into the beginning of the small intestine or colon causes reflexive propulsion of food toward the rectum.

The preterm infant experiences even more irregular and less predictable peristaltic waves along with antiperistaltic waves. These limitations further increase transit time and impair absorption. GI peristalsis develops gradually in the fetus from 33 to 40 weeks' gestation. Immaturity of peristalsis in the preterm infant is one reason that fetal passage of meconium is rarely seen before 34 weeks' gestation.

Intestinal Surface Area

The immature surface of the small intestine decreases absorptive area, especially in preterm infants. Numbers of intestinal villi and epithelial cells increase with gestation. In the mature intestine, epithelial cells in the crypts are undifferentiated and develop the ability to hydrolyze and transport nutrients as they migrate toward the top of the villus, replacing older cells. Turnover of intestinal epithelial cells is decreased in the newborn, impairing absorptive efficiency.

Alterations in the normal crypt-to-villous cell turnover rate lead to inadequate functional surface area along the brush border and glycocalyx and alter digestion, absorption, and host defense mechanisms. The surface area of the small intestine can be altered by ischemia, anoxia, and infection, further impeding absorption of nutrients. Enteric intake after birth induces epithelial hyperplasia, increasing cell turnover and stimulating production of microvillous enzymes such as pancreatic lipase, amylase, and trypsin.[46] Gut regulatory peptides and hormones increase at birth and have a trophic effect on the intestine (see Table 12-11).[134,169] Colostrum and human milk contain factors that stimulate epithelial cell turnover and maturation.[169] The gut mucosal immune system is still immature at term, increasing the risk of infection and other disorders.[46,254] Human milk contains substances that not only protect the infant from infection but also enhance maturation of this system ("gut closure"). Gut closure is discussed further in Chapter 13.

Intestinal Circulation

Intestinal circulation differs in newborns compared to adults. In the newborn, intestinal basal vascular resistance is low in the immediate postbirth period, probably mediated by nitric oxide production.[200] This lower resistance may alter the ability of the newborn to respond to arterial hypoxemia and hypotension, increasing the risk of ischemia and disorders such as NEC.[200]

Physiologic Limitations

Newborns are limited in their ability to digest and absorb certain nutrients due to decreased activity of specific enzymes and other substances as well as functional and anatomic limitations. However, newborns, especially if fed human milk, have mechanisms available that partially compensate for these alterations, resulting in relatively proficient digestion in term and many preterm infants.

A prominent difference in digestive processes between the neonate and adult is immaturity of exocrine pancreatic function, which forces the infant to use compensatory mechanisms that rely on nonpancreatic enzymes found in the lingual area and salivary secretions, intestinal brush border enterocytes, and human milk. Slow development of pancreatic exocrine function may be a protective mechanism to prevent degradation and loss of intestinal epithelial cells and brush border enzymes by the pancreatic proteolytic enzymes. Limitations of the newborn related to digestion and absorption of protein, carbohydrate, and fat and compensatory mechanisms are summarized in Table 12-13.

Table 12-13 **Physiologic Limitations in Digestion and Absorption of Protein, Carbohydrate, and Fat in the Neonate**

FACTOR	LIMITATION IN NEONATE	IMPLICATION	COMPENSATORY MECHANISMS
DIGESTION AND ABSORPTION OF PROTEIN			
Gastric acid	50% of adult values	Increased gastric pH Decreased pepsin activity Decreased gastric proteolysis	
Pepsinogen	50% of adult values	Decreased pepsin Decreased gastric proteolysis	
Trypsin	Near adult levels (but activity reduced)	Decreased proteolysis	
Enterokinase	10% of adult activity	Decreased activation of trypsin and other pancreatic peptidases	
Chymotrypsin	10%-60% of adult activity	Decreased proteolysis	
Carboxypeptidases	10%-60% of adult activity	Decreased proteolysis	
Intestinal mucosal dipeptidases	Adequate	Promote protein digestion	
Amino acid absorption	Adequate	Adequate absorption of amino acids and some intact proteins	
DIGESTION AND ABSORPTION OF CARBOHYDRATE			
Salivary amylase	⅓ of adult levels	Decreased starch digestion (infants ingest little starch)	Increased gastric pH helps retain activity in stomach Used to digest glucose polymers
Pancreatic amylase	0.2%-5% of adult levels	Decreased starch digestion	Mammary amylase
Sucrase, maltase, isomaltase	Adequate digestion of sucrose, maltose, isomaltose		
Glucoamylase	50%-100% of adult levels	Enhances digestion of glucose polymers	
Lactase	Term is 2-4 times greater than older children; preterm is 30% of term by 28-30 weeks	Term infant able to digest lactose well; preterm infant digests lactose adequately, especially lactose in milk	Colonic salvage
Glucose absorption	Term is 50%-60% of adult; lower in preterm	Adequate absorption at low levels; more problems in handling glucose load	
DIGESTION AND ABSORPTION OF FAT			
Pancreatic lipase	10%-20% of adult levels	Decreased fat digestion	Lingual and gastric lipase Human milk bile salt–stimulated lipase
Bile acids	Synthesis and bile acid pool	Decreased fat digestion and absorption	Human milk bile salt–stimulated lipase
	Term is 50% of adult values	Steatorrhea in preterm infants	
	Decreased reabsorption through the enterohepatic circulation	Decreased uptake and recirculation of bile acids	

Digestion and Absorption of Proteins

In spite of limitations in amounts and function of proteolytic enzymes, term and many preterm infants digest and absorb proteins relatively well.[136] The newborn's initial gastric pH is neutral or slightly alkaline.[136,174] Decreased secretion of gastric acid and prolonged buffering by the stomach contents due to delayed gastric emptying in newborns increase gastric pH. Amniotic fluid in the stomach also elevates gastric pH initially. Acid secretion is further decreased and gastric pH increased (5.5 to 7 versus 2 to 3 in adults) in preterm infants. Decreased gastric acid secretion can increase the risk of nosocomial infection since gastric acidity is a barrier to microorganisms.[171]

Gastric acid secretion increases within 24 hours of birth and doubles by 2 months, with varying findings in different studies.[70,89,174] Pepsinogen production is low (corrected for weight) for the first few months and is even lower in preterm infants.[136,174] The elevated pH reduces pepsin activity and gastric peptic hydrolysis in both term and preterm infants.[25,109,136,174] Although circulating levels of gastrin (which normally stimulates secretion of gastric acid and pepsin) are elevated, receptors for this hormone may be immature.[134,136] The decreased gastric acidity and pepsinogen levels may enhance development of gut host defense mechanisms by promoting activity of immunoglobulins and antigen recognition by the GI tract.[136]

Term and preterm infants have near adult levels of trypsin, but activity of trypsin and the other pancreatic proteolytic hormones is reduced. Chymotrypsin and carboxypeptidase B activity are 10% to 60% and enterokinase activity is 10% of adult values in preterm infants, increasing to 25% by term.[171] Because enterokinase catabolizes the conversion of trypsinogen to trypsin, which in turn activates the other pancreatic proteolytic enzymes, the level of enterokinase is the rate-limiting step for intestinal protein digestion.[136] This limitation does not seem to have a major impact on infants over 26 to 28 weeks' gestation, who are usually able to digest and absorb 85% of the dietary protein in human milk and most formulas.[25] However, preterm infants cannot handle formulas with excessive protein loads (greater than 5 g/kg/day). Intestinal brush border peptidase and cytosolic peptidase activity, along with the ability to transport and absorb amino acids, is well developed and efficient in term and preterm infants.[42,71,] The newborn's intestine absorbs more intact proteins and macromolecules, which may increase the risk for development of allergies (see Chapter 13) and NEC in infants fed formula.[136] In breast-fed infants, absorption of macromolecules from breast milk enhances passive immunity.[169,174]

Digestion and Absorption of Carbohydrates

Carbohydrate digestion in adults is dependent on salivary and pancreatic amylase and disaccharidases. Salivary amylase activity at birth is one third that of adults. Levels increase after 3 to 6 months of age and may be related to the addition of starch (solid foods) to the infant's diet.[89,135] Salivary amylase retains some activity in the infant's stomach and is effective in digestion of glucose polymers.[174,250]

Pancreatic amylase activity is decreased in term and preterm infants to 0.2% to 5% of adult values. Adequate levels are achieved after 4 to 6 months.[123] Cholecystokinin and secretin have little effect on pancreatic amylase secretion before 1 month. Amylase activity increases significantly after this time.

Mammary amylase in human milk compensates for the decreased pancreatic amylase. Mammary amylase is highest in colostrum, gradually decreasing after 6 weeks. Buffers in human milk and the higher gastric pH in the neonate help maintain mammary amylase activity.[135]

The term newborn has adequate levels of α-glucosidases such as sucrase, maltase, isomaltase, and glucoamylase. Sucrase and maltase attain maximal activity by 32 to 34 weeks' gestation or earlier. Glucoamylase is an intestinal brush border enzyme that digests glucose polymers found in many formulas.[25,135] Levels of glucoamylase are 50% to 100% of adult values and increase rapidly after birth.[136,250] Glucoamylase is less susceptible than disaccharidases to intestinal mucosal injury. This enzyme is evenly distributed along the small intestine, which, along with the prolonged transit time seen in infants, contributes to more efficient hydrolysis and mucosal uptake.[134,135] Digestion of glucose polymers depends on salivary amylase, glucoamylase, and human milk amylase. Neonates can effectively hydrolyze and absorb glucose polymers, especially those of short- to medium-chain length.

The major carbohydrate in human and cow's milk is lactose. Lactase activity increases rapidly in late gestation and is adequate after 36 weeks' gestation. At term, *lactase* levels are two to four times higher than in older infants. *Lactase* activity at 28 to 34 weeks' gestation is only 30% of term values, but increases after birth with exposure to *lactose*.[123,136,171] Despite low *lactase* activity, most preterm infants digest *lactose* adequately, especially *lactose* in human milk.[71,123,169,174] *Lactose* that is not absorbed in the small intestines is conserved by colonic salvage.

Colonic salvage involves bacterial fermentation of carbohydrate to hydrogen gas and short-chain fatty acids, which are absorbed by the colon, minimizing carbohydrate loss in stools (Figure 12-9).[71,123,171,174] These fatty acids are a source of calories, enhance fluid and electrolyte absorption by the colon, and promote cell replication in the gut.[123] In preterm infants, two thirds of the ingested lactose may reach the colon. Changes in colonic bacterial flora following antibiotic use or surgery may alter the infant's ability to conserve energy via colonic salvage. Lactase deficiency generally resolves when the preterm infant reaches a postmenstrual age of 36 to 40 weeks.[135] Infants need some lactose intake because lactose enhances calcium absorption.

Mechanisms for glucose, galactose, and fructose absorption develop early in gestation and are relatively mature. The capacity for mucosal glucose uptake at term is 50% to 60% of adult values.[135] Absorption of glucose is slower in preterm infants, with further reductions in SGA infants, suggesting that growth restriction may delay maturation of these processes. Infants seem to absorb glucose as well as adults at low glucose concentrations but have a maximal absorptive capacity about 20% that of the adult. Glucose

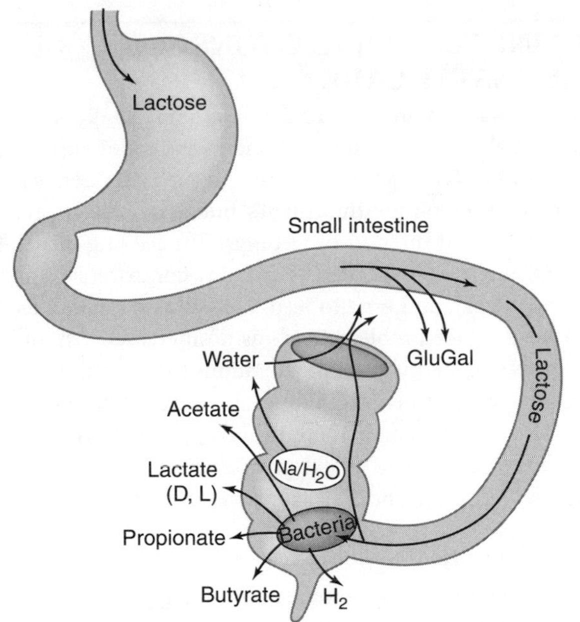

FIGURE 12-9 The two major fates of dietary lactose: (1) digestion in the small intestine with absorption of glucose (Glu) and galactose (Gal), or (2) fermentation in the colon to various gases such as H_2; lactate, and short-chain fatty acids including acetate, propionate, and butyrate. The absorption of short-chain fatty acids stimulates sodium and water absorption in the colon. Unfermented lactose may exert an osmotic stimulus causing fecal excretion of water. (From Kien, C.L. [1996]. Digestion, absorption, and fermentation of carbohydrates in the newborn. *Clin Perinatol*, 23, 213.)

transport increases by 2 to 3 weeks of age.[135] Hypoxia and ischemia decrease intestinal perfusion, altering the ultrastructure of intestinal cells, which decreases active transport and uptake of glucose.

Digestion and Absorption of Fats

Fat digestion in the adult relies on pancreatic lipase to break down triglycerides and bile acids to emulsify fat droplets before and during lipolysis. These processes are decreased in term and especially in preterm infants.[136,174,196] Lipase activity at term is 10% to 20% of that seen in older children, partly due to minimal responsiveness by pancreatic acinar cells to secretin and cholecystokinin during the first month. Term infants fail to absorb 10% to 15% and preterm infants 30% or more of ingested fat.[71,83] Lipase activity increases up to fourfold during the first week postbirth in healthy preterm infants.[174]

Bile acid synthesis is low due to lower bile synthesis and ileal absorption.[171] Bile acid pool size is one half of adult values in term infants, and one sixth of adult and one third of term infant values in preterm infants.[109,136,196,250] Because hepatic conjugation of bile acids in infants is taurine dependent (versus glycine dependent in the adult), adequate intake of taurine is essential in infancy.[136] The decreased bile acid pools are due to reduced hepatic synthesis and poorer recirculation and conservation of bile salts through enterohepatic shunting as a result of immaturity of liver and intestinal active transport processes.[25,136]

In preterm infants, concentrations of bile acids in the duodenal lumen may be below critical levels necessary for micelle formation (water-soluble aggregates of lipids and lipid-soluble substances).[25] Decreased micelle formation results in poor absorption of long-chain triglycerides (LCT), which are dependent on micelle formation for solubilization and subsequent hydrolysis. Infants are better able to absorb medium (MCT) and short-chain (SCT) triglycerides, which are not dependent on micelle formation. SCTs and MCTs are absorbed directly into the portal venous system, whereas LCTs must first be re-esterified to form chylomicrons before entering the lymphatics.[171]

Alternative pathways to compensate for the decreased levels of pancreatic lipase and bile acids include human milk bile salt–stimulated lipase (also called *mammary lipase* or *milk digestive lipase*), lingual lipase, and gastric lipase. Both gastric and lingual lipase have high activity at birth.[71,174] Gastric and lingual lipase activity is present by at least 26 weeks' gestation.[71] Lingual and gastric lipases hydrolyze 50% and mammary lipase 20% to 40% of dietary fat in infants.[83] Intragastric lipolysis by these extrapancreatic lipases breaks down triglycerides in the milk fat globule. As a result, the fat globule is a better substrate for the available pancreatic lipase and enhances action of bile salts. Hydrolysis of fat in the stomach can be documented in preterm infants as young as 26 to 32 weeks' gestation.

Mammary lipase is present in the milk of term and preterm mothers. This enzyme is stable at low pH (and not inactivated in the stomach) and hydrolyzes triglycerides at low concentrations of bile salts.[174] Mammary lipase works in the duodenum, and its activity is stimulated by bile salts at concentrations below those required for micelle formation such as are found in many preterm infants. Temperatures above 55° C (131° F) inactivate this enzyme; freezing does not seem to affect its activity. This lipase also produces monolauryl, a substance with antibacterial, antiviral, and antifungal activity.

Absorption of Other Substances

Alterations in fat absorption affect absorption of fat-soluble vitamins, especially in preterm infants who may need supplementation with water-soluble analogues. Absorptive capacity for folate is also lower. Lower gastric secretion of intrinsic factor may interfere with absorption of vitamin B_{12}.[136] Neonates are less able to adapt to changes in osmotic load in the large intestine, increasing the risk of diarrhea and electrolyte imbalance.

Mechanisms for absorption of iron are relatively well developed in term and preterm infants, with a high rate of iron absorption for the first 10 weeks postbirth.[136] Iron in human milk is absorbed better than iron in formula, with absorption of up to 50% of the iron in human milk, even in preterm infants.[136,250] For the first few months however, preterm infants may not absorb large quantities of iron due to saturation of transferrin with iron from turnover of red blood cells (see Chapter 8).

Calcium absorption is influenced by vitamin D, calcium, and phosphorus concentrations; fatty acids; and lactose (see Chapter 17). The complex relationship between calcium and lipid intake makes determining calcium concentrations for formulas difficult. A high calcium intake alters absorption and retention of fatty acids; a high lipid intake can decrease calcium absorption.[136] Calcium absorption is lower in infants than in adults when calcium concentrations are low, but it is more efficient at higher levels.[136] Zinc and copper are well absorbed in term infants but not in preterm infants, who may be in negative zinc or copper balance.[136,242] Mechanisms for absorption of many nutrients have not been well studied in human neonates.

Liver Function in the Neonate

Portal blood flow is lower in the fetus, with shunting of a portion of the blood away from the portal sinuses and liver parenchyma and into the inferior vena cava via the ductus venosus. Many excretory and detoxification functions of the fetal liver are assumed by the placenta and maternal liver. With removal of the placenta, blood flow through the ductus venosus ceases, with anatomic closure by proliferation of connective tissue by approximately 2 weeks in most term infants (see Chapter 9).

The newborn liver accounts for about 5% of the infant's weight. This physiologic enlargement is a result of the following factors (1) increased labile connective tissue (possibly in response to hypoxic stress with the abrupt shift in the oxygenation of blood supplying the liver at birth [i.e., from blood from the placenta to systemic venous blood]); (2) active liver hematopoiesis, which decreases by 6 weeks as liver metabolic functions increase; (3) increased liver glycogen; and (4) hepatic congestion due to changes in blood flow with removal of the placenta.[26,94]

Infants have a unique pathologic response to liver dysfunction, with active fibroblastic proliferation and early bile stasis that can alter the presentation of liver disorders. Decreased bile flow (cholestasis)—often in association with a direct (conjugated) hyperbilirubinemia—is seen with many liver disorders in infants. The cholestasis is due to disruption of the canalicular membrane, poor development of bile acid secretory mechanisms, and immaturity of bile acid synthesis.[94,124]

Birth results in induction of many liver enzyme systems; however, enzyme systems necessary for metabolism of some drugs are depressed in the newborn.[26] In the mature liver, oxidation and conjugation result in formation of water-soluble metabolites that are more readily excreted into bile. In the fetus, depression of these processes is an advantage, in that lipid-soluble metabolites are more readily transferred across the placenta where they can be handled by the maternal system. The liver's smooth endoplasmic reticulum (SER) is the location of many hepatic microsomal enzymes. The neonatal liver has little SER, and activities of microsomal enzymes are reduced or undetectable at birth, interfering with drug metabolism.[107] Hepatic metabolism of drugs is discussed in Chapter 7.

CLINICAL IMPLICATIONS FOR NEONATAL CARE

Food and warmth are "two of the most important controllable factors in determining survival and normal development."[187] Limitations of GI function in term and preterm neonates have major implications for the infant's nutritional needs and the composition and method of feedings. The feeding of sick and preterm infants is associated with many controversies, including when, what, and how to feed. Decisions regarding feeding can lead to other problems such as an increased risk of NEC and metabolic or nutritional alterations. This section reviews nutritional requirements of infants and implications of GI limitations for the selection of method and composition of feedings. Problems related to neonatal physiologic limitations such as reflux, dehydration, and NEC are also examined.

Infant Growth

Growth is controlled by complex hormonal, growth factor, and nutrient interactions.[263] Major regulating factors are growth hormone (somatostatin) and IGF-I. Thyroid hormones, insulin, glucocorticoids, leptin, and local growth factors also have important roles, especially in regulation of intermediary metabolism.[230,263] Pituitary growth hormone (GH) stimulates IGF-I (primarily from the liver, but also found in many other organs), which in conjunction with other growth factors stimulates cell differentiation and function.[263] Growth hormone resistance (characterized by increased GH and low IGF-I) has been reported in ELBW infants.[263]

Growth rates during the neonatal period are more rapid than at any other time. The method for growth assessment of term infants generally involves use of standardized charts from the National Center for Health and Statistics (http://www.cdc.gov/growthcharts). These charts have been revised to include a broader population base as well as more breastfed infants. Expected patterns and assessment of growth for preterm infants in the immediate postbirth period are controversial, especially regarding whether these infants should be expected to follow intrauterine or extrauterine patterns. Both intrauterine and extrauterine growth standards are available.

Generally recommendations have been that postnatal growth of preterm infants follow the pattern for intrauterine growth of a fetus of the same gestation, although it is unclear whether intrauterine rates are appropriate or realistic for these infants.[10,57,239] VLBW infants often do not grow at intrauterine rates and are at risk for postnatal growth restriction.[98,239,241] ELBW infants may not regain their birth weight for 2 to 3 weeks and are especially vulnerable for extrauterine growth restriction. Lower than optimal nutritional intake during the first week may result in a significant energy and protein deficit, which increases over the early weeks. This calculation of infant nutritional needs may need to take into account requirements for catch-up growth as well as the usual requirements for maintenance and growth.[57]

A variety of intrauterine growth charts are available, all of which have limitations in that they were developed from measurements of preterm infants at various gestations and thus may not represent a normal fetal population. Recently new intrauterine curves were published from U.S. data.[179] The growth chart used should be one that is most appropriate for the location and patient population (ethnic, socioeconomic, and demographic characteristics). General parameters for daily weight gain are in Table 12-14. Postnatal growth grids for LBW and VLBW infants for the first 3 years (using gestation-adjusted ages) have been developed for postdischarge care.

Nutritional Requirements of Term and Preterm Infants

Nutritional requirements of infants vary with gestational age and health status. Requirements for healthy term infants are assumed to be those found in human milk. For infants who are not breastfed, commercial formulas are alternatives for meeting nutritional needs. Nutritional requirements for preterm infants have been less clear. One problem has been the lack of knowledge and agreement on what is the optimal growth rate for the preterm infant and how closely this rate should parallel that of the fetus. Nutritional requirements for preterm infants are often estimated by assaying the body composition of fetuses at different gestational ages and examining fetal accretion of different nutrients. Water, energy, and caloric requirements are higher for preterm infants because of greater insensible water loss (see Chapter 11), increased exposure to stressors, and increased expectations for growth. Recommended nutritional requirements for preterm infants are available.[244]

Protein and energy are critical for growth and neurodevelopment.[17] Energy needs vary depending on the infant's age, thermal environment, activity, maturation, growth rate, and health status.[123] Maintenance caloric requirements are calculated based on resting energy expenditure, activity, cold stress, and fecal losses (Table 12-15). Growth requires additional calories (approximately 45 kcal for each 1-g weight gain).[123] The caloric (energy) maintenance and growth requirement for breastfed term newborns averages 85 to 100 kcal/kg/day, with 100 to 110 kcal/kg/day for formula-fed newborns.[83]

Preterm infants weighing less than 1000 g have maintenance requirements of approximately 50 to 70 kcal/kg/day, although this may be higher for some infants, depending on the infant's basal metabolic rate (increased with health problems), activity level (decreased in infants on morphine or fentanyl), cold stress (increases metabolic rate), specific dynamic action (efficiency of nutrient absorption), and fecal losses.[84] For growth these infants need an additional 45 to 70 kcal/kg/day.[66,123] Increasing the growth allowance above this level will increase weight gain, but not exponentially because the energy cost of weight gain also increases.[123] Most stable preterm infants achieve satisfactory growth on approximately 120 kcal/kg/day.[66,242] Caloric requirements for infants on parenteral feedings tend to be lower, averaging 80 to 110 kcal/kg/day, because activity level and fecal losses are lower.[71,83,123]

Fetal protein accretion is 3 to 4 g/kg/day.[84] The type of dietary protein affects daily protein requirements. For example, infants can achieve adequate growth with 2 to 2.5 g/kg/day of a whey-predominant feeding.[242] Inadequate protein leads to alterations in cardiorespiratory, liver, and renal function; decreased immunocompetence; altered brain growth; and poor weight gain and somatic growth. Term infants need 1.5 to 2.5 g/kg/day, whereas up to 4 g/kg/day has been used for preterm infants.[29,34,44,66,96,108,239] Preterm infants need protein intake early, beginning on days 1 or 2 of extrauterine life to

Table 12-14 Approximate Daily Weight Gain for Infants

AGE	WEIGHT
GESTATIONAL AGE	
24-28 weeks	15-20 g/kg/day
29-32 weeks	17-21 g/kg/day
33-36 weeks	14-15 g/kg/day
37-40 weeks	7-9 g/kg/day
CORRECTED AGE	
40 weeks-3 months	30 g/day
3-6 months	12 g/day
6-9 months	15 g/day
9-12 months	10 g/day
12-24 months	6 g/day

From Kalhan, S.C. & Price, P.T. (1999). Nutrition and selected disorders of the gastrointestinal tract. I: Nutrition for the high risk infant. In M.H. Klaus & A.A. Fanaroff (Eds.), *Care of the high risk neonate* (5th ed.). Philadelphia: Saunders.

Table 12-15 Estimated Energy Expenditure in a Growing Preterm Infant

EXPENDITURE	kcal/kg/DAY
Resting energy expenditure	47
Minimal activity*	4
Occasional cold stress*	10
Fecal loss of energy (1% to 16% of intake)	15
Growth† (includes dietary induced thermogenesis)	45
TOTAL	121

From Kalhan, S.C. & Price, P.T. (1999). Nutrition and selected disorders of the gastrointestinal tract. I: Nutrition for the high risk infant. In M.H. Klaus & A.A. Fanaroff (Eds.), *Care of the high risk neonate* (5th ed.). Philadelphia: Saunders.

*As infant matures, energy expended in activities, such as crying and breastfeeding, increases; at the same time, energy expended as a result of cold stress decreases.

†Calculated assuming 3.0 to 4.5 kcal/g weight gain at a rate of gain of 10 to 14 g/kg/day.

minimize loss of body stores and enhance growth.[44,66,239,263] Inadequate protein can alter IGF-I and other growth factors, increasing the risk of postnatal growth restriction in preterm infants. Serum IGF-I levels correlate with protein intake and nitrogen retention.[263] Current practices have moved toward earlier introduction of protein and use of minimal enteral feedings using colostrum or breast milk.[263] Excessive protein intake (greater than 5 g/kg/day) results in a metabolic overload with irritability and can lead to late metabolic acidosis, azotemia, edema, fever, lethargy, diarrhea, elevated blood urea nitrogen, and poorer developmental outcome.[29,94,194]

A major energy source in human milk and most formulas is fat, which accounts for 30% to 50% of the total calories.[10,190] Specific requirements include those for the essential fatty acids linoleic and α-linolenic acid (an omega-3 fatty acid), which are important for synthesis of other fatty acids and for growth and development, especially brain and vision development.[215] Approximately 3% (300 mg linoleic acid per 100 kcal) of the infant's energy intake should be essential fatty acids.[10,29] Inadequate fats or lack of essential fatty acids can lead to metabolic problems, skin disorders, and poor growth; excessive fats can lead to ketosis.

Carbohydrates make up 40% to 50% of the caloric content.[92] Inadequate carbohydrate can lead to hypoglycemia; excessive carbohydrate can lead to diarrhea. Infants, especially preterm infants who have poor stores and a higher growth rate, have increased needs for calcium, phosphorus, and vitamins to support growth and bone mineralization. Nutrient requirements for enteral and parenteral nutrition are available in neonatal texts.

Composition of Feedings

To maximize growth and reduce stress, the limitations of the neonate's GI, renal, and metabolic systems must be considered in selecting substances for feeding. This can be accomplished through analysis of the composition of human milk and commercial formulas and consideration of the advantages and disadvantages of each for that individual infant. This section discusses considerations in selecting feedings for term and preterm infants.

Protein

Milk protein consists of casein and whey proteins. Whey forms soft, flocculent curds. Casein forms tougher, more rubbery curds; it requires greater energy expenditure to digest and is more likely to be incompletely digested. Human milk has a whey-to-casein ratio around 70:30 (versus 20:80 in cow's milk). Whey is easier to digest in the presence of low levels of trypsin and pepsin and is associated with fewer imbalances in plasma amino acids in preterm infants.[212] Whey protein contains a different mixture of amino acids than casein, with increased levels of cystine and decreased methionine. Human milk contains less protein than cow's milk but has higher levels of nonprotein nitrogen with an amino acid composition that is easy for the infant to use.[53,190] The major whey protein in human milk is α-lactalbumin, which is high in amino acids that are essential for the infant. Other human milk proteins include lactoferrin, lysozyme, and secretory immunoglobulin A.

The amino acid composition of feedings is critical for optimal neonatal growth and development. Some amino acids are essential in the neonate that are not essential for adults due to the decreased ability of the infant to synthesize these amino acids.[123] For example, taurine is essential for central nervous system (CNS) growth, maintaining optimal retinal integrity and function, and bile acid synthesis. Intermediary metabolic pathways for synthesis of some amino acids are immature. The last enzyme in transsulfuration is absent in the fetus and develops slowly in preterm infants. These infants cannot synthesize cystine and have limited tolerance for methionine (which is normally converted to cystine). Similar limitations exist in the ability of the infant to oxidize tyrosine and phenylalanine. Transamination pathways are also not well developed, so histidine is an essential amino acid in the neonate but not in the adult.[136] Thus infants need a feeding that contains lower levels of methionine, phenylalanine, and tyrosine and adequate cystine, taurine, and histidine.[123] Glutamine is another important component in that it acts as a nitrogen transporter and enhances gut maturation, fat metabolism, and gut immune function in addition to producing glutamate, a neurotransmitter needed for CNS development (see Chapter 15).[44,92,170,190] Glutamine is a component of human milk. Glutamine supplementation of preterm infants has not proved to be of significant benefit in most studies.[245] Other amino acids such as threonine, aspartate, and proline may also be important in gut function and maturation.[45]

Carbohydrate

Immaturity of lactase activity in preterm infants may interfere with their ability to optimally use lactose-based formulas, although most infants have little difficulty digesting lactose. For example, preterm infants can absorb up to 90% of the lactose in human milk.[190,212] Carbohydrates other than lactose are often included in feedings if greater carbohydrate absorption is needed or if lactose is poorly tolerated.[136] Use of low-lactose feedings reduces the risk of overwhelming the infant's available lactase. Infants require some lactose for calcium and magnesium absorption. In addition, feedings containing lactose, especially breast milk, help stimulate lactase activity and lactose utilization.[190]

Glucose polymers are often used as an alternative carbohydrate substrate in formulas. Preterm infants hydrolyze and absorb glucose polymers in a manner similar to that with lactose in term infants.[136] Glucose polymers have several advantages: (1) ready availability from natural sources, including corn syrup solids; (2) high caloric density without significantly increasing the renal solute load (see Chapter 11); (3) incorporation into feedings without significantly increasing the osmotic load and risk of increased water loss and diarrhea; (4) more rapid emptying from the stomach of young infants than lactose or glucose; (5) independence from lactase and amylase; and (6) digestion by glucoamylase, which is present in adequate quantities in preterm infants and whose secretion is less likely to be altered by mucosal injury.[135,136]

Oligosaccharides are glucose polymers that prevent bacterial attachment to the intestinal mucosa, thus providing protection against infection. Oligosaccharides function as prebiotics and may play a role in gut host defense mechanisms. Oligosaccharides are a major component of human milk.[212] These substances are only partially digested in the small intestine, and when they reach the colon stimulate development of bifidogenic flora.[58]

Fat

Fats are the primary source of energy in human milk and many formulas. Fats provide a higher caloric density without significantly increasing osmotic load. Limitations in neonatal fat digestion and absorption can reduce the usefulness of this energy source. High-caloric-density formulas tend to be retained in the stomach for longer periods, thus delaying gastric emptying.

Infants need both saturated and unsaturated fatty acids in their diet. Human milk and vegetable oils (corn, coconut, and soy) are absorbed better than saturated fat (cow's milk or butter fat). Human milk fat is contained in fat globules that consist of fatty acids such as linoleic, linolenic, oleic, palmitic, arachidonic, and docosahexaenoic acids. The latter two acids are long-chain polyunsaturated fatty acids (PUFAs) that are sources of omega-6 fatty acids and are found in human milk. These PUFAs are precursors for prostaglandins and phospholipids and are important in neurologic and vision development.[113,190,212] Milk fat globules are more easily absorbed than other forms of fat in the presence of a reduced bile acid pool.[212] Human milk also contains long-chain polyunsaturates that are well absorbed and may enhance nervous system development.[123] Carnitine (synthesized from methionine and lysine) is important for fatty acid oxidation.[27,190] In formulas, unsaturated fats in vegetable oils are a source of the essential fatty acid linoleic acid. Short- and medium-chain fatty acids (MCFAs) can be absorbed intact across the gastric and intestinal mucosa. These triglycerides are not dependent on the reduced bile acid pools for emulsification and do not require carnitine, often low in preterm infants, for transfer into the mitochondria.[123] MCFAs are associated with more rapid gastric emptying and enhanced calcium and magnesium absorption.[190] About 10% to 50% of the fat in preterm formulas is in the form of MCFAs to enhance fat absorption. Infants need some long-chain fatty acids for integrity of cell membranes and brain development.[247] Excessive fat intake from MCFAs has been associated with a risk of essential fatty acid deficiency.[190]

Vitamins, Minerals, and Micronutrients

Infants need adequate amounts of essential vitamins, minerals, and micronutrients in their diet to support normal growth and development. Immature infants have decreased stores of most of these substances since stores accumulate late in gestation, and dietary supplementation may be needed. Specific requirements for many vitamins and micronutrients in preterm infants are unknown. Increased quantities of fat-soluble vitamins (A, D, E, K) and their water-soluble analogues compensate for the inadequate bile acid pools and poorer absorption of fat, especially in preterm infants. Requirements for B vitamins (coenzymes for metabolic processes and energy production) and folic acid (a cofactor for DNA synthesis) may also be increased because of the infant's greater growth rate and decreased intestinal absorption. Vitamin K is discussed in Chapter 8. Recommended daily intakes of minerals, vitamins, and micronutrients are available.[244]

Vitamin A. Vitamin A is needed for development of retina rod cells, light perception, tissue integrity, and repair and growth of epithelial tissue. Higher levels are needed in preterm infants due to poorer absorption and stores. Decreased vitamin A has been reported in infants with chronic lung disease (CLD).[83] This may be due to lowered intake or consumption of vitamin A in the repair of damaged lung epithelial tissue. Vitamin A levels should be monitored in infants on parenteral alimentation. Vitamin A in parenteral solutions decreases over 24 hours as a result of adherence of the vitamin to IV tubing and photodegradation.

Vitamin C. Vitamin C is water soluble, readily absorbed, and not stored in significant amounts. It is important in amino acid metabolism (needed for growth) and intestinal iron absorption. Deficiencies are associated with scurvy (rare) and transient hypertyrosinemia.[242]

Vitamin D. Vitamin D facilitates intestinal calcium and phosphorus absorption, bone mineralization, and calcium reabsorption from bone (see Chapter 17). Preterm infants have lower serum concentrations of vitamin D and increased needs due to more rapid growth and immaturity of enzymes involved in metabolism of dietary vitamin D to active substrates. These infants are at greater risk of osteopenia and, less often, rickets (see Chapter 17).[242]

Vitamin E. An important consideration related to both the fat and vitamin composition of feeding is the ratio of polyunsaturated fatty acid (especially linoleic acid) to vitamin E. The fat content of the red blood cell membrane is determined by dietary fat. Diets that contain high levels of PUFA or iron necessitate increased levels of vitamin E to protect red blood cells from oxidative injury and hemolysis. Recommended concentrations of vitamin E (α-tocopherol) to PUFA are 0.9 international unit vitamin E per gram of linoleic acid.[10,29] Preterm infants have lower vitamin E stores, poor absorption, and increased needs to protect cell membranes from peroxidative damage and prevent hemolytic anemia. Elevated serum vitamin E levels have been associated with NEC and cerebral hemorrhage, so high doses must be avoided.

Folate. Folate deficiency, which can lead to anemia, poor growth, and delayed CNS maturation, is seen more often in preterm infants. Folate needs are increased in VLBW infants, who have decreased stores and absorption and more rapid growth.[71] Supplementation has been recommended for preterm infants during the first 2 to 3 months, when intake is limited.[123,242]

Calcium, Phosphorus, and Magnesium. Calcium, phosphorus, and magnesium are essential in the neonate for bone mineralization and growth. The newborn with lower levels of parathyroid hormone (PTH) is less able to remove calcium from the bone, increasing the risk of hypocalcemia (see Chapter 17). Calcium levels in feedings may be increased to allow for calcium storage and support bone mineralization and growth. If calcium levels are altered, phosphorus intake also needs to be adjusted to maintain a homeostatic calcium-phosphorus balance. Vitamin D and magnesium are also needed for adequate bone mineralization and to prevent osteopenia and rickets.

Iron. Term and preterm infants develop a physiologic anemia during the first weeks after birth because of postnatal suppression of erythropoiesis (see Chapter 8). During this period, iron from destroyed red blood cells is stored for use when erythropoiesis resumes. Once the stored iron is used up, the infant's hemoglobin will again fall if adequate iron is not available from dietary sources or supplementation. Iron supplementation is usually started before the point of depletion to maintain and build up stores. Intestinal iron transport is lower in the neonate due to the inability to regulate iron absorption from the gut and up-regulate transport in response to low dietary intakes and down-regulate with high intakes.[56] Supplementation is started earlier in preterm infants, in that their iron stores are lower at birth and often further depleted by iatrogenic blood losses. Recommendations regarding iron supplementation are discussed in Chapter 8.

Micronutrients and Other Substances. Stores of micronutrients such as zinc, copper, iodine, chromium, selenium, and molybdenum are accumulated late in gestation. Requirements for micronutrients are often also increased in preterm infants due to poor stores and increased growth rates. Specific requirements and absorptive mechanisms for many of these elements are unknown. Concentrations in human milk are generally adequate, and commercial formulas are supplemented. Parenteral alimentation solutions are also supplemented with these elements so the infant does not become deficient. Other substances found in human milk are inositol, choline, and nucleotides and many anti-infective substances (see Chapters 5 and 13). Inositol is a lipotrophic growth factor that may enhance surfactant function and reduce cell damage by free radicals. Nucleotides enhance growth and development, GI function, and host defenses. Choline, a component of phospholipids and acetylcholine precursor, may enhance neural development and function. Anti-infective substances in human milk are summarized in Table 5-4.

Zinc. Zinc is an essential cofactor for over 70 enzymes needed for protein and nucleic acid synthesis. Zinc also is needed for neonatal immune system maturation and function.[63] Zinc deficiencies, usually characterized by an erythematous skin rash, inhibit uptake of fat-soluble vitamins and protein synthesis and can lead to growth restriction.[190] Deficiencies have been reported in preterm infants fed human milk and infants on parenteral nutrition with inadequate supplementation.[216] Excessive losses may occur in infants with ostomies or chronic diarrhea.[5,187]

Copper. Copper is also an enzyme co-factor and essential for hemoglobin synthesis, myelinization, and formation of antioxidant enzymes and collagen. Copper deficiency (failure to thrive, iron-resistant anemia, osteopenia, neutropenia, pallor, edema, seborrheic dermatitis, and hypotonia) has been reported in preterm infants fed formulas with low levels of copper and in infants with ostomies or chronic diarrhea.[5,190,216,247]

Electrolytes. Levels of potassium and sodium may be increased in preterm formulas to compensate for increased intestinal potassium and renal sodium losses and to support growth (sodium is co-precipitated in the bone during periods of active bone growth). Concentrations of specific electrolytes are also determined by fluid composition and levels of other electrolytes. Electrolytes are discussed in Chapter 11.

Calories and Renal Solute Load

The caloric level of the feeding should reflect the infant's energy needs, but at an osmolality that the infant's kidneys and other systems can handle without stress (see Chapter 11). Caloric content of human milk is generally around 20 kcal/oz but may vary considerably. Preterm human milk has a slightly higher caloric density, but it also varies. Standard formulas contain 20 kcal/oz and preterm formulas 24 kcal/oz. Higher calorie formulas may be used, but problems with osmotic and solute load often offset the advantages of extra calories. Osmolalities should be similar to those of physiologic fluids (250 to 300 mOsm per kg of water).

Human Milk

Human milk is an ideal, nutritionally adequate feeding for term and most preterm infants that meets the infant's unique nutritional needs and provides over 45 other enzymes, growth factors, and bioactive substances to enhance growth and development, protect the infant from infection, and enhance gut maturation.[11,139,170,236] Human milk also contains substances such as human milk bile salt–stimulated (mammary) lipase and mammary amylase, and has a low renal solute load (see Chapter 11), an amino acid composition ideal for the newborn, and lipids in a form that can be easily digested and absorbed. These and other characteristics of human milk compensate for the neonate's physiologic limitations. Preterm infants fed human milk have a lower incidence of NEC and infection, enhanced fat absorption, and more rapid gastric emptying.[139,155,170,236] Benefits of human milk in preterm infants also include a decreased rate of rehospitalization for illness after discharge and improved long-term sensorimotor and neurologic development.[213] Composition of human milk is described further in Chapter 5. The nutrient content of human milk can vary due to methods of expression and storage, portion of the milk used (i.e., foremilk versus hindmilk), and use of feeding tubes.[212,225]

Milk from mothers of preterm infants is different initially from that of term mothers and more closely approximates what are thought to be the nutritional needs of these infants (see Chapter 5).[89] The composition of this milk changes gradually over the first month after birth and by 1 month is similar to term milk. Preterm human milk is low (in terms of the preterm infant's nutrient requirements) in protein, calcium, phosphorus, iron, vitamins, and sodium, even though nutrients such as protein, iron, and calcium are in forms that are more readily absorbed by the infant. For example, it has been estimated that preterm infants fed human milk retain calcium and phosphorus equivalent to 15% to 20% of the calcium and 30% to 35% of the phosphorus accumulated by the fetus in utero. Most preterm infants fed their own mother's milk gain at rates similar to intrauterine rates or those of infants fed whey formulas.[123] VLBW infants fed human milk may need supplementation to promote growth and prevent deficiencies.

Human milk fortification is used to "increase the concentration of nutrients to such levels that at the customary feeding volumes infants receive amounts of all nutrients that meet the requirements."[17,p.234] Human milk fortifiers contain protein, carbohydrate, calcium, phosphate, vitamins, sodium, and other substances.[17,190,212] Use of these fortifiers results in short-term increases in weight gain, length, and head circumference.[127] However, standard fortification of human milk can lead to slower weight gain (than with formula feeding) in some preterm infants due to low protein intake (due to variable protein content of the breast milk for mothers of preterm infants and the decrease in protein content over the duration of lactation).[16,17,97,99] As a result individual fortification either via adjustable (protein intake is adjusted based on infant metabolic responses evaluated by periodic blood urea nitrogen levels) or targeted (periodic analysis of the protein content of the milk) fortification has been recommended.[17,72] The effect of fortification on anti-infective and other nonnutrient milk components has also been a concern.[190,212]

Parenteral Nutrition Solutions

Parenteral nutrition is the intravenous administration of a hypertonic solution containing amino acids, carbohydrates, fats, electrolytes, vitamins, minerals, and micronutrients in order to maintain positive nitrogen balance. Partial parenteral nutrition involves infusion of amino acids and carbohydrates with or without fats to supplement enteral feedings.[242] Infants generally cannot tolerate glucose loads over 6 to 8 mg/kg/min in the first 1 to 2 weeks. The usual range in solutions is 4 to 8 mg/kg/minute, although some infants may need higher amounts given gradually based on evaluation of energy needs and laboratory values.[84] Parenteral alimentation has been associated with nitrogen retention and weight gain in LBW infants.[123] Nutritional requirements of infants on parenteral feedings differ from those of infants on enteral feedings in that these solutions are infused directly into the blood rather than the immature gut.

Pediatric and neonatal mixtures are constituted for neonates with immature liver function and intermediary metabolic pathways for synthesis of some amino acids. These solutions, which contain higher levels of taurine, cytosine, and tyrosine and branched-chain amino acids, with reduced methionine and phenylalanine, improve nitrogen retention and normalize plasma values and approximate the amino acid pattern of human milk.[83,84,123,189] Early parenteral amino acid administration (within the first 1 to 2 days) seems to be well tolerated by most infants and is associated with greater nitrogen retention and a positive nitrogen balance.[29,83,194,237,240,241]

Lipid emulsions are isotonic with a high caloric density and can be used to provide adequate caloric intake through a peripheral infusion.[196,222] These emulsions are started within the first few days and gradually increased as tolerated. Lipid emulsions can lead to hyperlipidemia and hyperglycemia (reasons for alteration in glucose metabolism are unclear), especially with rates greater than 0.2 to 0.25 g/kg/hour (equivalent to 6 g/kg/day) or with use in VLBW and SGA infants with little adipose tissue.[29,83,240,241] The 20% emulsions are used, since 10% emulsions have a higher phospholipid content, which slows triglyceride clearance.[83,84,240] The 20% solutions also provide more calories without increasing fluid. Excess free fatty acids may compete with and displace bilirubin from albumin (see Chapter 18).[83] Although fats have been associated with decreased oxygenation and increased pulmonary vascular tone, these effects may be minimized by prolonging the infusion period and using rates less than 0.2 g/kg/hr.[84,123,240]

Issues in Infants with Various Health Problems

Immature infants generally tolerate feeding with preterm breast milk or preterm formulas better than standard formulas. Considerations discussed below for selecting feedings for preterm infants are also important in planning nutritional support for infants with specific health problems. These infants have individualized nutritional needs that may require use of specialized formulas or feeding methods. For example, critically ill infants may need to be fed via total or partial parenteral nutrition because of their inability to digest and absorb enteral feedings or the risk of complications. Nutrient needs of preterm and term infants with specific problems are summarized in Table 12-16.

Very Low–Birth Weight Infants

The considerations in selecting feedings are even more critical in planning for nutritional support of VLBW infants, whose body systems are even more immature. These infants are at risk for postnatal growth restriction.[98,241] Unique nutritional problems of these infants include the following:

1. Limited protein and energy reserves (e.g., a 1000-g preterm infant has only 10 g of stored fat versus 400 g in a term neonate). Energy needs may be increased by intermittent cold stress, infection, or stresses of the neonatal intensive care unit environment.
2. High ratio of surface area to body weight.
3. Small gastric capacity, which limits intake.
4. High water requirements due to increased insensible water losses and immature renal function. These factors limit the ability of the infant to tolerate high-caloric-density formulas due to risks associated with hyperosmolar solutions.
5. Immature digestive and absorptive capacities for fats, carbohydrates, vitamins, and micronutrients.

Table 12-16 Effect of Disease on Selected Nutrient Requirements in Preterm and Term Infants

	Preterm Infants			Term Infants			Both
NUTRIENT	RDS	CLD	NEC/SBS	CYANOTIC CHD	CHF	SEPSIS	IUGR
Free water	↓	↓	↑	↔	↓	↔	↑
Energy	↑	↑↑	↑↑	↑↑	↑↑	↑	↑
Fat	↔	↑	↑↑[a]	↑	↑	↔	↑
Carbohydrate	↑	↓	↑	↑	↑	↑	↑
Protein	↔	↑	↑	↑	↑	↑↑	↑
Calcium	↔	↑[b,c]	↑[a]	↑[d]	↑[c,d]	↔	↑
Iron	↔	↑[b]	↑	↑	↔	↓	↑

From Townsend, S.F., et al. (1998). Enteral nutrition. In G.B. Merenstein & S.L. Gardnêr (Eds.), *Handbook of neonatal intensive care* (4th ed.). St. Louis: Mosby.
CHD, Congenital heart disease; *CHF,* congestive heart failure; *CLD,* chronic lung disease; *IUGR,* intrauterine growth restriction; *NEC,* necrotizing enterocolitis; *RDS,* respiratory distress syndrome; *SBS,* short bowel syndrome.
[a]Particularly with loss of terminal ileum.
[b]In preterm infants less than 1500 g.
[c]Particularly with calciuric diurotics such as furosemide.
[d]Particularly if postoperative.

6. Immature brain and liver, which are vulnerable to damage from elevated plasma concentrations of amino acids such as tyrosine, methionine, and phenylalanine.[3]

Infants with Respiratory Problems

Infants with respiratory distress, including infants with bronchopulmonary dysplasia (BPD), may be unable to feed by breast or bottle due to rapid respiratory rates, fatigue, and inability to coordinate sucking, swallowing, and breathing. These infants need to be fed by other enteral (intragastric) or parenteral methods. Fluid and caloric requirements are often increased because of the increased metabolic demands, respiratory workload, oxygen consumption, and insensible water losses. Energy needs may increase up to 20% to 40% above baseline in infants with BPD. Oxygen consumption, energy expenditure, and work load are higher for infants with respiratory problems who are breathing spontaneously than for those on assisted ventilation. Intestinal disaccharidases may be diminished in infants following shock or ischemia, with a temporary carbohydrate intolerance.[94] Infants recovering from respiratory distress syndrome have been reported to have decreased functional residual capacity, with increases in respiratory rate and minute ventilation during nasogastric feedings.[94]

Infants with Cardiac Problems

Infants with cardiac problems often grow poorly due to increased metabolic demands and difficulty with feeding. Caloric requirements are increased because of hypermetabolism (higher metabolic rate and oxygen consumption secondary to increased cardiac and respiratory workload), tissue hypoxia, protein loss, increased frequency of infection, and poorer nutrient absorption due to decreased splanchnic blood flow. Infants with cardiac problems may be fluid and sodium restricted. Feeding problems may limit intake in that the infant may become fatigued, tachypneic, and stressed with feeding. Intervention strategies include use of higher-caloric-density and low-sodium formulas, frequent smaller feedings, feeding on demand and in an upright position, avoidance of feeding immediately after prolonged crying or when the infant is exhausted, and administration of oxygen with feeding as needed. Infants with renal problems may also need to be on low-sodium or solute-load formulas.

Infants with Short-Bowel Syndrome

Infants with reduction in the length of their small intestine, which usually results from surgical resection because of a congenital anomaly or NEC, are at very high risk for nutritional and growth problems due to reduction in intestinal absorptive surface area. In addition, the remaining sections of bowel may have been ischemic with villous atrophy. Loss of intestinal surface area results in loss of brush border enzymes such as the disaccharidases, resulting in carbohydrate intolerance and a pool of unabsorbed sugars that act as a rich substrate for bacterial growth. Infants who have less than 25 cm of residual small intestine (normal small intestinal length is 250 to 270 cm at term) if the ileocecal valve is intact or more than 40 cm without this valve are likely to eventually be able to tolerate enteral only feedings.[250] During resection, particular efforts are made to preserve the ileum (because of its critical role in bile acid and vitamin B_{12} absorption) and cecal valve.[94] Ileocecal resection is associated with gastric hypersecretion and hypersecretion of regulatory peptides (including motilin, enteroglucagon, and peptide YY) for several weeks.[250] Other problems in digestion and absorption of nutrients resulting from small bowel resection include disaccharide intolerance; decreased pancreatic and biliary secretions; impaired vitamin (especially folate and vitamin B_{12}), calcium, iron, zinc, and magnesium absorption; protein malabsorption; and bile salt depletion.[94]

With adequate enteral nutrition, the remaining bowel usually undergoes villous hyperplasia with increased cell proliferation and migration. This response is similar to maturational responses seen in the newborn following initiation of enteral feedings and is related to exposure of the gut to enteral feedings and to the trophic effect of GI hormones. Most infants receive parenteral nutrition immediately after surgery, but initiation of minimal enteral feedings—using an elemental lactose-free feeding as soon as the bowel has recovered—is important in enhancing villous hyperplasia.[136] Vitamin, mineral, and trace element supplementation is needed due to increased intestinal loss.

Considerations Related to Feeding Method

The healthy term infant is fed by breast or bottle depending on the parent's choice. The choice of feeding method for preterm or ill infants also depends on the parent's choice of breast milk or formula, as well as maturity, health status, growth pattern, and individual responses to specific methods. These infants can be fed by enteral or parenteral methods, each of which has specific advantages and disadvantages (Table 12-17). Factors related to oral feeding readiness in preterm infants have been reviewed.[152]

Clinically stable preterm infants can be breastfed. Infants as young as 32 weeks' gestation (approximately 1200 g) have been reported to have an organized sucking pattern at the breast, with 2 to 3 sucks per burst followed by a pause and stable transcutaneous oxygen pressures.[154] Infants who have not developed adequate suck-swallow, who fatigue easily, or for whom oral feeding is contraindicated due to health status require an alternative feeding method. With preterm infants this method is usually gavage (intragastric), given either as a bolus or in a continuous drip and using either breast milk or formula.

Intragastric gavage permits normal digestive processes and hormonal responses to occur. Tube insertion is generally easy because most infants who require gavage do not have a well-developed gag reflex. Infants who are fed intragastrically are generally able to tolerate higher osmotic loads than those fed transpylorically, with less distention, vomiting, and diarrhea. Risks of intragastric gavage such as regurgitation, aspiration, and gastric distention—which may compromise respiratory function—are reduced with transpyloric feedings. Transpyloric feeding tubes are harder to insert, and this feeding method is associated with complications such as impaired fat absorption, intestinal perforation, and ileus (see Table 12-17). Routine use of transpyloric feedings is not recommended due to the increased mortality risk.[153,193]

The benefits of continuous versus intermittent bolus feedings are not clear. The enteral feeding–induced surge of gut hormones following birth may be enhanced by bolus methods, although others have reported that continuous feeding

Table 12-17 Advantages and Risks of Various Feeding Methods

METHOD	ADVANTAGES	DISADVANTAGES
Peripheral venous nutrition	Not dependent on GI function No danger of aspiration Low infection risk	Repeated thermal and physiologic stress with replacement Effort to start and maintain Risk of tissue injury with extravasation Lack of nutrients into gut to promote intestinal growth and maturation
Central venous nutrition: percutaneous line	High concentration of infused glucose Not dependent on GI function No danger of aspiration Low risk of NEC No need of general anesthesia Lower risk of thrombosis than surgical line	Infection Lack of nutrients into gut to promote intestinal growth and maturation Perforation of vessel or heart
Central venous nutrition: surgical line	High concentration of glucose Possible when other methods fail Not dependent on GI function No danger of aspiration Low risk of NEC Avoids risk of peripheral vein	General anesthesia Vena cava thrombosis Infection Perforation of vessel or heart Lack of nutrients into gut to promote intestinal growth and maturation
Intermittent intragastric feeding	Promotes intestinal growth, gut hormone secretion, and bile flow Reliable nutrient delivery	Bypasses salivary and lingual enzymes
Continuous intragastric feeding	Larger volumes may be tolerated	Bypasses salivary and lingual enzymes Feeding components may be separated in tube
Transpyloric feeding	Does not rely on gastric emptying	Difficult tube placement Decreased fat absorption Possible increased mortality

Adapted from Bell, E.F. (2011). Nutritional support. In J.P. Goldsmith & E.H. Karotkin (Eds.), *Assisted ventilation of the neonate* (5th ed.). Philadelphia: Saunders.
GI, Gastrointestinal; *NEC*, necrotizing enterocolitis.

may enhance intestinal motility and GI tolerance.[19,31] No significant differences have been reported in growth, length of stay, or NEC incidence in VLBW infants fed by continuous nasogastric versus intermittent bolus feedings.[193] Bolus feedings stimulate cyclic responses in the secretion of gut hormones, insulin, and glucagon that are not seen in infants fed by continuous drip, although which response is best at this age is unknown.[19] Use of syringe pump infusion systems to deliver human milk by continuous infusion has been associated with loss of milk fat, decreased fat concentrations (especially at low infusion rates), and terminal delivery of a large fat load if fat in the tubing is recovered using an air infusion. Similar findings were not demonstrated with intermittent gavage or bolus feedings. The method and type of feeding will influence gastric emptying. Increasing caloric density decreases gastric emptying.

Parenteral solutions may be given via central or peripheral lines, which have advantages and risks (see Table 12-17). Infants on parenteral nutrition require careful monitoring because they are at greater risk for metabolic derangements, electrolyte imbalances, sepsis, anemia, and thromboembolic complications.

Regurgitation and Reflux

Newborns are more susceptible to regurgitation, vomiting, and gastroesophageal reflux (GER) due to anatomic and functional immaturity of their GI system. Regurgitation peaks at 3 months of age; 40% to 50% of infants regurgitate more than once a day.[80] Regurgitation is common in infants as a result of LES immaturity, transient LES relaxation, alterations in esophageal and gastric motility, delayed gastric emptying, entry of air into the stomach with swallowing, less acute esophageal-stomach angle, more time spent lying in a supine position, increased esophageal peristalsis, and a tendency toward reverse peristalsis.[80] These limitations and the frequency of regurgitation are more marked in preterm infants. Interventions to reduce regurgitation include frequent burping; feeding slowly in a semi-upright position to reduce air swallowing and passage of swallowed air into the duodenum; using small, frequent feedings; and placing the infant in a right lateral position after feeding to enhance gastric emptying.

Regurgitation does not mean that an infant has gastroesophageal reflux disease (GERD), although GERD is also seen more frequently in infants, particularly in preterm and ill neonates. GERD is the retrograde flow of gastric contents into the esophagus often accompanied by regurgitation, but it may occur in the absence of regurgitation.[94] Although this is a temporary phenomenon that generally resolves by 8 to 12 months, probably due to maturation of the GI system and introduction of solid food, GER can be severe enough to result in aspiration, esophagitis, and dysphagia.[80] Infants with reflux may present with choking, gagging, or other respiratory symptoms.

Reflux in preterm infants is related to immaturity: decreased LES tone, pressure, and size; intrathoracic LES position; delayed gastric emptying; and impaired intestinal motility, with abdominal distention and higher pressure. Altered esophageal motility and peristalsis lead to poor clearance of refluxed material and increased risk of aspiration.[25,84,151] Most infants with reflux respond to interventions such as positioning; small, frequent, or thickened feedings; or drugs that enhance gastric emptying or reduce acid secretion. Some infants may require pharmacologic management or surgical correction.[32]

Necrotizing Enterocolitis

NEC is a multifactorial disorder seen primarily in preterm infants, although the incidence is also increased in growth restricted infants secondary to altered placental function.[162] The incidence of NEC in preterm infants ranges from 5% (younger than 32 weeks) to 10% (younger than 28 weeks).[229] Although the entire gut can be involved, NEC is most prominent in the jejunum, ileum, and colon. Clinical manifestations range from signs of feeding intolerance (abdominal distention, residuals, gross or occult blood in the stools, vomiting) or general systemic signs (lethargy, apnea, respiratory distress, thermal instability) to sepsis, shock, and peritonitis, with intestinal perforation in about 30% of these infants.[83,123,264]

The cause of NEC is unclear, with no single etiologic factor found in all infants. "NEC appears to represent an overreaction of the immune system to some type of insult (for example, ischemia, infectious, related to introduction of enteric feeds, or response to translocation of normal enteric bacteria). This insult leads to disruption of intestinal epithelium, bacterial translocation, and overreaction of immature intestinal epithelial cells. There is activation of stress pathways and suppression of inhibitory pathways which lead to inappropriate mobilization of the host immune system and cytokine release. The result is an unfettered inflammatory response which has diffuse, harmful effects."[30,pp.145-146] An immature GI tract with immature immune and barrier function (including decreased mesenteric blood flow, increased local metabolic activity, reduced intercellular junction integrity with increased permeability, decreased mucous production, altered repair capacity and mobility, and altered antioxidant defenses), and luminal stasis that can lead to exaggerated inflammation and tissue injury also play a role in the pathogenesis of NEC.[48,162,172,264] These factors increase the risk of bowel ischemia, colonization with pathogenic organisms, and stimulation of cytokines and other proinflammatory mediators.[264] Genetic polymorphisms in toll-like receptors (TLRs) and abnormal TLR signaling and release of excessive proinflammatory cytokines such as interleukin-8, along with decreased or altered microbial colonization with altered species may also contribute to NEC (see Chapter 13).[4,163,172,219] Recently an association has been reported between packed red blood cell transfusion and necrotizing enterocolitis (NEC) in preterm infants.[33,50,186,149] The interaction of NEC and transfusion may be due to a transfusion-related acute reaction in the intestines, impaired blood flow to the intestines (and thus intestinal injury) from an anemia that led to the need for transfusion, or injuries to stored RBCs used for the transfusion that could increase the risk of vasoconstriction and ischemia in the intestinal microcirculation.[33,50,186]

Enteral feeding may be a key trigger for development of NEC since it leads to "increased metabolic demands, alteration of mucosal integrity, disturbance of optimal microbiological ecological balance (infection or overcolonization with pathogenic bacteria) and an exaggerated inflammatory response."[162, p.184] Early feeding per se does not necessarily predispose to an increased incidence of NEC. Although most infants have had enteral feedings before the development of symptoms, significant mortality from NEC has been reported in VLBW infants before the first feeding.[29,48]

With initiation of enteral intake, feedings remain in the intestinal lumen for extended periods (due to mucosal damage and limitations in absorptive function in immature infants) and serve as a substrate for further bacterial growth and intramural gas formation. The source of this gas is uncertain, but it may arise from bacterial fermentation of carbohydrates.[83,123] Rapid advances in feeding (especially increases of greater than 20 cal/kg/day) along with impaired absorptive function secondary to immaturity or ischemia may result in intraluminal accumulation of fermentation products and bacteria-derived peptides that lead to mucosal inflammation.[48,80,118] A large volume might further stress the mucosa (already injured from ischemia) and further impede blood flow by distention. This may lead to a local hypoxemia, vascular insufficiency, and accumulation of fermentation products due to impaired absorption.[250] Finally, hyperosmolar feedings may overwhelm the immature or damaged mucosa.

Human milk feedings have been demonstrated to reduce the risk of NEC[155,162,172,197,232] although current data are still insufficient to determine the feeding strategies that are most effective in preventing NEC.[34,160,161,162] Small enteral feedings (see Minimal Enteral Feedings) of human milk may protect the bowel from NEC by stimulating gut maturation, promoting mucosal integrity, providing substrate for intestinal enzymes, reducing pathogenic bacterial colonization, promoting growth of nonpathogenic microflora, reducing ileus, increasing perfusion, and ameliorating the proinflammatory response.[34,80,162] Use of probiotics (nonpathogenic lactobacilli and bifidobacteria) has been reported to decrease the incidence of NEC, but concerns remain due to methodologic limitations of current studies and about safety, particularly the risk of sepsis.[7,69,141,148,166,173,234]

MATURATIONAL CHANGES DURING INFANCY AND CHILDHOOD

Digestive and absorptive capabilities gradually mature over the first 6 months to 2 years following birth. An important aspect of intestinal maturation is gut closure, which provides protection against the transport of macromolecules across the intestinal mucosa, reducing the risk of infection and allergy development (see Chapter 13). The LES lengthens from 1 cm at birth to 2.5 cm by 6 months, with most of the increased length in the portion of the esophagus below the diaphragm.[107] LES basal tone increases after 6 months and is associated with resolution of reflux in most infants.[25] The esophagus, which is 10 cm (range, 7 to 14 cm) in length at term, grows about 0.65 cm per year, reaching an adult length of 25 cm in childhood.[124]

Pepsinogen levels reach adult levels by 3 months. Gastric acid production and pepsin activity do not reach adult levels until 2 years, limiting gastric proteolysis in infants. Levels of trypsin reach adult levels by 1 month.[136]

Pancreatic enzymes are minimal for the first 4 to 6 months; thus the infant is dependent on salivary and mammary amylase for initial digestion of carbohydrate. Pancreatic amylase activity increases after 4 to 6 months at about the time that starch (cereal) is introduced into the diet. Cereal is not efficiently digested before this time. Because hydrolysis of amylopectin (starch) is incomplete up to about 6 months, some neonates given formula thickened with cereal may develop diarrhea.[136]

Activity of maltase, isomaltase, and sucrase remains high into adulthood, with some decrease seen in older adults. Retention of lactase activity is variable and genetically controlled. Lactase activity usually decreases after 3 to 5 years to very low levels.[169] Significant lactase activity is retained primarily in individuals of northern European descent. Mucosal glucose transport is reduced until about 12 months.

Fat absorption does not approach adult efficiency until about 6 months. Lipase reaches adult levels by 2 years, so infants are dependent on lingual-gastric and mammary lipase. Lipolysis and micelle activity are minimal until 4 to 6 months; liver uptake of bile acids is decreased until 6 months.

Liver hematopoietic tissue generally disappears by 6 months.[26] Full expression of liver signaling pathways and amino acid transport pathways occurs by 2 years.[26] Development of enzyme systems needed for drug metabolism is described in Chapter 7.

Introduction of Solid Foods

Maturation of the intestinal system in infancy may be stimulated by weaning and the introduction of solid foods in a manner somewhat similar to changes induced by enteral feedings after birth.[136] Timing for introduction of solids should be based on development of neuromuscular processes involved in the ability of the infant to handle solids. The infant's ability to handle foods can be divided into three physiologic stages: (1) nursing (birth to 6 months), when the infant has excellent suck-swallow coordination and does best if fed human milk or formula; (2) transitional (4 to 8 months), when neuromuscular processes needed to swallow pureed solids develop; and (3) modified adult (6 to 12 months), when chopped foods can be swallowed without choking.[182]

There are no particular advantages, and some disadvantages, to introducing solid foods before 3 to 4 months in formula-fed or before 5 to 6 months in breastfed infants. Before 3 to 4 months, an extrusion reflex is present (extrusion of material placed on the anterior tongue) and GER may still be present. Contrary to what many parents and professionals believe, feeding cereal before bedtime in young infants has not been demonstrated to reduce the incidence of night awakenings and may contribute to dental caries and obesity.[146]

Introduction of solid foods is generally recommended at 4 to 6 months for formula-fed infants and after 6 months for breastfed infants. Infants fed foreign proteins before 6 months are thought to have a higher risk for developing food allergies, although data from controlled studies are limited (see Chapter 13). Cereal is usually the initial solid food given to infants. Rice and barley cereals are of low antigenicity and contain iron in a relatively easy to digest form. Early introduction of high-caloric-density foods is associated with an increased risk of obesity.

SUMMARY

Supporting nutritional needs and promoting nutritional status of infants are a challenge, but one that is critical for optimal outcome. Management of nutritional needs must be based on understanding of the anatomic and physiologic limitations of the GI system and the impact of these alterations on the infant's ability to consume, digest, and absorb various nutrients. Recommendations for clinical practice related to the GI system and perinatal nutrition are summarized in Table 12-18.

Table 12-18 Recommendations for Clinical Practice Related to the Gastrointestinal System and Perinatal Nutrition in Neonates

Assess feeding reflexes, suck-swallow coordination, cardiorespiratory and gastrointestinal (GI) function before initiating oral feedings (pp. 420-421).
Observe for regurgitation and GI reflux (p. 434).
Observe respiratory status after feeding (p. 432).
Evaluate for signs of dehydration and electrolyte imbalance (pp. 422, 430).
Monitor stools for reducing substance, blood, and consistency (pp. 434-435).
Record timing and appearance of first meconium stool (p. 420).
Know parameters used to measure growth and factors that alter accuracy of these parameters (pp. 426-427).
Monitor growth parameters using appropriate curves (pp. 426-427).
Counsel women regarding nutritional advantages of breastfeeding (p. 430 and Chapter 5).
Support breastfeeding in mothers of term and preterm infants (p. 430 and Chapter 5).
Initiate early enteral feeding as appropriate (pp. 418-420).
Promote early breastfeeding and colostrum intake (pp. 418-419 and Chapter 5).
Know limitations of gastrointestinal function in term and preterm infants (pp. 421-426 and Table 12-13).
Know the effects of health problems or surgery on digestion and absorption (pp. 431-433).
Evaluate composition of feedings (formula or human milk) in relationship to an individual infant's GI system limitations (pp. 427-430).
Avoid use of high solute load and caloric density formulas in immature infants (p. 430 and Chapter 11).
Evaluate renal function and fluid and electrolyte status in infants on high solute load or caloric density feedings (p. 430 and Chapter 11).
Recognize signs of liver dysfunction in infants (p. 426).
Know nutritional requirements for preterm and term infants (pp. 427-430).
Monitor nutritional intake to ensure that nutritional requirements are met (pp. 427-430).
Know energy requirements and factors that alter these requirements (pp. 427-428 and Table 12-15).
Monitor the caloric intake of infants (pp. 427-428).
Monitor neonates for signs of excessive or inadequate protein, carbohydrate, and fat intake (pp. 428-429, 431).
Monitor intake and ratio of vitamin E and linoleic acid (p. 429).
Ensure that term and preterm infants receive iron at the recommended times (p. 430 and Chapter 8).
Monitor intake of vitamins, minerals, and trace minerals (pp. 429-430).
Provide dietary supplementation (e.g., vitamins, minerals, trace elements, calories) as required (pp. 429-431).
Monitor infants for signs of vitamin, mineral, and micronutrient deficiencies (pp. 429-431).
Monitor preterm infants for signs of hypocalcemia (pp. 429-430 and Chapter 17).
Monitor very low–birth weight infants for alterations in serum sodium and potassium (p. 430 and Chapter 11).
Recognize the advantages and limitations of the use of human milk with preterm infants (pp. 430-431).
Assist mothers of preterm and ill infants in providing breast milk for their infants (pp. 430-431 and Chapter 5).
Recognize and monitor for signs of complications associated with parenteral nutrition (p. 431).
Recognize potential problems of infants with fetal growth restriction and the basis for these problems (p. 417 and Table 12-10).
Know the effects of specific health problems on nutritional intake, feeding method, and gastrointestinal function (pp. 431-433 and Table 12-16).
Use feeding techniques that promote adequate intake and reduce stress in infants with cardiorespiratory problems (p. 432).
Monitor infants following intestinal resection or with ostomies for adequacy of nutritional intake and excessive loss of nutrients (pp. 432-433).
Know the advantages and disadvantages of different feeding methods and monitor infants for potential complications (pp. 432-433 and Table 12-17).
Select feedings and feeding methods appropriate for an individual infant's maturity, age, and health status (pp. 427-434 and Table 12-17).
Identify infants at risk for necrotizing enterocolitis and monitor for signs (pp. 434-435).
Counsel parents regarding introduction of solids (pp. 435-436).

References

1. Abrams, B., et al. (2000). Pregnancy weight gain: Still controversial. *Am J Nutr, 71,* 1233.
2. Abu-Saad, K. & Fraser, D. (2010). Maternal nutrition and birth outcomes. *Epidemiol Rev, 32,* 5.
3. Adamkin, D.H. (1986). Nutrition in very low birth weight infants. *Clin Perinatol, 13,* 419.
4. Afrazi, A., et al. (2011). New insights into the pathogenesis and treatment of necrotizing enterocolitis: Toll-like receptors and beyond. *Pediatr Res, 69,* 183.
5. Aggett, P.J. (2000). Trace elements of the micropremie. *Clin Perinatol, 27,* 119.
6. Ahanya, S.N., et al. (2005). Meconium passage in utero: Mechanisms, consequences, and management. *Obstet Gynecol Surv, 60,* 45.
7. Alfaleh, K., Anabrees, J., & Bassler, D. (2010). Probiotics reduce the risk of necrotizing enterocolitis in preterm infants: A meta-analysis. *Neonatology, 97,* 93.
8. Allen, L.H. (2005). Multiple micronutrients in pregnancy and lactation: An overview. *Am J Clin Nutr, 81,* 1206S.
9. Amaizu, N., et al. (2008). Maturation of oral feeding skills in preterm infants. *Acta Paediatr, 97,* 61.
10. American Academy of Pediatrics Commit tee on Nutrition (2009). *Pediatric nutrition handbook* (6th ed). Elk Grove Village, IL: American Academy of Pediatrics.
11. American Academy of Pediatrics Section on Breastfeeding. (2005). Breastfeeding and the use of human milk. *Pediatrics, 115,* 496.
12. American College of Nurse-Midwives. (2008). Providing oral nutrition to women in labor. *J Midwifery Womens Health, 53,* 276.
13. American College of Obstetricians and Gynecologists. (2004). Clinical management guidelines for obstetrician-gynecologists: Nausea and vomiting of pregnancy. *Obstet Gynecol, 103,* 803.
14. Angelini, D.J. (1999). Obstetric triage: Management of acute nonobstetric abdominal pain in pregnancy. *J Nurse Midwifery, 44,* 572.
15. Armitage, J.A., Poston, L., & Taylor, P.D. (2008). Developmental origins of obesity and the metabolic syndrome: The role of maternal obesity. *Front Horm Res, 36,* 73.
16. Arslanoglu, S., Moro, G.E., & Ziegler, E.E. (2009). Preterm infants fed fortified human milk receive less protein than they need. *J Perinatol, 29,* 489.
17. Arslanoglu, S., Moro, G.E., & Ziegler, E.E. (2010). Optimization of human milk fortification for preterm infants: New concepts and recommendations. The WAPM Working Group On Nutrition. *J Perinat Med, 38,* 233.
18. Avsar, A.F. & Keskin, H.L. (2010). Haemorrhoids during pregnancy. *J Obstet Gynaecol, 30,* 231.
19. Aynsley-Green, A., et al. (1990). Gut hormones and regulatory peptides in relation to enteral feeding, gastroenteritis, and necrotizing enterocolitis in infancy. *J Pediatr, 117,* S24.
20. Baksu, A., et al. (2005). Serum leptin levels in preeclamptic pregnant women: Relationship to thyroid-stimulating hormone, body mass index, and proteinuria. *Am J Perinatal, 22,* 161.
21. Barak, S., et al. (2003). Common oral manifestations during pregnancy: A review. *Obstet Gynecol Surv, 58,* 624.
22. Barker, D.J. (2004). The developmental origins of adult disease. *J Am Coll Nutr, 23,* 588S.
23. Barker, D.J. (2005). The developmental origins of insulin resistance. *Horm Res, 64,* 2.
24. Barlow, S.M. (2009). Oral and respiratory control for preterm feeding. *Curr Opin Otolaryngol Head Neck Surg, 17,* 179.
25. Bates, M.D. & Balisteri, W.F. (2002). Development of the human digestive system. In A.A. Fanaroff & R.J. Martin (Eds.). *Neonatal-perinatal medicine: Diseases of the fetus and infant* (7th ed.). St. Louis: Mosby.
26. Beath, S.V. (2003). Hepatic function and physiology in the newborn. *Semin Neonatal, 8,* 337.
27. Beaulieu, D.B. & Kane, S. (2011). Inflammatory bowel disease in pregnancy. *Gastroenterol Clin North Am, 40,* 399.
28. Begum, K.S., Sachchithanantham, K., & De Somsubhra, S. (2011). Maternal obesity and pregnancy outcome. *Clin Exp Obstet Gynecol, 38,* 14.
29. Bell, E.F. (2011). Nutritional support. In J.P. Goldsmith & E.H. Karotkin (Eds.). *Assisted ventilation of the neonate* (5th ed.). Philadelphia: Saunders.
30. Berman, L. & Moss, R.L. (2011). Necrotizing enterocolitis: An update. *Semin Fetal Neonatal Med, 16,* 145.
31. Berseth, C.L. & Nordyke, C. (1993). Enteral nutrients promote postnatal maturation of intestinal motor activity in preterm infants. *Am J Physiol, 264,* G1046.
32. Birch, J.L. & Newell, S.J. (2009). Gastrooesophageal reflux disease in preterm infants: Current management and diagnostic dilemmas. *Arch Dis Child Fetal Neonatal Ed, 94,* F379.
33. Blau, J., et al. (2011). Transfusion-related acute gut injury: Necrotizing enterocolitis in very low birth weight neonates after packed red blood cell transfusion. *J Pediatr, 158,* 403.
34. Bombell, S. & McGuire, W. (2009). Early trophic feeding for very low birth weight infants. *Cochrane Database Syst Rev, 3,* CD000504.
35. Boone, S.A. & Shields, K.M. (2005). Treating pregnancy-related nausea and vomiting with ginger. *Ann Pharmacother, 39,* 1710.
36. Borrelli, F., et al. (2005). Effectiveness and safety of ginger in the treatment of pregnancy-induced nausea and vomiting. *Obstet Gynecol, 105,* 849.
37. Brawarsky, P., et al. (2005). Pre-pregnancy and pregnancy-related factors and the risk of excessive or inadequate gestational weight gain. *Int J Gynaecol Obstet, 91,* 125.
38. Brawarsky, P., et al. (2006). Fetal fatty acid oxidation defects and maternal liver disease in pregnancy. *Obstet Gynecol, 107,* 15.
39. Briana, D.D. & Malamitsi-Puchner, A. (2010). The role of adipocytokines in fetal growth. *Ann N Y Acad Sci, 1205,* 82.
40. Broach, J. & Newton, N. (1988). Food and beverages in labor. Part I: Cross-cultural and historical practices. *Birth, 15,* 81.
41. Broach, J. & Newton, N. (1988). Food and beverages in labor. Part II: The effects of cessation of oral intake during labor. *Birth, 15,* 88.
42. Broussard, D.L. & Altschuler, S.M. (2012). Development of the enteric nervous system. In R.A. Polin, W.W. Fox, & S.H. Abman (Eds.). *Fetal and neonatal physiology* (4th ed.). Philadelphia: Saunders.
43. Browning, M.F. (2006). Fetal fatty acid oxidation defects and maternal liver disease in pregnancy. *Obstet Gynecol, 107,* 115.
44. Brumberg, H. & La Gamma, E.F. (2003). New perspectives on nutrition enhance outcomes for premature infants. *Pediatr Ann, 32,* 617.
45. Burrin, D. (2012). Trophic factors and regulation of gastrointestinal tract and liver development. In R.A. Polin, W.W. Fox, & S.H. Abman (Eds.). *Fetal and neonatal physiology* (4th ed.). Philadelphia: Saunders.
46. Caicedo, R.A., et al. (2005). The developing intestinal ecosystem: Implications for the neonate. *Pediatr Res, 58,* 625.
47. Calkins, K. & Devaskar, S.U. (2011). Fetal origins of adult disease. *Curr Probl Pediatr Adolesc Health Care, 41,* 158.
48. Caplan, M.S. (2012). Pathophysiology and prevention of neonatal necrotizing enterocolitis. In R.A. Polin, W.W. Fox, & S.H. Abman (Eds.). *Fetal and neonatal physiology* (4th ed.). Philadelphia: Saunders.
49. Cetin, I., Alvino, G., & Cardellicchio, M. (2009). Long chain fatty acids and dietary fats in fetal nutrition. *J Physiol, 587,* 3441.
50. Christensen, R.D. (2011). Association between red blood cell transfusions and necrotizing enterocolitis. *J Pediatr, 158,* 349.
51. Christian, P. (2010). Micronutrients, birth weight, and survival. *Annu Rev Nutr, 30,* 83.
52. Chu, S.Y., et al. (2009). Gestational weight gain by body mass index among US women delivering live birth, 2004-2005: fueling future obesity, *Am J Obstet Gynecol, 200,* e1.
53. Chuang, C.K., et al. (2005). Free amino acids in full-term and pre-term human milk and infant formula. *J Pediatr Gastroenterol Nutr, 40,* 496.
54. Coad, J., Al-Rasasi, B., & Morgan, J. (2002). Nutrient insult in early pregnancy. *Proc Nutr Soc, 61,* 51.
55. Cogswell, M.E., Kettel-Khan, L., & Ramakrishnan, U. (2003). Iron supplement use among women in the United States: Science, policy and practice. *J Nutr, 133,* 1974S.

56. Collard, K.J. (2009). Iron homeostasis in the neonate. *Pediatrics, 123,* 1208.
57. Cooke, R. (2005). Postnatal growth in preterm infants: Have we got it right? *J Perinatol, 25,* 312.
58. Coppa, G.V., et al. (2004). The first prebiotics in humans: Human milk oligosaccharides. *J Clin Gastroenterol, 38,* S80.
59. Cornish, J., et al. (2007). A meta-analysis on the influence of inflammatory bowel disease on pregnancy. *Gut,* 56, 830.
60. Crowell, D.T. (1995). Weight change in the postpartum period. A review of the literature. *J Nurse Midwifery, 40,* 418.
61. Cunningham, G., et al. (2009). *Williams obstetrics* (23rd ed.). New York: McGraw-Hill.
62. Cunningham, J.T. (1998). Upper gastrointestinal tract disease. Small and large bowel disease. In N. Gleicher (Ed.). *Principles and practice of medical therapy in pregnancy* (3rd ed.). Stamford, CT: Appleton & Lange.
63. Cunningham-Rundles, S., et al. (2009). Role of nutrients in the development of neonatal immune response. *Nutr Rev, 67,* S152.
64. Davis, M. (2004). Nausea and vomiting of pregnancy: An evidence-based review. *J Perinat Neonatal Nurs, 18,* 312.
65. de Jong, E.M., et al. (2010). Etiology of esophageal atresia and tracheoesophageal fistula: "Mind the gap." *Curr Gastroenterol Rep, 12,* 215.
66. Denne, S.C. (2001). Protein and energy requirements in preterm infants. *Semin Neonatol, 6,* 377.
67. De-Regil, L.M., et al. (2010). Effects and safety of periconceptional folate supplementation for preventing birth defects. *Cochrane Database Syst Rev, 10,* CD007950.
68. Desai, M. & Ross, M.G. (2011). Fetal programming of adipose tissue: Effects of intrauterine growth restriction and maternal obesity/high-fat diet. *Semin Reprod Med,* 29, 237.
69. Deshpande, G., et al. (2010). Updated meta-analysis of probiotics for preventing necrotizing enterocolitis in preterm neonates. *Pediatrics, 125,* 921.
70. Dickinson, C.J. (2012). Development of gastric secretory function. In R.A. Polin, W.W. Fox, & S.H. Abman (Eds.). *Fetal and neonatal physiology* (4th ed.). Philadelphia: Saunders.
71. Dimmitt, R. & Sibley, E.O. (2012). Developmental anatomy and physiology of the gastrointestinal tract. In C.A. Gleason & S. Devaskar (Eds.). *Avery's diseases of the newborn* (9th ed.). Philadelphia: Saunders.
72. Di Natale, C., et al. (2011). Fortification of maternal milk for preterm infants. *J Matern Fetal Neonatal Med, 24,* 41.
73. Drozdowski, L.A., Clandinin, T., & Thomson, A.B. (2010). Ontogeny, growth and development of the small intestine: Understanding pediatric gastroenterology. *World J Gastroenterol, 16,* 787.
74. Dyer, J.S. & Rosenfeld, C.R. (2011). Metabolic imprinting by prenatal, perinatal and postnatal overnutrition: A review. *Semin Reprod Med, 29,* 266.
75. El-Haddad, M.A., et al. (2004). In utero development of fetal thirst and appetite: Potential for programming. *J Soc Gynecol Investig, 11,* 123.
76. Everson, G.T. (1992). Gastrointestinal motility in pregnancy. *Gastroenterol Clin North Am, 21,* 751.
77. Felix, J.F., et al. (2009). Genetic and environmental factors in the etiology of esophageal atresia and/or tracheoesophageal fistula: An overview of the current concepts. *Birth Defects Res A Clin Mol Teratol, 85,* 747.
78. Fernandez-Twinn, D.S., & Ozanne, S.E. (2010). Early life nutrition and metabolic programming. *Ann N Y Acad Sci,* 1212, 78.
79. Flaxman, S.M. & Sherman, P.W. (2000). Morning sickness: A mechanism for protecting mother and embryo. *Q Rev Biol, 75,* 113.
80. Friedman, J.R. & Liacouras, C.A. (2012). Pathophysiology of gastroesophageal reflux. In R.A. Polin, W.W. Fox, & S.H. Abman (Eds.). *Fetal and neonatal physiology* (4th ed.). Philadelphia: Saunders.
81. Fucile, S., Gisel, E.G., & Lau, C. (2005). Effect of an oral stimulation program on sucking skill maturation of preterm infants. *Dev Med Child Neurol, 47,* 158.
82. George, A., et al. (2011). Periodontal treatment during pregnancy and birth outcomes: A meta-analysis of randomised trials. *Int J Evid Based Healthc, 9,* 122.
83. Georgieff, M.K. (2005). Nutrition. In M.G. MacDonald, M.M.K. Seshia, & M.D. Mullett (Eds.). *Avery's neonatology: Pathophysiology and management of the newborn* (6th ed.). Philadelphia: Lippincott Williams & Wilkins.
84. Gewolb, I.H., et al. (2001). Developmental patterns of rhythmic suck and swallow of preterm infants. *Dev Med Child Neurol, 43,* 22.
85. Gicquel, C. & LeBouc, Y. (2006). Hormonal regulation of fetal growth. *Horm Res, 65,* 28.
86. Gluckman, P.D. & Hanson, M.A. (2004). Maternal constraint of fetal growth and its consequences. *Semin Fetal Neonatal Med, 9,* 419.
87. Gluckman, P.D., Hanson, M.A., & Pinal, C. (2005). The developmental origins of adult disease. *Matern Child Nutr, 1,* 1301.
88. Godfrey, K.M., Inskip, H.M., & Hanson, M.A. (2011). The long term effects of prenatal development on growth and metabolism. *Semin Reprod Med, 29,* 257.
89. Goldman, A.S. (2000). Modulation of the gastrointestinal tract of infants by human milk: Interfaces and interactions, an evolutionary perspective. *J Nutr, 130,* 426.
90. Goodwin, T. (2002). Nausea and vomiting of pregnancy: An obstetric syndrome. *Am J Obstet Gynecol, 186,* S184.
91. Gosche, J.R., et al. (2006). Midgut abnormalities. *Surg Clin North Am, 86,* 285.
92. Gregory, K. (2005). Update on nutrition for preterm and full-term infants. *J Obstet Gynecol Neonatal Nurs, 34,* 98.
93. Gross, T.L. & Kazzi, G.M. (1998). Maternal malnutrition and obesity. In N. Gleicher (Ed.). *Principles and practice of medical therapy in pregnancy* (3rd ed.). Stamford, CT: Appleton & Lange.
94. Gryboski, J.D. & Walker, W.A. (1983). *Gastrointestinal problems in the infant* (2nd ed.). Philadelphia: Saunders.
95. Han, Y.W. (2011). Oral health and adverse pregnancy outcomes—what's next? *J Dent Res, 90,* 289.
96. Hay, W.W. & Thureen, P. (2010). Protein for preterm infants: How much is needed? How much is enough? How much is too much? *Pediatr Neonatol, 51,* 198.
97. Hay, W.W. Jr. (2009). Optimal protein intake in preterm infants. *J Perinatol, 29,* 465.
98. Heird, W.C. (2001). Determination of nutritional requirements in preterm infants, with special reference to "catch-up" growth. *Semin Neonatol, 6,* 365.
99. Henriksen, C., et al. (2009). Growth and nutrient intake among very-low-birth-weight infants fed fortified human milk during hospitalization. *Br J Nutr, 102,* 1179.
100. Huxley, R.R. (2000). Nausea and vomiting in early pregnancy: Its role in placental development. *Obstet Gynecol, 95,* 779.
101. Hytten, F.E. & Chamberlain, G. (1980). *Clinical physiology in obstetrics.* Oxford: Blackwell Scientific.
102. Imdad, A. & Bhutta, Z.A. (2011). Effect of balanced protein energy supplementation during pregnancy on birth outcomes. *BMC Public Health, 11,* S17.
103. Institute of Medicine. (1990). *Nutrition during pregnancy.* Washington, DC: National Academy Press.
104. Institute of Medicine. (1997). *Dietary reference intakes for calcium, phosphorus, magnesium, vitamin D, and fluoride 1997.* Washington, DC: National Academy Press.
105. Institute of Medicine. (1998). *Dietary reference intakes for thiamin, riboflavin, niacin, vitamin B6, folate, vitamin B12, pantothenic acid, biotin, and choline 1998.* Washington, DC: National Academy Press.
106. Institute of Medicine. (2000). *Dietary reference intakes for vitamin C, vitamin E, selenium, and carotenoids 2000.* Washington, DC: National Academy Press.
107. Institute of Medicine. (2001). *Dietary reference intakes for vitamin A, vitamin K, arsenic, boron, chromium, copper, iodine, iron, manganese, molybdenum, nickel, silicon, vanadium, and zinc 2001.* Washington, DC: National Academy Press.

108. Institute of Medicine. (2002). *Dietary reference intakes for energy, carbohydrates, fiber, fat, protein, and amino acids (macronutrients) 2002*. Washington, DC: National Academy Press.
109. James, L.P. (2002). Pharmacology for the gastrointestinal tract. *Clin Perinatol, 29,* 115.
110. Jamjute, P., et al. (2009). Liver function test and pregnancy. *J Matern Fetal Neonatal Med, 22,* 274.
111. Jansson, T., Myatt, L., & Powell, T.L. (2009). The role of trophoblast nutrient and ion transporters in the development of pregnancy complications and adult disease. *Curr Vasc Pharmacol, 7,* 521.
112. Jarvis, S., et al. (2003). Cerebral palsy and intrauterine growth in single births: European collaborative study. *Lancet, 362,* 1106.
113. Jensen, C.L. & Heird, W.C. (2002). Lipids with an emphasis on long-chain polyunsaturated fatty acids. *Clin Perinatol, 29,* 261.
114. Jewell, D.J. & Young, G. (2003). Interventions for nausea and vomiting in early pregnancy. *Cochrane Database Syst Rev, 2,* CD00145.
115. Johnson, J.W. & Yancey, M.K. (1996). A critique of the new recommendations for weight gain in pregnancy. *Am J Obstet Gynecol, 174,* 254.
116. Kaiser, L. (2008). Position of the American Dietetic Association: Nutrition and lifestyle for a healthy pregnancy outcome. *J Am Diet Assoc, 108,* 553.
117. Kelly, T. F. & Savides, T.J. (2009). Gastrointestinal disease in pregnancy. In R.K. Creasy, et al. (Eds.). *Creasy & Resnik's Maternal-fetal medicine: Principles and practice* (6th ed.). Philadelphia: Saunders Elsevier.
118. Kennedy, K.A., et al. (2000). Rapid versus slow rate of advancement of feedings for promoting rapid growth and preventing necrotizing enterocolitis in parenterally fed low-birth-weight infants. *Cochrane Database Syst Rev, 2,* CD001241.
119. Kiess, W., et al. (2008). Adipocytes and adipose tissue. *Best Pract Res Clin Endocrinol Metab, 22,* 135.
120. King, J.C. (2000). Physiology of pregnancy and nutrient metabolism. *Am J Clin Nutr, 71,* 1218S.
121. King, J.C. (2001). Effect of reproduction on the bioavailability of calcium, zinc and selenium. *J Nutr, 13,* 1355S.
122. King, R., et al. (2011). Oral nutrition in labour: "Whose choice is it anyway?" A review of the literature. *Midwifery, 27,* 674.
123. Klaus, M.H. & Fanaroff, A.A. (2001). *Care of the high risk neonate* (5th ed.). Philadelphia: Saunders.
124. Kleinman, R., et al. (2008). *Walkers' pediatric gastrointestinal disease* (5th ed.). Hamilton, Ontario: B.C. Decker.
125. Kramer, M.S. & Kakuma, R. (2003). Energy and protein intake in pregnancy. *Cochrane Database Syst Rev, 4,* CD000032.
126. Kristal, A.R. & Rush, D. (1984). Maternal nutrition and duration of gestation: A review. *Clin Obstet Gynecol, 27,* 553.
127. Kuschel, C.A. & Harding, J.E. (2004). Multicomponent fortified human milk for promoting growth in preterm infants. *Cochrane Database Syst Rev, 2,* CD000343.
128. Ladyman, S.R., Augustine, R.A., & Grattan, D.R. (2010). Hormone interactions regulating energy balance during pregnancy. *J Neuroendocrinol, 22,* 805.
129. Lagiou, P., et al. (2003). Nausea and vomiting in pregnancy in relation to prolactin, estrogens, and progesterone: A prospective study. *Obstet Gynecol, 101,* 639.
130. Lappas, M., et al. (2005). Release and regulation of leptin, resistin and adiponectin from human placenta, fetal membranes, and maternal adipose tissue and skeletal muscle from normal and gestational diabetes mellitus-complicated pregnancies. *J Endocrinol, 186,* 457.
131. Lau, C., et al. (2000). Characterization of the developmental stages of sucking in preterm infants during bottle feeding. *Acta Paediatr, 89,* 846.
132. Lau, C. & Kusnierczyk, I. (2001). Quantitative evaluation of infant's nonnutritive and nutritive sucking. *Dysphagia, 16,* 58.
133. Lau, C., Smith, E.O., & Schanler, R.J. (2003). Coordination of suck-swallow and swallow respiration in preterm infants. *Acta Paediatr, 92,* 721.
134. Lebenthal, A. & Lebenthal, E. (1999). The ontology of the small intestinal epithelium. *J Parenter Enteral Nutr, 23,* S3.
135. Lebenthal, E. & Tucker, N.T. (1986). Carbohydrate digestion: Development in early infancy. *Clin Perinatol, 13,* 37.
136. Lebenthal, E. & Leung, Y.K. (1988). Feeding the premature and compromised infant: Gastrointestinal considerations. *Pediatr Clin North Am, 35,* 215.
137. Lebenthal, E. (1995). Gastrointestinal maturation and motility patterns as indicators for feeding the premature infant. *Pediatrics, 95,* 207.
138. Lee, N.M. & Saha, S. (2011). Nausea and vomiting of pregnancy. *Gastroenterol Clin North Am, 40,* 309.
139. Le Huërou-Luron, I., Blat, S., & Boudry, G. (2010). Breast- v. formula-feeding: Impacts on the digestive tract and immediate and long-term health effects. *Nutr Res Rev, 23,* 23.
140. Levin, B.E. (2006). Metabolic imprinting: critical impact of the perinatal environment on the regulation of energy homeostasis. *Philos Trans R Soc Lond B Biol Sci, 361,* 1107.
141. Lin, H.C., et al. (2008). Oral probiotics prevent necrotizing enterocolitis in very low birth weight preterm infants: A multicenter, randomized, controlled trial. *Pediatrics, 122,* 693.
142. Lindseth, G. & Bird-Baker, M.Y. (2004). Risk factors for cholelithiasis in pregnancy. *Res Nurs Health, 27,* 382.
143. Lopez-Jornet, P. & Bermejo-Fenoll, A. (2005). Gingival lesions as a first symptom of pemphigus vulgaris in pregnancy. *Br Dent J, 199,* 91.
144. Lucas, A. (2005). Long-term programming effects of early nutrition—implications for the preterm infant. *J Perinatol, 25,* S2.
145. Ludka, L.M. & Riberst, C.C. (1993). Eating and drinking in labor. A literature review. *J Nurse Midwifery, 38,* 199.
146. Mackin, M.L. (1990). Infant sleep and bedtime cereal. *Am J Dis Child, 143,* 1066.
147. Mahadevan, U., et al. (2011). The London Position Statement of the World Congress of Gastroenterology on Biological Therapy for IBD with the European Crohn's and Colitis Organisation: Pregnancy and pediatrics. *Am J Gastroenterol, 106,* 214.
148. Maharaj, D. (2009). Eating and drinking in labor: Should it be allowed? *Eur J Obstet Gynecol Reprod Biol, 146,* 3.
149. Mally, P., et al. (2006). Association of necrotizing enterocolitis with elective packed red blood cell transfusions in stable, growing, premature neonates. *Am J Perinatol, 23,* 451.
150. Marin, C.J., et al. (2005). Correlation between infant birth weight and mother's periodontal status. *J Clin Periodontol, 32,* 299.
151. Mazzotta, P. & Magee, L.A. (2000). A risk-benefit analysis of pharmacological and nonpharmacological treatments for nausea and vomiting of pregnancy. *Drugs, 59,* 781.
152. McGrath, J.M. & Braescu, A.V. (2004). State of the science: Feeding readiness in the preterm infant. *J Perinat Neonatal Nurs, 18,* 353.
153. McGuire, W. & McEwan, P. (2004). Systematic review of transpyloric versus gastric tube feeding for preterm infants. *Arch Dis Child Fetal Neonatal Ed, 89,* F245.
154. Meier, P. (1990). Nursing management of breast feeding for preterm infants. In S.G. Funk, et al. (Eds.). *Key aspects of recovery: Improving nutrition, rest, and mobility*. New York: Springer.
155. Meinzen-Derr, J., et al. (2009). Role of human milk in extremely low birth weight infants' risk of necrotizing enterocolitis or death. *J Perinatol, 29,* 57.
156. Mishkin, D.J., et al. (1998). Dental diseases. In N. Gleicher (Ed.). *Principles and practice of medical therapy in pregnancy* (3rd ed.). Stamford, CT: Appleton & Lange.
157. Monk, D. & Moore, G.E. (2004). Intrauterine growth restriction—genetic causes and consequences. *Semin Fetal Neonatal Med, 9,* 371.

158. Mook-Kanamori, D.O., et al. (2010). Risk factors and outcomes associated with first-trimester fetal growth restriction. *JAMA, 303,* 527.
159. Moore, K.L., Persaud, T.V.N., & Torchia, M.G. (2011). *The developing human: Clinically oriented embryology* (9th ed.). Philadelphia: Saunders Elsevier.
160. Morgan, J., Young, L., & McGuire, W. (2011). Slow advancement of enteral feed volumes to prevent necrotising enterocolitis in very low birth weight infants. *Cochrane Database Syst Rev, 3,* CD001241.
161. Morgan, J., Young, L., & McGuire, W. (2011). Delayed introduction of progressive enteral feeds to prevent necrotising enterocolitis in very low birth weight infants. *Cochrane Database Syst Rev, 3,* CD001970.
162. Morgan, J.A., Young, L., & McGuire, W. (2011). Pathogenesis and prevention of necrotizing enterocolitis. *Curr Opin Infect Dis, 24,* 183.
163. Morowitz, M.J., et al. (2010). Redefining the role of intestinal microbes in the pathogenesis of necrotizing enterocolitis. *Pediatrics, 125,* 777.
164. Moscandrew, M. & Kane, S. (2009). Inflammatory bowel diseases and management considerations: Fertility and pregnancy. *Curr Gastroenterol Rep, 11,* 395.
165. Moss, K.L., Beck, J.D., & Offenbacher, S. (2005). Clinical risk factors associated with incidence and progression of periodontal conditions in pregnant women. *J Clin Periodontol, 32,* 492.
166. Mshvildadze, M. & Neu, J. (2009). Probiotics and prevention of necrotizing enterocolitis. *Early Hum Dev, 85,* S71.
167. Muallem, M.M. & Rubeiz, N.G. (2006). Physiological and biological skin changes in pregnancy. *Clin Dermatol, 24,* 80.
168. Nelson, S.M., Matthews, P., & Poston, L. (2010). Maternal metabolism and obesity: Modifiable determinants of pregnancy outcome. *Hum Reprod Update, 16,* 255.
169. Neu, J. (1996). Nutrient absorption in the preterm neonate. *Clin Perinatol, 23,* 229.
170. Neu, J. & Bernstein, H. (2002). Update on host defense and immunomicronutrients. *Clin Perinatol, 29,* 41.
171. Neu, J. (2007). Gastrointestinal maturation and implications for infant feeding. *Early Hum Dev, 83,* 767.
172. Neu, J. & Walker, W.A. (2011). Necrotizing enterocolitis. *N Engl J Med, 364,* 255.
173. Neu, J. (2011). Routine probiotics for premature infants: Let's be careful!. *J Pediatr, 158,* 672.
174. Neu, J. & Mshvildadze, M. (2012). Digestion-absorption functions in fetuses, infants and children. In R.A. Polin, W.W. Fox, & S.H. Abman (Eds.). *Fetal and neonatal physiology* (4th ed.). Philadelphia: Saunders.
175. Nichols, A.A. (2005). Cholestasis of pregnancy: A review of the evidence. *J Perinat Neonatal Nurs, 19,* 217.
176. Niebyl, J.R. & Goodwin, T.M. (2002). Overview of nausea and vomiting of pregnancy with an emphasis on vitamins and ginger. *Am J Obstet Gynecol, 186,* S253.
177. Nikfar, S., et al. (2002). Use of proton pump inhibitors during pregnancy and rates of major malformations: A meta-1—I analysis. *Dig Dis Sci, 47,* 1526.
178. Nohr, E.A., et al. (2007). Obesity, gestational weight gain and preterm birth: A study within the Danish National Birth Cohort. *Paediatr Perinat Epidemiol, 21,* 5.
179. Olsen, I.E., et al. (2010). New intrauterine growth curves based on United States data. *Pediatrics, 125,* e214.
180. Olson, C.M., et al. (2003). Gestational weight gain and postpartum behaviors associated with weight change from early pregnancy to 1 year postpartum. *Int J Obes Relat Metab Disord, 27,* 117.
181. Olson, G. & Blackwell, S.C. (2011). Optimization of gestational weight gain in the obese gravida: A review. *Obstet Gynecol Clin North Am, 38,* 397.
182. Omari, T. & Rudolph, C.D. (2012). Gastrointestinal motility. In R.A. Polin, W.W. Fox, & S.H. Abman (Eds.). *Fetal and neonatal physiology* (4th ed.). Philadelphia: Saunders.
183. O'Sullivan, G., et al. (2009). Effect of food intake during labour on obstetric outcome: Randomised controlled trial. *BMJ, 338,* b784.
184. Ozkan, S., et al. (2005). Serum leptin levels in hypertensive disorder of pregnancy. *Eur J Obstet Gynecol Reprod Biol, 120,* 158.
185. Pan, C. & Perumalswami, P.V. (2011). Pregnancy-related liver diseases. *Clin Liver Dis, 15,* 199.
186. Paul, D.A., et al. (2011). Increased odds of necrotizing enterocolitis after transfusion of red blood cells in premature infants. *Pediatrics, 127,* 635.
187. Pereira, G.R. & Zucker, A. (1986). Nutritional deficiencies in the neonate. *Clin Perinatol, 13,* 175.
188. Picciano, M.F. (2003). Pregnancy and lactation: Physiological adjustments, nutritional requirements and the role of dietary supplements. *J Nutr, 133,* 1997S.
189. Poindexter, B.B. & Denne, S.C. (2012). Parenteral nutrition. In C.A. Gleason & S. Devaskar (Eds.). *Avery's diseases of the newborn* (9th ed.). Philadelphia: Saunders.
190. Poindexter, B.B. & Schanler, R.J. (2012). Enteral nutrition for the high-risk neonate In C.A. Gleason & S. Devaskar (Eds.). *Avery's diseases of the newborn* (9th ed.). Philadelphia: Saunders.
191. Polyzos, N.P., et al. (2009). Effect of periodontal disease treatment during pregnancy on preterm birth incidence: A metaanalysis of randomized trials. *Am J Obstet Gynecol, 200,* 225.
192. Portnoi, G., et al. (2003). Prospective comparative study of the safety and effectiveness of ginger for the treatment of nausea and vomiting in pregnancy. *Obstet Gynecol, 189,* 1374.
193. Premji, S. & Chessell, L. (2003). Continuous nasogastric milk feeding versus intermittent bolus milk feeding for premature infants less than 1500 grams. *Cochrane Database Syst Rev, 1,* CD001819.
194. Premji, S., Fenton, T., & Sauve, R. (2006). Does amount of protein in formula matter for low-birthweight infants? A Cochrane systematic review. *J Parenter Enteral Nutr, 30,* 507.
195. Premji, S.S. & Paes, B. (2000). Gastrointestinal function and growth in premature infants: Is non-nutritive sucking vital? *J Perinatol, 20,* 46.
196. Putet, G. (2000). Lipid metabolism of the micropremie. *Clin Perinatol, 27,* 57.
197. Quigley, M.A., et al. (2007). Formula milk versus donor breast milk for feeding preterm or low birth weight infants. *Cochrane Database Syst Rev, 4,* CD002971.
198. Rasmussen, K.M. & Yaktine, A.L. (2009). *Weight gain during pregnancy: Reexamining the guidelines. Institute of Medicine (US) and National Research Council (US) Committee to Reexamine IOM pregnancy weight guidelines.* Washington, DC: National Academies Press.
199. Rasmussen, K.M., et al. (2010). Recommendations for weight gain during pregnancy in the context of the obesity epidemic. *Obstet Gynecol, 116,* 1191.
200. Reber, K.M., Nankervis, C.A., & Nowicki, P.T. (2002). Newborn intestinal circulation. Physiology and pathophysiology. *Clin Perinatal, 29,* 23.
201. Resnik, R. (2004). The puerperium. In R.K. Creasy, R. Resnik, & J.D. Iams (Eds.). *Maternal-fetal medicine: Principles and practice* (5th ed.). Philadelphia: Saunders.
202. Resnik, R. & Creasy, R.K. (2009). Intrauterine growth restriction. In R.K. Creasy et al. (Eds.). *Creasy & Resnik's Maternal-fetal medicine: Principles and practice* (6th ed.). Philadelphia: Saunders Elsevier.
203. Richter, J.E. (2005). Review article: The management of heartburn in pregnancy. *Aliment Pharmacol Ther, 22,* 749.
204. Riely, C.A. & Fallon, H.J. (2004). Liver diseases. In G.N. Burrow, T.P. Duffy, & J.A. Copel (Eds.). *Medical complications during pregnancy* (6th ed.). Philadelphia: Saunders.
205. Robinson, J.S., et al. (2000). Origins of fetal growth restriction. *Eur J Obstet Gynecol Reprod Biol, 92,* 13.
206. Rollins, M.D., Chan, K.J., & Price, R.R. (2004). Laparoscopy for appendicitis and cholelithiasis during pregnancy: A new standard of care. *Surg Endosc, 18,* 237.
207. Rosso, P. (1990). *Nutrition and metabolism in pregnancy.* New York: Oxford University Press.
208. Rubin, P.H. & Janowitz, H.D. (1991). The digestive tract and pregnancy. In S.H. Cherry & I.R. Merkatz (Eds.). *Complications of pregnancy: Medical, surgical,*

gynecological, psychosocial, and perinatal (4th ed.). Baltimore: Williams & Wilkins.

209. Ruiz-Extremera, A., et al. (2005). Activity of hepatic enzymes from week sixteen of pregnancy. *Am J Obstet Gynecol, 193,* 2010.
210. Sadler, T.W. (2012). *Langman's medical embryology* (12th ed.) Philadelphia: Lippincott, Williams & Wilkins.
211. Schanler, R.J., et al. (1999). Feeding strategies for premature infants: Randomized trial of gastrointestinal priming and tube feeding method. *Pediatrics, 103,* 434.
212. Schanler, R.J. (2005). Human milk supplementation for preterm infants. *Acta Paediatr Suppl, 94,* 64.
213. Schanler, R.J. (2011). Outcomes of human milk-fed premature infants. *Semin Perinatol, 35,* 29.
214. Schneider, R.E., et al. (2000). Dental complications. In W.R. Cohen, S.H. Cherry, & I.R. Merkatz (Eds.). *Cherry & Merkatz's Complications of pregnancy* (5th ed.). Baltimore: Williams & Wilkins.
215. Scotland, N.E. (2009). Maternal nutrition. In R.K. Creasy, et al. (Eds.). *Creasy & Resnik's Maternal-fetal medicine: Principles and practice* (6th ed.). Philadelphia: Saunders Elsevier.
216. Shah, M.D. & Shah, S.R. (2009). Nutrient deficiencies in the premature infant. *Pediatr Clin North Am, 56,* 1069.
217. Shah, P.S. & Ohlsson, A. Knowledge Synthesis Group on Determinants of Low Birth Weight and Preterm Births. (2009). Effects of prenatal multimicronutrient supplementation on pregnancy outcomes: a meta-analysis. *CMAJ, 180,* E99.
218. Sharts-Hopko, N.C. (2010). Oral intake during labor: A review of the evidence. *MCN Am J Matern Child Nurs, 35,* 197.
219. Sherman, M.P. (2010). New concepts of microbial translocation in the neonatal intestine: mechanisms and prevention. *Clin Perinatol, 37,* 565.
220. Sibley, C.P., et al. (2010). Review: Adaptation in placental nutrient supply to meet fetal growth demand: implications for programming. *Placenta, 31,* S70.
221. Siega-Riz, A.M., Evenson, K.R., & Dole, N. (2004). Pregnancy-related weight gain—a link to obesity? *Nutr Rev, 62,* S105.
222. Simmer, K. & Rao, S.C. (2005). Early introduction of lipids to parenterally-fed preterm infants. *Cochrane Database Syst Rev, 2,* CD005256.
223. Simpson, J.L., et al. (2011). Micronutrients and women of reproductive potential: Required dietary intake and consequences of dietary deficiency or excess. Part II—vitamin D, vitamin A, iron, zinc, iodine, essential fatty acids. *J Matern Fetal Neonatal Med, 24,* 1.
224. Singata, M., Tranmer, J., & Gyte, G.M. (2010). Restricting oral fluid and food intake during labour. *Cochrane Database Syst Rev, 1,* CD003930.
225. Slutzah, M., et al. (2010). Refrigerator storage of expressed human milk in the neonatal intensive care unit. *J Pediatr, 156,* 26.
226. Smoleniec, J.S. & James, D.K. (1993). Gastrointestinal crises during pregnancy. *Dig Dis, 11,* 313.
227. Sohi, G., Revesz, A. & Hardy, D.B. (2011). Permanent implications of intrauterine growth restriction on cholesterol homeostasis. *Semin Reprod Med,* 29, 246.
228. Steinlauf, A.F., Chang, P.K. & Traube, M. (2004). Gastrointestinal complications. In G.N. Burrow, T.P. Duffy, & J.A. Copel (Eds.). *Medical complications during pregnancy* (6th ed.). Philadelphia: Saunders.
229. Stoll, B.J., et al. (2010). Neonatal outcomes of extremely preterm infants from the NICHD Neonatal Research Network. *Pediatrics, 126,* 443.
230. Styne, D.M. (2012). Endocrine factors affecting neonatal growth. In R.A. Polin, W.W. Fox, & S.H. Abman (Eds.). *Fetal and neonatal physiology* (4th ed.). Philadelphia: Saunders.
231. Suidan, J.S. & Young, B.K. (1986). The acute abdomen in pregnancy. In V.K. Rustgi & J.N. Cooper (Eds.). *Gastrointestinal and hepatic complications in pregnancy.* New York: John Wiley & Sons.
232. Sullivan, S., et al. (2010). An exclusively human milk-based diet is associated with a lower rate of necrotizing enterocolitis than a diet of human milk and bovine milk-based products. *J Pediatr, 156,* 562.
233. Symonds, M.E. & Ramsay, M.M. (2010). *Maternal-fetal nutrition during pregnancy and lactation.* Cambridge: Cambridge University Press.
234. Szajewska, H. (2010). Probiotics and prebiotics in preterm infants: Where are we? Where are we going? *Early Hum Dev, 86,* 81.
235. Tarnok, A. & Mehes, K. (2002). Gastrointestinal malformations, associated congenital abnormalities, and intrauterine growth. *J Pediatr Gastroenterol Nutr, 34,* 406.
236. Taylor, S.N., et al. (2009). Intestinal permeability in preterm infants by feeding type: Mother's milk versus formula. *Breastfeed Med, 4,* 11.
237. te Braake, F.W., et al. (2005). Amino acid administration to premature infants directly after birth. *J Pediatr, 147,* 457.
238. Thorn, S.R., et al. (2011). The intrauterine growth restriction phenotype: Fetal adaptations and potential implications for later life insulin resistance and diabetes. *Semin Reprod Med,* 29, 225.
239. Thureen, P. & Heird, W.C. (2005). Protein and energy requirements of the preterm/low birthweight (LBW) infant. *Pediatr Res, 57,* 95R.
240. Thureen, P.J. & Hay, W.W. (2000). Intravenous nutrition and postnatal growth of the micropremie. *Clin Perinatol, 27,* 197.
241. Thureen, P.J. & Hay Jr., W.W. (2001). Early aggressive nutrition in preterm infants. *Semin Neonatol, 6,* 403.
242. Trahms, C.M. (2001). Nutrition for the preterm and low-birth-weight infant. In *Nutrition in infancy and childhood* (7th ed.). New York: McGraw-Hill.
243. Tranmer, J.E., et al. (2005). The effect of unrestricted oral carbohydrate intake on labor progress. *J Obstet Gynecol Neonatal Nurs, 34,* 319.
244. Tsang, R.C., Uauy, R., Koletzko, B., Zlotkin, S.H. (2005). *Nutrition of the preterm infant. Scientific basis and practical guidelines.* Cincinnati, OH: Digital Educational Publishing, Inc.
245. Tubman, T.R., Thompson, S.W., & McGuire, W. (2008). Glutamine supplementation to prevent morbidity and mortality in preterm infants. *Cochrane Database Syst Rev, 1,* CD001457.
246. Tytgat, G.N., et al. (2003). Contemporary understanding and management of reflux and constipation in the general population and pregnancy: A consensus meeting. *Aliment Pharmacol Ther, 18,* 291.
247. Uauy, R., et al. (2000). Essential fatty acid metabolism in the micro premie. *Clin Perinatol, 27,* 71.
248. Uppal, A., et al. (2010). The effectiveness of periodontal disease treatment during pregnancy in reducing the risk of experiencing preterm birth and low birth weight: A meta-analysis. *J Am Dent Assoc, 141,* 1423.
249. Van Thiel, D.H. & Schade, R.R. (1986). Pregnancy: Its physiologic course, nutrient cost, and effects on gastrointestinal function. In V.K. Rustgi & J.N. Cooper (Eds.). *Gastrointestinal and hepatic complications in pregnancy.* New York: John Wiley & Sons.
250. Vanderhoof, J.A., et al. (2005). Gastrointestinal disease. In M.G. MacDonald, M.M.K. Seshia, & M.D. Mullett (Eds.). *Avery's Neonatology, pathophysiology and management of the newborn* (6th ed.). Philadelphia: Lippincott Williams & Wilkins.
251. Vedmedovska, N., et al. (2011). Placental pathology in fetal growth restriction. *Eur J Obstet Gynecol Reprod Biol, 155,* 36.
252. Verberg, M.E., et al. (2005). Hyperemesis gravidarum, a literature review. *Hum Reprod Update, 1,* 527.
253. Vutyavanich, T., et al. (2001). Ginger for nausea and vomiting in pregnancy: Randomized, double-masked, placebo-controlled trial. *Obstet Gynecol, 97,* 577.
254. Walker, W.A. (2000). Role of nutrients and bacterial colonization in the development of intestinal host defense. *J Pediatr Gastroenterol Nutr, 30,* S2.
255. Weaver, L.T. (1993). Development of bowel habit in preterm infants. *Arch Dis Child, 68,* 317.
256. Weigel, M.M., et al. (2006). Is the nausea and vomiting of early pregnancy really feto-protective? *J Perinat Med, 34,* 115.

257. Wells, J.C. (2011). The thrifty phenotype: An adaptation in growth or metabolism? *Am J Hum Biol, 23,* 65.
258. Williamson, S. & Mackillop, L. (2009). Diseases of the liver, biliary system, and pancreas. In R.K. Creasy, et al. (Eds.). *Creasy & Resnik's Maternal-fetal medicine: Principles and practice* (6th ed.). Philadelphia: Saunders Elsevier.
259. Wong, C.A., et al. (2007). Gastric emptying of water in obese pregnant women at term. *Anesth Analg, 105,* 751.
260. World Health Organization. (1997). *Care in normal birth: A practical guide. Report of a Technical Working Group*. Geneva: World Health Organization.
261. Xiong, X., et al. (2006). Periodontal disease and adverse pregnancy outcomes: A systematic review. *BJOG, 113,* 135.
262. Yarnada, H., et al. (2005). Genetic factors in fetal growth restriction and miscarriage. *Semin Thromb Hemost, 31,* 334.
263. Yeung, M.Y. & Smyth, J.P. (2003). Nutritionally regulated hormonal factors in prolonged postnatal growth retardation and its associated adverse neurodevelopmental outcome in extreme prematurity. *Biol Neonate, 84,* 1.
264. Yost, C.C. (2005). Neonatal necrotizing enterocolitis: Diagnosis, management, and pathogenesis. *J Infus Nurs, 28,* 130.
265. Yu, V.Y.H. & Upadhyay, A. (2004). Neonatal management of the growth-restricted infant. *Semin Fetal Neonatal Med, 9,* 403.

CHAPTER 13

Immune System and Host Defense Mechanisms

"Remarkable adaptations . . . allow a genetically and antigenically disparate conceptus to develop in direct contact with a fully competent maternal immune system."[100] Why doesn't the mother reject the fetus and placenta? Knowledge of maternal, fetal, and neonatal immune physiology and understanding of the immune relationship between a mother and her fetus are still evolving. Current theories regarding this question—along with alterations in host defense mechanisms in the mother and neonate and implications for clinical practice—are examined in this chapter.

The immune system is made up of organs and specialized cells whose primary purpose is to defend the body from foreign substances (antigens) that may cause tissue injury or disease. These defense mechanisms consist of nonspecific and specific factors. Nonspecific factors include physical and biochemical barriers including skin and mucosal barriers, bone marrow, lymphoid tissue, digestive enzymes, pH, temperature, proteins, and enzymes such as lysozyme, transferrin, and interferon. Specific factors include cellular and humoral components that respond to foreign substances. In addition, individual genetic susceptibilities affect both nonspecific factors and specific factors. Nonspecific and specific factors make up two arms of the immune response—the innate (also known as *natural* or *native immunity*) and the adaptive (also known as *specific* or *acquired immunity*) (Table 13-1). Mechanisms of innate and adaptive immunity work cooperatively through complex interactions to prevent, control, and eradicate foreign antigens in the body without doing harm to the host. Host immune mechanisms and terminology are summarized in Table 13-2 and Figures 13-1 and 13-2. Innate and adaptive immunity are summarized in Boxes 13-1 and 13-2 on page 446. Roles of cytokines (interleukins and interferons) in innate and adaptive immunity are summarized in Table 13-3.

MATERNAL PHYSIOLOGIC ADAPTATIONS

A general enhancement of innate immunity and suppression of adaptive immunity occur during pregnancy. Within adaptive responses, the cell-mediated (T helper 1, or Th1) response is less functional, the antibody-mediated (T helper 2, or Th2) response is enhanced, and the relation between the two is dysregulated. These alterations, which help prevent the mother's immune system from rejecting the semiallogenic fetus, increase her risk of developing certain infections and influence the course of chronic disorders such as autoimmune diseases. Because changes in both innate and adaptive immune responses occur, there is no overall trend toward immunosuppression or improved immune function in pregnant women and in general, immune function in pregnant women is similar to immune function in nonpregnant women.

Antepartum Period

"Pregnancy is an immunological balancing act in which the mother's immune system has to remain tolerant of potential major histocompatibility (MHC) antigens and yet maintain normal immune competence for defense against microorganisms."[167] The immune changes that occur systemically in the innate and adaptive systems and those that occur at the site of the fetal-maternal interface are described in this section.

Alterations in Innate Immunity

Mediators of the innate response are altered during pregnancy (Table 13-4). Chemotaxis (see the definition in Table 13-2) is decreased during pregnancy, which may delay initial maternal responses to infection.[48,107] In addition, production of interleukin (IL)-4 and interferon-γ (IFN-γ) may also be decreased.[107] Functionally, monocyte and granulocyte activity is enhanced, which results in faster and more efficient phagocytosis. This may help protect the mother so she does not mount a cell-mediated immune response to trophoblastic and fetal cells that appear in the maternal circulation. Natural killer (NK) cell activity is altered in a more complex manner. Systemic NK activity is down-regulated during pregnancy, secondary to the effects of progesterone, which appears to induce formation of a blocking factor that decreases lymphocyte proliferation and NK activity.[39] The result is that systemic NK cytolytic activity is normal in the first trimester but lower during the second and third trimesters and immediately after delivery.

Total white blood cell (WBC) volume increases slightly beginning in the second month and levels off during the second and third trimesters. The total WBC count in pregnancy

Table 13-1 **Components of Innate and Adaptive Immunity**

	CELLULAR COMPONENTS	HUMORAL COMPONENTS	MEDIATORS
Innate	Monocytes Macrophages Granulocytes NK cells Mast cells γδT cells* Endothelial cells	Complement Acute phase proteins (e.g., C-reactive protein)	Toll-like receptors Cytokines
Adaptive	Antigen presenting cells* T (lymphocyte) cells B (lymphocyte) cells	Antibodies	Cytokines

*These gamma delta T cells are found primarily in the gut mucosa. Antigen presenting cells are monocytes and/or macrophages that have engulfed a foreign object, processed it, and displayed it, within an MHC-I or MHC-II complex at the cell surface, to a T cell to initiate the adaptive immune response.

Table 13-2 **Definitions of Terms**

Active immunity: The response produced by an immunocompetent individual following exposure to foreign antigens (bacteria, viruses, attenuated or inactivated/killed viruses).

Adaptive immunity: Also known as "acquired immunity." The result of active immunity wherein specific antibody (humoral) and cell-mediated responses establish memory cells and antibodies that provide immunity during subsequent exposures to a specific antigen.

Allograft: Graft taken from an organism that is the same species as the recipient but not genetically identical. The fetus is a "semi-allograft."

Antibody: Proteins (immunoglobulins) that react with specific antigens. The five classes are IgA, IgD, IgE, IgG, and IgM.

Antibody (humoral)-mediated immunity: Adaptive immune mechanism mediated by B cells, which produces antibodies and protects the body from extracellular antigens.

Antigen: Substances perceived by one's host defense mechanisms as "foreign" (may include bacteria, viruses, pollutants, dust, certain foods, for example).

Antigen presenting cell (APC): A cell that displays MHC with antigen complexes on the surface of the cell. Any cell can be an APC in that all cells have class I MHC. The term *APC* is used to refer to cells that also express class II MHC and can activate T cells, dendritic cells, macrophages, and B cells.

Cell-mediated immunity: Adaptive immune mechanism provided by immune cells. $TCD4^+$ (T-helper cells), $TCD8^+$ (T-cytotoxic cells), and $TCD4^+/CD26^+$ (T-regulatory cells) provide protection against certain organisms, regulate B-cell function, defend against cancer, and mediate graft rejection.

Chemotaxis: Movement of neutrophils and other phagocytes in an organized fashion toward a site of antigenic invasion.

Complement: Thirty discrete plasma proteins that, as part of the innate immune response, function in a cascade of reactions to form a membrane attack complex that lyses cells. The effector response of the complement cascade also opsonizes antigen, increases vascular permeability, and stimulates chemotaxis to aid phagocytosis. The complement cascade can proceed via the classical pathway or alternate pathway.

Cytokines: Glycoproteins such as lymphokines, interleukins, interferon, and tissue necrosis factor that are produced by various components of the immune system, especially T lymphocytes and macrophages. Cytokines function as autocrine or paracrine agents to activate different arms of the immune response.

Cytotoxic/killer T cell (TCD8ᵀ): A type of T lymphocyte that acts directly on specific antigens or target cells that exhibit a specific antigen and induces cell lysis.

Fibronectin: Nonspecific opsonin, inhibitor of bacterial adherence to epithelial cells, and clot-stabilizing protein found in plasma and endothelial tissue.

Human leukocyte antigen (HLA): The major forms of specific tissue antigens found on tissue surfaces that are unique to each person (includes HLA-A, HLA-B, HLA-C, HLA-D, and in the placenta HLA-G).

Histocompatibility: The ability of tissue to accept a transplant from another individual.

Immunoglobulin: Antibodies produced by B lymphocytes (IgG, IgM, IgA, IgD, and IgE).

Innate immunity: Initial physical and nonspecific responses. Includes skin, mucosa, digestive enzymes. Primary effectors are polymorphonuclear neutrophils (PMNs), macrophages, monocytes, mast cells, natural killer (NK) cells, and complement. Innate immune response results in elimination of foreign substance or antigen and stimulation of the adaptive immune response.

Interleukin: A polypeptide member of the cytokine family. Produced by T cells, APCs, NK cells, and macrophages. Interleukins regulate and facilitate immune responses.

Interferon: Glycoprotein in the cytokine family. Primary role is in fighting viral infections.

Lymphokine: Subclass of cytokines. Mediators released by activated T cells that facilitate or act as costimulatory for immune reaction.

Memory cell: Form of B lymphocyte sensitized to specific antigens that has the ability to produce specific antibodies with subsequent stimulation by the specific antigen.

Major histocompatibility complex (MHC): Specific antigens found on tissue surfaces divided into two groups: MHC I (HLA-A, HLA-B, and HLA-C, which are found on most of a person's cells), and MHC II (found on surface of immune cells such as T and B lymphocytes).

Table 13-2 **Definitions of Terms—cont'd**

Natural killer (NK) cells: A subpopulation of lymphocytes in the innate immune response that form a first line of defense against cells infected with a virus and cancerous cells. NK cells have receptors that recognize class I MHC antigens and can attack without prior sensitization. They secrete cytokines that provide costimulation for T and B cells.
Opsonization: Processing and marking or altering the cell surface of an antigen by actions of immunoglobulin or complement; substances acting in this manner are called *opsonins.* This process is critical in allowing phagocytosis of organisms with capsular polysaccharide coats such as group B streptococci.
Passive immunity: Transfer of antibodies from an actively immunized to a nonimmunized person.
Plasma cell: Form of B lymphocyte able to secrete immunoglobulins.
Regulatory T cell: $TCD4^+/CD25^+$ cells. The exact function of these cells in unclear. They may inhibit production of interleukins (IL-10) that are necessary products and facilitators of the adaptive immune response. Thus they may help to slow or terminate immune response once the antigens are destroyed.
T helper cell ($TCD4^+$): A type of T lymphocyte that proliferates when in contact with an APC that exhibits class II MHC/antigen complexes (B cells, dendritic cells). $TCD4^+$ cells differentiate into Th1 or Th2 cells based on the cytokines produced. Th1 cells participate in cell-mediated immunity and Th2 cells participate in antibody-mediated immunity. These cells thus enhance the activity of B lymphocytes, other T cells, and macrophages via secretion of cytokines.
T suppressor cells: T lymphocytes that express $CD8^+$ cells and function to suppress the cellular immune response.
Th1 cells: A subset of $TCD4^+$ (T-helper cells) that facilitates cell-mediated immunity via secretion of interleukin-12 (IL-12), tumor-necrosis factor (TNF)-β, and interferon (IFN)-γ. The result is stimulation of macrophages and inflammation.
Th2 cells: A subset of $TCD4^+$ (T-helper cells) that facilitates antibody-mediated immunity via secretion of interleukin-4 (IL-4), interleukin-5 (IL-5), interleukin-12 (IL-12), and interleukin-13 (IL-13). The result is stimulation of B cells and production of antibodies.
Toll-like receptors (TLRs): Molecules on the surface of phagocytes and other cells that recognize the patterns of microbial products and generate signals to activate an innate immune response.

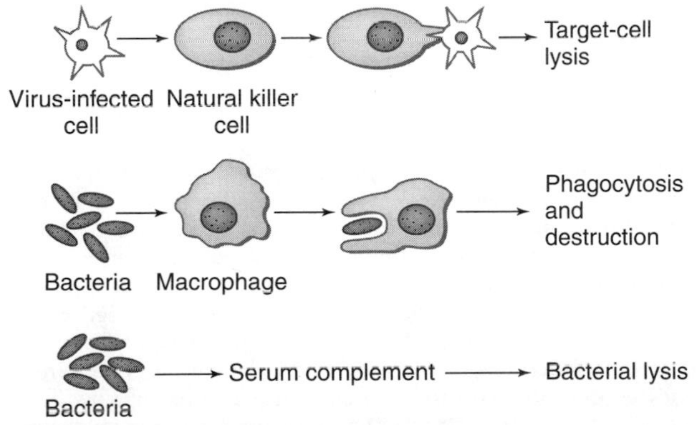

FIGURE 13-1 Summary of innate immunity. Surface antigens of viruses, bacteria, and tumors induce innate immune function. In this system, natural killer cells and phagocytes (e.g., macrophages) can recognize certain antigens in a nonspecific fashion and either lyse the offending infected cells or ingest and destroy the offending organism. Only the foreign nature of the antigen is required; antigen processing and major histocompatibility antigen participation are not necessary. (From Silver, R.M., Peltier, M.R., & Branch, D.W. [2004]. The immunology of pregnancy. In R.K. Creasy & R. Resnik [Eds.], *Maternal-fetal medicine: Principles and practice* [5th ed.]. Philadelphia: Saunders.)

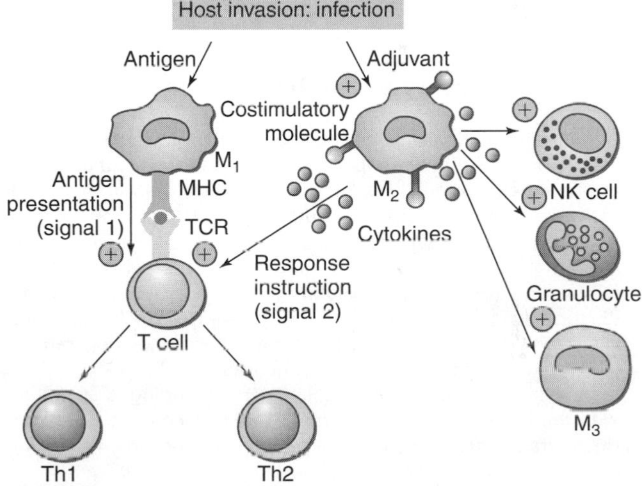

FIGURE 13-2 Summary of adaptive immunity. Adaptive immune responses initially require antigen processing and subsequent presentation in T cells. A T cell with a receptor specific for an inciting antigen will be activated and undergo differentiation into a Th1 or Th2 effector cell. In part, the type of cytokine produced by the activated T cell dictates the nature of the subsequent response. Interleukin (IL)-2 is the primary growth factor required for clonal proliferation of T cells; it stimulates the proliferation of cytotoxic and memory T cells. IL-4 and IL-5 stimulate B-cell proliferation, differentiation, and antibody production. (From Sacks, G., Sargent, I., & Redman, C. [1999]. An innate view of human pregnancy. *Immunol Today, 20,* 114.)

varies among individual women, ranging from 5000 to 12,000 per mm^3, with values as high as 15,000 per mm^3 reported (see Chapter 8).[129] The increase is primarily due to increased numbers of polymorphonuclear neutrophils (PMNs), monocytes, and granulocytes.[129] A slight shift to the left may occur, with occasional myelocytes and metamyelocytes seen on the peripheral smear. Changes in other WBC forms are minimal (see Chapter 8).

Alterations in PMN function have been reported.[48] PMN attachment, ingestion, and digestion of *Candida albicans* have been found to be increased, possibly secondary to the effects of human chorionic gonadotropin (hCG). Even so, pregnant women have higher rates of fungal infection, which may be secondary to the effects of estrogen on nutrient availability for fungal growth in the reproductive tract.[129] Estrogens may alter local mucosal barrier function, allowing adherence

BOX 13-1 Overview of Innate Immunity

The innate immune response, which includes inflammation, lysis of an antigen's cell membrane, and phagocytosis (see Figure 13-1) is the first-line defense mechanism that comes into play after exposure to a foreign antigen.[1,107] The innate immune response also has a crucial role in the activation of adaptive immune responses (see Figure 13-2). Innate immunity involves nonspecific inborn responses to a foreign antigen that are activated the first time the antigen is encountered. These defense mechanisms occur rapidly and only in response to microbes, not to noninfectious substances.[1] Important characteristics of innate immunity include the following: (1) a prior exposure to the antigen is not required for a response to occur; (2) repeated exposures to an antigen over time will not alter the host's innate immune response (i.e., immune responses do not become more vigorous); and (3) the ability to recognize molecular patterns shared by groups of microbes, but there is an inability to recognize fine distinctions between the microbes.[1] Innate immunity involves physical (e.g., epithelia, mucous membranes, secretions) and biochemical barriers.

Primary effector cells of an innate immune response are polymorphonuclear neutrophils, macrophages, monocytes, mast cells, and natural killer (NK) cells (a T-lymphocyte subpopulation).[107] In addition, toll-like receptors (TLRs) on cell surfaces (responsible for recognizing the molecular patterns of microbial products), endothelial cells, circulating factors (e.g., complement and acute phase proteins such as C-reactive protein), and cytokines and chemokines, which are secreted by macrophages and other cells, are actively involved in mediating the innate immune response and engaging the adaptive immune response (see Figures 13-1, 13-2, and 13-3).[1,107]

TLRs sense molecular patterns of pathogens and induce expression of cytokines and chemokines to activate defensive cells.[111] Recognition of molecular patterns occurs via pattern recognition receptors (PRRs). PRRs are found on cell surfaces, in intracellular vesicles, or in the cytoplasm. PRRs can recognize damaging molecular patterns such as cytokines, intracellular proteins, substances released by damaged cells, and pathogen-associated molecular patterns.[180] PRRs on TLRs "allow either the extracellular or liposomal (or endosomal) recognition of a wide range of microbes"[107] or via nucleotide binding oligomerization domain (NOD) proteins which are "cytoplasm bound receptors that facilitate responses to invasive intracellular bacteria."[107, p.92] Pathogens bind to TLR and other receptors on monocytes and macrophages, initiating a complement cascade with release of prostaglandins (which mediate fever with bacterial pathogens). The transcription factor NF-KB is released, which stimulates synthesis and release of both proinflammatory (such as IL-1B, IL-6, and TNF-α) and antiinflammatory cytokines (such as IL-1 and IL-10).[151]

BOX 13-2 Overview of Adaptive Immunity

Adaptive immunity is the development of a protective response to a specific foreign antigen that has been processed and presented by the innate system, and the establishment of an immunologic memory of that response.[107] There are six distinct characteristics of an adaptive immune response: (1) specificity (the ability to specifically respond to a distinct antigen or a part of an antigen); (2) diversity (the ability to respond to a wide variety of antigens); (3) memory (repeated exposures to an antigen will elicit more vigorous immune responses); (4) specialization (optimizing immune responses against different antigens); (5) self-limitation (ability to have immune responses decline after responding to an antigen with the immune system returning to a homeostatic state); and (6) nonreactivity to self (the ability to defend against foreign antigens while not harming the host).[1]

There are two types of adaptive immunity: humoral (antibody-mediated) and cell-mediated. Cellular components of the adaptive immune response include the following: (1) subpopulations of lymphocytes (e.g., B lymphocytes and T lymphocytes), (2) antigen presenting cells (APCs) (e.g., dendritic cells, monocytes, macrophages), and (3) effector cells (e.g., mononuclear phagocytes).[1,107]

The function of humoral, or antibody-mediated, immunity is to defend the host against extracellular microbes and other antigens. B lymphocytes (lymphocytes that originate in stem cells and mature in the bone marrow) are the mediators of humoral immune responses. Their primary function is the interruption of infection and the elimination of extracellular microbes. B lymphocytes secrete antibodies (immunoglobulins) that target specific foreign antigens for elimination. There are two types of antibody responses—primary and secondary. A primary antibody response involves the activation, proliferation, and differentiation of naive B lymphocytes into either antibody-secreting cells or memory cells. Some antibody-secreting cells may migrate to, and remain inactive in, the bone marrow. A secondary antibody response involves memory B lymphocytes that are activated to produce increasing amounts of antibodies. Often secondary antibody responses require B-lymphocyte stimulation by helper T lymphocytes. Typically, B cells are capable of producing antibodies to a specific antigen within 5 to 10 days after the initial exposure. With repeated exposures, immunologic memory allows B cells to respond to a specific antigen and produce antibodies sooner (i.e., within 1 to 3 days) with a more intense peak response.[1]

Cell-mediated immunity is responsible for the destruction of intracellular microbes and is mediated by T lymphocytes (lymphocytes that originate in stem cells in the bone marrow but mature in the thymus gland). The following steps are involved in this process: (1) presentation of a portion of a foreign antigen by major histocompatibility glycoprotein complexes (MHC-I or MHC-II) on the surface of APCs or B cells; (2) cell-associated antigen recognition by naive T cells (i.e., T cells whose function is to recognize microbial antigens); (3) activation of T cells to produce cytokines (e.g., interleukin [IL]-2) and express receptors for the cytokines; (4) T-cell proliferation and clonal expansion (i.e., a rapid increase in antigen-specific lymphocytes); (5) differentiation of the naive T cells into effector cells (whose function is to eliminate the microbe) or memory cells (whose function is to circulate in an inactive state until there is a repeat exposure to the microbe); and (6) inhibition of immune responses by suppressor or regulatory T cells when control or elimination of the foreign antigen has been accomplished.[1]

Subsets of T lymphocytes have different functions. $TCD8^+$ cells, also called *cytotoxic/killer T cells,* bind to MHC-I/antigen complexes (see Figure 13-4). All cells have MHC-I molecules that bind and present fragments of intracellular antigens on the cell surface. MHC antigens on the surfaces of cells classify the specific antigenic characteristics of that cell type. MHC-I molecules, present on most cells, can have three different types of MHC-I molecules: HLA-A, HLA-B, and HLA-C. MHC-II molecules, which are found on macrophages and B-cells, have HLA-D/DR proteins. The $TCD8^+$ binds to the MHC-I/antigen complex and then secretes molecules that lyse the infected target cell.[1]

BOX 13-2 Overview of Adaptive Immunity—cont'd

TCD4$^+$ cells, also called *T helper cells,* bind to MHC-II molecules, which are found on the surface of antigen presenting cells (APCs) such as macrophages. After binding to the APC, the TCD4$^+$ cell further differentiates into either a T helper (Th) 1 or Th2 cell. Th1 cells release lymphokines, tumor necrosis factor (TNF)-β, interferon (IFN)-γ, interleukin-2 (IL-2) and other interleukins, which facilitate cell-mediated immunity and initiate inflammation. Th2 cells secrete interleukins (IL-4, IL-5, IL-10, IL-13) that facilitate humoral immunity.[1,31,127]

Although most TCD4$^+$ cells belong to either Th1 or Th2 subsets, approximately 5% to 10% are T-regulatory cells. T-regulatory cells, also called *TCD4$^+$/CD25$^+$* or *suppressor cells,* secrete lymphokines (e.g., IL-10) that are immunosuppressants and inhibit the function of NK cells, Th1 cells, and Th2 cells. These regulatory cells play a role in inhibiting the immune response in the placenta at the fetal-maternal interface.[10]

In order for an adaptive immune response to antigens to occur, a process called *costimulation* must take place. Costimulation facilitates the identification of foreign or harmful antigens without jeopardizing the host's cells and tissues (see Figure 13-2). This process requires that two different signals be recognized by T lymphocytes in order for an adaptive immune response to occur. The "first signal" is the antigen binding to receptors on cell surfaces. For T lymphocytes, this process involves the binding of class I or class II MHC on the surface of an APC to T-cell receptors. The "second signal" involves costimulators that are expressed on APCs. Without costimulation, T lymphocytes are not able to respond to the antigen and they will remain in a state of unresponsiveness or experience apoptosis (i.e., cell death).[123]

Table 13-3 Cytokines: Interleukins and Interferons

CYTOKINE	PRINCIPAL SOURCE	ROLE IN INNATE IMMUNE RESPONSE	ROLE IN CELL-MEDIATED IMMUNE RESPONSE (Th1)	ROLE IN ANTIBODY-MEDIATED RESPONSE (Th2)
INTERLEUKIN (IL)				
IL-1	Macrophages and other antigen presenting cells (APCs)	Costimulation of APCs and T cells, production of prostaglandin, inflammation, acute phase response, hematopoiesis		
IL-2	Activated Th1 cells, NK cells		Proliferations of activated T cells, NK functions	Proliferation of B cells
IL-3	Activated T cells			Growth of hematopoietic progenitor cells
IL-4	Th2 and mast cells	Monokine production		B-cell proliferation, eosinophil and mast cell growth and function, IgE and class II MHC expression on B cells, inhibition of monocyte production
IL-5	Th2 and mast cells			Eosinophil growth and function
IL-6	Activated Th2 cells, APCs, other somatic cells	Acute phase response	Synergistic with IL-1 and TNF on T cells, thrombopoiesis	B-cell proliferation and differentiation into plasma cells and antibody production
IL-7	Thymic and marrow stromal cells	T and B lymphopoiesis		
IL-8	Macrophages, other somatic cells	Chemoattractant for neutrophils and T cells		
IL-9	T cells	Hematopoietic and thymopoietic effects		
IL-10	Activated Th2 cells, CD8$^+$ T and B cells, macrophages		Suppresses cellular immunity, mast cell growth	Inhibits cytokine production, promotes B-cell proliferation and antibody production
IL-11	Stromal cells	Synergistic hematopoietic and thrombopoietic effects		
IL-12	B cells, macrophages		Proliferation of NK cells, INF-γ production	
IL-13	Th2 cells			Similar to IL-4, promotes development of eosinophils

Continued

Table 13-3 Cytokines: Interleukins and Interferons—cont'd

CYTOKINE	PRINCIPAL SOURCE	ROLE IN INNATE IMMUNE RESPONSE	ROLE IN CELL-MEDIATED IMMUNE RESPONSE (Th1)	ROLE IN ANTIBODY-MEDIATED RESPONSE (Th2)
INTERFERON (IFN)				
IFN-α and IFN-β	Mononuclear phagocytes		Antiviral effects, induction of class I MHC on all somatic cells, activation of NK cells and macrophages	
IFN-γ	Activated Th1 and NK cells	Induces class I MHC on all somatic cells, induces class II MHC on APCs and somatic cells, activates macrophages, neutrophils, NK cells, promotes cell-mediated immunity, antiviral effects		

Modified from Silver, R.M., Peltier, M.R., & Branch, D.W. (2004). The immunology of pregnancy. In R.K. Creasy, R. Resnik, & J.D. Iams (Eds.), *Maternal-fetal medicine: Principles and practice* (5th ed.). Philadelphia: Saunders.

Table 13-4 Alterations in Host Defense Mechanisms during Pregnancy

ALTERATION	RESULT	IMPLICATION
INNATE IMMUNITY		
Increased PMNs	Increased available phagocytes	Protection of mother and fetus from infection
Altered metabolic activity and chemotaxis of PMNs	Delayed initial response to infection, especially gram-negative organisms	Increased risk of colonization, urinary tract infection
Decreased NK cell killer activity	Delayed initial response to infection	Increased risk of colonization with pathogens such as *Listeria* and toxoplasmosis Protect fetus and trophoblast from rejection
Increased fibronectin	Enhanced opsonization	Augmented maternal responses against bacterial infection
Increased total complement and C2, C3, and C3 split products	Enhanced chemotaxis and action of immunoglobulins through opsonization	Augmented maternal defenses against bacterial infection Protect fetus from infection
Decreased C1, C1a, B, and D	Delayed initial activation of complement system	Protect fetus and trophoblast from rejection
ADAPTIVE IMMUNITY		
Reduction in Th1 responses and inflammatory cytokine production	Reduction in cell-mediated responses and graft rejection	Increased risk of mycotic, fungal, and other opportunistic infections Protects semiallogenic fetus from rejection May result in improvement of rheumatoid arthritis
Enhanced Th2 response and production of antiinflammatory cytokines	Enhanced antibody-mediated responses Decrease in graft rejection Depressed reaction to tuberculin test	Protects mother against infection
Reduction in blood levels of immunoglobulins (IgG) in second half of pregnancy	Secondary to placental transfer to fetus and hemodilution Slower response to antigen stimulation in second half of pregnancy	Increased risk of colonization Protection for fetus/newborn

Table 13-4 Alterations in Host Defense Mechanisms during Pregnancy—cont'd

ALTERATION	RESULT	IMPLICATION
PLACENTA AND MEMBRANES		
Alterations in expression of class I and class II HLA antigens	Class I HLA antigens on cytotrophoblast do not stimulate graft rejection Syncytiotrophoblast does not express class I HLA antigens Class I HLA antigens actively inhibit activated T cells and activate inhibitory functions of NK cells Membranes do not have class II HLA antigens	Protects fetus from maternal immune response and rejection
Production of IDO	IDO catalyzes the degradation of tryptophan, which is essential for T-cell proliferation	Protects fetus from maternal immune response and rejection
Progesterone	Induces production of antiinflammatory cytokines that alter balance of TH1 and TH2 responses Stimulates lymphocytes to produce PIBF, which encourages B-cell production of asymmetric antibodies that function as blocking antibodies Alters NK cells to suppress killer activity	Protects fetus from maternal immune response and rejection
Complement regulatory molecules CD46, CD55 and CD59	Inhibits specific steps within the complement cascade	Protects fetus from maternal immune response and rejection

HLA, Human leukocyte antigen; *IDO,* indolamine 2,3 dehydrogenase; *NK,* natural killer cell; *PIBF,* progesterone-induced blocking factor; *PMN,* polymorphonuclear neutrophils; *Th1,* T helper 1; *Th2,* T helper 2.

of pathogenic organisms and increasing the risk of colonization. Conversely, improved PMN antibody expression during pregnancy may enhance phagocyte recognition and destruction of antigen-antibody complexes.

Toll-like receptors (TLR) are essential for the innate recognition of microorganisms and endogenous signals from tissue breakdown products, such as fetal fibronectin, hyaluronan, matrix proteins, and biglycans.[31] Both TLRs and the recently identified Nod-like receptors (NLR) are thought to be involved in regulating innate responses of the trophoblast to infections and tissue damage signals.[4] Changes in the cervix and fetal membranes with tissue remodeling near parturition may release these endogenous signals as part of the cascade leading to labor onset (Chapter 4).[31]

Alterations in the Inflammatory Response

Throughout pregnancy, the maternal circulation is seeded with small particles from the trophoblast. These cell clusters function as antigens of fetal origin and stimulate a systemic inflammatory response. The point of direct maternal contact with the placenta is at the junction with maternal endothelial cells in the uterine spiral arteries (see Chapter 3).[132] This contact activates endothelial cells and initiates an inflammatory response. However, a glycoprotein known as *pregnancy zone protein* (PZP) is produced during pregnancy, which has an inhibitory effect on the inflammatory process.[150] PZP levels increase 100- to 200-fold during pregnancy. PZP inhibits phagocytosis and suppresses inflammatory responses and IL-2 function near the decidua-trophoblast interface.[150,157]

Alterations in the Complement System

The complement system has a role in both innate and adaptive responses. Although pregnancy stimulates an overall activation of the complement system, this activation does not result in rejection of the fetus.[134] Alterations in the function of the complement system during pregnancy begin at 11 weeks' gestation with an increase (due to greater hepatic synthesis) in both total serum complement and specific proteins of the complement system, including C2, C3, and C3 split products (Figure 13-3).[92,134] These components enhance chemotaxis and actions of immunoglobulins through opsonization, thereby augmenting maternal defenses against bacterial infection. Other protein fragments of the complement system, such as C1, C1a, B, and D, are decreased.[134] C1q (involved in activation of the classic complement pathway, immune cell modification, cell processes, and maintenance of immune tolerance) is synthesized and secreted by decidual epithelial cells during pregnancy and is thought to have a role in changes in decidual blood vessels and mediation of cell-to-cell interaction between decidual and trophoblast cells.[115] Because complement fragments are involved in activation of the complement system, through either the classic or the alternative pathway, activity of the complement system early in the immune response may be delayed during pregnancy.

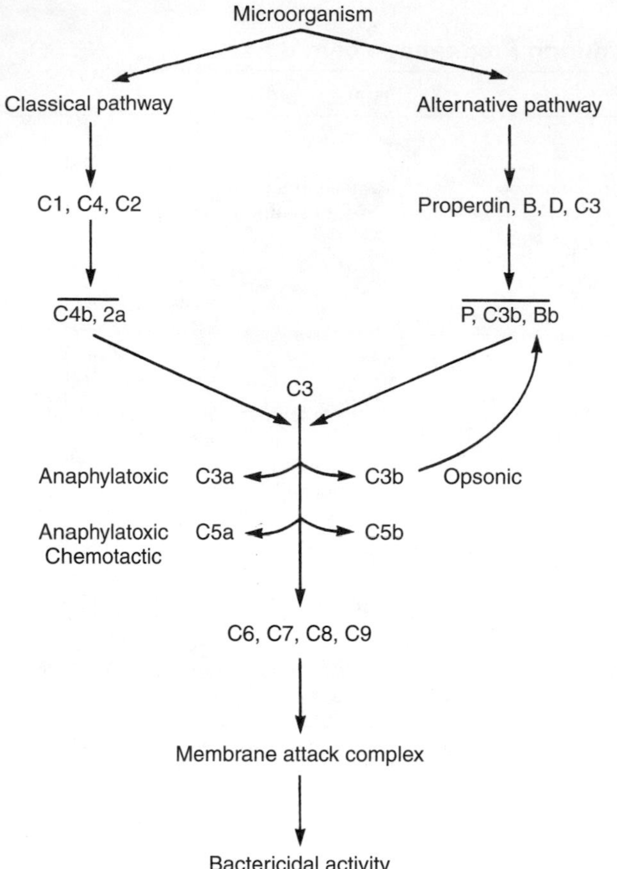

FIGURE 13-3 The complement system. The complement system involves a sequential series of discrete plasma proteins and their fragments that, when activated, enhance other parts of the immune system. Actions of complement include attraction of various cell types to the initial site of antigen invasion, promotion of chemotaxis and phagocytosis, enhancement of opsonization and other immunoglobulin functions, enhancement of histamine release and the inflammatory response, and direct destruction of antigens. Proteins of the complement system circulate in the plasma in an inactive state. Complement is activated through a sequential cascade. Activated molecules either act as enzymes to activate other proteins or fragments in the complement system or enhance actions of other parts of the immune system. There are two activation sequences. The classical pathway requires antibody or antigen-antibody complexes for activation, which occurs by C1 through C3. Complement activation and fixation are important for IgG and IgM function. Early in the immune response and during the initial inflammatory response, antibody may not be present, so an alternative activation sequence is needed. The alternative, or properdin, pathway is activated by factors B through C3 by substances such as bacterial products and circulating proteins. (From McLean, R.H. & Winkelstein, J.A. [1984]. Genetically determined variations in complement synthesis: Relationship to disease. *J Pediatr, 105,* 179.)

Alterations in Adaptive Immunity

Pregnancy is characterized by a switch in the balance of Th1 and Th2 cell subsets that results in enhanced Th2 function. This change is probably mediated by progesterone, which stimulates production of Th2 cytokines (e.g., IL-3, IL-4, IL-6, IL-10) and reduces the number of Th1 cytokines (e.g., IL-2, IFN-γ, tumor necrotic factor-β [TNF-β]) (see Table 13-3).[31,47] Because Th2 responses tend to enhance antibody-mediated responses and Th1 responses enhance cell-mediated immunity (Figure 13-4), this change alters the function of both antibody-mediated and cell-mediated responses. This has a potentially protective role in the maternal-fetal immune relationship.[31] Decreases in the number of Th1 cytokines may decrease maternal resistance to the spread of bacterial and viral organisms.[31,48] If there are alterations in this pattern so that Th1 predominates during pregnancy, inflammatory cytokine production increases, and is associated with spontaneous abortion, preeclampsia, preterm labor, and fetal growth restriction.[31,138] Alterations in adaptive immunity during pregnancy are summarized in Table 13-4.

Alterations in Cell-Mediated Immunity. Cell-mediated immunity is somewhat suppressed during pregnancy. Lymphocyte and macrophage synthesis, activation, and function are altered slightly in pregnancy secondary to influences from estrogens, corticosteroids, progesterone, α-fetoprotein (AFP), hCG, human placental lactogen (hPL), prostaglandins, and serum proteins.[47] Corticosteroids suppress activation of T-cell lymphokines, phagocytic activity, and lymphokine responsiveness of the macrophages.[47] Prostaglandins (especially PGE_1 and PGE_2), hPL, and AFP also appear to have an immunosuppressive role during pregnancy. AFP may induce production of regulatory T lymphocytes ($CD4^+/CD25^+$).[48]

Most investigators report that the total number of lymphocytes does not change significantly during pregnancy.[48,168] Some investigators have reported a decrease in the T-helper–to–T-suppressor ($CD4^+/CD8^+$) ratio. However, most reports indicate that the number of $TCD4^+$ (T-helper cells) decrease progressively to term, while the number of T-suppressor cells ($TCD8^+$) tend to remain relatively unchanged.[48]

Because $TCD4^+$ cells normally augment the cytotoxic responses involved in graft rejection, a decreased number of these cells may help protect the fetus from rejection by the mother. T-suppressor cell function may increase in late pregnancy and suppress B-cell function.[107] Decreased T-lymphocyte function and efficiency may increase the risk of viral and mycotic infections.

Alterations in Antibody-Mediated (Humoral) Immunity. Although a decreased response of B lymphocytes to antigen stimulation in late pregnancy and after birth has been reported by some authors and changes in levels of specific immunoglobulins have been documented, the antibody-mediated immune response is not significantly altered during gestation.

While a few studies have reported an increase in the number of B cells during pregnancy, most studies do not support this finding.[48] Some investigators have found that levels of maternal IgG fall as gestation progresses, with decreases ranging from 30% to 40% after 28 weeks.[48] However, others have found relatively little change. A decrease in IgG has been attributed to hemodilution of pregnancy, enhanced loss of IgG in the urine, and transfer of maternal IgG to the fetus in the last trimester. This relative decrease in IgG, along with alterations in the WBC population, may increase

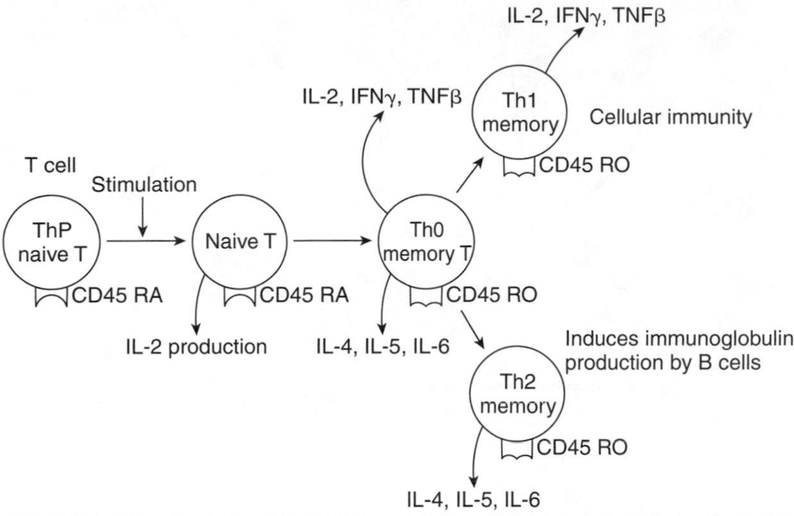

FIGURE 13-4 T-cell development from naive T cells to memory T cells. Cytokines released from different T-cell types are indicated as follows: *IL,* interleukin; *IFN,* interferon; *TNF,* tumor necrosis factor. (From Saito, S. [2000]. Cytokine network at the feto-maternal interface. *J Reprod Immunol, 47,* 92.)

the risk of bacterial colonization with certain pathogens (e.g., streptococci).

Immunoglobulin A (IgA) decreases or remains stable during gestation, immunoglobulin M (IgM) remains stable or may decrease slightly, immunoglobulin E (IgE) undergoes minimal or no change in levels, and immunoglobulin D (IgD) increases until term. The slight decrease in serum IgA may reflect increased levels of IgA found in saliva and other mucosal fluids.[48] The specific role of IgD in pregnancy is unknown.

Immune Function at the Fetal-Maternal Interface

The fetus is a semiallograft, that is, foreign tissue from the same species but with a different antigenic makeup. Because the fetus has maternal, paternal, and embryonic antigens, major antigenic differences may exist between the fetus and mother, including blood group antigens and tissue antigens such as human leukocyte antigen (HLA). Protection of the fetus from rejection seems to be predominantly a localized uterine response, although there are also systemic responses mediated primarily by endocrine factors.[158] Maternal tolerance of the fetal-placental unit has traditionally been believed to be secondary to elaboration of an immune "barrier" between the placenta and maternal tissue.[158] However, it is now understood that maternal immune systems are "aware of fetal antigens, that they respond vigorously to the presence of the fetus and that under normal circumstances they are tolerant to these antigens."[124] Thus tolerance of the fetus by the maternal immune system is "an active mechanism whereby fetal tissues are prevented from being recognized as foreign and/or from being rejected by the cells of the maternal immune system."[158] During pregnancy the trophoblast and maternal immune system have a regulatory and supportive interaction that is critical for both pregnancy maintenance and protection against infectious microorganisms.[107] Figure 13-5 illustrates interactions between the maternal immune system and the placental trophoblast.

Sperm are MHC class I– and II–negative, which usually protects them from recognition as foreign by the maternal immune system, although both sperm and seminal fluid carry other antigens. Seminal fluid also contains immunosuppressors. The woman responds to specific seminal fluid–induced cytokine and chemokine signals to increase immunosuppressive T-regulating (Treg) cells.[137,138] Exposure to paternal antigens on sperm and seminal fluid before pregnancy may lead to decreased responsiveness and maternal tolerance to paternal MHC antigens.[138,167]

How does trophoblast eliminate or evade the immune responses of B-cell and T-cell activation given the general enhanced innate and humoral immune function that is seen in the systemic circulation during pregnancy? Factors that are currently thought to have a role in maternal tolerance of the fetus include trophoblast HLA-G; progesterone, progesterone induced-blocking factor, altered NK cell function, a Th1/Th2 balance that favors Th2 responses; indolamine 2,3 dehydrogenase (IDO) (catalyzes tryptophan in lymphocytes, an amino acid needed for T-cell proliferation and survival); Fas ligand (immune modulating protein that induces apoptosis of maternal lymphocytes that are fetal antigen reactive); suppressor macrophages; annexin II; lowered complement activity; toll-like receptor (TLR) expression and function; local immune suppression (mediated by Fas/Fas ligand system), and possibly other mechanisms that hide trophoblastic antigens from the maternal immune system.[2,39,50,107,142,158]

Implantation, the first point of interaction between maternal and fetal tissues, involves an inflammatory process with cross-talk (molecular dialogues) between the decidua and conceptus that increases activity of innate immune cells and

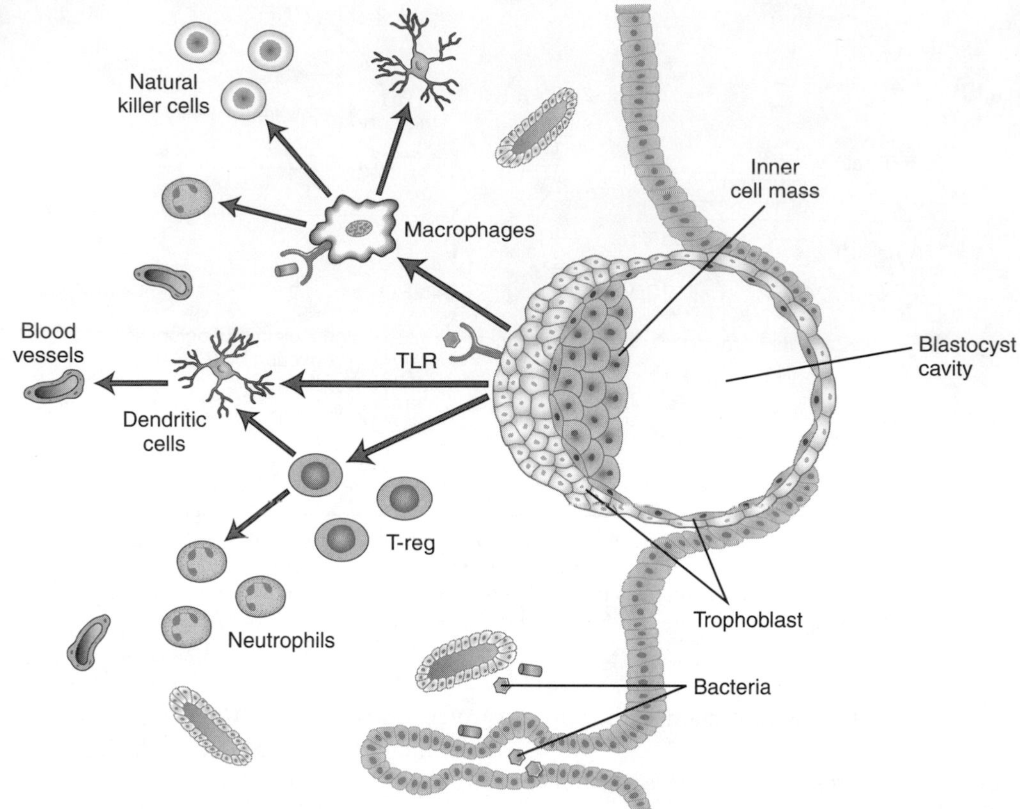

FIGURE 13-5 Trophoblast-immune interaction. This model summarizes a new perspective on trophoblast immune interaction, in which the placenta and the maternal immune system positively interact for the success of pregnancy. The trophoblast recognizes, through toll-like receptors (TLRs), microorganisms and the cellular components at the implantation site and responds to them with production of cytokines and chemokines. These factors coordinate the migration, differentiation, and function of maternal immune cells. (From Mor, G. & Abrahams, V.M. (2009). The immunology of pregnancy In R.K. Creasy, et al. (Eds.), *Creasy & Resnik's Maternal-fetal medicine: Principles and practice* (6th ed.). Philadelphia: Saunders, p. 91.)

is mediated by hormones, growth factors, cytokines, chemokines, adhesion molecules, extracellular matrix components and matrix metalloproteins.[51] The inflammatory process at the maternal-placental interface is most marked in the first and third trimesters. In the first trimester these changes occur with the initial contact between the embryonic trophoblast and maternal tissues with implantation and the remodeling of maternal blood vessels.[107] In the third trimester inflammation is a critical component of cervical changes in preparation for parturition and labor onset (see Chapter 4).[107]

After the placenta is established, the two points of contact between maternal and fetal tissues are the syncytiotrophoblast and the extravillous trophoblast. The syncytiotrophoblast is in contact with the endothelial cells of maternal spiral arteries and with the intervillous spaces, and is in direct contact with maternal blood. The extravillous trophoblast (primarily cytotrophoblast) forms the anchoring villi, which are in direct contact with maternal decidual tissue, and remodels maternal spiral arteries (see Chapter 3). Beginning in early pregnancy, small quantities of trophoblast cells detach and enter maternal blood through the uterine veins. These cells form minute emboli that eventually lodge in pulmonary capillaries and are cleared by proteolysis. This appears to be a normal process that does not lead to a maternal inflammatory response or other respiratory distress in women experiencing a normal pregnancy.

Trophoblast and Major Histocompatibility Antigens. The syncytiotrophoblast does not express either class I or class II MHC antigens, which are the main T cell targets in transplantation rejection.[124] The cytotrophoblast has a unique nonclassical MHC-I surface antigen, HLA-G, which does not stimulate the classic cytotoxic T-cell response.[85] HLA-G has a Fas/Fas ligand pathway for killing activated T cells and may help prevent maternal rejection of the fetus by inducing apoptosis of activated maternal T cells.[32,85] HLA-G inhibits NK cell cytotoxicity and dendritic cell (an antigen presenting cell) maturation.[50,176] HLA-G synthesis may be stimulated by IL-10 from the placenta. Extravillous trophoblast expresses HLA-G, HLA-C, and HLA-E (nonclassical MHC-I molecules that help these cells to evade maternal NK toxicity).[111,136,176] HLA-G acts on cells of both the innate and adaptive immune systems and has a major role in reprogramming maternal immune responses at the maternal-fetal interface.[136] Soluble HLA-G (sHLA-G) molecules are found in maternal plasma and increase from the first trimester on, peaking in the third trimester.[136] Decreased expression of

HLA-G on the extravillous trophoblast, seen in women with recurrent abortion and preeclampsia, alters conversion of the spiral arteries (see Chapter 3).[136,176] Decreased sHLA-G is found with placental abruption, miscarriage, and preeclampsia.[135]

Trophoblastic cells (specifically the villous cytotrophoblast and extravillous trophoblast) express TLRs and may be able to initiate an innate immune response in the presence of microorganisms at the site of implantation.[2,106] In addition, trophoblastic cells contain IDO, which enzymatically degrades tryptophan, a protein essential for T-cell proliferation, and TNF ligands that induce apoptosis. Together these molecules can kill activated immune cells.[158]

Natural Killer Cells. Two subsets of uterine NK cells are seen: endometrial NK cells, seen during the menstrual cycle, and decidual NK cells, which are seen during pregnancy.[124,182] Decidual NK cells are critical for pregnancy maintenance.[72] The first direct contact between maternal and fetal tissue occurs 6 to 7 days after conception at the time of implantation. Subsequently, the extravillous trophoblast cells invade the maternal endometrial lining and erode the endothelial tissues that line the maternal spiral arteries (see Chapter 3). NK cells in the pregnant decidua are phenotypically distinct from the NK cells in systemic circulation. Peripheral NK cells express $CD56^{dim}$, $CD16^{+}$, and $CD160^{+}$, a combination of characteristics that allow them to be highly cytotoxic. Conversely, decidual NK cells express $CD56^{bright}$, $CD16^{-}$, and $CD160^{-}$, which allows them to produce cytokines such as IL-8 and IL-10 that are beneficial for trophoblastic invasion.[69,72,95,111,131] These NK cells also secrete vascular epithelial growth factor (GF) and placental GF, which are angiogenic factors that promote trophoblast invasion and vascular remodling.[111,124] NK cells accumulate at the site of implantation and in the decidua. They recognize HLA-G, HLA-C, and HLA-E on the invading trophoblast and influence production of cytokines and cytolytic factors that facilitate decidualization and control of trophoblast invasion, angiogenesis, and growth.[86,95,107,119,176] Galectin-1 (Gal-1) is a carbohydrate binding protein with immunoregulatory functions that is found in high levels in uterine NK cells; Gal-1 is also found on trophoblast cells and may help reduce their cytotoxicity.[72,130] Up-regulation of Gal-1 induces differentiation of dendritic cells into a phenotype that dampens Th1 responses and suppresses autoimmune inflammation.[115] Trophoblast HLA-G can block receptors on the NK cell that initiate cell lysis. Thus the NK cell is altered to augment those functions that protect the conceptus while the general cytotoxic roles are down-regulated. Figure 13-6 illustrates how HLA-G on the trophoblast may inhibit maternal NK cells and block NK cytotoxicity toward fetal cells. Maternal stress, smoking, infection, and other factors can alter the NK phenotype and increase the risk of pregnancy complications.[72]

Decidual Macrophages. Macrophages cluster at the maternal-fetal interface and near the spiral arteries during trophoblast invasion (see Figure 13-5).[3] These macrophages produce IL-10, IDO, PGE_2, and other anti inflammatory molecules that trigger alloreactivity by the T cells to further protect the fetus.[113,158] Placental growth hormone (see Chapter 19) may also alter the maternal immune system.[158] Annexin II, a glycoprotein that binds to phospholipids, is produced by the placenta and may inhibit lymphocyte proliferation and IgG and IgM secretion at the placental site. Macrophages stimulated by Th1 cytokines or bacterial products develop a M1 phenotype and produce nitric oxide and free radicals to defend against microorganisms. Macrophages stimulated by

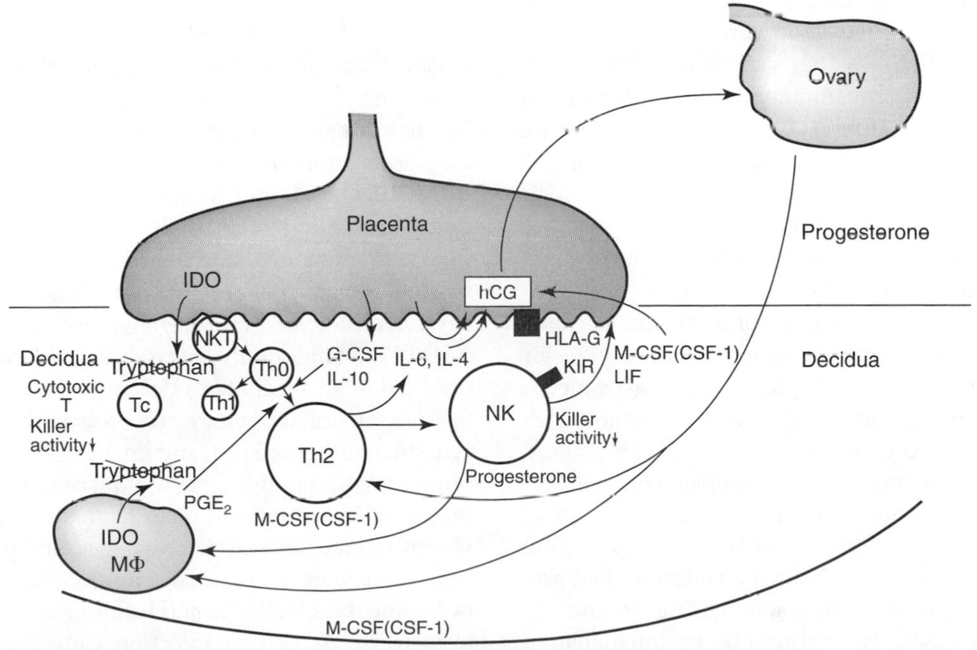

FIGURE 13-6 Cytokine and endocrine networks at the maternal-fetal interface. (From Saito, S. [2000]. Cytokine network at the feto-maternal interface. *J Reprod Immunol, 47,* 97.)

Th2 cytokines develop a, M2 phenotype and have immunosuppressive properties. M2 is the common phenotype of decidual macrophages involved in costimulatory signaling.[113]

T Cells and the Th1/Th2 Switch. Overall, there are more TCD8$^+$ cells than CD4$^+$ cells in the maternal decidua, which causes immunosuppressive activity to predominate.[107] Changes in the balance of the different T-helper subsets (Th1 versus Th2) result in strengthening of Th2 (antibody-mediated) responses and cytokines (IL-3, IL-4, IL-5, IL-6, and IL-10) and a reduction in Th1 (cell-mediated and graft rejection) responses and cytokines (IL-2, TNF-α, and IFN-γ). This distribution of cytokines at the maternal-fetal tissue interface (see Figure 13-6) is important in implantation, pregnancy maintenance, and maternal tolerance of the fetus. The Th2-specific cytokines IL-4, IL-5, and IL-10 inhibit inflammation and some macrophage functions, and down-regulate IFN-γ production, whereas the Th1 cytokines are the primary effectors of phagocytosis.[39,111,126,158] T-regulatory (Treg) cells (see Box 13-2 on page 446) normally account for 5% to 10% of peripheral CD4$^+$ T cells. These increase two- to threefold during pregnancy beginning prior to implantation, peaking in the second trimester, and decreasing by term (this decrease correlates with the decrease in progesterone).[111,127] Decreased Treg cells are seen with spontaneous abortion.[111,127] The maternal T cells interact with trophoblast cells to support remodeling of the uterine vasculature by removing apoptotic cells, producing matrix proteases, mediating immunotolerance of the fetus, and protecting the fetus from pathogens.[113]

Nevertheless, the mother initially creates a weak immune response to the fetus/placenta, as evidenced by production of antibody to paternal MHC antigens, production of specific T cells, and weak cellular sensitivity to paternal and fetal antigens.[75] This response usually results in an activation (facilitation) reaction rather than rejection response that is mediated by Th2 helper cells with release of Th2 cytokines, which down-regulate Th1 cytokines such as IL-2, IFN-γ, and TNF-α. As a result, maternal immune responses are down-regulated locally at the maternal-placental interface, but are not significantly affected at the systemic level.[39] Failure of Th2 responses to increase or of Th1 responses to decrease is associated with an increased risk of recurrent abortion.[25,101]

Role of Progesterone. Progesterone promotes production of IL-4 and IL-6, the Th1-to-Th2 switch, and IL-4.[31,50,126] Progesterone also stimulates activated lymphocytes and decidual cells to synthesize progesterone-induced blocking factor (PIBF).[39,155] PIBF stimulates B-cell production of asymmetric antibodies, which are antibodies that have a mannose-rich oligosaccharide group present on one of the Fab regions. Asymmetric antibodies cannot initiate complement or phagocytosis but they can combine with antigen. The result of this combination is an antigen-antibody complex that is univalent and functions as a "blocking antibody" that prevents further antigen-antibody interaction. PIBF also inhibits the cytotoxicity of NK cells.[39,59] Intrauterine inflammation and infection lead to decreased progesterone function and increased proinflammatory cytokines.[31] Progesterone may up-regulate TLR-4 and suppress TLR-2 to protect against preterm delivery.[31]

Transplacental Passage of Maternal Antibodies

Both protective and potentially damaging maternal antibodies cross the placenta. Maternal IgG antibodies are the only ones to cross in significant amounts. IgG has a specific carrier that facilitates active placental transport. Maternal antibody has multiple functions in the fetus and neonate including passive immunity against pathogens, epigenetic inheritance of immunologic memory, immunological imprinting, suppression of IgE responsiveness and suppression of tumor development.[87]

Fetal levels of IgG are low until 20 to 22 weeks' gestation, when passive and active transfer of IgG across the placenta increases.[164] All four IgG subclasses cross, although the IgG_1 and IgG_3 subclasses predominate and are transferred more efficiently.[164] A carrier attached to a trophoblast surface receptor that is specific for the Fc fragments of IgG (and does not bind to other immunoglobulins) mediates active transfer of IgG across the placenta.[70,164] This receptor has the greatest affinity for IgG_1 and IgG_3, followed by IgG_4 with low affinity for IgG_2; the receptor has no affinity for IgM or IgA.[81] Active transfer allows for movement of IgG to the fetus even when maternal levels are low.[70] IgG_1 crosses earliest in pregnancy and is the primary immunoglobulin transferred before 28 weeks. IgG_3 crosses later and does not reach maternal levels until after 32 to 33 weeks.[81] In most infants, IgG levels near term are higher than maternal levels.[57,82] Depending on maternal antibody complement, the newborn may have passive immunity against tetanus, diphtheria, polio, measles, mumps, group B streptococcus (GBS), *Escherichia coli,* hepatitis B virus (HBV), *Salmonella enterica*, and other pathogens.

Protection of the Fetus from Infection

Most viruses and many bacteria are capable of being transferred across the placenta, although relatively few are.[70] Immune factors that prevent maternal rejection of the fetus also protect the placenta from infectious agents.

All 10 TLRs found in humans are expressed in the placenta, primarily in the trophoblast.[107] The TLRs expressed vary with gestational age.[107,135] Each TLR is specific for the molecular pattern of certain organisms. For example TLR-4 has a receptor for gram-negative bacterial lipopolysaccharide; TLR-3 binds double-stranded viral DNA. TLRs help the trophoblast to recognize microorganisms. TLR simulation initiates an inflammatory response with up-regulation of cytokines and interferon, and up-regulation of antimicrobial proteins and peptides.[180] The placental trophoblast also secretes various antimicrobial factors to inhibit infectivity, recruit monocytes and macrophages, and prevent transmission to the fetus.[107] Aggressive microorganism invasion may overcome these defenses and lead to fetal infection and preterm labor. Ascending infection can result in a maternal immune response, production of PMNs in the amniotic fluid, and a fetal inflammatory response.[56,77,180] Altered TLR signal transduction is seen with preterm labor, preeclampsia, and intrauterine growth restriction.[77,107,135]

Occasionally organisms may reach the fetus by directly infecting placental tissue. Once the organism avoids cytokines at the maternal-placental interface, it must interact with trophoblast receptors to pass through the placental stroma and enter fetal blood. The primary placental defense is the Hofbauer (macrophage) cells. The placenta also contains phagocytes and lymphocytes and produces cytokines such as interferon.[39] The organisms most commonly transferred across the placenta are *Listeria monocytogenes*, *Treponema pallidum*, human immunodeficiency virus (HIV), parvovirus B19, rubella, *Toxoplasma gondii*, and cytomegalovirus (CMV).[114]

Amniotic fluid contains antibacterial and other protective substances similar to many of those found in human milk. These substances include transferrin, beta-lysin, peroxidase, fatty acids, IgG and IgA immunoglobulins, and lysozyme.[73,107] The antibacterial capacity of amniotic fluid improves with advancing gestation. Additionally, the fetal membranes provide barrier protection against ascending infection, although some organisms can penetrate intact membranes. Often pathogenic organisms enter the fetus via the respiratory tract, where surfactant protein (SP)-A and SP-D, alveolar macrophages, and PMNs provide additional defenses.[173,180,181]

Intrapartum Period

Initiation of labor, cervical ripening, membrane rupture, and myometrial contractility involve an inflammatory process (see Chapter 4).[31] Innate immune cells such as macrophages, dendritic cells, NK cells, and mast cells have roles in the onset of labor.[78] During labor and in the early postpartum period, the WBC count increases to values of up to 25,000 to 30,000 per mm^3. This increase is primarily due to an increase in neutrophils and may represent a normal response to physiologic stress.[35] Impairment in the functional activity of peripheral blood lymphocytes and a decrease in the absolute number of total $CD4^+$ and $CD8^+$ lymphocytes may be observed immediately after birth. Cytokines may also have a role in the initiation of labor (see Chapter 4) and in reversing the pregnancy-induced reduction of maternal immune responsiveness at the decidual-trophoblast barrier during labor and birth.[47] For example, IL-1 and IL-6 also increase with the onset of labor. TNF-α may assist in the initiation of contractions. IFN-γ may play a role in placental separation via activation of NK cells.[47]

Labor also has an effect on the fetal immune system. Labor alters neonatal neutrophil responses (see Neonatal Physiology). For example, newborns born vaginally exhibit leukocytosis, elevation of neutrophil count, and delayed apoptosis compared to infants born by cesarean section. These changes may be immunologically beneficial to the fetus.[104]

Postpartum Period

It is unclear how quickly the immune system returns to prepregnant function after delivery, with various studies reporting timelines from a few weeks to 3 to 9 months due to differences in measurement techniques.[153] The WBC count, which increases in labor and immediately after birth, gradually returns to normal values by 4 to 7 days. Progenitor cells from the fetus can be found in maternal tissue for many years postpartum.[111]

Immunologic Properties of Human Milk

The newborn is immunologically immature and therefore vulnerable to infection. Human milk contains many immunologic components, including leukocytes, immunoglobulins, and other proteins (see Table 5-4). Immunologic benefits for the breastfeeding child include lowered risk of developing asthma, cow's milk allergy, food allergy, gastrointestinal (GI) and respiratory infections, necrotizing enterocolitis, diabetes mellitus, and some immune disorders such as Crohn's disease, celiac disease, and multiple sclerosis.[45,87,116]

The leukocytes in human milk are primarily monocytic macrophages (85% to 90%) and lymphocytes (10% to 15%), with some neutrophils and epithelial cells.[45,116] Monocytic macrophages in human milk synthesize complement, lysozyme, and lactoferrin; transport immunoglobulin; and protect against necrotizing enterocolitis. These cells also have phagocytic activity against *Staphylococcus aureus*, *E. coli*, and *C. albicans* and may help regulate T-cell function.[116,175]

Similar concentrations of B and T lymphocytes are found in breast milk. B lymphocytes in human milk produce IgA, IgG, and IgM. T cells produce interferon, macrophage migration-inhibiting factor (MIF), and other cytokines. Because the neonate's own T cells are functionally immature, human milk may provide significant protection against gram-negative organisms. Human milk often contains antibodies against the O and K antigens of several *E. coli* serotypes, including K1, which has been associated with neonatal meningitis.

IgM levels are highest in colostrum, decrease after 5 days, and then remain constant for at least 180 days.[70] Levels of IgG in human milk are also consistent for at least the first 180 days. The immunoglobulin found in highest concentrations (90%) in colostrum and human milk is secretory IgA (sIgA). Levels of sIgA are highest in colostrum, fall gradually until 12 weeks, and then remain stable for the next 2 years of lactation.[90] The secretory component attached to the IgA monomer protects the IgA molecule from proteolytic digestion in the GI tract. sIgA does not enter the circulation from the gut but provides localized barrier protection by attaching to the mucosal epithelium and preventing attachment and invasion by specific infectious agents.[116] sIgA also neutralizes certain viruses and bacterial enterotoxins and inhibits intestinal absorption of proteins and other macromolecules found in foods.[116] The latter function may provide protection against the development of allergies. sIgA actions are enhanced by complement.

Human milk contains C3 and C4 and produces complement by the alternative pathway, which can be activated by factors such as bacterial products and circulating proteins. Most of the immunoglobulins in human milk are produced by sensitized antibody cells in the breast that have been transported to that site from gut-associated (i.e., maternal intestinal) lymphatic tissue and bronchotracheal-associated lymphatic tissue. Thus sIgA that is specific for a wide variety of respiratory and enteric bacterial and viral organisms can be found in human milk.[70] Depending on the mother's immunologic experience, the immunoglobulins in human milk may provide the infant with protection against pathogens such as diphtheria, pertussis, *Shigella, Salmonella*, poliovirus, and echoviruses.

Human milk contains other nonspecific protective factors that act synergistically with each other and sIgA to provide immunity to the newborn.[70,83,169,180] Lactoferrin, α-lactalbumin, and sIgA form the major whey proteins in human milk and constitute 60% to 80% of total human milk protein. Lactoferrin is an iron-binding protein that restricts the availability of iron needed for growth by certain fungi and bacteria such as *S. aureus* and *E. coli.* Folic acid and vitamin B_{12}-binding protein restrict available folate and vitamin B_{12} for bacterial and fungal growth.

Lysozyme is a bactericidal enzyme that lyses the cell walls of many bacteria and enhances *Lactobacillus* growth. Levels of lysozyme in human milk are several hundred times higher than in cow's milk. Lactoperoxidase inhibits bacterial growth and bifidus factor, a nitrogen-containing polysaccharide, promotes growth of anaerobic lactobacilli that compete with invasive gram-negative organisms. This factor also limits growth of *Shigella* and *Salmonella.* Lysozyme also acts with other substances to destroy *E. coli* and some strains of *Salmonella.* Factors in human milk that promote lactobacilli growth include lactose, low pH, and buffers.

Other immune components of human milk include. MIF; antiviral and antistaphylococcal factors; interferon (which prevents viral replication); lipase (which increases levels of free fatty acids and monoglycerides that may act against certain viruses); and oligosaccharides (which are complex carbohydrates that prevent attachment of bacteria and other antigens to gut epithelial receptors). Human milk acetic and lactic acid are two by-products of breast milk digestion in the gut. These acids decrease stool pH and inhibit growth of *Shigella* and *E. coli.* In addition, human milk can induce the production of immune factors such as sIgA by the infant. Maternal T cells in breast milk stimulate development of immune cells in the newborn thymus; thus the thymus gland of a breastfed infant is larger than the thymus in an infant receiving formula.[45,116]

In preterm infants, human milk may have a critical role in providing protection against infection and the development of allergies. The preterm infant's gastrointestinal tract lacks many intrinsic local host defense factors including sIgA, lysozyme, and gastric acid. In addition, the intestinal mucosal barrier function is more immature (see Gut Host Defense Mechanisms).[175] As a result, the preterm infant is at higher risk for bacterial penetration through the intestines and development of sepsis and necrotizing enterocolitis compared to term infants. The lack of sIgA and immaturity of the intestinal mucosa increase the likelihood of foreign macromolecules entering the circulation, which may increase the risk of allergies in genetically susceptible infants.[175] Human milk may enhance maturation of the intestinal mucosal barrier, thereby reducing the risk of both infections and allergies. Increased levels of sIgA, lactoferrin, and lysozyme have been found in milk from mothers of preterm infants.[175] Thus mothers of preterm infants may have an important immune adaptation that provides additional protection from infection for their infants.

CLINICAL IMPLICATIONS FOR THE PREGNANT WOMAN AND HER FETUS

Disruption and dysfunction of the immune system can result in disease processes (e.g., type 1 diabetes mellitus, rheumatoid arthritis, systemic lupus erythematosus [SLE], Graves' disease) the course of which can be influenced by pregnancy. In addition, immune dysfunction during pregnancy can be manifest in several ways that can adversely impact the outcome for the mother and her infant. For example, conditions such as infertility, spontaneous abortion, preeclampsia, and blood incompatibilities can be linked to immune dysfunction in the pregnant woman and/or fetus/neonate. Changes in maternal immune function during pregnancy can alter the course of preexisting disorders of the immune system and facilitate the development of some complications of pregnancy. Implications of these changes are reviewed in this section along with issues related to maternal-fetal interactions and immunization during pregnancy.

Spontaneous Abortion

There are multiple etiologies for spontaneous abortion. Immunologic factors include activation of an immune response secondary to microbial infection (e.g., chlamydia, listeriosis, parvovirus B19, or toxoplasmosis), an exaggerated maternal immune response to trophoblastic invasion (e.g., predominance of Th1 reactivity), a cytokine-induced failure of the ovary to produce sufficient progesterone, and the presence of autoimmune antibodies such as antiphospholipid antibodies that interfere with placentation.[138,142,176] Decreased expression of HLA-G on the extravillous trophoblast is seen in some women with recurrent abortion and is associated with altered conversion of the spiral arteries.[136,176] Decreased sHLA-G is also seen with spontaneous abortion.[135] Spontaneous abortion is also associated with decreased Treg cells in the decidua and increased peripheral T-cell activation.[30,111,127] Voisin suggests that some spontaneous abortions before 3 months in primiparous women may be secondary to a defect in active maternal tolerance of the fetus, whereas rejection after the third month or in women who have had a prior pregnancy may be due to excess rejection-type responses with increased levels of Th1 inflammatory cytokines such as IFN-γ, TNF-α, and TNF-β.[168]

Women who experience recurrent pregnancy loss, that is, three or more consecutive spontaneous abortions, exhibit decidual NK cell activity that is similar to the activity of NK cells in peripheral circulation, and a concomitant shift toward exaggerated Th1 immune responses instead of the usual pregnancy-exaggerated Th2 responses.[38] It is unclear whether the altered NK cells are the result of the Th1 predominance or whether the Th1 response is the result of a different population of decidual NK cells that cause spontaneous abortion instead of trophoblast expansion.

Recent evidence suggests that inadequate progesterone production occurs when the hypothalamic-pituitary-gonadal axis is inhibited by systemic immune activation that triggers a noninflammatory pathway for pregnancy failure.[43] This cytokine-induced failure of the ovary to produce progesterone results in resorption of the embryo. Both NK cells and TNF-α are effectors that can block this process by inhibiting the suppressor of cytokine signaling (SOCS) proteins, which are involved in the inhibition of progesterone production by the ovary.[43,142]

Risk of Maternal Infection

Even with alterations in host defense mechanisms, most women are not significantly immunocompromised during pregnancy nor do they experience a significant increase in the severity of bacterial infections during pregnancy.[107] However, suppression of maternal Th1 cell-mediated immunity may increase maternal susceptibility to, but not necessarily severity of, certain infections, especially viruses and certain opportunistic pathogens, including *C. albicans, Pneumocystis jiroveci* (formerly *Pneumocystis carinii*), *T. gondii, L. monocytogenes, Streptococcus pneumoniae, Neisseria gonorrhoeae, Mycobacterium tuberculosis,* polio, rubella, influenza, varicella, CMV, and herpes simplex virus (HSV).[40,47,107] Genetic polymorphisms in the genes that encode modulators of innate mucosal immunity, such as IL-6, IL-8, and TNF-α, may increase the risk of altered vaginal microflora.[52] Alterations in neutrophil chemotaxis and function also contribute to the persistence of infections during pregnancy.[48,129] Changes in the frequency of infections during pregnancy are also due to other reasons. For example, the increased incidence of urinary tract infections and pyelonephritis during pregnancy is primarily due to anatomic alterations in the urinary tract that result in urinary stasis (see Chapter 11).

Viral infections, however, are seen more frequently during pregnancy, especially during the second and third trimesters, and tend to be more severe. For example, in pregnant women, primary varicella is more likely to result in pneumonia and increased morbidity and the risk of complications with influenza is increased (see Chapter 10).[40]

Although methodological limitations are prevalent, most studies of HIV infection find that pregnancy does not appear to significantly increase the risk of death, disease progression, or $CD4^+$ counts below 200, although there are suggestive trends for these events to occur in some studies.[8] Antiviral therapies during pregnancy have significantly reduced perinatal transmission and improved outcomes for HIV-infected women and their infants.[8,40,104] Infected women experience a greater reduction in $TCD4^+$ cells during pregnancy and a longer time to return to normal after pregnancy than noninfected women, but the effects are equivocal.[8,80]

Fungal infections are also seen more frequently during pregnancy with an increase in symptomatic vulvovaginitis during the third trimester. The increased incidence of fungal infections is related to increased adherence of *Candida* to vaginal mucous membranes, increased glycogen in the vagina, enhanced proliferation of *Candida* under the influence of estrogen, and alterations in cell-mediated immunity.[40] The incidence of infection with protozoa (e.g., malaria, amebiasis) and helminthic (intestinal parasites) organisms is increased in countries where these organisms are prevalent. During pregnancy, malaria is more frequent and more severe, with an increased risk of sequelae. The malaria parasite has an affinity for placental tissue, leading to stillbirth and preterm birth. In addition, malaria is a major cause of low birth weight in endemic areas.[47] Latent malaria can be reactivated by iron overload during pregnancy.

Inflammation, Infection, and Preterm Labor

Inflammation (decidual, chorioamnionic, or systemic) is a significant etiologic factor in preterm labor (see Chapter 4 and Figure 4-7). "Preterm labor is a syndrome initiated by multiple mechanisms including intrauterine infection, utero placental ischemia or hemorrhage, uterine overdistention, cervical disease, stress, endocrine disorders, and other immunologically mediated processes."[31,p. 209] Many of these processes lead to inflammation at the maternal-fetal interface. Onset of labor involves inflammatory mediators, which these events can trigger.

Both acute and chronic maternal infections are associated with preterm labor. Intrauterine infection leads to activation of the innate immune system. Recognition of microorganisms by TLRs results in release of inflammatory chemokines and cytokines. Proinflammatory cytokines (IL-1β, TNF-α, IL-8, Il-6) in combination with microbial endotoxins increase prostaglandin production and release of matrix metalloproteases and other substances that can lead to cervical ripening, fetal membrane rupture, and increased myometrial contractility.[31]

Urinary tract infections have also been associated with preterm labor (see Chapter 11). Maternal fever can lead to maternal dehydration, resulting in increased uterine activity, which, along with elaboration of prostaglandins, may result in initiation of labor. In women with acute infections, high temperature alone may lead to the release of catecholamines and corticotropin-releasing hormone and increase uterine irritability. Preterm labor is discussed further in Chapter 4.

Although high levels of IgG and sIgA in maternal cervical mucus may provide protection against infection from vaginal pathogens, vaginal and cervical organisms have been linked with the initiation of preterm labor and premature rupture of membranes.[63,139] Both these events are probably mediated via inflammatory cytokines that stimulate prostaglandin $E_2\alpha$ production.[139]

Chorioamnionitis and Cerebral Palsy

Chorioamnionitis or inflammation of the placental membranes increases the risk that the fetus will develop cerebral palsy.[53,178] Although the exact mechanism has not been completely determined, several processes may contribute to the underlying pathophysiology. Elevated levels of fetal cytokines produced in response to maternal infection may directly injure the fetal brain or cause damage indirectly by increasing the permeability of the blood-brain barrier and facilitating passage of cytokines and microbial products into the brain. The presence of microbial products may induce an inflammatory process in the brain that damages the fetal brain and induces periventricular leukomalacia. Inflammation of the placental membranes may contribute to cerebral palsy by interfering with gas exchange and inducing a hypoxic-ischemic injury in the fetus (see Figure 6-4). Maternal fever may raise the core temperature of the fetus, which could be harmful to the fetal brain. Finally, maternal infection could cause direct infection of the fetal brain. Although the fetus is more susceptible to adverse effects of maternal infection early in gestation, the placenta is a poorer barrier against some pathogens late in gestation. Consequently, while adverse fetal effects of maternal infection are more likely at early gestational ages, the incidence of fetal infection is more likely late in pregnancy.[178] The attributable risk of cerebral palsy secondary to chorioamnionitis is estimated as approximately 12% in term infants and approximately 28% in preterm infants.[178]

Immunization and the Pregnant Woman

Alterations in the immune system during pregnancy do not seem to significantly alter the woman's responses to immunization.[42,47,49] Potential risks associated with immunization during pregnancy include fetal viremia, teratogenesis, interference with development of the infant's response to immunizations during childhood, and maternal side effects that might compromise uteroplacental function.[143]

Ideally, immunization of women of childbearing age should occur at least 3 months before conception (or immediately after delivery) to reduce the risk of infection and adverse fetal effects.[13,42] Immunity can be achieved by either passive or active means. At times, passive immunizations may be recommended during pregnancy after accidental or potential exposure to an organism associated with significant maternal or fetal risks.[13] Passive immunity involves transfer of antibodies from an actively immunized to a nonimmunized person and confers short-term protection until the antibodies are catabolized by the nonimmunized person's system. The physiologic transfer of antibodies from mother to fetus and injection of γ-globulin are both examples of passive immunity.

Active immunity involves exposure to some form of the antigen (attenuated or live organisms rendered noninfectious, inactivated or killed organisms, inactivated exotoxins or toxoids) that stimulates the production of antibodies and memory cells against that antigen by the nonimmunized person. Active immunization induces long-lasting or permanent immune responses.[42,143]

Immunization of pregnant women with live attenuated viruses or bacteria is not recommended because there is a small risk of transfer of the antigen to the fetus.[42,154] Immunization with measles (rubeola), mumps, and rubella vaccines is specifically contraindicated because of potential adverse fetal consequences. However, if a woman is accidentally vaccinated for rubella early in pregnancy, the risk of adverse fetal effects appears to be low, and therapeutic abortion is not recommended.[42] Inactive (i.e., dead) viruses (e.g., pneumococcal, influenza, diphtheria, tetanus, hepatitis B) are considered safe for use in pregnancy.[13,14,42,154] Since the risk of influenza-related morbidity is increased during pregnancy, influenza vaccinations are recommended for all pregnant women during flu season, regardless of trimester.[15,42] Administration of immunization for rubella during the first few days after birth is often recommended. The woman who receives rubella vaccine should be counseled to use methods to prevent conception for at least 4 weeks.[13,143]

Blood and blood products given within 14 days of active immunization may interfere with the effectiveness of the vaccine, because blood may contain antibodies against the antigens in the vaccine and therefore interfere with the woman's own immune response.[172] Although there is a small theoretic risk of transfer of antigens through breast milk or nasopharyngeal secretions from a recently immunized woman to her infant, this is a rare event without significant reported morbidity.[172] Current recommendations regarding specific immunizations during pregnancy can be found in several reviews.[13,49,143,154]

Malignancy and Pregnancy

Theoretically, alterations in the maternal immune system could increase the risk of malignancy because cell-mediated immunity, which is suppressed in the pregnant woman, normally protects against virally induced tumors. Some investigators have suggested that there is an increase in rate of progression and decreased survival times in women with breast and cervical cancer during pregnancy, but this has generally not been supported.[33] However, a delay in diagnosis (due to breast changes during pregnancy with increased engorgement and nodularity) may result in a more advanced stage at time of diagnosis.[33] Gestational breast cancer (diagnosis during pregnancy, lactation, or the first year postpartum) tends to involve "larger tumors, more frequent nodal involvement, metastasis and vascular invasion."[33, p. 893] The effect of pregnancy on malignant melanoma is also variable.[33] Melanoma may intensify during pregnancy and, then recede or disappear after delivery.[171] The basis for this change has been attributed to increased levels of melanocyte-stimulating hormone during pregnancy (see Chapter 14) and hormonal stimulation of estrogen receptors found on melanoma cells.

Immunologic Aspects of Preeclampsia

Preeclampsia is a complex, multifaceted disorder involving alterations in many major body systems (see Chapter 9 and Table 9-5). There is increasing evidence that vascular endothelial cell injury is an early event in the pathogenesis of preeclampsia.[132,133,148] The exact cause of this damage is unclear but an immunologic role has been suggested.[9,132,133,148] Factors that support an immunologic basis for preeclampsia include an increased incidence of the disorder in primigravidas or, in the case of multiparas, a pregnancy with a new partner or different sperm donor; an increase in pregnancies with a large placental mass (e.g., multiple pregnancies) or hydatidiform mole; a decreased incidence in repeat pregnancies (even if the previous pregnancy ended in a miscarriage) with the same father and consanguineous marriages; a decrease with longer cohabitation with the father before pregnancy (and thus exposure to paternal antigens in semen); and the presence of pathologic changes in the uterine vessels near the placental site that are similar to those with allograft rejection.[132,133,148]

Specific alterations in the immune system have been observed in women with preeclampsia. Many of these changes are exaggerations of the inflammatory changes normally found during pregnancy. However, women with preeclampsia have a further reduction of NK cell activity with increased peripheral and reduced decidual NK cells (which alters placental development and spiral artery remodeling), altered macrophage activation, more $TCD8^+$ cytotoxic cells, decreased $TCD4^+$-to-$TCD8^+$ ratio, more immune (antibody-antigen) complexes, increased levels of fibronectin, decreased IDO activity, and alterations in complement.[9,25,132,133,148] In women with preeclampsia the usual Th1/Th2 pattern during pregnancy is altered so that Th1 predominates with increased levels of inflammatory cytokines, including TNF-α, IL-2, IL-6, and IL-8, but reductions in IL-10.[9,31,133,138,148] In addition, increased expression of TLRs by the interstitial trophoblast or alterations in TLR signal transduction may contribute to local abnormal cytokine levels that lead to the development of preeclampsia.[9,77,107,135] Decreased placental HLA-G expression and sHLA-G are also reported.[100,133,136,148,176] These changes alters conversion of the spiral arteries and increase the risk of vascular endothelial injury, which appears to be the underlying mechanism that results in preeclampsia.

The Pregnant Woman with an Autoimmune Disease

The effect of pregnancy on autoimmune disorders is varied; individual women experience improvement, exacerbation, or no change depending on the disorder. These differences may be related to the immune mechanism involved in the specific disorder; that is, whether the disorder involves alteration in Th1 responses (which decrease during pregnancy) or Th2 responses (which increase). Autoimmune disorders are thought to impair T-suppressor cell activity, resulting in hyperactive B-lymphocyte response and production of autoantibodies that form immune (antibody-antigen) complexes with their target antigens.[122] Autoantibodies damage tissue either by directly reacting with antigens on the surface of cells or by combining with antigens to form immune complexes.[121,122] The immune complexes activate the complement cascade, which in turn stimulates phagocytosis, inflammatory responses, and tissue damage.

Because the usual changes in the immune system during pregnancy are the exact opposite of these events, women with autoimmune disorders may experience an improvement in their symptoms.[121,122] For example, 75% of women with rheumatoid arthritis experience improvement during pregnancy (which is associated with increased Th1 mediators, which are decreased in pregnancy), followed by a relapse within the first 3 months postpartum.[92,111,184] Other changes during pregnancy that might lead to this amelioration include changes in plasma levels of maternal humoral factors, depression of cell-mediated immunity, and suppression of inflammatory reactions.[92,97,111,122,184]

Pregnancy is unlikely to alter the natural history of SLE unless the woman has nephritis or is experiencing a flare at the time of conception.[97] However, SLE can adversely impact the course of pregnancy.[30] Women with mild disease that is under control for 6 to 12 months before and during pregnancy usually experience no exacerbation of SLE during pregnancy, and some may improve. Exacerbation, when it occurs, has been reported to be more frequent in early pregnancy and during the first 6 to 8 weeks after birth.[184] Postpartum exacerbation may represent a rebound phenomenon as suppression of cell-mediated activity is terminated.[122]

SLE involves production of autoantibodies of the IgG class and increases in Th2 mediators, which are increased in pregnancy normally.[122] Women with SLE who have anticardiolipin antibodies or lupus anticoagulant antibodies have an increased risk of thrombosis, spontaneous abortion, thrombocytopenia, preeclampsia, fetal growth restriction, and preterm birth.[92,97,159,170] Lupus anticoagulant factor is an immunoglobulin that binds to prothrombin-activating complexes and predisposes the woman to recurrent thrombosis in the spiral arteries and placental infarction. Some women with SLE who have anti-Ro/SS-A or anti-LA/SS-B will have a fetus with neonatal lupus erythematosus.[92,103] These infants have congenital heart block, cutaneous lupus rashes, cytopenia, and possibly other systemic manifestations. This syndrome is usually transient and resolves after birth, although complete heart block may not be transient.[92] Fetal heart block occurs because the anti-Ro/SS-A or anti-LA/SS-B antibodies lodge in the fetal cardiac conducting system and interfere with conduction pathways.[24]

Fetal and Neonatal Complications Associated with Transplacental Passage of Maternal Antibodies

Potentially damaging IgM class antibodies, such as the ABO antigens, and allergy-producing IgE antibodies generally do not cross the placenta. Smaller, potentially damaging maternal IgG antibodies may cross the placenta as a result of Rh incompatibility (see next section) or one of several maternal chronic diseases, leading to transient disorders in some neonates.[64] Neonatal effects from the passage of these IgG antibodies range from mild to severe. In general, if the disorder is not fatal during the perinatal period, manifestations are transient and regress as maternal antibody is catabolized.

Maternal Graves' disease may involve transplacental passage of a thyroid-stimulating immunoglobulin resulting in transient neonatal hyperthyroidism (in approximately 1% of offspring) that can persist for up to 2 to 6 months.[84,128] Myasthenia gravis is associated with passage of maternal IgG against acetylcholine receptors, resulting in transient myasthenia gravis in 10% to 20% of offspring. Symptoms can last from a few hours to up to 3 months.[152] Because symptoms usually develop after 12 hours of age, infants who appear healthy at birth may later develop respiratory failure.[18] The delay in symptom onset may be due to transfer of anticholinesterase drugs from the mother or elevated AFP.[152] Maternal antiplatelet antibodies induce fetal thrombocytopenia in up to 50% of the offspring of women with immune thrombocytopenia. The greatest neonatal risk is for severe hemorrhage in the perinatal period. In most infants, platelet levels reach lowest levels at 4 to 6 days after birth and return to normal by 1 to 2 months.[18] Risk to infants from antibody passage in women with SLE is described in the previous section.

Rho(D) Isoimmunization and ABO Incompatibility

Rho(D) isoimmunization can be used as a model to examine the application of immunologic principles and to illustrate how the interaction of maternal and fetal host defense mechanisms can result in pathophysiologic processes during the perinatal period. *Isoimmune hemolytic disease, hemolytic disease of the newborn (HDN),* and *erythroblastosis fetalis* are all terms for a disorder caused by transplacental passage of maternal IgG antibody that reacts with antigens on the fetal red blood cell (RBC) and leads to cell lysis. The fetal-neonatal effects include an increased risk of neonatal hyperbilirubinemia and, in severely affected infants, can include severe anemia, congestive heart failure, and death. Because maternal antibody remains in the infant's circulation, the hemolytic process continues after birth.

The Rh system involves a group of at least 45 different RBC surface antigens controlled by genes encoding Rh proteins (DCE). The Rh locus is on the short arm of chromosome 1.[102] A related protein, Rh glycoprotein, is essential for expression of the Rh antigen. Antigens of the D group are the ones usually involved in incompatibility between mother and fetus. Rho(D) isoimmunization occurs when an Rho(D)-negative mother carrying an Rho(D)-positive fetus produces antibody against the D antigen on the fetal RBC. Isoimmunization can also occur with other RBC antigens such as Kell, Duffy, Kidd, MNS, and the ABO system.

Rho(D) isoimmunization is of particular clinical importance because the D antigen is a potent antigen, is present in large amounts on the fetal RBC, appears as early as 6 weeks' gestational age, and stimulates formation of IgG-type antibody and memory cells in the mother.[62] The amount of antigen necessary to trigger an immune response in the mother varies for each person, as does the intensity of the response by the mother's immune system. The incidence of Rho(D) isoimmunization is relatively low, ranging from 10% to 14% if Rho(D) immune globulin (RhIG) is not given after birth to less than 2% if RhIG is given.[23,61] The R_2 phenotype (cDE) expresses the most D antigen and increases the risk of maternal sensitization.[162] Rho(D)-negative women are unlikely to have antibodies against the D antigen unless they have been immunized during a previous pregnancy or from a mismatched blood transfusion. As a result, isoimmunization is rare in first pregnancies. Normally during pregnancy the small amounts of fetal blood (less than 0.05 mL) that cross the placenta and enter the maternal circulation are too small to trigger production of antibodies by the mother's immune system. In a few women, however, as little as 0.01 mL of fetal blood has been reported to cause maternal immunization (sensitization).[23] Detectable fetal blood cells can be found in approximately 3% of pregnant women in the first trimester, 12% in the second trimester, and 45% in the third trimester.[62,162] Approximately 1% to 2% of Rho(D)-negative women develop anti-D antibodies during their first pregnancy.[23] This number can be reduced by prophylactic administration of RhIG during pregnancy.

At birth, larger quantities of fetal blood (0.5 mL or more) may enter the maternal circulation. This amount of fetal blood (if the fetus is Rho[D] positive) is sufficient to stimulate formation of both anti-D antibody and memory cells in many women (Figure 13-7, *A*). Formation of memory cells results in permanent immunization. During subsequent pregnancies, even a very small amount of blood from an Rho(D)-positive fetus entering the mother's system may be enough to trigger memory cells to produce antibodies against the D antigen on the fetal RBC. The antibodies that are produced in this secondary response are predominantly of the IgG_1 and IgG_3 subclasses and are thus actively transported across the placenta (see Transplacental Passage of Maternal Antibodies) to the fetal circulation where they hemolyze fetal RBCs (see Figure 13-7, *B*). With development of RhIG (a human γ-globulin concentrate of anti-D), initial active immunization of most Rh-negative women can be prevented. RhIG is given prophylactically at 28 weeks to prevent immunization during pregnancy; in the first 72 hours after birth if the newborn is Rh-positive; or after any potentially immunizing events such as an abortion, ectopic pregnancy, amniocentesis, or significant antepartal bleeding. A dose of RhIG at 28 weeks provides protection for approximately 12 weeks (i.e., until term).[62,102] The incidence of immunization during pregnancy is 1.6% to 2%, decreasing to 0.1% to 0.18% with administration of both antenatal and postpartum RhIG.[62,102,162] RhIG does not cause hemolysis in the fetus even though the majority of the antibodies are transported across the placenta.[61,93,162]

RhIG destroys fetal RBCs in the mother's system before the foreign D antigen on these cells can be recognized by her immune system and trigger formation of antibodies and, more importantly, memory cells (see Figure 13-7, *C*). However, the exact mechanism by which RhIG acts to prevent alloimmunization is unclear.[102] Three potential mechanisms have been suggested for the action of RhIG: (1) clearance of antigen from the mother's system; (2) antigen-blocking by attaching to antigenic sites on the fetal cells, thereby preventing interaction with maternal lymphocytes; or (3) central inhibition of antibody production.[23,26,62,162] The last theory suggests that RhIG forms immune complexes with the Rho(D) antigen. Immune complexes suppress the stimulating effect of helper T lymphocytes, which in turn suppresses antibody formation by B lymphocytes.[62,162]

The standard dose (300 mcg) provides protection for up to 15 mL of fetal RBCs.[62] Because development of an adequate antibody response to a specific antigen can take days or weeks

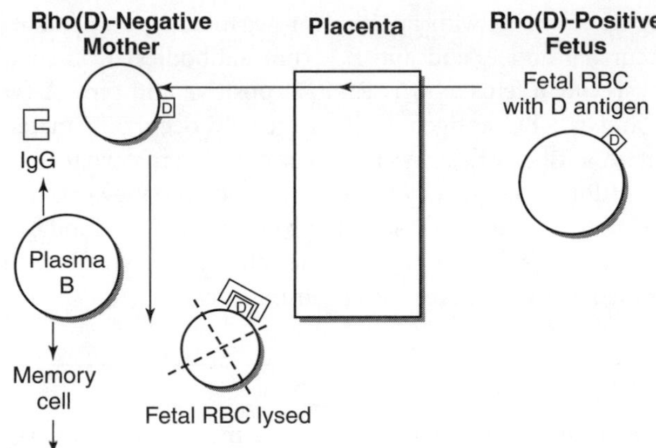

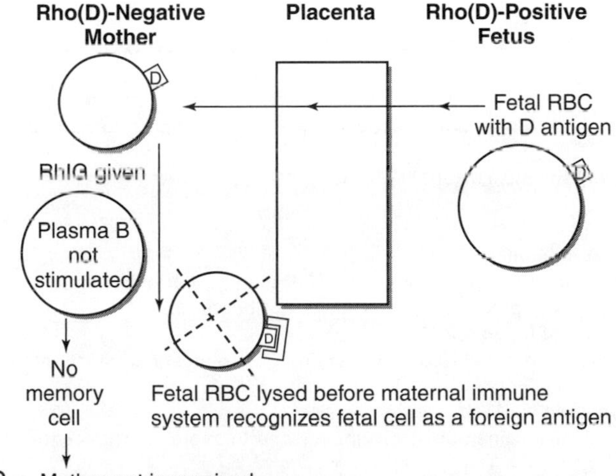

FIGURE 13-7 Rh isoimmunization. **A,** Process of immunization if Rho(D) immune globulin (RhIG) is not given to a previously nonimmunized woman. **B,** Action of maternal immune system in subsequent pregnancies once the mother has been immunized. **C,** Role of RhIG in prevention of maternal immunization.

in persons not previously sensitized, RhIG can probably be given up to at least 2 weeks after birth (possibly longer) if omitted earlier for some reason.[62] After antenatal administration of RhIG, some women may develop a low (1:4 or less) anti-D serum antibody titer. This positive titer reflects a passive immunity from the RhIG. The infant of a mother who received RhIG prophylaxis within 12 weeks may have a weakly positive direct Coombs test due to placental transfer of RhIG antibodies. Neither of these responses indicates maternal immunization, and postpartum RhIG administration is indicated.[23,62]

ABO Incompatibility

The potential for isoimmunization also exists with ABO incompatibility, although severe hemolytic disease in the fetus and newborn is rare even though ABO incompatibility is three times as common as Rho(D) incompatibility. Previous exposure and immunization are not necessary with ABO incompatibility because the mother already has naturally occurring antibodies against fetal RBC antigens. The most common situation in which ABO incompatibility occurs is with a type O mother and a type A (Figure 13-8, *A*) or, less frequently, type B infant. The A antigen seems to be more antigenic than the B antigen. The type O mother has naturally occurring anti-A and anti-B

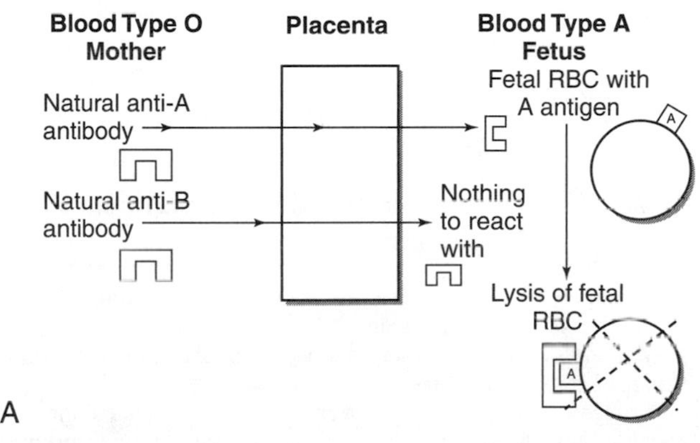

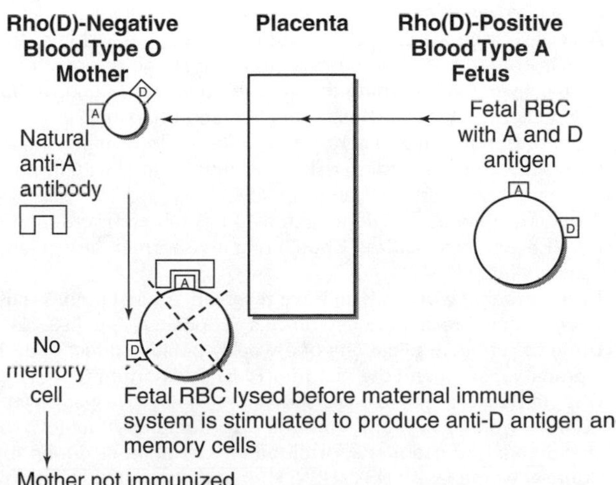

FIGURE 13-8 ABO incompatibility. **A,** Mechanisms of ABO incompatibility. **B,** Mechanism by which ABO and Rh incompatibility—occurring simultaneously—reduce the severity of Rh incompatibility.

antibodies in her serum that can react against the A or B antigens on the fetal RBCs. ABO incompatibility could also occur with a type AB infant but never with a type O infant (type O RBCs have neither A nor B antigens for maternal anti-A or anti-B antibodies to identify and react against).

Why is ABO incompatibility a relatively mild disorder compared with Rho(D) isoimmunization? The primary reason is that the antibodies of the ABO system are primarily IgM, which does not cross the placenta. However, rarely these antibodies may be of the IgG type. IgG antibodies of the ABO system are more common in persons with type O blood; hence ABO isoimmunization occurs most frequently between mothers who are type O and their type A or type B infants. Because A and B antigens also appear on somatic cells and are secreted into body fluids in most people, there is a large quantity of antigen to compete with the fetal RBCs for any maternal antibody. In addition, the fetus may have its own anti-A or anti-B antibodies that can neutralize maternal antibody. There are fewer A and B antigens than D antigens on the fetal RBCs, and these antigens are relatively weak, resulting in only a weakly positive Coombs test. ABO isoimmunization and probably Rho(D) isoimmunization do not occur in the opposite direction (i.e., from baby to mother) because fetal antibodies tend to be in a macroglobulin form that cannot cross the placenta.

The simultaneous occurrence of Rho(D) and ABO isoimmunization has a protective effect that reduces the likelihood of maternal Rho(D) sensitization. This is illustrated in Figure 13-8, *B*, with an Rho(D)-negative, type O (naturally occurring anti-A and anti-B serum antibodies) woman who is carrying a fetus who is Rho(D)-positive and type A (with A and B RBC antigens). The naturally occurring maternal anti-A antibody destroys fetal cells entering maternal circulation (during pregnancy or at delivery) before they can trigger the mother's immune system to produce anti-D antibodies and memory cells. If anti-D antibodies and memory cells are not formed, the woman remains unimmunized.[23,162]

SUMMARY

Alterations in maternal host defense mechanisms are critical for maintenance of the pregnancy, ensuring that the mother does not reject the fetus, and protecting the fetus against infection. Yet these same mechanisms may increase the risk of infection and other immune system disorders in the pregnant woman. Transplacental passage of maternal immunoglobulins provides protection against specific pathogens but can also lead to fetal disease. Concerns related to organisms that colonize the maternal genital tract (e.g., GBS) and sexually transmitted diseases such as HSV, HBV, and HIV have increased interest in host defense mechanisms and maternal-fetal interrelationships, and altered clinical practice in recent years. Recommendations for clinical practice based on changes in host defense mechanisms are summarized in Table 13-5. By recognizing the changes in maternal host defense mechanisms,

Table 13-5 Recommendations for Clinical Practice Related to Changes in Host Defense Mechanisms: Pregnant Woman

Recognize normal parameters for immune system components and patterns of change during pregnancy and the postpartum period (pp. 443, 445, 449-451, Table 13-4).
Obtain and evaluate complete history for possible exposure to infectious organisms, current illness, or presence of autoimmune disorders (pp. 456-459).
Recognize risk factors for development of specific infections (p. 457, Table 13-4).
Monitor and counsel women regarding early signs and symptoms of infection (p. 457).
Recognize clinical and laboratory changes during labor and delivery and postpartum that may mask signs of infection (p. 455 and Chapter 8).
Assess women with infections during the second and third trimesters for signs of preterm labor (p. 457 and Chapter 4).
Teach women methods to prevent or reduce the risk of infection while pregnant (pp. 456-459).
Counsel woman regarding the immunologic advantages of human milk and its potential role in preventing gastrointestinal infections and allergies (pp. 455-456, Table 5-4, and Chapter 12).
Monitor iron intake and serum ferritin levels in women with a history of malaria (p. 457).
Counsel women regarding risks of immunizations with live attenuated or killed vaccine during pregnancy and to avoid pregnancy for 3 months after immunization (p. 458).
Avoid giving immunizations within 14 days of administration of blood or blood products (except RhIG) (p. 458).
Give RhIG to unsensitized Rho(D)-negative women prophylactically at 24 to 30 weeks' gestation and after potentially immunizing events (pp. 460-461).
Recognize that women who have received antenatal RhIG may have low antibody titers for approximately 13 weeks yet may still need RhIG postpartum if the newborn is RH positive (pp. 460-461).
Understand the implications of a weakly positive direct Coombs' test in some infants of women who have received RhIG during the prenatal period and the need for RhIG postpartum (p. 461).
Give RhIG postpartum to unsensitized Rho(D)-negative women with a Rho(D)-positive newborn in the first 72 hours following birth (pp. 460-461).
Counsel women with autoimmune disorders about potential effects of pregnancy on course of disease (p. 459).
Use Standard Precautions for blood and body fluids during the perinatal period (pp. 457, 475).
Counsel women with HBV, HSV, HIV, and other viral infections regarding long-term effects on infant (including shedding of virus) and use of precautions to prevent spread of the infection (p. 457).
Counsel women with chronic disorders associated with transplacental passage of antibodies regarding the potential impact on their fetus and neonate (pp. 459-461).

health care providers can identify women and infants at risk and initiate appropriate interventions and counseling.

DEVELOPMENT OF HOST DEFENSE MECHANISMS IN THE FETUS

Cellular components of the immune system develop from precursor cells within blood islands of the yolk sac (see Chapter 8). Multipotential stem cells arise in these islands and migrate into the liver and spleen and later to the bone marrow and thymus. The mucosal immune system is developed by 28 weeks' gestation, but not activated until after birth, unless the infant is exposed to an intrauterine infection.[54]

B and T lymphocytes arise from common lymphoid stem cells. Pre–B cells are seen in the liver by 7 to 8 weeks; immature B lymphocytes with surface IgM receptors and complement are found in the fetal liver by 10 weeks.[70,82] By 12 weeks, B lymphocytes that have IgG and IgA cell surface receptors are seen in peripheral blood, bone marrow, liver, and spleen; numbers reach adult values by 15 weeks.[114,174] Fetal synthesis of immunoglobulins begins by 10 to 14 weeks; however, levels of fetal immunoglobulins produced by the fetus normally remain low throughout gestation.[66,174] Fetal serum IgG levels rise in the second and third trimesters primarily secondary to increased transplacental passage from the mother (see Transplacental Passage of Maternal Antibodies). Secretory IgA is not produced by the fetus/neonate until after birth. Elevated IgM levels in cord blood (greater than 20 mg/dL [greater than 0.20 g/L]) suggest intrauterine infection and may be seen in newborns with congenital cytomegalovirus (CMV), rubella, or toxoplasmosis. This IgM is of fetal origin as IgM does not cross from the mother.

Differentiation of the thymus begins at 6 to 7 weeks.[105] The thymus develops as an outgrowth of the third and fourth pharyngeal pouches. The rudimentary thymus on each side of the body grows toward midline. These structures fuse by 8 weeks and then gradually descend into the chest.[99] Stem cells from the liver and spleen migrate to the thymus to form thymocytes. T lymphocytes appear in the thymus by 7 weeks and in the blood by 12 weeks.[174]

Differentiation of $CD4^+$ and $CD8^+$ surface antigens begins around 10 weeks.[70] Mature $CD4^+$ and $CD8^+$ T lymphocytes are detected in the liver and spleen by 14 weeks, and in the fetal circulation by 15 to 16 weeks' gestation.[66,114] By midgestation, T cells are capable of secreting interleukin (IL)-2; tumor necrosis factor (TNF)-α; TNF-β; and, to a lesser extent, interferon (IFN)-γ, IL-3, IL-4, IL-5, and IL-6.[114] TNF, IL-1B, and IL-6 are found in amniotic fluid and increase to term; elevation of IL-6 is seen with intrauterine infection.[74,180] Surfactant protein (SP)-A and SP-D are elevated in amniotic fluid and may also have an immunoregulatory function.[173,181] Th1 responses tend to be inhibited by IL-10 from the placenta.[96] Innate responses are characterized by IL-23 directed immunity, which promotes development of Th17 $CD4^+$ and enhances defenses against extracellular pathogens.[176] Production of IL-12 , which induces IFN-γ production by $CD4^+$ T cells and NK cells, and differentiation of Th1 cells, is decreased.[176] Transplantation responses develop relatively early. Antigen recognition can be demonstrated by 12 weeks, and graft-versus-host reactions by 13 weeks' gestation. The fetus can increase production of proinflammatory cytokines with intrauterine infections and mount an inflammatory response. However, this may increase the risk of brain injury, especially white matter damage, and cerebral palsy (see section on Chorioamnionitis and Cerebral Palsy and Chapter 15).[74]

The fetal immune system is dominated by Th2 to "avoid proinflammatory Th1 type alloimmune responses to maternal tissue that may trigger preterm birth or spontaneous abortion."[125] IL-6, IL-10, and IL-23, and Th17 mediated immune responses are all up-regulated with increased production in response to bacterial lipopolysaccharide-binding protein.[176] TNF-α, IL-1B, and Th1 mediated immune responses are down-regulated in the fetus and amniotic fluid. This decreases the extent and duration of proinflammatory immune responses that can lead to preterm birth.[176] An exaggerated fetal immune response has been linked to periventricular leukomalacia and cerebral palsy in addition to preterm labor onset.[176]

White blood cells arise initially from yolk-sac stem cells (see Chapter 8). Neutrophils and macrophages arise from colony-forming unit–granulocyte-macrophage progenitor stem cells.[70] Myelopoiesis is 10 times more active in the fetus than in the adult and increases fourfold by the second trimester.[76] Granulocytic cells from which neutrophils arise can be found in fetal blood by 6 to 8 weeks and mature neutrophils by 14 to 30 weeks.[82,114] After 5 months, neutrophils are produced primarily in the bone marrow. Few granulocytes are found in peripheral blood during the first half of gestation (e.g., at 22 to 23 weeks' gestation, the fetus has approximately 2% of the neutrophils found in cord blood), but by term the number of granulocytes is similar to those observed in adults.[70]

Embryonic macrophages are found by 3 to 4 weeks in the yolk sac. By 4.5 weeks, approximately 70% of the blood cells in the liver are macrophages, decreasing to 1% to 2% over the next 6 weeks.[145] IL-1 produced by fetal macrophages up-regulates granulocyte colony stimulating factor production by fetal monocytes in the fetal liver and bone marrow.[82] True monocytes appear in the blood at 5 months, with levels increasing after 6 months when bone marrow hematopoiesis begins to predominate.[145]

Natural killer cells (which have a major role in surveillance against viral infection) are found in the liver and blood by 5 to 6 weeks; however, basal activity of these cells is almost undetectable until after 20 weeks' gestation and does not increase significantly until after 32 weeks.[108] "The fetus develops the capacity to recognize and respond to invading microorganisms through the action of toll-like receptor–initiated pathways and the production of proteins, such as antimicrobial peptides and lipopolysaccharide (LPS)-binding protein."[176, p. 141]

Complement protein synthesis by the fetal liver begins as early as 6 weeks, but individual components develop gradually and are not seen until 8 to 14 weeks; serum complement is seen after 20 to 22 weeks.[19] Complement increases rapidly after 26 to 28 weeks, but still may be only 50% to 75% of that of an adult by term.[70,174] Complement is not transferred across the placenta.

In summary, an innate immune response can be identified in the fetus early in gestation, while adaptive immune functions remain inactive until term. However, adaptive immune functions may be activated in some fetuses in the presence of fetal infection. In terms of the functional development of the immune system, 32 to 33 weeks' gestation seems to be a critical time. Before this point, the immune responses of the fetus or preterm infant are compromised in comparison with the term neonate.[108] However, after this time the preterm infant's immune system rapidly approaches that of term infants, although the immune system of these infants is still immature compared to that of adults.

NEONATAL PHYSIOLOGY

Newborns are vulnerable to infection because of (1) altered host defense mechanisms, particularly in the preterm infant, and (2) a lack of experience and exposure to many common organisms, resulting in delayed or diminished adaptive immune responses to foreign antigens. The newborn's immune system is adapted for fetal and early newborn life with decreased Th1 cytokine production and increased Th2 cytokines.[180] These adaptations are an advantage for the fetus, because the lower levels of Th1 cytokines reduce both the risk of alloimmune rejection between the mother and fetus and the risk of excessive inflammation that can lead to preterm birth, and during the early newborn period to allow for skin and gut colonization and induction of host defense functions.[125,177,180] However, after birth these adaptations increase the neonate's vulnerability to infection. Alterations in neonatal host defense mechanisms are found in innate immune system responses, inflammatory responses, antibody and cell-mediated immunity (i.e., adaptive immunity), and the complement system. (See Boxes 13-1 and 13-2 on page 446 for a review of innate and adaptive immunity.) Table 13-2 includes definitions of immune terminology. The newborn is also susceptible to infections as a result of other factors, including (1) entry of pathogenic organisms due to the breaks in mucosal or cutaneous barriers that may occur during birth; (2) gastrointestinal (GI) infections and potentially later development of allergies due to immaturity of the gut host defense mechanisms; and (3) disruption of skin barriers from invasive procedures, the use of tape and monitor leads, and intravenous catheters in infants who are born prematurely or who are ill.

Transitional Events

With the transition to extrauterine life, newborns move from the usually sterile, protected environment of the uterus into an environment filled with organisms, some of which are potentially pathogenic, and other antigens that challenge their still immature host defense mechanisms. During the initial days after birth, the newborn must contend with several challenges to the immune system, including (1) development of normal microorganism flora on mucosal surfaces (skin, respiratory system, and GI tract); (2) responding to bacterial colonization by potential pathogens; (3) processing exposure to dietary proteins that are potential allergens; (4) responding to exposures to other ingested or inhaled environmental agents with antigenic potential; and (5) beginning the transition from Th2-dominated fetal responses.

Skin Colonization

Newborns are initially colonized with organisms from the maternal genital tract acquired during the birth process. This is followed by colonization with maternal skin flora and other organisms present in the newborn's environment. The maternal genital tract flora at delivery normally includes *Lactobacillus, Escherichia coli,* and protective anaerobes, but it may also contain potentially dangerous organisms such as group B streptococcus (GBS) and *Chlamydia trachomatis.* Colonization occurs initially on the skin, umbilical cord, and genitalia, followed by mucous membranes of the eyes, ears, throat, and nares.[107] Skin flora is more extensive in infants with little or no vernix caseosa, which normally acts as a protective mechanical barrier.[107]

Intestinal Colonization

The normal intestinal microorganisms have both nutritional and immune system functions.[112,163] Immune functions include providing a barrier against pathogens, stimulating gut host defenses, and modulating inflammatory responses and intestinal permeability.[112,163] Nutritional functions include synthesis of vitamin K, short chain fatty acids, and biotin.[112]

Colonization of the GI system occurs in two stages. During the first stage (birth to 1 week), the infant is inoculated with organisms that he or she comes into contact with during and after birth. In the second stage (1 to 4 weeks), the infant's diet significantly influences the pattern of bacterial flora. The normal gut flora provides an important protective mechanism against GI infections by occupying potential pathogen-binding sites on intestinal mucosa. The upper small intestine is usually sterile or sparsely colonized, probably due to the gastric pH, or possibly due to the antibacterial properties of bile, secreted immunoglobulins, and normal intestinal motility (see Chapter 12). Coliform colonization of the upper small intestine can occur in very low–birth weight (VLBW) infants and infants who are intubated or fed by transpyloric tube. The decreased intestinal motility of preterm infants may predispose them to intestinal bacteria overgrowth.[27] Gut colonization occurs by attachment of organisms to glycoconjugate receptors in the intestinal mucosal surface. Oligosaccharides in human milk help prevent colonization with pathogenic organisms by competing for mucosal bacterial receptors.[46]

Meconium is usually sterile at birth, except perhaps after prolonged ruptured membranes. Bacteria can be found in meconium within a few hours of birth and increase rapidly over the next few days. Use of antimicrobial drugs during labor partially suppresses but does not prevent colonization and may result in a shift in the dominant gut flora and an increase in resistant flora.[160]

In the first few days after birth, the neonate may be further protected from potentially pathogenic gut organisms by the acidity of gastric secretions (which inhibits growth of gram-positive and gram-negative bacteria) and by immaturity of the gut epithelium (which alters attachment of pathogenic organisms). Infants for whom oral feedings are delayed are more likely to have no bacterial growth in fecal samples. The intestines of these infants are similar to the germ-free state. This state is associated with a slower mucosal cell turnover (which allows toxins to have a more profound effect), fewer lymphoid cells in the gut, and alterations in gut immune responses that may increase the risk of infection.[94]

Breastfed infants develop different colonization patterns from formula-fed infants. These different patterns may reflect physicochemical differences and the influence of antimicrobial factors in human milk.[46,110,139] The lower buffering capacity of human milk (due to lower concentrations of proteins and minerals) allows acids from bacterial metabolic end products to increase. The resulting acidic environment is one in which *Lactobacillus* and *Bifidobacterium* thrive, preventing growth of acid-sensitive organisms such as bacteroides and enterobacteria. The low protein and phosphate and high lactose contents of human milk also promote growth of these flora. Protective substances in human milk (see Table 5-4 and Immunologic Properties of Human Milk) may stimulate secretory IgA (sIgA), strengthen epithelial tight junctions, and possibly modify intestinal inflammatory and allergic responses.[116] Antimicrobial factors found in human milk may also alter gut colonization patterns. For example, lactoferrin is an iron-binding protein that is only 9% saturated in human milk. As a result, lactoferrin can bind iron entering the gut that is not absorbed and reduce the availability of iron for bacteria metabolism.[116]

Formula feedings buffer the acid produced by gut bacteria. This leads to an alkaline environment in which the bifidobacteria cannot compete with gut enterobacteria. Gram-negative enterococci become the dominant gut organism. As formulas become more similar to human milk, differences in colonization, although present, are less apparent.[34,46,139] Current research is examining the use of prebiotics such as galacto-oligosaccharides and fructo-oligosaccharides in formula-fed infants to stimulate intestinal flora similar to that of breastfed infants in order to enhance intestinal mucosal development.[118]

Alterations in Innate Immunity

The inflammatory response and phagocytosis (see Figures 13-1, 13-2, and Box 13-1 on page 446) in the newborn are different when compared with adult function because functional limitations of the infant's polymorphonuclear monocytes (PMNs) affect leukocyte metabolic activities, mobilization, chemotaxis, adhesion, opsonization, phagocytic activity, and intracellular killing. The neonate's PMNs are more rigid (due to an altered cytoskeleton), less deformable (due to generation of less actin), and have a poorer response to chemotactic stimulators and impaired receptor mobilization.[76,144] These limitations alter movement kinetics and orientation of the PMNs. The neonate's PMNs are less able to leave the blood vessel to reach the site of pathogen invasion because of the decreased deformability. The newborn's PMNs have less ability to adhere to the vascular epithelium, leading to poorer aggregation of PMNs along the vessel wall near the site of injury.[22,66,76] L-selectin expression, which is critical for initial neutrophil adhesion to vascular endothelium and migration, is low in neonates and decreases in the first 24 to 72 hours; levels are even lower in preterm infants.[22,76,144,180] Neonatal neutrophils have a three- to fourfold decrease in bactericidal permeability-increasing protein, which may increase the risk of gram-negative sepsis.[22]

Neonatal PMNs do not respond as readily as those of older individuals to chemotactic factors.[28,70] Chemotaxis (see the definition in Table 13-2) in neonates is about half as efficient as chemotaxis in adults, resulting in slower, more random movement of neutrophils and monocytes to the site of antigenic invasion.[28,76,180] This is secondary to the structural and functional limitations of neonatal PMNs and due to lower levels of chemotaxis stimulating substances in the neonate's blood. These limitations are exacerbated in septic infants.[180] The increased IL-6 production reduces PMN migration; however, IL-8 priming during labor improves PMN chemotaxis.[180,183] Other factors that alter chemotaxis include impaired PMN calcium metabolism, altered actin polymerization and adhesion defects.[76] In the fetus, the chemotaxis response is consistent from 24 weeks to term, decreases after birth, and then increases to reach adult levels in term infants by about 2 weeks of age.[28,22,140] In preterm infants, chemotaxis does not begin to respond efficiently until 2 to 3 weeks after birth and develops slowly.[28] The reason for this is unclear. Achievement of chemotaxis function at adult levels is delayed in more immature preterm infants, with less than two thirds of them achieving adult values by 42 weeks.[140] Therefore these infants remained at higher risk for infection even after reaching their due dates.

Newborns, particularly preterm infants, have decreased serum opsonic activity, resulting from low levels of immunoglobulins and complement components. In addition, neonates have difficulty recognizing and destroying encapsulated bacteria unless the pathogen is first opsonized by attaching complement fragments and immunoglobulins (see Table 13-2).[144]

Most studies report that phagocytic activity in the healthy term newborn is similar to phagocytic activity in adults, although newborn phagocytic cells are less responsive to stimulation by chemotaxic factors.[66,70] Thus phagocytosis is diminished to some extent by the decreased availability of neutrophils (the primary circulating phagocyte) at the invasion site due to altered chemotaxis. Macrophage (the primary tissue phagocyte) activity in response to cytokines (see Tables 13-2 and 13-3) from T cells is also decreased. Phagocytic activity and intracellular bactericidal activity of PMNs are probably not significantly different from the same function in adults in most healthy infants and are similar to adult levels by about

2 weeks.[18,28,70] However, some authors have reported that even healthy preterm infants born at less than 33 weeks' gestation have a poorer phagocytosis response for the first few months of life, possibly due to poor opsonization.[22]

Activated neutrophils normally undergo apoptosis within 24 to 48 hours. Neonatal neutrophils have a delay in apoptosis, prolonging their survival, possibly related to decreased expression of caspase-3, a component of several apoptosis pathways. The increased survival may be an advantage in fighting infection, but the elongated activation may increase the risk of chronic inflammation and disorders such as chronic lung disease.[76]

Phagocytosis has been found to be normal in most stressed neonates, although decreased phagocytosis toward some gram-negative bacteria has been reported. Infants who experience health complications either in utero or after birth (e.g., hypoxic-ischemic events, respiratory distress, meconium aspiration, sepsis, or hyperbilirubinemia) demonstrate significantly decreased bactericidal activity in response to both gram-positive and gram-negative organisms. Bactericidal activity may be reduced even further in VLBW infants who weigh less than 600 g.[18] The cause is unclear but may relate to developmental immaturity with intrinsic alterations or defects in leukocyte metabolic activity, or it may result from peroxidative damage to the cell.[66] There are several changes in cellular metabolism associated with phagocytosis including the respiratory "burst" with a rapid increase in oxygen consumption, the hexose monophosphate (HMP) shunt that is involved with glycolysis activity, and the production of toxic oxygen metabolites necessary for bactericidal activity. These activities are reduced in term infants with sepsis and in preterm infants of less than 34 weeks' gestation.[22,28,180] In preterm infants these metabolic processes remain low for the first 1 to 2 months of life.[22,28]

The number of neutrophils varies during the first few days after birth, with an increase after birth that peaks at 12 to 24 hours, declines to 72 hours, then remains stable during the neonatal period.[70,76] This increase is blunted and lower levels are seen in preterm infants.[76] The increase after birth is probably due to movement of marginated neutrophils into the main circulation.[76,144] PMN levels below 3000 m^3 in the first 3 days or below 1500 m^3 after the first 3 days are unusual in term infants; neutrophil levels may normally be as low as 1100 m^3 in preterm infants.[70] Although low PMN levels are normally associated with neonatal infection, they are also seen in infants born prematurely or after hypoxic-ischemic events, and in infants with intraventricular hemorrhage or Rh hemolytic disease.[70]

Bone marrow reserves, which are neutrophil storage pools (NSPs), are lower in the neonate, especially preterm infants. This is due to a reduction in granulocyte macrophage–colony-stimulating factor (GM-CSF).[28,76,82] Approximately one third of preterm infants have a functional neutropenia.[122] In neonates, especially preterm infants, the marrow is probably functioning at or near capacity for neutrophil proliferation. Therefore these infants are less able to increase production much further with infection and the NSP becomes exhausted more rapidly.[89,122,180] This may account for the neutropenia and shift to the left (release of immature forms of neutrophils) often seen with sepsis, especially in VLBW infants.[28]

Toll-like receptors (TLRs) and antigen presenting cells (APC) (see Box 13-1 on page 446) are different in neonates than adults. Neonatal TLR-mediated cytokine response is characterized by decreased Th1 proinflammatory cytokines (TNF-α, IL-12, IL-1B, IFN-γ) due in part to progesterone, PGE2, and plasma adenosine levels.[91,125,180] Plasma adenosine is increased with hypoxia and stress and inhibits TNF-α production by the monocytes and production of Th1 cytokines.[180] Labor up-regulates TLR-4 on monocytes and PMNs.[147,180] SP-A, SP-D, and alveolar macrophages act as pattern recognition and signaling molecules via interaction with TLRs, CD-14$^+$, and other components of the innate system.[173] TLRs may play a role in the pathogenesis of necrotizing enterocolitis, in particular, abnormal TLR-4 signaling in the intestines.[7,179] TLR-4 is a receptor for lipopolysaccharides (a component of the outer membrane of gram-negative bacteria). The altered signaling by TLR-4 limits innate responses to these organisms.[7]

APC function is decreased in the neonate resulting in increased reliance of the innate system for pathogen removal.[180] Cord blood dendritic cells have an immature phenotype and low chemokine levels, decreased endocytoxic activity, decreased antigen presenting and costimulatory capacity, and produce low levels of IL-12.[91] Neonatal dendritic cells require greater stimulation for activation and are poorer stimulants of T-cell proliferation with impaired IL-12 production.[180] Neonatal APCs express low levels of costimulatory molecules such as CD40, CD80, and CD86.[70] This characteristic, along with low IL-12 production by APCs and IFN-γ by neonatal T-helper cells reduces the infant's ability to induce Th1 responses and may lead to immune tolerance rather than response.[91,180]

The number of monocytes in infants is highest in the first 24 hours after birth and then decreases over the next month.[145] Neonatal monocyte chemotaxis and phagocytosis are altered during sepsis with a decreased delivery of these macrophages to infection sites.[70,82,89,125,180] Neonatal monocytes and dendritic cells have impaired expression of MHC II and costimulatory molecules, reducing antigen presentation to CH4$^+$ T cells.[180] Synthesis of interferon (IFN)-γ, interleukin (IL)-8, IL-10, extracellular matrix proteins, fibronectin, and leukotrienes by neonatal monocytic macrophages is reduced.[82] Monocyte antibody-dependent cellular cytotoxicity is about 50% of adult values.[82] Monocyte adhesion is similar to that of adults.[57] Monocytic bactericidal activity and processing of antigens are generally considered to be adequate.

Fibronectin, a glycoprotein found in plasma and tissues, inhibits bacterial adherence to epithelial cells; enhances antibody binding of bacteria such as staphylococci and GBS; and is involved in opsonization and clearance of fibrin, immune complexes, and platelets. Neonatal levels of plasma fibronectin average 50% of adult values, with the lowest levels seen in preterm infants and those with hypoxic-ischemic events or respiratory distress.[18,70,89] C-reactive protein (CRP) synthesis is similar in uninfected neonates and adults. A diminished CRP response has been observed in the first 12 to 24 hours after birth in infants infected with group B streptococcus.[67]

Numbers of natural killer (NK) cells, which provide protection against tumors or virus-infected cells, are similar to or greater than those in adults, but NK activity is reportedly decreased to 15% to 60% of adult activity.[58,70,89] Neonatal NK cells are phenotypically different from those of adults with a lower cytolytic capacity.[58] Most adult NK cells are $CD56^{high}$, whereas most neonatal NK cells are $CD56^{low}$, a more immature form.[57] Neonatal NK cells are less able to bind to target cells and have limited lytic ability.[89] The altered activity is probably mediated by the decreased levels of interferon and other cytokines that normally augment NK cell function. NK cells in preterm infants have decreased cytotoxic function.[57]

In general, the total number of circulating lymphocytes is similar to adult levels at birth but falls during the first 3 days and plateaus by 10 days of age. The ratio of T lymphocytes to B lymphocytes is lower in cord blood than in adult blood.[70] Neonatal mast cells secrete more histamine than adult cells, which alters dendritic cell cytokine production. Mast cells may play a role in development of erythema toxicum.[180]

APCs (including monocytes, macrophages, and dendritic cells) in the neonate "exhibit deficits in pathogen recognition, activation after stimulation, phagocytic function, bactericidal function and amplification of the immune response that may increase the risk for development and progression of EONS [early-onset neonatal sepsis]."[180, p. 314] The ability of neonates to localize infection is limited. As a result, septicemia is more likely to develop in neonates from spread of the pathogenic organism to the blood and cerebrospinal fluid. A major factor in this inability to localize infection is impaired chemotaxis. Adequate phagocytosis and killing of many pathogenic organisms such as GBS depend on complement (especially C3) and opsonic activity. Serum concentrations of C3 and thus opsonic activity are proportional to gestational age, further increasing the risk of sepsis in preterm infants.[70]

The inability to localize infection results in clinical manifestations of infection that are different in the newborn compared to the adult, and this can make the diagnosis of sepsis in the neonate difficult. Specifically, signs of sepsis in the neonate are often subtle and nonspecific, involving changes in activity, tone, color, or feeding. In addition, neonates have a poor hypothalamic response to pyrogens; therefore fever is not a reliable indicator of infection in the neonate. Alterations in innate immunity are summarized in Table 13-6.

Alterations in the Complement System

Newborns have decreased serum levels of both classical and alternative pathway components (see Figure 13-3), defective complement activation, and a decrease in complement receptors.[18,19,174,180] Components of the classical system in the term neonate are slightly reduced or comparable to adult values, whereas levels of these factors are significantly reduced in preterm infants and correlate with gestational age (see Table 13-7).[70] For example, levels of several key complement proteins (C1, C3, C4, C7, C9) are 55% to 75% of adult values in term infants, and 10% to 30% of adult levels in 28-week preterm infants. The lower levels of complement proteins result in decreased opsonization, decreased chemotaxic activity, and decreased cell lysis. Limited alternative pathway activity and marked reductions in properdin are seen in two thirds of newborns.[18,70] The classical and alternative pathways are further depressed in infants with documented sepsis.

Alterations in Adaptive Immunity

Cell-mediated and antibody-mediated (humoral) immunity is developmentally immature in both preterm and term neonates (see Table 13-6). Response of the adaptive system to APCs is less efficient than in adults.[180] Box 13-2 on page 446 and Figure 13-2 provide a review of adaptive immunity.

Alterations in Cell-Mediated Immunity

Absolute numbers of T lymphocytes in the newborn are higher than in adults, but the functional ability of newborn T cells is decreased, as is the diversity of specific T-cell receptors, which results in a delay in the response to specific organisms.[5,89] Cytotoxic activity of neonatal T cells is 30% to 60% less than in adults, and cytokine production is reduced.[101] Examples of cytokines and their roles are found in Table 13-3; cytokine production in the newborn is summarized in Table 13-8.

T-suppressor activity tends to dominate in the newborn.[108] Although Th2 (antibody-mediated) helper responses are the dominant response in the neonate, the T-helper cells provide relatively poor support of B cells.[144] For example, neonatal T cells do not induce neonatal B cells to produce some of the immunoglobulins that adult B cells would produce.[37] $CD4^+/CH25^{high}$ Treg cells are found in high levels in cord blood.[44,125] These cells suppress T-cell proliferation in response to cytokines and Th1 cytokine (especial IFN-γ) production thus limiting adaptive responses. This is an advantage in limiting autoimmunity but also limits responses to infection and vaccines.[125]

At birth most of the T lymphocytes are primary cells (i.e., naive cells) with few secondary memory T cells. Neonatal naive T cells differ from adult naive T cells in that the neonatal cells have a higher turnover rate and limited Th1 responses.[96] Primary T cells release less cytokine and have a diminished response to antigens.[37,114,139,144] The most prevalent T-cell phenotype in the neonate is the $CD45RA^+$ (naive) cell. These cells account for 90% of the neonate's T cells, decreasing to 50% (similar to adults) by 10 years of age. $CD45RA^+$ cells are "naive" because of the fetus's lack of exposure to foreign antigens. When exposed to a foreign antigen presented by a B lymphocyte or dendritic cell, the neonatal $CD45RA^+$ cells differentiate into $CD45RO^+$

Table 13-6 Alterations in Host Defense Mechanisms in the Neonate

ALTERATION	RESULT	IMPLICATION
INNATE IMMUNITY		
Structural alterations of PMNs	Altered movement kinetics and orientation of PMNs	Delayed initial response to invasion by pathogenic organisms
Altered PMN chemotaxis, adherence, and L-selectin expression	Slower movement to site of antigenic invasion Poorer PMN aggregation and adherence	Less able to localize infection Increased risk of generalized sepsis
Decreased NSP	Decreased ability to increase PMN production with sepsis	Neutropenia and more immature PMNs Increased risk of generalized sepsis
Decreased fibronectin	Delayed initial response to infection	Less able to localize infection Increased risk of generalized sepsis
Decreased NK activity	Decreased opsonization, lysis Delayed initial response to infection	Less able to localize infection Increased risk of generalized sepsis
Poor hypothalamic response to pyrogens	Fever is not a reliable sign of sepsis	Signs of sepsis often subtle and nonspecific
Altered respiratory "burst" and bactericidal activity in stressed and VLBW neonates	Decreases ability to destroy pathogens	Increased risk of severe infection
COMPLEMENT		
Decreased complement proteins C1, C3, C4, C7, and C9	Decreased opsonization	Decreased ability to localize infection
Deficient activity of alternative pathway	Decreased chemotaxis Decreased cell lysis	Decreased opsonization and ability to eliminate organisms with capsular polysaccharide coats such as GBS Increased risk and severity of bacterial sepsis
ADAPTIVE IMMUNITY: CELL–MEDIATED IMMUNITY		
Decreased T-cell function (reduced cytokine production, cytotoxic activity)	Reduced defenses against viral and fungal infections Alteration in B-lymphocyte function	Increased risk of severe infection and generalized septicemia
Down-regulation of Th1 responses	Decreased cell-mediated helper functions	Increased risk and severity of infection from herpes, CMV, and other TORCH organisms
Reduced levels of IL-4, IL-8, IL-12, and IFN-γ	Altered cell-mediated responses, immunoglobulin production, and innate responses	Increased risk of severe or overwhelming infection Less able to localize infection Increased risk of generalized sepsis
Naive T cells	Delayed responses to specific pathogenic organisms	Increased risk of viral and fungal infections
ADAPTIVE RESPONSES: ANTIBODY-MEDIATED IMMUNITY		
Decreased IgG in preterm infant due to lack of maternal transfer	Reduction in maternal antibodies that provide passive immunity against selected organism	Reduced defense against many pathogens
Decreased IgG_2 isotype	Decreased opsonization of organisms with capsular polysaccharide coats	Increased risk of bacterial sepsis, especially from gram-positive cocci (GBS)
Decreased IgA and absent sIgA	Reduced defense against GI and respiratory infections	Increased risk of respiratory and GI infections
Decreased IgM with less specificity	Reduced defense against viral and gram-negative organisms	Increased risk of *E. coli* sepsis and rubella, syphilis, toxoplasmosis, CMV, and other viral infections
Altered B-cell function due to altered T-cell activity and cytokine production	Slower switch from IgM to IgA and IgG production	Increased risk of severe infection and generalized septicemia
Lack of previous exposure of B cells to many organisms, with few memory cells	Delayed specific responses to pathogenic organisms	Increased risk of severe or overwhelming infection

CMV, Cytomegalovirus; *Ig*, immunoglobulin; *GBS*, group B streptococci; *GI*, gastrointestinal; *IFN*, interferon; *IL*, interleukin; *NK*, natural killer cells; *NSP*, neutrophil storage pool; *PMN*, polymorphonuclear neutrophils; *Th1*, T helper 1; *Th2*, T helper 2; *VLBW*, very low birth weight.

Table 13-7 Published Ranges of Complement Levels in Neonates

COMPLEMENT COMPONENT	Mean % of Adult Levels (Number of Studies)	
	TERM NEONATE	PRETERM NEONATE
CH*50*	56-90 (5)	45-71 (4)
AP*50*	49-65 (4)	40-55 (3)
Clq	61-90 (4)	27-58 (3)
C4	60-100 (5)	42-91 (4)
C2	76-100 (3)	67-96 (2)
C3	60-100 (5)	39-78 (4)
C5	73-75 (2)	67 (1)
C6	47-56 (2)	36 (1)
C7	67-92 (2)	72 (1)
C8	20-36 (2)	29 (1)
C9	<20-52 (3)	<20-41 (2)
B	35-64 (4)	36-50 (4)
9	33-71 (6)	16-65 (3)
H	61 (1)	—
C3bi	55 (1)	

From Lewis, D.B. & Wilson, C.B. (2001). Developmental immunology and role of host defenses in fetal and neonatal susceptibility to infection In J.S. Remington & J.O. Klein (Eds.), *Infectious diseases of the fetus and newborn infant* (5th ed.). Philadelphia: Saunders.

(memory) cells.[99] The neonatal CD45RO$^+$ cell is capable of producing significant amounts of cytokines (e.g., IFN-γ, TNF-α, GM-CSF) and acting as a helper cell for B-cell function.[37,114,139,144] However, because the newborn's T cells have no previous experience with most antigens until exposed and sensitized after birth, it probably takes 4 to 6 weeks for the newborn to achieve minimal adaptive immune protection.[18]

Impairment of cytokine production alters cell-mediated immunity, immunoglobulin production, and innate responses.[94,98] Although some cytokine production by neonatal T cells is altered, IL-1, IL-2, and IL-6 levels are normal or slightly reduced. However, levels of IL-4, IL-8, IL-12, and IFN-γ are reduced.[82,88,98] The decrease in IL-4 and IFN-γ is consistent with the "naive" state of CD45RA$^+$ cells.[55,96] IL-8 levels are markedly lower in preterm infants, limiting neutrophil mobilization and chemotaxis.[55] Development of necrotizing enterocolitis and bronchopulmonary dysplasia in preterm infants has been postulated to be related in part to unregulated cytokine production.[70] Genomic polymorphisms in gene encoding for production of cytokines may help explain individual differences in neonatal susceptibility to sepsis.

Neonates have down-regulation of Th1 responses with a decreased capacity to produce cytokines thus promoting Th1 (cell-mediated) responses with a blunted response to activation by IFN-γ, possibly due to decreased signal transduction.[6,17,88,96,99] This may increase susceptibility to oropharyngeal candidiasis.[98] Neonatal T cells are able to increase cytokine production when stimulated. For example, CD8$^+$ cytotoxic T cells can be stimulated and reach near adult levels of function in some cases with cytomegalovirus (CMV) exposure.[65,96] However, neonatal T cells require greater stimulation as well as stimulation from additional factors (e.g., accessory cells and signaling molecules) than adult cells to achieve full activity.[5,70,144] Cell-mediated immunity is further depressed in small-for-gestational-age (SGA) infants. These infants have a smaller proportion of T lymphocytes and altered lymphocyte function than appropriate-for-gestational-age (AGA) infants, perhaps secondary to alterations in thymic activity. The thymus of SGA infants is smaller in weight and volume and demonstrates histologic alterations and decreased activity of thymic inductive factors, which may contribute to immune dysfunction in these neonates.

Alterations in Antibody-Mediated (Humoral) Immunity

The fetal and neonatal differences in antibody-mediated immunity are primarily due to the alterations in T-cell activity, immature cytokine function, and the effects of passive immunization from immunoglobulins acquired transplacentally

Table 13-8 Production of Selected Cytokines in the Newborn

CYTOKINE	SOURCE	ACTIVITY	NEWBORN PRODUCTION
IL-1	Macrophage	T and B proliferation; Ig synthesis	Normal
IL-2	T cell	T and B proliferation; induction of IL-2 receptors	Normal to low
IL-4	T cell	B-cell proliferation; Ig switch	Low
IL-6	T and B cells, macrophages, endothelial cells	T and B activation; Ig production	Normal to low
IL-10	T cell	Inhibits T help; Ig production	Low
IL-12	T and B cells; macrophages	Promotes NK killing and antigen-dependent cytolysis	Low
IFN-γ	T cell	Inhibits Ig production; increases MHC expression; promotes antigen presentation	Low

From Schelonka, R.L. & Infante, A.J. (1998). Neonatal immunology. *Semin Perinatol, 22,* 7.
IFN, interferon; *Ig,* immunoglobulin; *IL,* interleukin; *MHC,* major histocompatibility complex; *NK,* natural killer cell.

and/or through breastfeeding. Activity of B cells requires signaling from the interaction of surface antigen and T-helper cells to amplify the immune response.[70] Because T-cell activity and cytokines are needed to enhance B-cell function, there is a reduction in fetal and neonatal production of immunoglobulins.[66,82] T-cell–dependent B responses have a delayed onset, peak at lower levels, are of shorter duration, and show different IgG isotypes than in adults.[70,96] T-cell–independent B responses are also deficient, especially in response to antigens with capsular polysaccharide coats such as group B streptococcus.[96,149] Neonatal B cells have fewer IL-5 receptors, decreased activation by IL-10, and poorer responses to Th2 antigens.[79,149] Many neonatal B cells have CD5+ surface antigens (B1a cells). B1a cells are not dependent on T-cell help for activation as are conventional B cells (B2).[79,114] However, neonatal T cells do not stimulate B cells to switch production of immunoglobulins from IgM to IgG or IgA. As a result, neonates produce primarily IgM and little IgG and IgA, even when exposed to bacteria with polysaccharide capsules.[79,144] Neonatal B cells in response to vaccine antigens tend to differentiate into memory B cells rather than antibody-producing plasma B cells.

The total amount of immunoglobulin at birth is 55% to 80% of adult values, and primarily consists of IgG from the mother.[82] Levels of serum immunoglobulins after birth are illustrated in Figure 13-9. Neonatal IgG values reflect the IgG acquired from the mother either transplacentally or via breast milk.[89] The newborn can produce IgG_1 in a manner similar to that of an adult; however, IgG_2 production is reduced to about 2 years. IgG_2 is important for defense against polysaccharide antigens such as are seen with GBS, K1 forms of *E. coli, Haemophilus influenzae,* pneumococcus, and meningococcus.[82] Development of antibody responses is primarily dependent on postbirth age rather than Postmenstrual age.[57]

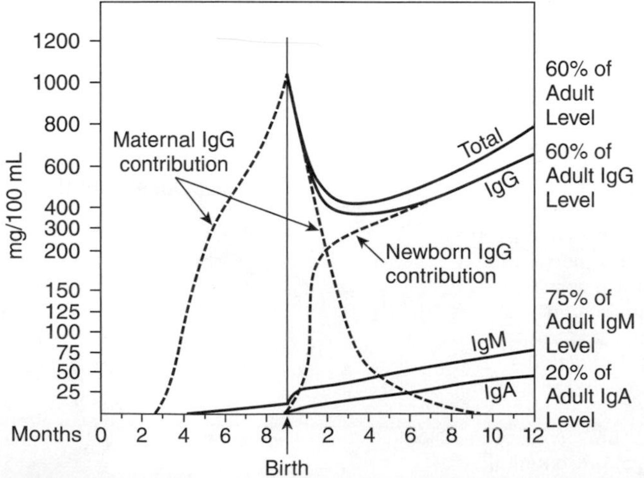

FIGURE 13-9 Immunoglobulin levels in the fetus, newborn, and infant. (From Stiehm, E.R. [1989]. *Immunologic disorders in infants and children* [3rd ed.]. Philadelphia: Saunders.)

IgG is important for immunity to bacteria, especially gram-negative organisms, bacterial toxins, and viruses.[70,174] Neonatal values depend on gestational age because placental transfer of IgG increases during the third trimester. Thus preterm infants may have inadequate protection. For example, cord blood values of IgG are minimal in infants born at 24 to 25 weeks' gestation and average 400 mg/dL (4.0 g/L) at 32 weeks and 1500 mg/dL (15 g/L) at term.[114,174,180] Term IgG levels are 90% to 95% of adult values and 5% to 10% higher than maternal values.[70,140] Levels of IgG are lower in SGA infants, possibly due to impaired placental transport of maternal IgG.[89] After birth, levels fall gradually as maternal IgG is catabolized. Because significant production of IgG by the infant does not occur until after 6 months, all infants experience a transient "physiologic hypogammaglobulinemia" (see Physiologic Hypogammaglobulinemia) in the first 6 months. However, as a result of IgG transfer in breast milk, the neonate continues to get antibodies against infectious agents for which the mother has circulating antibodies because of previous exposure or immunization (see Table 5-4).

IgA is important for localized immunity in the GI and respiratory tracts. As stated above, IgA does not cross the placenta in significant amounts. Neonatal (term and preterm) values are low (0.1 to 5 mg/dL [0.001 to 0.05 g/L], which is less than 2% of adult values). Elevated IgA is found in cord blood after maternal-fetal transfusion and occasionally with intrauterine infection, although IgM is seen more commonly after fetal infection.[114] sIgA is not found in neonates at birth but can be detected in saliva, tears, and intestinal mucosa by 2 weeks to 2 months.[82] sIgA occurs as a monomer or is attached to a polypeptide chain (secretory component). The polypeptide chain provides resistance to pH changes and protects the IgA molecule from proteolytic digestion in the GI tract.

IgM, which also does not cross the placenta, is important for protection against blood-borne infections and can trigger multiple effector functions of the classical complement cascade.[174] IgM is the major immunoglobulin synthesized in the first month of life.[5,66,122] IgM levels increase rapidly by 2 to 4 days after birth, probably secondary to stimulation from environmental antigens, although neonatal values are low (5 to 15 mg/dL [0.05 to 0.15 g/L]), with means of 6 mg/dL (0.06 g/L) at 28 weeks' gestation and 11 mg/dL (0.11 g/L) at term, which is approximately 10% of adult values.[70,89] The fetus is capable of producing significant IgM in response to exposure to certain antigens, such as the TORCH organisms, after 19 to 20 weeks' gestation, which may be due to activation of the fetal B1a cells.[114] However, neonatal IgM has less specificity than adult IgM in responding to specific antigens, which may hinder the initial recognition of pathogenic organisms. IgE and IgD do not cross the placenta in significant amounts, and newborn values are less than 10% of adult values.[66]

Few B cells that have differentiated into immunoglobulin-secreting cells (IgSCs) are seen in the first 5 days after birth, and those that are found are mostly IgM-secreting cells. By a month of age, two thirds of neonates have IgSCs, most of which are IgA-secreting cells. Increased IgSCs are more common in both term and preterm infants with intrauterine infection. Low serum concentrations of IgG in preterm infants may also be due to a decreased ability of their B cell to switch immunoglobulin isotype forms.[174]

Gut Host Defense Mechanisms

Maturation of the mucosal immune system occurs rapidly after birth in response to antigenic exposure and is well developed by 1 year of age in both preterm and term infants.[54] Host defense mechanisms in the gut involve both nonimmune and immune factors (Table 13-9). Many of these factors are initially immature in the neonate, which reduces the effectiveness of the gut mucosal barrier and increases the risk of GI disorders. Neonatal GI mucosal immaturity includes (1) increased permeability to macromolecules (all potential antigens), (2) altered immune tolerance, (3) decreased sIgA, and (4) decreased cytokine production. This allows entry of pathogenic organisms into systemic circulation and may increase the risk of development of allergic disorders. As defense mechanisms mature, GI barriers become more impermeable, offering greater protection against uptake of antigenic substances.[29,94] The development of gut defense mechanisms is sometimes referred to as *gut closure.*

Gut closure is influenced by ingestion of food, especially colostrum, which enhances maturation of the intestinal lining

Table 13-9 Alterations in Gut Host Defense Mechanisms in the Newborn

DEFENSE MECHANISM	MODE OF ACTION	ALTERATIONS IN NEWBORN
NONIMMUNE FACTORS		
Gastric acid	Decreased number of organisms entering intestines	Decreased in term and preterm infant until 4 weeks' postnatal age
Intestinal motility and peristalsis	Remove organisms and antigen	Decreased to 29 to 32 weeks' postconceptual age
Intraluminal proteolysis	Determines amount of macromolecular transport across intestinal epithelium	Decreased pancreatic enzyme function in preterm infant; some decrease in response in both term and preterm infants to 2 years; result is an increased absorption of intact proteins across small intestine
Mucosal surface		
Mucous coat	Provides physical barrier to attachment, uptake, and penetration of organisms and other antigens Carbohydrate moieties act as receptor inhibitors to protect against antigen penetration	Decreased and altered carbohydrate content and lack of mucus-specific receptor inhibition may interfere with surface defenses against organisms, toxins, and other antigens
Microvillous membrane	Carbohydrate composition influences specific adherence of organisms and other antigens to intestinal surface and prevents penetration	Altered membrane composition and incompletely developed surface leading to abnormal colonization, increased antigen penetration, and disease susceptibility
IMMUNOLOGIC FACTORS		
Secretory immunoglobulin A (sIgA)	Complexes with antigens to impede absorption from intestinal lumen Interferes with antigen attachment and uptake at mucosal surface	Low levels of IgA and especially sIgA result in increased transport of organisms, antigens, and other macromolecules across intestinal epithelium
Gut-associated lymphoid tissue (GALT)	Composed of Peyer's patches (aggregates of lymphoid tissue), plasma cells that are predominantly IgA producing, B and T lymphocytes, and specialized M epithelial cells. M cells bind and transport antigens to macrophages in lymphoid tissue	GALT develops more slowly than other lymphoid tissue and in newborns contains primarily T cells with few B cells Paucity of IgA-producing B cells (requires weeks to months to establish protective levels) Low levels of IgA Delayed response time to antigen penetration
Cell-mediated immunity	Includes activated T lymphocytes, mast cells, and macrophages along the intestinal lamina along with intraepithelial lymphocytes (cytotoxic T cells)	Immature and naive T lymphocytes, altered T suppressor function, and depression of responsiveness to specific antigens Decreased intestinal and intraepithelial lymphocytes in SGA and nutritionally deprived infants Respond to antigens with priming response versus tolerance

Compiled from references 46, 54, 94, 179.
SGA, Small for gestational age.

via introduction of factors such as thyroxine, transforming growth factor, insulin-like growth factors, neurotensin, cortisol, lactoferrin, bombesin, and epidermal growth factor.[94] Gut closure is delayed in preterm and SGA infants, who can absorb macromolecules across the intestinal epithelium for up to 8 to 12 months. Nonimmune factors that stimulate gut closure include maturation of gastric acid production, intestinal motility and peristalsis, intraluminal proteolytic activity, and the mechanical barrier properties of the gut mucosal surface.

The major specific immune factors that affect gut closure are sIgA and cell-mediated immunity. Fermentation of the prebiotic oligosaccharides contained in breast milk results in production of probiotic ("good") bacteria such as bifidobacteria and lactobacilli. These probiotics stimulate synthesis and secretion of sIgA and help produce a balanced Th1/Th2 response. sIgA also coats the mucosa to protect against bacterial invasion.[46]

Neonatal cell-mediated immunity, especially a localized depression of T-lymphocyte suppressor activity, and the decreased IgA hinder an effective response to antigens that can cross the intestinal barrier. The mature immune response to the presence of antigens in the gut is immune tolerance. With immune tolerance, the absorbed antigen elicits a localized IgA response that destroys most of the antigen. As a result, there are fewer antigens available to enter the systemic system. Immune tolerance appears to be enhanced by the presence of partially digested polypeptide fragments. These fragments may not be formed in the neonate secondary to immature proteolysis. With decreased IgA, greater amounts of antigen are absorbed. The presence of antigens also triggers T-suppressor cell activity, which interferes with and inhibits systemic responses to these antigens.[94] Decreased T-suppressor response can alter systemic immune responses and lead to inflammatory or allergic responses.

CLINICAL IMPLICATIONS FOR NEONATAL CARE

Neonates are more likely than adults to develop specific bacterial and viral infections and septicemia or meningitis if infection occurs. Immunodeficiency diseases are rarely manifested in newborns because maternally acquired IgG and sIgA in breast milk usually mask the effects of these disorders. However, immature neonatal immune responses are associated with the pathophysiology of several disorders. For example, the inflammatory response and cytokines play a role in tissue damage seen in bronchopulmonary dysplasia. Infection that causes cytokine-mediated injury to oligodendrocytes has been proposed as having a role in the pathogenesis of periventricular leukomalacia and brain injury following cerebral hypoxic-ischemic insults, which can lead to cerebral palsy (see Chorioamnionitis and Cerebral Palsy and Chapter 15).[117,120,141] Programming of the immune system in the fetal and neonatal period has long-term influences on immune system function and can increase or decrease the risk for later development of allergies and autoimmune disorders.[91,151]

Neonatal Vulnerability to Infection

Neonates are at increased risk of infection primarily because of their small NSP, reduced chemotaxis, decreased complement activity, decreased protective responses against capsular polysaccharide antigens, and large numbers of naive T cells, which reduce cell-mediated responses.[82,96,144] The chance of developing sepsis from exposure to gram-negative rods is increased because protection against these organisms is provided by IgM, IgA (against enteropathic *E. coli*), and T lymphocytes, all of which are present at decreased levels or have inefficient activity in the neonate. Similarly, markedly low values of IgA and the lack of sIgA increase vulnerability to respiratory and GI infections, whereas low IgM levels increase vulnerability to rubella, toxoplasmosis, CMV, and syphilis. The risk of GI infections is increased because of immaturity of the intestinal mucosal barrier and lack of gut closure.

Decreased complement activity, particularly the alternative pathway, leads to less opsonic activity. This may be a critical deficiency if the infant also lacks type-specific antibodies for organisms with a capsular polysaccharide coating, such as GBS or K1 *E. coli.* Altered activity of T lymphocytes along with their lack of antigen exposure increases the vulnerability to infection from herpes simplex virus (HSV), CMV, and *Candida.* Decreased production of IFN-γ (which inhibits viral replication) by the lymphocytes increases the risk of viral infection. In addition, IFN-γ is an important macrophage-activating factor that has an important role in destruction of intracellular pathogens such as *Toxoplasma gondii* and *Listeria monocytogenes.*

Immune Responses to Bacterial Infections

GBS and *E. coli* are common pathogens seen with neonatal sepsis. The pathophysiologic processes that lead to early-onset neonatal sepsis described below provide an example of how bacterial infection affects neonates: GBS is a β-hemolytic gram-positive cocci commonly found in the intestinal tract.

Newborns may acquire GBS via vertical transmission prior to or during birth. Although approximately 50% of newborns born to maternal carriers will be colonized at birth, passively acquired immunity derived from maternal antibodies protects the majority of healthy newborns from developing infection.[137] At birth, 1% to 2% of newborns born to colonized women will develop early-onset neonatal sepsis.[137] GBS sepsis is more likely to occur in infants deficient in type-specific IgG antibody. Neonates will lack these antibodies if their mother does not have the type-specific antibody to transfer to her infant, or if the infant is born prematurely before adequate maternal antibody has been transferred to the fetus. Maternal antibiotic prophylaxis given during the intrapartum period to women who are colonized with GBS reduces the risk of neonatal GBS sepsis.[165,166]

Once infected, the neonate may be unable to mount an appropriate response to GBS. When exposed to GBS, the B lymphocytes of most neonates do not produce adequate quantities of type-specific antibody critical for opsonization and phagocytosis.[89] Lower levels of complement in newborns, especially in preterm infants, further reduce opsonization of GBS and interfere with the phagocytic ability of the PMNs. In addition, optimal destruction of GBS depends on type-specific antibody, complement, and functional phagocytes. In infected neonates who do not have type-specific antibody, an increase in the time required for neutrophil migration to the invading organisms has been noted, along with a delay of 4 to 6 hours between the onset of infection and release of neutrophils from bone marrow storage pools (versus 2 hours in infants with type-specific antibodies).[70] This results in decreased complement activation (and thus opsonization and phagocytosis) and inability to localize the infection, and increases the risk of a rapidly progressing overwhelming septicemia.

Because of functional and structural alterations in PMNs that decrease chemotaxis, neonates are unable to rapidly deliver adequate numbers of phagocytes to the site of initial infection. Neutropenia, rarely seen in infected adults, is a frequent finding in neonatal septicemia. The reasons for this neutropenia include a small marrow storage pool of neutrophils and their precursors that is rapidly depleted with sepsis, inability of the marrow to increase production of neutrophils (stem cell proliferation rate is already at maximal activity), failure of the marrow to release additional neutrophils, sequestration of neutrophils along vessel walls (margination), and the short circulating half-life (4 to 7 hours) of neutrophils in the neonate.[89]

Neonates may also be deficient in local defense mechanisms in the lungs because of decreased numbers (and possibly altered function) of lung macrophages. This deficit may predispose the infant to GBS pneumonia. Immune responses of neonates against *E. coli* are similar to those described for GBS. However, anti-K1 *E. coli* IgG antibodies are much less common in the adult population, so the mother is less likely to provide protection to her fetus against this organism. In summary, the increased susceptibility of the neonate to bacterial pathogens results primarily from lack of type-specific antibody, alterations in the functional ability of PMNs (especially decreased chemotaxis), poor bone marrow response to maintain adequate numbers of neutrophils, and decreased complement, leading to ineffective opsonic activity necessary for phagocytosis and bactericidal activity (see Table 13-6).[89]

Immune Responses to Viral Infections

Viral infections tend to be more serious and devastating disorders in neonates than in older individuals. The major defense mechanisms against viral infections (cell-mediated immunity, NK cells, IgM, and the ability to localize infection) are all immature in the neonate. The decreased Th1 cytokines may also contribute to susceptibility to infection with intracellular pathogens.[180] In addition, most neonates have T lymphocytes that are not yet sensitized, that is, they are mostly still naive.

The neonate has varied responses depending on the characteristics and robustness of specific viruses. For example, the newborn produces mature $CD8^+$ T-cell responses after fetal exposure to CMV as early as 28 weeks' gestation, which may play a role in viral persistence after birth. However, the neonate has a low $CD8^+$ response to human immunodeficiency virus (HIV). The mechanisms underlying these differences are unclear but may be related to differences in cell priming or to low $CD4^+$ T-cell responses to HIV, or HIV may inhibit responses of young T cells or prevent development of $CD8^+$ responses.[96] Limitations in neonatal responses to selected infectious pathogens are summarized in Table 13-10. The

Table 13-10 Immune Responses to Vaccines and Infectious Pathogens in Early Life

VACCINE OR PATHOGEN	IMMUNE RESPONSES
Hepatitis B vaccine	Defective early Th1 and increased memory Th2 responses in newborns as compared to naive adults; higher antibody response than adults
Oral poliomyelitis vaccine	Defective Th1 response and similar antibody response in newborns as compared to immune adults
Mycobacterium bovis BCG vaccine	Adult-like Th1 response in newborns; promotes antibody, Th1, and Th2 responses to unrelated vaccines
Whole cell pertussis vaccine	Th1 response in 2-month-old infant
Measles vaccine	Lower Th1 response in 6- to 12-month-old infants as compared to immune adults
Human cytomegalovirus	Mature CD8 T-cell response and defective CD4 T-cell response in fetuses and infants as compared to adults
Human immunodeficiency virus	Defective CD4 and CD8 T-cell responses in newborns and infants as compared to adults
Trypanosoma cruzi	Adult-like CD8 T-cell response
Herpes simplex virus	Delayed IFN-γ response in infants as compared to adults
Bordetella pertussis	Th1 response in infants

Modified from Marchant, A. & Goldman, M. (2005). T cell-mediated immune responses in human newborns: Ready to learn? *Clin Exp Immunol, 141*, 12.

section below examines immunologic aspects of neonatal response to HSV and hepatitis B infection.

Herpes Simplex Virus (HSV) Infection

Neonates have impaired immune responses to both HSV1 and HSV2.[60,144] Consequently, neonatal HSV infection is often a rapidly progressing disorder that involves multiple body systems and has high morbidity and mortality rates. Severe systemic HSV infection is an age-related phenomenon, with the morbidity, mortality, and severity of illness decreasing after the first 4 weeks of life.[57] Susceptibility of neonates to severe HSV infection is due to immaturity of the immune system, alterations in neutrophil function, T-cell naiveté, fewer NK cells, and less efficient cell-mediated cytolysis.[60,89,144] Alterations in the neonate's immune system that increase the risk of HSV infection include decreased NK cell cytotoxicity, reduced ability of lymphocytes and monocytes to lyse HSV, decreased antibody-dependent cell-mediated toxicity, decreased or delayed production of and response to interferon, decreased diversity of specific receptors for HSV, delayed lymphocyte proliferation in response to antigens, blunted Th1 responses, and the inability of the neonate to generate a fever (HSV is a thermolabile organism).[57,89,144]

Eradication of HSV is dependent upon NK function and cell-mediated cytolysis, both of which are reduced in the newborn, probably as a result of decreased IL-12 and interferon activity.[144] Production of IFN-γ, IFN-α, and TNF-α are reduced and delayed in the neonate in response to HSV infection.[57] Since IFN-γ induces NK cells and other innate mechanisms, these responses are altered in the neonate.[158] The newborn develops antigen-specific T-cell responses to HSV more slowly due to altered function of T cells and myeloid dendritic cells. For example, it takes the neonatal $CD4^+$ cells 3 to 6 weeks to develop the same levels of antigen-sensitive cell response as the adult develops within 2 weeks.[57] Reduced complement and immature monocyte and macrophage responses to HSV also limit the infant's ability to respond to HSV. These changes enhance dissemination of the virus in the neonate.

Lack of maternal IgG antibodies, which are capable of neutralizing the virus and mediating antibody-dependent cell-mediated cytotoxicity, also increases the risk of neonatal HSV infection.[60] These maternal antibodies do not provide immunity to the neonate but are correlated with a lower infection rate in exposed newborns.[158] Women with primary HSV genital infection produce little IgG and their offspring are more likely to develop severe infection. A dose-dependent relationship has been observed between the amount of maternal anti-HSV antibody and the severity of neonatal infection, in which increasing levels of maternal antibody were associated with milder neonatal infection and a decreased incidence of disseminated infection or central nervous system involvement.[158]

Hepatitis B Virus Infection

Another virus that has become increasingly prevalent in perinatal care is hepatitis B virus (HBV). HBV can be transmitted from the mother to the fetus and newborn via vaginal secretions, amniotic fluid, maternal blood, saliva, and possibly breast milk. Most infants who develop HBV infection acquire the organism late in the third trimester or at delivery. Although clinical infection does not develop in many newborns exposed to HBV, fulminant neonatal disease will develop in some infants.[75] In addition, exposed infants may be at risk for the development of acute and chronic hepatitis, cirrhosis, and hepatocellular carcinoma as a result of perinatally acquired HBV infection.[71]

HBV is a DNA virus associated with three distinct antigen forms (surface, core, and e) and their respective antibodies (anti-HBs, anti-HBc, and anti-HBe). The outer protein surface contains a surface antigen (HBsAg), whereas the inner core of the virus contains the DNA genome (circular DNA form) and the core antigen (HBcAg). The third antigen (HBeAg) is a soluble serum antigen usually seen in association with HBsAg. Table 13-11 summarizes characteristics of these antigens and antibodies.

Table 13-11 Interpretation of the Presence of Combinations of Serologic Markers of Hepatitis B Virus

HBsAg	HBeAg	ANTI-HBe	ANTI-HBc	ANTI-HBS	INTERPRETATION	INFECTIVITY*
+	+	–	–	–	Incubation period for early acute HB	High
+	+	–	+	–	Acute HB or chronic carrier	High
+	–	+	+	–	Late during HB or chronic carrier	Low
–	–	+	+	+	Convalescent from acute HB infection	Low
–	–	–	+	+	Recovered from past HB infection	None
–	–	–	–	+	Immunized without infection; repeated exposure to HBsAg without infection; recovered from past infection	None
–	–	–	+	–	Recovered from past HB infection with undetectable anti-HBs; early convalescence or chronic carrier	??

From Hanshaw, J.B., Dudgeon, J.A., & Marshall, W.C. (1985). *Viral diseases of the fetus and newborn.* Philadelphia: Saunders, using data from Deinhardt, F., & Gust, L.P. (1982). Viral hepatitis. *Bull World Health Organ, 60,* 661.
HB, Hepatitis B; *HBV,* hepatitis B virus.
*Infectivity of blood.

HBeAg is a marker of infectivity and reflects ongoing viral replication. This antigen is usually seen in people with active disease and HBsAg-positive serum. HBsAg and HBeAg are detectable 1 to 3 weeks after HBV exposure but before onset of clinical symptoms. HBeAg may also be present after the active disease subsides, indicating either chronic disease or a carrier state. Women with HBeAg are usually infectious, and standard blood and body fluid precautions should be taken.

HBcAg is found only in hepatocytes and thus is not detectable in serum. However, antibodies to this antigen (anti-HBc) are seen during both acute infection and convalescence, making anti-HBc a reliable indicator of HBV infection. Immune response to HBcAg during an acute infection is primarily IgM-type antibody, which may persist for 4 to 6 months and indicates recent infection. IgG-type antibodies to HBcAg are also found in the carrier state.[75] The presence of anti-HBc in HBsAg-positive serum indicates low infectivity.

HBsAg can be found in the serum of people who have acute or chronic HBV infections or are carriers for the virus. Infants who acquire the virus during birth are seronegative initially but develop elevated serum HBsAg within 2 to 4 months.[70,71] The woman who is HBsAg-positive—regardless of whether she is a carrier or actively infected—can transmit the virus to her fetus and neonate and to others she comes in contact with. Therefore standard blood and body fluid precautions are recommended for health care personnel caring for the woman and her infant. The appearance of antibody against HBsAg (anti-HBs), in response to either active infection or immunization, reflects immunity to HBV.

The risk of maternal transmission of HBV to the neonate depends on the types of antigens and antibodies present. If the mother is positive for both HBsAg and HBeAg, there is a high likelihood of transmission to the fetus. Maternal anti-HBs antibodies do not provide significant protection of the infant from HBV infection because the amount of maternal antibody transferred provides only transient protection.[75] Women who are chronic carriers of HBsAg can transmit HBV to their infants after birth via breast milk if the infant is not vaccinated appropriately. This is especially true if the woman's serum is both HBsAg and HBeAg positive (indicating high infectivity), versus HBsAg and anti-HBe positive (indicating lower infectivity) or anti-HBc positive (indicating minimal likelihood of transfer).[75]

A combination of active and passive immunization is recommended for prevention of HBV infection in the neonate.[71] Thus HBV immune globulin (HBIG) and HBV vaccine are administered to infants of HBsAg-positive women. HBIG provides passive immunity by supplying antibodies to destroy HBV antigen that the infant may have acquired from the mother during the birth process. HBIG provides initial protection for the infant, although passive immunization may not completely suppress HBV infection.[71] Because infants of carrier mothers are at constant risk of reinfection, HBV vaccine is administered to provide immunization by stimulating the infant's system to produce its own antibodies against HBV.

Gut Immune Defenses and Necrotizing Enterocolitis

Immaturity of gut defense mechanisms has an etiologic role in the development of necrotizing enterocolitis (NEC). NEC is a multifactorial disorder that results in focal or diffuse ulceration and necrosis in the lower small intestine and colon (see Chapter 12). Factors involved in the development of NEC include intestinal ischemia, bacterial proliferation, and enteral feedings.[94] These stressors interact with the immature intestinal barrier to further increase mucosal permeability to enteric bacteria, toxins, and antigens.[94]

Human milk reduces the incidence and severity of NEC.[34] Human milk, particularly colostrum, facilitates gut closure by reducing antigen penetration, providing sIgA, and enhancing maturation of the mucosal epithelial cells and development of brush border enzymes such as lactase, sucrase, and alkaline phosphatase. Other factors contributing to the lower rate of GI infection in breastfed infants include antibacterial factors in human milk, stimulation of IgA, and the presence of ingested maternal antigen, which tends to promote immune tolerance responses.[34] With weaning and withdrawal of the immunosuppressive effect of human milk, the mucosal immune system is activated, with a physiologic inflammatory response followed by downregulation of responses.[34]

Diagnosis of Neonatal Infection

Although microbiologic techniques are the basic tools used in the diagnosis of infection, other parameters that reflect changes in components of the immune system can be useful. Newborns usually have low serum levels of IgM at birth. Thus elevated IgM levels (over 20 mg/dL [0.20 g/L]) in cord blood or in the first week are suggestive of an intrauterine or intrapartally acquired nonbacterial (fungal, viral, or parasitic) infection. Elevated IgM levels are not diagnostic of infection because an infant with an intrauterine infection may have normal IgM levels and a healthy infant may have elevated levels, especially if there was maternal bleeding into the fetal circulation during labor and birth. Generally IgM levels continue to rise in infected infants but remain stable or decrease in noninfected infants. Identification of specific IgM antibodies in cord blood to CMV, rubella, or spirochetes is evidence of intrauterine infection.[70]

The total number of white blood cells (WBCs) or percentages of individual WBC types are often not useful in diagnosing neonatal sepsis, but these values may provide evidence suggestive of infection. At birth the WBC count averages 15,000/mm^3 (range of 9000 to 30,000, although some healthy infants may have lower or higher values), falling to about 12,000 by the end of the first week. Total WBC counts below 4000 to 5000/mm^3 or above 25,000 to 30,000/mm^3 suggest infection but are not diagnostic.[18,70,89]

The neutrophil count varies significantly in normal newborns during the first few days, with lower counts seen in preterm infants. A transient neutrophilia usually occurs during this period, so neutrophil counts of 10,000 to 25,000/μL at this time are not necessarily suggestive of infection. Neutropenia can be a useful sign of sepsis in some neonates; however, a variety of clinical factors can also lead to neutropenia (Table 13-12). Mouzinho and colleagues proposed the following reference ranges for total neutrophil counts in VLBW infants less than 1500 g and 30 weeks' gestational age: 500 to 6000 at birth; 2200 to 14,000 at 18 hours; 1100 to 8800 at 60 hours; and 1100 to 5600 at 120 hours.[109]

The differential count can also be useful in the recognition of neonatal sepsis. Normally, in the first few days after birth, the majority of WBCs are PMN neutrophils (60%), with 20% to 40% of these neutrophils being band forms. Findings associated with infection include a relative absence of PMNs, an increased "shift to the left" (i.e., a predominance of immature forms of PMNs [bands, metamyelocytes, occasional myelocytes] due to an outpouring of immature cells from the bone marrow), an increase in toxic granulations in the PMNs, and an increase in the absolute number of bands or metamyelocytes (even with normal total neutrophil counts). Increased numbers of total immature neutrophils can be useful but are also influenced by infant variability and clinical factors (see Table 13-12). The absolute neutrophil count and the ratio of immature neutrophils to total neutrophils (I:T ratio) may also be useful. Maximum normal levels in term infants are 0.16 at 0 to 24 hours of age and 0.12 at 60 hours of age, with a maximum of 0.2 in preterm infants younger than 31 weeks' gestational age.[70] An increased I:T ratio suggests sepsis, but increases are also seen with other clinical conditions.

In some septic infants there is evidence of a marked decrease in the bone marrow NSP, which is normally reduced in the neonate. The decreased NSP probably arises from the release of stored neutrophils in response to sepsis, the increased need for phagocytes, and an inability of the bone marrow to significantly increase production of neutrophils because production is already near maximum capacity in the neonate.

Acute phase reactions involve proteins produced by the liver in response to inflammation due to sepsis, trauma, or other cell processes.[70] Examples of these substances are C-reactive protein (CRP), erythrocyte sedimentation rate (ESR), fibronectin, and fibrinogen. Most of these substances have not been useful in diagnosing neonatal infection due to low positive predictive values (e.g., if abnormal, the percentage of infants with infection).[70] Other investigators have examined the use of laboratory panels using combinations of these substances. Use of these panels has increased the negative predictive value (e.g., if normal, the percentage of infants without infection) but has not significantly increased the positive predictive value.[70] The acute phase reactant used most often in the neonate is CRP. In many infants, the CRP is normal at the onset of infection and then rises within the next day to peak at 2 to 3 days after the onset of an infection. CRP levels remain high until the infection is controlled and the inflammatory response begins to resolve, at which point the levels

Table 13-12 Clinical Factors Affecting Neutrophil Counts

	Neonates with Abnormal Values In:[a]				
	Total Neutrophils				
COMPLICATIONS	DECREASE	INCREASE	TOTAL IMMATURE INCREASE	INCREASED I:T RATIO[b]	APPROXIMATE DURATION (HOURS)
Maternal hypertension	++++	0	+	+	72
Maternal fever, neonate healthy	0	++	+++	++++	24
≥6 hours of antepartum oxytocin	0	++	++	++++	120
Asphyxia (5-minute Apgar ≤5)	+	++	++	+++	24-60
Meconium aspiration syndrome	0	++++	+++	++	72
Pneumothorax with uncomplicated hyaline membrane disease	0	++++	++++	++++	24
Seizures: no hypoglycemia, asphyxia, or CNS hemorrhage	0	+++	+++	++++	24
Prolonged crying (≥4 minutes)	0	++++	++++	++++	1
Asymptomatic blood glucose (≤30)	0	++	+++	+++	24
Hemolytic disease	++	++	+++	++	7-28 days
Surgery	0	++++	++++	+++	24
High altitude	0	++++	++++	0	6[c]

From Weinberg, J.A. & Powell, K.R. (2001). Laboratory aids for diagnosis of neonatal sepsis. In J.S. Remington & J.O. Klein (Eds.), *Infectious diseases of the fetus and newborn infant* (5th ed.). Philadelphia: Saunders.

CNS, central nervous system; *I:T ratio*, immature neutrophils to total neutrophils ratio.

[a]+, 0%-25% of neonates affected; ++, 25%-50%; +++, 50%-75%; ++++, 75%-100%.

[b]Immature forms/total neutrophil count.

[c]Not tested after 6 hours.

decline over the next 5 to 10 days.[107] A single CRP level generally has limited usefulness in initial diagnosis of infection, but serial levels may be useful in determining antibiotic effectiveness and duration of therapy.[107]

MATURATIONAL CHANGES DURING INFANCY AND CHILDHOOD

Infants and children remain at greater risk for infection because they have lower levels of immunoglobulins compared to adults. This risk is most marked during the first 6 months because of low levels of IgG associated with a physiologic hypogammaglobulinemia. Infancy is a time when hypersensitivity to food substances may develop because of immaturity of gut defense mechanisms. In this section, maturation of components of the host defense system is described followed by discussion of the physiologic hypogammaglobulinemia of infancy, immunizations, and the development of allergies.

Maturation of Host Defense Factors

Serum complement levels gradually increase to adult values by 6 to 18 months.[70] T-cell function is relatively mature by 3 to 6 months or sooner, although T-cell absolute numbers do not reach adult levels until 6 years.[144] Chemotaxis of neutrophils is underdeveloped until 2 years, and monocyte chemotaxis is less efficient than adult chemotaxis until 6 to 12 years.[89] IgG response to protein antigens is limited in infants less than 12 months and to polysaccharide antigens until 18 to 24 months.[149]

The immune responses to bacteria that have capsular polysaccharide do not reach adult capabilities until 1.5 to 2 years.[82,108] As a result, infants are more susceptible to infections from organisms such as *H. influenzae* type B, pneumococci, and meningococci. The exact age at which other components of the immune system reach maturity is unknown, although the risk of infection with many of the pathogens associated with neonatal infection decreases after 2 to 3 months of age. $CD45RO^+$ cells account for less than 5% of all T cells in the newborn, increasing to 35% to 45% by 16 years. Most of this increase is during the first year.[99] IFN-γ production is similar to that of adults by 2 years.[99] Weaning from human milk is associated with marked changes in the intestinal ecosystem.[16,27]

Physiologic Hypogammaglobulinemia

By 1 year of life, total levels of immunoglobulins are 60% of adult values (see Figure 13-9). During the first year of life, the infant's B cells secrete primarily IgM. IgM reaches 50% of adult values by 6 months and 75% to 80% by 1 year in both term and preterm infants. Adult levels of IgM are attained between 1 and 2 years.[70,122] IgA levels increase after birth and reach 20% of adult levels by 1 year. Levels of sIgA reach adult values by 10 years; serum IgA levels attain adult values during adolescence.[70,122,174] Salivary and gut IgA may reach adult levels by 5 years.[94] Because IgA protects against many respiratory and GI infections, young children are more predisposed toward developing these disorders.

IgG production by the infant is minimal during the first few months but increases significantly after 6 months of age, with a gradual increase toward adult levels in childhood.[70,122] The increase in IgG and other immunoglobulins is probably stimulated by exposure to environmental antigens. IgG_1 and IgG_3 reach 50% of adult values by 1 year and 100% by 8 years; IgG_2 and IgG_4 are 50% by 2 to 3 years and 100% by 10 to 12 years.[70,89] As a result, infants and toddlers are more susceptible to infection with *H. influenzae* type B, which is dependent on IgG_2 antibodies for opsonization of its capsular coating.[89] At term, IgG is 90% to 95% of adult values, which is greater than maternal values because maternal IgG is actively transferred across the placenta. After birth, IgG levels fall gradually as maternal IgG is catabolized. Maternally derived IgG reaches a nadir at 3 to 4 months at 400 mg/dL (4.0 g/L) and has generally disappeared by 9 months of age.[82] This fall, along with minimal IgG production by the infant, results in a "physiologic hypogammaglobulinemia" during the first year of life. Lowest levels of IgG occur at 2 to 4 months and remain low until at least 6 months (see Figure 13-9).

The initial 6 to 12 months is therefore a period of heightened vulnerability to infection in all infants, with a higher risk in preterm infants. Preterm infants have lower IgG levels at birth, reach lowest levels of IgG sooner, and remain at low levels longer because the ability to synthesize IgG is more closely related to conceptual age than to postbirth age.[66] VLBW infants may have IgG levels lower than 100 mg/dL (1.0 g/L) by 2 to 3 months of age. The lowest IgG levels during the first few months are directly proportional to gestational age and inversely proportional to postbirth age. The period of hypogammaglobulinemia is also exaggerated in SGA infants. These infants often have lower levels of maternal antibody, probably due to placental dysfunction.

Immunizations

Although immunizations have been part of well-baby care for many years, there is still controversy regarding timing, dosage, and side effects. Current recommendations for immunizations for infants and children are published each year by the Centers for Disease Control and Prevention (CDC) and the American Academy of Pediatrics and can be found on their websites. Contraindications and precautions for individual vaccinations are available on the CDC website. The American Academy of Pediatrics has recommended that immunizations be given to preterm infants at the same chronologic age as term infants.[11] However, hospitalized infants may receive blood or blood products, so vaccinations should not be given within 14 days of these treatments because blood or blood products may contain specific antibodies against the vaccine's antigen and interfere with the development of an appropriate immune response.[172] Preterm infants tend to be underimmunized and are often not immunized on schedule.

The ability of an infant to respond to antigens with production of specific antibodies improves after vaccination and is influenced by the stage of immune system development, type of vaccine, immunogenicity of the vaccine, number of doses, interval between doses, and maternal antibody.[36,177] Potential obstacles to effective neonatal immunization include "impaired antigen-presenting cell (APC) responses IFN-γ production to many (but not all) stimuli, a Th2 bias to immune responses, impaired antibody (Ab) affinity maturation, and the potential inhibitory effect of maternal antibody."[125] In some countries oral poliovirus, hepatitis B, and bacilli Calmette-Guerin (BCG) vaccinations are given at birth with good efficacy.[36,177]

Infant responses are not dependent on either birth weight or gestational age and are influenced more by exposure to antigens than by maturation of the immune system per se.[20] Bernbaum and colleagues examined antibody responses of term and preterm infants to diphtheria-tetanus-acellular pertussis (DTaP) vaccine injections at 2, 4, and 6 months after birth.[20] Before the first immunization, 84% of preterm and 100% of term infants had adequate antibody levels to diphtheria and tetanus (but only 16% of preterm infants and 86% of term infants to pertussis) from transplacental passage of maternal IgG. Thus preterm infants would have had fewer antibodies to protect them against these pathogens if they were exposed before being vaccinated. In addition in preterm infants antibody levels fall below protective cut-off values sooner for disorders such as measles, mumps, varicella-zoster, rubella, *Haemophilus influenzae* type-B, diphtheria, pertussis, and tetanus, increasing the risk for these disorders at earlier ages.[164] Adequate immune responses to diphtheria and tetanus were noted in term infants after one dose of this immunization, and in preterm infants after two doses. Both groups required two doses to mount adequate responses to pertussis. Fewer than half of preterm infants who received half-dose immunizations were able to mount an appropriate serologic response after three doses and required a fourth full dose to achieve this response.[21] Thus use of half-dose immunizations with preterm infants leaves about half of these infants unprotected. Consequently, preterm infants should receive full-dose vaccines.[21]

Preterm infants are reported to have fewer febrile or local reactions to DTaP injections, probably because of immature primary host defense mechanisms.[20,21] However, there have been several reports of transient adverse responses to immunizations in about 13% of hospitalized preterm infants with use of combination vaccinations containing either acellular or whole cell pertussis.[41,146] This response was primarily a transient increase in apneic and bradycardic episodes 8 to 12 hours after the immunization, possibly due to a vaccination-induced stimulation of the immune system; a few infants also had a fever.[146]

Passively acquired maternal antibody generally does not interfere with immunizations against diphtheria, pertussis, tetanus, or polio, perhaps because maternal antibody levels to these organisms are relatively low at the time vaccination occurs. By a month, infants respond adequately to tetanus and diphtheria and after 3 months, infants will respond well to pertussis. This may be why several doses of pertussis are required before an adequate antibody response is observed. Adult immunization to pertussis, which is included in the adult tetanus-diphtheria booster may change levels of passive immunization in newborns.

IgG acquired through placental transfer from the mother can interfere with live virus immunizations by neutralizing the viruses and preventing successful vaccination. The predominance of T-suppressor versus T-helper cells in the neonate may also interfere with the ability of the infant to respond appropriately. Therefore vaccination with live viruses is usually delayed until after the first year. Vaccination with HBV vaccine is effective early in infancy because this is an inactivated protein antigen.

Development of Allergic Disease

The etiology of allergic disorders is multifactorial. Hypersensitivity to cow's milk protein and foods is more frequent in infants than in older children. Alterations in APC function in infancy are associated with an increased risk of developing allergic disease in later life.[91,161] By 1 to 2 years, many children can tolerate substances to which they were "allergic" earlier.[66] However, exposure to potentially allergic substances in early infancy may sensitize susceptible infants to specific ingested proteins (via a process similar to that described earlier for Rh isoimmunization, although the antigen enters the infant through the gut in this case). Later exposure to even small quantities of that protein may invoke an allergic response. Therefore food substances known to have strong antigenic potential, such as egg white and nuts, are usually not recommended for young infants. However, data to support a relationship between early introduction of solid foods and the development of allergic disorders are limited with few controlled trials.[156]

Risk factors for the development of food allergies include "(1) genetic predisposition to atopy, (2) immature mucosal immune system, (3) inadequate normal gut flora, (4) increase in mucosal permeability, (5) IgA deficiency or other immunological defects, (6) gastrointestinal infections, (7) formula feeding, and (8) early introduction of solid foods before 4 months of age."[29,p. 397] Young infants are more at risk to develop food allergies because of immaturity of gut defense mechanisms, lack of gut closure, and the ability of the immature gut to absorb intact protein macromolecules.[17,29] Most infants fed cow's milk early develop IgG and IgA antibodies to cow's milk antigens. These antibodies are found from 3 to 9 months and then gradually decrease, but they may return (at lower levels) with later ingestion of cow's milk. The American Academy of Pediatrics recommends delaying introduction of solids until 6 months in infants who are exclusively breastfed and 4 to 6 months in infants fed formula.[12]

SUMMARY

The immune systems of the fetus and neonate are adaptive to the intrauterine environment and transition to the extrauterine environment. However, these alterations in their host defense mechanisms increase their risk of infection. This risk is particularly evident in relation to organisms that colonize the maternal genital tract, such as GBS and sexually transmitted diseases (e.g., HSV, HBV, HIV infections). Clinical recommendations for nurses working with neonates based on changes in host defense mechanisms are summarized in Table 13-13. By understanding the limitations of the immune system in the neonate and infant, nurses can appreciate neonatal vulnerabilities to infection from specific organisms and the risk for developing sepsis, develop increased understanding of the rationales behind specific infection control policies, and provide appropriate parent teaching.

Table 13-13 Recommendations for Clinical Practice Related to Host Defense Mechanisms in Neonates

Recognize normal parameters for immune system components and patterns of change during the neonatal period (pp. 465-447).
Obtain and evaluate maternal history of possible exposure to infectious organisms or potential for current illness (pp. 465-466).
Recognize risk factors for development and clinical manifestations of specific infections (pp. 472-475).
Recognize the subtle signs of infection in the neonate and that fever is an uncommon sign of infection (pp. 465-467).
Recognize laboratory findings associated with an increased likelihood of neonatal infection (pp. 475-477).
Monitor neonates for signs of infection, especially infants with disruption of their skin barrier; those who are preterm, ill, small for gestational age, or stressed; or those with delayed oral feedings (pp. 472-475).
Monitor for signs of necrotizing enterocolitis (p. 475 and Chapter 12).
Monitor for signs of group B streptococci (GBS) and *Escherichia coli* sepsis and for meningitis in infants of mothers colonized with these organisms, especially those women who do not have type-specific antibody (pp. 472-473).
Teach parents regarding methods to prevent or reduce the risk of infection in their infant (pp. 472-475, 477).
Monitor infants of women with chronic disorders associated with transplacental passage of antibodies for antibody-related clinical problems (pp. 459-462).
Monitor Rho(D)-positive infants of Rho(D)-negative women and A, B, or AB infants of type O mothers for jaundice and hyperbilirubinemia (pp. 460-461).
Recognize antigens and antibodies associated with hepatitis B virus (HBV) infection and institute hepatitis precautions for infants born to mothers who are HBsAg or HBeAg positive (pp. 474-475 and Table 13-11).
Give hepatitis B immune globulin (HBIG) and HBV vaccine to infants of mothers who are HBsAg positive (p. 475).
Use Standard Precautions for blood and body fluids during the perinatal period (pp. 473-475).
Know recommended schedule of immunizations (pp. 477-478).
Monitor infants to ensure that they receive immunizations as scheduled, especially preterm infants and infants with chronic problems (pp. 477-478).

References

1. Abbas, A.K., Lichtman, A.H., & Pillai, S. (2011). *Cellular and molecular immunology* (7th ed.). Philadelphia: Saunders.
2. Abrahams, V.M. & Mor, G. (2004). Toll-like receptors and their role in the trophoblast. *Placenta, 26*, 540.
3. Abrahams, V.M., et al. (2004). Macrophages and apoptotic cell clearance during pregnancy. *Am J Reprod Immunol, 51*, 275.
4. Abrahams, V.M. (2011). The role of the Nod-like receptor family in trophoblast innate immune responses. *J Reprod Immunol, 88*, 112.
5. Adkins, B. (2005). Neonatal T cell function. *J Pediatr Gastroenterol Nutr, 40*, S5.
6. Adkins, B., Leclerc, C., & Marshall-Clarke, S. (2004). Neonatal adaptive immunity comes of age. *Nat Rev Immunol, 4*, 55.
7. Afrazi, A., et al. (2011). New insights into the pathogenesis and treatment of necrotizing enterocolitis: Toll-like receptors and beyond. *Pediatr Res, 69*, 183.
8. Ahdieh, L. (2001). Pregnancy and infection with human immunodeficiency virus. *Clin Obstet Gynecol, 44*, 154.
9. Ahn, H., et al. (2011). Immunologic characteristics of preeclampsia, a comprehensive review. *Am J Reprod Immunol, 65*, 377.
10. Aluvihare, V.R. & Kallikourdis, M. (2005). Tolerance, suppression and the fetal allograft. *J Mol Med, 83*, 88.
11. American Academy of Pediatrics, Committee on Infectious Diseases. (2009). Immunization in special circumstances. Preterm and low birth weight infants. In L.K. Pickering, et al. (Eds.), *Red Book: 2009 Report of the committee on infectious disease* (28th ed.). Elk Grove Village, IL: American Academy of Pediatrics.
12. American Academy of Pediatrics Committee on Nutrition. (2009). *Pediatric nutrition handbook* (6th ed.). Elk Grove Village, IL: American Academy of Pediatrics.
13. American College of Obstetricians and Gynecologists. (2003). *Committee Opinion #282.* Immunization during pregnancy. Washington, DC: ACOG.
14. American College of Obstetricians and Gynecologists. (2009). ACOG Committee Opinion No. 438: Update on immunization and pregnancy: Tetanus, diphtheria, and pertussis vaccination. *Obstet Gynecol, 114* (2 Pt 1):398.
15. American College of Obstetricians and Gynecologists Committee on Obstetric Practice. (2010). ACOG Committee Opinion No. 468: Influenza vaccination during pregnancy. *Obstet Gynecol, 116*, 1006.
16. Bailey, M., et al. (2005). The development of the mucosal immune system pre and post-weaning: Balancing regulatory and effector function. *Proc Nutr Soc, 64*, 451.
17. Belderbos, M., Levy, O., & Bont, L. (2009). Neonatal innate immunity in allergy development. *Curr Opin Pediatr, 21*, 762.
18. Bellanti, J.A., Zeligs, B.J., & Pung, H.Y. (2005). Immunology of the fetus and newborn. In M.G. MacDonald, M.M.K. Seshia, & M.D. Mullett (Eds.), *Avery's Neonatology: Pathophysiology and management of the newborn* (6th ed.). Philadelphia: Lippincott Williams & Wilkins.
19. Berger, M. (2012). The complement system. In R.A. Polin, W.W. Fox, & S.H. Abman (Eds.), *Fetal and neonatal physiology* (3rd ed.). Philadelphia: Saunders.
20. Bernbaum, J., et al. (1984). Development of the premature infant's host defense mechanisms and its relationship to routine immunizations. *Clin Perinatol, 11*, 73.

21. Bernbaum, J., et al. (1989). Half-dose immunization for diphtheria, tetanus, pertussis: Response of preterm infants. *Pediatrics, 83*, 471.
22. Bhatia, M., et al. (2012). Neonatal neutrophil normal and abnormal physiology. In R.A. Polin, W.W. Fox, & S.H. Abman (Eds.), *Fetal and neonatal physiology* (3rd ed.). Philadelphia: Saunders.
23. Blackburn, S. (1985). *Rho(D) isoimmunization: Implications for the mother, fetus, and newborn. In NAACOG update series* (Vol. 3). Princeton, NJ: Continuing Professional Education Center.
24. Boh, E.E. (2004). Neonatal lupus erythematosus. *Clin Dermatol, 22*, 125.
25. Borzychowski, A.M., et al. (2005). Changes in systemic type 1 and type 2 immunity in normal pregnancy and pre-eclampsia may be mediated by natural killer cells. *Eur J Immunol, 35*, 3054.
26. Brinc, D. & Lazarus, A.H. (2009). Mechanisms of anti-D action in the prevention of hemolytic disease of the fetus and newborn. *Hematology Am Soc Hematol Educ Program*, 2009, 185.
27. Caicedo, R.A., et al. (2005). The developing intestinal ecosystem: Implications for the neonate. *Pediatr Res, 58*, 625.
28. Carr, R. (2000). Neutrophil production and function in newborn infants. *Br J Haematol, 110*, 18.
29. Chahine, B.G. & Bahna, S.L. (2010). The role of the gut mucosal immunity in the development of tolerance versus development of allergy to food. *Curr Opin Allergy Clin Immunol, 10*, 394.
30. Chakravarty, E.F. & Nelson, K.E. (2006). Obstetric hospitalizations in the United States for women with systemic lupus erythematosus and rheumatoid arthritis, *Arthritis Rheum, 54*, 899.
31. Challis, J.R., et al. (2009). Inflammation and pregnancy. *Reprod Sci, 16*, 206.
32. Chaouat, G., et al. (2010). Tolerance to the foetal allograft? *Am J Reprod Immunol, 63*, 624.
33. Cohn, D., Ramaswamy, B., & Blum, K. (2009). Malignancy and pregnancy. In R.K. Creasy, et al. (Eds.), *Creasy & Resnik's Maternal-fetal medicine: Principles and practice* (6th ed.). Philadelphia: Saunders.
34. Cummins, A.G. & Thompson, F.M. (1997). Postnatal changes in mucosal immune response: Physical perspective of breast feeding and weaning. *Immunol Cell Biol, 75*, 419.
35. Cunningham, G., et al. (2009). *Williams obstetrics* (23rd ed.). New York: McGraw-Hill.
36. Demirjian, A. & Levy, O. (2009). Safety and efficacy of neonatal vaccination. *Eur J Immunol, 39*, 36.
37. de Vries, E., et al. (1999). Analyzing the developing lymphocyte system of neonates and infants. *Eur J Pediatr, 158*, 611.
38. Dosiou, C. & Giudice, L.C. (2005). Natural killer cells in pregnancy and recurrent pregnancy loss. Endocrine and immunologic perspectives. *Endocr Rev, 26*, 44.
39. Druckmann, R. & Druckmann, M.A. (2005). Progesterone and the immunology of pregnancy. *J Steroid Biochem Mol Biol, 97*, 389.
40. Duff, P., Sweet, R.L., & Edwards, R.K. (2009). Maternal and fetal infections. In R.K. Creasy, et al. (Eds.), *Creasy & Resnik's Maternal-fetal medicine: Principles and practice* (6th ed.). Philadelphia: Saunders Elsevier.
41. Ellison, V.J., Davis, P.G., & Doyle, L.W. (2005). Adverse reactions to immunization with newer vaccines in the very preterm infant. *J Paediatr Child Health, 41*, 441.
42. Englund, J., Glezen, W.P., & Piedra, P.A. (1998). Maternal immunization against viral disease. *Vaccine, 16*, 1456.
43. Erlebacher, A., et al. (2004). Ovarian insufficiency and early pregnancy loss induced by activation of the innate immune system. *J Clin Invest, 114*, 39.
44. Fernandez, M.A., et al. (2008). T regulatory cells contribute to the attenuated primary CD8+ and CD4+ T cell responses to herpes simplex virus type 2 in neonatal mice. *J Immunol, 180*, 1556.
45. Field, C.J. (2005). The immunological components of human milk and their effect on the immune development in infants. *J Nutr, 135*, 1.
46. Forchielli, M.L. & Walker, W.A. (2005). The role of gut-associated lymphoid tissues and mucosal defense. *Br J Nutr, 3*, S41.
47. Formby, B. (1995). Immunologic response in pregnancy. Its role in endocrine disorders of pregnancy and influence on the course of maternal autoimmune diseases. *Endocrinol Metab Clin North Am, 24*, 187.
48. Gall, S.A. (1983). Maternal adjustments in the immune system in normal pregnancy. *Clin Obstet Gynecol, 26*, 521.
49. Gall, S.A. (2003). Maternal immunization. *Obstet Gynecol Clin North Am, 30*, 623.
50. Galofre, J.C. & Davies, T.F. (2009). Autoimmune thyroid disease in pregnancy: A review. *J Womens Health, 18*, 1847.
51. Garlanda, C., et al. (2008). Inflammatory reaction and implantation: The new entries PTX3 and D6. *Placenta, 29*(Suppl B), 129.
52. Genc, M.R. & Onderdonk, A. (2011). Endogenous bacterial flora in pregnant women and the influence of maternal genetic variation. *BJOG, 118*, 154.
53. Gibson, C.S., et al. (2003). Antenatal causes of cerebral palsy: Associations between inherited thrombophilias, viral and bacterial infection, and inherited susceptibility to infection. *Obstet Gynecol Survey, 58*, 209.
54. Gleeson, M. & Cripps, A.W. (2004). Development of mucosal immunity in the first year of life and relationship to sudden infant death syndrome. *FEMS Immunol Med Microbiol, 42*, 21.
55. Goldman, A.S. (2000). Back to basics: Host responses to infection. *Pediatr Rev, 21*, 342.
56. Gotsch, F., et al. (2007). The fetal inflammatory response syndrome. *Clin Obstet Gynecol, 50*, 652.
57. Guffey, M.B. & Kimberlin, D.W. (2012). Host defense mechanisms against viruses. In R.A. Polin, W.W. Fox, & S.H. Abman (Eds.), *Fetal and neonatal physiology* (4th ed.). Philadelphia: Saunders.
58. Guilmot, A., et al. (2011). Natural killer cell responses to infections in early life. *J Innate Immun, 3*, 280.
59. Gutierrez, G., et al. (2005). Asymmetric antibodies: A protective arm in pregnancy. *Chem Immunol Allergy, 89*, 158.
60. Gutierrez, K.M., Arvin, A.N., & Whitley, R.J. (2010). Herpes simplex virus infections. In J.S. Remington, et al. (Eds.), *Infectious diseases of the fetus and newborn infant* (7th ed.). Philadelphia: Saunders.
61. Harkness, U.F. & Spinnato, J.A. (2004). Prevention and management of RhD isoimmunization. *Clin Perinatol, 31*, 721.
62. Hartwell, E.A. (1998). Use of Rh immune globulin: ASCP practice parameter. *Am J Clin Pathol, 110*, 281.
63. Hein, M., et al. (2005). Immunoglobulin levels and phagocytes in the cervical mucus plug at term of pregnancy. *Acta Obstet Gynecol Scand, 84*, 734.
64. Hoftman, A.C., et al. (2008). Newborn illnesses caused by transplacental antibodies. *Adv Pediatr, 55*, 271.
65. Holt, P.G. (2003). Functionally mature virus-specific CD8(+) T memory cells in congenitally infected newborns: Proof of principle for neonatal vaccination? *J Clin Invest, 111*, 1645.
66. Holt, P.G. & Jones, C.A. (2000). The development of the immune system during pregnancy and early life. *Allergy, 55*, 688.
67. Jobe, A.H. (2010). "Miracle" extremely low birth weight neonates: Examples of developmental plasticity. *Obstet Gynecol, 116*, 1184.
68. Kai-Larsen, Y., et al. (2007). Antimicrobial components of the neonatal gut affected upon colonization. *Pediatr Res, 61*, 530.
69. Kalkunte, S.S., et al. (2009). Vascular endothelial growth factor C facilitates immune tolerance and endovascular activity of human uterine NK cells at the maternal-fetal interface. *J Immunol, 182*, 4085.
70. Kapur, R., Yoder, M.C., & Polin, R.A. (2011). Developmental immunology. In R.J. Martin, A.A. Fanaroff, & M.C. Walsh (Eds.), *Fanaroff and Martin's Neonatal-perinatal medicine: Diseases of the fetus and infant* (9th ed.). Philadelphia: Mosby Elsevier.
71. Karnsakul, W. & Schwarz, K. (2010). Hepatitis. In J.S. Remington, et al. (Eds.), *Infectious diseases of the fetus and newborn infant* (7th ed.). Philadelphia: Saunders.
72. Karimi, K. & Arck, P.C. (2010). Natural killer cells: Keepers of pregnancy in the turnstile of the environment. *Brain Behav Immun, 24*, 339.
73. Kim, Y.M., et al. (2005). Toll-like receptor 4: A potential link between "danger signals," the innate immune system, and preeclampsia? *Am J Obstet Gynecol, 193*, 921.

74. Kilpatrick, L. & Harris, M.C. (2012). Cytokines and inflammatory response in the fetus and neonate. In R.A. Polin, W.W. Fox, & S.H. Abman (Eds.), *Fetal and neonatal physiology* (4th ed.). Philadelphia: Saunders.
75. Klion, F.M. (1991). The liver in normal pregnancy. In S.H. Cherry & I.R. Merkatz (Eds.), *Complications of pregnancy: Medical, surgical, gynecological, psychosocial and perinatal* (4th ed.). Baltimore: Williams & Wilkins.
76. Koenig, J.M. & Yoder, M.C. (2004). Neonatal neutrophils: The good, the bad, and the ugly. *Clin Perinatol, 31,* 39.
77. Koga, K., Aldo, P.B., & Mor, G. (2009). Toll-like receptors and pregnancy: Trophoblast as modulators of the immune response. *J Obstet Gynaecol Res, 35,* 191.
78. Kumar, V. & Sharma, A. (2010). Mast cells: Emerging sentinel innate immune cells with diverse role in immunity. *Mol Immunol, 48,* 14.
79. Landers, C.D., Chelvarajan, R.L., & Bondada, S. (2005). The role of B cells and accessory cells in the neonatal response to TI-2 antigens. *Immunol Res, 31,* 25.
80. Landers, D.V., Martinez de Tejada, B., & Coyne, B.A. (1997). Immunology of HIV and pregnancy: The effects of each on the other. *Obstet Gynecol Clin North Am, 24,* 821.
81. Landor, M. (1995). Maternal-fetal transfer of immunoglobulins. *Ann Allergy Asthma Immunol, 74,* 279.
82. LaPine, T.R. & Hill, H.R. (2012). Host defense mechanisms against bacteria. In R.A. Polin, W.W. Fox, & S.H. Abman (Eds.), *Fetal and neonatal physiology* (4th ed.). Philadelphia: Saunders.
83. Lawrence, R.A. (2011). *Breastfeeding: A guide for the medical profession* (7th ed.). Philadelphia: Saunders.
84. Lazarus, J.H. (2005). Thyroid disease in pregnancy and childhood. *Minerva Endocrinol, 30,* 71.
85. Le Bouteiller, P. (2000). HLA-G in the human placenta: Expression and potential functions. *Biochem Soc Trans, 28,* 208.
86. Leftherioti, M.V. (2005). The significance of the women's repertoire of natural killer cell receptors in the maintenance of pregnancy. *Chem Immunol Allergy, 89,* 84.
87. Lemke, H., et al. (2009). Benefits and burden of the maternally-mediated immunological imprinting. *Autoimmun Rev, 8,* 394.
88. Levy, O. (2005). Innate immunity of the human newborn: Distinct cytokine responses to LPS and other Toll-like receptor agonists. *J Endotoxin Res, 11,* 113.
89. Lewis, D.B. & Wilson, C.B. (2010). Developmental immunology and role of host defenses in fetal and neonatal susceptibility to infection. In J.S. Remington & J.O. Klein (Eds.), *Infectious diseases of the fetus and newborn infant* (7th ed.). Philadelphia: Saunders.
90. Lilius, E.M. & Marnila, P. (2001). The role of colostral antibodies in prevention of microbial infections. *Curr Opin Infect Dis, 14,* 295.
91. Lisciandro, J.G. & van den Biggelaar, A.H. (2010). Neonatal immune function and inflammatory illnesses in later life: Lessons to be learnt from the developing world? *Clin Exp Allergy, 40,* 1719.
92. Lockshin, M.D., Salmon, J.E., & Erkan, D. (2009). Pregnancy and rheumatic diseases. In R.K. Creasy, et al. (Eds.), *Creasy & Resnik's Maternal-fetal medicine: Principles and practice* (6th ed.). Philadelphia: Saunders Elsevier.
93. Maatan-Metzger, A., et al. (2000). Maternal anti-D prophylaxis during pregnancy does not cause neonatal hemolysis. *Arch Dis Child Fetal Neonatal Ed, 84,* F60.
94. MacDonald, T.T., et al. (1996). The ontogeny of the mucosal immune system. In W.A. Walker, et al. (Eds.), *Pediatric gastrointestinal disease* (2nd ed.). St. Louis: Mosby.
95. Manaster, I. & Mandelboim, O. (2010). The unique properties of uterine NK cells. *Am J Reprod Immunol, 63,* 434.
96. Marchant, A. & Goldman, M. (2005). T cell-mediated immune responses in human newborns: Ready to learn? *Clin Exp Immunol, 141,* 10.
97. Märker-Hermann, E. & Fischer-Betz, R. (2010). Rheumatic diseases and pregnancy. *Curr Opin Obstet Gynecol, 22,* 458.
98. Marodi, L. (2012). Host-fungi interactions relevant to the newborn infant. In R.A. Polin, W.W. Fox, & S.H. Abman (Eds.), *Fetal and neonatal physiology* (4th ed.). Philadelphia: Saunders.
99. Marodi, L. & Notarangelo, L.D. (2012). T-cell development. In R.A. Polin, W.W. Fox, & S.H. Abman (Eds.), *Fetal and neonatal physiology* (4th ed.). Philadelphia: Saunders.
100. McMaster, M.T., Lim, K.H., & Taylor, R.N. (1998). Immunobiology of human pregnancy. *Curr Prob Obstet Gynecol Fertil, 21,* 1.
101. Mellor, A.L. & Munn, D.H. (2000). Immunology at the maternal-fetal interface: Lessons for T cell tolerance and suppression. *Annu Rev Immunol, 18,* 367.
102. Moise, K.J. (2009). Hemolytic disease of the fetus and newborn. In R.K. Creasy et al. (Eds.), *Creasy & Resnik's Maternal-fetal medicine: Principles and practice* (6th ed.). Philadelphia: Saunders Elsevier.
103. Mok, C.C. & Wong, R.W.S. (2001). Pregnancy in SLE. *Postgrad Med J, 77,* 157.
104. Molloy, E.J. (2004). Labor promotes neonatal neutrophil survival and lipopolysaccharide responsiveness. *Pediatr Res, 56,* 99.
105. Moore, K.L., Persaud, T.V.N. & Torchia, M. G. (2011). *The developing human: Clinically oriented embryology* (9th ed.). Philadelphia: Saunders Elsevier.
106. Mor, G., et al. (2005). Is the trophoblast an immune regulator? The role of toll-like receptors during pregnancy. *Crit Rev Immunol, 25,* 375.
107. Mor, G. & Abrahams, V.M. (2009). The immunology of pregnancy. In R.K. Creasy, et al. (Eds.), *Creasy & Resnik's Maternal-fetal medicine: Principles and practice* (6th ed.). Philadelphia: Saunders.
108. Moriyama, I., et al. (1987). Infection and the functional immaturity of the fetal immune system. In K. Maeda (Ed.), *The fetus as patient'*87 (Third International Symposium). Amsterdam: Excerpta Medica.
109. Mouzinho, A., et al. (1994). Revised reference ranges for circulating neutrophils in very-low-birth-weight neonates. *Pediatrics, 94,* 76.
110. Mshvildadze, M. & Neu, J. (2010). The infant intestinal microbiome: Friend or foe? *Early Hum Dev, 86,* S67.
111. Munoz-Suano, A., Hamilton, A.B., & Betz, A.G. (2011). Gimme shelter: The immune system during pregnancy. *Immunol Rev, 241,* 20.
112. Murgas Torrazza, R. & Neu, J. (*2011*). The developing intestinal microbiome and its relationship to health and disease in the neonate. *J Perinatol, 31,* S29.
113. Nagamatsu, T. & Schust, D.J. (2010). The immunomodulatory roles of macrophages at the maternal-fetal interface. *Reprod Sci, 17,* 209.
114. Nahmias, A.J. & Kourtis, A.P. (1997). The great balancing acts: The pregnant woman, placenta, fetus, and infectious agents. *Clin Perinatol, 24,* 497.
115. Nayak, A., et al. (2010). The non-classical functions of the classical complement pathway recognition subcomponent C1q. *Immunol Lett, 131,* 139.
116. Nelson, K.B. & Willoughby, R.E. (2000). Infection, inflammation, and the risk of cerebral palsy. *Curr Opin Neurol, 13,* 133.
117. Newburg, D.S., Ruiz-Palacios, G.M., & Morrow, A.L. (2005). Human milk glycans protect infants against enteric pathogens. *Annu Rev Nutr, 25,* 37.
118. Noetzel, M.J. & Burnstrom, J.E. (2001). The vulnerable oligodendrocyte, inflammatory observations on a cause of cerebral palsy. *Neurology, 66,* 1254.
119. Orange, J.S. & Ballas, Z.K. (2006). Natural killer cells in human health and disease. *Clin Immunol, 118,* 1.
120. O'Shea, T.M. & Dammann, O. (2000). Antecedents of cerebral palsy in very low-birth weight infants. *Clin Perinatol, 27,* 285.
121. Ostensen, M. (1999). Sex hormones and pregnancy in rheumatoid arthritis and systemic lupus erythematosus. *Ann N Y Acad Sci, 876,* 131.
122. Pappas, B.E. (1999). Primary immunodeficiency disorders in infancy. *Neonatal Netw, 18,* 13.

123. Petroff, M.G. & Perchellet, A. (2010). B7 family molecules as regulators of the maternal immune system in pregnancy. *Am J Reprod Immunol, 63,* 506.
124. Petroff, M.G. (2011). Review: Fetal antigens—identity, origins, and influences on the maternal immune system. *Placenta, 32,* S176.
125. Philbin, V.J. & Levy, O. (2009). Developmental biology of the innate immune response: Implications for neonatal and infant vaccine development. *Pediatr Res, 65,* 98R.
126. Piccinni, M.P., Maggi, E., & Romagnani, S. (2000). Role of hormone-controlled T-cell cytokines in the maintenance of pregnancy. *Biochem Soc Trans, 28,* 212.
127. Piccinni, M.P. (2010). T cell tolerance towards the fetal allograft. *J Reprod Immunol, 85,* 71.
128. Polak, M., et al. (2004). Fetal and neonatal thyroid function in relation to maternal Graves' disease. *Best Pract Res Clin Endocrinol Metab, 18,* 289.
129. Priddy, K.D. (1997). Immunologic adaptations during pregnancy. *J Obstet Gynecol Neonatal Nurs, 26,* 388.
130. Rabinovich, G.A. & Toscano, M.A. (2009). Turning "sweet" on immunity: galectin-glycan interactions in immune tolerance and inflammation. *Nat Rev Immunol, 9,* 338.
131. Rabot, M., et al. (2005). HLA class I/NK cell receptor interaction in early human deciduas basalis: Possible functional consequences. *Chem Immunol Allergy, 89,* 72.
132. Redman, C.W.G. & Sargent, I.L. (2003). Pre-eclampsia, the placenta and the maternal systemic inflammatory response—A review. *Placenta, 17,* S21.
133. Redman, C.W., & Sargent, I.L. (2005). Latest advances in understanding preeclampsia. *Science, 308,* 1592.
134. Richani, K., et al. (2005). Normal pregnancy is characterized by systemic activation of the complement system. *J Matern Fetal Neonatal Med, 17,* 239.
135. Riley, J.K. & Nelson, D.M. (2010). Toll-like receptors in pregnancy disorders and placental dysfunction. *Clin Rev Allergy Immunol, 39,* 185.
136. Rizzo, R., et al. (2011). The importance of HLA-G expression in embryos, trophoblast cells, and embryonic stem cells. *Cell Mol Life Sci, 68,* 341.
137. Robertson, S.A., et al. (2009). Activating T regulatory cells for tolerance in early pregnancy—the contribution of seminal fluid. *J Reprod Immunol, 83,* 109.
138. Robertson, S.A. (2010). Immune regulation of conception and embryo implantation—all about quality control? *J Reprod Immunol, 85,* 51.
139. Romero, R. & Lockwood, C.J. (2009). Pathogenesis of spontaneous preterm labor. In R.K. Creasy, et al. (Eds.), *Creasy & Resnik's Maternal-fetal medicine: Principles and practice* (6th ed.). Philadelphia: Saunders Elsevier.
140. Sacchi, F., et al. (1982). Differential maturation of neutrophil chemotaxis in term and preterm newborn infants. *J Pediatr, 101,* 273.
141. Saliba, E. & Henrot, A. (2001). Inflammatory mediators and neonatal brain damage. *Biol Neonate, 79,* 224.
142. Salmon, J.E. (2004). A noninflammatory pathway for pregnancy loss: Innate immune activation? *J Clin Invest, 114,* 15.
143. Samuel, B.U. & Barry, M. (1998). The pregnant traveler. *Infect Dis Clin North Am, 12,* 325.
144. Schelonka, R.L. & Infante, A.J. (1998). Neonatal immunology. *Semin Perinatol, 22,* 2.
145. Schibler, K.R. (2012). Mononuclear phagocyte system. In R.A. Polin, W.W. Fox, & S.H. Abman (Eds.), *Fetal and neonatal physiology* (3rd ed.). Philadelphia: Saunders.
146. Schulzke, S., et al. (2005). Apnoea and bradycardia in preterm infants following immunization with pentavalent or hexavalent vaccines. *Eur J Pediatr, 164,* 432.
147. Shen, C.M., et al. (2009). Labour increases the surface expression of two toll-like receptors in the cord blood monocytes of healthy term newborns. *Acta Paediatr, 98,* 959.
148. Sibai, B., Dekker, G., & Kupferminc, M. (2005). Pre-eclampsia. *Lancet, 365,* 785.
149. Siegrist, C.A. & Aspinall, R. (2009). B-cell responses to vaccination at the extremes of age. *Nat Rev Immunol, 9,* 185.
150. Skornicka, E., et al. (2004). Pregnancy zone protein is a carrier and modulator of placental protein-14 in T-cell growth and cytokine production. *Cell Immunol, 232,* 144.
151. Spencer, S.J., Galic, M.A., & Pittman, Q.J. (2011). Neonatal programming of innate immune function. *Am J Physiol Endocrinol Metab, 300,* E11.
152. Stafford, I.P. & Dildy, G.A. (2005). Myasthenia gravis and pregnancy. *Clin Obstet Gynecol, 48,* 48.
153. Stagnaro-Green, A., et al. (1992). A prospective study of lymphocyte initiated immunosuppression in normal pregnancy: Evidence of a T-cell etiology for postpartum thyroid dysfunction. *J Clin Endocrinol Metab, 74,* 645.
154. Stevenson, A.M. (1999). Immunizations for women and infants. *J Obstet Gynecol Neonatal Nurs, 28,* 534.
155. Szekeree-Bartho, J., et al. (2005). Progesterone dependent immunomodulation. *Chem Immunol Allergy, 89,* 118.
156. Tarini, B.A., et al. (2006). Systematic review of the relationship between early introduction of solid foods to infants and the development of allergic disease. *Arch Pediatr Adolesc Med, 160,* 502.
157. Tayade, C., et al. (2005). Functions of alpha 2 macroglobulins in pregnancy. *Mol Cell Endocrin, 245,* 60.
158. Thellin, O. (2000). Tolerance to the foeto-placental "graft": Ten ways to support a child for nine months. *Curr Opin Immunol, 12,* 731.
159. Tincani, A., et al. (2005). Pregnancy and autoimmunity: Maternal treatment and maternal disease influence on pregnancy outcome. *Autoimmunity Rev, 4,* 42.
160. Towers, C.J. & Briggs, G.G. (2002). Antepartum use of antibiotics and early-onset neonatal sepsis. *Am J Obstet Gynecol, 187,* 495.
161. Upham, J.W., et al. (2009). Plasmacytoid dendritic cells during infancy are inversely associated with childhood respiratory tract infections and wheezing. *J Allergy Clin Immunol, 124,* 707.
162. Urbaniak, S.J. & Greiss, M.A. (2000). RhD haemolytic disease of the fetus and the newborn. *Blood Rev, 14,* 44.
163. Vael, C. & Desager, K. (2009). The importance of the development of the intestinal microbiota in infancy. *Curr Opin Pediatr, 21,* 794.
164. van den Berg, J.P., et al. (2011). Transplacental transport of IgG antibodies to preterm infants: A review of the literature. *Early Hum Dev, 87,* 67.
165. Verani, J.R. & Schrag, S.J. (2010). Group B streptococcal disease in infants: Progress in prevention and continued challenges. *Clin Perinatol, 37,* 375.
166. Verani, J.R., et al. (2010). Prevention of perinatal group B streptococcal disease—revised guidelines from CDC, 2010. *MMWR Recomm Rep, 59,* 1.
167. Vince, G.S. & Johnson, P.M. (2000). Leukocyte populations and cytokine regulation in human uteroplacental tissues. *Biochem Soc Trans, 28,* 191.
168. Voisin, G.A. (1998). Immunology understood through pregnancy. *Am J Reprod Immunol, 40,* 124.
169. Walker, W.A. (2000). Role of nutrients and bacterial colonization in the development of intestinal host defense. *J Pediatr Gastroenterol Nutr, 30,* S2.
170. Warren, J.B. & Silver, R.M. (2004). Autoimmune disease in pregnancy: Systemic lupus erythematosus and antiphospholipid syndrome. *Obstet Gynecol Clin North Am, 31,* 345.
171. Weinberg, E.D. (1984). Pregnancy associated depression of cell-mediated immunity. *Rev Infect Dis, 6,* 814.
172. Weiner, C. & Buhimschi, C. (2009). *Drugs for pregnant and lactating women* (2nd ed.). London: Churchill Livingstone.
173. Whitsett, J.A. (2010). Review: The intersection of surfactant homeostasis and innate host defense of the lung: Lessons from newborn infants. *Innate Immun, 16,* 138.
174. Williams, C.B., Eisenstein, E.M., & Cole, F.S. (2012). Immunology of the fetus and newborn. In C.A. Gleason & S. Devaskar (Eds.), *Avery's Diseases of the newborn* (9th ed.). Philadelphia: Saunders.

175. Wilson, C.B. & Ogru, R. (2010). Human milk. In J.S. Remington & J.O. Klein (Eds.), *Infectious diseases of the fetus and newborn infant* (7th ed.). Philadelphia: Saunders.
176. Witkin, S.S., et al. (2011). Unique alterations in infection-induced immune activation during pregnancy. *BJOG, 118*, 145.
177. Wood, N. & Siegrist, C.A. (2011). Neonatal immunization: Where do we stand? *Curr Opin Infect Dis, 24*, 190.
178. Wu, Y.W. & Colford, J.M. (2000). Chorioamnionitis as a risk factor for cerebral palsy. *JAMA, 284*, 1417.
179. Wynn, J., et al. (2010). The host response to sepsis and developmental impact. *Pediatrics, 125*, 1031.
180. Wynn, J.L. & Levy, O. (2010). Role of innate host defenses in susceptibility to early-onset neonatal sepsis. *Clin Perinatol, 37*, 307.
181. Yadav, A.K., Madan, T., & Bernal, A.L. (2011). Surfactant proteins A and D in pregnancy and parturition. *Front Biosci (Elite Ed), 3*, 291.
182. Yagel, S. (2009). The developmental role of natural killer cells at the fetal-maternal interface. *Am J Obstet Gynecol, 201*, 344.
183. Yektaei-Karin, E., et al. (2007). The stress of birth enhances in vitro spontaneous and IL-8-induced neutrophil chemotaxis in the human newborn. *Pediatr Allergy Immunol, 18*, 643.
184. Zrour, S.H., et al. (2010). The impact of pregnancy on rheumatoid arthritis outcome: The role of maternofetal HLA class II disparity. *Joint Bone Spine, 77*, 36.

CHAPTER 14

The Integumentary System

The integumentary system consists of the skin and its appendages: eccrine, apocrine, apoeccrine, and sebaceous glands; hair; and nails. Functions of the skin include protection from physical and chemical injury, infection, and ultraviolet radiation; modulation of transepidermal water fluxes; prevention of fluid loss and fluid and electrolyte imbalances; and thermoregulation. The skin is also important in sensation (pain, pressure, touch, and temperature), tactile discrimination, contributes to maintenance of blood pressure by dilation or constriction of the peripheral capillaries, and contains precursor molecules for vitamin D.[49]

The skin and its associated structures are markedly altered during pregnancy. These changes are seen in most pregnant women, and although the changes themselves are seldom associated with serious physiologic consequences, they are of concern to most women because of the subsequent cosmetic alterations, some of which may persist following delivery. In addition, there are several dermatologic disorders that are seen almost exclusively in pregnant women that can cause severe physical discomfort and may be associated with increased fetal morbidity. For the neonate, the skin is a sophisticated and critical sensory organ for obtaining and receiving information about the environment. Because the neonate is an immunologically immature host, the integrity of the skin as a barrier to that same environment is essential to the survival and well-being of the infant. Immaturity of the skin alters its permeability, immunologic capacity, bonding of the epidermis to the dermis, and role in thermoregulation and fluid balance. As a result, neonates, especially preterm and ill infants, are at risk for toxicity from topical substances, infection, skin excoriation, fluid loss, and thermal instability.

MATERNAL PHYSIOLOGIC ADAPTATIONS

Physiologic changes in the skin and its appendages during pregnancy and the postpartum period include alterations in pigmentation; connective and cutaneous tissue; integumentary vascular system; hair, nails, and secretory glands; and pruritus. Some integumentary alterations regress completely during the postpartum period; others recede but never completely disappear. Most of these alterations are secondary to the hormonal changes of pregnancy.

Antepartum Period

The basis for changes in the skin, hair, and secretory glands during pregnancy are thought to be hormonal—especially the effects of estrogens and adrenocortical steroids. Similar alterations are often seen in women using oral contraceptives. There is a familial tendency or genetic predisposition for some of the cutaneous and vascular changes.[77,118]

Alterations in Pigmentation

Alterations in pigmentation are common during pregnancy and include hyperpigmentation of specific areas of the body and melasma (chloasma). In early pregnancy, hyperpigmentation is thought to be due to the effects of estrogens and progesterone on melanocytes. This finding is also consistent with reports of alterations in pigmentation associated with use of oral contraceptives.[31] Progression is also thought to be related to the effects of placental corticosteroid-releasing hormone and of pro-opiomelanocortin peptides such as adrenocorticotropic hormone (ACTH), melanocyte-stimulating hormone (MSH), β-endorphin (see Chapter 19), and possibly placental lipid stimulation of tyrosinase (enzyme involved in production of melanin).[77,85,90,93,96]

Hyperpigmentation. Hyperpigmentation is the most frequent integumentary alteration during pregnancy. Changes in pigmentation are seen in up to 91% of pregnant women, tend to be more frequent in women with dark hair or complexions, and are progressive throughout pregnancy.[62] Most women experience a mild, generalized increase in pigmentation that is especially prominent in areas of the body that tend to be naturally more intensely pigmented. These areas include the areolae, genital skin, axillae, inner aspects of the thighs, and linea alba.[23,28,61,77,93]

The linea alba is a tendinous median line that extends along the anterior of the abdomen from the umbilicus to the symphysis pubis and occasionally superiorly to the xiphoid process. Hyperpigmentation during pregnancy causes the linea alba to darken and become the linea nigra. Up to one third of women on oral contraceptives also develop a linea nigra. Pigmentary changes tend to fade during the postpartum period in fair-skinned women, but some pigmentary changes may remain in women with darker skin and hair. Hyperpigmentation may be exacerbated by sun exposure.[28,61,93,96]

Freckles, nevi, and recent scars may darken during pregnancy, perhaps due to an up-regulation of receptors for estrogens and progesterone on the nevus cell surface.[27] Existing melanocytic nevi may increase in size or new nevi may develop during pregnancy, although some have reported that existing melanocytic nevi do not change significantly during pregnancy.[57] Increased malignant degeneration of nevi is not seen during pregnancy.[57,85] Prophylactic removal of nevi following pregnancy may be considered. Any nevi showing signs suggestive of malignancy should be excised.[28,61,93,96]

Although rare, some women may develop pigmentary demarcation lines, which are areas of hypopigmentation that follow the distribution of peripheral cutaneous nerves, and disappear after delivery. The lines are thought to be due to prolonged uterine compression of these nerves, particularly at S1-S2, leading to a sharp demarcation between pigmented and hypopigmented areas.[2,89,93]

Melasma. Melasma (also known as *chloasma* or the "mask of pregnancy") is a common occurrence in pregnant women.[5,15,77,93,96] Melasma is characterized by irregular, blotchy areas of pigmentation on the face, usually bilateral and symmetrical and seen most commonly on the cheeks, chin, and nose.[77] The areas of altered pigmentation are not elevated and can range in color from light to dark brown. Three distribution patterns have been described: centrofacial (63%), involving the cheeks, forehead, upper lip, nose, and chin; malar (21%), over the cheeks and nose; and mandibular (16%), over the ramus of the mandible.[5] Three histological patterns have also been identified: epidermal (increased deposition of melanin in the melanocytes of the basal and suprabasal layers), which is seen in 70% of women; dermal (macrophages with large amounts of melanin can be found in both the papillary and reticular layers of the dermis), which is seen in 10% to 15%; and a mixed form, which is seen in 2%.[5,61] Although these pigmentary changes tend to fade completely within 1 year following pregnancy, they may persist (especially in dark-haired individuals).[63,93,96]

Melasma is associated with increased expression of α-melanocyte stimulating hormone in the involved skin area.[93] There is a genetic predisposition toward development of melasma.[5,100] Melasma is seen most frequently in women with dark hair and complexions, is exacerbated by the sun, and tends to recur (often with increased intensity) in subsequent pregnancies or with use of oral contraceptives.[10] Melasma has also been reported occasionally in nonpregnant individuals who are not on oral contraceptives or other hormonal medications.[54,93,96,118]

Avoidance of sun tanning during pregnancy, use of hats to avoid facial exposure to sun, and use of sunscreens with sun protective ratings greater than 15 may reduce the severity of melasma (Table 14-1). Because melasma often fades spontaneously following pregnancy, treatment is generally limited to the less than 10% of individuals with persistent pigmentation postpartum.[77] Various depigmenting formulas have been developed to treat persistent melasma, with varying success. These formulas tend to be relatively effective on epidermal-type melasma but have little effect on the dermal type. Treatment may need to be continued for 5 to 7 weeks before satisfactory results are achieved. Topical 2% to 5% hydroquinone with or without retinoic acid and corticosteroids has also been used postpartum, again with varying success. This treatment can result in complications such as hypopigmentation, hyperpigmentation, and contact dermatitis.[5,10,93,96,118]

Changes in Connective Tissue

Striae gravidarum (also called *linear striae, striae distensae,* or *linear stretch marks*) are linear tears in dermal collagen that are commonly seen during pregnancy. These markings initially appear as irregular, pink or purple, wrinkled linear streaks that gradually become white. Striae are most prominent by 6 to 7 months and occur in 50% to 80% of pregnant women.[93] They appear initially over the abdomen oriented in opposition to skin tension lines and later on the breasts, thighs, and inguinal area. Striae are seen more frequently in younger women with greater total weight gain during pregnancy, obese women, and women with larger birth weight infants.[12] In addition, there appears to be a familial tendency.[5,77,86,93,111,118]

Striae gravidarum usually fade following pregnancy but never completely disappear, remaining as depressed, irregular white bands. Some women report striae itching, although because both pruritus and striae formation are prominent over the abdominal area during pregnancy, these two phenomena may not be related. There is no effective treatment to prevent striae formation. Topical emollients and antipruritics may be used (see Table 14-1). However, the effectiveness of topical agents such as cocoa butter, vitamin E, tretinoin, and olive oil and of massage to prevent striae formation has not been substantiated in controlled studies.[77,96,102,120] Two recent studies found that cocoa butter did not prevent striae gravidarum or reduce its severity.[12,87]

Striae gravidarum are believed to arise from hormonal alterations—especially of estrogens, relaxin, and adrenocorticoids—along with alterations in the dermal support matrix with stretching.[87] The increased levels of estrogens, corticosteroids, and relaxin relax the adhesiveness between collagen fibers and foster formation of mucopolysaccharide ground substance, which causes separation of the fibers and striae formation. The increased glucocorticosteroids during pregnancy may decrease dermal fibroblasts and collagen synthesis. Mast cells, which contain hormonal receptors for estradiol, also increase. Mast cells release enzymes to lyse collagen.[5,61,96,102,118]

Vascular and Hematologic Changes

Vascular changes during pregnancy related to the integumentary system include development of spider nevi or angiomas, palmar erythema, nonpitting edema, cutis marmorata, purpura, hemangiomas, and varicosities. Purpura and scattered petechiae may be seen on the legs of some women and are due to decreased capillary integrity with increased hydrostatic

Table 14-1 **Nursing Management for Common Problems during Pregnancy Related to the Integumentary System**

ALTERATION	INTERVENTION
All alterations	Provide anticipatory teaching regarding appearance of alteration. Counsel regarding basis for alteration and course. Evaluate effect on body image and relationship with partner and provide counseling.
Hyperpigmentation	Avoid suntanning during pregnancy and use broad-spectrum (protective factor greater than 15) sunscreen. Use nonallergenic cover-ups.
Melasma	Avoid suntanning during pregnancy or when using oral contraceptives. Use broad-spectrum sunscreen (rating of 15 or greater). Use nonallergenic cover-ups. Counsel regarding the risk of similar changes with oral contraceptives. Counsel regarding alternative methods of birth control. Counsel regarding use of sunscreen and protection from sun with sunscreen use following pregnancy.
Striae gravidarum	Use topical emollients or antipruritics as required. Use supportive garments for breasts and abdomen.
Spider nevi	Reassure that most fade following pregnancy. Use cosmetic cover-up creams. Suggest considering electrocauterization if of great concern to patient.
Nonpitting edema	Elevate legs when sitting or lying down and when sleeping. Avoid prolonged standing or sitting. Rest in the left lateral decubitus position. Water immersion (standing or with exercise). Exercise. Avoid excessive added salt. Avoid tight clothing and girdles. Try elastic stockings (although their effectiveness is controversial).
Varicosities	Elevate legs when sitting or lying down and sleep in the Trendelenburg position. Avoid prolonged standing or sitting. Rest in the left lateral decubitus position. Exercise. Sitz bath for hemorrhoids. Avoid tight clothing. Wear elastic stockings or support hose.
Increased eccrine gland activity	Wear light, loose clothing. Increase fluid intake. Bathe or shower regularly.
Pruritus	Wear loose nonsynthetic clothing. Use cool compresses and take baths or showers. Use oatmeal baths. Use adequate skin lubrication. Consider topical antipruritics, emollients, and calamine lotion.

pressure.[5] These usually resolve postpartum. Vascular changes are a result of distention, instability, and proliferation of blood vessels mediated by changes in pituitary, adrenal, and placental hormones with increased release of angiogenic growth factors.[61,63,96] Other alterations in the vascular and hematologic systems are described in Chapters 8 and 9.

Vasomotor Instability. Vasomotor instability during pregnancy may result in flushing, feelings of hot or cold, and cutis marmorata.[5,44,89] Cutis marmorata is a transient bluish mottling of the legs that is exaggerated on exposure to cold. It arises from vasomotor instability secondary to elevated estrogens. Persistence postpartum is abnormal and may suggest underlying pathology such as collagen vascular disorder, systemic lupus erythematosus, or vasculitis. Other changes due to vasomotor instability during pregnancy include pallor, facial flushing, and heat and cold sensations. Purpura secondary to increased capillary fragility and permeability occurs during the last months of pregnancy in many women.[96,118]

Spider Nevi. Spider nevi (also called *spider angiomas, spider telangiectases,* or *nevus araneus*) are found in 10% to 15% of normal adults, in individuals with liver dysfunction, and in up to two thirds of pregnant women. These nevi are more common in white pregnant women (60% to 70% by term) than African-American pregnant women (10% by term).[44] Spider nevi consist of a central dilated arteriole that is flat or slightly raised with extensive radiating capillary branches. They are most prominent in areas of the skin drained by the superior vena cava (i.e., around the eyes, neck, throat, and arms). The basis for formation has been related to increased estrogen, because these structures are seen more frequently both during pregnancy and with use of oral contraceptives. However, many individuals with spider nevi associated with liver disorders do not have elevated estrogen levels.[61,118]

Spider nevi generally appear between 2 and 5 months of pregnancy and may increase in size and number as pregnancy progresses. These structures tend to regress spontaneously and fade within the first 7 weeks to 3 months following delivery, although they rarely completely disappear. They may recur or enlarge during subsequent pregnancies. Unresolved spider nevi can be treated by pulse-dye laser or electrodesiccation therapy.[93]

Palmar Erythema. Palmar erythema is seen with pregnancy, liver disease, estrogen therapy and collagen vascular diseases.[93] Two patterns of palmar erythema are seen during pregnancy: erythema of hypothenar and thenar eminences, palms, and fleshy portions of the fingertips; and diffuse mottling of the entire palm. The latter form is more common and similar to changes seen with hyperthyroidism and cirrhosis. Palmar erythema generally appears during the first two trimesters and disappears by 1 week after delivery. This phenomenon has a familial tendency and is seen in approximately two thirds of white pregnant women and one third of African American pregnant women. Spider nevi and palmar erythema often occur together, suggesting a common etiology generally believed to be elevated estrogen levels with increased skin blood flow.[5,28,44,61,90,93,118] No treatment is needed. Palmar erythema resolves after delivery.

Nonpitting Edema. Increased vascular permeability and sodium retention due to the effects of estrogens and corticosteroids result in transient nonpitting edema of the face, hands, and feet during late pregnancy.[44,89] In the lower extremities, this is aggravated by pressure from the growing uterus. Nonpitting edema occurs in the face, especially the eyelids in approximately 50% of women, and in the lower extremities in 70% and is not associated with preeclampsia.[96,118] Although most pronounced in the morning, it usually improves during the day. Interventions for non-pitting edema during pregnancy are listed in Table 14-1. Vulvar edema may also be seen.

Capillary Hemangiomas. Pre existing capillary hemangiomas may increase in size during pregnancy.[5,96] In up to one third of pregnant women, new hemangiomas appear by the end of the first trimester, with slight, slow enlargement during the remaining trimesters.[44,118] New hemangiomas usually appear on the head and neck and are unusual elsewhere.[96] Enlarged existing hemangiomas and new hemangiomas regress postpartum but may not completely disappear. Hemangioma development in pregnancy is related to elevated estrogen.[118]

Varicosities.[5,61,65,89,93,96,118] Varicosities develop in approximately 40% of pregnant women. Varicosities occur most commonly in the legs but may also appear in the pelvic vessels, vulva, and anal area with hemorrhoid formation. Varicosities arise from estrogen-induced elastic tissue fragility, vascular distension, relaxin-weakened collagen and elastin, increased venous pressure in the lower extremities and pelvis from pressure of the gravid uterus, and familial tendency for valvular incompetence. Varicosities generally regress postpartum but do not completely disappear. Thrombi are rare with leg varicosities but are more frequent with hemorrhoids. Hemorrhoids are discussed in Chapter 12.

Alterations in Cutaneous Tissue and Mucous Membranes

The most common mucous membrane alterations are changes in the vagina and cervix, which are seen in all pregnant women, and gingivitis, which is seen in many women. A less common oral finding is a cutaneous lesion of the gums known as *angiogranuloma,* or *epulis.* Epulis and gingivitis are discussed in Chapter 12. Increased flow to the nasal mucosa leads to rhinitis in up to one third of women.[37] Jacquemier-Chadwick and Goodell signs are vascular changes that are early signs of pregnancy. Jacquemier-Chadwick sign is characterized by erythema of the vestibule and vagina; Goodell sign is characterized by increased vascularity of the cervix.[61,63,96]

Another cutaneous change during pregnancy is the development of or increase in the number of existing skin tags called *molluscum fibrosum gravidarum* (also called *acrochordons* or, if large, *fibroepithelial polyps*).[5,77,90,96] These are soft, skin-colored or hyperpigmented skin tags, which are small (usually 1 to 5 mm), pedunculated fibromas that appear during the second half of pregnancy, primarily on the lateral aspects of the face and neck, upper axillae, groin, and between and underneath the breasts. The cause of fibromata molle is unknown but is thought to be hormonal. These skin tags are more common in the second half of pregnancy, when they may increase in size and number. These growths may regress or clear spontaneously following delivery, although many remain. Remaining skin tags can be excised.[61,63,77,90,93,96,118]

Alterations in Secretory Glands

Activity of the sebaceous, apocrine, and eccrine glands of the skin is altered during pregnancy. Sebaceous gland activity is generally reported to increase during pregnancy.[5,90,118] Many pregnant women report that their skin, especially on the face, feels "greasy." Some women may develop acne, often for the first time, although women with existing acne may or may not experience worsening of the acne.[5,61] These changes are due to increased ovarian and placental androgens.[61,93] Montgomery tubercles (small sebaceous glands on the areola) enlarge, beginning as early as 6 weeks' gestation. Changes in Montgomery tubercles and the breasts are described in Chapter 5.

Apocrine sweat gland activity decreases during pregnancy, possibly as a result of hormonal changes.[5,118] Eccrine sweat gland activity increases gradually during pregnancy, possibly because of increased thyroid activity along with increased body weight and metabolic activity.[89,90,118] Because eccrine glands are important (along with the cutaneous blood vessels) in thermoregulation at the skin surface (see Chapter 20), their increased activity reflects dissipation of excess heat produced by the increased metabolic activity of the pregnant woman and her fetus. Increased eccrine activity during pregnancy can lead to miliaria (prickly heat) or dyshidrotic eczema.[5,61,118] Palmar sweating is decreased in pregnancy, even though this is an area where eccrine glands are highly concentrated. The basis for this is unclear but may be related to increased thyroid or adrenocortical activity.[5,28,61] Interventions are listed in Table 14-1.

Alterations in Hair Growth

Estrogen increases the length of the anagen (growth) phase of hair follicles during pregnancy (see the Hair Loss section under Postpartum Period). This results in increased hair loss postpartum. The diameter of the hair shaft also thickens by late pregnancy in most women.[5,31,83] A mild hirsutism may develop, usually beginning around 20 weeks, with increased growth of hair on the upper lip, chin, and cheeks and in the suprapubic midline. Fine new hairs usually disappear by 6 weeks postpartum, but the coarser hairs usually remain.[13,61,77,93,96,113,118]

During late pregnancy and the early postpartum period, some women develop hair loss with frontoparietal recession of the hairline similar to changes seen in male-pattern baldness. This loss is rare and is usually associated with complete regrowth and not with later development of female-pattern alopecia.[61,96]

Alterations in the Nails

Changes in fingernails and toenails during pregnancy are uncommon and of unknown pathogenesis. Nail changes occur as early as 6 weeks and include transverse grooves, increased brittleness, distal separation of the nail bed (onycholysis), whitish discoloration (leukonychia), and subungual keratosis. These changes regress after delivery.[5,61,77,90,93,118] A faster toenail growth rate has been reported by some women during pregnancy, possibly due to increased peripheral blood flow due to estrogens, along with coarsening of the nail texture.[89]

Pruritus

Pruritus is the most common cutaneous symptom during pregnancy.[5] The itching may be localized, especially over the abdomen during the third trimester, or generalized. Abdominal pruritus at the end of the first trimester may be an isolated finding or an early sign of intrahepatic cholestasis of pregnancy with or without associated jaundice or one of the other specific dermatoses of pregnancy (Table 14-2). Pregnancy-associated pruritus always clears after delivery but may recur in subsequent pregnancies or with use of oral contraceptives.[93] Pregnant women with pruritus should also be assessed for other skin disorders, including pregnancy dermatoses, contact dermatitis, and drug reactions.[5,93,118]

Postpartum Period

Some of the changes in the integumentary system and its associated structures clear spontaneously following delivery; other alterations may regress or fade but do not disappear completely (see previous section for specific skin changes). Hyperpigmentation fades in many women; however, these changes may remain, especially in women with darker skin and hair. In addition melasma may persist for months postpartum in up to 30% of women.[93] After delivery, striae gravidarum and spider nevi fade and capillary hemangiomas, varicosities, and skin tags regress. However, these changes may not completely disappear.[61,93,96] Increased body and facial hair usually regresses by 6 months postpartum; thinning or regression of the hairline may not reverse completely.[77] Alterations in hair growth during pregnancy result in an increased hair loss during the postpartum period in many women.

Hair Loss

The scalp contains approximately 100,000 hair follicles. Hair fibers in each follicle independently cycle through three stages: anagen, catagen, and telogen. The anagen or growth stage lasts for 3 to 4 years and is characterized by intense metabolic activity. In this stage, hair grows an average of 0.34 mm/day.[93] Catagen is a transitional stage that lasts several weeks. During this stage, metabolic activity and growth slow as the hair bulb is retracted upward into the follicle. Growth of the hair fiber stops during telogen (resting stage). Eventually a new hair bulb begins growing, which ejects the previous hair.[93] Normally about 80% of hair follicles are in the anagen stage and 15% to 20% of hair fibers are in the telogen stage, with about 100 to 150 hairs shed per day.[96]

Under the influence of estrogen during pregnancy, the rate of hair growth slows and the anagen stage is prolonged. This results in an increased number of anagen hairs and a decrease in telogen hairs to less than 10% during the second and third trimesters. During the postpartum period, with the decline in estrogens, these anagen hairs enter catagen and then telogen and are shed. Since there are more anagen hairs (and thus eventually telogen hairs) than usual, most postpartum women experience an increased hair loss, beginning 4 to 20 weeks after delivery. During this time, 30% to 35% of the hairs may enter telogen. Generally, complete regrowth occurs by 4 to 6 months in two thirds of women and by 15 months in the remainder, although the hair may be less abundant than before pregnancy.[13,93,96,113] *Telogen effluvium* is the term used to describe the rapid transition of hair follicles into the telogen stage following delivery, surgery, or severe emotional or physical stress.[93,96,118]

CLINICAL IMPLICATIONS FOR THE PREGNANT WOMAN AND HER FETUS

The physiologic changes in the integumentary system during pregnancy and after delivery are common experiences for many women. These changes seldom significantly alter the function or structure of the integumentary system and are considered by some to be minor nuisances.[96] However, these changes may have significant psychological and cosmetic implications for the pregnant woman and can contribute to alterations in body image. General interventions include anticipatory counseling, education, and reassurance (see Table 14-1).

Dermatoses Associated with Pregnancy

In addition to the normal physiologic skin changes associated with pregnancy, there are several integumentary disorders that are unique to pregnancy. Specific dermatoses seen only during pregnancy include pemphigoid gestationis, impetigo herpetiformis, atopic eruptions of pregnancy/prurigo of pregnancy, pruritic urticarial papules and plaques of pregnancy (PUPPP) or polymorphic eruption of pregnancy (PEP), and intrahepatic cholestasis of pregnancy.[61,93,96] Several of these disorders have been associated with increased fetal morbidity and mortality (see Table 14-2). Most of these disorders resolve spontaneously within a few weeks after delivery, but can recur with subsequent pregnancies.[93]

The etiology of some of these disorders is unclear, although others have a hormonal or immunologic basis. For example, pemphigoid gestationis is an autoimmune disorder with production of anti–human leukocyte antigen (HLA) autoantibody against basal membranes that hold the epidermis and dermis together (see Table 14-2).[20,40,97] There has sometimes been confusion in classifying some of the rarer dermatoses, in that much of the literature regarding these disorders involves reports of small numbers of women, which may represent different variations of the same disorder. Treatment involves use of topical emollients, antipruritics, cold compresses, oatmeal baths (for relief of itching), and topical steroids. In women with moderate to severe eruptions, systemic steroids and antihistamines may be used. Cautions must be used in prescribing these and other dermatologic agents during pregnancy as some, such as retinoic acid, are teratogenic (see Chapter 7) and thus are contraindicated in pregnancy. There are limited data for most other agents on their use in pregnancy. Thus risk benefit must be carefully evaluated.[17,93]

Effects of Pregnancy on Pre existing Skin Disorders

The effects of pregnancy on pre existing skin disorders varies from no effect to marked improvement or worsening.[28,93,96,118] With disorders such as psoriasis, eczema, contact dermatitis, and acne vulgaris, this range of effects during pregnancy has been described within the same disease in different women.[93] Neurofibromas increase in size during pregnancy and new tumors may appear.[93] The effect of pregnancy on malignant melanoma is also variable.[22,93] No significant effect on survival in women with a diagnosis of localized melanoma (stage I or II) during pregnancy was found in an analysis of six case controlled studies.[27] Decreased survival or shorter disease-free survival for pregnant women with recurrent melanoma is reported in some studies.[22,27] Effects of pregnancy on other integumentary disorders are reviewed in the literature.[93,96]

SUMMARY

The effects of pregnancy on the integumentary system include physiologic changes in the skin and its appendages that are experienced by most pregnant women, skin disorders that are unique to pregnancy, and possible changes in pre existing skin disorders. Nursing management of the pregnant woman in relation to these effects includes preparation for the physiologic changes and their sequelae, and reassurance and support, as well as assessment for the specific dermatoses of pregnancy that are associated with maternal systemic symptoms and, if severe and untreated, with increased fetal mortality and morbidity. Clinical recommendations related to changes in the integumentary system during pregnancy are summarized in Table 14-3.

DEVELOPMENT OF THE INTEGUMENTARY SYSTEM IN THE FETUS

Anatomic Development

The basic structure of the skin develops during the first 60 days of gestation. Around the time of transition from embryo to fetus, the skin undergoes a series of rapid morphologic changes, including keratinization of the epidermal appendages (around 15 weeks) and interfollicular epithelium (around 22 to 24 weeks).[19] By the third trimester, the structure of the skin is similar to that of the adult. However, its barrier properties are still immature, especially in the infant born before term.[19] Further maturation of the skin occurs within the first weeks after birth and during infancy.[9,82,106,114]

The skin consists of the epidermis and dermis with an underlying subcutaneous layer (Figure 14-1). The epidermis consists of an outer stratum corneum, stratum granulosum, and the stratum germinativum, which consists of the stratum spinosum, and stratum basale (adjacent to the epidermal-dermal junction). The basal layer contaikns melanocytes (pigment-producing cells) and keratinocytes. Keratinocytes, the major cell of the epidermis, develop from stem cells in the basal layer and migrate outward to cornify the outer layer.[35] The stratum corneum is the barrier layer and consists of keratinocytes linked by lipids. Underneath the epidermis lies the dermis, formed from fibrous protein, collagen, and elastin fibers woven together. The dermis contains the nerves and blood vessels that nourish the skin cells and carry sensations from the skin to the brain (see Figure 14-1). Mechanical properties of the dermis include tensile strength, compressibility, resilience, and elasticity.[19] The subcutaneous layer is composed of fatty connective tissue that provides insulation and caloric storage.[71] The epidermis and dermis, along with their vascular and neural networks, develop concurrently.

Epidermis

Development of the epidermis "is characterized by coordinated establishment of increasing numbers of cell layers concomitant with expansion of skin surface area and cellular

Table 14-2 **Dermatoses of Pregnancy**

DISORDER*	INCIDENCE	ONSET AND ETIOLOGY	CHARACTERISTICS
Pemphigoid gestationis (herpes gestationis) (11, 20, 93, 96, 97, 98)	1/50,000-60,000 Seen most often in white women Has a familial tendency	Usually second and third trimesters Can appear as early as 2 weeks' gestation or up to 2 weeks postpartum (20%) May clear toward end of pregnancy and, then exacerbate postpartum Etiology: autoimmune disorder with production of anti-human leukocyte antigen (HLA) autoantibodies against basal membranes that hold the epidermis and dermis together seen in many women	Generalized, intense pruritus and erythematous urticarial plaques initially, followed by crops of fluid-filled vesicles and/or tense serum-filled bullae
Impetigo herpetiformis (93, 96, 98)	Very rare	First to third trimesters, with peak incidence in third trimester Etiology unknown; associated with hypocalcemia and hypoparathyroidism May be a form of pustular psoriasis	Small (1-2 mm), sterile, white pustules on irregular erythematous plaques; central pustules become crusted as new pustules develop in periphery of plaque
Atopic eruption of pregnancy/Prurigo of pregnancy (11, 93, 96, 97, 98)	1/300	Any trimester, usually by midgestation May be due to hypersensitivity to placental antigens Includes several disorders, including prurigo gestationis of Besnier, Nurse's prurigo of late pregnancy, and papular dermatitis of pregnancy (Spangler's)	Severe pruritus with small erythematous papules that are skin-colored; primary papules may be destroyed by scratching, leaving excoriated crusts as initial presentation
Pruritic urticarial papules and plaques of pregnancy (PUPPP), or polymorphic eruption of pregnancy (PEP) (11, 72, 93, 96, 97, 98)	0.6% of pregnant women (more common in primiparas)	Usually third trimester (at 36-39 weeks) or postpartum Self-limiting inflammatory disorder	Erythematous papules and urticarial plaques with excoriation usually absent
Intrahepatic cholestasis of pregnancy (11, 73, 81, 93, 97, 98)	0.02%-2.4% of pregnant women	Usually third trimester (rare before 25 weeks; persists to delivery) Cholestasis Multifactorial; related to genetic and environmental factors with alterations in estrogen clearance by liver and hepatocellular transport	Severe generalized pruritus without any skin lesions, especially on palms and soles, although excoriation may result from scratching; worse at night; 50% have darker urine and stools

*Numbers in parentheses refer to citations in reference list.

(keratinocyte) differentiation."[19] The epidermis develops from undifferentiated ectoderm at 5 to 8 weeks.[49] It initially consists of a single layer of cuboidal cells that develop from the outer germinal stratum (surface ectoderm) and can be identified during the third week of gestation (Figure 14-2, *A*). By 30 to 40 days, two layers are seen: the inner basal layer and the outer periderm (see Figure 14-2, *B*).[35,66] The definitive epidermis develops from the basal layer.

The periderm is a transient embryonic layer that disappears in the second half of gestation.[19,66] The periderm serves as the protective barrier for the embryo and fetus until the end of the second trimester and forms part of the vernix caseosa.[49,66] Until the underlying layers develop, active transport occurs across the periderm between the amniotic fluid and the embryo; thus the periderm acts as a nutrient interface with amniotic fluid.[49,66] The outer border of the periderm rapidly proliferates between 11 and 14 weeks with formation of blebs and microvillus projections, which are coated with very fine filaments.[35,49] Development of the epidermis is under the influence of epidermal growth factor (EGF); matrix adhesion is thought to be mediated by actin-associated α6B4 integrin.[49,66] Cell surface receptors for EGF are found on both the basal layer and periderm.[19]

LOCATION OF ERUPTIONS	COURSE	OTHER MATERNAL FINDINGS	EFFECT ON FETUS/NEONATE
Initially around umbilicus, then spreads over abdomen to chest, back, extremities, palms and soles; rarely involves face	Spontaneous resolution usually within first month postpartum May regress in late pregnancy; 75% flare at delivery or postpartum Often recurs in subsequent pregnancies (with earlier onset and increased severity) May reappear with menstrual cycle or with use of oral contraceptives	Pruritus, fatigue, fever, nausea, headache, and secondary infections May involve cyclic remissions and exacerbations	Severe forms have been associated with increased incidence of stillbirth, preterm birth, small-for-gestational-age (SGA) infants, and transient neonatal skin lesions; ncreased risks of SGA and preterm infants, probably due to placental insufficiency
Often appears initially in femoral or perineal areas; spreads to lower abdomen, to medial aspects of the thighs, and around the umbilicus; occasionally involves hands, feet, under nails, and tongue	Spontaneous resolution postpartum Tends to recur in subsequent pregnancies, with earlier onset and increased severity	Variable pruritus, associated with hypocalcemia, fever, lethargy, nausea, vomiting, and diarrhea	Increased incidence of abortion and stillbirth and possible placental insufficiency
Trunk (usually initial presentation) and/or extremities	Spontaneous resolution within 3-4 weeks after delivery May recur in subsequent pregnancies	Intense itching	None
Usually appear initially in abdomen, often in striae, then spread across abdomen to thighs, arms, and buttocks; rarely found above midthorax	Spontaneous clearing within 2-3 weeks after delivery Little tendency to recur	May have mild pruritus	None; twice as likely with male fetus or multiple pregnancy
Pruritus usually begins on abdomen, then spreads to other areas	Clears rapidly after delivery May recur with subsequent pregnancy (60%-70%) or use of estrogen medications (e.g., oral contraceptives)	May occur with or without jaundice (20%); serum alkaline phosphatase, serum glutamate oxaloacetate transaminase, and serum bilirubin are elevated High rate of recurrence with subsequent pregnancies	Associated with decreased birth weight, increased incidence of meconium staining, increased stillbirth, prematurity, and fetal hypoxia secondary to placental insufficiency Induction at 37 to 38 weeks to decrease the risk of stillbirth often recommended

By 60 days, the epidermis has three layers (see Figure 14-2, *D*): the basal layer, an intermediate layer, and the superficial periderm. The intermediate layer becomes more complex by the end of the fourth month, when the epidermis has stratified. The epidermal strata are the stratum basale; the stratum spinosum, which is made up of large polyhedral cells connected by tonofibrils; the stratum granulosum, which contains small keratohyalin granules; and the stratum corneum, which is made up of dead cells packed full of keratin.[101] Peridermal cells are replaced continuously until regression begins around 18 weeks. Shedding of peridermal cells begins in the scalp, plantar surfaces, and face, areas where keratinization first begins.[16] The periderm gradually undergoes regression and apoptosis as the stratum corneum and vernix caseosa develop (see Figure 14-2, *F*). The epidermis is keratinized in skin appendages at 11 to 15 weeks and in the interfollicular area at 22 to 24 weeks.[19] As stem cells in the stratum germinativum proliferate, they develop down growths (epidermal ridges) that extend into the dermis.

Protoplasmic fibers and cellular bridges begin to form. These make up the stratum spinosum, eventually protecting the neonate from dehydration and reducing permeability to noxious substances. From 11 to 18 weeks, this layer has an abundance of glycogen to provide energy for growth.[14]

Table 14-3 Recommendations for Clinical Practice Related to Changes in the Integumentary System in Pregnant Women

Recognize the usual changes involving the skin, hair, nails, and sebaceous and sweat glands during pregnancy and the postpartum period (pp. 484-488).
Provide anticipatory teaching regarding the usual alterations in the skin and its appendages during pregnancy (pp. 484-488).
Counsel pregnant women regarding the basis for integumentary alterations and their usual course, and whether or not the change will regress postpartum (pp. 484-488).
Evaluate the effect of integumentary changes on the woman's body image and relationship with her partner and provide counseling (pp. 484-488).
Counsel women regarding the potential for integumentary alterations during subsequent pregnancies or with use of oral contraceptives (pp. 484-488, Table 14-1).
Recommend specific interventions to reduce or ameliorate the effects of integumentary changes (Table 14-1).
Recognize the specific dermatoses associated with pregnancy (pp. 488, 491 and Table 14-2).
Avoid use of isotretinoin in pregnant women or sexually active women of childbearing age who are not using reliable, highly effective forms of birth control (p. 491 and Chapter 7).
Counsel women with chronic integumentary disorders regarding the effect of pregnancy on their disorder (p. 491).

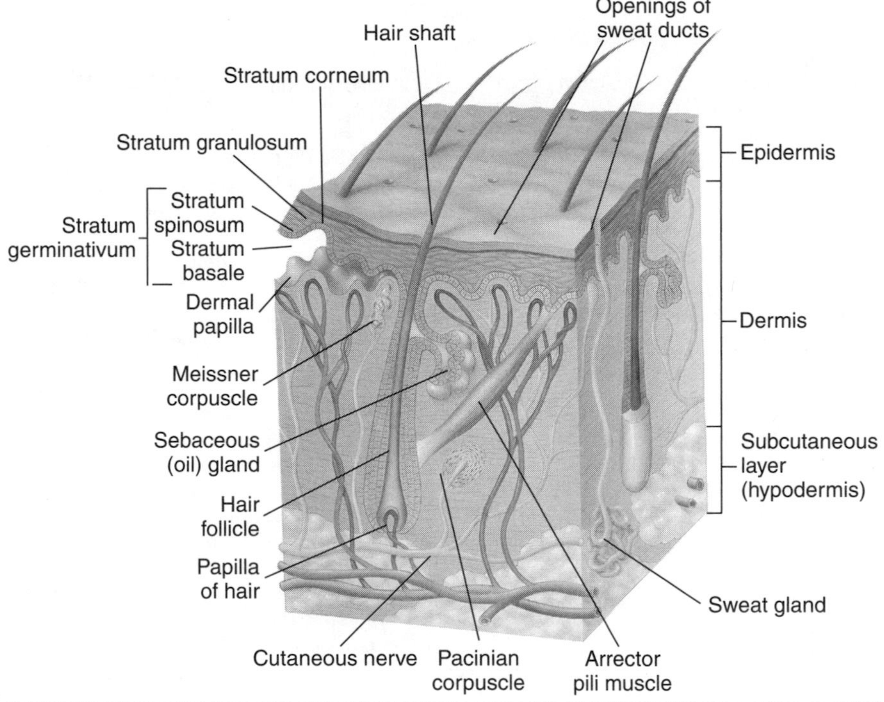

FIGURE 14-1 Structural components of the epidermis, dermis, and subcutaneous tissue. (From Thibodeau, G.A., & Patton, K.T. [2007]. *Anatomy and physiology* [6th ed.]. St. Louis: Mosby.)

Glycogen reserves decrease around 18 weeks.[49] Keratogenic structures become evident, leading to regional differences in epidermal thickness. By 24 weeks, the skin has largely concluded its period of histogenesis and moves into a period of structural and functional maturation.[19]

Ridge patterns (future fingerprints) are genetically determined, although modified by the intrauterine fluid environment, and can be seen on the surface of the hands and soles of the feet.[76] These ridges are seen between 11 and 17 weeks in the hands and between 12 and 18 weeks in the feet.[14] Chromosomal abnormalities such as Down syndrome modify the ridge pattern.

Keratins are produced in the stratum germinativum by 2 months and increase rapidly as the epidermis stratifies.[21] Keratinocytes are arranged in columnar fashion adjacent to the dermis.[19] Keratinocyte maturation is stimulated by several different growth factors, including EGF, transforming growth factors, insulin-like growth factors, and fibroblast growth factor.[14] The first signs of keratinization are seen by 22 to 24 weeks.[16,19]

As replacement keratinocytes mature, they rise and move through the stratum granulosum and acquire keratohyalin granules. As they continue to travel upward, the keratinocytes

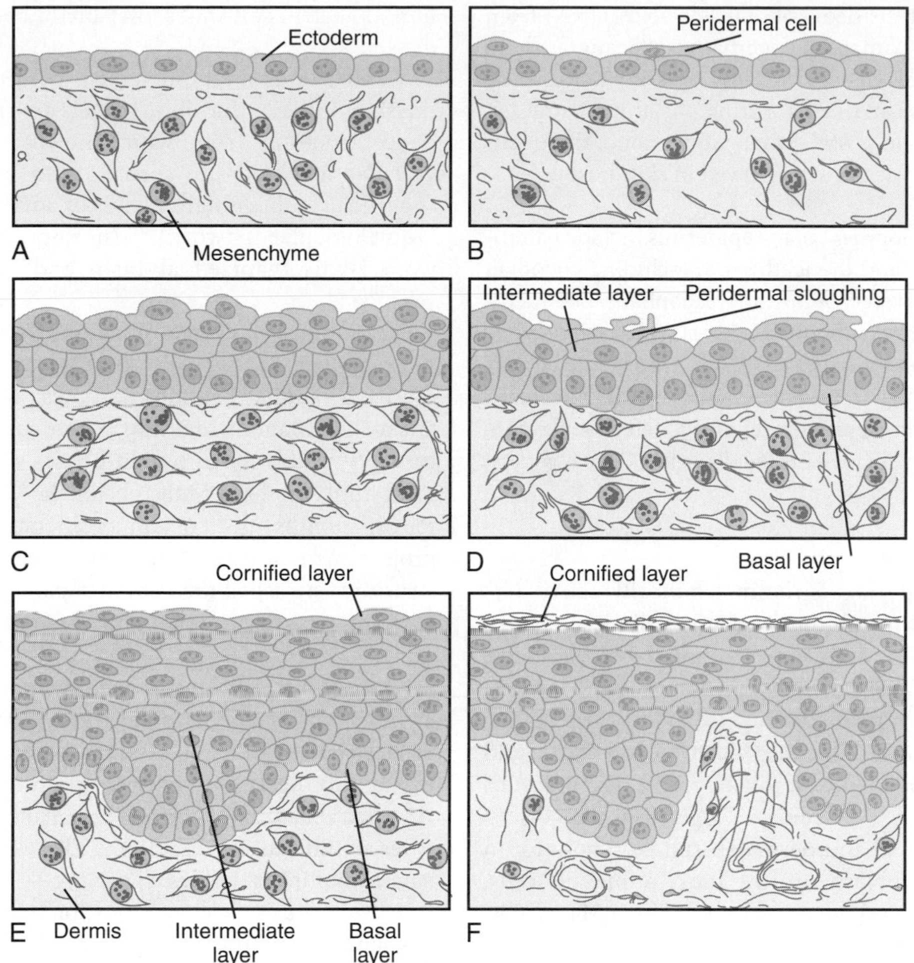

FIGURE 14-2 Stages in the histogenesis of human skin. **A,** At 1 month. **B,** At 2 months. **C,** At 2½ months. **D,** At 4 months. **E,** At 6 months. **F,** After birth. (From Carlson, B.M. [2004]. *Human embryology & developmental biology* [3rd ed.]. St. Louis: Mosby, as modified from Carlson, B. [1996]. *Patten's foundations of embryology* [6th ed.]. New York: McGraw-Hill.)

lose 85% of their water content and their organelles, which are replaced by keratin.[14,19,100] As the keratinocytes dehydrate and flatten, they adhere to each other to form a tough, resilient, and relatively impermeable membrane—the stratum corneum.[90] Transit time for a keratinocyte from the basal layer to the uppermost stratum takes approximately 28 days.[76] By 5 months, the periderm is completely shed, mixing with secretions from the sebaceous glands to form the vernix caseosa.[101]

The stratum corneum becomes thicker and more organized with increasing gestation, but it is not well defined until 23 to 24 weeks' gestation.[16,50] The stratum corneum is more fully developed by 34 weeks, but still immature compared to older children and adults.[9,32,82,106,114] Formation of the stratum corneum may be facilitated by vernix caseosa.[50] At 28 weeks, the stratum corneum consists of two to three cell layers, increasing to 15 or more layers (similar to the adult) after 32 weeks.[21]

During embryonic development, primitive Langerhans cells and melanocytes migrate into the epidermis.[49] Early in the second trimester, the epidermis is invaded by cells from the neural crest called *melanoblasts* or *dendritic melanocytes* because of their long processes much like dendrites. These cells come to lie adjacent to keratinocytes at the dermal-epidermal junction. By midgestation the melanoblasts have been converted to melanocytes, with formation of characteristic organelles or melanosomes and pigmentary granules, and gradually increase to adult numbers of cells.[19] Melanocytes transport melanin along their dendrites, from which it is taken up by the basal cells.[14,49]

Melanin production and transfer into surrounding keratinocytes occur by 4 to 5 months.[21] Production of melanin remains low in newborns, who have less pigmentation than older children.[66] Melanin is responsible for skin color; variations are due to the amount and color of the melanin. Prenatal pigmentation is seen in the nipples, axillae, and genitalia and around the anus. Racial variations are seen not in the number of melanocytes, but rather in the size, shape and activity of these cells and in the number of pigmentary granules per cell.[14,49] Melanin protects deoxyribonucleic acid (DNA) from ultraviolet radiation damage. Langerhans cells migrate into the epidermis by week 8, begin to develop CD1 antigens by 60 days, and increase markedly during the third trimester. Although their function is not entirely understood, these cells have phagocytic activity and are involved in skin host defense mechanisms.[14,19,21,49,66]

Alterations in development of the epidermis include palmoplantar keratodermas and the ichthyoses, including collodian babies (infants are covered by a shiny cellophane-like membrane) and infants with harlequin ichthyosis (characterized by thick, armor-like scales with fissures).[19,49,95] These disorders are characterized by a defective epidermal barrier with abnormalities in formation of the keratinocytes and a defective desquamation process. Many forms of these disorders have a genetic basis.[95,104]

Dermis

Lying below the epidermis is the metabolically active dermis, which exerts a symbiotic and controlling influence on the epidermis. The dermis is composed of connective tissue, amorphous ground substance, free cells, nerves, blood vessels, and lymphatic vessels (see Figure 14-1). The connective tissue consists of collagen (90%) and elastic and reticular fibers embedded in proteoglycans (ground substance) consisting of a protein with glycosaminoglycans such as hyaluronic acid and dermatan sulfate (chondroitin sulfate B).[49] The fibroblasts are the most numerous cells, producing collagen and glycosaminoglycans. Mast cells, histiocytes, macrophages, lymphocytes, and neutrophils are all present in the dermis.

The dermis originates from the somatopleuric mesenchyme and the somites.[35,76] Initially the dermis is a loose aggregate of interconnected mesodermal cells that secrete a liquid intercellular matrix rich in glycogen and hyaluronic acid.[26] Hyaluronic acid promotes cell migration.[19] With increasing age, dermatan becomes more prominent and dermal water content decreases.[49] The dermis in the eighth-week embryo has undifferentiated cells, appears myxedema-like (as seen in the umbilical cord), and contains no fibrils.[35] Eventually three layers form: superficial (adjacent to the epidermal basement membrane), papillary, and reticular.[49] The latter two layers are present by 4 months' gestation. Between 8 and 12 weeks, the fibroblasts form, leading to differentiation of connective tissue. During this time, fibrillae appear between dermal cells, which continue to grow, developing a network of collagenous and elastic fibers.[76,101] The fetal dermis contains all of the different types of collagens seen in the adult, although type III collagen is found in greater proportions in the fetus.[19] Elastin fibers are first seen around 20 weeks.[49]

With further maturation the dermal layer moves from an organ abundant in water, sugars, and hyaluronidase to one enriched with collagen and sulfated polysaccharides.[19,35] Immature skin may be edematous, a sign of the excess water and sodium contained within it and the continued immaturity of this system. Development of this fibrous matrix continues after birth, becoming thicker and denser.[7]

Capillaries and lymph vessels form simultaneously with the skin. Initially the blood vessels are simple endothelium-lined structures from which new capillaries grow. Two vascular networks are seen in skin by 60 to 70 days, a superficial (subpapillary plexus of adult) and a deeper layer (adult reticular network).[49] The subcapillary vascular network is disorganized at birth and matures in the first year.[19,32,84]

The dermal-epidermal junction is critical for skin integrity. The junction begins to develop in the first trimester as the basal lamina, hemidesmosomes, anchoring fibrils, and anchoring filaments develop.[19] This junction is still immature in very low–birth weight infants and is not fully developed until about 6 months postbirth.[21] During the third and fourth months, the corium proliferates to form papillary projections that extend into the epidermis. These irregular structures are called the *dermal papillae*. Some contain capillary loops that nourish the epidermis, and others have sensory nerve endings.

Disorders of the dermal-epidermal junction include various forms of epidermolysis bullosa (EB) that result in friction-induced cutaneous blistering, mucosal erosions, and wounds that do not heal.[19,49,95] EB is a group of inherited disorders classified according to the cleavage plane of the blisters. Major types are EB simplex, junctional EB, and dystrophic EB, each having multiple subtypes.[19,104]

Fat appears in the deeper portion of the dermis, becoming the subcorium (subcutaneous tissue). Most fat is laid down during the last trimester of pregnancy, and serves as a heat insulator, shock absorber, and calorie storage area.

Adipose Tissue

The hypodermis or subcutaneous tissue is a passive tissue that forms from mesenchymal cells. Subcutaneous tissue, which has a lobar structure surrounded by connective tissue, has its own blood supply. The first cells can be seen around 14 weeks; initially they are cytoplasmic and contain no fat droplets. With maturation, single or multiple fat granules develop.[76] Most adipose tissue is deposited in the third trimester.

Brown adipose tissue (BAT) differentiates from the hypodermal primitive cells between 26 and 30 weeks.[24,80] BAT accumulates in the neck; underneath the scapulae; and in the axillae, mediastinum, and perirenal tissues. BAT is critical for nonshivering thermogenesis, the major method of neonatal heat production (see Chapter 20).

Cutaneous Innervation

In the third month of gestation, free nerve endings connect with the papillary ridges of the finger and toe pads. By term these nerve endings are exceptionally well developed in the perioral area around the lips and sucking pads. Specialized nerve endings are less well developed and continue their maturation throughout infancy.[14,76]

The glands and muscles of the skin are innervated, and some are functional at birth; however, refinement of these responses continues after delivery. The arrector pili muscles, arterioles, and eccrine glands are innervated by the sympathetic nervous system to varying degrees. The sensory nerves may carry parasympathetic fibers to the vessel walls at birth; however, vasodilatory abilities are reduced until further innervation takes place. The axon reflex (stimulus in one branch of a nerve cell that is transmitted to an effector organ down another branch of the cell) is poorly developed even in term infants, so sweating is an unusual occurrence.

Epidermal Appendages

The structures that result from invaginations of epidermal germinative into the dermis or from the epidermis itself are the epidermal appendages.[49,66] These include the eccrine sweat, sebaceous, and apocrine sweat glands; lanugo and hair; and the nails.

Hair and Nails. The hair is an epidermal derivative that develops under mesodermal induction. Development of the hair follicle begins in the head area and then spreads caudally and ventrically.[66] All hair follicles develop prior to birth.[39] Follicular placodes can be seen by 75 to 80 days.[66] Hairs are first seen at 10 to 12 weeks.[14] Initially the hairs develop from solid epidermal proliferations, cylindrical downward growths of the stratum germinativum into the dermis, where dermal cells condense into dermal papillae (inducer cells). The base of these growths becomes the club-shaped hair bulb. The epithelial cells of the hair bulb form the follicular germinal matrix, which later gives rise to the hair itself. The lower part (dermal papilla) of the hair bulb becomes rapidly invaginated by the mesoderm, in which vessels and nerve endings develop. This forms the pilary complex.[14,18,21,76,101]

The central cells of each down growth (germinal matrix) form the hair shaft. As the epithelial cells continue to proliferate, the hair shaft is pushed upward toward the epidermal surface. The peripheral cells (epithelial hair sheath) become cuboidal and form the wall of the hair follicle.[18,101] By the end of the third month, extensive fine hairs (lanugo) have begun to develop. Hair on the eyebrows, upper lip, and chin regions appears around 16 weeks and is plentiful by 17 to 20 weeks.[14,53] Lanugo is shed before or after delivery and replaced by shorter, coarser hairs (vellus hairs) from new follicles.

Fetal scalp hair is visible by 19 to 21 weeks and the first complete hair cycles (anagen growth to catagen degeneration to telogen resting phases) are seen by 24 to 28 weeks with initiation of short catagen/telogen phases.[19,39,66] The onset of the hair cycle/anagen is mediated by papillary-derived insulin-like growth factor-1, fibroblast growth factor (FGF)-2, FGF-7, substance P, corticotropin, and capsaicin.[39] Hair growth is also influenced by other substances such as growth hormones, thyroid hormones, androgens, glucocorticoids, retinoids, and prolactin.[39] With subsequent hair cycles, the diameter of the hair shaft increases.

Melanoblasts migrate into the hair bulb and differentiate into melanocytes between 6 and 7 weeks.[39] During the second half of gestation, melanogenesis is active in the fetal hair follicle. Hair patterning and growth are influenced by central nervous system (CNS) development. Infants with neurologic abnormalities may have abnormal hair whorls or alterations in the direction of hair growth or amount of hair.[36] These differences may be related to tension on the epidermis during the period of hair follicle formation.[14]

Nails appear at 8 to 10 weeks and are the first tissue to keratinize, beginning around 11 weeks, and are completely formed by 5 months. During the remainder of gestation, nails continue to elongate.[19,49,66]

Sebaceous Glands. The sebaceous glands form within the epithelial wall of the hair follicle, usually as a small outpouching of ectodermal cells that penetrate the surrounding mesoderm at the hair follicle neck at 13 to 16 weeks.[66] These outgrowths branch to form the primordia of the glandular alveoli and ducts. The center cells degenerate to form a fatlike substance (sebum), which is secreted into the hair follicle or directly onto the skin. The sebum mixes with the desquamated peridermal cells to help form the vernix caseosa (see section on Vernix Caseosa).[49,53,101] Sebum is thought to be responsible for neonatal "acne."[66]

Most of the sebaceous glands differentiate at 13 to 15 weeks' gestation, immediately producing sebum in all hairy areas.[49] Each gland usually consists of several lobules filled with disintegrated cells that are extruded into an excretory duct. The rapid growth during gestation and immediately after birth is due to circulating maternal androgens and, possibly, endogenous steroid production by the fetus.[53]

Arrector Pili Muscle. Some of the surrounding mesenchymal cells differentiate to form the arrector pili muscle, which is made up of smooth muscle fibers that attach to the connective tissue sheath of the hair follicle and dermal papillary layer. These muscles are located a short distance from the follicular wall in a region where the ground substance is metachromatic. The connection of the muscle root sheath is a secondary event, with innervation occurring later.[101]

Eccrine and Apocrine Glands. The sweat glands are also appendages of the epidermal layer. There are three types of sweat glands. Only two are discussed here; less is known about the third type (apoeccrine), which develops in adolescence and is found only in adult axillae. The eccrine glands develop first and are distributed throughout the cutaneous barrier. The apocrine glands develop later and are more specialized. Both are down-growths of solid cylindrical epidermal tissue that invade the dermal layer and are innervated by sympathetic cholinergic nerves. No additional glands form after birth.[49]

The eccrine glands appear in the sixth week of embryogenesis and are innervated by the sympathetic nervous system. The epidermal tissue for this gland is more compact than that of the hair primordia, and it does not develop mesenchymal papillae. Once the bud reaches the dermis, it elongates and coils, developing a lumen at around 16 weeks.[19,76] Eccrine glands retain two layers of cells once the lumen is formed. The inner layer is made up of the lining and gland cells; the outer layer is specialized ectodermal smooth muscle cells that aid in the expulsion of secretions. Eccrine glands are seen on the volar surface of the hand at 3.5 months and in the axillae by 5 months.[18] All eccrine glands are present by 24 to 28 weeks, but do not function until after birth.[18,19]

The apocrine glands are large organs that develop after the eccrine glands. They are confined to the axillae, pubic area, and areolae of the mammary glands. Apocrine glands originate from and empty into the hair follicles, just above the sebaceous glands. By 7 to 8 months' gestation, they become transiently functional and produce a milky white fluid containing water, lipids, protein, reducing sugars, ferric iron, and ammonia.[49,76] Decomposition of this fluid by skin bacteria produces a characteristic odor.

Vernix Caseosa

"At birth the human infant is covered with a complex material [vernix caseosa] possessing endogenous anti-infective, antioxidative, moisturizing and cleansing capabilities."[49] Vernix caseosa forms as a superficial fatty film after 17 to 20 weeks. It is made up of sebaceous gland secretions and desquamated cells of the periderm or stratum corneum cells and is rich in triglycerides, fatty acids, cholesterol, ceramides (lipid-signaling molecules, which have a role in water regulation and barrier function), and unsaponified fats.[48,100] Vernix is composed of 80.5% water, 10.3% lipids, and 9.1% proteins.[52] After 36 weeks, the vernix thins and begins to disappear. Pulmonary surfactants in amniotic fluid mediate detachment of the vernix from the skin.[49] Both preterm and postterm infants have less vernix at birth than term infants. At term, the heaviest layers are found on the ears, shoulders, sacral region, and inguinal folds. The vernix has a tendency to accumulate at sites of dense lanugo growth.

The vernix is a biofilm that covers the fetus until birth and provides insulation of the skin during gestation, acts as an emollient to provide protection from amniotic fluid maceration, and minimizes friction at delivery. Vernix also prevents the loss of water and electrolytes from the skin to the amniotic fluid and contains antioxidants such as alpha-tocopheral.[94,108,115] Vernix has antimicrobial properties such as antifungal activity, opsonization capacity, inactivation of parasites, and protease inhibition that may protect the fetus from chorioamnionitis and contains substances such as lysozyme, lactoferrin, and defensins.[94,108,112,115] Vernix also optimizes stratum corneum hydration and may play a role in fetal wound healing.[32,50] Fetal wound healing differs from that of the adult (Table 14-4) and often the fetus heals without scarring.[21]

Functional Development

Intrauterine physiologic functioning of the skin is dependent upon the growth, development, and maturation of the fetus. The fluid environment of the uterus also has an impact on cutaneous functioning. The amniotic fluid ensures an even distribution of temperature and protection from trauma and injury, allowing for symmetric development of the fetus and providing a medium in which the fetus can move. Amniotic fluid composition and exchange are discussed in Chapter 3.

The longer the gestation, the more the skin contributes to the amniotic environment. As the fetus approaches 38 weeks, there is increased sloughing of anucleated cells and keratinized lipid-containing skin flakes. Increased numbers of lipid-laden cells are an indication of fetal maturation. The periderm provides the embryo with a barrier to the amniotic environment but does not eliminate the exchange of water and electrolytes between the amniotic fluid and the embryo.

Fetal skin permeability is dependent upon morphologic changes and maturation in the epidermis related to sulfhydrylation and keratinization. Permeability therefore does not decrease until the third trimester. Vernix caseosa contributes to this change. The decrease in permeability is also associated with a decrease in skin water content. A fetus at 22 weeks has

Table 14-4 Comparison of Fetal and Adult Wound Repair

VARIABLE	FETUS (<24 WEEKS)	ADULT
Tissue environment	Amniotic fluid rich in growth factors and hyaluronic acid Relative hypoxemia Sterile	Air
Inflammatory infiltrate	Limited neutrophils; lymphocytes predominate	Macrophages predominate
Extracellular matrix	Nonexcessive deposition of types III and IV collagen organized in a reticular pattern Increased amount of hyaluronic acid	Abundant type I collagen deposited into disorganized bundles

From Cohen, B.A. & Siegfried, E.C. (2012). Newborn skin: Development and basic concepts. In C.A. Gleason, & S. Devaskar (Eds.). *Avery's Diseases of the newborn* (9th ed.). Philadelphia: Saunders, p. 1364.

a skin water content close to 100%, which reduces to 92% in the term infant and 77% in adults. This decrease in water is associated with an increase in connective tissue, especially collagen.

NEONATAL PHYSIOLOGY

The physiology of the integumentary system in the neonate includes the barrier properties of the skin, permeability, transepidermal water loss, heat exchange between the environment and the infant, collagen instability, and the protective mechanisms of the skin. Along with these functions, the skin is the most sophisticated sensory organ system in the neonate. It accounts for about 13% of body weight in preterm infants, decreasing to 3% by adulthood.[47] The neonate obtains the vast majority of its information about the environment through the skin. Tactile development is discussed in Chapter 15.

Transitional Events

During the birth process the skin is subjected to the mechanical stress of the delivery process, changes in blood circulation, and the bacterial flora of the maternal genital tract. The skin also serves as a diagnostic barometer for systemic phenomena, especially those related to transition. Mechanical stresses include pressure from contractions, which alters blood flow to various regions and results in edema formation. Maternal structures (bony pelvis and musculature) can exert pressure on the presenting part, causing further edema and hematoma formation. Exertion of enough pressure may result in abrasions or cellular ischemia and tissue sloughing, threatening the integrity of the cutaneous barrier. In addition to natural forces, epidermal breaks can also be caused by obstetric interventions. Use of vacuum extraction and forceps can result in bruising, edema, tissue ischemia, tissue sloughing, subcutaneous fat necrosis, and nerve damage.

In the first hours following delivery, the infant develops an intense red color, which is characteristic of the newborn. This may remain for several hours; however, exposure to the cooler environment usually leads to a bluish mottling, which dissipates quickly upon warming. Newborn skin is relatively transparent and smooth looking and is soft and velvety to touch. This appearance is due to the lack of large skin folds and skin texture. The epidermis and stratum corneum of infant skin are thinner than in adults with smaller corneocytes and keratinocytes, more densely packed glyphics (island-like structures within the stratum corneum), and a denser microrelief network.[107] Localized edema may be seen, especially over the pubis and the dorsa of the hands and the feet. This edema decreases within the first few days of life, after which the skin lies loosely over the entire body.

Compared to the term infant, the preterm infant's skin is thinner, more transparent, and sometimes gelatinous, and has more lanugo. Transfer from the intrauterine amniotic fluid environment to the external air environment results in accelerated maturation of skin function in the preterm infant.

Newborns have less pigmentation than older children due to decreased melanin production (melanin acts as an ultraviolet light filter). The increased pigment in the ear tips, scrotum, linea alba, and areolae are due to maternal and placental hormones.[49] Because of their lack of pigmentation, young infants are more susceptible to damage from ultraviolet light.[107]

Lanugo hair is shed after birth and replaced with vellus hair.[18] The newborn has 10 times as many hair structures per unit of skin surface as adults.[106] At term hair follicles on the scalp are in different stages of the hair cycle depending on their location. Frontal and parietal hairs are moving to telogen; occipital are in anagen and move to catagen/telogen by 8 to 12 weeks post birth.[13] At birth the synchrony of hair growth (anagen) and hair loss (telogen) is transiently altered so hair may become thick and coarse or be lost (temporary alopecia).[49] The postnatal hair cycle lasts 2 to 6 months; length of an individual hair is determined by the length of the anagen phase.[39] Hair on the scalp at birth reflects metabolic activity from week 28 on and therefore may be useful for assessment of prenatal toxin exposures.[39]

Initially the skin is covered with the yellow-white vernix caseosa. This insulating layer is lost with the bathing that occurs in the nursery. Removal results in exposure of the stratum corneum to the much drier postnatal environment, with desquamation of the upper layers of the stratum corneum. After the first week, visible desquamation gives way to normal proliferation and flaking, signaling adaptation. This drying out of the skin is part of the natural maturational process. Any interference in this keratinization (e.g., use of lotions or creams) only delays the development of an effective barrier and prolongs the difficulties associated with an immature cutaneous surface, such as increased water loss and thermal instability. Common neonatal skin variations are summarized in Table 14-5.

Once these initial stages are complete the skin takes on the adult protective functions by providing the needed environmental barrier. This development includes the discharge of water and electrolytes, an acid mantle, resorptive capacities, generalized pigmentation, and regulation of blood circulation and nerve supply. Factors affecting infant skin condition are summarized in Figure 14-3.

Barrier Properties

The skin acts as a barrier to limit transepidermal water loss (TEWL), prevent absorption of drugs and other chemicals, and protect from invasion by pathogens.[16,18] The barrier properties of the skin are located almost entirely in the stratum corneum. The stratum corneum is thinner in the infant than the adult and in the preterm compared to the term infant, and it increases with increasing gestational and postnatal age.[18,51] Barrier maturation after birth is mediated by nuclear hormone receptors and their ligands (signal triggering and binding molecules).[32]

Table 14-5 **Normal Neonatal Skin Variations**

CONDITION	CHARACTERISTICS
Milia	1-mm yellow-white cysts Appears on cheeks, forehead, nose, and nasolabial folds Frequently occur in clusters Affect 40% of all infants
Miliaria	Develops within the first 12 hours Caused by obstructed eccrine sweat ducts Appears on forehead and skin folds Superficial, thin-walled grouped vesicles (miliaria crystallina) or deep, grouped red papules (miliaria rubra)
Erythema toxicum	Most common transient lesion Irregular erythematous macules or patches with yellow or white central papule Can affect any area of body except palms and soles Appears between 24 and 72 hours after birth; may continue to appear for up to 3 weeks; lesions dissipate in a few days More often affects full-term infants (30% to 70%)
Mongolian spots	Macular, gray-blue without sharp borders Most frequently occur in lumbosacral region Covers an area 10 cm or greater Caused by delayed disappearance of dermal melanocytes Affects up to 70% to 90% of African-American, Asian, and Native American infants and 5%-13% of white infants Gradually disappears over first few years of life
Harlequin color change	Transient color change usually appearing in first few days and sometimes up to 3 weeks of age, lasting a few minutes to ½ hour Midline demarcation; dependent side red; upper side pale Caused by temporary autonomic imbalance of cutaneous vasculature Nonsignificant More common in preterm infants
Ecchymoses	Subcutaneous hemorrhage Localized Usually seen over presenting part
Neonatal acne (cephalic pustulosis)	Small red papules and pustules on face Resolves spontaneously within 2 to 4 weeks Rarely associated with comedones or cysts
Café au lait spots	Brown macules or patches Less than 3 cm in diameter Occur occasionally in newborns; more common in African-American infants With six or more spots of greater than 0.5-cm diameter, the infant is at risk for underlying neurofibromatosis
Junctional (melanocytic) nevi	Flat, macular, purpura, or plaquelike pigmented lesions Brown to black Less than 1 cm Most develop later in childhood Neonatal risk minimal, with aging, risk for later melanoma, especially with large lesions
Hemangiomas	Relatively common Developmental vascular anomaly Capillary hemangiomas: dilated vessels Cavernous hemangiomas: large, dilated, blood-filled cavities; 65% are superficial; 15% are subcutaneous; 20% are mixed
Salmon patch hemangioma ("stork bites")	Occurs in up to 70% to 75% of normal newborns Flat macular hemangioma Appears on nape of neck, eyelids, and glabella area Indistinct borders Blanches with pressure Facial lesions disappear by 1 year of age; neck stains more permanent
Nevus flammeus	Port-wine stain hemangioma Sharply delineated Blanches only slightly Purple to red or jet black Does not involute If distributed over trigeminal territory of face, angiomatous malformation of the brain may occur (i.e., Sturge-Weber syndrome)

Table 14-5 **Normal Neonatal Skin Variations—cont'd**

CONDITION	CHARACTERISTICS
Strawberry hemangioma	Raised bright red capillary lesion with sharply demarcated borders Blanches with pressure Rarely seen immediately at birth; 90% manifest in neonatal period Increases in size for 4 to 9 months Most resolve spontaneously by early childhood Two times more frequent in females
Cavernous hemangioma	Deeper, less common Margins obscured by overlying epidermal tissue Reddish-blue Somewhat compressible Increases in size after birth
Cradle cap	Seborrheic eczema Reactive response to irritant Scaling lesions Greasy feeling

Components of barrier maturation include the thickness and organization of the epidermal layer. Organization of the epidermis has been compared to a brick wall with the corneocytes being the bricks and the lipid matrix the mortar.[47,50] In the mature stratum corneum, the corneocytes are arranged in an organized pattern (like bricks) with a lamellar lipid matrix (the mortar). The corneocytes are interconnected by dermatomes to form a stable barrier. The lipid matrix acts as a barrier to transepidermal water loss. In the immature infant, the matrix is less well developed, with increased transepidermal water loss; the corneocytes are arranged in a more disorganized fashion and there are fewer intercellular connections between corneocytes.[47,50]

Epidermal thickness and functional maturation increase rapidly until about 24 weeks' gestation.[18] From that point until term, there is progressive thickening, which is seen in dermoepidermal undulations.[100] In the term neonate the epidermis has marked regional variations in thickness, color, permeability, and surface chemical composition. As skin

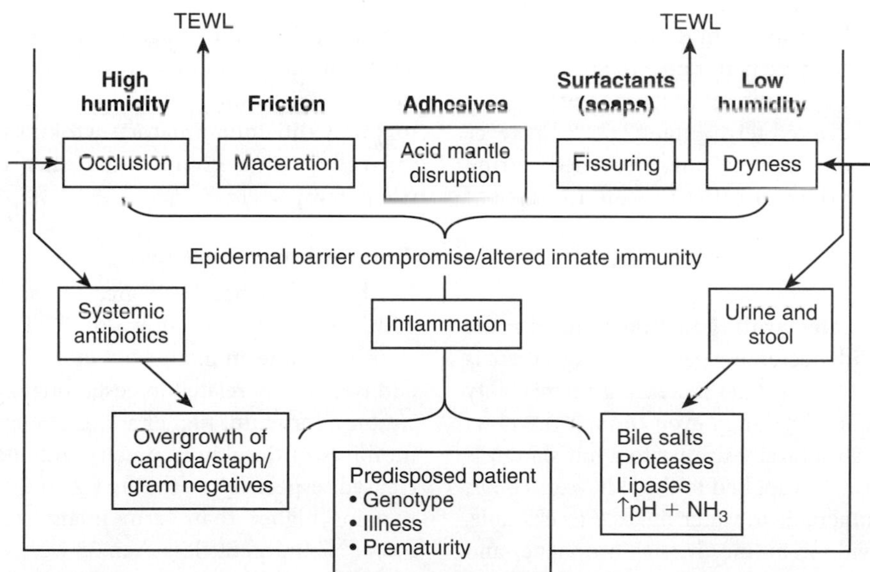

FIGURE 14-3 Factors affecting infant skin condition. The phenotype of infant skin results from the complex interplay of genotype and multiple environmental factors (humidity, friction, adhesive trauma, soap exposure). Considerations such as prematurity, illness (e.g., diarrhea), or the use of systemic antibiotics may affect regional skin health and lead to alterations in barrier function. *TEWL*, transepidermal water loss. (From Hoath, S.B. & Narendran, V. (2011). The skin. In R.J. Martin, A.A. Fanaroff, & M.C. Walsh (Eds.), *Fanaroff & Martin's Neonatal-perinatal medicine: Diseases of the fetus and infant* (9th ed.). St. Louis: Mosby Elsevier, p. 1735.)

matures, the thickness of the stratum corneum increases. In the term infant this is a relatively well-developed barrier that may be 10 to 20 layers thick, as in the adult. However, in the preterm infant (especially those younger than 30 weeks' gestation), the barrier is immature and may be only two to three layers thick. In infants younger than 24 gestational weeks, the stratum corneum is minimal.[32,107,116]

Skin hydration decreases immediately after birth, then increases as the stratum corneum adapts to the extrauterine environment.[116] Stratum corneum hydration is lower in infants of less than 30 weeks' gestation, related in part to incomplete development of the vernix caseosa (see Vernix Caseosa).[32,116] Stratum corneum hydration is higher in vernix covered areas. Extremely low–birth weight infants may exhibit an abnormal pattern of skin desquamation after several weeks of extrauterine life due to hyperproliferation of the stratum corneum.[114]

For both the term and preterm infant, consequences of barrier immaturity include increased permeability and increased TEWL. Each of these properties is a function of gestational and postnatal age. The thinness of the barrier layer leaves the preterm neonate with an increased transepidermal loss, an increased skin permeability to chemical substances and microbes, and a decreased ability to withstand mechanical forces of friction.[100] Rapid barrier maturation occurs over the first 10 to 14 days after birth in the term infant and 2 to 4 weeks in the preterm infant. Initial barrier maturation may take up to 8 weeks in the infant born at 25 to 27 weeks' gestational age, or until the infant reaches a postmenstrual age of 30 to 32 weeks.[56] Initial barrier maturation is mediated by exposure to the extrauterine environment. For example, an infant of 32 weeks' gestational age who is 2 weeks old has had significant epidermal development in the first 2 weeks of postnatal life. This infant may be better able to cope with the extrauterine environment in terms of integumentary system function than a newly delivered term infant.[43,76,100] However in all infants barrier maturation is not completed during the neonatal period, but is an ongoing process throughout infancy.[9,82,106,114]

Permeability

Skin permeability correlates with gestational age in the first few weeks of life. With decreasing gestational age, there is increasing permeability. Other factors increasing permeability are skin disease and injury.[16,100] Thus even though the newborn's skin may appear structurally similar to adult skin, it is more permeable to substances applied to the skin (e.g., drugs, chemicals) and more vulnerable to water fluxes. For example, antiseptics such as povidone-iodine, hexachlorophene, and isopropyl alcohol applied to an infant's skin are absorbed to a much greater extent than in adults.[16,100]

Protective Mechanisms

Although there are many immaturities in the cutaneous system, the accelerated maturation with birth (along with the pH of the infant's skin) results in a protective barrier to the environment as long as the skin stays intact. Natural moisturizing factors (NMFs) in the stratum corneum act as skin lubricants and humectants to help the skin retain moisture.[82] NMFs contain amino acids and their derivatives, organic acids, sugars, and ions. NMFs are lower in infants and altered with skin disorders and environmental factors.[82,107]

An acid skin surface with a pH lower than 5.0 enhances bacteriologic, chemical, and mechanical resistance and is needed for barrier maturation, repair, integrity, cohesion, and growth.[32,67,114] The acid mantle is formed from the uppermost layer of the epidermis, sweat, superficial fat, sebum, metabolic by-products of keratinization, and external substances (e.g., amniotic fluid, microorganisms). The acid mantle can be disrupted by bathing and by the use of soaps and other topical agents.[67]

Skin pH increases immediately after birth, from the fetal pH of 5.5 to 6, and then decreases over the first week to a pH of 5.0 to 5.5.[18,32,51] Skin pH reaches adult values by 3 to 4 weeks, although in some infants this may occur earlier or later.[18] The mechanism for this change remains unclear but may be due to changes in the composition of the surface lipids and the activity of the eccrine glands.[29] Vernix-covered areas have a more acidic pH than other areas in term infants.[32] The acid mantle forms more slowly in preterm infants, especially those weighing less than 1000 g.[33] Fox and colleagues reported that the skin pH in preterm infants (24 to 34 weeks' gestational age) increased to a mean of 6 on the first day after birth and then fell to 5.4 by 1 week and to 5 by 1 month.[33]

Immediately following delivery, microbial colonization also begins. These bacteria grow in a state of equilibrium, providing protection against invading pathogenic organisms. Surface biomarkers of epidermal innate immunity include structural proteins, albumin, both pro-inflammatory and anti-inflammatory cytokines and antigen processing cells.[79] Skin colonization after birth is discussed in Chapter 13.

Transepidermal Water Loss

Newborn skin has both greater water content and higher TEWL compared to adult skin.[106] TEWL decreases rapidly after birth in term infants but more slowly in preterm infants and is inversely related to gestational age. Due to the thinner stratum corneum, higher water content, and increased permeability of the skin in preterm infants, TEWL is greatly increased, especially in the first 2 to 3 weeks after birth, and remains higher than term infants for up to a month or more.[16,79] In infants less than 28 weeks' gestational age, there is a 10- to 15-fold increase in TEWL.[105] TEWL in infants less than 30 weeks' gestational age may exceed resting heat loss production.[99] As a result, fluid losses equivalent to 30% of their total body weight can occur. Even by 4 weeks post birth, TEWL in immature infants is still twice that of term infants.[105] TEWL in infants older than 34 weeks' gestational age approaches that of term infants. Other factors that increase

TEWL in very low–birth weight (VLBW) infants are their larger surface area in relation to body weight and increased blood supply that is closer to the skin surface.

These water losses can have a significant effect on fluid balance and the management and treatment of both preterm and term neonates (see Chapter 11). This may be compounded by environmental (e.g., radiant warmers) and therapeutic (e.g., phototherapy) modalities (see Chapters 18 and 20). An increase in caloric needs due to the excessive TEWL may account for up to 20% of energy expenditure of infants younger than 30 weeks' gestational age. Excess TEWL increases the risk of dehydration, intraventricular hemorrhage, hyperosmolar hypernatremia, and thermal instability due to evaporative heat loss.

The degree of TEWL is dependent upon the hydration of the stratum corneum, the skin surface temperature, ambient relative humidity, and the neural capability for control of sweating. Factors that may contribute to these losses include basal metabolic rate, body temperature, activity, use of radiant warmers, and conventional phototherapy.[32,41,45] Term infants show little regional differences in TEWL, except for increased losses from the palms and soles secondary to sweating. TEWL in preterm infants is lowest on the forehead, cheeks, palms, and soles—areas where keratinization occurs early. These infants also do not sweat. TEWL is 50% higher in the abdomen of these infants and higher with warm (versus cool) skin, increased ambient temperature, radiant heating, or skin damage.[16] Reduction of TEWL losses can be achieved through the use of thermal or plastic blankets or polyethylene skin wraps (see Chapter 20).[103]

Thermal Environment

Heat exchange between infant skin and the environment is dependent on the thermal gradient between the body surface and environment. Studies have found minimal oxygen consumption when the body surface and environmental temperature gradient does not exceed 1.5° C (2.5° F). Use of incubators, radiant warmers, and phototherapy modifies the environment, either reducing or accelerating oxygen consumption. The rate of thermal exchange between infant and environment is dependent upon relative humidity, wind velocity, radiant surfaces, and ambient air temperatures. In neonates, 50% to 75% of heat loss occurs through radiation and is therefore dependent upon both ambient (incubator) and environmental (room) temperature (see Chapter 20). Higher humidity underneath diapers may down-regulate barrier competence in that area, increasing the risk of diaper dermatitis.[32]

Phototherapy (see Chapter 18) is an added radiant heat source. Infants receiving phototherapy have increased insensible water loss (IWL), respiratory rate, peripheral blood flow, and heel skin temperature. Absorption of infrared light waves increases kinetic energy, producing a degradation of the radiant energy to heat and leading to these clinical changes. The increased IWL is a compensatory mechanism to dissipate heat through hyperpnea and peripheral vasodilation. Careful temperature control can reduce some of these effects.

TEWL and heat loss via the skin are intimately linked (increased environmental temperature increases TEWL). Sweating is an important mechanism for heat regulation when thermal stress occurs and is a source of IWL.[35] However, the ability to sweat in response to thermal or emotional stressors is dependent upon gestational and postnatal age.[43]

Infants of 36 weeks' gestational age or older are able to generate sweat with a thermal stimulus, but generally require a greater stimulus than an adult.[21] Term infants demonstrate emotional (palmar or plantar) sweating with an abrupt increase in palmoplantar sweating with exposure to a painful stimulus by the third day.[43,49,50,100] The onset of sweating is delayed in preterm infants more than 28 weeks' gestation; sweating is minimal or nonexistent in infants less than 28 weeks' gestation, due to inadequate sweat gland development.[100] Infants of 28 weeks' gestation will sweat in response to a thermal challenge by 2 weeks post birth.[100] These infants will have mild background palmar sweating with arousal but do not have the abrupt increase seen in term infants.[100] Emotional sweating is weak or absent in preterm infants and develops from 36 weeks postmenstrual age.[32]

Sweating appears first on the forehead, and that may be the only place where it does occur, and then on the chest and upper arms.[32] Gestational age and the number of sites where sweating is found during the first week of life are correlated.[43,50] After that period, this correlation disappears. The amount of water loss varies with the state of arousal, the site of sweating, and the ambient and body temperatures, with the highest loss occurring from the forehead and then from the chest and the upper arms.[43,50]

Although the density of sweat glands is greatest at birth, many glands are inactive; adult function is not achieved until 2 to 3 years of age.[19,50] The ability to respond to thermal stress matures between 21 and 33 days in more mature preterm infants and by 5 days in term infants. The actual water loss due to perspiration in the term infant is low, and although the preterm infant has greater losses, most are due not to perspiration but to TEWL.

Maturation of the sweat response may be a function of gland development (anatomic and functional) or maturation of the nervous system. In the fetus at 28 weeks the full complement of sweat glands is in place, many having formed lumina. The cholinergic fibers of the sympathetic nervous system are also in place. Chemical maturation, however, has not occurred, contributing to the absence of the sweat response in these infants.[43]

Cohesion Between Epidermis and Dermis

Increased fluid losses may occur due to stripping of the stratum corneum through the repeated removal of tape. This problem is due to decreased cohesion between the epidermis and dermis. The epidermis firmly adheres to the underlying dermis in the adult at the dermoepidermal junction. The basal layer is anchored to the basement membrane by hemidesmosomes, anchoring filaments, and fibers that protrude from the undersurface of the basal cells. The undulations encountered in its structure enhance resistance to shearing stress at the junction.[105]

The skin of the preterm infant has decreased anchoring structures, higher water content, and widely spaced collagen fiber bundles in the dermis. This structural liability makes their skin integrity fragile and more susceptible to trauma from shearing and frictional or adhesive forces.[19,67] For the preterm infant, cutaneous injury may occur with very little manipulation. The bond between the epidermis and the adhesive may be stronger than the bond between the infant's epidermis and dermis.[71] Denuded and damaged skin increases TEWL and may be a site of entry for bacterial infection until healing occurs. Extreme care when applying and removing tape or monitoring devices is therefore warranted, especially in the VLBW infant.

Collagen and Elastin Instability

The connective tissue of the dermis is composed of collagen and elastin fibers embedded in a mucopolysaccharide gel. Collagen makes up more than 90% of the connective tissue, with fibroblasts being the most numerous cells. Like epidermal-dermal cohesion, collagen stability also increases with gestational and postnatal age. Collagen maintains the tensile properties of skin, and the elastic fibers allow elastic recoil of the stretched skin. Because the elastin fibers are finer and less mature in the neonate, the skin stretches less and is more susceptible to damage from shearing forces. These liabilities are compounded in preterm infants.

Large amounts of glycosaminoglycans, proteoglycans, and glycoproteins in newborn skin bind large amounts of water. This provides a gel-like composition, which increases the compressibility of the newborn skin and decreases the potential for skin breakdown in the term infant.

Lack of connective tissue can result in increased trauma to the cutaneous layers in the VLBW infant. In addition, decreased collagen and elastic fibers may contribute to edema formation in the dermal layer, with concomitant increases in fluid loss due to increased fluid availability. This tendency toward water fixation decreases with increasing gestational age as collagen stability increases. Heat loss may be enhanced and thermal stability jeopardized due to the decreased insulative capabilities of the fibrous elements of the dermal layer.[71]

Cutaneous Blood Flow

The skin microcirculation is important in temperature maintenance, fluid balance regulation, tissue nutrition, and oxygen supply.[32] The skin microvascular architecture is poorly developed and disorganized at birth with a horizontal dense plexus.[19,32] Capillary loops are seen only in nailbeds, palms, and soles until after the first 2 weeks and not seen in all areas until 14 to 17 weeks after birth.[32] Decreased skin capillary density is reported in some studies.[84] Significant changes in blood vessel diameter are not noted until after the first month.[60] During the first year the adult structure forms and vasomotor tone control is refined. Vasomotor tone is achieved through a complex series of nervous and chemical control mechanisms. These involve the sympathetic nervous system, norepinephrine, acetylcholine, and histamine. Other possible chemical influences include serotonin, vasoactive polypeptides, corticosteroids, and prostaglandins. VLBW preterm infants have immature vasomotor control even with low temperatures (see Chapter 20).[32,58]

CLINICAL IMPLICATIONS FOR NEONATAL CARE

Clinical implications for the neonate due to the limitations of the integumentary system include skin care, absorption of substances through the skin, the use of adhesives, and thermal stability. Thermal stability and evaporative water loss are discussed in Chapter 20. The Association of Women's Health, Obstetric and Neonatal Nurses/National Association of Neonatal Nurses Skin Care Guidelines are based on research evidence and expert opinion and provide guidance for skin assessment, bathing, cord care, reducing transepidermal water loss (TEWL), use of adhesives and emollients, and care of skin breakdown, intravenous line infiltration, and diaper dermatitis.[3,68,70]

Bathing

There is little consensus about the frequency of bathing. The timing of the first bath is delayed until the infant's temperature and condition are stabilized and is influenced by cultural and family preferences.[9] Standard precautions should be used before and during the first bath to avoid heat loss. Investigators have reported that it takes an average of an hour for the infant to return to prebath temperature.[75] Others have found that the timing of the first bath did not significantly affect temperature.[6] Term infants do not need daily bathing. Bathing, versus cloth or sponge washing, has been reported to be less stressful with less TEWL heat loss and better maintenance of stratum corneum hydration, with no differences in infection or bacterial colonization rates.[9,38]

Frequent baths are not needed for VLBW infants. Less frequent bathing has not been associated with an increase in infection or other adverse effects.[34,92] Bathing can be a stressful experience for VLBW infants, with alterations in blood pH, hypoxemia, respiratory distress, increased oxygen consumption, crying, and behavioral stress cues.[64,88,109,121] Bathing may also alter skin barrier properties.

Soaps are not generally needed in infants because of the low output of their sebaceous glands. Washing infants with alkaline soap destroys the acid mantle by neutralizing the pH. For the term infant, it takes 1 hour for the pH to return to baseline; for preterm infants it takes even longer. Due to concerns about increased skin permeability to other solutions, warm water only is recommended for preterm infants younger than 32 weeks' gestation.[71]

Mild neutral pH soaps should only be used if needed for highly soiled areas. Because of concerns about human immunodeficiency virus and other pathogens, some institutions use a dilute antiseptic solution for the initial bath for term infants. The efficacy of this procedure is not clear.[71] The solution should be thoroughly rinsed off the infant's skin. Both antiseptic soaps and plain water decrease skin colonization of the infant, but only for about 4 hours, by which time the skin has re-colonized.[71] No differences in skin bacterial colonization have been found after bathing with warm water versus mild soap and water.[25]

To facilitate rapid epidermal maturation following delivery, manipulation (handling) should be minimized, especially with preterm infants. Routine use of lubricants should be avoided and dry skin care practices instituted. Dry skin care includes the use of cotton sponges and water to remove blood from the face and head as well as meconium from the perineum. The remainder of the skin should be left untouched unless grossly soiled.

Creams, emollients, and lotions are not recommended for routine use, although there is a lack of evidence to support this recommendation.[117] Not only do these substances affect the acid mantle; they may also be absorbed percutaneously. The optimal skin condition for the neonate is dry and flaking, without cracks and fissures. If cracking does occur, a thin application of nonperfumed, preservative-free emollient can be used.

Umbilical Cord Care

Cord care practices are often embedded in institutional tradition. Practices range from no care to cleansing with triple dye (brilliant green, gentian violet, and proflavine hemisulfate), povidone-iodine, chlorhexidine, isopropyl alcohol, or antimicrobial ointments. There are few data on the most effective method.[55,71,105]

Aseptic cord care decreases cord bacterial colonization but not necessarily the risk of infection, and delays cord separation.[4,30,55,78] The current trend in both developed and developing countries is toward dry cord care. The World Health Organization recommends dry cord care in developing countries with soap and water cleaning of visibly soiled cords.[119] Developing countries have a high cord infection rate; however, few studies demonstrate that antiseptic cord care reduces this rate.[78] A Cochrane review by Zupan and colleagues of 21 studies (with 8959 subjects primarily from developed countries) found no difference in infection rates between dry cord care, placebo, and antiseptic use and also found that the use of antiseptics prolonged the time to cord separation.[122] Similar findings have been reported in preterm infants.[30] Aseptic care has been associated with decreased maternal concerns about the cord.[122] However, Zupan and colleagues also concluded that "there appears to be no good reason to stop use of antiseptics in situations where bacterial infection remains high."[122]

Use of Adhesives

The epidermis is pulled off when adhesives are removed and can strip up to 70% to 90% of the stratum corneum in immature infants. In adults it takes 10 adhesive removals to disrupt the skin barrier versus only one removal of plastic tape, pectin barrier, or adhesive tape to do so in the preterm infant.[69] Lund and colleagues compared plastic tape, pectin barrier, and hydrophilic gel use in the first week after birth in infants born at 24 to 40 weeks' gestation.[69] They found that pectin barriers and plastic tape had the highest colorimeter and vaporimeter scores, suggesting greater epidermal injury with these products than with hydrophilic gels. Skin barrier function returned to baseline by 24 hours. Although gel adhesives seemed preferable, they did not adhere as well to the skin as other products and thus required more frequent replacement.[69]

Denuded areas are a potential source of infection; they are also uncomfortable and are areas of increased fluid loss. Use of transparent semipermeable occlusive dressings, water-activated gel electrodes, and minimal tape to secure monitoring equipment and intravenous lines may reduce injury. Transparent dressings are impermeable to water and bacteria while also providing protection to abrasions and skin irritation. These dressings can also be used to cover line insertion sites or incision sites from invasive procedures. The advantages of this type of dressing include providing an optimal moist environment for healing, allowing serous exudate to form over the wound, facilitating migration of new cells across the wound area, and preventing cellular dehydration.[46]

The use of skin-bonding agents such as benzoin or Mastisol to promote adhesion should be avoided due to the already significant cohesion that occurs with tape.[71] These substances increase tape-epidermis adhesion and potentiate epidermal stripping upon tape removal. In addition, benzoin is absorbed through the skin, allowing acids to be released into the bloodstream. Adhesive removal products should also be avoided in immature infants because of concerns about increased skin permeability.

Protection from Infection

Protection from infection requires that the skin, as the first line of defense against infection, stay intact. Current monitoring modalities require manipulation and attachment of equipment to the infant's epidermal layer. Careful handling can reduce shear damage and epidermal sloughing. Application of noninvasive monitoring equipment needs to be done such that pressure or constriction of blood flow does not occur. Crater formation may occur in preterm infants with very thin skin. The use of heated electrodes can lead to local hyperthermia and erythema. Increasing the frequency of site changes may also reduce skin damage. Extreme care should be used when removing the adherent ring or using equipment that allows for electrode site changes without moving the ring each time.

Transepidermal Absorption

Percutaneous absorption of substances can occur through two pathways: via the cells of the stratum corneum (the transepidermal route) and via the hair follicle–sebaceous gland complex (the transappendageal route). The major pathway is most likely the transepidermal route, with diffusion of a substance through the stratum corneum and epidermis into the dermis and microcirculation. In addition, the subepidermal circulation is readily accessible, enhancing rapid absorption.

Neonates are at increased risk for toxic reactions from absorption of topically applied substances for the reasons listed in Table 14-6. Along with these differences, skin metabolism is different in neonates, so drugs applied topically may result in the release of metabolites different from those that would occur if the drugs were given by other routes. This increases the risk of toxicity. Occlusion of the skin (e.g., placement against the mattress) permits more complete absorption, with longer contact enhancing absorption of the substance. In preterm infants, percutaneous absorption occurs even more rapidly and completely as a result of their increased skin permeability.

The history of neonatal practice demonstrates the problems with the use of topical agents. For example, hexachlorophene was formerly used to prevent coagulase-positive staphylococci colonization; this practice was later found to increase the risk of central nervous system damage.[59] Eventually the Food and Drug Administration modified the allowable uses of hexachlorophene. Current practices also can lead to detrimental effects if not monitored carefully. Topical application of povidone-iodine yields significantly elevated levels of iodine in blood plasma if not removed completely from the skin after completion of invasive procedures (e.g., chest tube insertion, percutaneous line insertion).[1,91] Chlorhexidine at 0.5% has been reported to be superior to 10% povidone-iodine in decreasing colonization of peripheral catheters, possibly due to skin residues that prolong the half-life of the latter. Gentle cleansing of the skin with water removes these residues and reduces this risk. In addition to risks of epidermal stripping with use of benzoin, this substance contains many different acids, all of which can be absorbed, causing either immediate or delayed reactions.

Table 14-6 Factors Placing Neonates at Risk for Toxic Reactions Secondary to Absorption of Topically Applied Substances

Increased permeability of the skin
Increased surface area–to–body weight ratio
Lower blood pressure
Variable skin blood flow patterns
Greater proportion of body weight being made up of brain and liver
Incomplete kidney development resulting in changes in drug excretion
Different body compartment ratios
Larger total body water content
Elevated ratio of intracellular to extracellular water
Decreased adipose tissue

From West, D., Worobec, S., & Solomon, L. (1981). Pharmacology and toxicology of infant skin. *J Invest Dermatol, 76,* 147.

Isopropyl alcohol is also absorbed through the skin. Alcohol use can result in dry skin, skin irritation, and skin burns. The concentration of the solution, duration of exposure, and condition of the exposed skin determine the effects of alcohol use. Tissue destruction occurs with the de-esterifying of the skin and the disruption of the cell structure. Exposure, pressure, and decreased perfusion can contribute to the development of burns from alcohol, complicating fluid management and providing portals for infection.[42]

Extremely Immature Infants

The extremely low–birth weight (ELBW) infant has edematous, friable, gelatinous skin that is covered with abundant lanugo. These infants have decreased subcutaneous tissue and increased water content. This is compounded by a greater ratio of surface area to body weight. All of these characteristics create difficulties in fluid balance and temperature control due to the high TEWL.[99,100] TEWL increases the risk of dehydration, hypothermia, and fluid and electrolyte imbalances. Double-walled incubators, plastic or thermal blankets, and polyethylene skin wraps reduce TEWL and promote thermal stability (see Chapter 20). Polyethylene wraps and bags are recommended for use with preterm infants to reduce heat loss after birth and in the early days postbirth.[8,15,74] These wraps enhance radiant heat gain and reduce evaporative losses, insensible water loss (IWL), and TEWL by creating a microenvironment under the wrap.[8] Unwrapping the infant disrupts this microenvironment, so it should be minimized.[8]

Humidity also decreases TEWL. Increasing the ambient humidity to 85% eliminates almost all evaporative losses, although use of very high humidity is often accompanied by concerns of infection from water borne organisms. Other products to prevent or manage barrier compromise in the preterm infant include gel-filled mattresses or pads, transparent semiocclusive dressings, and hydrocolloid dressings.[46,110]

The preterm infant's skin is exceedingly sensitive. Skin permeability and collagen instability increase with decreasing gestational age. Cohesion at the dermoepidermal junction is also markedly reduced, which can cause stratum corneum and epidermal stripping with handling and attachment of monitoring devices. Careful handling and policies about skin adhesive practices should be employed. The maintenance of skin integrity should be the goal. Denuded areas may benefit from transparent dressings, thereby reducing further damage, providing protection from microbial invasion, and reducing fluid losses.

The stratum corneum is extremely thin; therefore cutaneous permeability is greater, providing little protection against topical substances. Percutaneous absorption occurs more rapidly and completely, placing these infants at greater risk for toxic reactions.[59] The use of harsh de-esterifying substances (soaps and alcohol) should be kept to an absolute minimum. The acid mantle is easily disrupted, and cellular destruction is possible. Avoid use of 70% isopropyl alcohol with these infants, since alcohol is more irritating and less effective than povidone-iodine and chlorhexidine.[67] Use of any of these products should be judicious and followed by complete removal with sterile water.

Collagen instability and incomplete dermal structures result in increased cutaneous edema and decreased resiliency. This may result in skin necrosis due to edema pressure within the dermis. The use of gentle handling with little compression force or friction, careful regular turning, and gentle range-of-motion exercises may help to reduce this tendency.

MATURATIONAL CHANGES DURING INFANCY AND CHILDHOOD

Although the term infant's skin is functionally comparable to adult skin, loss of water content, desquamation, and drying of the stratum corneum enhance further maturation of skin function within the first few days. The stratum corneum and epidermis remain thinner than that of the adult throughout infancy.[106,107] Skin barrier function development is reflected in maturation of skin water-handling (the water transport and storage properties of the stratum corneum) characteristics. For at least the first year after birth differences between infants and adults are reported in the distribution and transport of water in superficial skin layers.[9,82,106,114] Stratum corneum hydration is similar to or higher than that of the adult from 3 to 48 months with higher skin surface water content for at least the first year.[32]

Collagen stability results in a decreased ability to retain fluid within the dermis. This improves with increasing gestational age and in the early postnatal period. Most of the other components of the dermis are not formed until after birth and may not be mature until 3 years of age. Skin resiliency is therefore affected and is low in term infants and even lower in preterm infants.

Melanin production and pigmentation are low during neonatal life, although high circulating maternal and placental hormones can lead to deep pigmentation of certain areas (i.e., linea alba, areolae, and scrotum). This decrease in production is even greater in the preterm infant. Given that melanin protects the skin from the ultraviolet rays of the sun by absorbing their radiant energy, neonates have an increased sensitivity to sunlight.[24] Sunburn can damage the barrier effectiveness of the skin by causing dehydration and desquamation and can increase the risk of later development of skin cancer.

Although the sweat glands are functional within a short time of birth, activating influences are different in the infant than in the adult. For the first 2½ years of life, the sweat glands function irregularly and the total number of glands that are active is small. Emotionally induced eccrine sweating is much less marked in the prepubertal period than in adults. The sebaceous glands are also somewhat dormant until puberty.

The sebaceous glands are large and active in utero, contributing to the lipid content of the vernix caseosa. After birth, these glands rapidly decrease in size between 2 months and 2 years, and remain small and quiescent until puberty. At puberty, they once again become active structures.[19,49] The free fatty acids in the gland secretions have a fungistatic effect and provide immunity against scalp infections from these pathogens. Sebum secretion increases after birth, reaching adult values by 1 month and then decreasing after 6 months to values below adults until puberty.[32]

The vasculature also changes over the first year of life. Initially the cutaneous capillary network is underdeveloped and disorganized; a progression to an orderly mature pattern occurs during infancy.[49]

SUMMARY

The skin plays a major role in the protection of neonates from the environment into which they are born. The development of the acid mantle and microbial colonization provide protection against pathogenic organisms. The thickness of the stratum corneum determines the effectiveness of this protection and reduces permeability to the loss of fluids and absorption of topical substances.

Gestational age is the major determinant of collagen and elastin stability, the thickness of the stratum corneum barrier, and thermal regulatory abilities. Delivery results in a rapid proliferation of the stratum corneum in the preterm infant in an attempt to compensate for some of the liabilities with which these infants must cope. The fragility of the premature infant's skin results in denuded areas due to friction and shearing forces, as well as separation of the epidermis through adhesive stripping.

Understanding the normal developmental processes that the integumentary system undergoes as well as the goal of each of these processes provides the basis for nursing therapeutics. Careful assessment of skin integrity, knowledge of normal neonatal variations, and conservative therapeutics can result in appropriate and timely interventions. The care of the skin can enhance integumentary capabilities and contribute to the infant's ability to assimilate information from the environment. Clinical implications for nursing practice are summarized in Table 14-7.

Table 14-7 Recommendations for Clinical Practice Related to the Integumentary System in Neonates

GENERAL CONSIDERATIONS FOR SKIN CARE
Know normal development and limitations of the neonatal integumentary system (pp. 497, 499-502).
Know the normal integumentary variations encountered in the neonate (Table 14-5).
Monitor skin integrity on a routine basis (pp. 497, 499-502).
Maintain a neutral thermal environment (pp. 501-502 and Chapter 20).
Evaluate intake, output, and hydration status (pp. 500-501 and Chapter 11).
Avoid routine use of lubricants (pp. 502-503).
Bathe only as needed using plain water (or neutral soaps if needed for highly soiled areas) (pp. 502-503).
Counsel parents to use caution in exposing the infant to direct sunlight (p. 505).

FLUID AND HEAT LOSS
Use thermal blankets or plastic wrappings to reduce losses (pp. 500-501, 504-505 and Chapter 20).
Monitor phototherapy equipment use and position (p. 501 and Chapter 18).
Monitor environmental and body temperature regularly (pp. 500-502 and Chapter 20).
Avoid removing vernix (pp. 496, 500).
Assess skin for stratum corneum stripping and institute measures to reduce it (pp. 502, 505).
Maintain appropriate humidity levels within the nursery (pp. 500-501 and Chapter 20).

BARRIER MAINTENANCE
Implement minimal tape-use policies (pp. 502, 505).
Avoid using adhesive bandages (pp. 502, 505).
Remove tape carefully, using warm water to facilitate process (pp. 502, 505).
Avoid benzoin preparations (pp. 502, 505).
Implement plain-water bathing of preterm infants (pp. 502-503).
Ensure appropriate positioning, avoiding pressure on bony prominences and friction stress points (pp. 504-505).
Use alcohol sparingly (pp. 500, 503-505).
Promote careful handling of preterm infants (pp. 504-505).
Recognize activities that produce friction, shearing, or stress, and implement interventions to reduce them (pp. 502, 504-505).

PERMEABILITY
Avoid routine lubrication (pp. 502-503).
Know the factors that place neonates at risk for toxic responses to topically applied substances (p. 504 and Table 14-6).
Practice conservative treatment of integumentary disruptions (pp. 499-502, 504).
Counsel parents regarding the use of topical emollients and powders (pp. 502-503).
Avoid the use of benzoin (p. 503).
Ensure immediate cleansing of skin prepped with povidone-iodine or chlorhexidine following invasive procedures (p. 503).
Use alcohol sparingly on skin (pp. 500, 503-505).

References

1. Afsar, F.S. (2009). Skin care for preterm and term neonates. *Clin Exp Dermatol, 34,* 855.
2. Amichai, B. & Grunwald, M.H. (2007). Pigmentary demarcation lines of pregnancy. *Eur J Obstet Gynecol Reprod Biol, 131,* 239.
3. Association of Women's Health, Obstetric and Neonatal Nurses. (2007). *Neonatal skin care: Evidence-based clinical practice guideline* (2nd ed.). Washington, DC: AWHONN.
4. Aygun, C., Subasi, A., & Kucukoduk, S. (2005). Timing of umbilical cord separation and neonatal intensive care unit practices. *Am J Perinatol, 22,* 249.
5. Barankin, B., Silver, S.G., & Carruthers, A. (2002). The skin in pregnancy. *J Cutan Med Surg, 6,* 236.
6. Behring, A., Vezeau, T.M., & Fink, R. (2003). Timing of the newborn first bath: A replication. *Neonatal Netw, 22,* 39.
7. Bell, E.F. & Oh, W. (2005). Fluid and electrolyte management. In M.G. MacDonald, M.M.K. Seshi, & M.D. Mullett (Eds.), *Avery's Neonatology: Pathophysiology and management of the newborn* (6th ed.). Philadelphia: Lippincott Williams & Wilkins.
8. Bissinger, R.L. & Annibale, D.J. (2010). Thermoregulation in very low-birth-weight infants during the golden hour: Results and implications. *Adv Neonatal Care,* 10, 230. Erratum in: *Adv Neonatal Care* (2010), *10,* 351.
9. Blume-Peytavi, U., et al. (2009). Bathing and cleansing in newborns from day 1 to first year of life: Recommendations from a European round table meeting. *J Eur Acad Dermatol Venereol, 23,* 751.
10. Bolanca, I., et al. (2008). Chloasma—the mask of pregnancy. *Coll Anthropol, 32,* 139.
11. Bremmer, M., Driscoll, M.S., & Colgan, R. (2010). The skin disorders of pregnancy: A family physician's guide. *J Fam Pract, 59,* 89.
12. Buchanan, K., Fletcher, H.M., & Reid, M. (2010). Prevention of striae gravidarum with cocoa butter cream. *Int J Gynaecol Obstet, 108,* 65.
13. Camacho-Martínez, F.M. (2009). Hair loss in women. *Semin Cutan Med Surg, 28,* 19.
14. Carlson, B.M. (2008). *Human embryology & developmental biology* (4th ed.). St. Louis: Mosby Elsevier.
15. Carroll, P.D., et al. (2010). Use of polyethylene bags in extremely low birth weight infant resuscitation for the prevention of hypothermia. *J Reprod Med, 55,* 9.
16. Cartlidge, P. (2000). The epidermal barrier. *Semin Neonatol, 5,* 273.
17. Chi, C.C., et al. (2010). Systematic review of the safety of topical corticosteroids in pregnancy. *J Am Acad Dermatol, 62,* 694.
18. Chiou, Y.B. & Blume-Peytavi, U. (2004). Stratum corneum maturation. A review of neonatal skin function. *Skin Pharmacol Physiol, 17,* 57.
19. Chu, D.H. & Loomis, C.A. (2012). Structure and development of the skin and cutaneous appendages. In R.A. Polin, W.W. Fox, & S.H. Abman (Eds.), *Fetal and neonatal physiology* (4th.). Philadelphia: Saunders.

20. Cobo, M.F., et al. (2009). Pemphigoid gestationis: Clinical and laboratory evaluation. *Clinics (Sao Paulo), 64,* 1043.
21. Cohen, B.A. & Püttgen, K.B. (2012). Newborn skin: Development and basic concepts. In C.A. Gleason & S. Devaskar (Eds.). *Avery's Diseases of the newborn* (9th ed.). Philadelphia: Saunders.
22. Cohn D. (2009). Malignancies and pregnancy. In R.K. Creasy, et al. (Eds.), *Creasy & Resnik's Maternal-fetal medicine: Principles and practice* (6th ed.). Philadelphia: Saunders.
23. Cunningham, F.G., et al. (2009). *Williams obstetrics* (23rd ed.). New York: McGraw-Hill.
24. Cypess, A.M. & Kahn, C.R. (2010). The role and importance of brown adipose tissue in energy homeostasis. *Curr Opin Pediatr, 22,* 478.
25. da Cunha, M.L. & Procianoy, R.S. (2005). Effect of bathing on skin flora of preterm newborns. *J Perinatol, 25,* 375.
26. Dinulos, J.G.H. & Darmstadt, G.L. (2005). Dermatologic conditions. In M.G. MacDonald, M.M.K. Seshia, & M.D. Mullett (Eds.), *Avery's Neonatology: Pathophysiology and management of the newborn* (6th ed.). Philadelphia: Lippincott Williams & Wilkins.
27. Driscoll, M.S. & Grant-Kels, J.M. (2009). Nevi and melanoma in the pregnant woman. *Clin Dermatol, 27,* 116.
28. Elling, S.V. & Powell, F.C. (1997). Physiological changes in the skin during pregnancy. *Clin Dermatol, 15,* 35.
29. Esterly, N.B. (1998). pH patterns in newborns. In R.A. Polin & W.W. Fox (Eds.), *Fetal and neonatal physiology* (2nd ed.). Philadelphia: Saunders.
30. Evens, K., et al. (2004). Does umbilical cord care in preterm infants influence cord bacterial colonization or detachment? *J Perinatol, 24,* 100.
31. Farage, M.A., Neill, S., & MacLean, A.B. (2009). Physiological changes associated with the menstrual cycle: A review. *Obstet Gynecol Surv, 64,* 58.
32. Fluhr, J.W., et al. (2010). Functional skin adaptation in infancy—almost complete but not fully competent. *Exp Dermatol, 19,* 483.
33. Fox, C.E., et al. (1998). The timing of skin acidification in very low birth weight infants. *J Perinatol, 18,* 272.
34. Franck, L.S., et al. (2000). Effect of less frequent bathing of preterm infants on skin flora and pathogen colonization. *J Obstet Gynecol Neonatal Nurs, 29,* 584.
35. Freinkel, R.K. & Woodley, D.T. (2001). *Biology of the skin.* New York: Parthenon.
36. Furdon, S.A. & Clark, D.A. (2003). Scalp hair characteristics in the newborn infant. *Adv Neonatal Care, 3,* 286.
37. Gani, F., et al. (2003). Rhinitis in pregnancy. *Allerg Immunol (Paris), 35,* 306.
38. Garcia Bartels, N., et al. (2009). Influence of bathing or washing on skin barrier function in newborns during the first four weeks of life. *Skin Pharmacol Physiol, 22,* 248.
39. Gareri, J. & Koren, G. (2010). Prenatal hair development: Implications for drug exposure determination. *Forensic Sci Int, 196,* 27.
40. Ghasemi, A., et al. (2007). Striae gravidarum: Associated factors. *J Eur Acad Dermatol Venereol, 21,* 743.
41. Grunhagen, D.J., et al. (2002). Transepidermal water loss during halogen spotlight phototherapy in preterm infants. *Pediatr Res, 51,* 402.
42. Harpin, V.A. & Rutter, N. (1982). Percutaneous alcohol absorption and skin necrosis in a premature infant. *Arch Dis Child, 57,* 477.
43. Harpin, V.A. & Rutter, N. (1982). Sweating in preterm babies. *J Pediatr, 100,* 614.
44. Henry, F., et al. (2006). Blood vessel changes during pregnancy: A review. *Am J Clin Dermatol, 7,* 65.
45. Hey, E.N. & Katz, G. (1969). Evaporative water loss in the newborn baby. *J Physiol, 200,* 605.
46. Hoath, S.B. (1997). The stickiness of newborn skin: Bioadhesion and the epidermal barrier. *J Pediatr, 131,* 338.
47. Hoath, S.B. & Narendran, V. (2000). Adhesives and emollients in the preterm infant. *Semin Neonatol, 5,* 289.
48. Hoath, S.B., Pickens, W.L., & Visscher, M.O. (2006). The biology of vernix caseosa. *Int J Cosmet Sci, 28,* 319.
49. Hoath, S.B. & Narendran, V. (2011). The skin. In R.J. Martin, A.A. Fanaroff, & M.C. Walsh (Eds.), *Fanaroff & Martin's Neonatal-perinatal medicine: Diseases of the fetus and infant* (9th ed.). St. Louis: Mosby.
50. Hoath, S.H. (2012). Physiologic development of the skin. In R.A. Polin, W.W. Fox, & S.H. Abman (Eds.), *Fetal and neonatal physiology* (4th ed.). Philadelphia: Saunders.
51. Hoeger, P.H. & Enzmann, C.C. (2002). Skin physiology of the neonate and young infant: A prospective study of functional skin parameters during early infancy. *Pediatr Dermatol, 19,* 256.
52. Hoeger, P.H., et al. (2002). Epidermal barrier lipids in human vernix caseosa: Corresponding ceramide pattern in vernix and fetal skin. *Br J Dermatol, 146,* 194.
53. Irmak, M.K., Oztas, E., & Vural, H. (2004). Dependence of fetal hairs and sebaceous glands on fetal adrenal cortex and possible control from adrenal medulla. *Med Hypotheses, 62,* 486.
54. Jadotte, Y.T. & Schwartz, R.A. (2010). Melasma: Insights and perspectives. *Acta Dermatovenerol Croat, 18,* 124.
55. Janssen, P., et al. (2003). To dye or not to dye: A randomized, clinical trial of a triple dye/alcohol regime versus dry cord care. *Pediatrics, 111,* 15.
56. Kalia, Y.N., et al. (1998). Development of skin barrier function in preterm infants. *J Invest Dermatol, 111,* 320.
57. Katz, V.L., Farmer, R.M., & Dotters, D. (2002). Focus on primary care: From nevus to neoplasm: Myths of melanoma in pregnancy. *Obstet Gynecol Surv, 57,* 112.
58. Knobel, R.B., et al. (2009). Extremely low birth weight preterm infants lack vasomotor response in relationship to cold body temperatures at birth. *J Perinatol, 29,* 814.
59. Kopelman, A.E. (1973). Cutaneous absorption of hexachlorophene in low-birth-weight infants. *J Pediatr, 82,* 972.
60. Kroth, J., et al. (2008). Functional vessel density in the first month of life in preterm neonates. *Pediatr Res, 64,* 567.
61. Kroumpouzos, G. & Cohen, L.M. (2003). Specific dermatoses of pregnancy: An evidence-based systematic review. *Am J Obstet Gynecol, 188,* 1083.
62. Kumari, R., Jaisankar, T.J., & Thappa, D.M. (2007). A clinical study of skin changes in pregnancy. *Indian J Dermatol Venereol Leprol, 73,* 141.
63. Lawley, T.J. & Yancy, K.B. (1999). Skin changes and diseases of pregnancy. In I.M. Freedberg, et al. (Eds.), *Fitzpatrick's dermatology in general medicine* (5th ed.). New York: McGraw-Hill.
64. Lee, H.K. (2002). Effects of sponge bathing on vagal tone and behavioral responses in premature infants. *J Clin Nurs, 11,* 510.
65. Lim, C.S. & Davies, A.H. (2009). Pathogenesis of primary varicose veins. *Br J Surg, 96,* 1231.
66. Loomis, A.C., et al. (2008). Fetal skin development. In Eichenfield, L.F., et al. (Eds.), *Neonatal dermatology* (2nd ed.). Philadelphia: Saunders.
67. Lund, C., (1999). Prevention and management of infant skin breakdown. *Nurs Clin North Am, 34,* 907.
68. Lund, C., et al. (1999). Neonatal skin care: The scientific basis for practice. *J Obstet Gynecol Neonatal Nurs, 28,* 241.
69. Lund, C.H., et al. (1997). Disruption of barrier function in neonatal skin associated with adhesive removal. *J Pediatr, 131,* 367.
70. Lund, C.H., et al. (2001). Neonatal skin care: Clinical outcomes of the AWHONN/NANN evidence-based clinical practice guideline. Association of Women's Health, Obstetric and Neonatal Nurses and the National Association of Neonatal Nurses. *J Obstet Gynecol Neonatal Nurs, 30,* 41.
71. Maayan-Metzger, A., et al. (2004). Effect of radiant warmer on transepidermal water loss (TEWL) and skin hydration in preterm infants. *J Perinatol, 24,* 372.
72. Matz, H., Orion, E., & Wolf, R. (2006). Pruritic urticarial papules and plaques of pregnancy: Polymorphic eruption of pregnancy (PUPPP). *Clin Dermatol, 24,* 105.
73. Mays, J.K. (2010). The active management of intrahepatic cholestasis of pregnancy. *Curr Opin Obstet Gynecol, 22,* 100.
74. McCall, E.M., et al. (2008). Interventions to prevent hypothermia at birth in preterm and/or low birthweight infants. *Cochrane Database Syst Rev* 1, CD004210.
75. Medves, J.M. & O'Brien, B. (2004). The effect of bather and location of first bath on maintaining thermal stability in newborns. *J Obstet Gynecol Neonatal Nurs, 33,* 175.

76. Moore, K.L., Persaud, T.V.N., & Torchia, M.G. (2011). *The developing human: Clinically orinted embryology* (9th ed.). Philadelphia: Saunders.
77. Muallem, M.M. & Rubeiz, N.G. (2006). Physiological and biological skin changes in pregnancy. *Clin Dermatol, 24,* 80.
78. Mullany, L.C., Darmstadt, G.L., & Tielsch, J.M. (2003). Role of antimicrobial applications to the umbilical cord in neonates to prevent bacterial colonization and infection: A review of the evidence. *Pediatr Infect Dis J, 22,* 996.
79. Narendran, V., et al. (2010). Biomarkers of epidermal innate immunity in premature and full-term infants. *Pediatr Res, 67,* 382.
80. Nedergaard, J. & Cannon, B. (2012). Brown adipose tissue: Development and function. In R.A. Polin, W.W. Fox, & S.H. Abman (Eds.), *Fetal and neonatal physiology* (4th ed.). Philadelphia: Saunders.
81. Nichols, A.A. (2005). Cholestasis of pregnancy: A review of the evidence. *J Perinat Neonatal Nurs, 19,* 217.
82. Nikolovski, J., et al. (2008). Barrier function and water-holding and transport properties of infant stratum corneum are different from adult and continue to develop through the first year of life. *J Invest Dermatol, 128,* 1728.
83. Nissimov, J. & Elchalal, U. (2003). Scalp hair diameter increases during pregnancy. *Clin Exp Dermatol, 28,* 525.
84. Norman, M. (2008). Low birth weight and the developing vascular tree: A systematic review. *Acta Paediatr, 97,* 1165.
85. Nussbaum, R. & Benedetto, A.V. (2006). Cosmetic aspects of pregnancy. *Clin Dermatol, 24,* 133.
86. Osman, H., et al. (2007). Risk factors for the development of striae gravidarum. *Am J Obstet Gynecol, 196,* 62.e1.
87. Osman, H., et al. (2008). Cocoa butter lotion for prevention of striae gravidarum: A double-blind, randomized and placebo-controlled trial. *BJOG, 115,* 1138.
88. Peters, K.L. (1998). Bathing premature infants: Physiological and behavioral consequences. *Am J Crit Care, 7,* 90.
89. Ponnapula, P. & Boberg, J.S. (2010). Lower extremity changes experienced during pregnancy. *J Foot Ankle Surg, 49,* 452.
90. Powell, F. & Powell, B. (1987). Cutaneous changes during pregnancy. *Ir Med J, 80,* 50.
91. Pyati, S.P., et al. (1977). Absorption of iodine in the neonate following topical use of povidone iodine. *J Pediatr, 91,* 825.
92. Quinn, D., Newton, N., & Piecuch, R. (2005). Effect of less frequent bathing on premature infant skin. *J Obstet Gynecol Neonatal Nurs, 34,* 741.
93. Rapini, R.P. (2009). The skin and pregnancy. In R.K. Creasy, et al. (Eds.), *Creasy & Resnik's Maternal-fetal medicine: Principles and practice* (6th ed.). Philadelphia: Saunders.
94. Rissmann, R., et al. (2008). Temperature-induced changes in structural and physicochemical properties of vernix caseosa. *J Invest Dermatol, 128,* 292.
95. Rogers, M. (2005). Neonatal dermatology. In J.M. Rennie (Ed.), *Roberton's textbook of neonatology* (4th ed.). Edinburgh: Churchill Livingstone.
96. Rosen, C.F. (2004). The skin in pregnancy. In G.N. Burrow, T.P. Duffy, & J.A. Copel (Eds.), *Medical complications during pregnancy* (6th ed.). Philadelphia: Saunders.
97. Roth, M.M. (2009). Specific pregnancy dermatoses. *Dermatol Nurs, 21,* 70.
98. Roth, M.M. (2011). Pregnancy dermatoses: diagnosis, management, and controversies. *Am J Clin Dermatol, 12,* 25.
99. Rutter, N. & Hull, D. (1979). Water loss from the skin of term and preterm babies. *Arch Dis Child, 54,* 858.
100. Rutter, N. (2000). Physiology of the newborn skin. In J. Haper & A. Oranje (Eds.), *Textbook of pediatric dermatology.* Oxford: Blackwell Scientific.
101. Sadler, T.W. (2012). *Langman's Medical embryology* (12th ed.). Philadelphia: Lippincott Williams & Wilkins.
102. Salter, S.A. & Kimball, A.B. (2006). Striae gravidarum. *Clin Dermatol, 24,* 97.
103. Sedin, G. (2004). To avoid heat loss in very preterm infants. *J Pediatr, 145,* 720.
104. Shwayder, T. & Akland, T. (2005). Neonatal skin barrier: Structure, function, and disorders. *Dermatol Ther, 18,* 87.
105. Siegfried, E.C. (1998). Neonatal skin and skin care. *Dermatol Clin, 16,* 437.
106. Stamatas, G.N., et al. (2010). Infant skin microstructure assessed in vivo differs from adult skin in organization and at the cellular level. *Pediatr Dermatol, 27,* 125.
107. Stamatas, G.N., et al. (2011). Infant skin physiology and development during the first years of life: A review of recent findings based on in vivo studies. *Int J Cosmet Sci, 33,* 17.
108. Tansirikongkol, A., et al. (2008). Equilibrium water content in native vernix and its cellular component. *J Pharm Sci, 97,* 985.
109. Tapia-Rombo, C.A., Morales-Mora, M., & Alvarez-Vazquez, E. (2003). Variations of vital signs, skin color, behavior and oxygen saturation in premature neonates after sponge bathing. Possible complications. *Rev Invest Clin, 55,* 438.
110. Taquino, L.T. (2000). Promoting wound healing in the neonatal setting: Process versus protocol. *J Perinat Neonatal Nurs, 14,* 104.
111. Thomas, R.G. & Liston, W.A. (2004). Clinical associations of striae gravidarum. *J Obstet Gynaecol, 24,* 270.
112. Tollin, M., et al. (2005). Vernix caseosa as a multi-component defense system based on polypeptides, lipids and their interactions. *Cell Mol Life Sci, 62,* 2390.
113. Tosti, A., et al. (2009). Hair loss in women. *Minerva Ginecol, 61,* 445.
114. Visscher, M., et al. (2009). Skin care in the NICU patient: Effects of wipes versus cloth and water on stratum corneum integrity. *Neonatology, 96,* 226.
115. Visscher, M.O., et al. (2005). Vernix caseosa in neonatal adaptation. *J Perinatol, 25,* 440.
116. Visscher, M.O., et al. (2011). Neonatal skin maturation-vernix caseosa and free amino acids. *Pediatr Dermatol, 28,* 122.
117. Walker, L., Downe, S., & Gomez, L. (2005). Skin care in the well term newborn: Two systematic reviews. *Birth, 32,* 224.
118. Wong, R.C. & Ellis, C.N. (1989). Physiologic skin changes in pregnancy. *Semin Dermatol, 8,* 7.
119. World Health Organization. (1998). *Care of the umbilical cord: WHO/FHE/MSM-Cord care*. Geneva: WHO.
120. Young, G.L. & Jewell, D. (2000). Creams for preventing stretch marks in pregnancy. *Cochrane Database Syst Rev* 2, CD000066.
121. Yung-Weng, W. & Ying-Ju, C. (2004). A preliminary study of bottom care effects on premature infants' heart rate and oxygen saturation. *J Nurs Res, 12,* 161.
122. Zupan, J., Garner, P., & Omari, A.A. (2004). Topical umbilical cord care at birth. *Cochrane Database Sys Rev* 3, CD001057.

Neurologic, Muscular, and Sensory Systems

CHAPTER 15

The neurologic, muscular, and sensory systems are three of the most complex systems in the human body. Normal function of the central nervous system (CNS) is critical for functioning of individual organs and integration of organ systems to achieve coordinated physiologic and neurobehavioral processes. Alterations in neuromuscular and sensory processes during pregnancy give rise to common experiences such as musculoskeletal discomforts, sleep disturbances, and alterations in sensation. Discomforts and pain during the antepartum, intrapartum, and postpartum periods influence maternal adaptation and the course of labor. Newborn and particularly preterm infants must respond to the extrauterine environment with neuromuscular and sensory systems that are still immature. Neurologic dysfunction during the neonatal period due to insults before, during, or after birth can affect the infant's ability to survive the perinatal and neonatal periods and has implications for later developmental and cognitive outcome. This chapter examines physiologic adaptations in the mother, implications for healthy pregnant women and those with chronic health problems, neurodevelopmental processes in the fetus and newborn, and clinical implications for these infants.

MATERNAL PHYSIOLOGIC ADAPTATIONS

During pregnancy the neurologic, muscular, and sensory systems are influenced by the altered hormonal milieu and by alterations in other systems. The effects of these changes on the muscular and sensory systems are well documented. Many of the hormones of pregnancy also have CNS activity, although their specific effects on neurologic function are not as well understood as their effects on other body systems. As a result, there is little known about specific changes in the function of the neurologic system during pregnancy, other than effects on endocrine glands (see Chapter 19). During the intrapartum period, maternal physiologic and psychologic responses are altered by the discomfort and pain of labor. These responses can have a significant impact on fetal homeostasis in addition to having important implications for management of the woman in labor.

Antepartum Period

This section examines specific alterations during pregnancy in ocular and otolaryngeal function, sleep, and the musculoskeletal system.

Ocular Changes

The eyes of the pregnant woman undergo several alterations during pregnancy that result from physiologic and hormonal adaptations. The pregnant woman develops a mild corneal edema, particularly during the third trimester. The cornea becomes slightly thicker, which (along with the fluid retention) changes its topography and may slightly alter the refractory power of the eye. Corneal hyposensitivity may sometimes also develops during this period, probably because of the increased thickness and fluid retention.[172,182,217,238] A few women experience an increase in corneal epithelial pigmentation (known as *Krukenberg spindles*), possibly secondary to increases in estrogens, progesterone, adrenocorticotropic hormone (ACTH), and melanocyte-stimulating hormone.[45,182] The composition of tears changes slightly with an increase in secretion of lysozyme.[172] Disruption of lacrimal acinar cells can lead to dry eyes.[182]

Most studies report that intraocular pressure falls about 10%, especially during the second half of gestation (after 28 weeks), although variations are seen among women in the degree of change.[45,54,77,182,196,217] This change is believed to be due to the effects of progesterone, relaxin, and human chorionic gonadotropin combined with an increase in aqueous outflow and decreased episcleral pressure.[45,224,238] Similar findings have been reported for women on oral contraceptives. The decrease in intraocular pressure is greater in multiparas than primiparas.[196] Changes in intraocular pressure are independent of changes in systemic blood pressure.[77] An increase in intraocular pressure has been reported in women with preeclampsia. This increase is not correlated with blood pressure, but may be due to increased extracellular fluid volume and decreased aqueous humor outflow in the preeclamptic woman.[77]

Ptosis, usually unilateral, occasionally develops for unknown reasons, but may be related to changes in the levator aponeurosis due to hormonal and fluid changes or stress.[172,182,238] Ptosis may also occur as a complication of lumbar anesthesia, either as an isolated finding or as part of Horner syndrome. Horner syndrome is characterized by ptosis, miosis, and anhidrosis secondary to interruption of sympathetic innervation.[238] Some women experience an increased pigmentation of the face and eyelids known as *melasma* (see Chapter 14).

During pregnancy there is a progressive decrease in blood flow to the conjunctiva, which is sensitive to estrogen. This change is most marked in women with preeclampsia as a result of spasm and ischemia.[11] In these women, changes in the conjunctival vessels may occur earlier than in the retinal vessels. Subconjunctival hemorrhages may occur spontaneously during pregnancy or in labor, with spontaneous resolution.

Otolaryngeal Changes

Changes in the ear, nose, and larynx are related to modifications in fluid dynamics and vascular permeability, increased protein synthesis, vasomotor alterations of the autonomic nervous system, and increased vascularity, along with hormonal (especially estrogen) influences.[65,135,208,215] As a result of these alterations, the nasal mucosa becomes congested and hyperemic. The pregnant woman experiences nasal stuffiness and obstruction associated with serous rhinorrhea or postnasal discharge. Altered olfactory perception with increased sensation to smell has also been reported.[35,129]

Pregnancy rhinitis (defined as nasal congestion that lasts 6 or more weeks without signs of infection or allergy) is seen in up to 30% of all pregnant women and in approximately two thirds of those who smoke.[65,129,183] These symptoms may appear anytime but usually begin in the second trimester and parallel increasing estrogen levels.[65,195,242] The symptoms may interfere with sleep and the sense of smell. The cause is unknown, but placental growth hormone has been implicated as a stimulator of nasal mucosal growth.[65] The rhinitis may also be due to increased sensitivity to allergens in women with subclinical allergy.[129] Vascular congestion may result in epistaxis from rupture of superficial blood vessels. External nasal alar dilators or nasal washings with a saline solution may provide some relief.[65] Systemic antihistamines should be used with caution and only for short periods. Pseudoephedrine should be avoided, especially in the first trimester due to a reported increase in the risk of gastroschisis.[215] Prolonged use (over 3 to 5 days) of topical sympathomimetic nasal sprays should be avoided because they can cause rebound congestion.[65,135,195,242]

The pregnant woman may also complain of ear stuffiness or blocked ears unrelieved by swallowing. This change is believed to result from estrogen-induced changes in mucous membranes of the eustachian tube, edema of the nasopharynx, and alterations in fluid dynamics and pressures of the middle ear.[129,135,195,242] Some women may experience a transient, mild hearing loss, and an increased risk of serous effusion. Management is usually supportive. Increased estrogen and progesterone leads to transient vertigo in some women.[129,216,242] Tinnitus is more common during pregnancy, possibly due to hyperdynamic circulation, increased peripheral lymphatic fluid, and hormonal changes.[129,216] Symptoms resolve with delivery. Ménière's disease may be exacerbated during pregnancy because of fluid retention.[242]

Laryngeal changes during pregnancy are hormonally induced and include erythema and edema of the vocal cords accompanied by vascular dilation and small submucosal hemorrhages.[139,195,242] The woman may note hoarseness, deepening or cracking of the voice, persistent cough, or other vocal changes. Some women report the quality of their voice improves during the first two trimesters due to better lubrication of the vocal cords.[94] Laryngeal changes can complicate administration of endotracheal anesthesia. Similar changes are reported in women premenstrually and with use of progesterone-dominated oral contraceptives.[195] Maximal phonation time decreases and vocal fatigue is more prevalent during pregnancy, possibly due to the decreased thoracic cage volume with uterine growth.[94] The airway becomes hyperemic with mucosal edema and a decreased diameter of the upper airway, which may increase snoring and sleep disorders.[29,75] The edema arises from the increased plasma volume and capillary congestion.[29,139]

Musculoskeletal Changes

Pregnancy is characterized by changes in posture and gait. Relaxin and progesterone affect the cartilage and connective tissue of the sacroiliac joints and the symphysis pubis. This, along with external rotation of the femurs, increases the mobility of these joints and leads to the characteristic "waddle" gait seen in many pregnant women.[71,116,165] Widening and increased mobility of the sacroiliac synchondroses and symphysis pubis begins by 10 to 12 weeks.[103] The symphysis pubis may widen up to 10 mm.[26,116]

Musculoskeletal changes during pregnancy may also be due to changes in gait to compensate for the increase in and redistribution of body mass.[71] The altered gait in pregnancy may increase the load on the lateral side of the foot and hindfoot, leading to lower limb pain. Ligamentous laxity increases due primarily to the effects of estrogen.[26,203] Estrogen and progesterone receptors on fibroblasts within the walls of the blood vessels supplying the anterior cruciate ligaments increase during pregnancy, with decreased collagen synthesis and increased relaxin. Relaxin remodels collagen fibers and reduces their diameters.[26] The risk of ligament injury is increased during pregnancy.[116] Muscle cramps are more frequent in pregnant women, especially during the second half of pregnancy and at night (see Chapter 17).[105,116]

Pregnant women often experience back pain and other discomforts (see section on Musculoskeletal Discomforts). Distention of the abdomen with growth of the fetus tilts the pelvis forward, shifting the center of gravity. The woman compensates by developing an increased curvature (lordosis) of the spine that may strain muscles and ligaments of the back. Stretching and decreased tone of the abdominal muscles also contribute to the lordosis. Diastasis of the rectus abdominis muscles in the third trimester may persist after delivery. Breast tenderness, heaviness, tingling, and occasionally pain occur by 6 weeks. These changes are due to estrogens, progesterone, human placental lactogen (hPL), increased blood volume, and venous stasis. Long-term bed rest can lead to muscle atrophy and change gastrocnemius muscle metabolism.[20,154] Muscle recovery postpartum can take more than six weeks.[20,154]

Sleep

Sleep patterns are altered during pregnancy and the postpartum period. Sleep quality and insomnia tend to be most prominent in the first and third trimesters.[59,106,123,137,212,218] With advancing gestation total sleep hours progressively decrease.[123] Sleep time also decreases prior to labor onset with an increase in night awakenings reported beginning about 5 days prior to labor onset.[17] Both hormonal and mechanical factors alter the pregnant woman's sleep-wake patterns (Figure 15-1).[209,212] Sleep is divided into rapid eye movement (REM) and non–rapid eye movement (NREM) or deep sleep, which is subdivided into four stages. Hormonal changes alter sleep during pregnancy. Progesterone has a sedative effect and increases NREM sleep.[209,212] Estrogens and cortisol decrease REM, whereas prolactin increases both REM and NREM sleep.[61,212] Changes in sleep stages are seen by 11 to 12 weeks.[139] In general, pregnant women tend to have less deep and lighter sleep and more awakenings (from less than 5% to 10% by the third trimester).[139]

During the first trimester, total sleep time increases, as does napping. By the second half of gestation, pregnant women have less overall sleep time and more night awakenings than nonpregnant women do. The pregnant woman has decreased REM sleep in the third trimester, along with increased awakenings and napping, and diminished alertness during the day.[59,104,106,137,212] Early-onset REM sleep is reported in pregnant women with depression or mood disorders.[139] Alterations in NREM sleep with an increase in stage 1 (sleep latency or transition between wakefulness and sleep) and a decrease in stages 2 and 4 (delta sleep or deep sleep stage) during late pregnancy have also been noted.[122,137] The decrease in stage 4 NREM sleep has implications for the pregnant woman's functioning, because this stage is important for basic biologic processes such as tissue repair and recovery from fatigue.[140] In summary, changes to sleep reported during the first trimester include increased total sleep, napping, daytime sleepiness and insomnia, and decreased REM, and stage 3 and stage 4 NREM sleep; changes during the second trimester included increased awakenings with normal total sleep times and decreased REM, stage 3 NREM, and stage 4 NREM sleep; third trimester changes included increased daytime sleepiness, insomnia, nocturnal awakenings, and stage 1 NREM sleep, and decreased REM, stage 3 NREM, and stage 4 NREM sleep.[59,106,122,137,212,218,236] During pregnancy, night awakenings are often associated with nocturia, dyspnea, heartburn, uterine activity, nasal congestion, muscle aches, stress, and anxiety and can lead to sleep disturbances and insomnia. The major reasons given by women for sleep alterations include urinary frequency, backache, leg cramps, restless legs, heartburn, and fetal activity.[61,104,139,236] Interventions include establishing regular sleep-wake habits

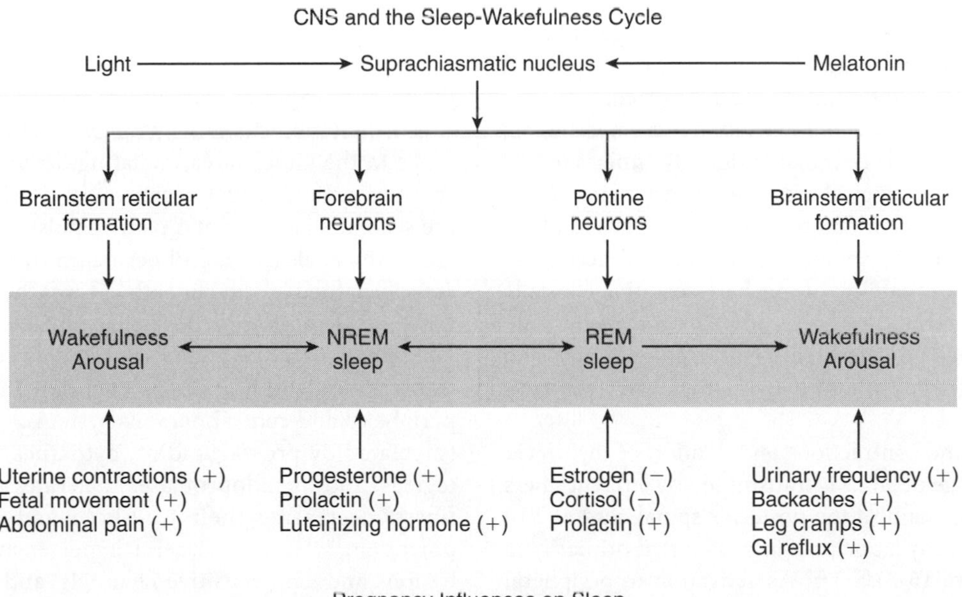

FIGURE 15-1 Central nervous system (CNS) structures involved in the sleep-wakefulness cycle and pregnancy influences on this cycle. The biological clock (suprachiasmatic nucleus), influenced by light and melatonin, interacts with neurons to generate a circadian timing for wakefulness and arousal and for rapid eye movement (REM) and non-REM (NREM) sleep. Bidirectional changes in physiologic states can occur, except in the REM and wakefulness stages. Physiologic and hormonal events in pregnancy promote (+) or reduce (−) time spent in each state through as yet unclear neural mechanisms. (From Santiago, J.R., et al. [2001]. Sleep and sleep disorders in pregnancy. *Ann Intern Med, 134,* 397.)

and periods, avoiding caffeine, relaxation techniques, massage, heat and support for lower back pain, modifying the sleep environment, and limiting fluids in the evening.[212] Sleep medications should be avoided because these drugs alter the physiologic mechanisms of sleep by suppressing REM and NREM stages 3 and 4 and may cross the placenta to the fetus. Sleep loss (i.e., sleeping less than 6 hours per night) in the last 3 to 4 weeks of pregnancy may increase labor length and need for cesarean birth.[76,94,138,259]

A pregnancy-associated sleep disorder has been described by the American Sleep Disorders Association.[9] Individuals with sleep disorder breathing may have an increase in severity during pregnancy due to partial airway obstruction by otolaryngeal changes.[29,208,209] Increases are also reported in snoring and possibly obstructive sleep apnea (OSA), although the prevalence of OSA during pregnancy is not well documented.[29,75,208,209] The prevalence of snoring during pregnancy is 15% to 30% by the third trimester.[139] An increase in hypertension, preeclampsia, gestational diabetes, and fetal growth restriction has been reported in pregnant women who snore.[28,29,75,168]

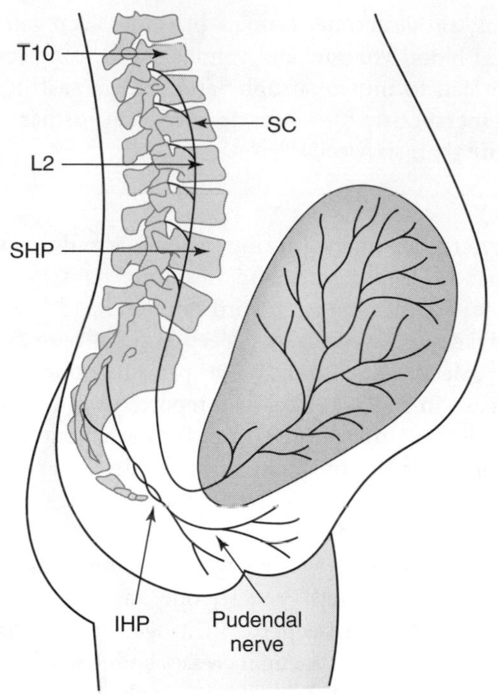

FIGURE 15-2 Neural pathways. The uterus, including the lower uterine segment and the cervix, is supplied by nociceptive afferents that pass to the spinal cord accompanying sympathetic nerves in the inferior hypogastric plexus (IHP), the superior hypogastric plexus (SHP), and the hypogastric nerve. They then pass through the lumbar and lower thoracic sympathetic chain (SC) and enter the spinal cord through the posterior nerve roots of T10, T11, T12, and L1. The pudendal nerve supplies structures in the pelvis. (From Rowlands, S. & Permezel, M. [1998]. Physiology of pain in labour. *Baillieres Clin Obstet Gynaecol, 12*, 350.)

Intrapartum Period

Pain and Discomfort during Labor

The woman in labor experiences two types of pain: visceral and somatic. Visceral pain is related to contraction of the uterus and dilation and stretching of the cervix. Uterine pain during the first stage of labor results from ischemia caused by constriction and contraction of the arteries supplying the myometrium. Somatic pain is caused by pressure of the presenting part on the birth canal, vulva, and perineum. Visceral pain is experienced primarily during the first stage of labor; somatic pain is experienced during transition and the second stage.[68] Somatic pain is more intense and localized.

The corpus of the uterus is relatively denervated by late pregnancy while the cervix remains densely innervated.[240] This suggests that the cervical area maybe the major site of pain in labor.[240] Near term numbers of nerve cells and fibers in the sensory area of the spinal column decrease accompanied by increased excitability of mechanosensitive efferents in the cervix.[125,181] The pain threshold may be altered in late pregnancy, enhanced by elevated β-endorphins, leading to a proposed "pregnancy-induced hypoanalgesia" (see next section).[79,125,181]

Pain from uterine contractions and dilation of the cervix during the first stage of labor is transmitted by afferent fibers to the sympathetic chain of the posterior spinal cord at T10 to T12, and L1. In early labor, pain is transmitted primarily to T11 to T12 (Figure 15-2).[68,79,206] As activation of peripheral small A-delta (myelinated) and C afferent (unmyelinated) nerve fibers of these nerve terminals (by kinin-like substances released from the uterine and cervical tissues) intensifies, transmission spreads to T10 and L1. Pain during the first stage may be referred; that is, the nerve impulses from the uterus and cervix stimulate spinal cord neurons, innervating both the uterus and the abdominal wall. As a result, the woman experiences pain over the abdominal wall between the umbilicus and symphysis pubis, around the iliac crests to the gluteal area, radiating down the thighs, and in the lumbar and sacral regions.[79,231] During transition and the second stage, somatic pain impulses from distention of the birth canal, vulva, and perineum by the presenting part are transmitted by the pudendal nerves through the posterior roots of the parasympathetic chain at S2, S3, and S4.[41,79]

Peripheral tissue injury and inflammation change the transcription and function of channels and receptors in the peripheral and central nervous systems.[102,240] Inflammation (mediated by prostaglandins, cytokines, granulocytes, integrins, and metalloproteases) activates nociceptive nerve fibers, decreasing their threshold and increasing action potentials.[102,127] This visceral hypersensitivity is mediated by ion- and acid-sensitive channels, and by prostaglandin E_2, *N*-methyl-D-aspartate (NMDA), and other receptors.[102] Stimulation of dorsal root NMDA receptors mediates central hypersensitivity.[127]

As the A-delta and C nerve fibers enter the dorsal horn of the spinal cord, they synapse and ascend to the brainstem by the spinothalamic tract (see Figure 15-2). The pain impulses entering the brain stimulate a variety of neurons, including cortical neurons and those of the brainstem reticular formation (integrative function), thalamus, hypothalamus, and limbic system.[206] The result is a conscious sensation of pain as well as a variety of ventilatory, circulatory, and metabolic responses. Spatial and temporal summation is processed in the cortex.[151,206] These responses include increases in ventilation, cardiac output, peripheral resistance, gastric acid secretion, metabolic rate, oxygen consumption, and catecholamine release.

The perception of pain is influenced by physiologic, psychologic, and cultural factors. Pain can lead to anxiety and influence maternal physiologic responses and the course of labor. For example, physical manifestations of anxiety may include muscular tension, hyperventilation, increased sympathetic activity, and norepinephrine release, which can lead to increased cardiac output, blood pressure, metabolic rate, and oxygen consumption and impaired uterine contractility (Figure 15-3).[18,119,205] Anxiety can also increase fear and tension, reducing pain tolerance, which decreases uterine contractility.[18,119,151] Relaxation techniques such as progressive muscle relaxation, touch, breathing, imagery, and autosuggestion help reduce anxiety and prevent or stop this cycle.[119]

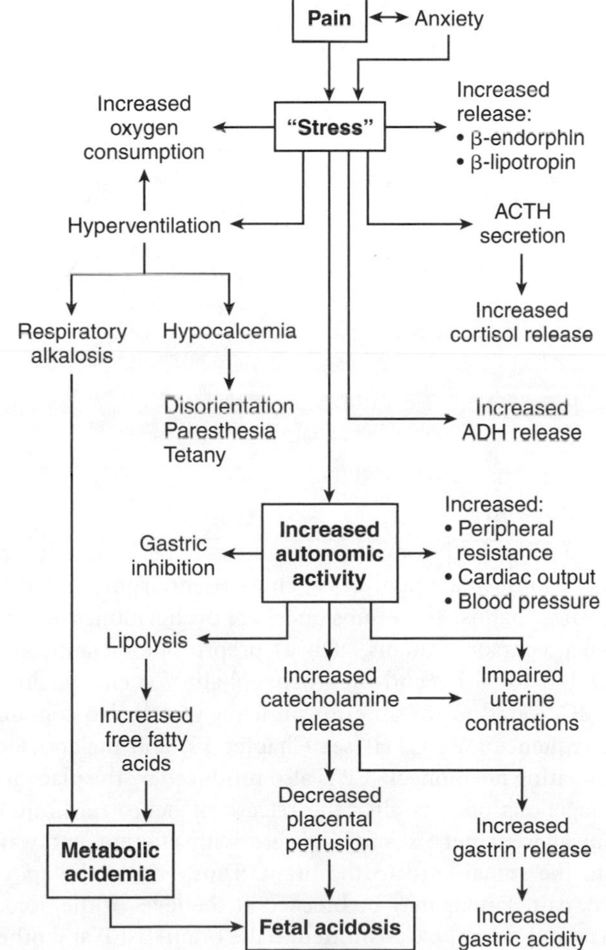

FIGURE 15-3 Physiologic changes secondary to pain in labor. (From Brownridge, P. & Cohen, S. [1988]. Neural blockade for obstetric and gynecologic surgery. In M.J. Cousins & P.O. Bridenbaugh [Eds.], *Neural blockade* [2nd ed.]. Philadelphia: Lippincott.)

Descending spinal tracts in the dorsal horn modulate nociception via input from the cortex and limbic system with release of endogenous opioids such as β-endorphins and enkephalins (see next section).[205] These modulating factors are produced by the placenta as well as the mother and may include an opioid-enhancing factor.[205] Other modulating factors include analgesia induced by mechanical stimulation of the hypogastric (uterine mechanical stimulation) and pelvic (vaginal distention) nerves.[206] Exogenous modification of labor pain includes both pharmacologic (opioids, sedatives, analgesics, anesthetics) interventions and nonpharmacologic cognitive, behavioral, and sensory techniques.[70,156] These techniques include relaxation, cognitive and behavioral childbirth preparation, hypnosis, acupuncture, movement, positioning, vocalizations, touch, massage, music, biofeedback, transcutaneous electrical nerve stimulation (TENS), and hydrotherapy (Table 15-1).[13,15,18,41,62,70,113,119,206,225,227,229]

The gate control theory postulates that nervous stimuli can be inhibited at the level of the substantia gelatinosa and dorsal horn of the spinal cord from reaching the thalamus and cerebral cortex:

> "The theory proposes that a neural mechanism in the dorsal horns of the spinal cord acts like a gate which can increase or decrease the flow of nerve impulses from peripheral fibers to the central nervous system. Somatic input is therefore subjected to the modulating influence of the gate before it evokes pain perception and response. The degree to which the gate increases or decreases sensory transmission is determined by the relative activity in large-diameter (A-beta) and small diameter (A-delta and C) fibers and by descending influences from the brain. When the amount of information that passes through the gate exceeds a critical level, it activates the neural areas responsible for pain experience and response."[163, p. 222]

Techniques to close the gate (inhibit) include stimulation of large nerve fibers to block impulses from the smaller pain fibers. This provides a basis for use of massage and effleurage during labor. With continued use of these techniques, the large nerve fibers become habituated and stimuli from smaller fibers are no longer blocked. Thus, as labor progresses, the woman needs to stimulate other fibers (using techniques such as heat, pressure with change of position, and massage of other areas). Because descending fibers may also inhibit transmission to the brain, concentration techniques may also be useful.[41,119,157]

The neuromatrix theory of pain expands on the gate control theory and emphasizes that pain is a multi-dimensional, whole body-mind-spirit experience that may underlie the basis for the efficacy of nonpharmacologic pain interventions during labor.[114,162,243]

> "The neuromatrix theory incorporates many of the same elements of the gate control theory. Both theories view the brain as the ultimate arbitrator of the

Table 15-1 Proposed Mechanisms of Labor Pain Reduction with Various Nonpharmacologic Measures

MECHANISMS	ACUPUNCTURE/ACUPRESSURE	AROMATHERAPY	BREATHING/FOCUS	CHILDBIRTH EDUCATION	COLD	EMOTIONAL SUPPORT	HEAT	HYDROTHERAPY	HYPNOSIS	INTRADERMAL WATER BLOCK	MASSAGE/TOUCH	MOVEMENT AND POSITIONING	MUSIC/AUDIOANALGESIA	RELAXATION	TENS
Counterirritation analgesia (brief intense stimulation of trigger points)					X					X					X
Increases endorphins	X									X			X		X
Provides stimuli from peripheral sensory receptors to inhibit pain awareness		X			X		X	X			X		X		X
Increases joint mobility							X	X				X			
Alters pressures within pelvis and on soft tissues								X			X	X			
Improves energy flow along meridians crucial to labor progress and comfort	X				X										
Decreases muscle tension	X				X		X	X	X		X			X	
Alters nerve conduction velocity (slows pain transmission to CNS)					X										
Decreases anxiety/fear, provides reassurance		X	X	X		X			X		X	X	X	X	
Increases woman's sense of control, reducing pain perception			X	X		X			X			X	X	X	X
Distraction of attention from pain		X	X		X	X	X	X	X		X	X	X		X
Enhances or changes mood, reducing pain perception		X				X			X		X		X	X	
Cues rhythmic activity and rituals			X			X					X	X		X	

From Simkin, P. & Bolding, A. (2004). Update on nonpharmacologic approaches to relieve labor pain and prevent suffering. *J Midwifery Womens Health*, 49, 491.
CNS, Central nervous system; *TENS*, transcutaneous electrical nerve stimulation.

multiple dimensions of pain. However, the gate control theory emphasizes the opening or closing of a gate at the level of the spinal cord as the preeminent mechanism controlling the ultimate perception of pain. The neuromatrix theory of pain recognizes the simultaneous convergence of a panoply of influences, including one's past experiences, cultural factors, emotional state, cognitive input, stress regulation, and immune systems, as well as immediate sensory input . . . The multiple influences that create pain perception are generated from 3 parallel processing networks: sensory-discriminative (somatosensory components), affective-motivational (limbic system components), and evaluative-cognitive (thalamocortical components). Additional contributions of the autonomic nervous system, the stress response system, and immune system modulation are also recognized in this model."[243,p.483]

β-Endorphins

Pain during the intrapartum period may be modulated by endogenous opiate peptides such as β-endorphins (B-EPs) and enkephalins. These substances are prohormones derived from precursor proteins such as prepro-opiomelanocortin (POMC) for B-EP and preproenkephalin for enkephalin.[78] POMC, found in the anterior pituitary gland, also contains the sequence for ACTH (see Chapter 19) and melanocyte-stimulating hormone. B-EP is also produced by the placenta. Endogenous opioids alter the release of neurotransmitters from afferent nerves and interfere with efferent pathways from the spinal cord to the brain. Thus, within the spinal cord, pain signals may be blocked at the level of the dorsal horns and never be transmitted to the brain. B-EP and other endogenous opioids, in addition to their analgesic role, may also alter mood during pregnancy and have a role in regulation of secretion of pituitary hormones.[78] For example, B-EP appears to modulate release of luteinizing hormone, prolactin, growth hormone, and follicle-stimulating hormone by the anterior pituitary and arginine vasopressin from the posterior pituitary gland.[78]

Maternal plasma B-EP levels increase during pregnancy, especially from 28 weeks on, and are significantly elevated during late pregnancy and labor.[46,78] Increased levels may be related to the increase in corticotropin-releasing hormone near term (see Chapters 4 and 19).[46] Maximum levels of B-EP are found during parturition and decrease postpartum.[260] Levels correlate with uterine muscle contraction and cervical effacement. B-EP release may be stimulated by stress as an adaptive response. Endorphins may increase the pain threshold, are associated with feelings of euphoria and analgesia, and may enable the woman to tolerate the pain of labor and delivery.

The increased levels of B-EP during labor may contribute to the decreased doses of anesthetic drugs generally required in pregnant women compared with nonpregnant women.[46,79] Women with low B-EP levels at term may have a greater need for pain medication during labor.[46,79] The variable decrease in doses of local anesthetics for epidural and spinal blocks is also caused by vascular congestion within the spinal canal and progesterone as well as the altered neuronal sensitivity. Increased progesterone levels also contribute to the decreased doses of inhalation anesthetics needed for pregnant women through their effect on the respiratory system.

Postpartum Period

B-EP levels decrease by 24 hours after birth. Levels are higher after vaginal versus cesarean birth.[260] Levels of B-EP are twice as high in colostrum as in maternal plasma and may assist the newborn in the transition to extrauterine life and mediate the stressful events of labor and delivery.[260]

During the postpartum period the ocular and otolaryngeal changes resolve as the physiologic and hormonal adaptations of pregnancy are reversed. Sensitivity of the cornea returns to the usual parameters by 6 to 8 weeks postpartum.[172] Intraocular pressure returns to prepregnancy levels by 2 to 3 months postpartum.[224] Both ptosis and subconjunctival hemorrhages disappear spontaneously.[172] Nasal congestion, ear stuffiness, tinnitus, and laryngeal changes and related discomforts usually disappear within a few days after delivery.[65,94,129,215,216] Head aches, generally bilateral and frontal, are a common discomfort in the first week after delivery. Postpartum headaches tend to begin around the time of postpartum weight loss and have been attributed to alterations in fluid and electrolyte balance.

Sleep during the Postpartum Period

Sleep is altered during the immediate postpartum period. Most of these changes normalize after the first weeks postpartum, but primiparas may experience altered sleep for up to 3 months.[61,137] Stage 1 NREM sleep is longer immediately after birth than before birth. Stage 4 NREM sleep is also longer immediately after birth than before birth, with a gradual change to prepregnancy levels by about 2 weeks. REM sleep is decreased and awake time increased on the first postpartum night, with a reversal of these findings by 3 days.[112,122] These changes are probably related to the initial euphoria and discomfort after childbirth, followed by fatigue and restoration. Postpartum women have less overall sleep time and more night awakenings than nonpregnant women do. These night awakenings are often associated with urination, discomfort, activity by roommates or nursing staff, and infant feeding. Opportunities for restorative sleep after delivery and during the first postpartum night are often impeded by the environment and interruptions for nursing care activities.[112,140] Disturbances in maternal sleep lead to fatigue and a perceived lack of sleep effectivensss.[207]

The main reasons for night wakening postpartum are newborn sleep and feeding patterns.[112] Maternal night wakefulness decreases significantly from weeks 3 to 12.[178] This decrease is related to development of the infant's sleep-wake rhythm. Women who breastfeed have more deep sleep and overall sleep, possibly related to prolactin secretion, less arousal due to closer infant proximity, and infant sleep-wake patterns.[24,139,247]

Sleep medications alter sleep physiology and suppress REM sleep and NREM stages 3 and 4 and thus should be avoided. OSA and sleep disorder breathing generally resolve postpartum as the changes in the airway and larynx resolve.[29,209]

Postpartum Discomfort

During the first few days to weeks of the postpartum period, the woman may experience considerable discomfort. The discomfort and pain can arise from a variety of sources, including an episiotomy, lacerations, perineal trauma, incisions, uterine contractions after delivery (afterpains), hemorrhoids, breast engorgement, and nipple tenderness. Breast engorgement initially occurs in both the lactating and nonlactating woman because of stasis and distention of the vascular and lymphatic circulations. In the breastfeeding woman, secondary engorgement occurs because of distention of the breast with milk as lactation is established. Alterations in comfort not only cause physical and emotional stress but can also interfere with the ability of the woman to interact with and care for her infant. Back pain generally disappears within a few weeks or months after delivery, although 8% to 10% of women continue to report pain 1 to 2 years later.[90,247]

CLINICAL IMPLICATIONS FOR THE PREGNANT WOMAN AND HER FETUS

Changes in the neurologic, sensory, and musculoskeletal systems may result in common alterations and discomforts of pregnancy such as backache. In addition, the physiologic and hormonal changes of pregnancy—along with mechanical forces during pregnancy, labor, and delivery—can lead to specific neurologic disorders in the pregnant woman. These disorders are primarily peripheral neuropathies and compression/entrapment disorders that arise late in gestation or during the intrapartum and postpartum periods. The usual physiologic and hormonal changes of pregnancy can also alter the course of preexisting neurologic disorders such as epilepsy, myasthenia gravis, and migraine headaches. Finally, pregnancy may occasionally be associated with the initial presentation of symptoms of disorders such as brain tumors, arteriovenous malformations, and multiple sclerosis, which can affect both the woman and her infant.

Ocular Adaptations

Although ocular alterations during pregnancy generally do not have major clinical significance, they can result in minor discomforts, particularly for women who wear contact lenses. Some women may be unable to tolerate their lenses and may occasionally develop corneal edema. The basis for this intolerance is believed to be retention of water by the cornea, changes in the composition of tears, and alterations in corneal topography.[182,224] Changes in tear composition can make the contact lenses feel greasy shortly after insertion and cause blurring of vision.[172,182] Pregnancy may also alter healing following photorefractive keratectomy. Myopic regression and corneal haziness are reported in about 10% of postpartum women.[222] Alterations in refractory power along with occasional transient insufficiency of accommodation can cause difficulty in reading and in near vision or blurred vision in someone who is farsighted.[172,217,238] These alterations resolve in the postpartum period. New prescriptions for glasses or contact lenses should be delayed until several weeks after delivery.

Women with specific disorders such as preeclampsia and diabetes mellitus may have ocular complications associated with their disease process. Preeclampsia is associated with vasospasm of the conjunctival vessels and narrowing of the retinal arterioles. The latter may progress to severe arteriolar spasm or multiple retinal hemorrhages. Most of these changes reverse within 3 weeks postpartum.[224,238] In severe disease retinal detachment may occur.[238] Mild to moderate visual disturbances are most common; severe or complete loss of vision is rare.[238] However, up to 15% of women with severe preeclampsia develop cortical blindness that is almost always transient, lasting 4 hours to 8 days.[224] The changes that occur with preeclampsia may be related to vascular changes, endothelial damage, coexisting systemic vascular disease, altered cerebral autoregulation, and hypoperfusion with ischemia or hyperperfusion with edema.[224]

Development and progression of diabetic retinopathy in pregnant women are more closely correlated with the duration of the disorder, severity of the diabetes, coexisting hypertension or preeclampsia, and degree of glycemic control.[182,217,224] Pregnant diabetic women (particularly those with established proliferative retinopathy) often demonstrate deterioration related to the metabolic and hormonal changes of pregnancy. Some women without diabetic retinopathy at the onset of pregnancy may develop mild nonproliferative diabetic retinopathy (NPDR) during pregnancy and those with NPDR may have progression.[217,224] Although reversal of these pregnancy-induced changes usually occurs over the first 6 to 12 months postpartum, some women, especially those with preexisting retinopathy, do not experience complete return to their prepregnant status.[54,217,224,238] Careful baseline assessment and surveillance during pregnancy are essential. Women with gestational diabetes are not at increased risk for retinopathy during pregnancy.[54,217]

Because intraocular pressure falls during pregnancy, the pregnant woman with glaucoma may experience an improvement with a decreased need for medications.[54,182,238] This has an additional advantage of reducing fetal exposure to these agents, which should be used with caution and carefully monitored.[217] Many ocular inflammatory disorders improve during pregnancy, possibly because of increased cortisol and other glucocorticosteroids, with exacerbation postpartum.

Any symptoms of eye infections in the pregnant woman must be assessed, because some sexually transmitted organisms such as herpes simplex virus and chlamydia may cause concurrent ocular infections. The presence of these organisms can have adverse consequences for the neonate if the mother also has a genital infection. For example, genital chlamydia can cause conjunctivitis and pneumonia in the newborn, and genital herpes simplex virus can cause disseminated or localized neonatal infection. Treatment of maternal ocular disorders during pregnancy should be done cautiously and with attention paid to the possible effects of the medication on the fetus. Even topical eye ointments must be used with caution because they can be absorbed systemically and cross the placenta to the fetus.[238] If these agents must be used, nasolacrimal occlusion after instillation may reduce systemic absorption.[224]

Musculoskeletal Discomforts

The pregnant woman may experience discomfort or pain associated with breast changes or stretching of the round ligament with growth of the uterus, pressure of uterine nerve roots, or pressure of the presenting part on the perineum. The latter type of pain is most prominent close to the onset of labor and is aggravated by vascular engorgement of these tissues. Increased joint mobility can result in muscle and ligament strain and discomfort. Pregnant women also have an increased risk of falls.[103,159,193] Falls are reported in 27% of pregnant women and are the leading cause of emergency department visits during pregnancy.[158,159] The increased risk of falls is related to weight gain, shift in the center of gravity, edema, deceased abdominal muscle strength, changes in mechanical load, ligament laxity, and changes in joint kinetics.[158,159] Regular exercise may be useful in reducing the risk of falls.[159]

Hip and knee joint pain may occur due to ligamentous laxity, joint strain, and weight gain.[26,203] A 20% weight gain increases the force on weight-bearing joints by 50% to 100%

during pregnancy.[203] Knee pain is due to patellofemoral dysfunction from ligamentous laxity, increased femoral torsion, and increased pelvic width.[203] Preexisting knee pain may increase or pain may occur for the first time. These changes are usually benign and reverse postpartum.[203] Pubic pain results from inflammation of the symphysis pubis and usually responds to rest and ice.[203]

Many pregnant women experience low back pain (including lumbar pain and pelvic girdle pain) during pregnancy due to a combination of hormonal and mechanical factors including exaggeration of the lumbar lordotic curve due to shifting of the center of gravity, weight gain, and relaxation of ligaments, or from muscle spasm due to pressure on nerve roots.[26,95,247] The sacroiliac ligaments, which usually resist femoral rotation, are less likely to do so during pregnancy. This along with the lumbar lordosis "shifts the center of gravity anteriorly, causing a strain on the lower back and sacroiliac joint. As the strong sacroiliac ligaments become increasingly lax during pregnancy, this allows an increase in the forward shift of the uterus, thereby placing more strain on the pelvic floor and back."[203]

Backache occurs in about 45% to 50% of women, most commonly after 18 weeks of pregnancy, although high backache earlier may result from breast alterations.[57,90,95,103,116,165,247,254] Approximately 10% of these women experience severe back pain, peaking in intensity during the evening and night, and localized to the lower back or sacroiliac region.

An increased frequency of backache is reported in multiparas, in individuals with a history of back pain before pregnancy or with a previous pregnancy, and with increasing maternal age.[103,116,203,254] Backache has not been associated with weight gain in pregnancy, height, or infant birth weight.[26,103,116,203,247] Women tend to experience less pain if they are physically fit before pregnancy, exercise during pregnancy, and have had education on postural adjustments (e.g., upright posture, tucking the pelvis, rotating shoulders) to reduce back pain.[247] Other recommendations include avoiding anything that increases the lordosis (e.g., high-heeled shoes), application of local heat, exercises to increase lower abdominal and back muscle tone beginning early in pregnancy, abdominal pillows, backrubs, use of a firm mattress, bed board, or back support, pelvic tilt exercise, aerobic exercise such as swimming, and conditioning before subsequent pregnancies.[57,116,188,247] Acupuncture has also been found to provide relief.[131,228] Backache, round ligament pain, or other discomfort should be assessed to distinguish "normal" discomfort from other processes such as preterm labor.

Exacerbation of intervertebral disk disorders is seen during pregnancy and the immediate postpartum period, probably because of postural changes and an increase in mechanical stress.[11,26,230] The most frequently affected areas are the fifth lumbar and first sacral nerve roots. Management usually involves bed rest. Spondylolisthesis (slipping of one lumbar vertebra forward onto the vertebra below) especially at L4 to L5 or at L5 to S1 is aggravated.[203] True herniation of the disk is rare.[95,203,230]

During the third trimester, the woman may experience numbness and tingling of the arms, fingers, legs, and toes. Paresthesia of the upper extremities may be caused by marked lordosis along with anterior flexion of the neck and slumping of the shoulders, placing traction on the brachial, ulnar, and median nerves. In the legs and toes, paresthesia may be caused by pressure of the uterus on the blood vessels and nerves supplying the lower extremities. Painful legs are experienced by many pregnant women and arise either from the mechanical effects of the uterus (e.g., the altered gait and posture during pregnancy and compression of the inferior vena cava and iliac veins when supine) or from systemic alterations. Systemic alterations that can lead to painful legs include musculoskeletal changes, reduced serum albumin (decreasing colloid osmotic pressure and increasing dependent edema), changes in coagulation, and alterations in calcium and phosphorus metabolism and diet. These causes must be differentiated from thromboembolic disorders, which are also more prevalent during pregnancy (see Chapter 8). Leg cramps during the last few months of gestation are common. These cramps may be related to alterations in calcium and phosphorus metabolism (see Chapter 17) or to pressure of the enlarged uterus on pelvic blood vessels or nerves supplying the lower extremities.

Restless Legs Syndrome

Restless legs syndrome is an idiopathic disorder seen in up to 26% of pregnant women (2 to 3 times the risk in the general population) by the third trimester and may interfere with sleep.[57,64,105,239] This syndrome is often mistaken for leg cramps, and neuromuscular findings may be similar to those associated with excess caffeine consumption.[57] Restless legs syndrome usually occurs 10 to 20 minutes after the woman gets into bed. It is characterized by an urge to move the legs accompanied by unpleasant sensations, a "creeping, wormy, burning ache [that] develops within their legs. The more the urge to allow the legs to fidget is resisted, the greater the urge becomes until it can no longer be withstood."[57] Restless legs syndrome is usually bilateral and symmetric, occasionally involving the arms as well.[64] This transient disorder generally appears in the third trimester and disappears shortly after delivery.[64,239] The neurologic examination is negative.

The cause of restless legs syndrome is unknown. It may have a genetic basis or be related to the hormonal changes of pregnancy or may be related to alterations in dopamine metabolism.[64,139] If the woman is iron deficient, improvement in the symptoms of restless legs syndrome may occur with treatment of the anemia. Women who are supplemented with folic acid have been reported to be less likely to develop this disorder.[57,64,96,139] Restless legs syndrome may also be associated with polyneuropathy and vascular insufficiency. Usually no treatment is indicated, other than ensuring adequate iron and folate intake. Walking may relieve some symptoms. If the disorder is severe, pharmacologic therapy may be considered; however, these may have potential risk to the fetus so risk-benefit must be carefully evaluated.[57,105,239]

Chorea Gravidarum

Chorea gravidarum is a disorder involving rapid, brief, nonrhythmic, involuntary, jerky movements of the limbs, nonpatterned facial grimacing, and slurred speech.[57] Mild cases may involve only persistent restlessness and clumsiness.[11] This disorder is seen both in pregnancy (incidence of 1 in 139,000) and in women on oral contraceptives.[11,57] Symptoms usually begin in the first trimester and may persist to the postpartum period.[57] Approximately 30% of pregnant women with this disorder become asymptomatic by the third trimester; the remainder become asymptomatic shortly after delivery.[57] A recurrence rate of 20% has been reported with subsequent pregnancies.[11]

The cause of chorea gravidarum is unknown, although it is related to streptococcal infection and is most common in women with a history of rheumatic fever or heart disease.[11] This disorder has also been related to hormonal changes during pregnancy or contraceptive use, in that estrogen can stimulate postsynaptic dopamine receptors (inhibitory transmitters with effects in the motor cortex and basal ganglia).[57] Chorea gravidarum may also have a hematologic or immunologic basis. Changes in these systems during pregnancy may exacerbate a preexisting basal ganglia disturbance.[11] There are no fetal effects reported.

Headache

Heacaches are common complaints during pregnancy and the postpartum period.[126] The most common forms of headaches in pregnant and breastfeeding women are those caused by muscular contraction/tension or migraines without aura.[57,155] Tension headaches are characterized by a persistent bandlike or viselike pain extending from the base of the neck to the forehead. The woman often notices the headache on awakening, with worsening of symptoms during the evening.[11,57] The discomfort may be aggravated by postural changes or stress. Tension headaches during pregnancy may also be due to hormonal influences, eye strain secondary to ocular changes, nasal congestion, emotional tension, muscle spasm, fatigue, altered cerebral fluid dynamics, or the mild respiratory alkalosis characteristic of pregnancy (see Chapter 10). Reproductive hormones, especially estrogens, interact with the trigeminovascular system to alter cerebral blood flow and neurochemical release.

Because headaches may also be a symptom of disorders such as preeclampsia, however, any pregnant woman complaining of headaches must be carefully evaluated. Management includes massaging neck and shoulder muscles, application of heat or ice to the neck, rest, warm baths, and minimal use of simple analgesics (acetaminophen).[57] Sedatives and hypnotics are not recommended for routine use in pregnant or lactating women because they are ineffective and metabolites cross the placenta and the blood-milk barrier and are excreted more slowly by the fetus and infant.[11]

Migraine Headaches

Migraine headaches occur in 3% to 5% of the general population. Migraines are more common in women and often occur with menses, with the initial development of migraine headaches associated with onset of menses. Migraines may also occur for the first time during the first 2 to 3 months postpartum. Although the frequency of headaches decreases with age, migraines may flare up or start with menopause.[57] Headaches are also more frequent and severe in women on oral contraceptives, especially pills with higher estrogen content.[11,57]

Both migraines with and without aura are vascular headaches caused by cerebral vasodilation and cranial artery dilation. The severe throbbing during the initial phases is attributed to intense cerebral vasoconstriction with subsequent vasodilation.[57] Migraines with and without aura may be different clinical entities.[175,241] Migraines without aura (MO) are seen most frequently; migraine with aura (previously called classic migraine) are less common.[155] Migraines with aura (MA) are characterized by 20 to 30 minutes of sensorimotor prodromal symptoms followed by a severe unilateral headache accompanied by nausea. The prodromal symptoms usually involve visual phenomena but may also include aphasia, hemiplegia, and paresthesia. MO is unilateral less often and not associated with prodromal symptoms.

MO generally improve or disappear during pregnancy.[175,241] During pregnancy, approximately 48% to 80% of women with a history of MO experience complete remission or decreased frequency, particularly during the second and third trimesters as estrogen and progesterone levels increase.[107,155,241] This change is particularly notable in women with a history of menstrual migraine (i.e., migraine associated with estrogen withdrawal). Migraines usually return within a few hours or days after delivery or with the first postpregnancy menses.[155] Return of headaches is delayed in women who breastfeed, probably due to the altered hormonal milieu.[175,241]

MA may occur for the first time during pregnancy, usually during the first trimester, although they can occur in any trimester, and some women may experience a worsening of their migraines.[57,107,241] Over 20% of women with MA have their first headache during pregnancy and about 50% of women with MA continue to have attacks during pregnancy.[241]

The basis for remission of migraine headaches during pregnancy is unclear. Although the cause of migraines is unknown, migraines have been attributed to estrogen deficiency, excessive gonadotropins, fluid and salt retention, and increased red blood cell (RBC) mass. Migraines are associated with periods of estrogen withdrawal such as menses or menopause, which involve changes in estrogen and progesterone levels and patterns of circulating estrogens.[11] Thus migraine remission during pregnancy may be related to changes in estrogen (particularly the sustained estrogen levels), progesterone, and aldosterone, or to hematologic and cardiovascular alterations.[175,241] The progressive increase in B-EP during pregnancy may also contribute to remissions.[241] Migraines have been linked to an increased risk of developing gestational hypertension, preeclampsia and vascular complications.[4,175]

Dietary and lifestyle interventions for migraines include a balanced diet, avoidance of dietary triggers, alcohol and smoking, exercise, and relaxation. The efficacy of nonpharmacological interventions such as relaxation techniques, including biofeedback, and acupuncture for migraine prophylaxis has also been documented.[3]

MA headaches are often treated with ergot alkaloids. Because these compounds have oxytocic properties and are Food and Drug Administration pregnancy category X, they should not be used during pregnancy because of the risk of miscarriage, fetal distress, preterm labor, and possibly birth defects (especially intestinal atresia and Moebius syndrome).[57,72,155,260] Analgesics (acetaminophen) are used for symptomatic relief. As noted above, other interventions include avoidance of triggers, biofeedback, analgesics, sedatives, and β-blockers. Propranolol has been used as a prophylactic treatment for frequent MA but its use during pregnancy is controversial because this drug has been associated with altered fetal growth as well as fetal and neonatal β-adrenergic blockade with subsequent decreased responsiveness to stress during asphyxia.[11,57,155] Sumatriptan (serotonin agonist) has been used with great caution due to concerns about effects on the fetus, although specific adverse effects have generally not been reported to date in most studies.[11,72,107,150,232]

The Pregnant Woman with a Chronic Neurologic Disorder

The physiologic and hormonal changes of pregnancy can influence the course of chronic neurologic and neuromuscular disorders such as epilepsy, myasthenia gravis, and multiple sclerosis. These disorders also have ramifications for the health and well-being of the mother and her infant. The implications of epilepsy and selected other neurologic and neuromuscular disorders during pregnancy are summarized in Table 15-2.

The Pregnant Woman with Epilepsy

Epilepsy is one of the most common neurologic disorders seen in pregnant women. The course of epilepsy is affected by the hormonal and physiologic changes of pregnancy, as well as by psychologic stress. Estrogens and progesterone alter seizure thresholds—estrogens by activating seizure foci, inhibiting γ-amino butyric acid (an inhibitory neurochemical), and potentiating glutamate (an excitatory neurotransmitter); and progesterone by potentiating barbiturate-like ligands at the γ-amino butyric acid channel and thus dampening activity.[11,149] These responses may account for the exacerbation of seizure activity with menses in many women with severe epilepsy.[57] Seizure activity or susceptibility to seizures may also be affected by water and sodium retention, sleep alterations, and the mild respiratory alkalosis of pregnancy.[187] The decreased seizure activity seen in some women may also be due to improved compliance in taking their medication.[11,97] The frequency of seizures before pregnancy tends to be predictive of seizure activity during pregnancy.[57,97,223]

An important factor affecting the pregnant epileptic is the effect of the usual physiologic changes of pregnancy on the metabolism of antiepileptic drugs (AEDs). The goal in managing the pregnant epileptic is to keep the mother free of seizures and to minimize the effects of epilepsy on both the pregnant woman and fetus, including fetal teratogenic effects.[57,98,187] Fetal anomalies and an increased risk of developmental delay syndrome has been described for AEDs. Congenital anomalies seen with increased frequency in infants of women with epilepsy include neural tube defects (especially with valproic acid), cleft lip and palate, congenital heart defects, and urogenital defects.[98,187] Some AEDs cause a mild folate deficiency so folate supplementation is especially important for the woman with epilepsy.[11,99,149] However, excess folate should be avoided because this may alter hepatic microsomal enzyme activity and decrease AED levels.[149] Use and risks of AEDs are discussed further in Chapter 7.

Peripheral Neuropathies

Pregnancy, labor and delivery, and lactation are associated with an increased incidence of a variety of peripheral neuropathies. Most of these disorders, although uncomfortable, do not alter the course of pregnancy, nor are they associated with maternal or fetal and neonatal complications. Other peripheral neuropathies develop secondary to trauma or pressure injury during the intrapartum or postpartum periods. Table 15-3 summarizes these disorders and their implications.

The Woman with a Spinal Cord Injury

Successful pregnancies are not uncommon for women who are paraplegic or quadriplegic. The usual physiologic changes of pregnancy place the woman with a spinal cord transection at increased risk for certain problems, however, including increased urinary incontinence, urinary tract and other infections, constipation, and pressure ulcers.[11] Most of these problems can be prevented or minimized with good care. Management of the paralyzed pregnant woman usually includes careful attention to bladder and skin care, high-bulk diet, adequate fluid intake, prevention of anemia, stool softeners, and acidification of the urine with vitamin C supplements.[11,57]

Labor and delivery present unique challenges and risks. Since contraction of the myometrium is relatively independent of neuronal influence (see Chapter 4), uterine contractions are usually normal. However, the level of the lesion influences the woman's perception of contractions. Sacral anesthesia is present in all of these women. Women with cauda equina lesions have relaxed perineal muscles. Women with lesions below T10 to T11—the level at which the uterine sensory nerves enter the spinal cord—experience labor pain.[57] Women with lesions at T10 and T11 may perceive contractions as abdominal discomfort or muscle spasm.

If the lesion is above T9, labor will be painless, the onset of contractions will not be felt, and delivery may be precipitous.[116] These women need careful monitoring of the cervix and contractions from about 24 weeks' gestation on because preterm labor is common.[11] If the woman also has spasticity, local somatic reflex arcs may be activated by labor contractions. This may result in painful extensor and flexor muscle spasms and sustained ankle clonus.[11,57]

Table 15-2 **Implications for Selected Neurologic and Neuromuscular Disorders for the Pregnant Woman and Her Infant**

DISORDER AND BASIS	IMPLICATIONS FOR PREGNANT WOMAN	IMPLICATIONS FOR FETUS/NEONATE
EPILEPSY		
Heterogeneous disorder associated with sudden alterations in brain electrical activity, producing involuntary motor or sensory phenomena. One of the most common neurologic disorders seen in pregnant women (incidence of 0.3% to 0.6%).	Effect of pregnancy on the course of epilepsy is variable and unpredictable. Seizure frequency may increase, decrease, or stay the same. Seizures may appear for the first time during pregnancy or reappear after many seizure-free years. Most women return to their prepregnant pattern after delivery. Usual physiologic changes of pregnancy alter the metabolism of anticonvulsant drugs with a risk of subtherapeutic plasma concentrations and increased risk of seizures. May need increase in AED dosages (see Chapter 7), especially during the second half of pregnancy (reversed by 6 weeks postpartum). Higher incidence of stillbirth and possibly preterm labor, but risks of other complications are not necessarily increased. Maternal bleeding may occur secondary to deficiency of vitamin K–dependent clotting factors, which may be associated with phenytoin or phenobarbital use.	Major risks are from pathophysiologic consequences of maternal seizures and the use of antiepileptic drugs (AEDs). Each AED has potential fetal and neonatal risks (see Chapter 7), such as fetal anticonvulsant syndrome, congenital anomalies, hemorrhagic disease of the newborn, folic acid deficiency, and neonatal addiction and withdrawal. Increased frequency of congenital anomalies in both epileptic women who are on AEDs and those who are not. The risk of anomalies is also increased if the father has epilepsy but the mother does not. Teratogenicity related to specific AEDs is described in Chapter 7. Risk of hemorrhagic disease of the newborn may be increased due to a deficiency of vitamin K–dependent clotting factors secondary to competitive inhibition of the formation of precursor molecules by AEDs (see Chapter 8).
MYASTHENIA GRAVIS		
Autoimmune disorder involving an IgG antibody against acetylcholine receptors on striated muscle. Reduction of available acetylcholine at postsynaptic receptors of the neuromuscular junction. Results in muscular weakness and fatigue.	May improve, worsen, or stay the same (effects are variable with each pregnancy). Most often exacerbates in first trimester and improves in second and third trimesters, possibly due to effects of blocking of IgG antibodies by immunologic changes of pregnancy (see Chapter 13) or α-fetoprotein. Increased frequency of exacerbation in first few months postpartum. No effect on smooth muscle and thus myometrium, so labor is not prolonged, although the woman may have difficulty with expulsive efforts. Long-term maternal outcome is not altered. Avoid use of muscle relaxants; magnesium sulfate for preeclampsia (can lead to apnea because hypermagnesemia inhibits release of acetylcholine); inhalation anesthetics and narcotics (because these pregnant women tend to hypoventilate if they have a bulbar muscle weakness); procaine if on pyridostigmine or neostigmine, which inhibit hydrolysis of procaine and can result in seizures (can use lidocaine); extensive regional blocks (may compromise respiration); and azathioprine (potential teratogenic effects).	Fetal myasthenia gravis does not occur, possibly due to blocking of the IgG antibody by α-fetoprotein. About 10% to 20% of neonates develop transient myasthenia gravis due to passage of maternal IgG antibody against the acetylcholine receptors of striated muscle (see Chapter 13). Symptoms appear within 12 to 72 hours of birth and resolve spontaneously by 3 months (usually in 1 to 3 weeks). Infants with transient myasthenia gravis often feed poorly, have a weak cry, are hypotonic, and are at risk for respiratory difficulty and aspiration. Many of these infants require anticholinesterase therapy and some will need assisted ventilation. Neonatal effects do not correlate with maternal disease severity or antibody titer.

Table 15-2 Implications for Selected Neurologic and Neuromuscular Disorders for the Pregnant Woman and Her Infant—cont'd

DISORDER AND BASIS	IMPLICATIONS FOR PREGNANT WOMAN	IMPLICATIONS FOR FETUS/NEONATE
MYOTONIC DYSTROPHY		
Progressive autosomal dominant disorder that appears as a congenital form (possibly requiring an additional maternally transmitted factor) or, more commonly, with onset in young adulthood. Muscular weakness and myotonia affect both striated and smooth muscle, including the myometrium.	Muscular weakness and myotonia may worsen, often in the second half of pregnancy (possibly due to effects of progesterone on cell membranes). Delayed gut motility with increased constipation in pregnancy. Increased risk of spontaneous and habitual abortion, and preterm labor. Abnormal uterine contractions, prolonged first stage, poor voluntary expulsive efforts in second stage, poor involution with risk of postpartum hemorrhage. Avoid the use of inhalation anesthetics (often hypoventilate with chronic respiratory acidosis) and depolarizing muscle relaxants (succinylcholine) that can cause myotonic spasms and hyperthermia.	Presence of maternal disorder does not affect infant per se. If fetus has inherited myotonic muscular dystrophy, severe fetal and neonatal myotonia may occur. Fetal effects may include poor swallowing with hydramnios and arthrogryposis from inactivity; neonates may have respiratory distress and feeding problems.
MULTIPLE SCLEROSIS (MS)		
Multifocal central nervous system demyelinating disorder with disseminated inflammatory lesions of cerebral myelin. Onset in early adulthood with unpredictable exacerbations and remissions over many years with increasing disability.	Tendency for remission during pregnancy; rate of relapses decreases with each trimester, possibly owing to immunosuppressant effects of α-fetoprotein and estrogens with decreased proinflammatory cytokines. Twofold to threefold increase in relapses in first 3 to 6 months postpartum, possibly due to decreased estrogens and reversal of immune changes of pregnancy. Usually minimal effect on course of pregnancy or incidence of complications. May experience worsening of bowel and bladder problems and urinary tract infection; for paraplegic or quadriplegic care and risks similar to those for a woman with a spinal cord injury. Medications need to be reviewed to evaluate if changes are needed. Long-term course of disease unaffected by pregnancy.	None reported.

Compiled from references 11, 19, 27, 57, 97, 98, 99, 149, 223, 233.
IgG, Immunoglobulin G.

Autonomic hyperreflexia or dysreflexia (also called *autonomic stress syndrome*) may occur during labor in women with complete cord lesions above T5 to T6 (above the outflow of the splanchnic autonomic nerves). This syndrome is characterized by hyperstimulation of the autonomic system with brief periods of severe hypertension, throbbing headaches, reflex bradycardia, sweating, nasal congestion, cutaneous vasodilation with flushed skin, and piloerection above the level of the lesion.[11,57,116,189] Symptoms generally occur with uterine contractions and are most prominent immediately before delivery. Symptoms may be mistaken for preeclampsia.[11,57] Autonomic hyperreflexia occurs because of the sudden release of large amounts of catecholamines during uterine contractions. This syndrome can result in life-threatening complications including intracranial hemorrhage and cardiac arrhythmias. Treatment includes regional anesthesia, antihypertensive agents, and perhaps use of α_1-adrenergic blockers or peripheral vasodilators.[57,116,189]

Forceps may be required during delivery if the muscles used for expulsion during the second stage are paralyzed or if severe hyperreflexia occurs.[57] During the postpartum period, care involves prevention of complications of the elimination and integumentary systems. Poor wound healing is a concern and may be aggravated by anemia. Paraplegic and

Table 15-3 Peripheral Neuropathies during Pregnancy and Lactation

DISORDER	DESCRIPTION	IMPLICATION
NEUROPATHIES ASSOCIATED WITH PREGNANCY		
Bell's palsy (idiopathic facial paralysis)	Acute unilateral neuropathy of the seventh cranial nerve leading to facial paralysis with weakness of the forehead and lower face	Three times more frequent during pregnancy, possibly because of an inflammatory reaction with entrapment of the medial and occasionally ulnar nerve with soft tissue edema Most often occurs in the third trimester or first 2 weeks postpartum; associated with preeclampsia Onset late in pregnancy usually associated with full recovery (but may take months) and generally requires no treatment if partial or mild
Transient carpal tunnel syndrome	Entrapment and compression of the medial nerve at the wrist, more prominent in dominant hand	May develop in pregnancy because of excessive fluid retention Onset usually in second or third trimester Nocturnal hand pain reported by 20% to 40% of pregnant women, with electromyographic (EMG) evidence of this syndrome in about 5% Supportive treatment (splinting of wrist at night); a few may require surgery Most cases resolve by 3 months postpartum; may recur with later pregnancies
de Quervain tenosynovitis	Compression and irritation of tendons of extensor pollicis brevi and abductor pollicis longus of wrist	Seen in late pregnancy and lactation May be associated with fluid retention during pregnancy or child care activities postpartum Mild symptoms in late pregnancy increase after delivery and rapidly cease after weaning
Meralgia paresthesia (lateral femoral cutaneous neuropathy)	Unilateral or bilateral entrapment and compression of lateral femoral cutaneous nerve as it passes beneath the inguinal ligament	Associated with obesity and rapid weight gain in pregnancy; also related to trauma and stretch injury Lumbar lordosis in pregnancy may make nerve more vulnerable to compression Develops in third trimester, resolves spontaneously over first 3 months postpartum
NEUROPATHIES OCCURRING IN THE INTRAPARTUM AND POSTPARTUM PERIODS		
Postpartum footdrop	Compression of the lumbosacral trunk against the sacral ala by the fetal head or of the common peroneal nerve between leg braces and the fibular head	Most common intrapartum nerve injury Seen most often in women of short stature with large infants Clinical manifestations may not appear until 24 to 48 hours postpartum Prognosis is good if only the myelin sheath has been distorted, with improvement in 2 to 3 months
Other traumatic neuropathies	Compression of the lumbosacral plexus or obturator, femoral, or peroneal nerves against the pelvic wall, leading to muscular weakness and palsy	Associated with obstetric practices including use of lithotomy position, application of forceps, prolonged pressure from the fetal head, or trauma or hematomas from cesarean delivery Prognosis is good if only the myelin sheath has been distorted, with improvement in 2 to 3 months
Neuropathies associated with breastfeeding	Pressure on the nerves of the axilla Pain and tingling with flexion of the elbow Transient carpal tunnel syndrome	Occurs during engorgement with numbness and tingling of flexor surface of arms to ulnar distribution of hands that abates as the infant sucks. Disappears as engorgement resolves. Seen in women using a hand pump Develops about 1 month after delivery and resolves within a month of weaning

Compiled from references 11, 26, 27, 57, 79, 101, 103, 134, 153, 203, 223.

quadriplegic women have let-down reflexes and can successfully breastfeed.

The Woman with a Brain or Spinal Cord Tumor

Brain tumors, especially meningiomas, may enlarge during pregnancy because of stimulation of tumor estrogen receptors that stimulate growth of neoplastic cells, increased vascularity and blood volume, and increased extracellular volume.[177] As a result of these changes, many tumors become symptomatic during the second half of pregnancy. Tumors may temporarily regress postpartum. Brain tumors account for approximately 10% of all maternal deaths.[57]

Spinal cord tumors tend to exacerbate with pregnancy and menstruation. The most common spinal cord lesions in pregnant women are arteriovenous malformations (AVMs) and angiomas. An AVM is characterized by rapid shunting of blood between an artery and vein without any intervening capillaries, thus depriving adjacent areas of oxygen and nutrients. Exacerbations during pregnancy may be related to (1) mechanical pressure of the gravid uterus on the vena cava, causing partial outflow obstruction with shifting of blood flow to vertebral and epidural veins and engorgement of the venous side of the malformation; (2) increased vascularity and blood volume; or (3) dilation of the shunt by estrogens.[57]

Cerebral Vascular Disorders

The physiologic and hormonal changes of pregnancy also increase the risk of certain cerebral vascular disorders with life-threatening consequences. Although most individual disorders are relatively rare, cerebral vascular disorders as a group are not uncommon during pregnancy.[11] The basis for and risks of subarachnoid hemorrhage, cerebral ischemia, and cerebral venous thrombosis during pregnancy are summarized in Table 15-4.

Preeclampsia and Eclampsia

CNS changes occur in both preeclamptic and eclamptic women. The more severe changes markedly increase the risk of fetal and maternal mortality. CNS manifestations of preeclampsia and eclampsia may include cerebral irritability (e.g., hyperreflexia, headache, clonus, altered consciousness), visual disturbances, cerebral edema, cerebral hemorrhage, and convulsions (with eclampsia). These events are the result of arteriolar vasospasm and vasoconstriction, fluid shifts from the vascular to intravascular space, and possibly a failure of cerebral autoregulation with localized capillary rupture.[57] Most changes are reversible, but some women with eclampsia may have permanent changes, although few long-term studies have been done.[244]

Eclampsia is the development of seizures in a pregnant woman with signs and symptoms of preeclampsia. Convulsions may be focal, multifocal, or generalized. Potential etiologic factors for seizures and coma in these women include cerebral vasospasm, hemorrhage, ischemia, edema, and hypertensive or metabolic encephalopathy. Donaldson and Duffy suggest that the cerebral manifestations of eclampsia are primarily due to severe vasoconstriction in association with failure of cerebral autoregulation to limit perfusion and pressure within the thin-walled cerebral capillaries.[57] This leads to a pressure-induced rupture of thin-walled capillaries

Table 15-4 Cerebrovascular Disorders: Possible Basis for Increased Risk during Pregnancy

DISORDER	RISK	BASIS
Subarachnoid hemorrhage (SAH)	1 to 2 in 10,000 deliveries	Risk increased due to hormonal effects on arterial and venous intima and media organization, increased plasma volume.
	Accounts for about 5% of all maternal deaths, usually due to arteriovenous malformation (AVM) or berry aneurysm.	May be related to alterations of arterial and venous intima by hormonal changes during pregnancy.
	Risk due to aneurysm increases with each trimester and postpartum.	Bleeding during pregnancy may be associated with enlargement or increased shunting during pregnancy related to altered hemodynamics, increased cerebral blood flow (CBF), changes in coagulation, or hormonal influences altering integrity of blood vessels.
	AVMs most often bleed in the second trimester or in the intrapartum period.	
	One third of SAHs occur with bearing down and Valsalva maneuvers.	Bleeding during labor in women with these anomalies may be initiated by rapid pressure and flow changes associated with Valsalva maneuver.
	Mortality is higher if due to aneurysm.	
Cerebral ischemia	Fivefold to 10-fold increase during pregnancy (a similar increase is noted with oral contraceptives).	Hormonal changes, anemia, and altered blood coagulation during pregnancy may be factors predisposing to emboli formation.
	Most occur in second and third trimesters and during the first week postpartum.	Often occurs secondary to other disorders such as mitral valve prolapse, hypertension, subacute bacterial endocarditis, hypotension, or sickle cell anemia, or with use of anticoagulants.
Cerebral venous thrombosis	1 in 2500 to 1 in 10,000 deliveries.	Hematologic changes and alterations in blood coagulation in pregnancy may increase risk.
	Most occur from 3 days to 1 month postpartum (most frequent at 2 to 3 weeks).	Increased risk of preeclampsia and cesarean section.
	May be arterial (most common in first week) or venous in origin.	

Compiled from references 11, 38, 57, 79, 177, 202, 223.

Table 15-5 Recommendations for Clinical Practice Related to the Neurologic, Muscular, and Sensory Systems in Pregnant Women

Recognize the usual ocular, otolaryngeal, and neuromuscular changes during pregnancy (pp. 509-512).
Provide anticipatory teaching regarding usual ocular, otolaryngeal, and neuromuscular changes during pregnancy (pp. 509-512).
Counsel women regarding intervention strategies for common problems related to ocular changes (pp. 509-510, 516).
Counsel women, when possible, to delay getting new prescriptions for glasses or contact lenses until several weeks postpartum (p. 516).
Counsel women to avoid cycloplegic or mydriatic agents and topical ophthalmic ointments during pregnancy and, if necessary, to use nasolacrimal occlusion after use (p. 516).
Counsel women regarding intervention strategies for common problems related to otolaryngeal changes (p. 510).
Counsel women regarding intervention strategies for common problems related to musculoskeletal changes (pp. 510-511, 516-517).
Assess posture and lifting techniques used by pregnant women (pp. 510-511, 516-517).
Teach pregnant women relaxation techniques and exercises to reduce muscle strain and tension (pp. 516-517).
Recognize and assess for factors associated with painful legs during pregnancy (pp. 517-518).
Assess sleep patterns of pregnant and postpartum women and implement interventions to enhance rest and sleep (pp. 511-512, 515).
Avoid use of sleep medications during pregnancy (p. 515).
Assess women complaining of backache, headache, round ligament pain, or other discomfort for signs of other disorders (pp. 516-519).
Understand the basis for maternal feelings of pain and discomfort during labor and delivery and implement appropriate interventions (pp. 512-515, Figure 15-3, and Table 15-1).
Counsel women during the postpartum period regarding alterations in comfort and implement appropriate interventions (p. 515).
Assess and counsel women with diabetes mellitus and preeclampsia regarding potential ocular complications (p. 516).
Assess eye infections in pregnant women and evaluate for pathogenesis by organisms implicated in sexually transmitted disorders (p. 516).
Counsel women with migraine headaches regarding effects of pregnancy on their disorder and remission postpartum (pp. 518-519).
Know and counsel women regarding the side effects of drugs used to treat specific neurologic disorders and potential toxicity to the woman and fetus (pp. 518-519 and Chapter 7).
Counsel women with chronic neurologic disorders regarding the impact of their disorder on pregnancy and of pregnancy on the disorder (pp. 519, 521, 523 and Table 15-2).
Know the effects of physiologic alterations during pregnancy on metabolism of anticonvulsants (p. 519, Table 15-2, and Chapter 7).
Monitor epileptic women during pregnancy and postpartum for levels of and responses to anticonvulsants (p. 519, Table 15-2, and Chapter 7).
Evaluate the infant of an epileptic woman for congenital anomalies, folate deficiency, drug withdrawal, bleeding, and feeding behaviors (p. 519 and Table 15-2).
Ensure that vitamin K is administered to newborns of epileptic women who are on anticonvulsants (p. 519 and Chapter 8).
Recognize signs and symptoms of peripheral neuropathies and implement appropriate preventive and intervention strategies (p. 519 and Table 15-3).
Evaluate the woman with a spinal cord injury for bowel, bladder, and integumentary complications and implement appropriate interventions (pp. 519, 521).
Monitor the woman with a spinal cord lesion for initiation of contractions, progression of labor, and autonomic hyperreflexia (pp. 519, 521).
Recognize the basis for and risks of cerebral vascular disorders during pregnancy (p. 523 and Table 15-4).
Recognize the cerebral manifestations of preeclampsia and eclampsia and implement appropriate interventions (pp. 523-524).

with vasogenic edema and hemorrhage. "In physiologic terms the upper limit of the autoregulation of cerebral perfusion of blood pressure, which is proportional to mean arterial blood pressure [and thus not standard diastolic or systolic values], has been exceeded. Cerebral eclampsia is hypertensive encephalopathy in previously normotensive women."[57] Magnesium sulfate, which may selectively increase cerebral blood flow and oxygen consumption, has been found to be more effective than AEDs in preventing recurrent seizures in these women.[180] Hypertensive disorders in pregnancy are discussed in Chapter 9.

SUMMARY

The neurologic system and mediation of discomfort and pain are often of major concern for women during the intrapartum period. This system is probably the one about which least is known regarding specific effects of pregnancy. The pregnant woman experiences alterations in her neuromuscular and sensory systems related to the hormonal and physiologic adaptations of gestation. These changes may result in common experiences and discomforts of pregnancy—including backaches and headaches, ocular and voice changes, nasal stuffiness, epistaxis, sleep disturbances, postpartum blues, and peripheral neuropathies—and alter the course of neurologic disorders. Recommendations for clinical practice related to the neuromuscular and sensory systems during pregnancy are summarized in Table 15-5.

DEVELOPMENT OF THE NEUROLOGIC, MUSCULAR, AND SENSORY SYSTEMS IN THE FETUS

The neurologic, muscular and sensory systems undergo a series of complex structural and functional changes to reach maturation. The central nervous system (CNS) is one of the earliest systems to begin development and the latest to completely mature. Table 15-6 summarizes CNS development and the timing and origin of specific anomalies. This section examines anatomic and functional development of the fetal nervous,

Table 15-6 Major Stages of Human Brain Development and Related Disorders

TIME OF OCCURRENCE (WEEKS' GESTATION)	STAGE OF HUMAN DEVELOPMENT	MAJOR EVENTS		MAJOR ANOMALIES DURING STAGE
3 to 4	Neurulation	Notochord (gives rise to neural plate, neural tube, and neural crest cells)		
		Neural plate		
		Neural tube	Brain differentiation of prosencephalon, mesencephalon, and rhombencephalon at 20 days	Anencephaly Encephalocele Meningocele Meningomyelocele Myeloschisis
			Spinal cord	Arnold-Chiari malformation
			Dura	
		Neural crest cells	Dorsal root ganglia Pia and arachnoid Schwann cells Autonomic ganglia	
4 to 7	Caudal neural tube formation	Canalization followed by regressive differentiation		Spina bifida occulta
5 to 6	Ventral induction (prosencephalon development)	Prechordal mesoderm	Face and forebrain	Dermal sinus
		Prosencephalon	Cleavage of prosencephalon into cerebral vesicles forms two cerebral hemispheres at 33 days' gestational age	Faciotelencephalic malformations
8 to 16	Neuronal proliferation	Cellular proliferation in the ventricular and subventricular zones Proliferation of vascular tree, particularly venous Interkinetic nuclear migration Neuroblasts Glioblasts	Differentiation of the hypothalamus Optic vesicles Olfactory bulbs and tracts First fibers in internal capsule at 41 days' gestational age Thalamus and basal ganglia	Microencephaly (microencephaly vera and radial microbrain) Macrencephaly
12 to 20	Migration	Radial migration in cerebrum Radial tangential migration in the cerebellum	Cortical lamination Neuronal migration in the cerebral cortex is completed at about 5 months Neuronal migration in the cerebellum is completed at about 1 year postnatally	Schizencephaly Agenesis of the corpus callosum Hirschsprung's disease
24 to postnatal	Organization	Late neuronal migration in cerebrum and cerebellum Alignment, orientation, and layering of cortical neurons Synaptic contacts Proliferation of glia and differentiation		Mental retardation Down syndrome Perinatal insults
Peak at birth to years postnatal	Myelinization	Bulbospinal tracts	24 weeks' gestational age to postnatal	Cerebral white matter hypoplasia
		Motor roots	24 weeks' gestational age to postnatal	
		Medial lemniscus	24 weeks' gestational age to postnatal	
		Pyramidal tract	38 weeks' gestational age to 2 years postnatally	
		Frontopontine tract	7 to 8 months to 2 years postnatally	
		Corpus callosum	4 months to 16 years postnatally	

Adapted from Hill, A. & Volpe, J.J. (1989). *Fetal neurology.* New York: Raven.

sensory, and motor systems and development of sensory abilities in preterm infants. CNS development occurs via the interaction of multiple genes and signaling molecules, including *Wnt*, neurotropic proteins such as transforming growth factors (especially sonic hedgehog), fibroblast growth factors, platelet-derived growth factors and other neurotropins.[37,194] Other factors involved in CNS development are vitamins (especially vitamin A and folic acid), essential fatty acids, thyroid hormones (see Chapter 19), and steroid hormones.[194]

Anatomic Development of the Central Nervous System

Embryonic Development of the Central Nervous System

The development of the nervous system begins approximately 18 days after fertilization.[173] The process by which the beginnings of the nervous system are laid down is called *primary neurulation* and includes formation of the neural plate, neural folds, and neural tube (Figure 15-4). This process occurs on the dorsal surface of the embryo and leads to formation of the brain and spinal cord (dorsal induction).[50,249]

The neural plate develops an invagination in its center, called the *neural groove*, beginning 22 to 23 days after fertilization. Bulges on both sides of the neural tube groove, called the *neural folds*, accompany the invagination process. The neural folds continue to enlarge, enveloping the neural groove, and fuse to form the neural tube, an entity separate from the overlying ectodermal layer.[173] The neural tube forms the CNS, with the rostral (anterior) portion developing into the brain (Figure 15-5) and the caudal (posterior) portion into the spinal cord. The neocortex forms in the dorsolateral wall of the rostral portion of the neural tube.[53] The ventricles and canal of the spinal cord are derived from the lumen of the

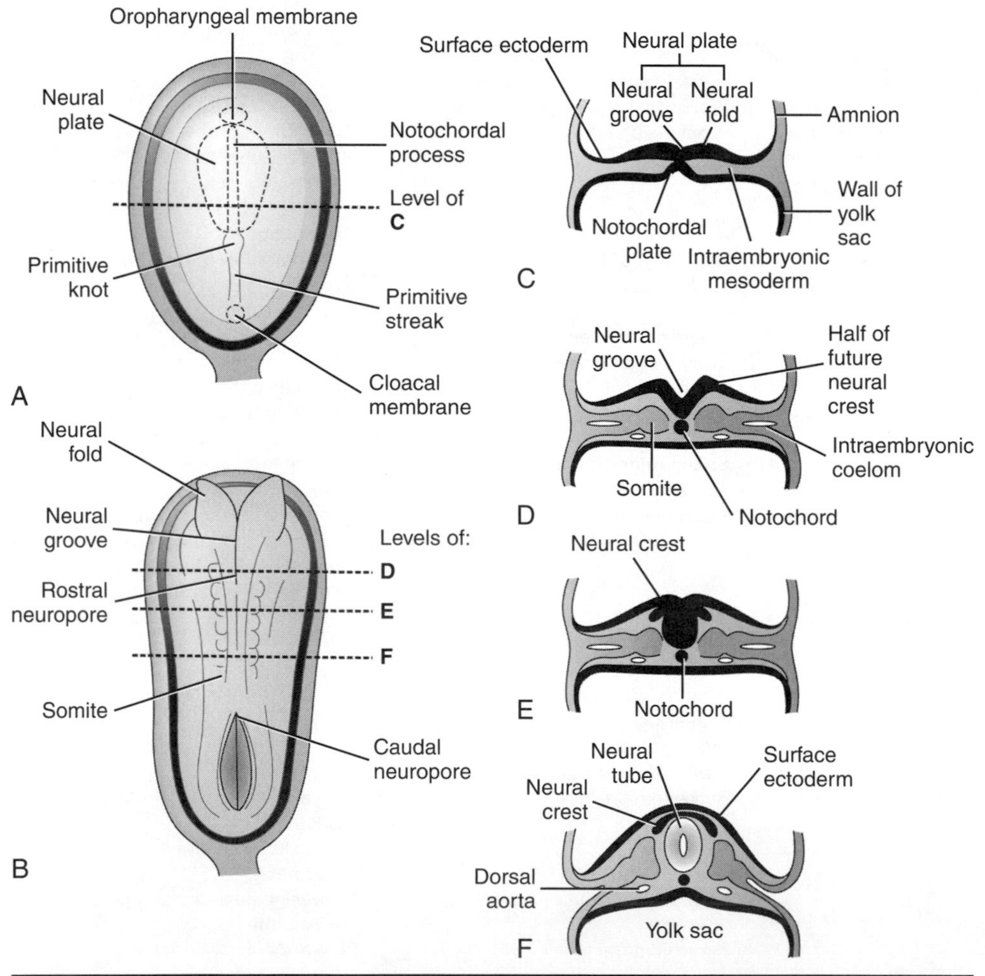

FIGURE 15-4 Embryonic formation of neural plate and neural tube. **A,** Dorsal view of an embryo of about 18 days, exposed by removing the amnion. **B,** Transverse section of this embryo, showing the neural plate and early development of the neural groove. The developing notochord is also shown. **C,** Dorsal view of an embryo of about 22 days. The neural folds have fused opposite the somites but are widely spread out at both ends of the embryo. The rostral and caudal neuropores are indicated. Closure of the neural tube occurs initially in the region corresponding to the future junction of the brain and spinal cord. **D** to **F,** Transverse sections of this embryo at the levels shown in **C,** illustrating formation of the neural tube and its detachment from the surface ectoderm. (From Moore, K.L. & Persaud, T.V.N. [2003]. *The developing human: Clinically oriented embryology* [7th ed.]. Philadelphia: Saunders.)

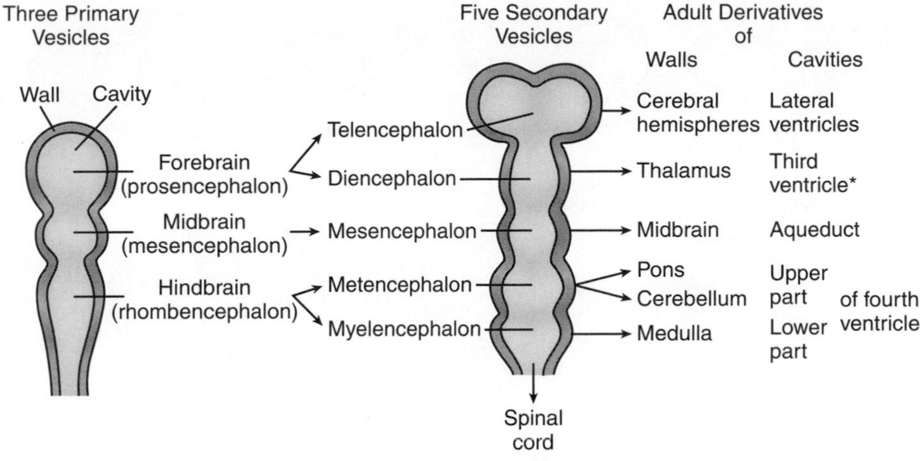

FIGURE 15-5 Embryonic development of the brain vesicles and adult derivatives. *The rostral (anterior) part of the third ventricle forms from the cavity of the telencephalon; most of the third ventricle is derived from the cavity of diencephalon. (From Moore, K.L., & Persaud, T.V.N. [2003]. *The developing human: Clinically oriented embryology* [7th ed.]. Philadelphia: Saunders.)

neural tube.[173] Closure of the neural tube begins in the area of the future lower medulla at 22 days and proceeds in cephalad and caudal directions. The rostral opening (neuropore) closes by approximately 24 days; the caudal neuropore (at L1 to L2) closes 2 days later at approximately 26 days at the level of the upper sacrum.[249] Failure of these neuropores to close gives rise to neural tube defects (NTDs).

Formation of the caudal portion of the neural tube in the lower sacral and coccygeal areas begins at 28 to 32 days. This process is known as *secondary neurulation.* Vacuoles develop in the caudal cell mass at the end of the neural tube. These vacuoles coalesce and fuse with the end of the neural tube. This process continues until 7 weeks, followed by a regression of much of the caudal mass that continues until after birth.[249]

As the neural tube is forming, neuroectodermal cells at the edge of the neural plate near the border with the ectoderm migrate into the neural folds located on both sides of the developing neural groove, forming the neural crest. Neural crest cells later migrate into different areas of the developing embryo to form the craniofacial skeleton, connective tissue, and neurons; peripheral nervous system, including the cranial and spinal nerve sensory ganglia; autonomic nervous system; Schwann cells; pigment cells; the pia and arachnoid layers of the meninges; and the peripheral nerves.[50,173,210] Induction of the neural crest cells occurs via signaling molecules from the mesoderm and endoderm, such as transforming growth factors (including bone morphogenetic proteins), fibroblast growth factors, and Wnt.

Ventral induction (prosencephalon development) refers to processes occurring on the ventral portion of the embryo, leading to formation of the face and forebrain, including eye formation, olfactory formation, and forebrain structures. Thus, errors of ventral induction often produce both facial and nervous system anomalies.[249] Sonic hedgehog signaling (see Chapter 3) is the prominent molecular pathway in prosencephalon development.[249] After closure of the rostral portion of the neural tube, three vesicles form that are the precursors of the brain. These vesicles, the forebrain (prosencephalon), midbrain (mesencephalon), and hindbrain (rhombencephalon), develop in the fourth week. With further differentiation the forebrain becomes the telencephalon and diencephalon, while the hindbrain becomes the metencephalon and myelencephalon, creating five vesicles. Adult derivatives of the vesicles are shown in Figure 15-5.

In the caudal portion of the neural tube, the alar (dorsal) and basal (ventral) plates develop. These structures are the beginning formation of the motor and sensory tracts that develop in the ventral and dorsal areas, respectively, of the cord.[173] In conjunction with formation of the spinal cord from the caudal neural tube, cells from the neural crest break into groups along the length of the cord, forming spinal and cranial ganglia and ganglia of the autonomic nervous system. Further differentiation and migration of neural crest cells and their fibers result in formation of the peripheral nerves (somatic and visceral, sensory and motor) and their connections. The primitive brain structures also go through a series of flexures or foldings (Figure 15-6, *A*).

Common Embryonic Anomalies of the Central Nervous System

The most common CNS anomalies arise in the embryonic period during the period of primary neurulation and result from failure of neural tube closure. These anomalies include anencephaly, myelomeningocele, encephalocele, and spina bifida occulta. NTDs are usually accompanied by alterations in vertebral, meningeal, vascular, and dermal structures and arise from a complex interaction of environmental and genetic factors. NTDs have a familial pattern with an increased recurrence rate. Approximately 2% to 16% of infants with isolated NTDs have cytogenic abnormalities. NTDs also occur in infants with other congenital defects. These infants may have normal or abnormal karyotypes. A small number of NTDs occur secondary to teratogen exposure.[171]

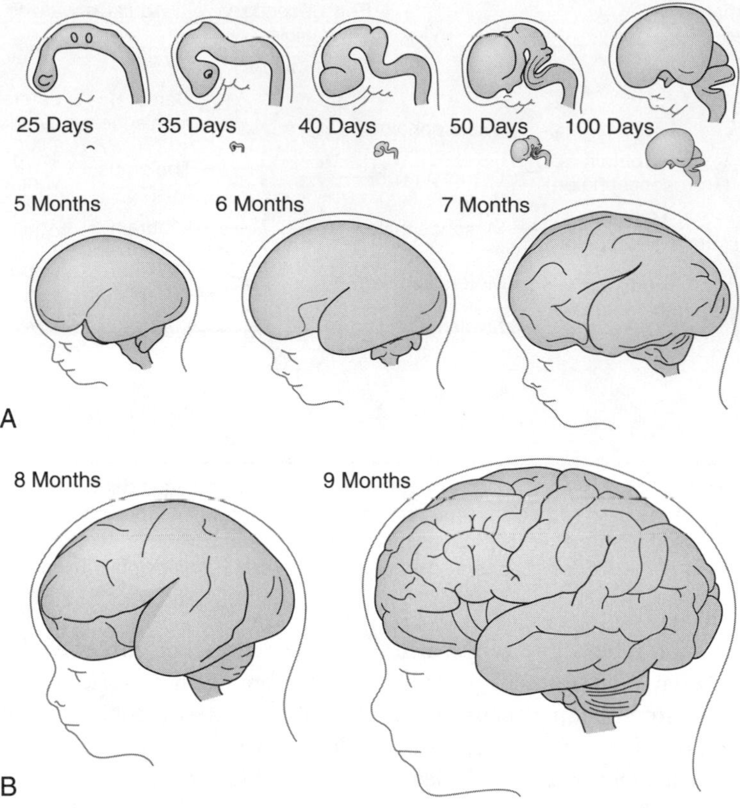

FIGURE 15-6 Folding of embryonic brain and formation of gyri. **A,** Folding during embryonic development. **B,** Development of sulci and gyri during fetal period. (From Cowan, W.M. [1979]. The development of the brain. *Sci Am, 241,* 116.)

Periconceptional folic acid supplementation significantly reduces the risk of NTDs in women with a history of a previous infant with an NTD and in the general public.[161,171] Current recommendations are that women of childbearing age consume 0.4 mg of folic acid daily, with higher recommendations (4 mg beginning 3 months before pregnancy and lasting through the first trimester) for women who have previously had a child with an NTD.[8] Research continues regarding folate-related and other metabolic pathways and NTDs, the role of gene polymorphisms, and the roles of other nutrients such as vitamin B_{12}.[50,171]

α-Fetoprotein leaks into the amniotic fluid and maternal serum in infants with open NTDs. Maternal serum screening at 16 to 18 weeks is used to identify infants at risk for NTDs, with follow-up ultrasound screening for diagnostic confirmation (see Chapter 3).

Anencephaly is due to failure of the neural tube to fuse in the cranial area. Because this area forms the forebrain, anencephalic infants have minimal development of brain tissue above the midbrain. Tissue that does develop is poorly differentiated and becomes necrotic with exposure to amniotic fluid. This results in a mass of vascular tissue with neuronal and glial elements and a choroid plexus with partial absence of the skull bones.[173] Because anencephaly arises from failure of the neural tube to close cranially, the insult occurs at or before 24 days.[249]

Encephaloceles also arise from failure of closure of part of the caudal portion of the neural tube and occur no later than 26 days.[249] About 70% to 80% of these defects occur in the occipital region, with the sac protruding from the back of the head or base of the neck.[23,249] The protruding sac varies considerably in size, but the size does not correlate with the presence of neural elements. Ten percent to 20% of encephaloceles contain no neural elements.[249] Hydrocephalus occurs in up to 50% of occipital encephaloceles due to alterations in the posterior fossa.[249] Hydrocephalus may be present at birth or develop after repair of the defect. Encephaloceles may occur in association with meningomyelocele.

Spina bifida is a general term used to describe defects associated with malformations of the spinal cord and vertebrae that usually arise from defects in closure of the caudal neuropore. Approximately 80% occur in the lumbar area, which is the final area of neural tube fusion. Thus, spina bifida, arising from defects in primary neurulation, occurs at or before 26 days.[249] Defects range from minor malformations to disorders that result in paraplegia or quadriplegia and loss of bladder and bowel control. The degree of sensory and motor neurologic deficit depends on the level and severity of the defect. The two major forms of spina bifida are spina bifida occulta and spina bifida cystica.

Spina bifida occulta (occult dysraphic state) is a vertebral defect at L5 or S1 that arises from failure of the vertebral arch to grow and fuse.[23,246] These are defects of secondary neurulation during formation of the caudal portion of the spinal cord. Most people with this defect have no problems and the defect may be unrecognized. A few have underlying abnormalities of the spinal cord or nerve roots, which are manifested externally by a hemangioma, dimple, tuft of hair, or lipoma in the lower lumbar or sacral area.

Spina bifida cystica describes NTDs characterized by a cystic sac, containing meninges or spinal cord elements, along with vertebral defects, covered by epithelium or a thin membrane, and usually occurring in the lumbar or lumbosacral area. Spina bifida cystica is usually due to alterations in primary neurulation. The three main forms of spina bifida cystica are meningocele, meningomyelocele, and myeloschisis. Meningocele (5% of infants with spina bifida cystica) involves a sac containing meninges and cerebrospinal fluid (CSF) but with the spinal cord and nerve roots in their normal position. These infants usually have minimal residual neurologic deficit if the defect is covered with skin and is managed appropriately.

With a meningomyelocele, the most common (80% to 90%) form of spina bifida cystica, the sac contains spinal cord or nerve roots in addition to meninges and CSF. During development, nerve tissues become incorporated into the wall of the sac, impairing differentiation of nerve fibers.[23] These infants have a neurologic deficit below the level of the sac. Most infants have hydrocephalus and an Arnold Chiari malformation in which the medulla protrudes downward below the foramen magnum and overlaps the spinal cord.[246]

Myeloschisis is a severe defect that occurs no later than 24 days.[249] With this disorder there is no cystic covering; the spinal cord is an open, exposed, flattened mass of neural tissue. These infants have a high mortality rate and significant neurologic deficits and are at great risk for infection. This defect can involve the entire length of the spinal cord and can occur in association with anencephaly.[23]

Intrauterine repair of meningomyelocele has been associated with short-term benefits including reversal of hindbrain herniation, which may enhance brain growth and reduce hydrocephalus. Some studies have found improved lower extremity function; other have not.[33] However, intrauterine repair is also associated with risks, including increased perinatal mortality, and most all infants are preterm.[2,171] A large trial randomizing infants to prenatal (before 26 weeks) or postnatal repair with follow-up to 30 months was recently completed.[2] Intrauterine surgery significantly reduced the need for shunting after birth and improved outcomes at 30 months, but was associated with an increased risk of preterm delivery and uterine dehiscence at delivery.[2]

Disorders of ventral induction are thought to arise no later than 5 to 6 weeks' gestation. Disorders of forebrain development often have concurrent facial anomalies and include holoprosencephaly (failure of the brain to divide into 2 cerebral hemispheres) and holotelencephaly (see Table 15-6).

Fetal Neurodevelopment

The earliest growth of the brain occurs in structures such as basal ganglia, thalamus, midbrain, and brainstem, whereas structures such as the cerebrum and cerebellum form somewhat later. Once the embryologic formations are established, CNS development is characterized by overlapping processes involved in formation of the neocortex and myelinization. These processes include neuronal proliferation (neurogenesis), neuronal and glial cell migration, organization, and myelinization. Organization and myelinization continue past birth.

Neuronal Proliferation

Neuronal proliferation (neuronogenesis) is a period of massive production of neurons and their precursors. The maximal rate of neuronal proliferation occurs between 12 and 18 weeks' gestation.[249] During proliferation the walls of the neural tube thicken, forming layers. The ependyma is the interior lining of the neural tube that later becomes the lining of the ventricles and the central canal of the spinal cord. In the subependymal layer the neurons and glial cells of the CNS are formed in the ventricular and subventricular zones of the germinal layer (germinal matrix).[249] Neuronal proliferation begins at 6 weeks in the ventricular zone and at 7 weeks in the subventricular zone; both zones reach their peak proliferation by 12 weeks.[39] In conjunction with the proliferation of neurons, glial cells also increase in number; however, with the exception of radial glial cells, the peak in glial cell numbers occurs roughly from 5 months' gestational age through the first year of life.[249] Radial glia have two major functions. First they serve as guides during neuron migration (see next section) and secondly they are neuronal progenitors in the ventricular zone.[249] Thus neurons arise from both neuronal and radial glial cell progenitors. Although most of the neuronal complement is formed early in fetal life, a few areas, notably the cerebral subventricular zone and the external granular layer of the cerebellum, continue to acquire neurons during the early months after birth (see Development of the Cerebellum).[249] This pattern of neuronal formation produces a particular vulnerability in the preterm infant. In late gestation the ventricular and subventricular zones disappear almost completely (a subventricular zone remnant persists to adulthood) and proliferation shifts to intermediary and subplate zones for continued production of glial cells.[39]

Alterations in neuronal proliferation can lead to increases or decreases in number and size of cells in the brain and associated structures. Micrencephaly arises from a decrease in size (micrencephaly vera) or number (radial microbrain) of neuronal-glial stem cell units.[246,249] Micrencephaly vera may be due to unknown causes; have a familial basis; or be associated with teratogens such as alcohol, cocaine, radiation, and maternal phenylketonuria.[249] Excessive proliferation (macrencephaly) may also be due to unknown causes, have a familial basis, or occur with growth disturbances (e.g., achondroplasia or Beckwith-Wiedemann syndrome) and chromosomal disorders (fragile X and Klinefelter syndromes). Macrencephaly is also seen with neurocutaneous syndromes (such as multiple hemangiomas and neurofibromatosis) that involve excessive proliferation of cells within the central nervous system and of mesodermal structures.[249]

Migration

Once formed, neurons travel from the germinal layer in the subependymal region below the lateral ventricles to the areas of the nervous system where they will further differentiate, forming the gray matter, and take on unique and individual functions.[249] The bulk of migration occurs from 10 to 20 weeks' gestation (usually completed by 22 weeks; Figure 15-7).[53,167,249] Two types of neuron migration are seen in the cerebrum and cerebellum: radial and tangential. Radially migration accounts for much of the cortex and involves radial glia, which appear by 10 weeks' gestation (Figure 15-8).[115,167,249] The nuclei of the radial glia are in the germinal matrix. The basal process of each cell is attached to the ventricle and the apical process is attached to the pia matter.[115] These processes extending from the radial glia guide the neuron to its respective site. Radial glia also act as progenitors for neuron and astrocyte generation.[249] Migration is mediated by signaling proteins, surface molecules, and receptors on both the neurons and the radial glia.[249] Cajal-Retzius cells in the external cortical layer secrete reelin, an extracellular matrix glycoprotein. Reelin is thought to exert a stop signal for the migrating neurons.[167,249] Radial glial–assisted migration also occurs in the cerebellum. Cortical and cerebellar neurons migrate tangentially without radial glia guidance.[167]

The neocortex develops in six zones, which are, from innermost to outermost, the ventricular zone, subventricular zone, intermediate zone, subplate, cortical plate, and marginal zone. Neurons forming in the ventricular and subventricular zones migrate through the cortical plate to form more and more superficial layers. The initial neurons migrate toward the cerebral walls to form the preplate. The next neurons migrate to areas deep within the cortex, whereas later neurons migrate further to the surface of the cortex. As a result, neurons formed early come to lie in deeper layers of cortex and subcortex; those formed later end at more superficial layers.[249] Thus neocortex formation follows an "inside-first-outside-last" pattern, except for the early neurons of the subplate.[198,249] The subplate and marginal zone are transient structures that develop in parallel with the cortical plate, and then regress after the cortex is formed.[167] Most cortical neurons have reached their sites by 20 to 24 weeks' gestation.[249]

The subplate zone and subplate neurons are critical structures in neocortex development. The roles of the subplate are listed in Table 15-7. The subplate is the first place where synapses form within the cortex and receive input from thalamic and other regions.[40] The subplate, located just below the developing cortex, serves as a "waiting room" or temporary site for thalamocortical and corticocortical projections and helps guide axons to cortical and subcortical targets and in establishing functional connections between brain regions.[48,53] For example, thalamic fibers enter the subplate area before their target neurons are in place and transiently form synaptic connections with subplate neurons.[249] These are held in the subplate until the cortical plate is ready.

Subplate formation begins at 12 weeks, and reaches its maximum size at 27 to 30 weeks.[49,53,252] Thalamic afferents develop at 12 to 16 weeks and reach the subplate by 20 to 24 weeks.[118,252] Between 24 and 32 weeks axonal growth to the subplate and cortex increases and thalamocortical afferents move from the subplate to the cortex. Callosal and corticocortical axons enter the subplate from 24 to 32 weeks and enter the cortex from 32 to 26 weeks as the subplate begins to regress.[249,252] Thus the subplate is "a significant reservoir of functional connectivity in the preterm infant."[53] The subplate is vulnerable to perinatal injury in these infants.

The subplate undergoes programmed cell death after birth, although subplate neurons remain as interstitial neurons.[128,249] Interstitial neurons are embedded in superficial white matter. Alterations in interstitial neurons or in their role in cortical circuitry may play a role in some forms of schizophrenia.[128]

Disorders of migration alter gyral development and lead to hypoplasia or agenesis of the corpus callosum. Gyral development is most prominent during the last 3 months of gestation (see Figure 15-6,), with the most rapid increase between 26 and 28 weeks. The increased gyri result in a change in head shape (from oval to biparietal prominence). Gyral disorders arise secondary to inborn errors of metabolism, such as fatty acid oxidation defects, chromosomal anomalies, and exogenous insults, especially in preterm infants.[172,246,249]

Organization

Organization refers to the processes by which the nervous system takes on the capacity to operate as an integrated whole. This phase of neurodevelopment begins at approximately 6 months' gestation (see Figure 15-7) and extends many years after birth, and probably continues into adulthood. Neuron growth and connections lead to development of sulci and gyri (see Figure 15-6), with a brain growth spurt seen from 26 to 30 weeks. With increasing organization, fetal and infant behaviors become more complex.[6,249] Alterations in organization are seen in infants with Down, fragile X, and Angelman syndromes; periventricular leukomalacia (PVL); inflammation and infection; and hypothyroxinemia.[199,200,249] Injury to the cortex and subcortical area white matter can lead to disorders such as cerebral palsy. Focal lesions in the immature brain can lead to reorganization of sensory, motor, and related tracts.[40]

During the period of organization, six processes occur.[249] The first is differentiation and development of subplate neurons (see Migration). These neurons migrate to cortex early and guide ascending and descending projections to target neurons. Subplate neurons provide a connection site for axons ascending from the thalamus and other sites, until the neurons that these axons will eventually connect with have

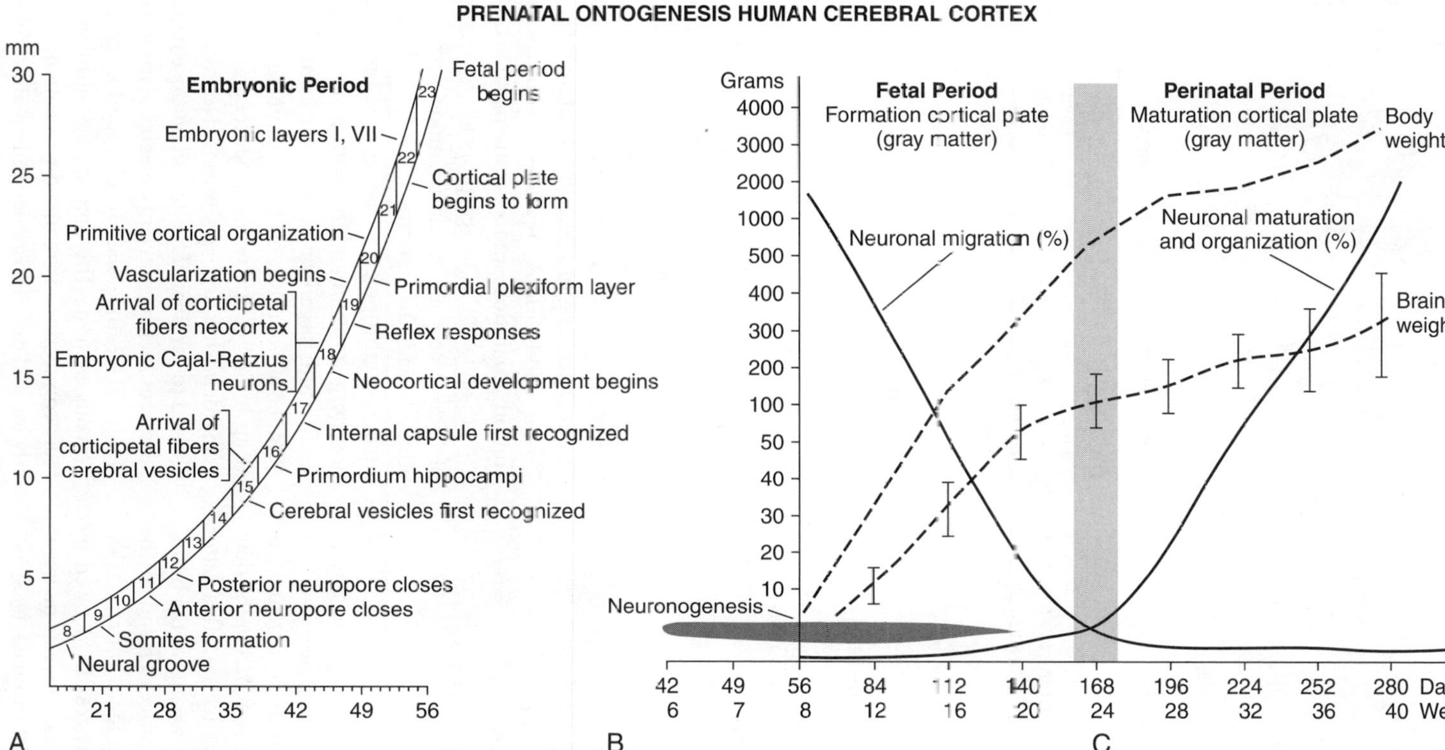

FIGURE 15-7 Major events in the early development of the cerebral cortex. **A,** Embryonic period: appearance of cerebral vesicles, arrival of corticopetal fibers, and establishment of the primordial plexiform layer. **B,** Fetal period: neuronal migration and formation of the cortical plate. **C,** Perinatal period: ascending neuronal differentiation and maturation of the cortical plate (gray matter). (From Marin-Padilla, M. [1993]. Pathogenesis of later-acquired leptomeningeal heterotopias and secondary cortical alterations: A Golgi study. In A.M. Galabruda [Ed.], *Dyslexia and development.* Cambridge, MA: Harvard University Press.)

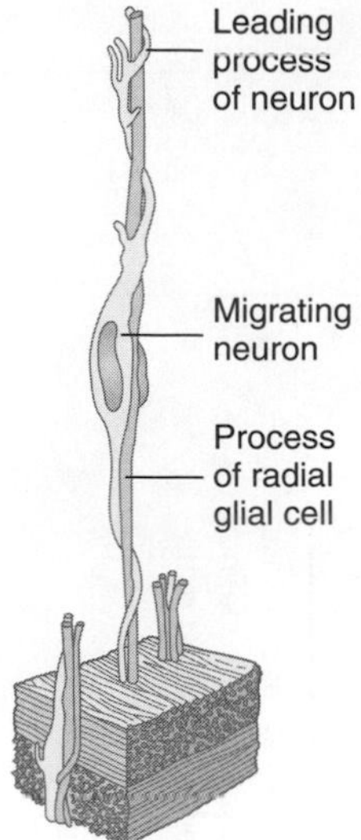

FIGURE 15-8 Radial glial cells and their associations with peripherally migrating neurons during the development of the brain. (Based on Rakic, P. [1975]. Cell migration and neuronal ectopias in the brain. *Birth Defects Orig Article Series, 11,* 95.)

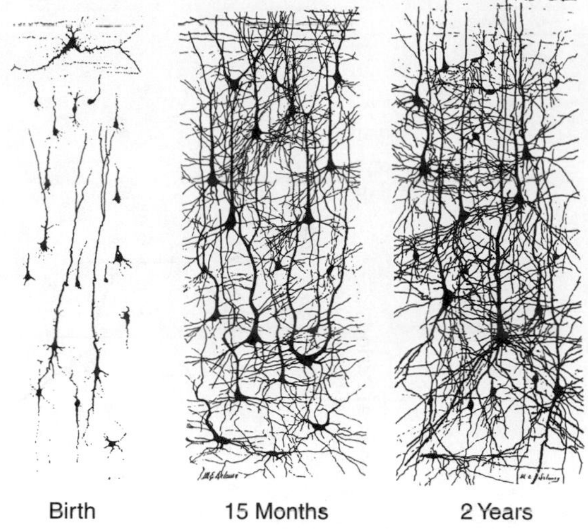

FIGURE 15-9 Dendritic growth. (From Dobbing, J. [1975]. Human brain development and its vulnerability. In *Biologic and clinical aspects of brain development.* [Mead Johnson Symposium on Perinatal and Developmental Medicine, no. 6.] Evansville, IN: Mead Johnson.)

Table 15-7 Major Roles of Subplate Neurons

Serve as sites of synaptic contact for "waiting" thalamic, commissural, and association (corticocortical) afferents
Establish a functional link between waiting afferents and their cortical targets
Provide axonal guidance into cerebral cortex for the ascending afferents
Facilitate cerebral cortical organization and synaptic development
Provide "pioneering" axonal guidance for efferent projections from the cortex to subcortical targets, e.g., thalamus

From Volpe, J.J. (2009). The encephalopathy of prematurity—brain injury and impaired brain development inextricably intertwined. *Semin Pediatr Neurol, 16,* p. 172.

migrated from the germinal matrix. The subplate reaches its peak from 22 to 34 weeks.[249]

The second and third processes involve arrangement of cortical neurons in layers and arborization, wherein the dendrites and axons undergo extensive branching. This latter process is sometimes referred to as the "wiring of the brain" (Figure 15-9). The increase in cellular processes and in the size of the neuronal field is prerequisite for communication throughout the nervous system. This process is followed by the formation of connections or synapses between neurons, the fourth component of organization. The intracellular structures and enzymes that will produce neurotransmitters also develop at this time. Connections between cells are critical for integration across all areas of the nervous system. Throughout development, synapses continue to restructure; this process is believed to be the basis for memory and learning. Impulse conduction provides for functional validation of connections. Evidence suggests that use of conduction pathways may increase or alter connections.[249] Characteristics of early neuronal activity include poor spontaneous neuronal activity, slow conduction velocity, slow synaptic potentials, and synaptic transmission uncertainty. Immaturity of neurotransmitters and hypersensitivity of NMDA receptors increases the risk of receptor overstimulation with hypoxic-ischemic events (see Hypoxic-Ischemic Encephalopathy).

Synaptogenesis is mediated by excitatory neurotransmitters such as glutamate.[73,132] Glutamate acts on *N*-methyl-D-aspartate (NMDA) receptors to enhance neuronal proliferation, migration, and synaptic plasticity. During the brain growth spurt, NMDA receptors are hypersensitive. Blockage of these receptors in animal models by substances such as ethanol leads to apoptosis.[73,115,132,211,249] Other substances, such as erythropoietin, may also be important in enhancing brain organization and for neuroprotection.[130,160,211,258]

The fifth organizational process entails reduction in the number of neurons and their connections through the death of up to half of the original neurons as well as regression of many dendrites and synapses.[249] Neuronal survival has been likened to survival of the fittest, because neurons compete for resources such as nutrients, electrical impulses, and synapses. Neuronal death assists in elimination of errors within the nervous system. The appropriate number of neurons and their connections is retained while neurons that are improperly located or fail to achieve adequate connections are eliminated. Numbers of neurons are maximal in the fetus and survival is dependent on neurons or groups of neurons getting appropriate numbers of connections. From 8 months' gestation to adulthood, numbers of neurons and synapses decrease. For example, there are an estimated 620,000/m^3

neurons in the visual cortex at 7 months' gestation versus 100,000/m^3 at term and 40,000/m^3 in the adult.[150]

Cell death and selective elimination of neuronal processes is important in adjusting the size of individual neurons to their anticipated need and in brain plasticity in infants. In the developing brain, neuronal processes targeted for elimination can be saved if they are needed, for example, because of damage to other processes in order to preserve functional ability. Excitatory neurotransmitters, such as glutamate, mediate neural development and organization by acting on NMDA receptors.[23]

The final organizational process is differentiation of glia from the general precursor cells into specific types and glia proliferation. The increase in glia begins at approximately 30 weeks' gestation, continues into the second year, and then plateaus. There are three main types of glia: myelin-building (oligodendrocytes and Schwann cells), guiding (radial glia [for neuron migration], and Schwann cells), and "clean-up" (astroglia and microglia). The astroglia and microglia remove waste and dead tissue and occupy space left by neurons that have died, among other functions. Astrocytes also provide support for neurons. Astrocytes undergo rapid proliferation from 24-32 weeks (peak 26 weeks).[226,249] These glia are found primarily in deep cortical layers and white matter. They assist with axonal guidance, growth, brain structural development, and functioning of the blood-brain barrier.[226] Astrocytes can release transmitters (such as glutamate) to send signals to neighboring neurons. Each astrocyte may interact with several neurons and hundreds to thousands of synapses to integrate information.[226,249] Microglia are the brain macrophages and immune cells. They also have a role in brain development with increased numbers seen in the third trimester. Activated microglia with white matter injury can lead to cellular injury initiated by ischemia and inflammation (mediated by reactive oxygen species, cytokines, and glutamate).[226,249] Oligodendrocytes produce myelin in the CNS. During the premyelinating period (before 32 weeks' gestation), oligodendrocytes are especially vulnerable to hypoxic-ischemic injury. Damage to these glial cells is a prominent feature in brain injury in preterm infants (see White Matter Injury).[253] Schwann cells produce myelin for the peripheral nerves. Schwann cells also act as guiding glia following peripheral nerve injury to guide regenerating axons to their targets.[249]

Myelinization

Myelinization refers to the laying down of myelin, the lipoprotein insulating the covering of nerve fibers. Myelinization increases the speed of transmission along axons by 100-fold.[150] This process occurs in both the central and peripheral nerve systems. Glia migrate to locations along the developing nerve fibers. Myelin is formed as the glia (either Schwann cells in the peripheral nervous system or oligodendroglia in the CNS) wrap around the nerve fiber. The glia's cellular membrane, once wrapped around the fiber, fuses to become myelin.

Myelinization begins during the second trimester and continues into adulthood.[249] The process of myelinization occurs at differing times in areas throughout the nervous system. For example, myelinization of somatosensory and auditory areas is nearly complete by term, whereas prefrontal lobe myelinization is not completed until after 20 years.[150] Myelinization of the forebrain is most rapid after birth. Myelinization first begins in the peripheral nervous system, with motor fibers becoming myelinated before sensory fibers. In the CNS, myelinization of sensory areas precedes that of motor areas, with the primary sensory areas becoming myelinated relatively early in development. Incomplete myelinization does not prevent function. However, because incomplete myelinization affects nerve conduction, it does alter the speed of impulse conduction. The order of myelinization parallels overall nervous system functional development and generally precedes mature function.[173] Areas of the brain that support higher-level functions, such as cognition and learning, myelinate later in life.[249] Some brain areas continue to lay down myelin well into adulthood. Because myelin is a lipoprotein, dietary adequacy of fats and protein is important for normal myelinization. Disorders of myelinization are seen with amino and organic acidopathies, hypothyroidism, undernutrition, and perinatal insults such as PVL.[249]

Cerebellar Development

The cerebellum is one of later brain structures to mature. The cerebellum undergoes a rapid growth spurt from 24 to 40 weeks with a fivefold increase in volume reflecting underlying histogenic and cytogenic changes; the cerebellar cortex increases more than 30-fold during this period.[36,146] Prior to 20 weeks two proliferation zones are established that give rise to the major cerebellar structures. Between 20 and 40 weeks increased external surface foliation is seen with development of the external granular layer, Purkinje cell (neuron) differentiation, and migration.[36,146] The lateral hemispheres of the cerebellum are involved in cognitive and motor function; the middle layers in regulation of emotion, social behavior, and affect.[148] The cerebellum is important in cognition and acts as a node in distribution of neural networks with interconnections with thalamus, parietal, and prefrontal cortex.[184] Cerebellar damage (see Cerebellar Injury in Preterm Infants) can alter language development, behavioral function and cognitive function.[36,146,148,184,249]

Development of Specific Systems

Autonomic Nervous System. The autonomic nervous system has both central and peripheral components. Peripheral portions develop from neural crest cells. Ganglia are formed from neural crest cells that migrate beyond the neural tube. Sympathetic ganglia are derived from neural crest cells that collect along either side of the developing spinal cord at about 5 weeks' gestational age.[173] The parasympathetic ganglia and plexi also form by migration.[173] Once they reach their respective sites, neurons in the autonomic ganglia continue to differentiate. Nerve fibers, originating in the cord, grow out and make connections with the ganglia. The autonomic nervous system regulates many endocrine functions through nerve impulses. The embryonic origins of some autonomic end organs demonstrate a structural basis for these regulatory actions. The pituitary, a primary source of autonomic regulation, is derived from two forms of tissues. The adenohypophysis is formed from ectoderm and the neurohypophysis is formed from neuroectoderm. Similarly, the adrenal gland is derived from two types of tissues. The adrenal cortex is derived from mesoderm, whereas the medulla, which secretes catecholamines, is derived from neuroectoderm (specifically neural crest cells) and is controlled by the sympathetic nervous system.

Peripheral Nervous System. The peripheral nervous system is derived from the neural crest. Through migration and specialization, cells of the neural crest develop into cranial, spinal, and visceral nerves and ganglia. Neural crest cells are precursors of the adrenal medulla chromaffin cells that secrete epinephrine.[173] Support cells of the peripheral nervous system also derive from the neural crest. Nerve fibers that eventually innervate skeletal motor fibers emerge from the spinal basal plate, combine into bundles to form the ventral root, and migrate to the developing motor fibers.[173] Sensory fibers form the dorsal root in a similar manner.

Functional Development

Studies of fetal neural activity in utero are limited to external monitoring of CNS electrical activity or noninvasive detection of fetal responses using measures of fetal movement or ultrasonography. The knowledge of fetal neural capabilities has been augmented by an accident of nature, that is, preterm birth. Much of our understanding of fetal function comes from the study of preterm infants, who technically are not fetal. However, the behavior of these infants provides one means of appreciating fetal behaviors at various gestational ages. Studies of preterm infants have greatly increased information concerning operation of the fetal nervous system. The following section describes the neural function of the fetus, defined as gestational age less than 38 weeks. In many instances, information pertains to the "fetal infant" or preterm infant. Appreciation of fetal neural development provides a basis for anticipation of the many capabilities of the preterm and term infant.

Sensory Abilities

Generally the somatic sensory and special sensory systems develop in the following chronologic order: touch, proprioception, vestibular, chemoreception (smell and taste), hearing, and vision.[92] As noted in the section on Myelinization, in the peripheral areas, motor fibers myelinate before sensory fibers, whereas in the central nervous system sensory fibers myelinate before motor fibers. Thus in terms of rate of impulse transmission, differences in myelinization are one basis for limited integration of sensory and motor actions in the fetus.

The early fetus has been shown to respond to touch around the mouth at around 2 months of gestational age; hands become touch sensitive by 10 to 11 weeks.[245] Touch in utero entails contact with amniotic fluid that is approximately at body temperature and contact with body parts or the wall of the uterus. Maternal movement and buoyant amniotic fluid provide rich vestibular stimulation for the fetus in utero.

Nociceptors appear at 6 to 8 weeks' gestation, initially around the mouth; by 11 weeks in the face, palms, and soles; by 15 weeks in the trunk, arms, and legs; and by 20 to 22 weeks are abundant throughout the fetus (Table 15-8).[49,118,152,167,245] The fetus can process pain at the subcortical level before cortical structures are in place.[245] Sensory fibers to dorsal interneuron areas may develop as early as 6 weeks with development and differentiation of dorsal horn afferents beginning at 12 to 13 weeks.[1,152] Afferent synapses in the dorsal spinal cord

Table 15-8 Anatomic and Functional Development of the Different Parts of the Pain System

PART OF THE SYSTEM	DEVELOPMENTAL EVENT	TIMING (WEEKS)
Nociceptors	Nociceptors appear (starting around the mouth and later developing over the entire body).	7-20
Peripheral afferents	Synapses appear to the spinal cord.	10-30
Spinal cord	Stimulation results in motor movements.	7.5
	Spinothalamic connections are established.	20
	Myelinization of pain pathways.	22
	Descending tracts develop.	Postnatally
Thalamocortical tracts	First axons appear to the cortical plate.	20-22
	Functional synapse formation of the thalamocortical occurs.	26-34
Cerebral cortex	Cortical neurons migrate (cortex develops).	8-20
	First EEG burst may be detected.	20
	Symmetric and synchronic EEG activity appears.	26
	Sleep and wakefulness patterns in EEG become distinguishable.	30
	Evoked potential becomes detectable.	29

From Vanhatalo, S. & van Nieuwenhuizen, O. (2000). Fetal pain? *Brain Dev, 22,* 146.
EEG, Electroencephalogram.

and peripheral receptors start as early as 8 weeks' gestation.[152] Connections to the thalamus begin at 14 weeks and are complete by 20 weeks; thalamocortical connections are seen by 13 weeks and are more developed by 26 to 30 weeks.[49,152,1] These connections are myelinated by 29 weeks.[245] By at least 24 weeks noxious stimuli cause a response in the primary sensory cortex. Completion of these connections stimulates development of axons and synaptogenesis with selective elimination of excess connections and cell populations.[49]

Proprioception, which is involved with perception of joint and body movement and the position of the body, is interrelated with tactile and vestibular receptors. Vestibular sensation is a form of proprioceptive sensation involved in balance and postural control. Vestibular sensation, mediated by receptors in the ear, detects changes in direction and rate of head movement. Vestibular receptors mature by 14 to 15 weeks.[136]

Smell is mediated by three groups of receptors that bind fragrant molecules: (1) main ciliated neuroreceptors (seen by 11 weeks), (2) trigeminal nerve endings (respond by 7 to 10 weeks), and (3) vomeronasal (appear by 5 to 6 weeks and are maximal by 20 weeks).[145,256] Olfactory marker protein is present by 28 weeks.[43] Odor molecules in amniotic fluid stimulate the fetal smell receptors by the third trimester.[256] The fetus may detect aromatic substances and flavors from the maternal diet in amniotic fluid. This stimulation may have a role in programming later dietary preferences.[16,43,118,133,164] Responsiveness to odors is observed in preterm infants beginning at approximately 28 weeks and is readily documented by 32 weeks' gestation in most infants.[43]

Taste occurs by activation of the taste buds and stimulation of the trigeminal nerve. Taste buds appear by 7 to 8 weeks and are morphologically mature by 13 to 15 weeks.[43] Taste receptors are present by 16 weeks, reaching adult numbers by term.[136] The fetus ingests amniotic fluid (see Chapter 3). Although variations occur in the composition of the amniotic fluid, it is unknown to what extent the fetus experiences taste. However, injection of a sweet substance increases fetal swallowing, whereas a bitter substance decreases swallowing.[43] Preterm infants respond to sweet taste by as early as 24 weeks and consistently by 28 to 32 weeks.[43]

The structures of the auditory system, including the inner ear and cochlea, are mature enough to support hearing by approximately 20 weeks' gestation; fetal hearing begins at 24 to 25 weeks.[93] At this point the fluid spaces in the cochlea are still poorly developed, the basal membrane is thick, hair cell innervation and arrangement are immature, and sensitivity to sound is poor. Sound sensitivity matures rapidly from 24 to 35 weeks.[255] The tympanic membrane is similar to that in the adult by 28 weeks.[255] The cochlea matures slowly during the third trimester, undergoing "tuning" during this period. Tuning of the cochlea so that areas are frequency-specific involves mechanical maturation of the basilar membrane and outer hair cells.[255] Tuning begins in the base (high-frequency sounds) and proceeds toward the apex (low-frequency sounds). Changes in the sound environment, as occurs with preterm birth, may alter this process.

Auditory evoked potentials can be recorded as early as 25 to 26 weeks' gestation, but are not reliable until after 28 weeks.[91,93,255] The fetus in the third trimester can discriminate between maternal live voice and tape-recorded voice and familiar versus novel sounds.[85] Responses to sound are observed in preterm infants at approximately 25 to 28 weeks' gestational age.[91] The preterm infant can be observed to orient to sound, with evidence of arousal and attention. The hearing threshold decreases with gestational age. For example, in infants of 28 to 34 weeks' gestational age, the hearing threshold is approximately 40 decibels, whereas in term infants the hearing threshold is approximately 20 decibels.

Intrauterine recordings demonstrate that sounds in the external environment are audible to the fetus. High-frequency sounds are attenuated, whereas low-frequency sounds are not. External sound is reduced by about one-half its strength by the time it reaches the fetus.[133] For example, a 90-dB sound in a midrange frequency would be decreased to 45 dB by the time it reached the fetus.[85] The intrauterine auditory environment includes sounds within the mother such as breathing, movement of blood through the umbilical cord, and intestinal peristalsis and differs significantly from the sound environment of the preterm infant.[83] Hearing in preterm infants of different gestational ages is summarized in Table 15-9.

Table 15-9 Development of Hearing in Preterm and Term Infants

GESTATIONAL AGE	ANATOMIC AND FUNCTIONAL DEVELOPMENT
Preterm infants <28 weeks	Fetal hearing begins by 23 to 24 weeks Threshold about 65 db, with a range of 500-1000 Hz Auditory brainstem responses by 26 to 28 weeks
Preterm infants 28-30 weeks	Rapid maturation of cochlea and auditory nerve Responses rapidly fatigue Initial auditory processing by 30 weeks Threshold 40 db with an increased frequency range
Preterm infants 32-34 weeks	Outer hair cells mature by 32 weeks Rapid maturation of cochlea and auditory nerve
Preterm infants >34 weeks	Increased speed of conduction Ossicles and electrophysiology complete by 36 weeks Hearing threshold 30 db, with increasing range Increasing ability to localize and discriminate
Term infants	Localize and discriminate sounds Hearing threshold of 20 db, with a range of 500-4000 Hz

Compiled from references 22, 31, 80, 92, 93, 136, 191.
db, Decibels; *Hz*, Hertz.

Formation of the eyes begins during embryonic development. The fovea can be identified by 14 weeks' gestation but maturation of the foveal region is not complete until late childhood.[169] Rod differentiation and retinal vascularization begin by 25 weeks' gestation and myelinization of the optic nerve begins at 24 weeks.[80,91] The choroid vasculature (vessels that underlie the retina and pigment epithelium) are mature by 21 weeks. Retinal vessels that supply the inner retina develop in parallel with the retina. These vessels begin to develop from the optic disk at the base of the hyaloid artery and extend peripherally to the ora serrata.[169] Growth is particularly rapid from 24 to 28 weeks and, then continues at a slower pace. Zone III, the most peripheral retina, has minimal vessel development in preterm infants at 29 weeks; by 36 weeks about half of the vessels have developed, and almost all are developed by 45 to 49 weeks.[169]

The neurons forming the visual cortex are in place at 26 weeks. Between 28 and 34 weeks' gestation, visual neuronal connections and processes undergo rapid development.[91] Visual evoked potentials can be recorded between 25 and 30 weeks.[91] Visual attention begins at about 30 to 32 weeks' gestation, although it is fleeting at this age. Development of vision in preterm infants at different gestational ages is summarized in Table 15-10.

The natural sensory environment of the uterus is developmentally appropriate for the fetus. This environment provides stimuli that are rich, varied, and rhythmical. Intrauterine sensory stimulation programs have not been studied extensively and cannot be assumed to be beneficial or without risk. Because the normal uterine sensory environment is already rich, the benefits of programs to supplement intrauterine stimulation are unclear at this time.

Motor Abilities

The development of motor activity in the fetus is a function of both neural and muscular maturation. Muscle cells develop from mesoderm. Innervation during development is critical for muscle fiber development.[249] Muscle cells, as well

Table 15-10 Development of Vision in Preterm and Term Infants

GESTATIONAL AGE	ANATOMIC AND FUNCTIONAL DEVELOPMENT
Preterm infants 24-28 weeks	Eyelid: unfuses at 24-26 weeks Lens: cloudy; second of four layers forming Cornea: hazy until 27 weeks Retina: rod differentiation by 25 weeks; vascularization begins Visual cortex: rapid dendritic growth No pupillary response Eyelid tightening to bright light but quickly fatigues VER to bright light but quickly fatigues Very myopic
Preterm infants 30-34 weeks	Lens: clearing; second layer complete, third forming Retina: rod complete except for fovea by 32 weeks; cone differentiation begins Visual cortex: rapid dendritic and synapse development VER more complex, latency decreases Bright light causes sustained pupil closure Abrupt reduction may cause eye opening Pupillary response sluggish but more mature Spontaneous eye opening, with brief fixation in low light
Preterm infants 34-36 weeks	Pupils: complete pupillary reflex by 36 weeks Retina: cone numbers in fovea increase Blood vessels reach nasal retina Visual cortex: morphologically similar to term Increased alertness; less sustained than in a term infant VER resembles that of term infant with longer latency Spontaneous orientation toward soft light Beginning to track and show visual preferences Less myopic
Term infants	Still immature, with much development from birth to 6 months Retinal vessels reach periphery of temporal retina Lens transmits more short-wave light than adult Acuity approximately 20/200 to 20/1600 Attend to form, object, and face; track horizontally and some vertically Can see objects to at least 2½ feet; attends best at 8-12 inches

Adapted from Glass, P. (1999). The vulnerable neonate and the neonatal intensive care environment. In G.B. Avery, M.A. Fletcher, & M.G. MacDonald (Eds.), *Neonatology: Pathophysiology and management of the newborn* (5th ed.). Philadelphia: Lippincott Williams & Wilkins.
VER, Visual evoked response.

as neurons, undergo migration and differentiation during development. Mature myocytes are present at approximately 38 weeks; muscle cells increase in size postnatally.[249]

The pattern of fetal motor development includes differences in both emergence of muscle tone and the amount of movement over time.[91] Development of muscle tone follows a caudocephalad and distal-proximal pattern; that is, lower extremities precede upper extremities and extremities precede axial or truncal muscle tone. Motor development is associated with increased flexor tone, with lower extremities demonstrating flexion before upper extremities. In the lower extremities, passive flexor tone is noticed at 29 weeks' gestation and active flexor tone becomes apparent at 31 weeks. Tone in the upper extremities develops later, with flexor tone demonstrated in the upper extremities by 34 weeks.[10] Active tone develops before passive tone; that is, muscle tone is seen during movement or action before resting muscle tone. Both tone and flexion increase with gestational age. Motor movement also shows increasing coordination with gestational age, with less tremor, smoother movement, and more coordination.[91] More complex motor movements are observed after 24 weeks' gestation.[91] Muscle tone is used as one criterion in scoring gestational age.

Muscle tone is limited before 28 weeks' gestation. By 32 weeks, flexor tone can be observed in the lower extremities; it is observable in the upper extremities by 36 weeks. The term infant demonstrates flexion.[249] Movement changes with development. At 28 to 32 weeks' gestation, movement is slow and may appear uncoordinated, with flailing- or writhing-type movements.[249] By 32 weeks' gestation, flexion movements are somewhat more coordinated.[249] Neonates of this age can turn their head, but head control is lacking. With continued development there is increasing strength: alternating movements may be seen in the lower extremities, and head control improves.[249] Fetal movements are episodic and cyclical with cycles increasing in duration and regularity from midgestation to term.[186]

During pregnancy the pattern of fetal movements is one of increasing frequency of movements, followed by a reduction in movement close to term. Spontaneous movements begin at 7 to 8 weeks' gestation with slow flexion-extension of the vertebral column and passive displacement of the extremities, followed by discrete limb movements at 9 weeks. The earliest reflex is tilting of the head with perioral touch (7.5 weeks); legs demonstrate reflexive movement by 14 weeks.[245] The development of movement involves twitching-type movement before 10 weeks, followed by independent limb movement (10 to 12 weeks); hand to face movement (12 to 13 weeks); limb, head, and torso movement (12 to 16 weeks); sucking on fingers (15 weeks); and increasingly complex hand, face, and respiratory movements after 24 weeks.[91,249]

All types of movements seen after birth are present by about 18 weeks' gestation. Maternal perception of fetal movement occurs at approximately 16 weeks' gestation in multiparas, and slightly later in primiparas. Before this time, fetal movements are too fine to be noticed. Fetal movements increase during gestation, reaching a maximum between 26 and 32 weeks; after this time the constraints of the uterine environment reduce fetal movement. Movements are largely spontaneous but can be stimulated.

The developing motor activity of the fetus reflects integration of nervous system activity as well as general fetal well-being. Changes in fetal movement may reflect placental insufficiency, hypoxemia, or other evidence of fetal distress. Daily fetal movement monitoring has been used as a screening tool for fetal well-being during the third trimester (see Chapter 6). In addition to changes in tone and frequency of movement during pregnancy, fetal movements provide evidence of fetal sleep-wake or state patterns.

Fetal State Patterns

Although the constancy of the uterine environment may suggest similar consistency in fetal behavior, this assumption is untrue. Fetal behaviors exhibit regular patterns of occurrence, particularly sleep-wake behaviors or behavioral states in the third trimester. In the adult, sleep-wake behaviors demonstrate a diurnal pattern of activity and sleep. Sleep in the fetus and infant does not follow this pattern. Sleep changes with maturation of the central nervous system. Because sleep is qualitatively and quantitatively different in the young compared with adults, fetal and infant sleep-wake patterns are more commonly described as *states*. In the infant, state is determined by characteristics of heart and respiratory regularity, eyes open or closed, motor activity, and presence or absence of rapid eye movements (REM). Although not all of these parameters can be observed in the fetus, fetal state can be determined by regularity of heart rate, presence of eye movements, and fetal movement.[56]

In the fetus as well as the infant, motor activity and irregular heart rate occur during REM sleep. Motor movement also occurs during awake periods. During quiet sleep, regular heart rate and minimal motor movement are noted. Alteration of quiet and active periods in fetal movement have been reported as early as 21 weeks' gestation; however, there is little evidence of regular, rhythmic pattern and limited coordination among state parameters at this time.[234] Fetal movement is largely continuous in early pregnancy, but with increasing maturation, quiet periods emerge. For example, at 24 to 26 weeks' gestation there is almost continual motor activity of the fetal extremities; by 28 weeks distinct periods of quiescence and activity alternate; by 32 weeks' gestation, alteration of activity and quiet periods becomes more regular and rhythmic.[58] Between 28 and 32 weeks (and possibly as early as 27 weeks), heart rate cycles in conjunction with activity/nonactivity cycles are noted.[186] By 32 weeks' gestation, patterns of fetal heart rate, eye movement, and gross body movements also begin to show coordination.[248] This periodic function is credited with being a prenatal version of the alteration of REM (fetal state 2F) and quiet sleep (fetal state 1F), representing an underlying rest-activity cycle.[196] Duration of state 2F is longer than state 1F. An agitated state (4F), seen infrequently and primarily near term, is associated with decreased time in state 2F.[56] The fetal state cycle is approximately 40 minutes long.[234] With continuing development, the length of quiet periods and the integration among state behaviors increase.[185] These changes continue after birth.

NEONATAL PHYSIOLOGY

Transitional Events

At birth, the transition from intrauterine to extrauterine life entails a number of changes in the nervous system. The nervous system does not "turn on" at birth; rather, nervous system activity has increased steadily during pregnancy, producing a term gestation infant whose nervous system is prepared to receive and process information and respond in ways suited to neonatal development. In examining transition, it is useful to identify the behavioral abilities of the neonate, experiences of the fetus in the intrauterine environment, and differences between the intrauterine and extrauterine environments. The change in environment is the major challenge for the neonate's nervous system. The transitional characteristics of four areas of nervous system function are examined here: autonomic, motor, sensory, and state regulation.

Autonomic Regulation

During fetal life, placental circulation provides a steady flow of oxygen and nutrients supporting the metabolic needs of the fetus. At birth, the first challenge faced by the neonate is initiating and sustaining respiration. In addition to an intact pulmonary and cardiovascular system, nervous system control of respiration and heart activity is required. Although fetal respiratory movements are preparation for this action, the fetus has no experience breathing independently or in regulating cardiac and pulmonary functions to produce stable blood oxygen requirements in ambient air. The fetus has had experience monitoring autonomic functions and, to a degree, regulating vegetative behaviors. These capabilities are evidenced by fetal responses to hypoxemia or hypoglycemia, such as changes in activity, heart rate, and blood pressure.

In extrauterine life, nutrient intake must be derived independently from an outside source. Two primary changes in feeding occur: route of intake and pattern of intake. The neonate must switch to oral intake, which is achieved through sucking. In the uterus, the fetus has had sucking and feeding experiences in which amniotic fluid has been ingested, but the fetus has not needed to coordinate breathing with sucking and swallowing (see Chapter 12). Second, neonatal feeding is periodic, rather than the continuous supply of nutrients provided to the fetus. Hunger, thirst, and satiety centers must regulate food intake and the neonate must exhibit appropriate hunger cues to elicit feeding from the caregiver and must be able to end feeding with cues indicating satiety.

In the uterus the fetal temperature varies little. Thus, a major challenge at the time of birth is initiation of thermoregulation. Although thermoregulatory abilities begin at approximately 30 weeks' gestation, the fetus has not been required to independently monitor body temperature and adjust metabolic rate to meet thermal needs (see Chapter 20).

Motor Functions

Beginning early in fetal development, skeletal muscles are involved in movement. These experiences with motor activities provide a means of promoting motor development as well as an opportunity to test out motor innervation. Within the uterus, however, motor activities are enacted in an environment that reduces the effects of gravity and provides confinement. The buoyant amniotic fluid and uterine walls are replaced by the extrauterine environment, in which motion is not confined and gravity has a greater effect. Although movements of the fetus may have been smooth and limited in scale, movements of the neonate are often erratic or flailing. The neonate must exert energy to maintain body position against the pull of gravity.

Sensory Functions

The sensory input provided by the extrauterine environment is markedly different from that of the uterus. Before looking at these differences, however, it is important to recognize the sensory experience of birth itself. Although the fetus has experienced Braxton-Hicks contractions, the steady, rhythmic contractions of the uterus and resultant pressure changes are a new experience. The continuous flow of oxygen and nutrients through the placenta may be altered during contractions, providing intense autonomic input. The descent into the birth canal increases pressure, perhaps to the degree of being uncomfortable. During labor, the mother's activity pattern may change and the sounds from the mother's body may be altered, such as rapid or heavy breathing or heart rate increase. Concurrent with the experiences of labor, changes in the extrauterine environment (e.g., noise) may be sensed by the infant. It would seem that the process of birth is one of being bombarded with stimuli. After birth a number of new sensory experiences await. In general, sensations in the extrauterine environment are different in nature, more intense, and lack the pattern experienced in the intrauterine environment.

Whereas the uterus is dark, the extrauterine environment provides more, often intense light in the immediate postbirth period. In the uterus, the fetus was bathed in amniotic fluid that exhibited rare temperature variation, but the extrauterine environment is much cooler and can exhibit great variability. Until birth the fetus has never experienced cold stimulation. In the intrauterine environment, the sounds were relatively constant and rhythmical. Sounds from the mother's environment did reach the fetus, but were muted to a degree by body tissue and the amniotic fluid. The sounds in the external environment vary from silence to an overwhelming din and include many new sounds the neonate has not previously experienced.

For the fetus, touch consisted of warm amniotic fluid and the smooth wall of the uterus. After birth, for the first time the newborn infant has dry skin. Forms of touch increase dramatically after birth, including input from handling, stroking, rubbing, and possibly pain. The newborn has never worn clothing; even the touch of fabric against the skin is a new sensation. Taste sensations had been limited to amniotic fluid ingested in utero, and breast milk, formula, and possibly oral medications provide new taste and smell experiences. Breast odors are preferred from birth.

Sleep-Wake Pattern

After birth the neonate must manage sleep and activity patterns. Caregivers are important timekeepers for the neonate, but infants and their mothers may be separated. In animals, the mother has an important influence on establishing biorhythms in her offspring. There is evidence that state organization is disturbed in the first few days after birth; there may be increased alertness in the first few days, followed by the infant's beginning to establish his or her own individual pattern.[91]

Neural Connections and Conduction of Impulses

Gestational age determines the level of brain maturation, including acquisition of neuronal component, dendritic and axonal branching, formation of connections between neurons, and myelinization. Although at term gestation most neurons have formed and migrated to their respective sites, a number of cerebellar neurons are completing this process and are at particular risk during hypoxic-ischemic events. For the preterm infant, depending on the degree of prematurity, the extrauterine environment poses risks for the developing brain.

Although the elaboration of dendritic and axonal branches and connections between neurons begins in fetal life, these processes continue into adulthood. The ability of a neuron to change structure and function has been called *plasticity*. The more immature the infant is at birth, the greater the impact of central nervous system (CNS) plasticity (see Neural [Brain] Plasticity). There is considerable evidence in animal studies that sensory input influences later neuronal structure and function. In human infants, a rich environment during infancy improves developmental outcome by maximizing brain potential. This plasticity is both an advantage and a liability. Although sensory input may increase cellular processes and interconnections, the sensory environment may also produce undesired changes in structure and function.[21,44,55,111] The preterm infant in the neonatal intensive care unit may be particularly vulnerable to these alterations.

Myelinization occurs predominantly in fetal and infant life but continues through the fourth decade and beyond. Brain areas governing high-level functions myelinate later in life. In the fetus and infant, myelinization involves both sensory and motor fibers and pathways. The primary effect of myelinization is on speed of transmission or conduction, because the presence of myelin insulates the nerve fiber, increasing conduction rate. Because myelin is being laid down at varying rates throughout the central and peripheral nervous systems, rate of conduction potentially affects the integration of sensory information and effector response. In terms of sensory perception, the difference in conduction speed (msec) is not appreciable at the conscious level; however, even seemingly minor differences in transmission have an impact on integration of information. Speed of transmission is important in spatial (number of impulses coming into the CNS from various sites) and temporal (rapidity with which impulses are being sent) summation. Thus systems in which summation is required for neuronal firing may react less quickly. Conduction rate is inversely related to postmenstrual age, becoming similar to that in adults by 3 to 4 years.[249]

Circulation in the Neonatal Brain

The brain of the neonate demonstrates differences in circulation compared with that of the adult. These differences produce vulnerability to damage by hypoxemia and pressure.

Blood-Brain Barrier

Early in embryonic life, circulation is conducted by a rudimentary capillary network. Development is accompanied by proliferation of blood vessels, increasing the blood supply to meet the increasing metabolic demands of the growing CNS. The complexity of the brain's vascular system increases in the last trimester. There is a rapid increase in the number and size of cerebral blood vessels after 26 weeks, peaking by 35 weeks.[100] Developmental aspects of blood brain barrier properties, which include anatomic, transport, and metabolic functions, are summarized in Table 15-11.

Sources of the anatomic blood-brain barrier include the tight junctions between the endothelial cells forming the capillaries, which limit diffusion of substances into the brain tissue; the basement membrane of the endothelial cells; and the astrocyte foot processes surrounding the capillary, which help to maintain the integrity of the barrier.[48,42] In the fetus and neonate, the tight junction between the capillary endothelial cells is not as well formed as that of the adult. However, the tight junctions develop early and are probably quite effective barriers to proteins, but are probably more permeable to small lipid-soluble molecules.[42,214] Endothelial tight junctions can be altered by hypoosmolar conditions, hypercarbia, asphyxia, and intracranial infection leading to vasculitis with increased permeability and potential for rupture.[249] A second component of the blood-brain barrier is the basement membrane supporting capillary endothelial cells. In the neonate and infant this basement membrane is not fully developed.[70] Additionally, the astrocyte feet, which normally surround the capillary, are not completely developed in the neonate. These three alterations in the blood-brain barrier predispose to capillary leakage and hemorrhage. Because cellular junctions are not well formed, the brain capillaries are sensitive to osmolar (and hence volume) changes of the blood.

Cerebral Autoregulation

Cerebral blood flow (CBF) is regulated by both systemic factors (e.g., $PaCO_2$, pH, PaO_2, and blood glucose) and autoregulation. *Cerebral autoregulation* refers to the local control

Table 15-11 Maturation of the Blood-Brain Barrier

BARRIER PROPERTY	DEVELOPMENTAL CHANGE
ANATOMIC	
Endothelial-astrocyte association	↑
Complexity of interendothelial tight junction	↑
Interendothelial clefts	↓↓
Endothelial fenestrations	↓↓
Vesicular transports	↓↓ (?)
Basement membrane	↑
TRANSPORT SYSTEMS	
Large neutral amino acid transporter (LAT1)	↓
Small neutral amino acid transporter (AIA2)	↑↑
Hexose transporter (GLUT1)	↑
Amine	↓
Monocarboxylic acid transporter (MCT1)	↓
Insulin	↓
METABOLISM	
Aromatic amino acid decarboxylase	↑
Monoamine oxidase	↑
γ-Glutamyl transpeptidase	↑
Alkaline phosphatase	↓

From Laterra, J. & Goldstem, G.W. (2004). Development of the blood-brain barrier. In R.A. Polin, W.W. Fox, & S.H. Abman (Eds.), *Fetal and neonatal physiology* (3rd ed.). Philadelphia: Saunders, p. 1699.

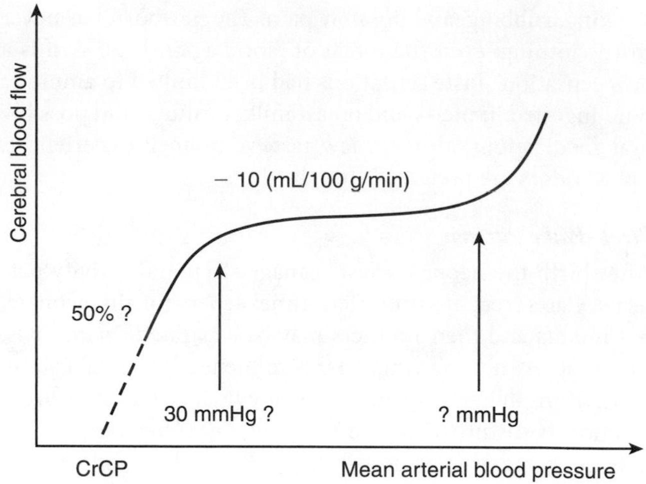

FIGURE 15-10 A schematic drawing of the blood flow/mean arterial pressure relation of the normal cerebral circulation in a preterm newborn infant. The flat portion represents the autoregulatory plateau. Below the lower threshold, blood flow falls more than in proportion to pressure. The critical closing pressure (CrCP) depends on the intracranial pressure and on arterial elasticity. The lower threshold is 30 mmHg (3.99 kPa) or less. There are no good estimates of the upper threshold, although it is assumed that the ischemic threshold is around 50% of resting blood flow. (From Greisen, G. [1997]. Cerebral blood flow and energy metabolism in the newborn. *Clin Perinatol, 24,* 424.)

of brain blood flow, modifying resistance to compensate for changes in pressure, thus sustaining consistent flow over a range of pressures.[82] In adults, cerebral blood flow is constant from an arterial pressure of 50 to 175 mmHg (6.65 to 23.75 kPa).[190] Cerebral autoregulation is mediated by vasoactive factors such as H^+ and K^+ ions, adenosine, prostaglandins, osmolality, and calcium.[249] These factors are all operative in the neonate.[89,201,249] The autoregulatory capabilities of the fetal and neonatal brain are limited, although pressure flow autoregulation is present even in very low–birth weight (VLBW) infants.[87] The range (specific figures have not been determined) for cerebral autoregulation is narrower in the newborn, who is less able to limit CBF with hypertension (Figure 15-10).[100,190] In utero this is not a severe limitation, in that metabolic demands of the brain are less and the cardiovascular system is not required to act independently. In the neonate, however, restriction of autoregulation predisposes the neonate to inadequate or excess pressure, resulting in too little or too much blood flow. Consequences are risk of bleeding from vascular rupture, increased intracranial pressure, and hypoxia/ischemia.

Cerebral perfusion pressure is a function of gestational age, and CBF increases with maturation.[249] Compared with that in the adult, however, cerebral perfusion pressure is low in the term infant and even lower in the preterm infant. Preterm infants have an extremely narrow range of autoregulation. Normal blood pressure in the preterm infant is slightly above the lower limit of autoregulation (approximately 30 mmHg [3.99 kPa], although a mean of 23 ± 11 mmHg [3.05 ± 1.46 kPa] has also been reported).[88,100,249] Thus in the preterm infant, CBF is close to the level at which oxygen and nutrient delivery is potentially compromised.[87,249]

Low CBF and limited autoregulation combine to place the neonate in a position where there is a fine balance between cerebral ischemia and potential rupture of vessels or increased intracranial pressure.[100] The lower the gestational age, the greater the vulnerability.[249] Autoregulation additionally exhibits a lag in responsiveness. A sudden intense rise or drop in cerebral blood pressure or flow may not be immediately controlled through autoregulatory efforts.

By itself, autoregulation of CBF creates a high-risk situation that is magnified by the influence of hypoxemia. Hypoxemia abolishes autoregulation.[249] Thus during hypoxemia, CBF becomes pressure-passive. Autoregulation is further influenced by hypercarbia and acidosis, conditions that frequently occur in conjunction with hypoxemia. The nature of respiration in preterm infants predisposes to hypoxemia, hypercarbia, and acidosis. Because autoregulation exhibits a lag, even transient alterations in oxygen and carbon dioxide can have deleterious results as autoregulation is compromised.

Effects of autoregulation are a consequence of alterations in cerebral blood pressure and flow. Pressure, resistance, and flow are related physical processes. When blood flow is pressure-passive, a rise in blood pressure produces an increase in flow. The fragile capillaries of the immature brain possess neither tight junctions between endothelial cells nor a strong basement membrane; therefore increased blood pressure and flow increase intracranial pressure. This increased pressure and flow may rupture the delicate capillaries, leading to bleeding.

Impairment of autoregulation may also produce damage through inability to respond to low blood pressure. Under normal circumstances, cerebral perfusion in the neonate is marginally adequate. Given any reduction in blood pressure, autoregulatory abilities do not support maintenance of blood flow. As a result, reduction in blood pressure may reduce cerebral perfusion, producing ischemia and hypoxia and damage to brain tissue. Hypoxia is therefore a critical concern because brain tissue may be injured by lack of oxygen as well as a reduction in CBF.

The nature of the distribution of the vascular system in the brain and the different types of tissues (white or gray matter) are associated with risk for hypoxic damage. Blood flow is linked to metabolism. Gray matter has a higher metabolic rate than does white matter; consequently, perfusion of gray matter exceeds that of white matter.[249] The lower blood flow in white matter predisposes this form of nervous tissue to the effects of limited autoregulation and hypoxemia.[249] An area in the neonate that is particularly vulnerable to pressure- and hypoxia-related injury is the periventricular white matter. The subependymal germinal matrix layer, located in ventricular and subventricular areas, has a dense capillary network. The immaturity of the vasculature and extracellular matrix in this area increases the risk for hemorrhage, although the role of impaired autoregulation in the pathogenesis of intraventricular hemorrhage in the preterm infant is unclear.[82]

Neonatal Sensory Function

In general, the rate of nerve transmission continues to increase with postmenstrual age. Evidence from animal experiments suggests that active use of sensory receptors and pathways is required for further development. Sensory deprivation results in degeneration of neural structures, leading to permanent damage and long-term implications for sensory function. In most circumstances, however, sensory deprivation does not occur. Sensory stimulation that is excessive and the quality and pattern of stimulation that is inappropriate for the neonate may also alter sensory system development.

A second consideration is the need for attention as a prerequisite for sensory input. The neonate's level of alertness and arousal determines attention to sensory stimulation. Thus any condition affecting neurologic control of alertness interferes with reception and processing of sensory input. The autonomic nervous system mediates responsiveness to the external environment. Alertness and arousal are functions of the infant's sleep-wake patterns or state, as well as the infant's physiologic status. Sensory input must always be considered in light of the infant's state.

Sensory Modalities

Neonates possess well-developed sensitivity to vestibular and kinesthetic stimulation. Rocking motions produce soothing and quieting of the neonate and infant. Use of vestibular stimulation with preterm infants has been associated with increased rhythmicity and organization, decreased apnea, improved weight gain, sleep promotion, and increased alertness and attention.[22] Somatosensory evoked responses to median nerve stimulation can be measured from at least 7 months' gestation (meaning that "the somatosensory pathways can conduct impulses to the cortex and that the cortex is developed enough to produce the responses"), although latency is increased with a smaller and wider response.[193]

The term neonate can detect, localize, and discriminate various distinct odorants and respond to noxious odors. Neonates and infants can differentiate breast pads soaked with their mother's breast milk from those soaked with water or other substances. They habituate to repeated presentation of the same odor and show a preference for odors associated with positive reinforcements.[136,256] Term neonates exhibit a preference for sweet taste, showing aversion to sour or bitter tastes, and can differentiate between tastes.[240,256] Newborns are most responsive to sweet and sour tastes, less to bitter, and they show little response to salty taste.[16,54] Preterm infants respond to taste and smell by 26 to 27 weeks' gestational age and possibly earlier, in that this has not been extensively studied.[43] Flavors in breast milk reflect the maternal diet and may play a role in programing later dietary preferences.[16,164]

Term newborns can hear and discriminate sounds (see Table 15-9). Hearing acuity is best in the low and mid-range frequencies, with high-frequency selective hearing developing in later infancy.[191,255] Additionally, hearing sensitivity increases and hearing threshold decreases with development.[191] Term infants differentiate among complex sounds, although with less sensitivity than adults, attending to sounds of interest and showing aversion to noxious sounds, and may have a preference for speech sounds to which they were exposed in utero.[133] They can distinguish their mothers' voices and preferentially turn toward the direction of the mother's voice.[85] Neonates and infants demonstrate a preference for high intonation and the rhythmic, sing-song vocalization that is called "motherese." The auditory system in preterm infants prior to 34 weeks' gestation is characterized by rapid maturation of the cochlea and auditory nerve. Environmental noise may alter development and tuning of the cochlea during this time. Responses to sounds tend to rapidly fatigue. They can hear sounds as soft as about 40 dB. Preterm infants are at risk for both conductive (problems with transmission of sound to cochlea) and sensorineural (damage to inner ear and auditory nerve) hearing loss as well as auditory processing deficits. Auditory capabilities of VLBW infants are discussed further on p. 535 and summarized in Table 15-9.

Although vision in the term neonate is qualitatively different from that of the adult, the visual abilities of these infants are adept. Visual function depends on development of visual pathways, the lateral geniculate nucleus (LGN) in the thalamus and linkages between the LGN and the visual cortex.[32] The LGN is immature at birth with a rapid increase in synaptogenesis within the visual cortex after birth and in linkages between the many sections of the visual cortex.[30,32] Vision is functional at birth, but marked changes occur in the first 2 years of life.[63] The retina continues to mature after birth. The fovea, the most sensitive area of the retina and associated with high-level discrimination, is not as sensitive in the neonate as in adults.[80,92] Newborns are myopic (20/400).[63] The neonate's limited accommodation ability decreases the ability to focus on objects that are extremely close to or far from the face. Accommodation improves during the first 3 months of life.[92] Visual acuity is only 1/40 of that of adults.[118] Infants see objects to a distance of at least 2½ feet but attend best to objects that are within 8 to 12 inches from their eyes and have high contrast or contours.[92] Neonates can follow movement of an object. Visual function in term infants is summarized in Table 15-10).

Preterm infants demonstrate pupillary light responses and blinking to light by 29 weeks' gestation with awake visual attention by 30 weeks. These infants fix briefly on the human face after 26 weeks and on simple patterns by 30 weeks' gestation, and demonstrate pattern preferences by 31 to 32 weeks. Visual scanning with cessation of sucking is seen from 30 weeks and is active after 36 weeks.[91,133,249] Preterm infants take longer to fixate on an object and are less responsive to visual stimuli than term infants and have poorer visual acuity and ability to accommodate. Most of the visual stimuli to which VLBW infants are exposed during their brief awake states are probably inappropriate to the infants' visual capabilities.[22,91] Visual capabilities of VLBW infants are discussed further on p. 536 and summarized in Table 15-10. Structural and growth alterations of the eye are seen in higher incidence in preterm infants, including retinopathy of prematurity (ROP), strabismus, myopia, amblyopia, and astigmatism.[32] Myopia is a common finding in children with regressed ROP. Alterations in vision function (visual acuity, color vision, contrast sensitivity, problems with visual processing, visual attention, pattern discrimination, visual recognition memory, and visual-motor integration) are also seen in preterm infants.

Sensory Processing

The neonate is readily capable of receiving sensory information. The neonate also demonstrates the ability to discriminate sensory information and to attend to sensory input. Knowledge of the neonate's sensory reception abilities must be balanced with appreciation of sensory processing abilities, since in this area the neonate demonstrates developmental differences within the nervous system that have implications for long-term outcomes. Although reception of sensory input is grossly intact, the ability to process information and respond in an organized fashion is limited. Adaptation, habituation, and inhibition limit responsiveness to stimuli; without these processes, people would be bombarded with input. In the brain of the neonate, the structures and processes that underlie the ability to modulate sensory input are not well developed.

The neonate's brain continues to develop connections between neurons and to lay down myelin. The degree of connectedness between neurons and speed of electrical conduction affect integration and organization of overall nervous system function. Behaviors of the neonate reflect these underlying maturational differences in the CNS. Neonates may exhibit differences in arousability, the extensiveness of responses, attention, tolerance to stimulation, soothability, regularity of state, motor tone, activity, synchrony, and rhythmicity.[6,58] Although stimulation is required for normal development, the neonate can also be overwhelmed by sensory input because of the level of brain development. Just as environmental temperature for the neonate must be neither too warm nor too cool, so too the sensory input for a neonate must be balanced to the infant's individual needs and tolerance. Provision of a developmentally appropriate sensory environment is based on "stimuli that have sensory or affective properties that are consistent with developmental capabilities and thus most likely to be appropriately incorporated into neural processes."[55] For extremely immature infants, this means delaying auditory and visual input until the infant is stable and has more mature neurosensory capabilities.[22] Studies with animal models demonstrate that out-of-sequence stimulation of one system interferes with development of not only that system but also other systems that are still immature.[23,84,143,144] For example, inappropriate visual stimulation while hearing and vision are still developing may alter not only vision but also hearing development.[23,81,84,143,144]

Neural (Brain) Plasticity

The brain changes in response to external experiences (plasticity) and changing environments. Development involves gene-environment interaction. The environment affects how genes work and genes affect how environment is interpreted. Neuronal differentiation and organization are controlled by the interaction of genes and the environment. Animal studies demonstrate that environmental input influences the fate and neural capabilities at the cellular level both before and after birth. Permanent alterations in neuronal networks, wiring, function, and behavior may arise with exposure to early inappropriate sensory input.[83,144,147,226] During early infancy there is rapid growth, differentiation, and organization of neurons, axons, dendrites, and synapses with a surge in brain connectivity and efficiency of neuronal circuitry.[147,249] These changes are due to "interplay between a predetermined genetic program and the modifications of positive and negative environmental influences."[147]

Each neuron has many synaptic connections that allow the brain to integrate and organize information. Initially there is an overproduction of neurons and nerve connections. Many of the extra neurons and connections are later eliminated based on early environment and experiences.[21,55,174] The brain is thought to strengthen and retain connections that are used repeatedly and is more likely to eliminate underused connections. Thus improper sensory input (too much or too little) or input that is inappropriate in terms of timing may alter brain development.[21] The environment of immature infants in the neonatal intensive care unit (NICU) and in the early months following discharge is critical for brain development and later cognitive function.[144,147,226] The brain in the neonate is still under construction with enhanced plasticity. During this time there are periods when development is particularly sensitive to experience or environmental influences. "Enhanced plasticity of the developing brain allows it to be influenced more strongly by the environment, than is the adult brain. However, this increased plasticity also creates selective brain vulnerability [and is more sensitive to deprivation]."[147,p. 94]

Greenough and Black postulated two types of neural plasticity: experience-expectant and experience-dependent.[21,86] Experience-expectant plasticity is thought to be linked to the brain developmental timetable; that is, specific sensory experiences and input are needed at specific times for neural development and maturation. This stage requires appropriate timing and quality of input for normal development. Thus altered sequences or types of sensory inputs can alter or disrupt development. Experience-dependent plasticity involves interaction with the environment to develop specific skills for later use. This form of plasticity involves memory and learning and allows development of flexibility, adaptation, and individual differences in social and intellectual development.[21,86]

Neonatal Motor Function

Movement may be reflexive or volitional in nature. In adults, as in neonates, volitional motor activity entails movement under the control of the cortex and other higher-level control. In the neonate, however, control of motor function is emerging and demonstrates increasing integration and organization of the CNS. Reflexes in the neonates are somewhat different from those seen in the adult. Some of the reflexes exhibited by the neonate reflect both development of the muscles themselves as well as CNS control. Additionally, some reflexes normally observed only in the neonate and infant indicate the effects of development on motor control mechanisms. In general, motor activities include muscle tone, motor abilities, the quality of movement, and presence and strength of reflexes.[73] Motor control is critical to further development. Through movement and reflexes, infants are capable of expressing needs, eliciting care, taking in oral nutrients, and experiencing and manipulating their environment.

Muscle Development

The motor abilities of the neonate demonstrate a characteristic pattern of development that reflects underlying changes in both nervous system control and maturation of the muscle cells themselves. Muscle is derived from mesoderm. During embryonic development, formation of muscle cells is dependent on innervation by the nervous system. The full complement of muscle cells is generally achieved at approximately 38 weeks' gestational age, with formation of few muscle cells after this time. After birth, muscle cells increase in size by increasing the diameter of the muscle fibers and also grow in length.[173] Muscle strength in particular is an outcome of muscle enlargement and growth.

Developmental changes in the innervation of muscle include myelinization of afferent fibers and pathways; increasing activity in the motor cortex; and increasing coordination of system-modifying motor actions within the cerebellum, basal ganglia, and reticular activating system. Myelinization improves the speed of motor nerve conduction. Maturation of the motor cortex allows conscious control of motor activities. The increasing integration of all levels of motor control results in smooth, coordinated movements; balance; and appropriate motor tone. Neonates exhibit a characteristic pattern of tone and flexion that undergoes predictable change throughout development.

The term neonate demonstrates strong muscle tone, which is largely passive.[249] After birth, active motor tone, which is the tone during use of muscles, increases and passive tone decreases. Alterations in muscle tone interfere with motor activities. Hypertonicity (excessive muscle tone) and hypotonicity (inadequate muscle tone) affect the underlying muscle tension that normally supports motor function. The predominant flexed position of the term neonate shows innervation of flexor muscles and reciprocal relaxation of extensor muscles. The flexed position is not only protective but also assists in conservation of energy by reducing motor movements and assists in thermoregulation by reducing the surface area for heat loss. Motor development entails inhibition of flexion and increasing extensor activity. These changes occur in part because of increasing control by the motor cortex. When cortical innervation is interrupted, as in pathologic conditions, loss of extensor innervation results in flexion. Increasing sophistication of control by the CNS improves coordination of movement, control and accuracy of movement, and synchrony and rhythmicity of movement. These capabilities support ongoing motor development including head control, turning over, reaching, and grasping.

Neonatal Reflexes

Reflexes are automatic, built-in motor behaviors occurring at the spinal level. Reflexes therefore provide information about muscle tone and lower level motor function. Reflexes serve many neonatal needs in interacting with the extrauterine environment and provide valuable information regarding the neonate's motor and neural status. Although reflexes are automatic rather than volitional, the reflexive responses of the neonate provide evidence to parents and other caregivers of the neonate's motor capabilities, responsiveness, and individual needs. The development and strength of reflexes vary with gestational age.

Many reflexes characteristic to the neonate seemingly disappear with development. Some reflexes (such as the Babinski reflex) are masked by higher-order functions but are observed in the adult when pathologic conditions interfere with higher-level control. Other reflexes considered abnormal in the adult are seen in the neonate. For instance, clonus of the knee and ankle is commonly observed in the neonate, as is the Babinski reflex.

The Moro reflex involves abduction of the arms at the shoulder with the elbows in extension and the hands open, followed by adduction of the arms at the shoulder into an embrace position with flexion of the elbows. Crying often accompanies the Moro reflex. Portions of the Moro reflex can be observed as early as 28 weeks' gestational age, with a mature reflex seen at approximately 36 to 37 weeks.[10]

Neonates exhibit a strong palmar grasp reflex with fingers tightly flexed and curled into the palm. The palmar grasp reflex is so strong that infants can grasp, although not consciously, items placed in the hand. The palmar grasp may also be assessed in the pull-to-sit maneuver. Although the palmar grasp is first observed at approximately 28 weeks' gestational age, full strength is not achieved until approximately 32 weeks.[10]

The tonic neck reflex (also termed the *fencing position*) is stimulated by rotation of the head to the side. The reflex movements include extension of the arm and leg on the side to which the head is turned, and flexion of the arm and leg on the side opposite to which the head is turned. The movements of the extremities are similar to the crossed extensor reflex. Portions of the tonic neck reflex appear during later fetal development, but the reflex is often not well established until several weeks after birth.[249] Like the Moro reflex, the tonic neck reflex stabilizes position, preventing rolling.

Neonates demonstrate a rhythmic stepping motion of their lower extremities. When the neonate is held upright with the feet touching a solid surface, an alternating stepping motion is observed. There is some evidence that coordination exhibited in the stepping reflex may be predictive of later developmental outcomes.

The sucking and rooting reflexes are essential for oral intake of nutrients by the neonate. Rooting assists the neonate in locating and latching on to the nipple and occurs at about 32 weeks' gestation. Stimulation of the perioral region results in turning of the head in the direction of the stimulus and mouthing actions in search of the nipple. The sucking reflex is present at 28 weeks' gestation, but is weak and uncoordinated with swallowing. Some suck-swallow synchrony is seen by 32 to 34 weeks, and synchrony is complete by 36 to 38 weeks.[10]

Sleep-Wake Pattern

Fetal activity records document fluctuating periods of activity and quiescence that increase in duration and regularity from midgestation to term.[186] After birth the infant exhibits alternating periods of sleep and wakefulness that initially reflect fetal activity/inactivity patterns. Sleep in neonates and infants exhibits developmental differences from that of the adult. As a result, sleep is not as well defined and definitions are less precise than in the adult. Consequently, neonatal and infant sleep is described in terms of state—that is, a group of physiologic and behavioral characteristics that regularly recur together.[22]

Neonates and young infants spend a large portion of the 24-hour day sleeping. Sleep therefore does not initially follow a light-dark pattern and is not diurnal, as in the adult. A major accomplishment in the development of the infant is the ability to sleep through the night and adapt to the diurnal pattern of activity and sleep-wake behaviors of the family. The sleep-wake pattern is an indicator of neurologic status and the neonate's ability to organize behavior.

Definition of Infant States

A number of systems have been developed to code or score neonatal and infant sleep-wake states. The major difference between conventional definitions of infant states is the number of subtypes of states and therefore the specificity and precision of the various states. Generally, the more immature the neonate is according to gestational and postmenstrual age, the grosser or less precise the definitions of state, because the quality of state and consistency among indicators improve with age. The six categories of infant state described by Wolff and Brazelton are discussed here.[31,257] Each state is complete unto itself, representing a particular form of neural control. The six sleep-wake states are as follows: quiet (deep) sleep, active (light) sleep, drowsy, awake (quiet) alert, active alert, and crying. The ability to clearly differentiate these states is dependent on the infant's postmenstrual age. The proportion of time spent in each of these states also varies with postmenstrual age. Immature infants in particular have what is termed *intermediate sleep* in which electroencephalographic (EEG), physiologic, and behavioral parameters meet neither active nor quiet sleep criteria.[47]

Quiet (deep or NREM) sleep is deep, restful sleep with the eyes closed, little body or facial movement, except for an occasional startle or twitch, regular respiration and heart rate, and no movement of the eyes.[185] Quiet sleep is restorative and anabolic. An increase in cell mitosis and replication occurs during this state. Oxygen consumption reaches the lowest levels during quiet sleep. In addition, the release of growth hormone is associated with quiet sleep, as are high levels of serotonin and low levels of glucocorticoid.

During active (light) sleep, the eyes are closed but there are movements of the extremities and face, mouthing, grimacing, and sucking movements. Respiration and heart rate are irregular and penile erections occur. Active bouts of REM occur in association with dreaming; the fine, rapid movement of the eyes can be observed beneath the lid. Active sleep is also called *paradoxical sleep* or *REM sleep* and has been likened to "wide-awake asleep" because the level of brain activity is similar to that of the awake state. Information is processed during active sleep and entered into memory; thus active sleep has been linked to learning. Restructuring of synapses and changes in protein synthesis increase during active sleep.

During the drowsy state, the infant seems partially awake and partially asleep. Drowsiness usually indicates a state transition between awake and sleep states. In the quiet alert state, the infant is awake, the eyes are open, and there is little motor movement. The infant is alert and shows interest or attention by focusing on visual stimulation. The infant appears to be "drinking in" information from the surrounding environment and processing this information. This state is characterized by limited motion and activity associated with the infant attending to sensory information.

The neonate or infant's motor activity escalates in the active awake state. The eyes are less bright than in the quiet alert state. There may be spitting up or hiccoughing. Respiration often becomes increased and irregular and skin color changes may occur. The active alert state often precedes crying. In healthy infants, crying is easily recognizable. Crying behaviors include closed eyes with facial characteristics and the vocalization of cry sounds. In preterm infants the motor actions associated with cry sounds are evident, but because of the infant's immaturity and weakness, the sounds may be weak or absent.

Sleep-Wake States Related to Brain Maturation

Sleep is required for brain development. "Sleep is not merely a state of rest but also is a period of intense brain activity involving higher cortical functions."[47] Sleep-wake patterns change with CNS maturation. Postnatal development of the sleep-wake state pattern reflects the underlying maturation of the reticular activating system, brainstem, and related circadian rhythms. The developmental changes in state include both alterations in temporal pattern and the integration of variables within the state. Inhibitory ability increases with CNS maturation. Increased inhibitory ability results in smoother muscle movements, reduces global responses, improves habituation and adaptation, and generally acts to improve the infant's attentional abilities as well as bring about specific changes in sleep. These sleep changes include increasing duration of sleep periods, consolidation of sleep into nighttime hours, and maturation of the sleep states themselves. Within each state, synchrony among the state variables increases.

Infant development entails increasing amounts of quiet sleep as well as increasing periods of quiet alertness. Both of these states reflect sophisticated neural control. Sustaining a state consistently or making a transition from one state to another requires tremendous neural organization. Thus sleep-wake patterns are an excellent window to the infant's neurologic status. Alterations in sleep-wake patterns are observed in infants with Down syndrome, biochemical disturbances, and brain malformations, and following asphyxia.[91]

Sleep is necessary for somatic and brain growth and development. As described earlier, restorative and growth processes are facilitated during quiet sleep. REM sleep is important for learning and memory. Attention behavior development parallels development of quiet sleep, indicating both inhibition and maturity.[185] The amount of quiet awake time parallels quiet sleep, and both increase with development.[91]

Development of Infant States

Before 28 to 30 weeks' gestational age, the preterm infant shows minimal pattern of state activity either by behavioral or EEG characteristics. Active or (REM) sleep appears at 28 to 30 weeks' gestation with evidence of cycling of states at 32 weeks.[58,91] Well-developed quiet sleep appears much later in development, initially becoming apparent at approximately 36 weeks of gestational age.[185] With maturation, intermediate or transitional sleep decreases, accompanied by an increase in quiet sleep; active sleep stays relatively stable.[170,249] General trends in sleep development include increasing quiet sleep, decreasing active sleep, and putting sleep cycles together consecutively, which yields longer sleep periods.[110]

The EEG of the infant is not always consistent with the behavioral expression of state. State is evidenced behaviorally before it is apparent on the EEG. Before 30 weeks' gestation, EEG activity is present but is discontinuous and of low amplitude. At 30 to 36 weeks' gestational age, active sleep can be determined by EEG.[249] Between 36 and 40 weeks' gestational age, both active and quiet sleep can be determined by EEG. Maturation of EEG activity includes differentiation of discontinuous activity into mature EEG waveforms and an increase in the amplitude of EEG waves.[170] The EEG of the newborn frequently shows paroxysmal activity, asymmetry of the left and right portions of the brain, and considerable individual variation.[170]

Continued development of sleep-wake patterns after birth also involves changes in the temporal pattern of sleep and the integration of variables within states. In the first month, neonates sleep an average of 12 to 16 hours per day.[14] Periods of sleep occur around the clock. Periods of sleep are short, typically not extending beyond 3 or 4 hours. The sleep cycle is roughly 50 minutes, compared with the 90-minute adult sleep cycle. Sleep begins with active (REM) sleep versus NREM sleep in adults.[47] Initially, a sleep period may be only one to two cycles.[47] Over the first weeks, the amount of active sleep during the day decreases and active sleep increases during the nighttime hours.[186]

Circadian rhythmicity matures after birth with development of the sleep-wake rhythms and hormonal secretion prominent in the first 2 to 3 months.[205,220] Timing of sleep and wake is regulated by circadian clocks (entrained to light-dark cycles) and homeostatic processes (need for sleep after a certain time awake referred to as *sleep pressure*).[186] Homeostatic mechanisms are modified in early infancy; that is, infants spend relatively little time in waking before the need to sleep intervenes, thus sleep pressure accumulates more rapidly.[186] Evidence of a circadian sleep rhythm emerges at 5 to 6 weeks with progressive maturation over the next few months.[204] By 1 month, infants start to slowly shift toward more sleep at night than in the day, but they continue daytime napping for up to 4 to 5 years.[204]

State Modulation

Some infants seem to "sleep like babies," whereas some are difficult to soothe, awaken easily, and sleep for short intervals and at unpredictable times. Other infants are overly drowsy, difficult to arouse, and sleep excessive periods of time. Differences in sleep-wake patterns reflect differences in neurologic development and the infant's ability to modulate state. *State modulation* refers to the infant's ability to make smooth transitions between states, arouse when appropriate, and sustain sleep states. By modulating or regulating state, infants can control sensory input to some extent and modulate their responses to the environment.[31] In addition, the infant can use state behaviors to guide caregiving and to modify social interactions. Problems with state modulation, therefore, entail problems regulating sensory input and responses. Infants who cannot use state changes to turn stimulation on or off may be either missing important input or become sensory overloaded. State modulation is therefore an asset in the infant's adaptation to the environment. Problems with state modulation may emanate from the infant or environment. Infant factors influencing state modulation include immaturity, pain, stress, maternal substance abuse, and illness. Environmental factors that affect state regulation and interfere with the infant's sleep-wake pattern include noise, light, temperature, and caregiver actions.

Neurobehavioral Organization

The concept of neurobehavioral organization is a means of holistically viewing the infant's response capabilities. The connectedness between elements of the nervous system is the basis for integration and organization of overall function. Neurobehavioral organization captures the essence of neonatal and infant function in the extrauterine environment and determines the infant's interaction with the surrounding physical and social environment.

What does neurobehavioral organization encompass? Als's synactive theory of development defines five subsystems governing the infant's interaction with the environment: autonomic/physiologic, motor, state organizational, attentional/interactive, and self-regulatory capacity (synactivation is the process by which these fives subsystems interact and influence each other).[5] These subsystems are interdependent and hierarchical; that is, the order of development begins with autonomic/physiologic stability, followed in succession by motor, state, and attentional/interactive, and finally development of self-regulatory capacity. The level of organization is determined by development and is largely dependent on postmenstrual age; however, illness or injury may alter neurologic function and therefore neurobehavioral organization. In addition, organization at any level is determined by the previous levels. Thus, state organization is dependent on organization and stability of the motor and autonomic/physiologic subsystems; attentional/interactive behaviors require organization of the state, motor, and autonomic/physiologic subsystems. An infant's behavioral responses or cues are indicative of the level of organization.

Autonomic organization entails regulation of cardiorespiratory activity, gastrointestinal peristalsis, and peripheral skin blood flow. Motor organization includes skeletal muscle tone, posture, and quality of movement. State organization involves orderly progression of sleep-wake states, the ability to sustain a state, and smooth state transitions. The culmination of neurobehavioral organization is in the infant's attentional/interactive and self-regulatory abilities. The attentional/interactive subsystem involves the infant's ability to orient and focus on stimuli and achieve well-defined periods of alertness. Self-regulatory capacity is the ability of the infant to maintain integrity and balance between subsystems, integrate all the subsystems, and modulate state.[5]

Neurobehavioral organization thus refers to the ability to modulate state, control internal reactions, control motor responses, self-regulate, respond to people and events in the external environment, and maintain an appropriate degree of alertness.[31] Neurobehavioral organization is critical to energy consumption, oxygen and calorie requirements, and growth, as well as the foundation for development and interactions with parents and other caregivers. Components of neurobehavioral organization include the ability to regulate sensory input, feed efficiently and effectively, coordinate sucking and swallowing, self-console, exhibit smooth coordinated movement, maintain muscle tone, and elicit caregiving through appropriate cues. Tools to assess neurobehavioral organization rely on observation of the infant in interaction with both the physical and social environments. For example, the Newborn Behavioral Assessment Scale (NBAS) is an assessment of the infant's ability to organize and modulate states, habituate to external stimulation, regulate motor activity in the face of increasing sensory input, respond to reflexive testing, alert and orient to visual and auditory stimuli, interact with a caregiver, and self-console.[31] The Assessment of Preterm Infants' Behavior (APIB) is a neurobehavioral tool based on Als's synactive theory of development and geared to the assessment of the preterm infant and high-risk term infant.[7] The purpose of the APIB assessment is to determine how the infant is coping with the intense environment of the NICU and the degree of CNS organization.[7]

CLINICAL IMPLICATIONS FOR NEONATAL CARE

During the neonatal period, glial proliferation, myelinization, cell differentiation, dendrite expansion, and synapse formation and remodeling are occurring within the nervous system. The developing CNS is vulnerable to a number of influences, including the effects of the environment, handling, and caregiving. In addition, the immature CNS produces variations in seizure activity and influences the diagnosis and treatment of pain. These concerns are particularly important when considering the infant born prematurely, since development of the nervous system is not consistent with demands posed by the extrauterine environment. The preterm infant is usually a third trimester fetus, and, with the increasing survival of extremely premature infants, viability is extending into the second trimester.

Risks Posed by the Caregiving Environment

Healthy term infants are well equipped to adapt to life outside the uterus. When neonates are compromised by illness or prematurity, adaptive abilities are challenged. The extrauterine environment is a critical factor in the development of the immature CNS and may alter developmental outcomes. The hospital care environment has been viewed as providing a deficient or inappropriate sensory environment for the immature infant. Caregiving should always be individualized and based on recognition of infant cues (Table 15-12).[5,6,22] Emphasis has been placed on controlling the physical environment, including noise and light, and caregiving interactions such as pacing and individualizing caregiving to fit the infant's level of neurobehavioral maturation.[5,6,22,67,147,237]

Stability or engagement cues demonstrate organization and reflect the infant's readiness for interaction (see Table 15-12). Distress or disengagement cues (see Table 15-12) indicate disorganization and signal the caregiver to provide supportive measures and time for recuperation. Supportive measures include interventions such as positioning, environmental modifications, providing boundaries, swaddling, and reducing stressful stimuli.[5,22] The Neonatal Individualized Developmental Care and Assessment Program (NIDCAP) is a specialized training program for high-risk infant care providers that focuses on sensitive recognition of infant behavioral cues and individualized intervention strategies to promote and support neurobehavioral organization (http://www.nidcap.org/) in collaboration with families.[6]

Table 15-12 Infant Neurobehavioral Cues

DISTRESS/DISENGAGEMENT CUES	STABILITY/ENGAGEMENT CUES
Bradycardia, apnea	Facial gaze
Rapid heart or respiration rate	Smiling
Grunting	Vocalization
Stooling	Feeding posture
Mottled skin	Flexion of arms and legs
Dusky color	Eyes alert
Cyanosis	Stable heart rate
Tremor	Stable respiratory rate
Finger splay	Smooth movements
Fingers interlaced	Hand to mouth
Arching	Finger folding
Hyperalert face	Smooth state transitions
Facial grimace	Sucking and mouthing
Limb extension	Consolable
Gaze aversion	"Ooh" face
Eyes closed	Alert
Slack jaw	Eye-to-eye contact
Open mouth	Grasping
Tongue thrusting	
Sighing	
Regurgitation	
Jitteriness	
Flaccid	
Vomiting	
Hand to ear	
Worried face	
Rapid state change	
Eyes floating	
Staring	
Hyperextension	
Glassy eyed	
Tongue protrusion	
Flushed	
Hiccough	
Startle	
Yawn	
Flaccidity	
Sneezing	

Compiled from references 5, 6, 22, 176.

Vulnerability to Brain Injury in Preterm and Term Infants

Systemic hypoxemia and decreased cerebral perfusion leading to hypoxic-ischemic damage to the brain with hemorrhage and edema. The site of injury varies with maturational changes in the vascular anatomy and metabolic activity of the brain. In preterm infants, the neuropathology consists of multiple lesions including germinal matrix-intraventricular hemorrhage (IVH) that may include periventricular hemorrhagic infarction with posthemorrhagic hydrocephalus, and periventricular leukomalacia (PVL; *leukomalacia* refers to change in the brain's white matter reflective of softening) with accompanying neuronal/axonal abnormalities (referred to as the *encephalopathy of prematurity*).[249,252] PVL accompanied by neuronal and axonal alterations is the most common brain injury in preterm infants.[48,120,249,250,252] Preterm infants are also at increased risk for cerebellar injury.[146,148,166,249,250] Reductions in both gray and white matter volume are seen in preterm infants. These reductions are seen even without documented injury (PVL or IVH) and persist into childhood.[120] In term infants the site of injury usually involves the cerebral cortex with neuronal loss.[48] In older preterm and term infants, insults of this type result in hypoxic-ischemic encephalopathy (HIE) in the cerebral cortex and other areas.

Germinal Matrix and Intraventricular Hemorrhage

Germinal matrix hemorrhage (GMH) and intraventricular hemorrhage (IVH) are common forms of intracranial hemorrhage in the preterm infant. The consequences of intracranial hemorrhage include direct neuronal damage due to pressure and inflammation and the risk of developing posthemorrhagic hydrocephalus; severe hemorrhage may result in death.[249] Long-term outcomes are variable but include motor and sensory disabilities as well as cognitive delay.

The occurrence of GMH/IVH is related to structural and functional differences in the immature CNS, including the nature of the subependymal germinal matrix, differences in regulation of CBF, and venous pressure. The hemorrhage usually begins as a microvascular event that spreads, presumably due to overperfusion of the area. The site of GMH/IVH is developmentally related. In term infants IVH occurs predominantly in the ventricular choroid plexus and trauma is more often a precipitating factor.[249] In preterm infants, bleeding occurs more often in the subependymal germinal matrix located adjacent the lateral ventricles in the subependymal layer (GMH), with subsequent extension of the hemorrhage into the ventricles (IVH).[249] GMH in preterm infants occurs most often in the area of the caudate nucleus and foramen of Monro. Blood may also be found in the white matter with severe IVH because of an associated hypoxic-ischemic insult. The highest risk of GMH/IVH is during the period of germinal matrix prominence (i.e., in infants less than 34 weeks' gestation). The more immature the neonate is, the greater the risk of GMH/IVH.[249]

The germinal matrix is a highly cellular, high metabolic area characterized as gelatinous in structure.[249] The germinal matrix receives a rich blood supply chiefly through a large bed of irregular vessels (immature vascular rete) that are fragile due to a thin basement membrane and are prone to disruption.[100] In addition, the venous drainage in the area of the germinal matrix entails a distinctive U-shaped curve, and venous tributaries merge and flow into the vein of Galen, which is predisposed to stasis and increased venous pressure. After about 35 to 36 weeks, the germinal matrix involutes and the blood vessels become true capillaries.[100,142]

The physical characteristics of the germinal matrix, along with its highly vascular nature and potential limits in venous drainage, predispose to bleeding. These characteristics interact with cerebral autoregulation and the effects of hypoxia on autoregulation. During episodes of hypoxemia, autoregulation is abolished and blood flow becomes pressure-passive. Hypercarbia and acidosis also disrupt autoregulation. Thus any condition that reduces blood oxygen levels may alter autoregulation and contribute to the development of GMH/IVH. Although cardiorespiratory problems are easily recognized as sources of hypoxia, any factor that increases oxygen demand beyond the supply capabilities (i.e., increased metabolic rate) is also suspect in producing hypoxia, altered autoregulation, and GMH/IVH. Examples include thermoregulatory requirements, effects of handling, environmental disruptions, pain, or motor activity. During periods of pressure-passive flow, fragile capillaries of the germinal matrix may rupture if CBF or pressure increases. Once capillary disruption occurs, alterations in coagulation—which are thought to accompany perinatal complications—potentially perpetuate the hemorrhage.

Factors that produce fluctuating, decreased, or increased CBF also contribute to GMH/IVH.[25,249] If autoregulation of CBF is compromised, alterations in systemic blood pressure may also be causative factors. Examples of conditions thought to contribute to GMH/IVH include the pressure effects of ventilatory assistance, infusion of volume-expanding fluids, hypercarbia and other causes of cerebral vasodilation, increase in central venous pressure, or respiratory distress.[249]

Many of the health care procedures experienced by preterm infants (e.g., handling or suctioning) alter oxygen level and blood pressure. Research on the effects of procedures has shown that blood pressure initially drops, followed by a rise; the more intensive the care is, the greater the initial drop and the greater the rebound.[25] Prevention of GMH/IVH requires sensitivity regarding the fragile nature of the capillaries within the CNS and recognition of the effects of hypoxemia on autoregulation, as well as the role of autoregulation and pressure in cerebral perfusion.

White Matter Injury (Periventricular Leukomalacia)

White matter hypoxic-ischemic injury (WMI) is the most common severe neurologic insult seen in preterm infa nts.[48,51,249,252,253] The primary insult is destruction of brain tissue with injury to the cerebral white matter (PVL) usually accompanied by secondary developmental disturbances (associated axonal and neuronal alterations in gray matter).[48,120,249,250,252] PVL can involve both focal necrotic lesions deep in white matter with loss of all cellular elements and diffuse injury in central cerebral white matter with damage to pre-myelinating oligodendrocytes (pre-OL) that may delay or alter their maturation, astrogliosis, and microglia infiltration.[253] PVL focal lesions can be either a cystic form (lesions are several millimeters or more and evolve to cysts) or a noncystic form (lesions are microscopic and evolve to glial scars).[48,120,249,250,252] Noncystic PVL is the major form and is seen in 50% of VLBW infants; the cystic form of PVL is seen in less than 5%.[253] The associated axonal and neuronal alterations in the gray matter can affect multiple areas including cerebral white matter (axons and subplate neurons), thalamus, basal ganglia, cerebral cortex, cerebellum, and brainstem.[252,253] The pathogenesis of PVL is illustrated in Figure 15-11. Table 15-13 summarizes the mechanisms in the development of PVL and major maturation-dependent factors.

During peak vulnerability for PVL, cerebral white matter axons are undergoing rapid growth and synaptogenesis, and are vulnerable to damage.[53,132] Two principal neuron types are seen in the cerebral white matter at this time: subplate neurons (in subcortical white matter) and late-migrating GABAergic neurons (in central white matter).[53,250,252] Both types of neurons are critical for cerebral cortical and thalamic development.[53,252] Injury to the subplate neurons alters both afferent and efferent axons. Damage to afferent axons alters pre-OL generation and decreases cortical and thalamic development.[250] Damage to efferent axons alters cortical development.[250] Injury to the thalamus decreases axon generation and alters pre-OL development, myelinization, thalamic development, and cortical development.[256] Pre-OL damage in both cystic and noncystic PVL leads to inadequate myelin-producing oligodendrocytes and cerebral hypomyelinization.[48,253]

The brain is most vulnerable to WMI at 24 to 32 weeks' gestation when the white matter is immature and poorly vascularized.[48] WMI is associated with cerebral ischemia, altered cerebral autoregulation, infection/inflammation, and the vulnerability of the pre-OL in the VLBW infant (Table 15-13).[250,252,253] Necrotic changes subsequent to ischemia occur in the white matter in the area of the ventricles.[51,249] WMI may be seen in association with GMH/IVH, but it is a separate lesion that may occur in the absence of GMH/IVH.[23]

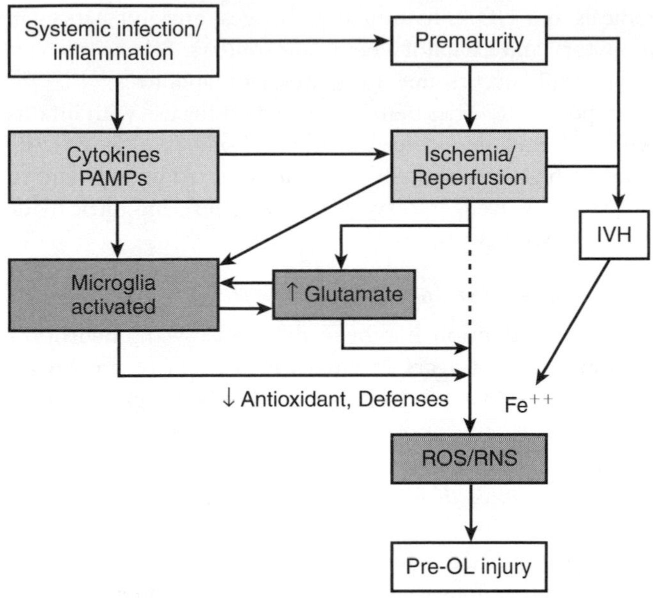

FIGURE 15-11 Pathogenesis of PVL. The two major upstream mechanisms (light gray) are ischemia and systemic infection/inflammation, activating three major downstream mechanisms (dark gray): microglial activation, glutamate excitotoxicity, and ultimately, free radical attack. *IVH,* intraventricular hemorrhage; *OL,* oligodendrocyte; *PAMPS,* pathogen associated molecular patterns; *ROS/RNS,* reactive oxygen species/reactive nitrogen species (From Volpe, J.J., et al. [2011]. The developing oligodendrocyte: Key cellular target in brain injury in the premature infant. *Int J Dev Neurosci, 29,* 426.

Table 15-13 Pathogenesis of Periventricular Leukomalacia: Major Interacting Factors

CEREBRAL ISCHEMIA
- Pressure-passive cerebral circulation
- Hypocarbia

SYSTEMIC INFECTION/INFLAMMATION
- Propensity for maternal intrauterine infection or postnatal neonatal infection
- Potentiation of cerebral ischemic injury

MATURATION-DEPENDENT INTRINSIC VULNERABILITY OF PRE-OLs
- Microglial activation
- Excitotoxicity
- Free radical (ROS/RNS) attack

From Volpe, J.J., et al. (2011). The developing oligodendrocyte: Key cellular target in brain injury in the premature infant. *Int J Dev Neurosci, 29,* 425.
OLs, oligodendrocytes; *ROS/RNS,* reactive oxygen species/reactice nitrogen species.

Vascular structure and factors influencing CBF place the preterm infant at risk for PVL. Areas of blood flow near the lateral ventricles is impaired by hypotension.[82,249] Underperfusion of these areas leads to ischemia and necrosis. Reduction of blood oxygen decreases delivery of oxygen to these vulnerable regions, leading to hypoxic-ischemic injury. Cerebral autoregulation is immature, leading to a pressure-passive state that further alters cerebral perfusion.[252,253] Hypocarbia as a consequence of ventilator management can lead to cerebral vasoconstriction and further decreases in cerebral blood flow.[250,252,253] The pathogenesis of hypoxia-ischemia is described in the section on Hypoxic-Ischemic Encephalopathy.

Perinatal infection and immune-mediated inflammatory response with release of proinflammatory cytokines is thought to play a prominent role in PVL pathogenesis.[23,48,201,250,252,253] Infection/inflammation may arise from intrauterine or postnatal infection. Intrauterine infection is also an important mediator of preterm labor (see Chapter 4). Infection activates the immune system including the brain microglia with production of cytokines, free radicals, and glutamate that result in excitotoxicity and can injure the pre-OL and other brain cells (see Table 15-13).[48,253] Hypoxia and inflammation may have potentiating effects.[253] Infants with hypoxic-ischemic events, prolonged rupture of the membranes, and chorioamnionitis are at increased risk for PVL.[249]

The pre-OL are vulnerable to damage by cytokines, glutamate, adenosine, and free radicals, which can lead to alterations in cognitive, visual, and motor function.[124,249] Pre-Ols have low levels of antioxidant enzymes and a high oxidative metabolism, so they are vulnerable to oxidative stress with hypoxic-ischemic events.[48] Damage includes impairment of OL development and survival, altered myelinization, and axonal damage and disruption (Figure 15-11).[199]

WMI and its associated neuronal and axonal alteration (the encephalopathy of prematurity) are the leading causes of neurological disability in preterm infants. Sequelae may include cerebral palsy and motor, cognitive, learning, and behavioral deficits.[48,179,249,250] Preventative interventions being used or investigated include reducing hypoxia-ischemia, infection/inflammation, and microglia activation; increasing antioxidant defenses; and decreasing excitability.[48,201,253]

Cerebellar Injury in Preterm Infants

Preterm infants are also at risk for injury to the cerebellum. The cerebellum is one of the later brain structures to mature, is important in cognition, and acts as a node in distribution of neural networks with interconnections with the thalamus, parietal and prefrontal cortex.[148,184] A series of developmental events occur at the end of the second/beginning of the third trimester that are essential for the structural and functional integrity of the cerebellum.[146] Cerebellar abnormalities in preterm infants include those that are primarily destructive (i.e., hemorrhage and infarction) and those that are primarily a consequence of impaired development. Cerebellar underdevelopment is the most common alteration and is seen primarily in infants born at 24 to 32 weeks' gestation (and especially in those born at 24 to 28 weeks).[146,250,251] Infants have a bilateral, usually symmetrical, decrease in cerebellar volume.[146] Cerebellar injury often occurs with PVL or IVH.[146,250]

Insults may lead to the altered sequences of motor development seen in some preterm infants and may contribute to alterations in language (especially expressive) and social-behavioral and cognitive function.[146,251] Motor disturbances include a range of findings from incoordination to cerebral palsy and deficits in motor planning and execution; cognitive deficits usually involve visual-spatial abilities, verbal fluency, reading, memory, and learning; attentional deficits involve regulation of shifts in attention; and social/affective disturbances include mood abnormalities and autistic behaviors.[146,166,251]

Hypoxic-Ischemic Encephalopathy

After 33 to 34 weeks' gestation, blood flow and brain metabolic activity is less prominent in the periventricular area and shifts to the cortical area. As a result, hypoxia and ischemia in older preterm and term infants are more likely to damage areas of the peripheral and dorsal cerebral cortex. The primary lesion in hypoxic injury is necrosis of neurons in the cortices of the cerebrum and cerebellum, and possibly the brainstem. The primary ischemic injury occurs in the posterior (boundary area) portion of the parasagittal region. This area is farthest from the original blood supply of the major cerebral vessels and with systemic hypotension or hypoperfusion receives the least blood. With asphyxia and systemic hypotension, cerebral perfusion is maintained at first by cerebral vasodilation and redistribution of blood flow to the brain from other organs. If the asphyxia continues, brain water balance and CBF are altered and ischemia and edema develop.

The primary mechanisms for cell damage with hypoxic-ischemic encephalopathy (HIE) are excitotoxicity, inflammation, and oxidative stress, which deplete energy reserves. The pathophysiology of HIE is illustrated in Figure 6-4. Damage occurs in two phases. During the first phase, damage from the initial hypoxic insult leads to cell death secondary to (1) depolarization and influx of sodium, chloride, and water leading to cell edema and lysis; (2) interference with the cell's ability to produce an action potential, leading to failure of the sodium-potassium pump and cell edema; (3) accumulation of calcium due to activation of NA/K channels and *N*-methyl-D-aspartate (NMDA) glutamate-mediated receptors; and (4) movement of calcium into the cell via voltage-dependent ion channels opened by the changes in the sodium-potassium pump.[23] These events may initially have a neuroprotective effect by reducing neuronal excitability and conserving oxygen. However, with reperfusion and reoxygenation, free oxygen radicals can accumulate, causing primary neuronal death. Persistence of hypoxia and ischemia activates NMDA receptors, leading to further increases in intracellular calcium via glutamate-controlled ion channels. Glutamate and nitric oxide (NO) are released and accumulate. Glutamate at high levels is neurotoxic. NO, which at normal levels promotes vasodilation and increased blood flow, at toxic levels leads to production of excess free oxygen radicals, further activation of NMDA receptors, and production of peroxynitrates, which cause further cell damage. The reperfusion phase usually begins 6 to 12 hours or more after the initial insult and is characterized by hyperexcitability, cytotoxic edema, and damage from the release of free oxygen radicals and NO, inflammatory changes, and imbalances in inhibitory and excitatory neurotransmitters. Secondary neuronal death occurs due to necrosis or apoptosis.[23,142,249,253] Therapeutic strategies being investigated for use with infants with HIE include induced head and body cooling, calcium channel blockers, antioxidants, xanthine oxidase inhibitors, free radical scavengers, erythropoietin (Epo), and nitric oxide synthetase inhibitors.[34,60,66,130,213,219,221,253,258,261]

Neuroprotection Strategies

Increasing attention has been directed toward neuroprotection in recent years in efforts to prevent or ameliorate neurological insults. Neuroprotection strategies include preventive, rescue, and reparative interventions.[147] Limperopoulos defines these:

> "A *preventive therapy* is initiated before a potential insult results in injury, and requires advance knowledge of a likely or imminent insult. An example of a preventive intervention is the infant undergoing open-heart repair of complex congenital heart disease that is managed with deep hypothermia during the high-risk procedure. On a different scale is the use of individualized neonatal developmental care to optimize brain development in premature infants by reducing the discrepancy between the premature extrauterine and fetal environments; this optimization is achieved largely through a program that reduces excessive stimulation and attempts to promote an appropriate physiological milieu for the developing brain. In a different category is neural *rescue* therapy, which is initiated at, or soon after, a potential brain insult occurs, but before injury becomes irreversible. An example of a rescue strategy is induced mild hypothermia in full-term infants who suffer a hypoxic-ischemic insult during perinatal asphyxia. Finally, a neural *reparative* strategy is one that attempts to exploit the restructuring potential of the developing brain to maximize recovery in the aftermath of irreversible brain injury."[147,p. 95]

Developmental care focuses on providing an environment for the infant that is individualized for that infant and supports brain development, family adaptation, and long-term developmental needs, while reducing the effects of stress in the NICU.[141,192,237] "The goal is to conserve the infant's energy for growth, facilitate physiological stability and the infant's recovery from illness and promoting neurobehavioral development and family integration."[141,p. 11] Interventions include family-centered care, NIDCAP, skin-to-skin holding (kangaroo care), positioning strategies, clustering caregiving, multisensory interventions, parent collaboration in care, enhancing feeding experiences, and modifying the NICU physical and caregiving environment.[141,192,237]

Mild induced hypothermia is a neuroprotective strategy to reduce secondary reperfusion injuries in infants who are at risk for post-asphyxial hypoxic-ischemic encephalopathy.

Studies report beneficial effects in terms of improved survival and outcome with no significant adverse effects; however, even with cooling, mortality and morbidity remain high (see Chapter 20).[60,219,221] Epo has anti-inflammatory, antioxidant, angiogenic, antiepileptic, and neurotropic effects.[130,258] Although much of the work to date has been with animal models, trials of recombinant Epo with term infants with HIE have demonstrated potential efficacy in improving neurodevelopmental outcomes.[66,261] Neural tissues have Epo receptors that when activated lead to cell division, maturation, and inhibition of apoptopsis.[130,258] Endogenous Epo is produced in the brain, primarily by astrocytes, but also by oligodendrocytes, endothelial cells, neurons, and microglia.[130] Production is up-regulated by hypoxia, so Epo may have a protective role with hypoxic-ischemic encephalopathy (HIE), PVL, and hyperoxic brain injury.[130]

Neonatal Seizures

Seizure activity is the most frequent sign of neurologic problems in the neonate and infant.[249] Seizures result from an abnormal neuronal electrical discharge. Thus seizures are caused by a number of conditions in which the environment of neurons, which support normal electrical activity, is altered. These conditions include hypoxemia, ischemia, hypoglycemia, hypocalcemia, hyperkalemia, hypomagnesemia, hyponatremia or hypernatremia, acidosis, and meningitis.[132,249] In general, seizure activity may entail eye movements, oral movements, changes in posture, motor movements such as bicycling or rowing actions, and apnea. Types of seizures and their description are listed in Table 15-14. The timing of seizure onset and type of seizure are related to pathology and gestational age.[249]

Table 15-14 **Types of Neonatal Seizures**

SUBTLE SEIZURES
Premature and full-term infants
Ocular-tonic horizontal deviation of the eyes ± jerking; and sustained eye opening with ocular fixation
Eyelid blinking or fluttering
Sucking, smacking, drooling, or other oral-buccal-lingual movements
"Swimming," "rowing," and "pedaling" movements

GENERALIZED TONIC SEIZURES
Primarily premature infants
Tonic extension of upper and lower limbs (mimics decerebrate posturing)
Tonic flexion of upper limbs and extension of lower limbs (mimics decorticate posturing)

MULTIFOCAL CLONIC SEIZURES
Primarily full-term infants
Multifocal clonic movements, either simultaneous or in sequence
Nonordered ("non-Jacksonian") migration

FOCAL CLONIC SEIZURES
Full-term more than premature infants
Well-localized clonic jerking
Infant usually not unconscious

From Volpe, J.J. (2001). *Neurology of the newborn* (4th ed.). Philadelphia: Saunders.

Seizure activity is determined by brain maturation. Thus seizures are expressed differently based on gestational age and postbirth age and often do not resemble the seizure activity of adults.[108,249] These differences in seizure activity result from the structural and functional differences in the immature CNS. Lower rate of nerve conduction, limited myelinization, and reduced connectivity between neurons reduce the threshold for neuron firing and the decreased ability to propagate a seizure.[108,249,262] Consequently, the signs of seizure in the neonate are often subtle and more localized than in the adult. In adults there is a balance between the excitatory neurotransmitters (such as glutamate) and inhibitory neurotransmitters (such as γ-amino butyric acid [GABA]). In the neonate, GABA is initially excitatory, with a mismatch, with increased glutamate and a delay in maturation of the inhibitory system.[108,109,132] GABA is altered in the early weeks after birth and may alter neonatal responses to antiepileptic drugs (e.g., phenobarbital and phenytoin) that enhance GABA function.[132,197,211] In addition NMDA receptors, which respond to glutamate, are increased in the neonatal brain and spinal cord because glutamate is needed for synaptogenesis (see section on Organization).[69,73,109,132,262] Seizure activity in the neonate is more likely to be generated in areas of the brain that are more mature, such as the temporal lobe and subcortical structures such as the limbic area. This area is involved with behaviors such as sucking, drooling, chewing, swallowing, oculomotor deviations, and apneic episodes, behaviors typical of those seen with subtle seizures in the neonate.[249]

Because seizures involve massive discharge of neurons, a seizure is associated with an intense increase in energy consumption by the neurons. Additionally, the seizure activity may interfere with adequate oxygenation of the blood. Hypoxia, as well as hypoglycemia and other metabolic changes, may occur within the CNS during seizures.[249] Although the neonatal brain is less susceptible than the adult brain to seizure-induced injury, seizures are related to developmental problems, particularly the effects of repeated seizures on the developing nervous system.[108]

Neonatal Pain

That pain occurs in the neonate and infant is unequivocal. In the history of infant care, the understanding of pain in infants was determined largely by conceptualization of brain function at this age. For many years the infant's central nervous system was believed to have minimal function above the level of the brainstem, so the infant's ability to perceive and respond to pain was ignored. It was also believed that the infant's level of myelinization prevented pain perception and therefore attenuated the effects of pain. Discrediting of pain was further rationalized because it was assumed that the infant had no memory for painful experiences. Although a mass of data confirms the occurrence of pain in neonates and infants, some practices in the care of infants continue to be colored by previous thinking. Objectively assessing pain in infants and determining appropriate management are still challenges to neonatal care.

Pain Perception in Neonates and Infants

A number of reviews summarize studies that document the presence of pain in the fetus, neonate, and infant.[69,121,231,245] Because of the neurologic development of the neonate, pain may be qualitatively different from that experienced later in life, but it does exist. Table 15-8 summarizes anatomic and functional development of the different parts of the pain system. Pain receptors are in place and in fact the density of pain receptors (nociceptors) is comparable to or greater in the neonate than in adults.[1,12] The fibers that conduct pain stimuli to the spinal cord are in place early in fetal life. Nociceptive receptors are among the first fibers to grow into the spinal cord in the fetus. The density of nociceptive nerve endings in the skin is similar to that in adults until 28 weeks' gestation and then increases to exceed adult density until approximately 2 years of age.[245] Receptive fields are wider in neonates (with increased width with decreasing gestational age) leading to more widespread sensitivity. Thus non-noxious stimuli may also be perceived as painful by the immature infant.[121]

In the neonate, transmission of pain occurs primarily along the C fibers, which are unmyelinated fibers, rather than along the A-delta myelinated fibers, as occurs in older individuals.[74] Ascending mechanisms develop earlier than descending mechanisms.[121] In the spinal cord, the pathways that carry pain stimuli to the brain (anterolateral pathways) are undergoing myelinization (Figure 15-12). Peripheral pain fibers are unmyelinated; therefore myelinization with development does not alter transmission of pain messages to the spinal cord. The pain pathways are myelinated by 30 weeks' gestation, and thalamic fibers that relay information to the cortex are myelinated by 37 weeks' gestation.[249] Thus the rate of transmission may be altered (slower), but this is offset by the shorter distance that impulses must travel to reach the brain. These factors may be particularly important in temporal and spatial summation (see Neural Connections and Conduction of Impulses). Myelinization may have an effect on central processing and integration of pain information. Neonates, both term and preterm, have all the anatomic and functional requirements for pain perception.[69] Neonates possess the ability to produce endogenous opiates; increased levels of these substances are found after birth, and levels increase with difficult births and during times of stress (see Chapter 19).[69,245] However, levels of these endogenous opioids are usually lower than needed to produce analgesia.[69,74] Pain management involves both pharmacologic and nonpharmacologic interventions such as containment/swaddling, positioning, sucrose, nonnutritive sucking, maternal holding and touch, auditory and olfactory interventions, and skin-to-skin care.[121,235]

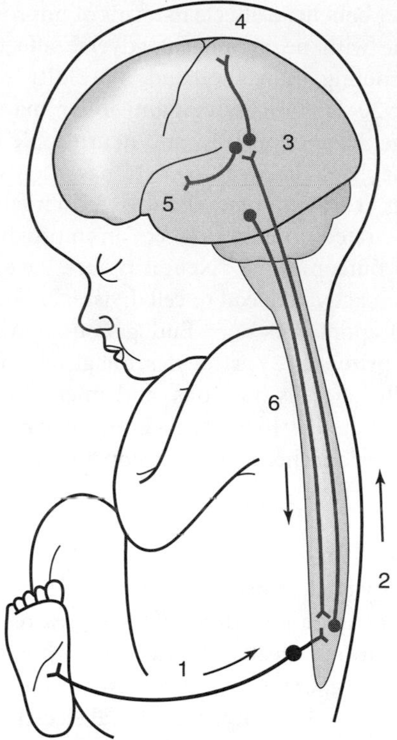

FIGURE 15-12 The neuronal pathways participating in pain. (1) Peripheral afferent nerve transmits signal to (2) the ascending tract neuron in the spinal cord dorsal horn, which synapses with (3) the next neuron in the hypothalamus. Here the pain impulse is distributed to two systems, which bring the signal to (4) somatosensory cortex (pain perception) and (5) limbic cortex (affective component). In addition there are (6) a number of descending neuronal pathways to the dorsal horn of the spinal cord, which modulate the ascending pain impulses. (From Vanhatalo, S., & van Nieuwenhuizen, O. [2000]. Fetal pain? *Brain Dev, 22,* 146.)

Consequences of Pain in the Neonate

Physiologic responses to pain are similar in the adult and the neonate (Table 15-15).[69] Neonates and infants may have severe consequences in terms of health status and outcomes. Although the infant's ability to verbally describe pain is limited, physiologic responses evidence distress. In general, responses to pain include release of catecholamines and cortisol. Heart rate changes and respiratory rate are linked to increased oxygen consumption. Blood glucose levels rise and the increase in metabolic rate increases energy requirements. A rise in blood pressure produces an elevation in intracranial pressure. Each of these responses may have adverse effects for the neonate, including increased oxygen and ventilatory requirements, changes in blood osmolarity, hypoxia, and the risk of intracranial hemorrhage. Furthermore, the energy demands of the stress response to pain have implications for growth and wound healing.

Infants may be more vulnerable to the effects of pain because of their level of neurobehavioral organization and limited coping skills. Neonates have virtually no control over the pain experience and cannot cognitively appreciate what

Table 15-15 Pain Responses of Neonates and Infants

MOTOR RESPONSES	
Generalized motor activity	Reflexive withdrawal from pain
Swiping movements	Positioning
Increased/decreased motor tone	Fist clenching
Kicking	Wiggling
Guarding	Thrashing
Pulling away	
FACIAL EXPRESSIONS	
Grimace	Furrowed brow
Chin quiver	Wincing
Frowning	Cry face
Tears in eyes	Gazing
VOCALIZATIONS	
Cry	Whimper
Groan	
SLEEP-WAKE/ACTIVITY DISTURBANCE	
Rapid state changes	Inability to sustain state
Increased or decreased activity	Fussiness
Decreased consolability	Irritability
Agitation	Restlessness
Lethargy	
AUTONOMIC RESPONSES	
Pallor	Palmar sweating
Diaphoresis	Hyperglycemia
Dilated pupils	Shallow respirations
Increased/decreased heart rate	Apnea
Increased/decreased respiratory rate	Increased ventilatory needs
Decreased oxygen level	Increased/decreased carbon dioxide level
Increase in blood pressure	Increase in intracranial pressure
Cyanosis	Increase in serum cortisol
Flushing	

Compiled from references 1, 74, 121, 249.

is happening or why. Of great concern are the long-term effects of early pain experiences on later development and psychologic outcomes. Although this area has not been thoroughly studied, evidence of memory capacities in the neonate augments this concern. Early stress and pain in the fetus and neonate may alter pain thresholds and produce permanent changes in neural pathways, increasing the risk of later disorders such as adult psychopathology, altered pain sensitivity, altered responses to stress, and stress-related disorders.[12,121]

MATURATIONAL CHANGES DURING INFANCY AND CHILDHOOD

Brain growth and maturation continue after birth into childhood and adolescence, with some processes continuing to mature into adulthood. Thus infancy and childhood are times for "nurturing the brain."[117,150] The neonatal period and early infancy are periods of increased vulnerability to insults because of the rapid brain growth during this period. The brain reaches 90% of adult weight by 2 years because of increases in nerve fibers and development of nerve tracts. Synaptic density is greatest at 3 years of age. The rate of synapse development differs between brain regions. For example, synaptogenesis in the prefrontal lobe increases from 8 months to a maximum at 2 years; the cortex from 2 years to 12 to 13 years. Brain growth spurts occur at 10 to 12 years (with frontal lobe development and development of logic processes and ability to plan), 13 to 15 years in areas of brain that control perception and motor function, and from 17 years on in frontal lobes of cortex. White matter increases linearly during development. Gray matter increases during pre-adolescence, peaks early in the frontal cortex during adolescence, decreases during post-adolescence. More complex cognitive functions, however, such as organized and abstract thought, self-control, interference inhibition, and cognitive flexibility develop throughout adolescence with progressive myelinization with higher-order association cortices. Cognitive development is a major function of the prefrontal cortex, which reaches maturity in late adolescence and the transition into adulthood.[117,249]

Myelinization continues through late adolescence and early adulthood. Nociceptive receptor density gradually decreases to adult levels by 2 years. The cerebellar growth spurt begins later (about 30 weeks' gestation) and ends earlier (about 1 year) than in other areas and thus is particularly vulnerable to nutritional and other insults during infancy. CBF and metabolism increase to 6 years and then decline.[100]

The cranial bones are not fully fused until 16 to 18 months of age. With increasing gestational age, conduction rates increase. The speed of transmission becomes similar to that of adults by 3 to 4 years of age.[249] At 8 months, electrical responses after stimulation become like those observed in the adult. By 8 months of age, the six EEG patterns observed in the mature brain are found in the EEG of the infant.[185] The Moro reflex disappears by 6 months, palmar grasp by 2 months, and tonic neck reflex by 7 months of age.

Postnatal changes in eye structure, which begin around 6 weeks and continue to 8 months, include maturation of the retina macula (responsible for color, contrast, visual acuity, and stereoscopic vision) and fovea (responsible for central vision).[32] Sensory abilities are similar to those of the adult at approximately 2 years of age. Visual acuity is adult-like at 2 years of age, changing from 20/400 at birth to 20/50 by 1 year and 20/20 by 2 years.[63] Three-dimensional vision begins by 6 months and reaches adult levels by 7 years.[63] Color vision is present to some degree by 2 months of age and increases to adult levels by 6 months.[63] By 4 to 5 months, visual-motor neuroconnections begin to develop, although the prehensile stage is not reached until 6 to 7 months. By 5 to 6 months, visual impulses begin to be retained (memory), with recognition of familiar and strange objects and faces. The foveal region is not completely developed until several years of age and cone density does not reach adult numbers until about 10 years.[169] The macular region also matures by about 10 years.[169]

Infants sleep a mean of 14 to 15 hours per day by 1 month of age.[14] As the infant develops, total sleep time (the total number of hours spent asleep) per day decreases to a mean of 13 to 14 hours per day by 12 months with individual variations.[14] By 3 months, the infant has changed to quiet sleep as the initial state at sleep onset, at least with some sleep episodes, but a portion continues to start with active sleep until up to 6 to 9 months.[52,186] Sleep cycles increase in length, reaching the adult length in roughly the late school-age years. The infant is increasingly capable of linking together two or more sleep cycles, leading to increased duration of sleep periods.[110] Sleep first exhibits longer periods and then gradually becomes consolidated into the nighttime hours. The percentage of sleep time spent in active sleep decreases as wakefulness increases; the percentage of time in quiet sleep remains relatively stable.[52,186] By 3 months, REM sleep is seen more often in early portions of sleep cycles and NREM in later (similar to adult patterns), and motor activity in active sleep decreases.[47,52] Circadian rhythms emerge by 2 to 3 months as infants become more responsive to light-dark cycles and social and other environmental cues.[47]

SUMMARY

Transition from intrauterine to extrauterine life involves numerous changes in the nervous system as the infant adapts to his or her new environment and caregivers. The term newborn has the ability to receive and process information and respond in ways suited to neonatal development. These abilities are less well developed in the preterm infant. In the past two decades our knowledge of response patterns, interactive abilities, and cues used by term and preterm infants to communicate with caregivers has expanded dramatically. An understanding of the level of maturation and organization of these systems in the neonate is critical for providing appropriate environments, promoting neurobehavioral organization, and influencing parent teaching. Recommendations for clinical practice related to the neuromuscular and sensory systems in the neonate are summarized in Table 15-16.

Table 15-16 Recommendations for Clinical Practice Related to the Neurologic, Muscular, and Sensory Systems in Neonates

Know the major stages for development of the neuromuscular and sensory systems (pp. 526-535).
Provide parent counseling and teaching regarding development of central nervous system (CNS) defects (pp. 526-533 and Table 15-6).
Recognize the stages of CNS development and vulnerabilities in preterm infants (pp. 530-533).
Recognize the processes of fetal neurosensory development (pp. 534-536).
Recognize the sensorimotor capabilities of the term infant and provide appropriate interventions (pp. 538-539, 541-542 and Tables 15-9 and 15-10).
Recognize the sensorimotor capabilities of the preterm infant and provide appropriate interventions (pp. 534-536, 538-539, 541-542 and Tables 15-9 and 15-10).
Promote neurosensory adaptations during transition to extrauterine life (pp. 538-539).
Protect term and preterm infants from overstimulation (pp. 541-543, 546).
Recognize implications of differences in cerebral blood flow and autoregulation within the neonate (pp. 539-541).
Implement interventions to prevent or minimize changes in oxygenation and intracranial pressure (pp. 539-541, 547-550).
Position term and preterm infants to enhance motor development (pp. 536-537, 538, 543-544).
Assess reflexes, motor tone, and sensory capabilities (pp. 536-537, 538, 543-544 and Tables 15-9 and 15-10).
Recognize normal and abnormal neonatal reflex responses (pp. 543-544).
Recognize different states and their implications (pp. 539, 544-546).
Interact with infants appropriate to their state (pp. 544-546).
Promote state modulation in term and preterm infants (p. 546).
Promote neurobehavioral organization in term and preterm infants (p. 546).
Recognize stress, stability, engagement, and disengagement cues and respond appropriately (pp. 546-547 and Table 15-12).
Modify the neonatal intensive care unit environment to reduce sensory overload (pp. 546-547).
Teach parents to recognize infant states, stress, stability, engagement, disengagement cues, and sensorimotor capabilities (pp. 546-547 and Table 15-12).
Recognize factors that may increase the risk of germinal matrix hemorrhage (GMH), intraventricular hemorrhage (IVH), white matter injury (WMI), and hypoxic-ischemic encephalopathy (HIE) (pp. 547-551).
Implement interventions to reduce the risk of GMH, IVH, WMI, cerebellar injury, and HIE (pp. 547-551).
Recognize signs of seizure activity (p. 551 and Table 15-14).
Recognize consequences of pain in the neonate (pp. 552-553).
Assess infants for signs of pain (pp. 551-553 and Table 15-15).
Use pharmacologic and nonpharmacologic interventions to treat neonatal pain (pp. 552-553).

References

1. Ades, A.M. & Myers, M. (2012). Developmental aspects of pain. In R.A. Polin, W.W. Fox, & S.H. Abman (Eds.), *Fetal and neonatal physiology* (4th ed.). Philadelphia: Saunders.
2. Adzick, N.S., et al. (2011). A randomized trial of prenatal versus postnatal repair of myelomeningocele. *N Engl J Med, 364,* 993.
3. Airola, G., et al. (2010). Non-pharmacological management of migraine during pregnancy, *Neurol Sci, 31,* S63.
4. Allais, G., et al. (2010). The risks of women with migraine during pregnancy. *Neurol Sci, 31(Suppl. 1),* S59.
5. Als, H. (1986). A synactive model of neonatal organization: Framework for the assessment of neurobehavioral development in the premature infant and for support of infants and parents in the neonatal intensive care unit. *Phys Occup Ther Pediatr, 6,* 3.
6. Als, H. (1999). Reading the premature infant. In F. Goldson (Ed.), *Nurturing the premature infant: Developmental interventions in the neonatal intensive care nursery*. New York: Oxford University Press.
7. Als, H., et al. (1982). Toward a research instrument for the assessment of preterm infants' behavior (APIB). In H.B. Fitzgerald, B.M. Lester, & M.W. Yogman (Eds.), *Theory and research in behavioral pediatrics (Vol. 1).* New York: Plenum Press.
8. American Academy of Pediatrics Committee on Genetics. (1999). Folic acid for the prevention of neural tube defects. *Pediatrics, 104,* 325.
9. American Academy of Sleep Medicine. (2005). *International classification of sleep disorders* (2nd ed.). Chicago: American Academy of Sleep Medicine.
10. Amiel-Tison, C. (1977). Evaluation of the neuromuscular system of the infant. In A. Rudolph (Ed.), *Pediatrics*. New York: Appleton-Century-Crofts.
11. Aminoff, M.J. (2009). Neurologic disorders. In R.K. Creasy, et al. (Eds.), *Creasy & Resnik's Maternal-fetal medicine: Principles and practice (6th ed.).* Philadelphia: Saunders.
12. Anand, K.J.S. (2000). Effects of perinatal pain and stress. *Prog Brain Res, 122,* 117.
13. Anderson, F.W. & Johnson, C.T. (2005). Complementary and alternative medicine in obstetrics. *Int J Gynaecol Obstet, 91,* 116.
14. Barnard, K.E. (1999). *Beginning rhythms: The emerging process of sleep-wake behaviors and self-regulation.* Seattle: Nursing Child Assessment Satellite Training, University of Washington.
15. Barragán Loayza, I.M., Solà, I., & Juandó Prats, C. (2011). Biofeedback for pain management during labour. *Cochrane Database Syst Rev 6,* CD006168.
16. Beauchamp, G.K. & Mennella, J.A. (2011). Flavor perception in human infants: Development and functional significance. *Digestion, 83,* S1.
17. Beebe, K.R. & Lee, K.A. (2007). Sleep disturbance in late pregnancy and early labor. *Perinat Neonatal Nurs, 21,* 103.
18. Benfield, R.D., et al. (2010). The effects of hydrotherapy on anxiety, pain, neuroendocrine responses, and contraction dynamics during labor. *Biol Res Nurs, 12,* 28.
19. Bennett, K.A. (2005). Pregnancy and multiple sclerosis. *Clin Obstet Gynecol, 48,* 38.
20. Bigelow, C. & Stone, J. (2011). Bed rest in pregnancy. *Mt Sinai J Med, 78,* 291.
21. Black, J.E. (1998). How a child builds its brain: Some lessons from animal studies of neural plasticity. *Prev Med, 27,* 168.
22. Blackburn, S. & VandenBerg, K. (1997). Assessment and management of neonatal neurobehavioral development. In C. Kenner, J.W. Lott, & A.A. Flandermeyer (Eds.), *Comprehensive neonatal nursing care: A physiologic perspective.* Philadelphia: Saunders.
23. Blackburn, S.T. & Ditzenberger, G. (2007). Neurologic system. In C. Kenner & J.W. Lott (Eds.), *Comprehensive neonatal care: An interdisciplinary approach* (4th ed.). Philadelphia: Saunders.
24. Blyton, D.M., Sullivan, C.E., & Edwards, N. (2002). Lactation is associated with an increase in slow-wave sleep in women. *J Sleep Res, 11,* 297.
25. Bonfacio, S.L., Gonzalez, F. & Ferriero, D.M. (2012). Central nervous system injury and neuroprotection. In C.A. Gleason & S. Devaskar (Eds.). *Avery's Diseases of the newborn* (9th ed.). Philadelphia: Saunders.
26. Borg-Stein, J., Dugan, S.A., & Gruber, J. (2005). Musculoskeletal aspects of pregnancy. *Am J Phys Med Rehabil, 84,* 180.
27. Borg-Stein, J. & Dugan, S.A. (2007). Musculoskeletal disorders of pregnancy, delivery and postpartum. *Phys Med Rehabil Clin N Am, 18,* 459.
28. Bourjeily, G., et al. (2010). Pregnancy and fetal outcomes of symptoms of sleep-disordered breathing. *Eur Respir J, 36,* 849.
29. Bourjeily, G., Ankner, G., & Mohsenin, V. (2011). Sleep-disordered breathing in pregnancy. *Clin Chest Med, 32,* 175.
30. Bourne, J.A. (2010). Unravelling the development of the visual cortex: Implications for plasticity and repair. *J Anat, 217,* 449.
31. Brazelton, T.B. & Nugent, J.K. (2011). *Neonatal behavioral assessment scale* (4th ed.). London: MacKeith.
32. Brémond-Gignac, D., et al. (2011). Visual development in infants: Physiological and pathological mechanisms. European Network of Study and Research in Eye Development. *Curr Opin Ophthalmol, 22,* S1.
33. Bruner, J.P., & Tulipan, N. (2005). Intrauterine repair of spina bifida. *Clin Obstet Gynecol, 48,* 942.
34. Calvert, J.W. & Zhang, J.H. (2005). Pathophysiology of an hypoxic-ischemic insult during the perinatal period. *Neurolog Res, 27,* 246.
35. Cameron, E.L. (2007). Measures of human olfactory perception during pregnancy. *Chem Senses, 32,* 775.
36. Carletti, B. & Rossi, F. (2008). Neurogenesis in the cerebellum. *Neuroscientist, 14,* 91.
37. Cayuso, J. & Marti, E. (2005). Morphogens in motion: Growth control of the neural tube. *J Neurobiol, 64,* 376.
38. Chalmers, E.A. (2005). Perinatal stroke—risk factors and management. *Br J Haematol, 130,* 333.
39. Chan, W.Y., et al. (2002). Proliferation and apoptosis in the developing human neocortex. *Anat Rec, 267,* 261.
40. Clowry, G., Molnár, Z., & Rakic P. (2010). Renewed focus on the developing human neocortex. *J Anat, 217,* 276.
41. Cluett, E.R., et al. (2009). Immersion in water in pregnancy, labour and birth. *Cochrane Database Syst Rev 2,* CD000111.
42. Cohen, S.S., et al. (2012). Development of the blood-brain barrier. In R.A. Polin, W.W. Fox, & S.H. Abman (Eds.), *Fetal and neonatal physiology* (4th ed.). Philadelphia: Saunders.
43. Cowart, B.J., Beaucaup, G.K., & Mennella, J.A. (2012). Development of taste and smell in the neonate. In R.A. Polin, W.W. Fox, & S.H. Abman (Eds.), *Fetal and neonatal physiology* (4th ed.). Philadelphia: Saunders.
44. Crespi, E.J. & Denver, R.J. (2005). Ancient origins of human developmental plasticity. *Am J Hum Biol, 17,* 44.
45. Cunningham, G., et al. (2009). *Williams obstetrics* (23rd ed.). New York: McGraw-Hill.
46. Dabo, F., et al. (2010). Plasma levels of beta-endorphin during pregnancy and use of labor analgesia. *Reprod Sci, 17,* 742.
47. Davis, K.F., Parker, K.P., & Montgomery, G.L. (2004). Sleep in infants and young children: Part one: Normal sleep. *J Pediatr Health Care, 18,* 65.
48. Deng, W. (2010). Neurobiology of injury to the developing brain. *Nat Rev Neurol, 6,* 328.
49. Derbyshire, S.W. (2010). Foetal pain? *Best Pract Res Clin Obstet Gynaecol, 24,* 647.
50. Detrait, E.R., et al. (2005). Human neural tube defects: Developmental biology, epidemiology, and genetics. *Neurotoxicol Teratol, 27,* 515.
51. De Vries, L.S. & Rennie, J.M. (2005). Neurological problems of the neonate: Preterm brain injury: Preterm cerebral hemorrhage. In. J.M. Rennie (Ed.), *Roberton's textbook of neonatology* (4th ed.). Edinburgh: Churchill Livingstone.
52. de Weerd, A.W. & van den Bossche, R.A. (2003). The development of sleep during the first months of life. *Sleep Med Rev, 7,* 179.
53. Diaz, A.L. & Gleeson, J.G. (2009). The molecular and genetic mechanisms of neocortex development. *Clin Perinatol, 36,* 503.
54. Dinn, R.B., Harris, A., & Marcus, P.S. (2003). Ocular changes in pregnancy. *Obstet Gynecol Surv, 58,* 137.
55. DiPietro, J.A. (2000). Baby and the brain: Advances in child development. *Annu Rev Public Health, 21,* 455.

56. DiPietro, J.A. (2005). Neurobehavioral assessment before birth. *Ment Retard Dev Disabil Res Rev, 11,* 4.
57. Donaldson, J.O. & Duffy, T.P. (2004). Neurologic complications. In G.N. Burrow, T.P. Duffy, & J.A. Copel (Eds.), *Medical complications during pregnancy* (6th ed.). Philadelphia: Saunders.
58. Dreyfus-Brisac, C. (1975). Neurophysiological studies in human premature and full-term newborns. *Biol Psychol, 10,* 485.
59. Driver, H.S. & Shapiro, C.M. (1992). A longitudinal study of sleep stages in young women during pregnancy and postpartum. *Sleep, 15,* 449.
60. Drury, P.P., Bennet, L., & Gunn, A.J. (2010). Mechanisms of hypothermic neuroprotection. *Semin Fetal Neonatal Med, 15,* 287.
61. Dzaja, A., et al. (2005). Women's sleep in health and disease. *J Psychiatr Res, 39,* 55.
62. Eappen, S. & Robbins, D. (2002). Nonpharmacological means of pain relief for labor and delivery. *Int Anesthesiol Clin, 40,* 103.
63. Edward, D.P. & Kaufman, L.M. (2003). Anatomy, development, and physiology of the visual system. *Pediatr Clin North Am, 50,* 1.
64. Ekbom, K. & Ulfberg, J. (2009). Restless legs syndrome. *J Intern Med, 266,* 419.
65. Ellegard, E.K. (2003). The etiology and management of pregnancy rhinitis. *Am J Respir Med, 2,* 469.
66. Elmahdy, H., et al. (2010). Human recombinant erythropoietin in asphyxia neonatorum: Pilot trial. *Pediatrics, 125,* e1135.
67. Fielder, A.R. & Moseley, M.J. (2000). Environmental light and the preterm infant. *Semin Perinatol, 24,* 291.
68. Fishman, S.M., Ballantyne, J.C., & Rathmell, J.P. (2009). *Bonica's Management of pain* (4th ed.). Philadelphia: Lippincott.
69. Fitzgerald, M. & Jennings, E. (1999). The postnatal development of spinal sensory processing. *Proc Natl Acad Sci U S A, 96,* 7719.
70. Florence, D.J. & Palmer, D.G. (2003). Therapeutic choices for the discomforts of labor. *J Perinat Neonatal Nurs, 17,* 238.
71. Foti, T., et al. (2000). A biomechanical analysis of gait during pregnancy. *J Bone Joint Surg Am, 82,* 625.
72. Fox, A.W., Diamond, M.L., & Spierings, E.L. (2005). Migraine during pregnancy: Options for therapy. *CNS Drugs, 19,* 465.
73. Fox, K., et al. (1996). Glutamate receptor blockage at cortical synapses disrupts development of thalamocortical and columnar organization in somatosensory cortex. *Proc Nat Acad Sci U S A, 93,* 5584.
74. Franck, L.S., et al. (2000). Pain assessment in infants and children. *Pediatr Clin North Am, 47,* 487.
75. Franklin, K.A., et al. (2000). Snoring, pregnancy-induced hypertension, and growth retardation of the fetus. *Chest, 117,* 137.
76. Gay, C.L., Lee, K.A., & Lee, S.Y. (2004). Sleep patterns and fatigue in new mothers and fathers. *Biol Res Nurs, 5,* 311.
77. Giannina, G., et al. (1997). Comparison of intraocular pressure between normotensive and preeclamptic women in the peripartum period. *Am J Obstet Gynecol, 176,* 1052.
78. Gianoulakis, C. & Chretien, M. (1998). Endorphins in fetomaternal physiology. In N. Gleicher (Ed.), *Principles of medical therapy in pregnancy* (3rd ed.). Stamford, CT: Appleton & Lange.
79. Gibbs, R.S., et al. (2008). *Danforth's Obstetrics and gynecology* (10th ed). Philadelphia: Lippincott Williams & Wilkins.
80. Glass, P. (1999). The vulnerable neonate and the neonatal intensive care environment. In G.B. Avery, M.A. Fletcher, & M.G. MacDonald (Eds.), *Neonatology: Pathophysiology and management of the newborn* (5th ed.). Philadelphia: Lippincott Williams & Wilkins.
81. Glass, P. (2005). The vulnerable neonate and the neonatal intensive care environment. In M.G. MacDonald, M. Seshia, & M. Mullett (Eds.), *Avery's Neonatology: Pathophysiology and management of the newborn* (5th ed.). Philadelphia: Lippincott Williams & Wilkins.
82. Gleason, C.A., Hohimer, A.R. & Back, S.A. (2012). Developmental physiology of the central nervous system. In C.A. Gleason & S. Devaskar (Eds.). *Avery's Diseases of the newborn* (9th ed.). Philadelphia: Saunders.
83. Graven, S.N. (2000). Sound and the developing infant in the NICU: Conclusions and recommendations for care, *J Perinatol, 20,* S88.
84. Graven, S.N. (2004). Early sensory visual development of the fetus and newborn. *Clin Perinatol, 31,* 199.
85. Gray, L. & Philbin, M.K. (2004). Effects of the neonatal intensive care unit on auditory attention and distraction. *Clin Perinatol, 31,* 243.
86. Greenough, W.T., et al. (1987). Experience and brain development. *Child Dev, 58,* 539.
87. Greisen, G. (1997). Cerebral blood flow and energy metabolism in the newborn. *Clin Perinatol, 24,* 531.
88. Greisen, G. (2005). Autoregulation of cerebral blood flow in newborn babies. *Early Hum Dev, 81,* 423.
89. Greisen, G. (2009). To autoregulate or not to autoregulate—that is no longer the question. *Semin Pediatr Neurol, 16,* 207.
90. Gutke, A., Ostgaard, H.C., & Oberg, B. (2008). Predicting persistent pregnancy-related low back pain. *Spine, 33,* E386.
91. Hack, M. (1987). The sensorimotor development of the preterm infant. In A.A. Fanaroff & R.J. Martin (Eds.), *Behrman's neonatal-perinatal medicine* (4th ed.). St. Louis: Mosby.
92. Haith, M.M. (1986). Sensory and perceptual processes in early infancy. *J Pediatr, 109,* 158.
93. Hall, J.W. (2000). Development of the ear and hearing, *J Perinatol, 20,* S12.
94. Hamdan, A.L., et al. (2009). Effect of pregnancy on the speaking voice. *J Voice, 23,* 490.
95. Han, I.H. (2010). Pregnancy and spinal problems. *Curr Opin Obstet Gynecol, 22,* 477.
96. Happe, S. & Trenkwalder, C. (2004). Role of dopamine receptor agonists in the treatment of restless legs syndrome. *CNS Drugs, 18,* 27.
97. Harden, C.L., et al. (2009). Practice parameter update: Management issues for women with epilepsy—focus on pregnancy (an evidence-based review): Obstetrical complications and change in seizure frequency: Report of the Quality Standards Subcommittee and Therapeutics and Technology Assessment Subcommittee of the American Academy of Neurology and American Epilepsy Society. *Neurology, 73,* 126.
98. Harden, C.L., et al. (2009). Practice parameter update: Management issues for women with epilepsy—focus on pregnancy (an evidence-based review): Teratogenesis and perinatal outcomes: Report of the Quality Standards Subcommittee and Therapeutics and Technology Assessment Subcommittee of the American Academy of Neurology and American Epilepsy Society. *Neurology, 73,* 133.
99. Harden, C.L., et al. (2009). Practice parameter update: Management issues for women with epilepsy—focus on pregnancy (an evidence-based review): Vitamin K, folic acid, blood levels, and breastfeeding: Report of the Quality Standards Subcommittee and Therapeutics and Technology Assessment Subcommittee of the American Academy of Neurology and American Epilepsy Society. *Neurology, 73,* 142.
100. Hardy, P., et al. (1997). Control of cerebral and ocular blood flow autoregulation in neonates. *Pediatr Clin North Am, 44,* 137.
101. Hart, M.A. (2005). Help! My orthopaedic patient is pregnant! *Orthop Nurs, 24,* 108.
102. Harvey, V.L. & Dickenson, A.H. (2008). Mechanisms of pain in nonmalignant disease. *Curr Opin Support Palliat Care, 2,* 133.
103. Heckman, J.D. & Sassard, R. (1994). Musculoskeletal considerations in pregnancy. *J Bone Joint Surg Am, 76,* 1720.
104. Hedman, C., et al. (2002). Effects of pregnancy on mothers' sleep. *Sleep Med, 3,* 37.
105. Hensley, J.G. (2009). Leg cramps and restless legs syndrome during pregnancy. *J Midwifery Womens Health, 54,* 211.
106. Hertz, G., et al. (1992). Sleep in normal late pregnancy. *Sleep, 15,* 246.
107. Hilaire, M.L., Cross, L.B., & Eichner, S.F. (2004). Treatment of migraine headaches with sumatriptan in pregnancy. *Ann Pharmacother, 38,* 1726.
108. Holmes, G.L. & Ben-Ari, Y. (2001). The neurobiology and consequences of epilepsy in the developing brain. *Pediatr Res, 49,* 320.
109. Holmes, G.L. (2009). The long-term effects of neonatal seizures. *Clin Perinatol, 36,* 901.
110. Hoppenbrouwers, T., et al. (1988). Sleep and waking states in infancy: Normative studies. *Sleep, 11,* 387.
111. Horton, T.H. (2005). Fetal origins of developmental plasticity: Animal models of induced life history variation. *Am J Hum Biol, 17,* 34.

112. Hunter, L.P., Rychnovsky, J.D., & Yount, S.M. (2009). A selective review of maternal sleep characteristics in the postpartum period. *J Obstet Gynecol Neonatal Nurs, 38,* 60.
113. Huntley, A.L., Coon, J.T., & Ernst, E. (2004). Complementary and alternative medicine for labor pain: A systematic review. *Am J Obstet Gynecol, 191,* 36.
114. Iannetti, G.D. & Mourax, A. (2010). From the neuromatrix to the pain matrix (and back). *Exp Brain Res, 205,* 1.
115. Ikonomidou, C., et al. (2001). Neurotransmitters and apoptosis in the developing brain. *Biochem Pharmacol, 62,* 401.
116. Ireland, M.L. & Ott, S.M. (2000). The effects of pregnancy on the musculoskeletal system. *Clin Orthop, 372,* 169.
117. Ito, M. (2004). "Nurturing the brain" as an emerging research field involving child neurology. *Brain Dev, 26,* 429.
118. Jensen, F.E. (2009). Neonatal seizures: An update on mechanisms and management. *Clin Perinatol, 36,* 881.
119. Jimenez, S.L.M. (1983). Application of the body's natural pain relief mechanisms to reduce discomfort in labor and delivery. *NAACOG Update Series, 1,* 1.
120. Jobe, A.H. (2010). "Miracle" extremely low birth weight neonates: Examples of developmental plasticity. *Obstet Gynecol, 116,* 1184.
121. Johnston, C.C., Fernandes, A.M., & Campbell-Yeo, M. (2011). Pain in neonates is different, *Pain, 152,* S65.
122. Karacan, I., et al. (1968). Characteristics of sleep patterns during late pregnancy and the postpartum periods. *Am J Obstet Gynecol, 10,* 579.
123. Kennelly, M.M., et al. (2011). Effects of body mass index on sleep patterns during pregnancy. *J Obstet Gynaecol, 31,* 125.
124. Kinney, H.C. (2005). Human myelinization and perinatal white matter disorders. *J Neurolog Sci, 228,* 190.
125. Kirby, M.A., Groves, M.M., & Yellon, S.M. (2010). Retrograde tracing of spinal cord connections to the cervix with pregnancy. *Reproduction, 139,* 645.
126. Klein, A.M. & Loder, E. (2010). Postpartum headache. *Int J Obstet Anesth, 19,* 422.
127. Kojić, Z., et al. (2007). Labor pain—physiological basis and regulatory mechanisms (Abstract). *Srp Arh Celok Lek, 135,* 235.
128. Kostović, I., Judaš, M., & Sedmak, G. (2011). Developmental history of the subplate zone, subplate neurons and interstitial white matter neurons: Relevance for schizophrenia. *Int J Dev Neurosci, 29,* 193.
129. Kumar, R., Hayhurst, K.L., & Robson, A.K. (2011). Ear, nose, and throat manifestations during pregnancy. *Otolaryngol Head Neck Surg, 145,* 188.
130. Kumral, A., et al. (2010). Erythropoietin in neonatal brain protection: The past, the present and the future. *Brain Dev, 33,* 632.
131. Kvorning, N., et al. (2004). Acupuncture relieves pelvic and low-back pain in late pregnancy. *Acta Obstet Gynecol Scand, 83,* 246.
132. Lagercrantz, H. & Changeux, J.P. (2009). The emergence of human consciousness: From fetal to neonatal life. *Pediatr Res, 65,* 255.
133. Lagercrantz, H. & Changeux, J.P. (2010). Basic consciousness of the newborn. *Semin Perinatol, 34,* 201.
134. Lawrence, R.A. (2011). *Breastfeeding: A guide for the medical profession* (7th ed.). Philadelphia: Saunders.
135. Lawson, W., Reino, A.J., & Biller, H.F. (2000). Ear, nose & throat disorders in pregnancy. In Cohen, W.R., Cherry, S.H., & Merkatz, I.R. (Eds.), *Cherry and Merkatz's Complications of pregnancy* (5th ed.). Philadelphia: Lippincott Williams & Wilkins.
136. Lecanuet, J.P. & Schaal, B. (1996). Fetal sensory competencies. *Eur J Obstet Gynecol, 68,* 1.
137. Lee, K.A., et al. (2000). Parity and sleep patterns during and after pregnancy. *Obstet Gynecol, 95,* 14.
138. Lee, K.A. & Gay, C.L. (2004). Sleep in late pregnancy predicts length of labor and type of delivery. *Am J Obstet Gynecol, 191,* 2041.
139. Lee, K.A., et al. (2008). The influence of reproductive status and age on women's sleep. *J Womens Health (Larchmt), 17,* 1209.
140. Lentz, M.J., & Killien, M.G. (1991). Are you sleeping? Sleep patterns during postpartum hospitalization. *J Perinatal Neonatal Nurs, 4,* 30.
141. Lester, B.M., et al. (2011). Infant neurobehavioral development. *Semin Perinatol, 35,* 8.
142. Levene, M. & Evans, D.J. (2005). Neurological problems of the neonate: Hypoxic-ischemic brain injury. In J.M. Rennie (Ed.), *Roberton's Textbook of neonatology* (4th ed.). Edinburgh: Churchill Livingstone.
143. Lickliter, R. (2000). Atypical perinatal sensory stimulation and early perceptual development: Insights from developmental psychobiology, *J Perinatal, 20,* S45.
144. Lickliter, R. (2000). The role of sensory stimulation in perinatal development: Insights from comparative research for care of the high-risk infant. *J Behavioral Dev Pediatr, 21,* 437.
145. Liem, K.D. & Greisen, G. (2010). Monitoring of cerebral haemodynamics in newborn infants. *Early Hum Dev, 86,* 155.
146. Limperopoulos, C., et al. (2007). Does cerebellar injury in premature infants contribute to the high prevalence of long-term cognitive, learning, and behavioral disability in survivors? *Pediatrics, 120,* 584.
147. Limperopoulos, C. (2010). Advanced neuroimaging techniques: Their role in development of future fetal and neonatal neuroprotection. *Semin Perinatol, 34,* 93.
148. Limperopoulos, C. (2010). Extreme prematurity, cerebellar injury, and autism. *Semin Pediatr Neurol, 17,* 25.
149. Liporace, J. & D'Abreu, A. (2003). Epilepsy and women's health: Family planning, bone health, menopause, and menstrual-related seizures. *Mayo Clin Proc, 78,* 497.
150. Loder, E. (2003). Safety of sumatriptan in pregnancy: A review of the data so far. *CNS Drugs, 17,* 1.
151. Lowe, N.K. (1996). The pain and discomfort of labor and birth. *J Obstet Gynecol Neonatal Nurs, 25,* 82.
152. Lowery, C.L., et al. (2007). Neurodevelopmental changes of fetal pain. *Semin Perinatol, 31,* 275.
153. Mabie, W.C. (2005). Peripheral neuropathies during pregnancy. *Clin Obstet Gynecol, 48,* 57.
154. Maloni, J.A. (2010). Antepartum bed rest for pregnancy complications: Efficacy and safety for preventing preterm birth. *Biol Res Nurs, 12,* 106.
155. Martin, S.R. & Foley, M.R. (2005). Approach to the pregnant patient with headache. *Clin Obstet Gynecol, 48,* 2.
156. McCool, W.F., Packman, J., & Zwerling, A. (2004). Obstetric anesthesia: Changes and choices. *J Midwifery Womens Health, 49,* 505.
157. McCool, W.F., Smith, T., & Aberg, C. (2004). Pain in women's health: A multi-faceted approach toward understanding. *J Midwifery Womens Health, 49,* 473.
158. McCrory, J.L., et al. (2010). Dynamic postural stability during advancing pregnancy. *J Biomech, 43,* 2434.
159. McCrory, J.L., et al. (2010). Dynamic postural stability in pregnant fallers and non-fallers. *BJOG, 117,* 954.
160. McPherson, R.J. & Juul, S.E. (2010). Erythropoietin for infants with hypoxic-ischemic encephalopathy. *Curr Opin Pediatr, 22,* 139.
161. Medical Research Council Vitamin Study Research Group. (1991). Prevention of neural tube defects: Results of the Medical Research Council Vitamin Study. *Lancet, 338,* 131.
162. Melzack, R. (2005). Evolution of the neuromatrix theory of pain. The Prithvi Raj Lecture: Presented at the Third World Congress of World Institute of Pain, Barcelona 2004. *Pain Pract, 5,* 85.
163. Melzak, R. & Wald, P.D. (1983). *The challenge of pain.* New York: Basic Books.
164. Mennella, J.A., et al. (2011). The timing and duration of a sensitive period in human flavor learning: A randomized trial. *Am J Clin Nutr, 93,* 1019.
165. Mens, J.M., Pool-Goudzwaard, A., & Stam, H.J. (2009). Mobility of the pelvic joints in pregnancy-related lumbopelvic pain: A systematic review. *Obstet Gynecol Surv, 64,* 200.
166. Messerschmidt, A., et al. (2008). Disrupted cerebellar development in preterm infants is associated with impaired neurodevelopmental outcome. *Eur J Pediatr, 167,* 1141.

167. Meyer, G. (2001). Human neocortical development: The importance of embryonic and early fetal events. *Neuroscientist, 7,* 303.
168. Micheli, K., et al. (2011). Sleep patterns in late pregnancy and risk of preterm birth and fetal growth restriction. *Epidemiology, 22,* 738.
169. Mintz-Hittner, H.A. (2012). Retinal development and the pathophysiology of retinopathy of prematurity. In R.A. Polin, W.W. Fox, & S.H. Abman (Eds.), *Fetal and neonatal physiology* (4th ed.). Philadelphia: Saunders.
170. Mirmiran, M., Maas, Y.G., & Ariagno, R.L. (2003). Development of fetal and neonatal sleep and circadian rhythms. *Sleep Med Rev, 7,* 321.
171. Mitchell, L.E. (2005). Epidemiology of neural tube defects. *Am J Med Genet C Semin Med Genet, 135,* 88.
172. Mogil, L.G. & Friedman, A.H. (2000). Ocular complications of pregnancy. In W.R. Cohen, S.H. Cherry, & I.R. Merkatz (Eds.), *Cherry and Merkatz's Complications of pregnancy* (5th ed.). Philadelphia: Lippincott Williams & Wilkins.
173. Moore, K.L., Persaud, T.V.N & Torchia, M.G. (2011). *The developing human: Clinically oriented embryology* (9th ed.). Philadelphia: Saunders.
174. Murphy, K.M., et al. (2005). Development of human visual cortex: A balance between excitatory and inhibitory plasticity mechanisms. *Dev Psychobiol, 46,* 209.
175. Nappi, R.E., et al. (2011). Headaches during pregnancy. *Curr Pain Headache Rep, 15,* 289.
176. *NCAST learning resource manual.* (1987). Seattle: Nursing Child Assessment Satellite Training, University of Washington Child Development and Mental Retardation Center.
177. Ng, J. & Kitchen, N. (2008). Neurosurgery and pregnancy. *J Neurol Neurosurg Psychiatry, 79,* 745.
178. Nishihara, K., et al. (2000). Mothers' wakefulness at night in the post-partum period is related to their infants' circadian sleep-wake rhythm. *Psychiatry Clin Neurosci, 54,* 305.
179. Northam, G.B., et al. (2011). Total brain white matter is a major determinant of IQ in adolescents born preterm. *Ann Neurol, 69,* 702.
180. Norwitz, E.R., Hsu, C.D., & Repke, J.T. (2002). Acute complications of preeclampsia. *Clin Obstet Gynecol, 45,* 308.
181. Ohel, I., et al. (2007). A rise in pain threshold during labor: A prospective clinical trial, *Pain, 132,* S104.
182. Omoti, A.E., Waziri-Erameh, J.M., & Okeigbemen, V.W. (2008). A review of the changes in the ophthalmic and visual system in pregnancy. *Afr J Reprod Health, 12,* 185.
183. Osur, S.L. (2005). The management of asthma and rhinitis during pregnancy. *J Womens Health, 14,* 263.
184. Parker, J., et al. (2008). Cerebellar growth and behavioral & neuropsychological outcome in preterm adolescents. *Brain, 131,* 344.
185. Parmelee, A.H. & Stern, E. (1972). Development of states in infants. In C.D. Clemente, D.P. Purpura, & F.E. Mayer (Eds.), *Sleep and the maturing nervous system.* New York: Academic Press.
186. Peirano, P., Algarin, C., & Uauy, R. (2003). Sleep-wake states and their regulatory mechanisms throughout early human development, *J Pediatr, 143,* S70.
187. Pennell, P.B. (2003). The importance of monotherapy in pregnancy, *Neurology, 60,* S31.
188. Pennick, V.E. & Young, G. (2007). Interventions for preventing and treating pelvic and back pain in pregnancy. *Cochrane Database Syst Rev 2,* CD001139.
189. Pereira, L. (2003). Obstetric management of the patient with spinal cord injury. *Obstet Gynecol Surv, 58,* 678.
190. Perlman, J.M. (2012). Cerebral blood flow in premature infants: Regulation, measurement, and pathophysiology of intraventricular hemorrhage. In R.A. Polin, W.W. Fox, & S.H. Abman (Eds.), *Fetal and neonatal physiology* (4th ed.). Philadelphia: Saunders.
191. Philbin, M.K. & Klaas, P. (2000). Hearing and behavioral responses to sound in full-term newborns, *J Perinatol, 20,* S68.
192. Pickler, R.H., et al. (2010). A model of neurodevelopmental risk and protection for preterm infants. *J Perinat Neonatal Nurs, 24,* 356.
193. Pihko, E., & Lauronen, L. (2004). Somatosensory processing in healthy newborns, *Exp Neurol, 190,* S2.
194. Pleasure, J., & Pleasure, D. (2012). Trophic factor and nutritional and hormonal regulation of brain development. In R.A. Polin, W.W. Fox, & S.H. Abman (Eds.), *Fetal and neonatal physiology* (4th ed.). Philadelphia: Saunders.
195. Portugal, L.G. & Applebaum, E.L. (1998). Otolaryngology: Head and neck problems in pregnancy. In N. Gleicher (Ed.), *Principles of medical therapy in pregnancy* (3rd ed.). Stamford, CT: Appleton & Lange.
196. Qureshi, I.A., et al. (2000). The ocular hypotensive effect of late pregnancy is higher in multigravidae than in primigravidae. *Graefes Arch Clin Exp Ophthalmol, 238,* 64.
197. Rakhade, S.N. & Jensen, F.E. (2009). Epileptogenesis in the immature brain: Emerging mechanisms. *Nat Rev Neurol, 5,* 380.
198. Rash, B.G. & Grove, E.A. (2006). Area and layer patterning in the developing cerebral cortex. *Curr Opin Neurobiol, 16,* 25.
199. Rees, S. & Harding, R. (2004). Brain development during fetal life: Influences of the intra-uterine environment. *Neurosci Lett, 361,* 111.
200. Rees, S. & Inder, T. (2005). Fetal and neonatal origins of altered brain development. *Early Hum Dev, 81,* 753.
201. Rees, S., Harding, R., & Walker, D. (2011). The biological basis of injury and neuroprotection in the fetal and neonatal brain. *Int J Dev Neurosci, 29,* 551.
202. Ringelstein, E.B. & Knecht, S. (2006). Cerebral small vessel diseases: Manifestations in young women. *Curr Opin Neurol, 19,* 55.
203. Ritchie, J.R. (2003). Orthopedic considerations during pregnancy. *Clin Obstet Gynecol, 46,* 456.
204. Rivkees, S.A. (2003). Developing circadian rhythmicity in infants. *Pediatrics, 112,* 373.
205. Rivkees, S.A. & Hao, H. (2000). Developing circadian rhythmicity. *Semin Perinatol, 24,* 232.
206. Rowlands, S. & Permezel, M. (1998). Physiology of pain in labour. *Baillieres Clin Obstet Gynaecol, 12,* 347.
207. Rychnovsky, J. & Hunter, L.P. (2009). The relationship between sleep characteristics and fatigue in healthy postpartum women. *Womens Health Issues, 19,* 38.
208. Saaresranta, T. & Polo, O. (2003). Sleep-disordered breathing and hormones. *Eur Respir J, 22,* 161.
209. Sahota, P.K., Jain, S.S., & Dhand, R. (2003). Sleep disorders in pregnancy. *Curr Opin Pulm Med, 9,* 477.
210. Sakai, D. & Wakamatsu, Y. (2005). Regulatory mechanisms for neural crest formation. *Cells Tissues Organs, 179,* 24.
211. Sanchez, R.M. & Jensen, F.E. (2001). Maturational aspects of epilepsy mechanisms and consequences for the immature brain. *Epilepsia, 42,* 577.
212. Santiago, J.R., et al. (2001). Sleep and sleep disorders in pregnancy. *Ann Intern Med, 134,* 396.
213. Saugstad, O.D. (2001). Resuscitation of the asphyxic newborn infant: New insight leads to new therapeutic possibilities. *Biol Neonate, 79,* 258.
214. Saunders, N.R. (1999). Barrier mechanisms in the brain. II: Immature brain. *Clin Exp Pharmacol Physiol, 26,* 85.
215. Schatz, M. (1998). Special considerations for the pregnant woman and senior citizen with airway disease, *J Allergy Clin Immunol, 101,* S373.
216. Schmidt, P.M., et al. (2010). Hearing and vestibular complaints during pregnancy. *Braz J Otorhinolaryngol, 76,* 29.
217. Schultz, K.L., Birnbaum, A.D., & Goldstein, D.A. (2005). Ocular disease in pregnancy. *Curr Opin Ophthalmol, 16,* 308.
218. Schweiger, M.S. (1972). Sleep disturbance in pregnancy: A subjective survey. *Am J Obstet Gynecol, 114,* 879.
219. Selway, L.D. (2010). State of the science: Hypoxic ischemic encephalopathy and hypothermic intervention for neonates. *Adv Neonatal Care, 10,* 60.
220. Seron-Ferre, M., et al. (2002). Perinatal neuroendocrine regulation. Development of the circadian time-keeping system. *Mol Cell Endocrinol, 186,* 169.

221. Shah, P.S. (2010). Hypothermia: A systematic review and meta-analysis of clinical trials. *Semin Fetal Neonatal Med, 15,* 238.
222. Sharif, K. (1997). Regression of myopia induced by pregnancy after photorefractive keratectomy, *J Refract Surg, 13,* S445.
223. Shehata, H.A. & Okosun, H. (2004). Neurological disorders in pregnancy. *Curr Opin Obstet Gynecol, 16,* 117.
224. Sheth, B.P. & Mieler, W.F. (2001). Ocular complications of pregnancy. *Curr Opin Ophthalmol, 12,* 455.
225. Simkin, P. & Bolding, A. (2004). Update on nonpharmacologic approaches to relieve labor pain and prevent suffering. *J Midwifery Womens Health, 49,* 489.
226. Sizun, J. & Browne, J.V. (2006). *Research on early developmental care in preterm neonates.* New Barnet, UK: John Libbey Publishing.
227. Smith, C.A., et al. (2006). Complementary and alternative therapies for pain management in labour. *Cochrane Database Syst Rev 4,* CD003521.
228. Smith, C.A. & Cochrane, S. (2009). Does acupuncture have a place as an adjunct treatment during pregnancy? A review of randomized controlled trials and systematic reviews. *Birth, 36,* 246.
229. Smith, C.A., et al. (2011). Acupuncture or acupressure for pain management in labour. *Cochrane Database Syst Rev 7,* CD009232.
230. Smith, M.W., Marcus, P.S., & Wurtz, L.D. (2008). Orthopedic issues in pregnancy. *Obstet Gynecol Surv, 63,* 103.
231. Smith, R.P., et al. (2000). Pain and stress in the human fetus. *Eur J Obstet Gynecol Reprod Biol, 92,* 161.
232. Soldin, O.P., Dahlin, J., & O'Mara, D.M. (2008). Triptans in pregnancy. *Ther Drug Monit, 30,* 5.
233. Stafford, I.P. & Dildy, G.A. (2005). Myasthenia gravis and pregnancy. *Clin Obstet Gynecol, 48,* 48.
234. Sterman, M.B. (1972). The basic rest-activity cycle and sleep: Developmental considerations in man and cats. In C.D. Clemente, D.P. Purpura, & F.E. Mayer (Eds.), *Sleep and the maturing nervous system.* New York: Academic Press.
235. Stevens, B., Yamada, J., & Ohlsson, A. (2010). Sucrose for analgesia in newborn infants undergoing painful procedures. *Cochrane Database Syst Rev 1,* CD001069.
236. Suzuki, S., et al. (1994). Sleeping patterns during pregnancy in Japanese women. *J Psychosom Obstet Gynecol, 15,* 19.
237. Symington, A., Pinelli, J. (2006). Developmental care for promoting and preventing morbidity in preterm infants. *Cochrane Database Syst Rev* 2006 Apr *19*;(2): CD001814.
238. Teich, S.A. (1998). Common disturbances of vision and ocular movement and surgery of the eye. In N. Gleicher (Ed.), *Principles of medical therapy in pregnancy* (3rd ed.). Stamford, CT: Appleton & Lange.
239. Thorpy, M., et al. (2000). Restless legs syndrome: Detection and management in primary care: National Heart, Lung, and Blood Institute Working Group on Restless Legs Syndrome. *Am Fam Physician, 62,* 108.
240. Tingåker, B.K. & Irestedt, L. (2010). Changes in uterine innervation in pregnancy and during labour. *Curr Opin Anaesthesiol, 23,* 300.
241. Torelli, P., Allais, G. & Manzoni, G.C. (2010). Clinical review of headache in pregnancy, *Neurol Sci, 31,* S55.
242. Torsiglieri, A.J., et al. (1990). Otolaryngologic manifestations of pregnancy. *Otolaryngol Head Neck Surg, 102,* 293.
243. Trout, K.K. (2004). The neuromatrix theory of pain: Implications for selected nonpharmacologic methods of pain relief for labor. *J Nurs Midwifery, 49,* 482.
244. van Pampus, M.G. & Aarnoudse, J.G. (2005). Long-term outcomes after preeclampsia. *Clin Obstet Gynecol, 48,* 489.
245. Vanhatalo, S. & van Nieuwenhuizen, O. (2000). Fetal pain? *Brain Dev, 22,* 145.
246. Verity, C., Firth, H., & French-Constant, C. (2003). Congenital abnormalities of the central nervous system, *J Neurol Neurosurg Psychiatry, 74,* i3.
247. Vermani, E., Mittal, R., & Weeks, A. (2010). Pelvic girdle pain and low back pain in pregnancy: A review. *Pain Pract, 10,* 60.
248. Visser, G.H.A., et al. (1987). Fetal behavior at 30 to 32 weeks' gestation. *Pediatr Res, 22,* 655.
249. Volpe, J.J. (2008). *Neurology of the newborn* (5th ed.). Philadelphia: W.B. Saunders.
250. Volpe, J.J. (2009). Brain injury in premature infants: A complex amalgam of destructive and developmental disturbances. *Lancet Neurol, 8,* 110.
251. Volpe, J.J. (2009). Cerebellum of the premature infant: Rapidly developing, vulnerable, clinically important. *J Child Neurol, 24,* 1085.
252. Volpe, J.J. (2009). The encephalopathy of prematurity—brain injury and impaired brain development inextricably intertwined. *Semin Pediatr Neurol, 16,* 167.
253. Volpe, J.J., et al. (2011). The developing oligodendrocyte: Key cellular target in brain injury in the premature infant. *Int J Dev Neurosci, 29,* 423.
254. Wang, S.M. (2004). Low back pain during pregnancy: Prevalence, risk factors, and outcomes. *Obstet Gynecol, 104,* 65.
255. Werner, L. (2012). Early development of the human auditory system. In R.A. Polin, W.W. Fox, & S.H. Abman (Eds.), *Fetal and neonatal physiology* (4 ed.). Philadelphia: Saunders.
256. Winberg, J., et al. (1998). Olfaction and human neonatal behaviour: Clinical implications. *Acta Paediatr, 87,* 6.
257. Wolff, P.H. (1966). The causes, controls, and organization of behavior in the neonate. *Psychol Issues, 5,* 1.
258. Xiong, T., et al. (2011). Erythropoietin for neonatal brain injury: Opportunity and challenge. *Int J Dev Neurosci, 29,* 583.
259. Zafarghandi, N., et al. (2011). The effects of sleep quality and duration in late pregnancy on labor and fetal outcome. *Med,* 2011 Aug *10.* [Epub ahead of print.]
260. Zanardo, V., et al. (2001). Labor pain effects on colostral milk beta-endorphin concentrations of lactating mothers. *Biol Neonate, 79,* 87.
261. Zhu, C., et al. (2009). Erythropoietin improved neurologic outcomes in newborns with hypoxic-ischemic encephalopathy, *Pediatrics, 124,* e218.
262. Zupanc, M.L. (2004). Neonatal seizures. *Clin Perinatol, 51,* 961.

CHAPTER 16

Carbohydrate, Fat, and Protein Metabolism

Metabolism comes from the Greek word meaning "to change" and is the totality of chemical reactions within a living organism. Four principles that underlie and guide metabolic functions in humans are "(1) plasma glucose must be maintained within normal limits; (2) an optimal source of glycogen must be maintained as an emergency fuel; (3) an optimal supply of protein must be maintained for use in enzymatic mechanisms of metabolism as well as muscular mobility; excess protein is converted to fat and the nitrogen released is excreted in urine; and (4) protein must be conserved when it is scarce and stored fat used in time of caloric need."[47,p.2]

Metabolic processes in the pregnant woman, fetus, and neonate are closely linked with and mediated by the function of various endocrine glands. Major alterations in metabolic processes arise during pregnancy. These changes are essential for the mother to provide adequate nutrients to support fetal growth and development. Maternal metabolic changes also alter the course of pregnancy in women with chronic disorders such as diabetes mellitus. After birth, major changes occur in both the sources of nutrients and the use of substrates by the infant. Limitations in metabolic processes and related endocrine function during this period can compromise extrauterine adaptation and health. This chapter examines alterations in carbohydrate, fat, and protein metabolism and related endocrinology during pregnancy and in the fetus and neonate.

MATERNAL PHYSIOLOGIC ADAPTATIONS

Metabolic adaptations during pregnancy are directed toward (1) ensuring satisfactory growth and development of the fetus; (2) providing the fetus with adequate stores of energy and substrates needed for transition to extrauterine life; (3) meeting maternal needs to cope with the increased physiologic demands of pregnancy; and (4) providing energy and substrate stores for the demands of pregnancy, labor, and lactation.[6] The first two demands compete with the third and fourth demands. As a result, alterations in maternal metabolic processes can significantly affect maternal and fetal health status.

Pregnancy involves a "coordinated series of physiologic adjustments which act in concert to preserve maternal homeostasis while at the same time providing for fetal growth and development."[47] Pregnancy is primarily an anabolic state in which food intake and appetite are increased, activity is decreased, approximately 3.5 kg of fat is deposited, energy reserves of approximately 30,000 kcal (125,550 J) are established, and 900 g of new protein is synthesized by the mother, fetus, and placenta. The overall energy cost of reproduction is estimated at 75,000 to 85,000 kcal (313,875 to 355,725 J).[6,80,82] Anabolic aspects are most prominent during the first two trimesters when, due to enhanced lipogenesis, accumulation of maternal fat and increased blood volume lead to maternal weight gain (Figure 16-1).[19,78] Protein and glycogen synthesis increase in muscle with increased glycogenolysis (breakdown of glycogen to form glucose) and decreased glycolysis in the liver.[78] Insulin increases in response to glucose with a normal or slight increase in peripheral insulin sensitivity and serum glucose levels. This results in uptake of nutrients and maternal fat accumulation. During the third trimester, the woman's metabolic status becomes more catabolic as stored fat is used (see Figure 16-1). Gluconeogenesis (formation of glucose from amino acids and glycerol) in the liver decreases and intestinal dietary fat absorption increases.[78] Lipolytic activity within adipose tissue is enhanced with increases in plasma free fatty acids and glycerol. Maternal ketone production is increased. Counterinsulin hormones increase, leading to insulin resistance. During this phase, maternal weight gain is primarily due to the growing fetus and placenta; the fetus gains 90% of its growth in the last half of pregnancy.[12,19,57,80,82]

Antepartum Period

Pregnancy is associated with major changes in metabolic processes and endocrine function. Pregnancy has been characterized as a metabolic "tug of war" between the competing needs of the mother and the fetus.[47] The fetus and placenta influence maternal metabolic alterations in that these tissues become an additional site for metabolism of maternal hormones as well as new sites for hormonal biosynthesis. Many of the metabolic changes during pregnancy are aimed at providing substances (especially glucose, lipids, and amino acids) for the growth and

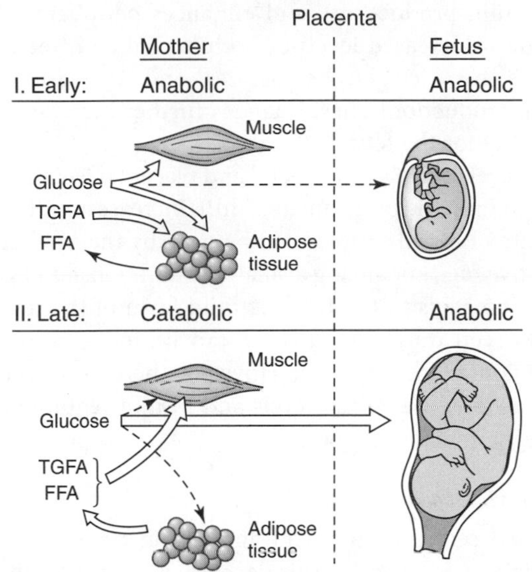

FIGURE 16-1 Fuel disposition in pregnancy during early (I) and late (II) gestation. (From Knopp, R.H., Childs, M.T., & Warth, M.R. [1979]. Dietary management of the pregnant diabetic. In M. Winick [Ed.], *Nutritional management of genetic disorders*. New York: Wiley-Interscience.)

development of the fetus. As the fetus and placenta grow, maternal fuel economy is altered to support this growth.[38,109]

Human placental lactogen (hPL), estrogen, progesterone, and possibly leptin influence metabolic processes during pregnancy, primarily by altering glucose utilization and insulin action. These changes contribute to the diabetogenic effects of pregnancy, stimulate alterations in lipid and protein metabolism, and increase the availability of glucose and amino acids for transfer to the fetus, while at the same time providing an alternative energy substrate (free fatty acids) to meet maternal needs and maintain homeostasis. The changes in carbohydrate and lipid metabolism parallel the energy needs of the mother and fetus, whereas the changes in maternal nitrogen and protein metabolism occur early in pregnancy, before fetal demand.

Basal Metabolic Rate

The basal metabolic rate (BMR) increases during pregnancy (Figure 16-2). The rate of change varies with maternal prepregnant nutritional status and fetal growth. Significant variations are seen among individual women with up to an eightfold increase reported. Similar variations are reported for fat accretion.[17,79,91] If a woman has low energy reserves at conception, there is less of an increase in the BMR and energy is conserved.

The total energy required for pregnancy can be divided into three parts: (1) obligatory energy needed for the fetus, placenta, uterus, and breasts (which is the smallest part); (2) energy for maternal fat storage; and (3) energy maintenance of these new tissues.[79] If a woman has lower energy stores, less of the maternal energy intake is needed to maintain new tissues and energy is conserved for maternal basic needs and the fetal-placental unit.[79,80,107,109] For example, in undernourished women, fetal weight accounts for 60% of the pregnancy weight gain, versus 25% in a well-nourished woman.[109] This energy-sparing response may allow the woman to sustain the pregnancy but is often at the expense of fetal growth, with decreased birth weight and risk of fetal growth restriction.[109] Prentice and Goldberg suggest that leptin might monitor a woman's prepregnancy energy stores and adjust or coordinate maternal metabolic resources.[109] Women with large-for-gestational-age (LGA) infants tend to have increased BMR with less maternal energy storage.[79,111]

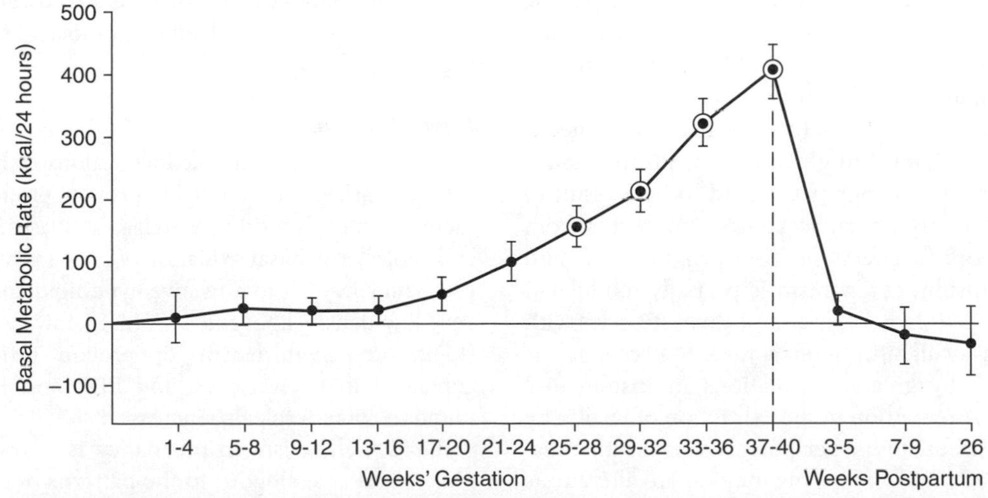

FIGURE 16-2 Changes in basal metabolic rate (BMR) throughout pregnancy and during the first 6 months postpartum for 96 women (means and confidence intervals). (From Durnin, J.V. [1991]. Energy requirements of pregnancy. *Diabetes, 40*, 152.)

The pregnant woman meets the energy demands of pregnancy by increasing her intake, decreasing her activity, or limiting fat storage.[80,107] King and colleagues propose three examples of how women in different situations might alter their energy to sustain pregnancy.[79] First, an underweight impoverished woman with limited food, poor fat stores, and need for physical work cannot increase food intake or limit physical activity during pregnancy. Her body responds by decreasing basal energy expenditures so that pregnant energy needs are similar to prepregnant needs. Second, a normal weight woman in a developed country with fat stores before pregnancy and adequate nutrition during pregnancy increases fat stores in pregnancy and increases her BMR slightly. Finally, an overweight woman in a developed country increases her BMR by 20% or more, perhaps to reduce additional fat deposition.[79]

Carbohydrate Metabolism

Basal endogenous hepatic glucose production remains sensitive to insulin and increases up to 30% by the third trimester to meet fetal and placental needs.[12,16,72,98] Endogenous glucose production increases with gestational age, paralleling fetal and maternal needs.[72] Maternal glucose levels are generally 10% to 20% lower than in nonpregnant women. In addition, during the overnight fasting period, maternal plasma glucose values fall to levels 15 to 20 mg/dL (0.8 to 1.1 mmol/L) lower than in nonpregnant women.[88] This decrease in glucose leads to lower insulin levels during the postabsorptive state (between meals and overnight) and a tendency toward hypoglycemia and ketosis. The decreased glucose level in the postabsorptive state is due to increased plasma volume in early pregnancy and later to placental transport of glucose to the fetus, which increases during gestation as fetal glucose needs increase.[98,101]

During the first two trimesters, the pregnant woman is in an anabolic state. Insulin secretion increases with increased peripheral glucose use without increases in insulin resistance.[47] As pregnancy progresses, peripheral glucose use by the mother decreases because of increasing insulin resistance. This reduces maternal glucose utilization and makes glucose more readily available to the fetus. The mother compensates by using fat stores to meet her energy needs with breakdown of glycerol to glucose.[57] Insulin resistance in the latter part of pregnancy is believed to be a result of a decrease in sensitivity of cell receptors that results from the insulin antagonism effects of hPL, progesterone, and cortisol.[16,47] The insulin antagonism is partially modulated by pancreatic β-cell hyperplasia and hypertrophy with increased insulin availability after a meal.[16] Pregnancy is also characterized by greater oscillations in insulin and glucagon levels.[47] A reduction in the extraction of insulin by the liver may contribute to the peripheral hyperinsulinemia. Variations in hepatic insulin binding may lead to alterations in the ratio of insulin to glucagon.[6]

Progesterone augments insulin secretion, decreases peripheral insulin effectiveness, and increases insulin levels after a meal. Estrogen increases the level of plasma cortisol (an insulin antagonist), stimulates β-cell hyperplasia (and thus insulin production), and enhances peripheral glucose utilization. Increased levels of both bound and free cortisol decrease hepatic glycogen stores and increase hepatic glucose production. These changes further increase glucose availability for the fetus.[88,98]

hPL levels correlate with fetal and placental weight and are higher in multiple pregnancies.[16] hPL increases synthesis and availability of lipids. Lipids can be used by the mother as an alternative fuel, enhancing availability and transfer of glucose and amino acids to the fetus. A mild form of the metabolic changes seen during pregnancy can be induced by giving hPL to nonpregnant women. However, there is no consistent relationship between hPL levels and insulin requirements in the pregnant diabetic woman.

Protein Metabolism

Decreased serum amino acid and serum protein levels are found in pregnancy.[6,42,72] This decrease is related to increased placental uptake, increased insulin levels, hepatic diversion of amino acids for gluconeogenesis, and transfer of amino acids to the fetus.[6,42] The fetus uses some of these amino acids for glucose formation. Maternal plasma levels of glucogenic amino acids (e.g., those that can be converted into glucose), such as alanine, threonine, glutamate, and serine, are reduced due to placental transfer of these amino acids.[31,72] Maternal plasma alanine levels, in particular, are lower because alanine is a key precursor for glucose formation (via gluconeogenesis) by the fetal liver.[72]

Alterations in protein metabolism during pregnancy have a biphasic pattern.[72] During the first half of gestation, maternal protein storage increases, with a net retention of 1.3 g/day of nitrogen.[80] Most of this is transported to the fetus, but some is retained in maternal tissues. During the second half, maternal protein use is more economic, with decreased urinary nitrogen excretion, thus conserving protein.[86] These changes may be mediated by decreased activity of hepatic enzymes involved in amino acid deamination and urea synthesis.

Lipid Metabolism

Pregnancy results in marked alterations in lipid metabolism with a markedly different lipoprotein profile, with marked increases in triglycerides, as well as increases in phospholipids and cholesterol. Basal oxidation of fatty acids increases 70% in pregnancy leading to a relative hyperlipidemia.[27] Synthesis of very-low-density lipoprotein (VLDL), low-density lipoprotein (LDL), and high-density lipoprotein (HDL), which are contained in triglycerides, and LDL and HDL, which are found in cholesterol, also increase.[59]

Lipid metabolism in pregnancy is characterized by two phases and is analogous to the patterns of change in carbohydrate and protein metabolism.[19,57] During the first two trimesters, triglyceride synthesis and fat storage increase. VLDL increases threefold in the second and third trimesters.

LDL decreases slightly initially, followed by a progressive rise.[100] HDL increases progressively to 24 weeks, then decreases to 32 weeks and stabilizes for the remainder of pregnancy.[100] Triglycerides increase 40% by 18 weeks and 250% by term.[87] Phospholipids and cholesterol levels also increase; the triglyceride-to-cholesterol level remains stable since cholesterol also increases.[59,58] By late pregnancy, cholesterol levels are 50% higher than prior to pregnancy, regardless of maternal dietary intake.[42] These changes enhance the availability of substrates for the fetus.[57]

Maternal fat storage is most prominent from 10 to 30 weeks, before the peak of fetal energy demands.[79] Promotion of lipogenesis and suppression of lipolysis during this phase are mediated by progressive increases in insulin responsiveness and enhanced by progesterone, cortisol, leptin, and prolactin.[6,16,30,42,59] Estrogens decrease lipoprotein lipase activity.[18] During this period the pregnant woman experiences a physiologic ketosis with a twofold to threefold increase in baseline ketone body production, with an acute increase after fasting, suggesting enhanced fat utilization.[116,130]

Lipid metabolism in late pregnancy is illustrated in Figure 16-3. The third trimester is characterized by both lipogenesis and lipolysis, with increased breakdown of fat deposits.[19,32,57,58] These changes are mediated by increased adipose tissue lipolytic activity and decreased lipoprotein lipase (LPL) activity (due to estrogens).[19,58] LPL, which is present in the capillary endothelium of extrahepatic tissues, hydrolyzes circulating triglycerides, including VLDL, producing free fatty acids and glycerol.[58] Adipose tissue is broken down into free fatty acids and glycerol, which circulate to the liver and are converted to active forms (acyl-CoA and glycerol-3-phosphate) and re-esterified into triglycerides (circulate as VLDL).[19,58] Glycerol can also be used for glucose synthesis (gluconeogenesis). The increased lipolysis is due to the rise of hPL levels with its antiinsulinogenic and lipolytic effects, as well as the effects of cortisol, glucagon, and prolactin, resulting in increased lipolytic activity in adipose tissue.[16,19,57,58,78] Enhanced ketogenesis in the liver is a consequence of increased oxidation of free fatty acids for energy and release of ketone bodies.[58] The fat mobilization is associated with increased glucose and amino acid uptake by the fetus. Thus fats are used by the mother as an alternative energy substrate, allowing the mother to conserve glucose for the fetus and her central nervous system (CNS) during the second half of gestation.[6,16,59,58] Fetal glucose and ketone uptake increases. Ketones are used by the fetus for oxidative metabolism, lipogenesis, triglyceride production, and as substrate for brain lipid synthesis.[58,78,116,130]

The changes in lipid metabolism during pregnancy are reflected in changes in maternal serum free fatty acid concentrations as well as plasma triglyceride, cholesterol, and phospholipid levels. These changes may be exaggerated in obese women.[27] The minimal change in free fatty acids during early pregnancy is probably due to increased fat storage and augmented fat utilization. As maternal fat stores are mobilized, serum levels of triglycerides, free fatty acids, glycerol, and triglyceride-rich lipoproteins (VLDL) increase to peak near

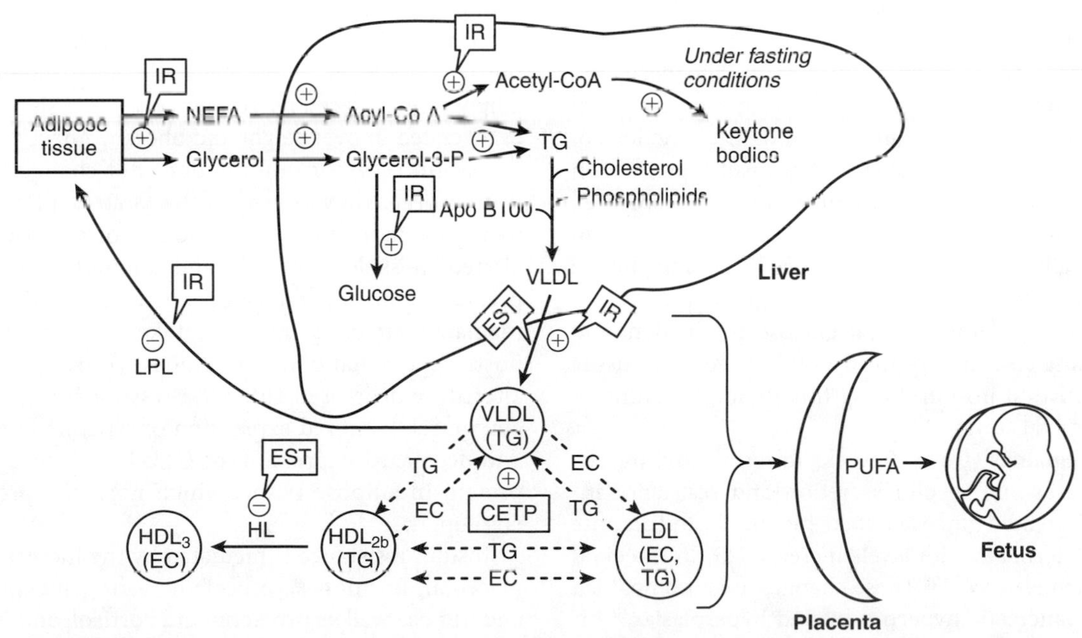

FIGURE 16-3 Major lipid metabolism interactions during late pregnancy, with indications of control roles of insulin resistance (IR) and enhanced estrogen (EST). +, activated steps; −, inhibited steps; *HL*, hepatic lipase; *LPL*, lipoprotein lipase; *NEFA*, nonesterified fatty acids; *TG*, triglyceride. (From Herrera, E., & Ortega-Senovilla, H. [2010]. Disturbances in lipid metabolism in diabetic pregnancy—Are these the cause of the problem? *Best Pract Res Clin Endocrinol Metab*, *24*, 517.)

term.[19,58,59] Because elevations in free fatty acids are due to catabolism of stored triglycerides (into free fatty acid and glycerol), changes in free fatty acids are mirrored by changes in glycerol.[6] Hypertriglyceridemia during the third trimester is primarily due to increases in VLDLs and decreased peripheral clearance.[16,19,58,59] The increase is due to reduced VLDL clearance secondary to decreased activity of LPL in the liver and adipose tissue, enhanced activity of cholesterol ester transferase, increased gastrointestinal absorption of lipids, and increased hepatic triglyceride production.[16,32,58,59] The decrease in lipoprotein lipase is due to increases in estrogens in late pregnancy and the increasing insulin resistance.[58,78] Near term, lipoprotein lipase activity increases in the mammary glands. This enhances availability of triglycerides for milk production.[57]

Changes in lipid metabolism are accompanied by functional and morphologic changes in the adipocytes. Hypertrophy of these cells accommodates the increased fat storage during the first two thirds of pregnancy. In the last trimester, maximal glucose transport, glucose oxidation, and lipogenesis within the adipocytes decrease.[42] The number of insulin receptors on the adipocytes increases in the first part of pregnancy and returns to prepregnant levels by term.[6,42] Because responsiveness of adipose tissue to insulin is not diminished as much as that of other tissues, these changes in the adipocytes facilitate fat storage.[42] After a meal, maternal fat stores are replenished by increased glucose uptake, incorporation of glucose into glycerol, and esterification of fatty acids by adipocytes.[6]

Table 16-1 Metabolic Effects of Insulin and Glucagon

HORMONE	METABOLIC ACTIONS
Insulin	Acts in the liver to:
	Increase glycogen synthesis from carbohydrate (glycogenesis) or fat and protein (glyconeogenesis)
	Decrease formation of glucose from fats and protein (gluconeogenesis)
	Increase protein synthesis
	Acts in muscle to:
	Increase glucose uptake
	Increase glycogen and protein synthesis
	Retard proteolysis
	Acts in adipose cells to:
	Increase glucose uptake
	Increase conversion of carbohydrate to fat
	Decrease lipolysis
	Increase uptake of free fatty acids
Glucagon	Acts in the liver to:
	Decrease glycogen synthesis and increase conversion of glycogen to glucose (glycogenolysis)
	Increase uptake of amino acids
	Increase conversion of alanine to glucose
	Increase ketogenesis
	Acts in adipose tissue to:
	Increase lipolysis

Compiled from Guyton, A.C., & Hall, J.E. (2010). *Textbook of medical physiology* (12th ed.). Philadelphia: Saunders Elsevier; Widmaier, E., Raff, H., & Strang, K.T. (2005). *Vander's Human physiology: The mechanism of body function* (10th ed.). New York: McGraw-Hill.

Insulin

Insulin levels and responsiveness of tissues to insulin change dramatically during pregnancy, leading to peripheral insulin resistance. Peripheral insulin resistance is "the decreased ability of insulin to affect glucose uptake, primarily in skeletal muscle and to a lesser degree in adipose tissue."[98] Actions of insulin are summarized in Table 16-1.[40] Insulin production and sensitivity during pregnancy differ in early compared to later pregnancy.[16] During early pregnancy (up to 12 to 14 weeks), insulin responses are enhanced, sending glucose to the embryo and young fetus. The pregnant woman has a normal glucose tolerance, basal glucose production, and peripheral muscle sensitivity to insulin.[16,110] Adipose tissue is more sensitive to insulin during this period, resulting in lipogenesis and fat storage.[110]

In later pregnancy (from 20 weeks to term), insulin sensitivity decreases and insulin secretion and resistance increase with decreased glucose uptake by muscle and adipose tissue.[16,131] Maternal insulin levels increase 2.5- to threefold by the third trimester.[47,78,98] These changes are accompanied by maternal pancreatic hypertrophy and hyperplasia.[110] Increased insulin secretion ensures adequate maternal protein synthesis in the face of increasing resistance of peripheral tissues to the effects of insulin. With increasing gestation, mean insulin sensitivity decreases up to 50% to 70%.[78] Tissue resistance is most prominent in liver, adipose, and muscle cells, and is further altered in women with preeclampsia.[119] The increasing insulin resistance promotes nutrient flux from the mother to the fetus and promotion of adipose tissue accumulation.[78] Insulin resistance is often exaggerated in overweight and obese women.[27]

Insulin receptor binding does not change significantly during pregnancy, however, the postreceptor insulin signaling cascade, and thus handling of glucose by cells, is altered in skeletal muscle and adipose tissue.[110] During pregnancy insulin receptor substrate-1 (IRS-1) is downregulated, affecting insulin uptake and use by cells.[98] The postreceptor handling of glucose during pregnancy is altered by decreased IRS-1 expression (especially in skeletal muscle), altered expression of tyrosine kinase activity, and decreased expression of GLUT-4 glucose transporter protein in adipose tissue, which normally promotes glucose uptake.[98,110]

Insulin resistance is mediated by the increasing levels of placental hormones, especially estrogens, progesterone, and hPL, as well as prolactin and cortisol, and is minimally affected by changes in blood glucose levels.[98] Other factors that play an important role in the insulin resistance of pregnancy are tumor necrosis factor-α and other cytokines, circulating free fatty acids, leptin, and placental growth hormone, which stimulates insulin-like growth factor-I (IGF-I).[15,78,197,124] In late pregnancy, although basal insulin levels are elevated, maternal blood glucose values are similar to prepregnant levels.[6] Increased insulin secretion after a meal (in response to the higher blood glucose) offsets the contrainsulin effects of the placental hormones and facilitates movement of nutrients to the fetus. The insulin resistance of late pregnancy enhances maternal fat breakdown and increased gluconeogenesis and ketogenesis in the postabsorptive state, the state in which changes in insulin response are most apparent.[16,47,58] If the pregnant woman is not able to elevate her insulin secretion to overcome the increasing pregnancy-induced insulin resistance, maternal and fetal hyperglycemia will result and metabolic abnormalities such as gestational diabetes may develop or existing metabolic problems such as diabetes will be aggravated.

Alterations in insulin production and responsiveness are critical in integrating changes in carbohydrate and fat metabolism throughout the course of pregnancy. Baird summarizes these interactions as follows: During early pregnancy, increased insulin in response to glucose, minimal changes in insulin sensitivity, and increased number of insulin receptors on the adipocytes result in normal or slightly enhanced carbohydrate tolerance. The increased hepatic synthesis and secretion of triglycerides during this period, along with a normal or slightly elevated removal of triglycerides from the circulation, lead to a net storage of fat. During late pregnancy, the elevated plasma insulin, decrease in numbers of adipocyte insulin receptors to prepregnant levels, and increasing insulin resistance result in reduced assimilation of glucose and triglycerides by maternal tissues, greater transfer of these substances to the fetus, and increased lipolysis. The net result is a decrease in maternal blood glucose, increased glucose turnover, and greater maternal reliance on lipid catabolism for energy.[6] Changes in lipid, carbohydrate, and protein metabolism are summarized in Table 16-2.

Absorptive versus Postabsorptive States

In addition to phasic changes in metabolic processes in early versus late pregnancy, metabolism of amino acids, carbohydrates, and fats also varies on a daily basis depending on whether the mother is in the absorptive (fed) or postabsorptive state (Figures 16-4 and 16-5). As a result of these changes, pregnancy has been characterized as a time of both "accelerated starvation" and "facilitated anabolism."[96]

Absorptive State. During the absorptive (fed) state, ingested nutrients (amino acid, glucose, triglyceride) are entering the blood from the gastrointestinal tract (see Chapter 12) and must be oxidized for energy, used for protein synthesis, or stored. The average meal takes 4 to 6 hours for complete absorption. In this state anabolism exceeds catabolism and glucose is the major energy source. Small amounts of amino acid and fat are converted into energy or used to resynthesize body proteins or for structural fat. Most of the amino acid and fat and any extra carbohydrate are transformed into adipose tissue; carbohydrate is also stored as glycogen.

Insulin has an anabolic and anticatabolic role during this state.[78] Insulin secretion increases and plasma insulin levels rise. Insulin promotes glucose uptake by the hepatocytes and peripheral tissues, inhibits glycogen breakdown, and inhibits lipolysis in adipose tissue. Glucose is converted to glycogen for storage in the liver, cardiac muscle, and skeletal muscle. Muscle amino acid uptake is enhanced and proteolysis inhibited.[78]

After a meal the pregnant woman has higher glucose, insulin, and triglyceride levels and suppression of glycogen compared to nonpregnant women. Thus the absorptive state during pregnancy (see Figure 16-4, *A*) is characterized by relative hyperinsulinemia (related to decreased insulin sensitivity), hyperglycemia (due to failure of liver glucose uptake), insulin resistance (especially in skeletal muscle), hypertriglyceridemia, and lipogenesis (more glucose is converted to triglyceride for storage).[6,16,78,119,129] Pregnancy has been called a state of facilitated anabolism to describe

Table 16-2 Maternal Metabolic Processes during Pregnancy: Relationship between Hormonal and Metabolic Changes

HORMONAL CHANGE	EFFECT	METABOLIC CHANGE
Increased hPL	Diabetogenic Decreased glucose tolerance	Facilitated anabolism during feeding Accelerated starvation during fasting
Increased prolactin	Insulin resistance	Facilitated anabolism during feeding Accelerated starvation during fasting
Increased bound and free cortisol	Decreased hepatic glycogen stores Increased hepatic glucose production	Ensures glucose and amino acids to fetus
Increased estrogen, progesterone, and insulin during early pregnancy	Increased fat synthesis Fat cell hypertrophy Inhibition of lipolysis	Anabolic fat storage during early pregnancy
Increased hPL in late pregnancy	Lipolysis	Catabolic fat mobilization in late pregnancy

Adapted from Moore, T.R. (2004). Diabetes and pregnancy. In R.K. Creasy, R. Resnik, & J.D. Iams (Eds.), *Maternal-fetal medicine: Principles and practice* (5th ed.). Philadelphia: Saunders. *hPL,* human placental lactogen.

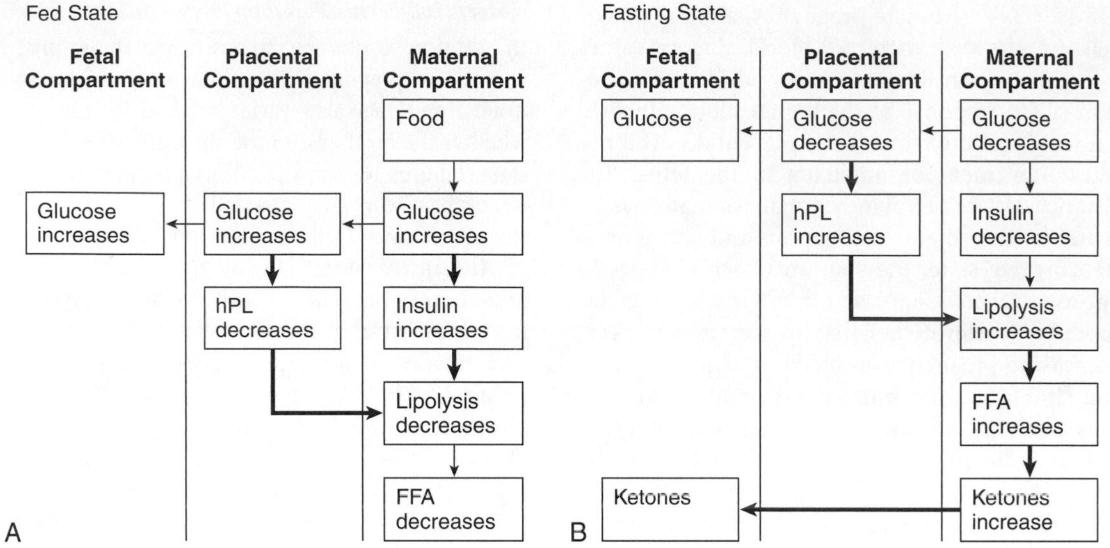

FIGURE 16-4 The absorptive and postabsorptive states during pregnancy. **A,** Absorptive or fed state. **B,** Postabsorptive or fasting state. (From Speroff, L., Glass, R.H., & Kase, N.G. [1999]. *Clinical gynecologic endocrinology and fertility* [6th ed.]. Baltimore: Williams & Wilkins.)

these metabolic alterations that conserve energy, especially during early pregnancy.[94] These changes increase glucose availability for transport to the fetus; increase availability of an alternate energy source (triglycerides) for maternal needs; and provide fewer stimuli for maternal gluconeogenesis, glycogenolysis, and ketogenesis.[42,47]

Maternal blood glucose levels may rise transiently to 130 to 140 mg/dL (7.2 to 7.8 mmol/L) (see Figure 16-5). Gluconeogenesis and circulating free fatty acids are decreased. Under the influence of placental hormones, resistance of the liver and peripheral tissues to insulin is increased by as much as 60% to 70%.[119,129] The hyperinsulinemic response is most marked during the third trimester because of hypertrophy and hyperplasia of islet β cells. These cells become more responsive to alterations in blood glucose and amino acid levels. The increased insulin levels after eating overcome the insulin resistance to allow glucose uptake by muscles for storage as glycogen.[119] Even with increased production of insulin, however, overall glucose levels are maintained, although at a relatively lower level than in nonpregnant women because of the counterbalancing effects of estrogen, progesterone, and hPL.

Postabsorptive and Fasting State. In the postabsorptive state (i.e., when nutrients are not entering the blood from the intestines, beginning 4 to 6 hours after a meal) and fasting state (12 or more hours after the last meal), energy must be supplied by body stores. Insulin levels are low. Fat and protein synthesis are decreased and catabolism exceeds anabolism. Gluconeogenesis (production of new glucose from lactate, amino acids [especially alanine], and glycerol) and catabolism of fat are the main sources of energy.[78] Plasma glucose levels are maintained during the postabsorptive state by use of these alternate sources of glucose and glucose-sparing or fat-utilization reactions.[16,42] The CNS continues to use glucose, while other organs and tissues become glucose sparing, depending on fat as the primary energy source.

During the fasting state (e.g., overnight between the evening meal and breakfast), plasma glucose levels decline. The magnitude of the decline is greater in pregnant women than in nonpregnant women, due to the continuous transfer of glucose to the fetus, and is associated with a more rapid conversion to fat metabolism. Fatty acids are liberated by breakdown of triglycerides. Lipolysis yields glycerol (converted to glucose by the liver) and free fatty acids, which are catabolized to ketone bodies (oxidized for energy). Under homeostatic conditions ketones do not accumulate in the body to produce ketoacidosis because excess ketones not needed for energy are rapidly cleared by the kidneys.[78]

This response is an exaggeration of the changes normally seen during the overnight fast in nonpregnant women. These changes would normally raise blood glucose levels, but in the pregnant woman the fasting glucose level tends to be lower because of the limited availability of substrate for gluconeogenesis. For example, as early as 15 weeks' gestation, maternal glucose levels after a 12- to 14-hour overnight fast are 15 to 20 mg (0.8 to 1.1 mmol/L) lower than levels in nonpregnant women. The decrease in glucose during the overnight "fasting" period is especially prominent during the second and third trimesters.[6,78]

The exaggerated maternal responses during the fasting state are influenced by (1) continuous placental uptake of glucose and amino acids from the maternal circulation; (2) decreased peripheral utilization of glucose as plasma concentrations of ketones and free fatty acids increase; (3) decreased renal absorption of glucose; and (4) decreased

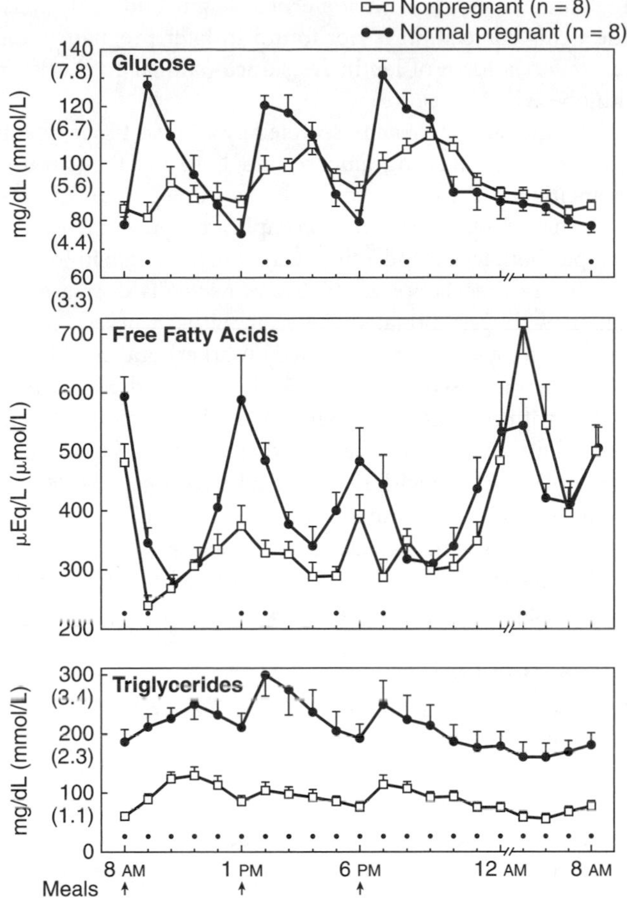

FIGURE 16-5 Glucose and insulin response to 24 hours of feeding and fasting in the third trimester of pregnancy (closed circles) and the nonpregnant state (open squares). In the fed state, pregnancy is associated with elevated levels of both circulating glucose and insulin. In the fasting state, pregnancy is associated with decreases in glucose below those seen in the nonpregnant state. (From Phelps, R.L., et al. [1981]. Carbohydrate metabolism in pregnancy. *Am J Obstet Gynecol, 140,* 730.)

hepatic glucose production. This response, seen primarily in late pregnancy, is characterized by lower fasting glucose and amino acid levels, increased blood glucose levels after eating, and increased plasma free fatty acids, triglycerides, ketones, and insulin secretion in response to glucose.[12,42,78] Thus the postabsorptive fasting state in pregnancy is characterized by a relative hypoglycemia (due to the fetal siphon, increased renal losses, and decreased liver production), hyperketonuria (ketones used as an alternative energy source), hypoaminoacidemia (due to placental transfer for use in fetal glucose production), and hypoinsulinemia (see Figures 16-4, *B*, and 16-5).[12,24,57,72,78,98] Hypoalaninemia also develops because maternal protein stores can provide only limited substrate, which is insufficient to meet both maternal and fetal amino acid needs.[47] Increased insulin during the postabsorptive state enhances uptake of glucose into the maternal skeletal muscle and adipose tissue. In lean women, this leads to suppression of hepatic glucose production in late pregnancy. Less suppression is seen in obese women, therefore the alteration in insulin sensitivity is greater in obese than nonobese women.[98]

Levels of lipoprotein lipase are increased, enhancing triglyceride breakdown with release of free fatty acids and glycerol (which is broken down into glucose) and production of ketone bodies to provide energy when plasma glucose supply is low.[16] Glycerol is a source for hepatic gluconeogenesis. The elevated free fatty acids prevent glucose uptake and oxidation by maternal cells, thus preserving glucose for the maternal CNS and the fetus.[12] In the nonpregnant woman this switch to fat oxidation occurs after 14 to 18 hours of fasting; during pregnancy the switch occurs after 2 to 3 hours and has been termed accelerated starvation.[12,19,42,96]

Metabolic changes characteristic of this state are primarily due to hPL, which promotes lipolysis to increase free fatty acid levels and opposes insulin action, thus increasing glucose availability to the fetus. Other factors influencing this response include increased glucose utilization by the fetus ("the fetal siphon") and mother, along with an increase in the volume of distribution for glucose (i.e., hemodilution).[78] During the second half of pregnancy, effectiveness of insulin in translocating glucose into cells is reduced.[78] Because insulin is the ultimate arbitrator of both the absorptive and postabsorptive states, alterations in insulin secretion alter substrate availability to the mother and fetus.[47] The insulin antagonism in pregnancy is progressive, paralleling the growth of the fetoplacental unit, and disappears immediately after delivery. Placental hormones and other substances are major factors in producing this insulin antagonism.

Drainage of glucose and amino acids by the fetus may lead to increased maternal appetite and a feeling of faintness sometimes experienced in pregnancy. Pregnant women may experience more rapid development of ketosis and fasting hypoglycemia after food deprivation. With greater maternal reliance on fat utilization during pregnancy, production of ketone bodies and risks of abnormalities such as acidosis are increased. Dieting and caloric restriction during pregnancy should be considered potentially dangerous to both the mother and fetus.[37]

Effects of Placental Hormones and Other Substances

The phasic changes in carbohydrate, lipid, and protein metabolism during pregnancy are due to the interplay of placental hormones, especially estrogen, progesterone, hPL, and leptin.[75,98] During the first half of pregnancy, metabolism is affected primarily by estrogens and progesterone. In late pregnancy the influences of increasing concentrations of hPL and leptin become more prominent. Maternal metabolic changes are also influenced by prolactin and cortisol.[12]

Estrogen stimulates islet β-cell hyperplasia and insulin secretion, enhances glucose utilization in peripheral tissues, and increases plasma cortisol, an insulin antagonist. As a result, particularly in the first half of gestation, estrogen decreases fasting glucose levels, improves glucose tolerance, and increases glycogen storage.[78] Progesterone augments insulin secretion, increases fasting plasma insulin concentrations, and diminishes peripheral insulin effectiveness. Cortisol mediates these changes by inhibiting glucose uptake and oxidation, increasing liver glucose production, and possibly augmenting glucagon secretion.[12] Cortisol increases to 2.5 times normal levels by late pregnancy.[12,131] Prolactin increases fivefold to 10-fold and stimulates insulin production and, at least in animal models, increases the number of β-cell receptors.[131]

Human placental lactogen (hPL), also called human chorionic somatomammotropin (hCS), is a polypeptide hormone produced by the syncytiotrophoblast (see Chapter 3). hPL is the most potent insulin antagonist of the placental hormones. This hormone is secreted primarily into the maternal circulation although some is also secreted into fetal circulation after around 6 weeks.[43] Levels of hPL increase markedly after 20 weeks. Because effects of hPL are similar to those of growth hormone, it has been called the "growth hormone" of the second half of pregnancy.[12] hPL action increases availability of maternal glucose and amino acids to the fetus. Other effects of hPL include diminished tissue response to insulin; increased β-cell mass; lipolysis, which increases plasma free fatty acids; enhanced nitrogen retention; decreased urinary potassium excretion; and increased calcium excretion. The major effect is sparing of maternal carbohydrate (glucose) by providing alternative energy sources such as free fatty acids for the mother.[16]

Several adipokines, including leptin, adiponectin, and retinal binding protein 4 (RBP4), are also important for ensuring adequate substrate for fetal growth.[58] Leptin, a protein product of the obese (ob) gene, was identified in 1994. It is produced and secreted by adipose tissue and other tissues, including the placenta during pregnancy. Leptin is involved in regulating appetite and food intake and enhancing energy expenditure, and may also be important in signaling readiness for sexual maturation at puberty.[128] Leptin receptors are found in the hypothalamus, placenta, muscle, liver, lymphoid tissue, uterus, chorion, amnion, pancreas, ovary, and adipose tissue.[78,124] Placental leptin is secreted into both maternal and fetal circulations.[86]

Leptin plays a role in maturation and regulation of reproduction and "may serve as a detector of long-term metabolic fuel availability signaling the presence of significant maternal fat stores to initiate reproduction."[16] Leptin modulates glucose metabolism, insulin sensitivity, and adipose tissue lipolysis during pregnancy, enhancing breakdown of maternal fat stores in the second half of pregnancy and availability of glucose and lipids for the fetus.[58] Other roles of leptin in pregnancy may be to mediate changes in appetite, thermogenesis, and lipid metabolism.[16,49] Leptin may also modulate fetal growth. Concentrations of leptin increase from 6 to 8 weeks' gestation, rising further in the second and (especially) third trimesters.[81] The increase is probably primarily due to increased placental leptin production. Levels in early pregnancy correlate with maternal weight and body mass index; this correlation is not found in later pregnancy and may reflect a form of leptin resistance (similar to that seen with obesity).[16,81]

Adiponectin is a protein, secreted by adipose tissue, that is involved in modulating glucose and lipid metabolism and enhancing insulin sensitivity.[58] Changes in leptin and adiponectin have been reported in complicated pregnancies. For example, both leptin and adiponectin are increased in women with severe preeclampsia.[7,84,86] Adiponectin is decreased in women with gestational diabetes mellitus, whereas tumor necrosis factor-α (an inflammatory marker) and cord blood leptin are increased.[55,58,90,112] Low levels of adiponectin in women with gestational diabetes may play a role in the increased insulin resistance seen in these women.[58] Low leptin levels are associated with spontaneous abortion.[83] RBP4 may also have a role in glucose metabolism and insulin sensitivity. RBP4 increases with increasing gestational age (probably due to placental production) and is increased in pregnancies complicated by gestational diabetes.[58]

Intrapartum Period

The processes of parturition are dependent on an available supply of glucose and triglycerides as energy sources. In addition, essential fatty acids are important as precursors of prostaglandins (arachidonic acid, from which prostaglandins are derived, is a derivative of essential fatty acid), which are critical to the onset of labor. These relationships are described in Chapter 4.

During labor and delivery, maternal glucose consumption increases markedly to produce the energy required by the uterus and skeletal muscles.[47] As a result, maternal insulin requirements fall. Oxytocin may augment or supplant insulin during this period. In animals, oxytocin has been demonstrated to act similarly to insulin; that is, oxytocin stimulates glucose oxidation, lipogenesis, glycogen synthesis, and protein formation.[47]

Postpartum Period

With removal of the placenta, concentrations of placental hormones such as hPL, estrogens, and progesterone fall rapidly within hours after delivery (see Chapter 5). The postpartum woman is in a state of relative hypopituitarism with blunted production of gonadotropins and growth hormone.[47] This hypopituitarism may result from the feedback effects of elevated hPL and prolactin levels during pregnancy on the pituitary gland. hPL is similar to growth hormone, and its disappearance with removal of the placenta leaves the woman without its contrainsulin effects during a period of relative deficiency of growth hormone.[47] Plasma leptin levels decrease by 24 hours after delivery.[83]

Fasting plasma glucose levels fall within a few days, then increase reaching late pregnancy fasting levels by 5 days.[42] It is unclear when these levels return to prepregnant values.[42] The insulin resistance of late pregnancy is reversed soon after delivery.[98]

Plasma free fatty acids fall to prepregnant levels by 3 days; triglycerides by 2 weeks.[18,42] During the first week the decrease in triglycerides coincides with the fall in hPL. This fall is more rapid in women who are breastfeeding.[18,58] In these women, free fatty acids rise to late pregnancy levels by 6 weeks, followed by a decrease to prepregnant levels by 3 to 6 months.[6] The increasing levels of fatty acids from 1 to 6 weeks postpartum may reflect maternal use of other nutrients for milk production.[6] Cholesterol levels slowly decrease to prepregnant levels over the first few weeks postpartum.[42] Maternal plasma amino acid levels return to prepregnant values of approximately 4.3 mg/dL (0.043 g/L) (versus pregnant values of 3.5 mg/dL [0.35 g/L]) by several days after birth.[1,35]

CLINICAL IMPLICATIONS FOR THE PREGNANT WOMAN AND HER FETUS

The metabolic adaptations of pregnancy safeguard against variations in maternal caloric intake, changes in activity, increased metabolic efficiency, and changes in the metabolism of carbohydrates, fats, and proteins.[6] These metabolic changes occur in a phasic pattern—probably programmed by placental hormones—that spreads the energy costs and protein requirements of pregnancy over the entire 9 months of gestation. In early pregnancy, energy is conserved (facilitated anabolism), followed by later redirection of energy (glucose) to the fetus ("accelerated starvation"), whereas throughout pregnancy the mother uses protein more economically to provide adequate amino acids for development of the fetal brain and other organs.[6,47] Pregnancy has also been characterized as a diabetogenic state. This state is reflected in the elevated blood glucose levels in association with increasing insulin resistance. This state is described in this section along with the basis for alterations in the glucose tolerance test (GTT) and the effects of the normal metabolic changes of pregnancy on the diabetic woman and her fetus.

The diabetogenic effects of pregnancy are reflected by alterations in the GTT, with higher glucose values after a meal reflecting an acquired resistance to insulin. The alterations in carbohydrate metabolism are most evident during late pregnancy in the absorptive state (see Figure 16-4, *A*). When the woman is in this state and glucose is being added to the plasma from the gut, her blood glucose levels do not drop as rapidly as usual, even in the face of higher circulating insulin levels. This response results from decreased maternal sensitivity to insulin due to the action of hormones such as hPL, progesterone, and cortisol. Secretion of these hormones increases during the second half of pregnancy; therefore diabetogenic effects are most prominent during this period. Insulin resistance is somewhat compensated for by increased plasma insulin concentrations.[78]

The changes in insulin sensitivity tend to protect the fetus if the mother is fasting by keeping glucose in the blood and thus available for placental transfer. hPL decreases insulin effectiveness (and thus movement of glucose out of the blood into maternal cells) by decreasing tissue sensitivity and mobilizes free fatty acids and amino acids. The result is an increase in available glucose and amino acids for transfer to the fetus and increased free fatty acids for maternal energy.

Effects of Metabolic Changes on Glucose Tolerance Tests

The alterations in carbohydrate metabolism in the absorptive state during pregnancy result in an elevated blood glucose response to a carbohydrate load. The progressive decrease in glucose tolerance is reflected in the criteria for an abnormal GTT in pregnancy. These changes are most marked in the third trimester.

Two methods commonly used to evaluate glucose tolerance in pregnancy are (1) a one-step 75-g, 2-hour test (recommended by the World Health Organization); and (2) a two-step test with a 1-hour 50-g glucose challenge (screening test) followed by a 100-g, 3-hour oral glucose tolerance test (OGTT) if challenge levels are either 135 mg/dL (7.5 mmol/L) or greater (more women meet criteria for the 3-hour test, but a greater proportion of women with gestational diabetes mellitus [GDM] are identified) or 140 mg/dL (7.8 mmol/L).[78,98] The one-step testing has a lower detection rate for GDM.[97] The two-step test has been used most commonly in the United States, whereas the one-step test is used most commonly in other countries.[95,98] The Fifth International Workshop Conference on Gestational Diabees Mellitus recommended the two-step test.[95] However, following the Hyperglycemia and Adverse Pregnancy Outcome (HAPO) study, the International Association of Diabetes and Pregnancy Study Groups (IADPSG) recommended use of a 75-g glucose load followed by fasting, 12-, and 2-hour plasma glucose concentrations.[64]

During pregnancy, the initial fasting blood glucose value is lower than in nonpregnant individuals, because of decreased glucose utilization and increased fat utilization by the mother (making increased glucose available to the fetus) and the subsequent effects of the fetal siphon. Blood glucose levels tend to remain high after ingestion of carbohydrates for a longer period of time secondary to insulin antagonism and decreased insulin sensitivity. Normally the magnitude of the increase in blood glucose after a carbohydrate feeding is a reflection of failure in glucose uptake by the liver. During pregnancy the increased glucose response in the face of increased endogenous insulin confirms the relative insensitivity and resistance of the liver (as well as peripheral tissues such as muscle and adipose tissue) to insulin.[78,98]

Maternal-Fetal Relationships

Growth and development of the fetus is dependent upon the availability of a constant supply of glucose, amino acids, and lipids from the mother for energy, protein synthesis, and production of new tissues. The fetus must also develop adequate stores of these substances to meet the demands of the intrapartum period and transition to extrauterine life. Placental transfer of selected nutrients and hormones is summarized in Figure 16-6. Fetal requirements for substrates

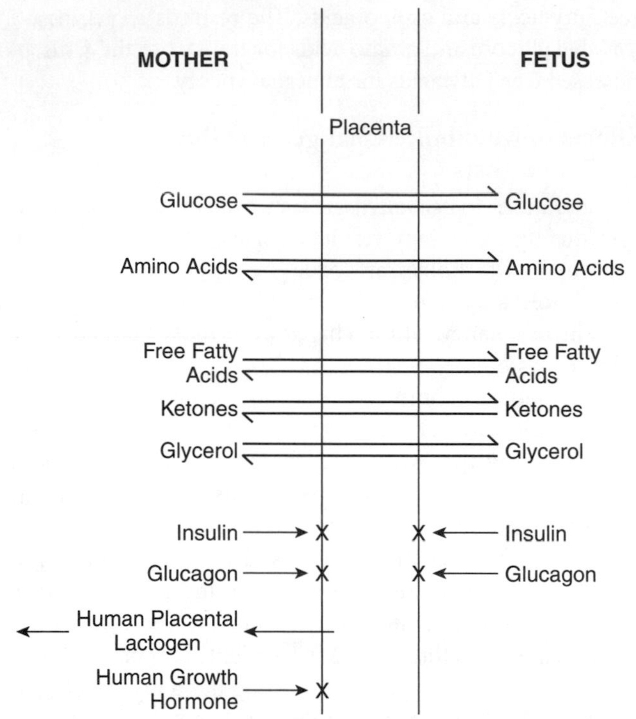

FIGURE 16-6 Maternal-fetal substrate, hormone relationships. (From Kalhan, S., & Parimi, P.S. [2006]. Disorders of carbohydrate metabolism. In A.A. Fanaroff, R.J. Martin, & M.C. Walsh [Eds.], *Fanaroff and Martin's Neonatal-perinatal medicine: Diseases of the fetus and infant* [8th ed.]. St. Louis: Mosby.)

involved in carbohydrate, fat, and protein metabolism are discussed in the next section.

Alterations in maternal metabolic processes or in placental transfer of essential nutrients that increase the availability of specific substrates are usually an advantage to the fetus but can be a disadvantage in altered maternal metabolic states. For example, because fetal energy requirements are met almost exclusively by glucose, the metabolic changes in pregnancy increase availability of glucose in maternal plasma for placental transfer by reducing the efficiency of maternal glucose storage. If the usual metabolic changes of pregnancy or placental function are altered, however, variations in fetal growth—such as occur in the infant of a diabetic mother or the an infant with fetal growth restriction—may develop.[122] Maternal glucose infusions during the intrapartum period can lead to a fetal hyperglycemia that stimulates insulin and inhibits glucagon secretion. This may delay gluconeogenesis after birth and increase the risk of neonatal hypoglycemia.

The placenta is a highly metabolic organ with its own substrate needs. Placental metabolic activities include glycolysis, gluconeogenesis, glycogenesis, oxidation, protein synthesis, amino acid interconversion, triglyceride synthesis, and alterations in the length of fatty acid chains (see Chapter 3). The placenta can modify nutrient uptake to meet fetal growth demands.[115] The degree of glucose uptake by the placenta is similar to that of the brain. Cholesterol from the mother is essential for placental synthesis of estrogens and progesterone. Fatty acids are needed by the placenta for oxidation and membrane formation.[16] Leptin may have a role in coordinating placental metabolism.[81]

Glucose is the nutrient that crosses the placenta in highest concentrations. The increased maternal reliance on fats as an alternative energy source, especially during the maternal postabsorptive fasting state, conserves maternal glucose for transfer to the fetus. The fetal-placental unit uses approximately 50% of the total maternal glucose needed for pregnancy.[57] Glucose crosses via facilitated transport by insulin dependent glucose transporters.[81] Amino acids are transferred via active transport because levels are higher in the fetus than in the mother. Amino acids are removed from maternal circulation and concentrated in the placental intercellular matrix. As fetal amino acid levels fall, these placental stores are transferred to the fetus. Mechanisms for amino acid transfer include direct transfer from mother to fetus without modification in the placenta, metabolism of maternally derived amino acids by the placenta to produce other amino acids (which are then transferred to the fetus), and production of new amino acids by the placenta for fetal transfer.[57,61] Maternal lipoproteins do not cross the placenta directly, but are taken up by the placenta where placental lipoprotein lipase along with other lipases, enzymes, receptors, and fatty acid binding proteins facilitate transfer of fatty acids to the fetus.[57,58,59,78] Essential fatty acids and long-chain polyunsaturated fatty acids needed for fetal growth and development cross the placenta.[59] Free fatty acids are transferred to the fetus according to maternal-fetal concentration gradients mediated by specific fatty acid carriers. The pattern of essential and other fatty acids in the fetus reflect maternal concentrations.[57,61] Ketones, especially acetoacetate and β-hydroxybutyrate, diffuse readily across the placenta; concentrations are similar in the mother and fetus.[78] Inadequate maternal dietary fatty acids such as docosahexaenoic acid (DHA) increase the risk of altered neurologic and vision development in offspring.[18,44]

The Pregnant Diabetic Woman

The classification system for diabetes proposed by the National Diabetes Data Group and adopted by the American Diabetic Association includes (1) type 1 diabetes ("β-cell destruction, usually leading to absolute insulin deficiency"), (2) type 2 diabetes ("ranging from predominantly insulin resistance with relative insulin deficiency to predominantly an insulin secretory defect with insulin resistance"), (3) other specific types of diabetes (including genetic defects, pancreas alterations, or endocrine, drug-induced, or infectious etiologies), and (4) gestational diabetes mellitus.[3] Individuals with impaired fasting glucose and/or impaired glucose tolerance are referred to as having "pre-diabetes."[3]

The metabolic changes during pregnancy contribute to alterations in insulin requirements in insulin-dependent pregnant diabetic women. Because the metabolic changes in pregnancy normally lead to increased insulin availability by the end of pregnancy, it is not surprising that pregnant diabetic women experience an increase in insulin requirements by this time.[47,78,98]

Management of the pregnant diabetic woman and the woman who develops gestational diabetes is complex. There are many controversies regarding screening, diagnosis, treatment, and outcomes of women with gestational diabetes.[46,70,78,87] Guidelines for screening and diagnosis of gestational diabetes from various groups around the world were summarized by Leary et al. in a recent article.[87] Some of the current controversies relate to the findings and subsequent recommendations from the HAPO study.[41,45,46,87] The HAPO study was a prospective, randomized controlled multinational study of 25,000 pregnant women in 10 countries who did not have a diagnosis of diabetes on study entry.[45,46] This study examined the relationship between maternal glucose concentrations lower than those diagnostic of diabetes and adverse perinatal outcomes.[45,85] Findings demonstrated a linear association between findings on the 75-g OGTT and the following fetal/maternal outcomes: birth weight greater than 90th percentile, increased cord blood C-peptide level, and risks of neonatal hypoglycemia, fetal shoulder dystocia, neonatal hyperbilirubinemia, and maternal preeclampsia.[45,46] In the HAPO study, both fasting and post 75-g OGTT levels were correlated to maternal and neonatal outcomes.[26,41,45,85] In response to the HAPO study, an IADPSG consensus panel recently published new guidelines on screening and diagnosis of GDM at the first prenatal visit for all or high-risk women and screening all women at 24 to 28 weeks. With the IADPSG recommendations women would be diagnosed with GDM earlier on the basis of an initial fasting glucose of 92 to 126 mg/dL (5.1 to 7.0 mmol/L) or an abnormal fasting (92 mg/dL or 5.1 mmol/L), 1-hour (180 mg/dL or 10.0 mmol/L), or 2-hour (153 mg/dL or 8.5 mmol/L) 75-g OGTT with a single abnormal glucose considered adequate for the diagnosis.[64] Recommendations are controversial and their effect on current practice and policies is unclear.[41,87,132]

GDM is defined as "carbohydrate intolerance of various degrees of severity with onset or first recognition during pregnancy."[98] GDM occurs in 3% to 9% of pregnancies in the United States.[98] Women with GDM have a pronounced peripheral insulin resistance, decreased numbers of insulin receptors, and decreased binding of insulin to target cells, which results in a progressive alteration in glucose tolerance.[16] Fasting, postprandial, and 24-hour glucose, and lipid and amino acid concentrations are altered.[16] Possible etiologies include an autoimmune defect in the β cells, impaired β-cell function, increased insulin degradation, and decreased tissue sensitivity to insulin, either due to impaired insulin-receptor binding or intracellular insulin signaling.[110] Two to 13% of women with GDM have specific antibodies against β-cell antigens.[98] Most women with GDM have impaired β-cell function and adaptation during pregnancy with chronic insulin resistance, which has an additive effect in pregnancy.[98] It is unclear if insulin resistance occurs prior to alterations in β-cell function or if these events occur together.[98] A decrease in IRS-1 concentration and decreased ability of insulin receptor-B (found inside skeletal muscle cells) to be phosphorylated by tyrosine have been reported.[98] These changes further alter insulin signaling and reduces glucose transport activity. In late pregnancy, the pregnant woman normally increases insulin secretion, but the woman with GDM, because of underlying chronic insulin resistance, has even greater insulin resistance, producing less insulin compared to the amount of resistance.[98]

During the postpartum period, women with GDM continue to show defects in insulin action and sensitivity, even after glucose tolerance tests have normalized.[2] Women with GDM have an increased risk for later development of diabetes, primarily type 2.[16] Approximately 10% develop diabetes in the first months postpartum, 50% by 5 years postpartum, and 70% by 10 years postpartum.[2,16,17] The risk is greater with weight gain after pregnancy or GDM in a subsequent pregnancy.[2,16] Several studies suggest that infant outcomes, including macrosomia and shoulder dystocia, could be reduced by treating women with mild hyperglycemia who did not reach diagnostic criteria for GDM.[26,85]

Pregnant women with type 1 diabetes may experience no change or decreased insulin requirements during the first trimester because of increased glucose siphoning by the fetus, which decreases maternal blood glucose levels. Maternal food intake may also decrease during this period because of the nausea and vomiting of pregnancy. Because circulating glucose levels are reduced, maternal insulin requirements are often lowered. As pregnancy progresses, the diabetogenic actions of increasing amounts of placental hormones and the increasing insulin insensitivity outweigh the effects of the fetal siphon. Women with type 1 diabetes appear to have similar alterations in insulin sensitivity during pregnancy to woman with normal glucose tolerance.[98] Thus maternal insulin requirements usually increase during the second half of gestation to levels two to three times higher than prepregnancy values.[47,78,98]

The diabetic woman may have altered insulin requirements during labor, probably because of an increase in energy needs (and thus glucose utilization) and the presence of oxytocin, with its insulin-like effects. After delivery and removal of the placenta, levels of estrogens, progesterone, and hPL fall rapidly. This quickly reverses the insulin insensitivity of pregnancy. Maternal insulin requirements usually fall rapidly to prepregnancy levels or even below (due to a rebound phenomenon). Oxytocin may also contribute to these changes. As a result, the insulin-dependent diabetic woman may need little or no exogenous insulin the first few days after delivery. Insulin requirements generally return to prepregnancy levels by 4 to 6 weeks postpartum.[37]

Levels of glycosylated hemoglobin and other glycosylated proteins are useful in monitoring glucose concentrations over time and in genetic counseling and have been used to evaluate fetal and maternal risks for complications in a pregnancy complicated by maternal diabetes. Glycosylated hemoglobin is formed slowly over the lifespan of the red blood cell and represents an overall measure of glycemia. The parameters used most frequently are hemoglobin A1c (the most abundant component of hemoglobin A) and total amounts of hemoglobin A. Levels of glycosylated hemoglobin A reflect ambient glucose concentrations over the previous 4 to 6 weeks and have been used to monitor maternal glycemic control on a monthly basis. Hemoglobin A1c is higher in pregnant diabetic women than in other pregnant women, but lower than in nonpregnant diabetic women. Maternal levels of hemoglobin A1c correlate with development of fetal anomalies, with the lowest levels having the least risk.[98,111] Hemoglobin A1c is not as useful as an independent measure of glycemic control in pregnancy, because these levels may not be a good predictor of capillary blood glucose levels in the woman.

Fetus of a Diabetic Mother

Maternal metabolic abnormalities, particularly hyperglycemia during the period of embryonic organogenesis (3 to 8 weeks' gestation), have been associated with an increased risk of congenital anomalies.[1,78,81,98] The most common anomalies involve the cardiovascular system (especially atrial septal defects, ventricular septal defects, and transposition of the great vessels) and central nervous system (neural tube defects), with urinary tract malformations, anal/rectal atresias, and caudal regression syndrome also seen with increased frequency.[78] The risk is increased four- to eight-fold in women with overt diabetes prior to conception, with no increase in women who develop GDM after the first trimester or in offspring of diabetic fathers.[98] Rigid glycemic control before conception and during early pregnancy has been associated with a reduction in the frequency of congenital anomalies, but the risk is still higher than in the nondiabetic woman.[62,98] Preconceptional counseling and glycemic control are critical for improving pregnancy outcome in a diabetic mother. Using data from a meta-analysis, Ray and colleagues reported that mean fasting capillary glucose levels of 70 to 130 mg/dL (3.9 to 7.2 mmol/L) and a glycosylated hemoglobin level less than 4 standard deviations above normal during the periconceptional period minimized the risk of glycemia-related anomalies.[111] The basis for the increase in anomalies is not completely understood. Possible etiologies include excessive formation of free oxygen radicals in the mitochondria; inhibition of prostacyclin formation resulting in an excess of thromboxane A2, as compared to prostacyclin (thromboxane A2 is a potent vasoconstrictor that alters vascularization of tissues); altered levels of arachidonic acid and myoinositol; lipid peroxidation; increased somatomedin inhibitors; accumulation of sorbitol and trace metals; and hyperglycemia-induced apoptosis with exaggerated programmed cell death (glucose alters the expression of regulating genes).[78,98,104]

Macrosomia is seen in up to 20% of infants of women with GDM and 35% of women with other forms of diabetes.[116] This phenomenon is generally thought to arise from increased fetal production of insulin and other growth factors, especially IGF-I and leptin, in response to fetal hyperglycemia.[66,98,105] This leads to excessive transfer of nutrients across the placenta. Because maternal insulin does not cross the placenta (see Figure 16-6), fetal hyperinsulinemia arises as a response to increased placental transfer of substrates, particularly glucose. Maternal hyperglycemia increases fetal insulin, IGFs, and leptin, which up-regulates glucose transporters (GLUT) that move glucose across the placenta and into fetal cells.[41,58,62,103] Up-regulation of these glucose transporters in women with type 1 diabetes may lead to excessive transfer of glucose to the fetus even with good maternal glucose control.[32] Hyperglycemia in pregnant diabetic women results in fetal hyperglycemia and subsequent hyperplasia of the fetal pancreatic islet cells, with increased production of insulin, enhanced glycogen synthesis, lipogenesis, and increased protein synthesis.[98,129]

Increased levels of other substances ("mixed nutrients"), particularly amino acids and fatty acids, are also thought to be important in the development of fetal macrosomia, because fetal overgrowth remains a problem even with strict glycemic control.[58,67] Maternal diabetes alters lipid metabolism and increases transfer of fatty acids to the fetus and the amount of triglyceride stored in the placenta.[58] These changes are secondary to alterations in several factors that influence fatty acid transfer, including maternal and fetal blood flow and concentrations of serum proteins and placental fatty acid–binding protein. Elevated levels of triglycerides in the pregnant diabetic woman also enhance lipid availability to the fetus.[58] Maternal triglycerides and nonesterified fatty acid levels in women with well controlled GDM correlated with fat mass and weight in the newborn.[117] Increased intrauterine fat deposition may also be due to altered fat metabolism in the fetus of women with GDM.[103]

Levels of endogenous insulin and IGF-I in the fetus are correlated with the development of macrosomia.[67] Insulin and IGF-I are major mediators of fetal growth; therefore fetal hyperinsulinemia leads to increased body fat and organ size. The major organs affected are the heart, lungs, liver, spleen, thymus, and adrenal gland. The brain and kidney are not significantly affected. The organomegaly probably arises from increased protein synthesis. Even short-term fetal hyperinsulinemia promotes storage of excess nutrients. Stringent maternal glucose control, especially during the third trimester, when fetal growth peaks, reduces the risk of macrosomia, primarily be reducing fetal adipose tissue mass.[105] However, the accelerated growth velocity seen in these infants may continue into childhood and adulthood.

The placenta is also affected, especially in women whose diabetes is poorly controlled, with increased peripheral and capillary surface area and intervillous space volume. These changes may result from the increased glucose load and abnormal metabolic environment with fetal hyperinsulinemia or as a compensatory mechanism to increase oxygen delivery. The fetus of a diabetic mother shows increases in metabolic rate and oxygen consumption due to metabolism of excessive glucose and other substrates.[6] The risk of later development of type 1 diabetes in infants whose mother has type 1 diabetes is 1.3%. The risk of later development of type 2 diabetes is 15% if one parent (up to 60% if both parents) has type 2 diabetes.[78] Additional morbidities in infants of diabetic women are discussed on pp. 583-584

SUMMARY

Maternal adaptations during pregnancy alter the woman's metabolic processes. These changes are critical for protection of the mother and promote her ability to adapt to pregnancy. Maternal adaptations are essential to ensure that the fetus obtains an adequate supply of nutrients to support growth and development. Alterations in metabolic processes in the mother also interact with the course of disorders such as diabetes mellitus. An understanding of the normal metabolic changes during pregnancy increases understanding of the alterations seen in the pregnant diabetic woman, the fetus, and the newborn. Implications for clinical practice are summarized in Table 16-3.

DEVELOPMENT OF CARBOHYDRATE, FAT, AND PROTEIN METABOLISM IN THE FETUS

The placenta and fetal liver function as a "coordinated multiorgan system for the exchange of nutrients and for ensuring the production of nutrients sufficient to meet fetal requirements."[9] Fetal metabolic processes are dominated by anabolism and governed primarily by glucose with little oxidation of fat. The fetus must produce energy and maintain oxidative phosphorylation in the face of a low-oxygen environment. Although energy is produced in the fetus under aerobic conditions, the fetus has a greater capacity for anaerobic metabolism and is efficient in using lactate. Oxygen consumption in the fetus is 8 mL/kg/min. Glucose contributes more than half of the substrate for oxygen consumption.[9,108]

The fetal caloric requirement has been estimated to average 90 to 100 kcal/kg/day. Almost all of the fetal fuel requirements are met by metabolism of glucose; lactate; and amino acids such as alanine, glutamate, and serine.[9,51] The fetus also uses these substrates as major precursors for storage of fuels (e.g., fatty acids, glycogen). The stored fuels are critical energy sources during the intrapartum period and transition to extrauterine life. By term, the fetus has increased its weight 175-fold, protein content 400-fold, and fat content 5000-fold. Fetal nutrient uptake and growth is influenced by maternal nutrition and health; uterine blood flow; placental nutrient uptake, metabolism, and transfer; umbilical blood flow; and the fetal endocrine system.[38]

Substances are transported across the placental syncytiotrophoblast from maternal to fetal circulations. The syncytiotrophoblast is "the transporting epithelium of the human placenta,"[32] consisting of two polarized plasma membranes. The microvillous membrane (MVM) faces maternal blood in the intervillous space; the basal membrane (BM) faces the fetal capillary epithelium.[32]

Insulin-like growth factors (IGF-I and IGF-II) are the dominant endocrine regulators of fetal growth and cord blood levels correlated with birth weight.[14,20] IGF-I and IGF-II levels increase longitudinally to about 33 weeks, then increase twofold to threefold more to term. IGF-I is thought to be the primary controller of fetal size in the second half of pregnancy. IGF-I (but not IGF-II) is significantly lower in infants with fetal growth restriction.[20] Cord blood IGF-I levels are also lower in women who smoke.[20]

Fetal leptin, adiponectin, and other adipokines (resistin, visfatin, and apelin) are involved in controlling fetal growth.[15,] Leptin may act by modulating growth hormone secretion and may also have a role in hematopoiesis and angiogenesis. Leptin has been found in immature subcutaneous fat cells by 6 to 10 weeks' gestation.[4] Circulating levels of leptin, an adipostatic hormone, increase after 32 to 34 weeks' gestation,

Table 16-3 Recommendations for Clinical Practice Related to Changes in Carbohydrate, Protein, and Fat Metabolism in Pregnant Women

Recognize the usual changes in carbohydrate, protein, and fat metabolism during pregnancy (pp. 560-567 and Table 16-2).
Assess and monitor maternal nutrition in terms of carbohydrate, protein, and fat intake (pp. 560-567 and Chapter 12).
Counsel women regarding nutrient and energy requirements to meet maternal and fetal needs during pregnancy (pp. 560-567, 569-570).
Monitor maternal glucose and ketone status (pp. 562, 569-570).
Monitor fetal growth (pp. 569-570, 572-573).
Understand the implications of changes in the absorptive and postabsorptive states for the pregnant woman and her fetus (pp. 565-567 and Figures 16-4 and 16-5).
Monitor maternal energy status during the intrapartum period (p. 568).
Counsel women regarding changes in appetite and weight during pregnancy (pp. 560-562 and Chapter 12).
Know how glucose tolerance test parameters are altered during pregnancy (p. 569).
Recognize the effects of metabolic changes on insulin requirements of diabetic women during the prenatal, intrapartum, and postpartum periods (pp. 570-572).
Evaluate and monitor metabolic and insulin status in the pregnant diabetic woman (pp. 570-572).
Counsel diabetic women regarding the effects of diabetes on pregnancy and the fetus and of pregnancy on diabetes (pp. 570-572 and Figure 16-11).
Counsel diabetic women regarding strategies prior to pregnancy to optimize maternal and fetal outcomes (pp. 570-572).
Recognize the potential effects of diabetes on the fetus and newborn (pp. 570-572 and Figure 16-11).

around the time of increasing body fat mass.[102,105] Levels of leptin decrease rapidly after birth and may help limit energy expenditure and conserve the infant's nutrient reserves for later growth and development.[55] Leptin levels at birth have been reported to correlate with intrauterine growth and be a predictor of neonatal bone mass.[20,69] Concentrations of leptin are higher in large-for-gestational-age (LGA) infants than in infants of appropriate size for gestational age; concentrations are also higher in LGA infants than in small-for-gestational-age (SGA) infants.

The nutritional, metabolic, and hormonal status during fetal and early postbirth life can alter organ development including the hypothalamus and other endocrine structures (see Chapter 19).[18,99] The mechanisms by which the fetal environment influences later status are thought to be related to placental adaptive responses to the intrauterine environment. After birth these adaptations may no longer be appropriate for the extrauterine environment and lead to altered glucose-insulin metabolism, lipid metabolism, and endocrine programming. Alterations in fetal and early neonatal nutrition "result in neuroendocrine, pancreatic, skeletal muscle, and adipose tissue dysfunction, and increased food intake and decreased energy expenditure. This leads to increased adiposity and adult disease."[18] These adult onset disorders include insulin resistance and type 2 diabetes, obesity, hypertensive disorders, coronary artery disease, and osteoporosis.[18,28,33,36,39,99]

Carbohydrate Metabolism

The fetus has been described as a "glucose-dependent parasite" and uses glucose from the mother as the major substrate for energy production.[82] Eighty percent of fetal energy comes from carbohydrate (glucose) oxidation.[71,114] Fetal glucose utilization rates (averaging 5 mg/kg/min) are higher than in adults (2 to 3 mg/kg/min).[51,71] Even with fetal growth restriction, maternal glucose is the major energy substrate for the fetus, although the placenta can produce alternate substrates such as lactate and ketone bodies for use as energy and for glycogen synthesis.[71]

Glucose is transported across the placenta via sodium-independent carrier-mediated facilitated diffusion.[68,116] The placenta has a high facility for glucose uptake and transport via a family of membrane transport proteins (GLUTs, which is the gene symbol for facilitated glucose transporter) on the microvillous membrane facing maternal blood and fetal-facing basal membrane of the placenta.[62,68,108] Various GLUT isoforms are expressed in the syncytiotrophoblast, including GLUT-1, -3, -4, and -12. GLUT-4 and -12 are sensitive to insulin.[68] GLUT-1 and GLUT-2 are expressed early in development and are found on both the trophoblast and blastocyst.[104] GLUT-1 is the major fetal glucose transporter; fetal GLUT-2 levels remain low.[118] GLUT-1 is expressed on almost all fetal tissues, enhancing cellular glucose uptake.[121] In animal models maternal hyperglycemia during early gestation down-regulates these receptors, increasing the risk of apoptosis and neural tube and limb defects. There is a fivefold greater increase in GLUT-1 on the microvillous membrane facing maternal blood than on the fetal-facing basal membrane during the first trimester.[62,68,108] This increases the movement of maternal glucose into the placenta, where approximately 30% to 40% is used by the placenta for oxidation or converted to glycogen and lactate to meet its energy needs.[68]

Basal membrane glucose transport is the rate-limiting step in fetal glucose transfer.[8,68] In the second half of pregnancy, basal membrane GLUT-1 receptors increase at least twofold and their activity increases 50% to meet increasing demands with fetal growth in late pregnancy.[62,108] If the uteroplacental nutrient supply is diminished, the fetus consumes nutrients and oxidizes them at the usual rate, but the placenta reduces consumption of both nutrients and oxygen. Increased placental GLUT-1 receptors with increased glucose transport to the fetus have been found in diabetic women with hyperglycemia.[120] Placental glucose transport is summarized in Figure 16-7.

During the first few days after fertilization, the zygote has a limited ability to metabolize glucose. After the embryonic genome is activated, glucose metabolism increases.[29] Both glucose and pyruvate uptake increase initially; glucose uptake remains high throughout pregnancy, while pyruvate uptake falls.

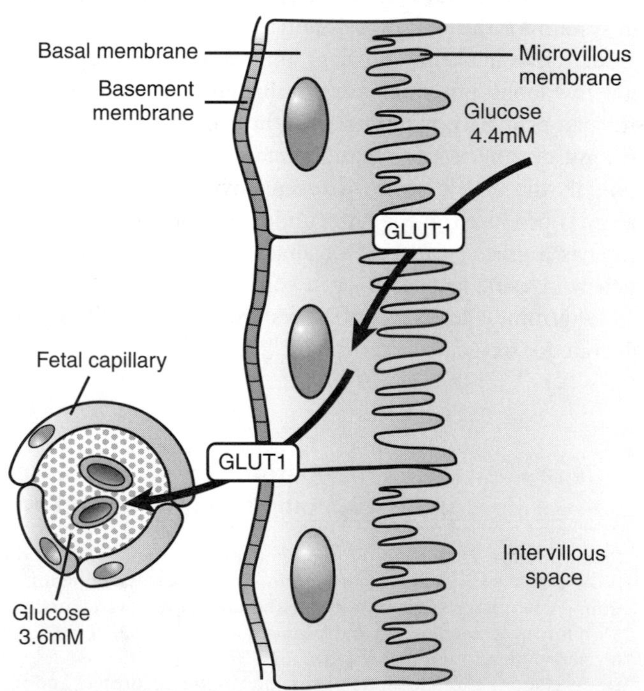

FIGURE 16-7 Principles for placental glucose transport. Glucose transport across the placental barrier is primarily mediated by glucose transporter 1 (GLUT-1), an isoform of the family of facilitated glucose transporters. Despite the high glucose consumption of the placenta itself, the glucose concentrations in the umbilical vein are only approximately 1 mM lower than in the intervillous space, indicating a large transport capacity for glucose. Due to the facilitated nature of glucose transport net transfer is sensitive to changes in the concentration gradient. (From Jansson, T., Myatt, L., & Powell, T.L. [2009]. The role of trophoblast nutrient and ion transporters in the development of pregnancy complications and adult disease. *Curr Vasc Pharmacol*, *7*, 524.)

The major regulators of fetal growth are IGF-I and IGF-II, which stimulate cell proliferation, differentiation, and metabolism.[38] IGFs act via cell membrane receptors and are modulated by a group of binding proteins. The liver is the main source of IGFs, which have autocrine, paracrine, and endocrine functions. IGF-I can be detected in fetal tissue by 9 weeks' gestation and in fetal circulation by 15 weeks' gestation.[34] Both IGF-I and IGF-II increase with gestational age. In early gestation, IGF-II activity, which is not significantly affected by nutritional factors, is predominant. In late pregnancy, IGF-I, which is regulated by nutrient availability, is predominant. Fetal growth in later gestation is regulated by the interaction of glucose, insulin, and IGF-I.[38] Glucose transfer across the placenta stimulates fetal insulin release. Insulin in turn stimulates lipogenesis and IGF, which increases fetal anabolism and placental uptake of glucose and other nutrients for fetal (versus placental) use.

Lower levels of IGF-I are seen in preterm and growth-restricted infants.[89] Levels are also reduced in infants of mothers who smoke.[113] Even though glucose and insulin concentrations are lower with fetal growth restriction, the fetus maintains glucose uptake and utilization due to increased insulin sensitivity, enhancing movement of glucose into cells. This is mediated by increased expression of GLUT and insulin-responsive glucose transporters.[116] With chronic substrate deprivation, the growth restricted fetus will develop systems for glucose production, initially by glycogenolysis (breakdown of glycogen to glucose) and later by gluconeogenesis (production of new glucose from lactate, amino acids [especially alanine], and glycerol) along with the reduction in fetal growth.[116] Poor fetal nutrition may alter the ability to produce and respond to insulin in adulthood, increasing the risk of type 2 diabetes, or may alter fetal low-density lipoprotein metabolism, increasing the risk of later coronary artery disease.[18,36,89,74,131]

Under basal, nonstressed conditions, the fetal glucose pool is in equilibrium with the maternal pool.[132] Enzymes for fetal gluconeogenesis are present by 3 months' gestation, but fetal glucose production is minimal and maternal glucose remains the source of fetal glucose.[52,71,116] Ambient fetal glucose levels are generally 20 to 40 mg/dL (1.1 to 2.2 mmol/L) less than maternal levels (or 70% to 80% of maternal values) and increase slightly toward the end of gestation.[71,78] This gradient is regulated by the placenta and favors transfer of glucose across the placenta from the mother through carrier-mediated facilitated diffusion (GLUTs) (Figure 16-7).

The usual lower limit for fetal glucose is 54 mg/dL (3 mmol/L), especially after 30 weeks.[51] If fetal glucose supply decreases, then placental glucose uptake increases, and vice versa, as seen with the infant of a diabetic mother.[68,71] Extra glucose is stored by the fetus as glycogen and triglycerides.[73] The levels at which glucose carriers become saturated are significantly above the usual maternal blood glucose level, which promotes a constant supply of glucose to the fetus.[82] There is no net transfer of insulin or glucagon to the fetus (see Figure 16-6). With adequate maternal nutrition, gluconeogenesis and ketogenesis are not seen in the fetus.[93,116] If the placental supply of glucose is inadequate, the fetus can use ketone bodies and other substrates as alternative energy sources.[116] As noted above, with prolonged glucose deprivation, the fetus can produce some glucose initially by glycogenolysis and later by gluconeogenesis, probably mediated by cortisol.[51,116]

Fetal glucose utilization is independent of maternal glucose availability. The linear relationship between maternal and fetal glucose levels is maintained during maternal euglycemia, hypoglycemia, and hyperglycemia.[73] The mother meets this demand by an increasing reliance on fat metabolism for her own fuel needs. If the maternal system is not able to meet the fetal demand for gluconeogenic precursors, hypoglycemia can result. Because fetal blood glucose levels are 70% to 80% of maternal values, maternal hypoglycemia leads to even lower fetal blood glucose levels.[78] Placental glucose transfer increases with increasing gestational age not only by increases in GLUT, but also by increases in insulin receptors on fetal tissues particularly adipose tissue and skeletal muscle. Glucose is also needed by the fetus for protein synthesis, as a precursor for fat synthesis, for conversion to glycogen for storage, and as the primary substrate for oxidative metabolism. Most of the transferred glucose is oxidized to carbon dioxide and water with release of energy by the tricarboxylic acid cycle and oxidative phosphorylation.

The fetus has an active capacity for anaerobic metabolism, which has a greater role in fetal metabolic processes than it does in adults. The fetus has increased amounts of glycolytic isoenzymes such as hexokinase, glucose-6-phosphate dehydrogenase (G6PD), and pyruvate dehydrogenase, which favor anaerobic glycolysis.[73] Fetal and especially placental tissues actively metabolize glucose to lactate. The lactate generated by the placenta serves as an important fuel for the fetus.[51] Lactate is a major precursor of fetal hepatic glycogen and fatty acid synthesis.[73] Under aerobic conditions the fetus is a net consumer of lactate. The placenta produces large amounts of lactate and ammonia, which may help in regulating metabolic activities in the fetal hepatocytes.[51] The fetus can also use ketone bodies produced from β-oxidation of fatty acids as another alternative fuel source.[116]

The fetal liver contains enzymes needed to both synthesize and catabolize glycogen to store and release glucose. The fetus can also synthesize glycogen from pyruvate, acetate, and alanine.[73] Glycogen synthesis is greater than glycogenolysis in the fetus. Glycogen synthetase and other gluconeogenic enzymes can be found in the liver from the eighth week and increase to term, with a rapid increase seen after 36 weeks' gestation.[73,93] Deposition of hepatic glycogen during the perinatal period is regulated by glucocorticoids and insulin. Glucocorticoids may induce glycogen synthetase, which is then activated by insulin. Fetal cells have increased insulin receptors, greater receptor affinity for glucose, and delayed maturation of hepatic glucagon receptors. These changes promote storage of glucose as glycogen and fat. Glycogen can be synthesized from lactate, pyruvate, alanine, and glycerol as well as glucose.[108]

Glycogen is stored in fetal tissues from 9 weeks' gestation on and increases slowly from 15 to 20 weeks, then more rapidly during the third trimester.[71] Until 20 to 24 weeks, the fetal liver is the main glycogen storehouse; after that time, glycogen is stored in cardiac and skeletal muscle, and to a lesser extent in the kidneys, intestines, and brain (primarily in the astrocytes).[107,108] Liver and skeletal muscle glycogen concentrations peak at term.[108] Compared with adults, the term fetus has significantly more liver, skeletal muscle, and cardiac muscle glycogen stores. Liver glycogen synthesis is regulated by fetal insulin, the hypothalamic-pituitary axis, and thyroid hormones.[108]

Immunoreactive insulin is present in fetal plasma and islet tissue as early as 8 weeks' gestation.[71,120] Insulin levels are dependent upon fetal glucose levels.[51] Insulin production is stimulated by increasing glucose and amino acid concentrations, especially after 20 weeks.[71] Fetal glucose metabolism is relatively independent of the insulin-glucagon regulatory mechanisms seen after birth, however. Acute changes in glucose concentrations leading to hypoglycemia or hyperglycemia do not significantly alter fetal insulin or glucagon secretion.[118] However, secretion of these hormones is markedly altered by chronic changes such as long-term hyperglycemia in a diabetic woman, which augments insulin secretion by β-cell hyperplasia and suppresses glucagon, or by chronic maternal malnutrition, which depresses insulin and stimulates release of fetal glucagon.[71,132] Because insulin is a fetal growth hormone, fetal hyperinsulinemic states are associated with fetal and neonatal macrosomia.[57,71]

Glucagon is found in fetal plasma by 15 weeks' gestation and reaches peak concentrations at 24 to 26 weeks. In comparison with adults, the number of fetal hepatic glucagon receptors is decreased and insulin receptors are increased. Fetal liver cells, erythrocytes, monocytes, and lung cells have an increased affinity for insulin. These attributes promote insulin-mediated anabolic processes such as glycogen formation and decrease glucagon-mediated catabolism.[132]

The fetal liver receives the highest net flux of maternal glucose because it is the first organ system encountered by blood returning from the placenta (see Chapter 9). Fetal hepatic enzymes for glycogenesis (carbohydrate to glycogen) are increased, whereas enzymes for glycolysis (carbohydrate to pyruvate and lactate) and gluconeogenesis (fat and protein to glucose) are present but decreased. For example, glucose-6-phosphatase, an enzyme involved in gluconeogenesis and inhibited by glucose and amino acids, is at 20% to 50% of adult levels at midgestation. These relationships are maintained until birth, when decreased glucose availability and onset of high-fat feedings stimulate decreases in glycogenolytic enzymes.

Lipid Metabolism

Lipids are a critical component of brain development, of retinal development, and for structural and functional integrity of neuronal and glial membranes, and are the main component of the myelin sheath.[32,58,63,127] Fetal fat content increases during gestation from 0.5% of body weight in early gestation to approximately 3.5% by 28 weeks and 16% by term or by approximately 3.4 g/kg/day in the third trimester.[127] This increase is due to transfer of fatty acids from the mother and active lipogenesis in the fetal liver and other tissues. Lipogenesis is primarily through the fatty acid synthetase pathway, which is highly active in the fetus. The placenta modulates the fatty acid supply for its use and for fetal use.[19] Placental leptin stimulates lipolysis and is excreted to both maternal and fetal circulations. As a result the placenta may have a role in modulating fatty acid supply based on fetal demands.[44]

Long-chain polyunsaturated fatty acids in the mother are primarily found in the form of esterified fatty acids such as triglycerides, phospholipids, and esterified cholesterol. Maternal lipoproteins do not cross the placenta but are taken up by the placenta where they are broken down and their products used for energy or steroid hormone production or released to the fetus.[59] The placenta contains various tissue receptors, enzymes, and fatty acid binding proteins to upload these lipoproteins and to transport polyunsaturated fatty acids and nonesterified fatty acids to the fetus.[32,68] Free fatty acids cross by diffusion in limited amounts, with a net flux of unesterified fatty acids to the fetus.[58,59,125] These fatty acids are derived primarily from maternal circulating free fatty acids or cleavage of maternal triglycerides by lipoprotein lipase.[56] The maternal diet is reflected in the fatty acid content of fetal tissues.[59] Ketone bodies and glycerol also cross the placenta.[59] Placental lipid transport is illustrated in Figure 16-8. Because transport of fatty acids is partly controlled by maternal concentrations, increased maternal levels are associated with increased transfer and fetal storage.[16,19,62,123,125] Other factors influencing free fatty acid transfer include serum albumin level, fatty acid chain length, lipid solubility, uteroplacental and umbilical blood flow, α-fetoprotein, placental proteins that bind fatty acids, and binding affinity.[58,71,125]

Essential fatty acids (EFA), such as linoleic and α-linolenic acids, cannot be synthesized by the fetus and must be transported across the placenta.[32,58,59,68] These substances can then be desaturated by the fetus to form other fatty acids.[58] Transfer of essential fatty acids increases in late pregnancy, when demand for brown and white adipose tissue development and for vascular and neural growth increases; however, some early transfer is needed for uteroplacental vascular development.[125] Long-chain polyunsaturated fatty acids (LCPUFA) from the mother are critical for development of the brain and retinal and brain growth.[44,58] The fetus has limited capacity to synthesize LCPUFA due to low levels of desaturating enzymes.[44,58] In the third trimester when fetal neuronal and vascular growth is high, selective transport of LCPUFA derivatives such as arachidonic acid and docosahexaenoic acid (DHA) increases.[58,59,126] The preterm infant thus needs a diet that includes these critical substances.[44] Linoleic acid is converted to arachidonic acid, the main precursor for prostaglandins, thromboxanes, and leukotrienes; α-linolenic acid is converted

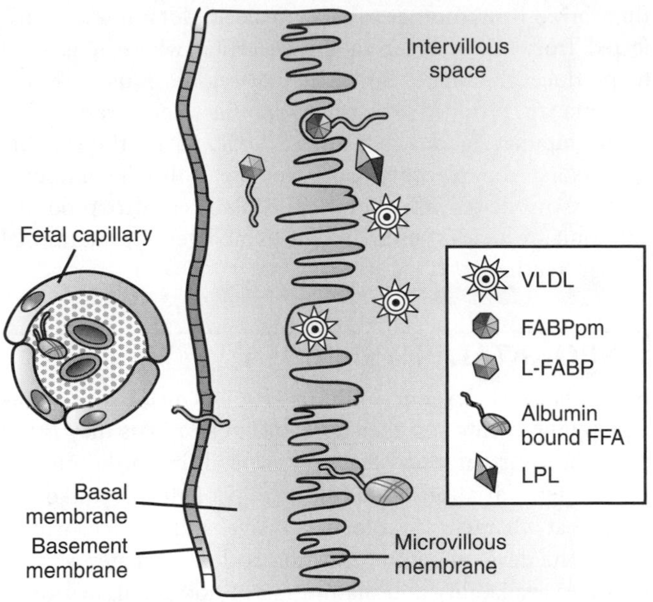

FIGURE 16-8 Principles for placental lipid transport. In the maternal blood there are two major sources for free fatty acids (FFA) that can be transported to the fetus: FFA bound to albumin and triglycerides in lipoproteins. Albumin-FFA complexes can interact with fatty acid binding proteins in the microvillous plasma membrane (MVM), resulting in the uptake of FFA into the syncytiotrophoblast cell. Triglycerides in maternal lipoproteins, in particular very-low-density lipoproteins (VLDL), are hydrolyzed into FFA by lipoprotein lipase (LPL) expressed in the MVM. FFA is subsequently transferred across the MVM. Alternatively, maternal lipoproteins interact with LDL/VLDL receptors in MVM resulting in endocytosis and intracellular hydrolysis, which releases FFA. Intracellularly, FFA are transported bound to fatty acid binding proteins. The mechanisms for FFA transfer across the basal plasma membrane are not well established. (From Jansson, T., Myatt, L., & Powell, T.L. [2009]. The role of trophoblast nutrient and ion transporters in the development of pregnancy complications and adult disease. *Curr Vasc Pharmacol, 7,* 526.)

to DHA (needed for fetal growth and development) and eicosapentaenoic acid (precursor of prostaglandins that inhibit platelet aggregation).[19]

Increased fat deposition during the third trimester is associated with increasing fetal weight and decreased serum triglycerides because these are used in fat deposition.[23] Most (80%) of the fetal fat accretion during this period is due to de novo synthesis from acetyl coenzyme A (CoA) with formation of palmitic acid, especially in the brain and liver.[56,125]

Fetal lipid metabolism is characterized by early development of mechanisms for cholesterol metabolism and lipogenesis with decreased lipolytic activity throughout gestation, except in the liver.[101] Fetal fatty acid synthesis occurs through lipogenesis and desaturation of essential fatty acids. Lipogenesis is dependent upon substrate availability. Lipogenic precursors include glucose, lactate, and ketone bodies; the latter two are the most important.[56,109]

The rate of synthesis is primarily controlled by the ratio of plasma insulin-to-glucagon levels. Insulin stimulates and glucagon inhibits fatty acid synthesis. The action of glucagon is mediated by cyclic adenosine monophosphate (cAMP), which inhibits acetyl-CoA enzymes.[56] The high insulin-to-glucagon ratio in the fetus promotes fatty acid synthesis. Lipogenesis is increased by glucose, fatty acids, and T4 (see Chapter 19) and reduced by catecholamines.[125] The fetal liver and brain contain enzymes for ketone oxidation as an alternative energy substrate; the fetal brain can use ketones for energy by 10 to 12 weeks' gestation.[59,108] Lipolytic activity becomes active after delivery, when the infant can no longer rely on a constant glucose supply from the mother and must cope with a relatively high fat intake.

By 15 weeks the fetus has developed enzymes to convert acetate or citrate to fatty acid and thus the potential to use fat as an alternative source of energy. Blood lipid and free fatty acid levels are relatively stable after about 26 weeks but remain low until after delivery. The free fatty acids that cross the placenta are used by the fetus in organ development; synthesis of pulmonary surfactant, other phospholipids, bile, and serum lipoprotein; formation of cell membranes; precursors for prostaglandins; and as second messenger precursors. Fatty acids needed by developing neuronal and glial cells and in formation of the myelin sheath are synthesized within the brain.[56]

The fetus needs cholesterol for cell membranes, bile acid synthesis, embryogenesis (cell proliferation and differentiation), synaptogenesis, production of steroid hormones, and cell-cycle regulation.[58] The fetus obtains cholesterol from endogenous biosynthesis and placental transport.[59] Fetal cholesterol levels are high in early pregnancy, decrease, then rise, peaking in the third trimester.[59,101] Fetal and maternal cholesterol levels are not correlated.[59] Activity of the pentose phosphate intermediary metabolic pathway is also high in the fetus. Activity of this pathway is associated with cell proliferation and an increased requirement for ribose phosphate precursors of nucleic acids and provision of nicotinamide adenine dinucleotide (NADH) for synthesis of long-chain fatty acids.

Protein Metabolism

At least 10 amino acids are essential for the fetus, including those essential for adults plus cysteine and histidine, with a dependency on arginine and tyrosine. Arginine and leucine are insulin secretogogues; arginine may also enhance vascular development. Taurine helps regulate metabolism and is needed in development of the heart, eye, and brain. Because of the relative inactivity of hepatic enzymes such as cystathionase and phenylalanine hydroxylase, the fetus cannot synthesize tyrosine and cysteine from phenylalanine and methionine. The fetus uses amino acids for protein synthesis or oxidation because organ development involves continuous remodeling (breakdown and resynthesis) of tissue. The availability of glucose and other substances influences fetal amino acid catabolism and protein accretion.[54]

There is a net flux of most amino acids from the mother to the fetus.[82] Because concentrations of most amino acids are higher in fetal than maternal blood, amino acids are actively transported from maternal blood across the placental microvillous membrane.[68] Amino acid levels in the syncytiotrophoblast are higher than in either maternal or fetal circulations. Facilitated diffusion moves substances across the syncytiotrophoblast basal membrane to fetal blood.[68] There are at least 15 different amino acid transporters, each mediating uptake of several different amino acids, and each amino acid may use multiple transport systems.[68]

Placental amino acid transport is illustrated in Figure 16-9. Fetal-to-maternal amino acid nitrogen ratios average 1.03 to 3.0, with a net active transfer of nitrogen to the fetus of 54 nmol/day and a total accumulation of about 400 g of protein by term.[6,54,82] Amino acid transport is not significantly affected by fluctuations in uterine or placental blood flow.[54] Transport may be down-regulated in the growth restricted fetus.[68]

Amino acids are supplied to the fetus in greater amounts than are needed for nitrogen accretion. The fetus uses the carbon from excess amino acids for oxidation and to make nonessential amino acids.[54] Some critical amino acids are not transferred across the placenta directly but are, instead, produced in the placenta. For example, glutamate, which is needed for neurotransmitters and brain development, is not transferred from mother to fetus. Instead glutamine is transferred from the mother to the placenta, where it is used to produce glutamate. Similarly asparagine is used by the placenta to produce aspartate, another neurotransmitter. Both glutamate and aspartate are toxic, so by transferring precursors, the placenta can produce only the amounts that are needed by the fetus. The placenta also produces ammonia, which is used by the fetal liver for additional protein synthesis.

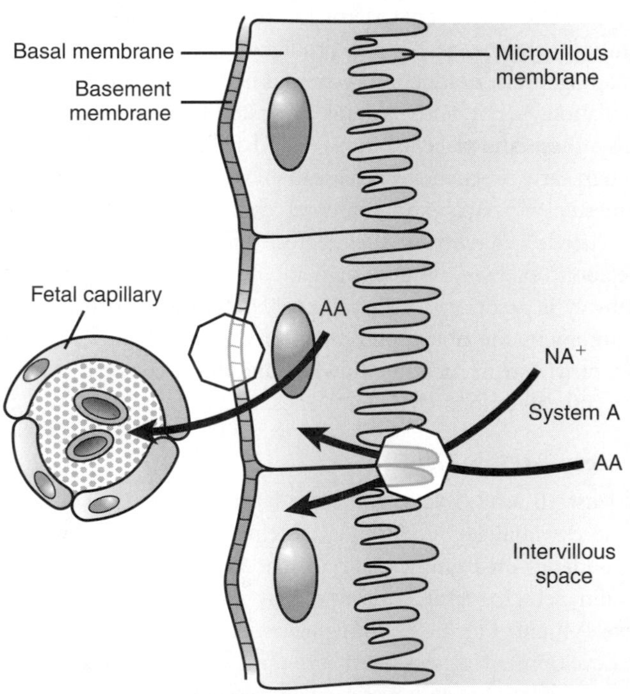

FIGURE 16-9 Principles for placental amino acid transport. Amino acid (AA) transport across the placenta is an active transport resulting in higher concentrations of AA in fetal blood as compared to the maternal circulation. The transport across the syncytiotrophoblast microvillous plasma membrane constitutes the active step, often energized by the inwardly directed Na^+-gradient (via the System A transporter). As a consequence, AA concentrations in the syncytiotrophoblast cytoplasm are much higher than in maternal and fetal blood. The transport across the basal plasma membrane is facilitated by specific transporters and driven by the outwardly directed concentrations gradient for AA. (From Jansson, T., Myatt, L., & Powell, T.L. [2009]. The role of trophoblast nutrient and ion transporters in the development of pregnancy complications and adult disease. *Curr Vasc Pharmacol, 7,* 525.)

NEONATAL PHYSIOLOGY

Neonates must develop a homeostatic balance between energy requirements and the supply of substrates as they move from the constant glucose supply of fetal life to the normal intermittent variations in the availability of glucose and other fuels that characterize the absorptive and postabsorptive states. The development of this homeostasis is dependent on substrate availability and maturation of hormonal, neuronal, and enzymatic systems and is influenced by gestational age, health status, and intake.

Transitional Events

Metabolic transition is characterized by a shift from the anabolic-dominant fetal state to the catabolic state of the neonate. This transition is influenced by genetic, environmental, and endocrine factors as well as by major alterations in energy metabolism within the mitochondria. Changes in metabolism with birth are regulated by the expression of specific genes and gene products that alter the activity of various enzymes.[23] Shortly prior to term birth, induction of hepatic glucose production begins and is enhanced postbirth by increased glucocorticoids and glucagon.[116] The ability of the fetus to use glucose anaerobically and to readily metabolize lactate may be important in maintaining homeostasis during the stresses of labor and delivery. The fetus prepares for this transition during the last weeks of gestation by increasing fuel storage in the form of glycogen and lipids. Glycogen is critical in order to maintain glucose homeostasis immediately after birth, whereas the fat stores, through lipolysis of fatty acids and ketone bodies, serve as an alternate energy source. Postnatal changes in metabolism involve the transition from the almost exclusive reliance on glucose for energy production in the fetus to markedly increased use of fatty acid oxidation and ketone body use for energy production in the neonate. An increase in epinephrine, norepinephrine, and glucagon and a decrease in insulin at birth promote mobilization of fatty acids and glycogen metabolism.[73]

Carbohydrate Metabolism

Birth results in the loss of the maternal glucose source. As a result, neonatal blood glucose normally falls after birth, reaching a nadir at 30 to 90 (generally around 60) minutes after birth (Figure 16-10).[71] This fall in glucose is thought to be necessary for activating postnatal glucose production processes.[116] Glucose values then rise and stabilize by 2 to 3 hours

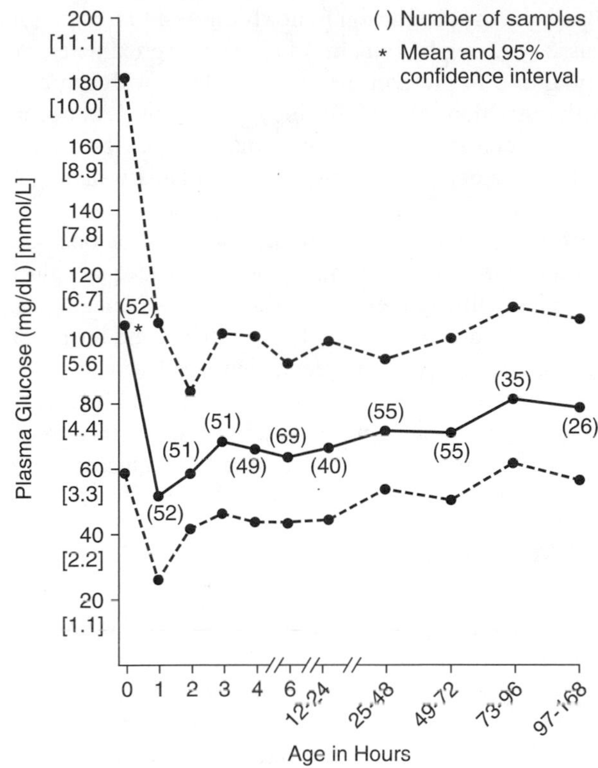

FIGURE 16-10 Plasma glucose levels in healthy term neonates delivered vaginally with birth weights between 2.5 and 4 kg. (From Srinivansan, G., et al. [1986]. Plasma glucose values in normal neonates: A new look. *J Pediatr, 109,* 114.)

after birth.[52,71] The glucose nadir and timing of the nadir are influenced by maternal glucose infusion during the intrapartum period.[71] Steady-state hepatic release of glucose at 4 to 6 mg/kg/min is seen by 2 to 3 hours in term infants.[40,107] Mean glucose levels in term healthy infants in the first week average 80 mg/dL.[71] The basis for the fall in blood glucose is summarized in Table 16-4.

The newborn responds to the decrease in blood glucose in several ways. The rapid glycogenolysis (liberation of glucose from glycogen) after birth is stimulated by a fall in the insulin-to-glucagon ratio and sluggish insulin secretion (because of the decreased blood glucose with removal of the placenta), increased serum glucagon, stimulation of the sympathetic nervous system with catecholamine release, increased thyroid stimulating hormone, and increases in hepatic cAMP.[23,107,118] Because insulin promotes transfer of glucose out of the blood into cells, the lowered levels decrease transfer and elevate blood glucose levels. Glucagon stimulates conversion of glycogen into glucose, also raising blood glucose levels.

Table 16-4 **Basis for Changes in Blood Glucose Levels Immediately after Birth**

CHARACTERISTIC	BASIS
Immature liver enzyme systems	Promotes glucose storage rather than release
Larger brain in proportion to body size	Obligatory glucose user
Increased red blood cell volume	Obligatory glucose user
Decreased liver response to glucagons	Limits release of glucose from glycogen stores
Increased energy needs	Increased metabolic and motor activity with birth

Hepatic glycogen stores decrease markedly during this period. In the term infant, glycogen stores only last an estimated 10 hours after birth before glucose must be produced by gluconeogenesis (production of new glucose from lactate, amino acids [especially alanine], and glycerol).[40] As glycogen falls, the newborn responds by mobilizing fat stores with release of free fatty acids. This response is stimulated by the catecholamine release associated with cooling at birth (see Chapter 20), which rapidly increases free fatty acids.[121] Increased secretion of catecholamines at birth increases glucagon secretion (together these activate hepatic glycogen phosphorylase and glycogenolysis), suppresses insulin, reverses the fetal insulin-to-glucagon ratio, increases lipolysis to provide an alternate energy source, activates enzymes needed for gluconeogenesis, and augments growth hormone secretion.[116,121,132] Healthy infants are able to readily mobilize free fatty acids and oxidize ketones to maintain their blood glucose levels.

Breastfed infants have lower blood glucose levels and higher ketone bodies than bottle-fed infants.[52,116] The elevated ketone bodies may provide an alternate fuel during the period of lower nutrient intake as breastfeeding is being established. This may be especially important for the brain, which can readily use ketones as an alternate energy source.[23,52,116,121] Production of glucose from amino acids, especially alanine, increases and accounts for 4% to 10% of the glucose used for energy in term infants.

Gluconeogenesis also contributes to systemic glucose production after birth. Substrates metabolized by the liver to produce glucose include glycerol, lactate, alanine, and pyruvate.[40,71,73,121] Lactate may account for up to 30% of hepatic glucose production, with 5% to 10% from alanine and glycerol via gluconeogenesis.[94] Gluconeogenic enzyme activity increases after birth. Both glycogenolysis and gluconeogenesis pathways are dependent on the hepatic microsomal glucose-6-phosphatase (G6PD) enzyme system, which has only about 10% of adult activity at birth.[60] The cortisol surge with birth stimulates G6PD activity in the liver and hepatic glucose release.[116] Adult values are reached by about 3 days in term infants, but take longer in preterm infants.[60] By 12 to 24 hours after birth, both gluconeogenesis and ketogenesis are active.[93,121] From late fetal life to 3 days after birth, blood glucose regulation is glucose dominant. As a result, gluconeogenesis is diminished during this period. After this period, blood glucose regulation becomes insulin dominant (the adult pattern). The increased gluconeogenesis after birth is regulated by changes in the serum insulin-to-glucagon ratio, catecholamine secretion, fatty acid oxidation, and activation of hepatic enzyme systems.[121] The very low–birth weight (VLBW) infant is able to produce glucose to meet basal metabolic needs with appropriate responses to exogenous glucose and amino acid infusions, although hepatic glucose production may be sluggish or incomplete. In the first day after birth in term infants, about 50% of glucose is produced via glucogenolysis and 30% to 40% by gluconeogenesis (primarily from glycerol, but also from alanine and lactate).[52]

After birth, GLUT-1 glucose transporters decrease, whereas GLUT-2 (involved in uptake of glucose by liver, pancreatic β cells, and intestinal and renal epithelium) and GLUT-3 (involved in uptake by neurons, especially in the cerebellum, skeletal muscle, and other tissues) increase rapidly.[35,52,120,122] Activity of GLUT-4 (involved in uptake by muscle and adipose tissue) and other GLUTs increases more slowly.[120,122] GLUT-1, although lower in the neonate than in the fetus, remains active and needed for transfer of glucose into red blood cells and across the blood-brain barrier.[126] Both GLUT-1 and GLUT-3 are important in regulating brain glucose supply and are prominent in the blood-brain barrier epithelial cells, astrocytes, oligodendrocytes, choroid plexus, and cerebral cortex.[52] Major alternative fuels for the brain are pyruvate, lactate, and ketones. These are transported across the blood-brain barrier by monocarboxylate transporters.[52]

Increased glucagon concentrations and norepinephrine are important in subsequent activation of the hepatic gluconeogenic enzymes.[71,73,77,122] The predominant enzymes activated during this period are hepatic glycogen phosphorylase, glucose-6-phosphate dehydrogenase (G6PD), and phosphoenolpyruvate carboxykinase (PEP-CK). Hepatic glycogen phosphorylase is activated by norepinephrine and glucagon and stimulates glycogenolysis.[40,116] G6PD activity increases markedly after birth, increasing hepatic release of glucose.[116] This is probably due to surges of glucagon and cAMP, which help shift the activity of the liver from glycogen storage to glucose production. PEP-CK, which is inhibited by insulin, is the rate-limiting enzyme for gluconeogenesis.[40,116] With changes in the insulin-to-glucagon ratio after birth, this enzyme increases about 20-fold, reaching adult levels by 24 hours after birth and thus increasing gluconeogenesis.[40,121]

The resumption of a carbohydrate source (i.e., feeding) generally stabilizes the infant's glucose concentration, and most neonates achieve a steady-state in their glucose concentrations by about 5 days. The first enteral feeding immediately increases blood glucose levels. This increase is accompanied by an increase in plasma insulin levels in term infants and development of cyclic changes in insulin and blood glucose levels. In preterm infants the initial feeding is not accompanied by similar hormonal changes and the cyclic responses in insulin and blood glucose take 2 to 3 days to develop (and longer in VLBW infants or infants who are not fed). Enteral feeding stimulates production of digestive hormones and secretion of peptides critical for induction of gastrointestinal tract maturation and development of the enteroinsular axis (see Chapter 12). These changes lead to additional modifications of hepatic metabolism.

Basal glucose production in newborns is 4 to 6 mg/kg/min versus 2 to 3 mg/kg/min in adults and approximately 6 to 8 mg/kg/min in preterm infants and infants with symmetric growth restriction.[40,51,52,116] The high glucose needs in neonates reflect the increased brain-to-body mass, in that the brain has a high obligatory glucose use.[62,73] For infants weighing less than 1000 g, glucose is the major energy source for most of the neonatal period.[35] Newborns are able to use ketone bodies and lactate for brain energy metabolism if inadequate glucose is available, although excess levels can be damaging. This mechanism is present in term, large preterm, and term small-for-gestational-age (SGA) infants but is absent in VLBW infants and other intrauterine growth–restricted infants who are at risk for hypoglycemia.[50] Glycogen stores in astrocytes may provide another alternative source of glucose for the neurons during periods of low glucose.[50]

Lipid Metabolism

The inability of the fetus to readily oxidize fatty acids is rapidly reversed at birth because of changes in the functional ability of enzymes such as carnitine palmitoyltransferase. During this period the levels of glucose and free fatty acids are mirror images of each other. Lipolysis, with enhanced oxidation of free fatty acids and ketogenesis, increases quickly after birth, reaching a maximum within a few hours.[36,56,76,107] This increase is reflected in changes in plasma free fatty acid levels, which rise rapidly beginning 4 to 6 hours after birth and reach adult levels by 24 hours. By this time, 60% to 70% of the infant's energy is produced from oxidation of fat.[114]

Fat is the major form of stored calories in the newborn, and the preferred energy source for tissues such as the heart and adrenal cortex, which have high energy demands. Fat stores are significantly reduced in low–birth weight infants. After birth, mobilization of fatty acids from these stores is reflected in the rise in serum levels over the first few hours. This process is initiated by the increase in catecholamines and glucagon, resulting in increased cAMP followed by an increase in protein kinases, phosphorylation, and activation of adipose tissue lipase with release of fatty acids.[36,56]

The transition from glucose to fatty acid oxidation after birth is reflected in the fall of the respiratory quotient from 0.9 to less than 0.8 by 2 hours.[76,114] This indicates that the infant has moved from obtaining nearly two thirds of its energy from oxidation of glycogen immediately after birth, to deriving most of its energy from fat metabolism, conserving glucose to ensure an adequate glucose supply for the central nervous system.[40,71,107] This transition reflects increasing dependence on oxidative metabolism and is associated with an increase in the number of mitochondria and enzymes of the Krebs cycle and changes in serum free fatty acid levels. This shift to fat metabolism is delayed in infants of diabetic mothers with hyperinsulinemia.[71,73] The neonate's brain may use free fatty acids, along with branched-chain amino acids and ketones, as additional energy sources.[40]

The increase in fatty acid oxidation and ketogenesis after birth, stimulated by the thyroid stimulating hormone surge and increased thyroid hormones with birth, is related to increased enzyme activity, especially of carnitine palmitoyltransferase. Carnitine activity enhances fatty acid oxidation. Concentrations of carnitine are high in human milk for 2 to 3 days after delivery. Another factor influencing this change is alteration in the insulin-to-glucagon ratio with increased glucagon. This increases the availability of substrates such as acetyl-CoA and carnitine for fatty acid oxidation in the mitochondria.

Serum cholesterol levels in cord blood are 50 to 75 mg/dL (1.3 to 1.9 mmol/L), about one-half adult values, and serum triglycerides average 30 to 50 mg/dL (0.3 to 0.6 mmol/L).[101] Cholesterol in preterm infants may be as high as 100 mg/dL (2.6 mmol/L) if they are born during the time of the normal fetal cholesterol peak in the third trimester.[101] Low-density lipoprotein cholesterol concentrations decrease with increasing gestational age and are 25 to 30 mg/dL (0.5 to 0.8 mmol/L, about one fifth adult values) at term; high-density lipoprotein cholesterol is 25 mg/dL (0.6 mmol/L) at term (about one-half adult values).[101] Very-low-density lipoprotein (VLDL) transports less than one third of the total serum triglycerides in the term infant, versus that in the adult in whom VLDL is the major transporter of triglycerides.[101] Serum cholesterol and lipoprotein increase rapidly after birth, especially in breastfed infants.[101]

Protein Metabolism

Serum amino acid levels are higher during the first few weeks of life.[92] Urinary amino acids are elevated immediately after birth, with excretion of 8.8 mg/day in preterm and 7.6 mg/day in term infants versus 2.5 mg/day in older children. The average body nitrogen content at birth is 2%.[92]

The newborn has a limited capacity to synthesize protein, primarily because of the relative inactivity of several hepatic enzymes. This limitation is especially marked in preterm infants, whose capacity to use excess amino acid is reduced. Preterm infants who receive excess protein or an unbalanced amino acid intake are at risk for hyperammonemia, azotemia, metabolic acidosis, and altered plasma amino acid profiles. The latter changes are associated with altered protein synthesis, growth, central nervous system (CNS) function, and bile acid uptake. The ability to metabolize excess amino acids may also be altered in the newborn depending on maturity of enzyme systems in the liver and skeletal muscle and activity of the urea cycle to eliminate nitrogen.

CLINICAL IMPLICATIONS FOR NEONATAL CARE

The newborn's transitional state in relation to glucose homeostasis can result in problems even for healthy newborns as they attempt to provide adequate energy for maintenance and growth. Alterations in metabolic processes in the newborn can result in clinical problems, most notably hypoglycemia. The status of metabolic function in the newborn also influences nutritional needs (see Chapter 12).

Neonatal Hypoglycemia

The neonate may develop hypoglycemia if glycogen stores are insufficient to provide fuel during transition until production of energy by fat oxidation is adequate, or if the infant fails to adequately mobilize available glycogen stores. The physiologically optimal range for plasma glucose is given as 70 to 100 mg/dL (3.9 to 5.6 mmol/L).[77,122] Plasma glucose levels (whole blood glucose levels are 10% to 15% lower than plasma levels) below 40 mg/dL (2.2 mmol/L) are uncommon in the first few hours after birth in healthy infants with early feeding, and the lowest optimal level of glucose is probably around 60 mg/dL (3.3 mmol/L).[24,71,77,122] Arterial samples are slightly higher than venous samples (by 10% to 15%) with capillary samples intermediate.[10] Elevated hematocrits can lead to lower glucose levels due to the high glucose utilization by the red blood cells. Newer technologies for continuous interstitial glucose monitoring, currently being investigated for use in the neonate, have identified more episodes of intermittent blood glucose levels than previously recognized, however the physiologic significance and long-term significance of these episodes are unknown.[48,53]

Four approaches have been used to define hypoglycemia.[23,25] These include approaches based on appearance of clinical manifestations, measured glucose value ranges, acute metabolic changes and endocrine responses, and long-term neurologic outcomes.[23] None have been satisfactory. Aynsley-Green and Hawdon note that "hypoglycemia is a continuum, no single blood glucose concentration reflecting functional changes in every infant at that level."[5] Similarly, an expert panel concluded that the "rational definition of hypoglycemia is clearly not a specific value but a continuum of falling blood glucose values, creating thresholds for neurologic dysfunction, which may vary from one cause of hypoglycemia or clinical circumstance to another."[22]

Focus should be on promoting normoglycemia with prompt intervention for less optimal values.[22,104] The optimal glucose value and risk for neurologic sequelae probably varies from infant to infant depending on their brain maturity, glycogen stores, presence of hypoxia or ischemia, activity of gluconeogenic pathways, glucose transport status, and brain glucose demand.[24] Most sources cite levels below 40 to 45 mg/dL (2.2 to 2.5 mmol/L) as cutoff values for neonatal hypoglycemia.[48,52,71,77,116] There is no evidence that the preterm infant is able to tolerate low glucose better than term infants.[5,122] Infants who are very immature or ill (hypoxia, ischemia, sepsis) may have greater glucose needs and be more vulnerable to the effects of hypoglycemia.[24] The American Academy of Pediatrics Committee on Fetus and Newborn recently published a practice guideline and algorithm for screening and management of hypoglycemia in late preterm and term newborns.[21] This guideline suggests that for these infants, a "reasonable (although arbitrary) cutoff for treating symptomatic infants is 40 mg/dL. This value is higher than the physiologic nadir and higher than concentrations usually associated with clinical signs. . . . A reasonable goal is to maintain plasma glucose concentrations in symptomatic infants between 40 and 50 mg/dL."[21,p.678]

Clinical signs of hypoglycemia include tremors, jitteriness, irregular respiration, hypotonia, apnea, cyanosis, poor feeding, high-pitched cry, lethargy, irritability, hypothermia, and seizures. Because hypoglycemic infants may be symptomatic or asymptomatic and signs of hypoglycemia are often nonspecific, careful monitoring of infants at risk for development of hypoglycemia is critical. Multiple factors influence the outcome of infants with hypoglycemia, including severity and duration of the episode, cerebral blood flow and central nervous system (CNS) glucose levels, rates of glucose uptake, maturity, availability of alternative substrates, response to intervention, and type of clinical manifestation.[22,24,50,93,116]

Glucose is critical for the brain and hypoglycemia increases the risk of brain injury. Decreased glucose availability increases release of glutamate, free radicals, and other toxic metabolites that can lead to mitochondrial damage, altered ATP-dependent ion transport across neuronal membranes, changes in cell membranes, cellular edema, and neuronal necrosis (see Chapter 15). Unfortunately many studies on the outcome of infants with hypoglycemia have significant methodologic limitations and there have been no controlled prospective studies.[13,107,116] Infants with persistent and recurrent hypoglycemia have the poorest neurologic outcomes.[116] Hypoglycemia and hypoxic ischemic events may have an additive effect on neuronal injury.[116] Brain neuroprotective responses to hypoglycemia include increased epinephrine, increased cerebral blood flow, use of alternative fuels such as ketone bodies and lactate, and degradation of glycogen stored in astrocytes.[107,115] This may contribute to the lack of clinical signs even with low blood glucose levels.[40] Kalahan and Devaskar concluded that "transient asymptomatic hypoglycemia in an otherwise healthy neonate has been associated with a good prognosis. Several studies of small groups of subjects have suggested that symptomatic hypoglycemia in the infant results in long-term neurologic damage. However, these data should be interpreted with caution because of a number of confounding variables."[71]

Neonatal hypoglycemia can arise from an inadequate supply of glucose, alterations in endocrine regulation, or increased glucose regulation.[24,25,71,77] Preterm and SGA infants tend to develop hypoglycemia because of insufficient glycogen and fat stores and a decreased rate of gluconeogenesis. Normally with hypoglycemia, brain glucose utilization decreases by up to 50%, with increased reliance on ketones and lactate for energy. Preterm infants may be limited in their ability to mobilize these responses and thus more vulnerable to the effects of hypoglycemia.[35] Infants of diabetic mothers usually have sufficient stores; however, glycogenolysis is prevented by their high insulin levels and inability to secrete glucagon despite falling blood glucose levels. Infants at risk for neonatal hypoglycemia and associated mechanisms are summarized in Table 16-5.

Table 16-5 Causes and Time Course of Neonatal Hypoglycemia

MECHANISM	CLINICAL SETTING	EXPECTED DURATION
Decreased substrate availability	Fetal growth restriction	Transient
	Prematurity	Transient
	Reduced glycogen storage	Transient
	Reduced fat stores	Transient
	Reduced ketogenesis	Transient
	Glycogen storage disease	Prolonged
	Inborn errors of metabolism	Prolonged
Endocrine disturbances: hyperinsulinemia	Infant of a diabetic mother	Transient
	Persistent hyperinsulinism of infancy	Transient
	Congenital hyperinsulinism	Prolonged
	Beckwith-Wiedemann syndrome	Prolonged
	Erythroblastosis fetalis	Prolonged
	Exchange transfusion	Transient
	Islet cell dysplasia	Transient
	Maternal β-sympathomimetics	Transient
	Improperly placed umbilical artery catheter	Transient
	Inadvertent insulin administration	Transient
Other endocrine disorders	Immaturity of hepatic enzymes necessary for glucose production	Transient
	Reduced or failed counter-regulation	Prolonged
	Hypopituitarism	Prolonged
	Hypothyroidism	Prolonged
	Adrenal insufficiency	Prolonged
Increased utilization	Increased brain to body and live weight with increased brain consumption of glucose	Prolonged
	Asphyxia	Transient
	Hypothermia	Transient
Miscellaneous or multiple mechanisms	Sepsis	Transient
	Congenital heart disease	Transient
	Central nervous system abnormalities	Prolonged

From McGowan, J.E., et al. (2011). Glucose homeostasis. In S.L. Gardner, et al. (Eds.), *Merenstein & Gardner's Handbook of neonatal intensive care* (7th ed.). St. Louis: Mosby Elsevier, p. 360.

The Preterm Infant

Hypoglycemia is a common problem of preterm infants. Preterm infants usually develop hypoglycemia secondary to inadequate intake or decreased hepatic glucose production. These infants have decreased glycogen and fat reserves (accumulation of these stores occurs during the third trimester), and immature hepatic function, with low levels of gluconeogenic and glycogenolytic enzymes, especially glucose-6-phosphatase, which is important in glycogenolysis and gluconeogenesis.[60,71] Their initial hormonal response to low glucose levels may be limited.[60] Preterm infants are less able to produce alternate substrates such as ketone bodies. These infants may also have altered metabolic demands from tachypnea, respiratory distress syndrome, hypoxia, hypothermia, or other events that increase glucose use. Infants of mothers treated long term with β-adrenergic agonists for preterm labor (these agents are now being used less frequently) may develop hypoglycemia secondary to hyperinsulinemia.[104] These agents rapidly cross the placenta and stimulate β-cell receptors on the fetal pancreas, with subsequent insulin release and altered glucose homeostasis in the fetus and newborn. Maternal treatment with benzothiazide diuretics can also stimulate fetal β-cell receptors and increase maternal and thus fetal glucose levels.[71] Maternal propranolol, which can interfere with the catecholamine surge at birth, may also increase the risk of hypoglycemia.[71]

The Growth Restricted Infant

Growth restricted infants are at risk for hypoglycemia primarily because of alterations in hepatic glucose production and increased glucose utilization.[71,77] These infants may have reduced glycogen stores due to altered placental transport of substrates during fetal life, delayed maturation of gluconeogenesis, and a tendency toward hyperinsulinemia.[93] Insulin sensitivity is decreased in the liver and increased in the peripheral cells. Growth restricted infants have increased energy demands due to their greater brain-to-body mass size, increased metabolic rate, and tendency toward polycythemia, but smaller energy stores. Because the brain and red blood cells are obligatory glucose users, these factors can markedly increase glucose needs even in nonstressed infants. Glucose utilization may be further increased by chronic or acute perinatal hypoxia. Secretion of hepatic gluconeogenic enzymes (especially PEP-CK) is impaired in these infants, further limiting their ability to increase glucose production to meet metabolic demands.[116] Growth restricted infants are at risk for later obesity and other long-term health risks (see Chapter 12).[11,74,131]

The Infant of a Diabetic Mother

Although improved preconceptional care and careful metabolic control of pregnant diabetic women have reduced the incidence of significant macrosomia and improved perinatal mortality, infants of a diabetic mothers (IDMs) continue to be at risk for these as well as other health problems.[130] The cause of these problems relates to fetal and neonatal responses to maternal metabolic alterations and consequences to the neonate of cessation of placental transfer of substrates after birth. Many IDMs are LGA, lethargic, poor feeders, and at risk for the problems summarized in Figure 16-11 (see also pp. 572-573 for a discussion of the proposed basis for macrosomia and risk of congenital anomalies in IDMs). Infants born to diabetic mothers with significant vascular involvement are often SGA, but with more mature liver enzyme systems and lungs due to the effects of intrauterine stress. This group of infants is at particular risk for problems associated with chronic hypoxia such as asphyxia and polycythemia.

A prominent problem seen in IDMs is hypoglycemia. Hyperinsulinemia and a blunted glucagon response, aggravated by decreased hepatic responsiveness to glucose, are responsible for the hypoglycemia.[118] Levels of epinephrine and norepinephrine are also elevated, suggesting that hypoglycemia in these infants also may be related to adrenal medullary exhaustion.[25,] In addition exposure in utero to marked increases in glucose (due to higher maternal glucose levels) up-regulates insulin secretion and alters glucose disposal. This

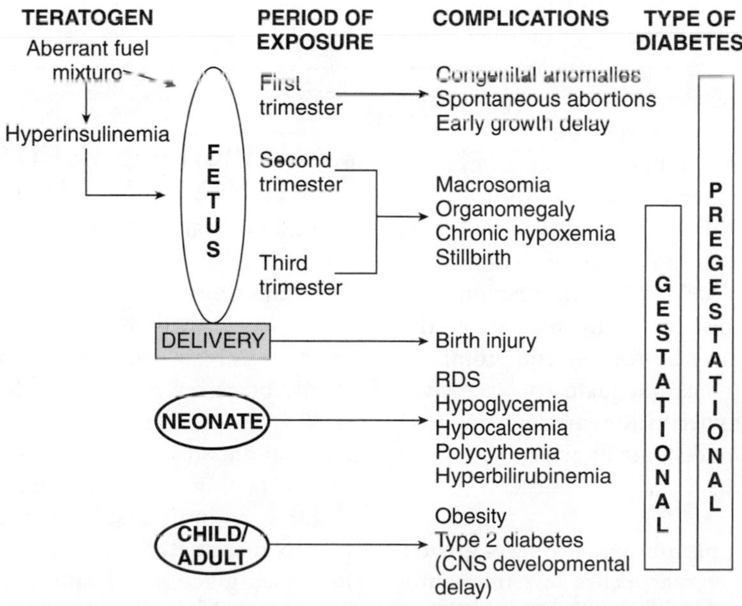

FIGURE 16-11 Diagrammatic representation of the multiple deleterious effects of the pregnancy of a diabetic patient on the offspring during the various periods of fetal and postnatal life. *CNS,* central nervous system; *RDS,* respiratory distress syndrome. (Adapted from Hod, M., et al. [1995]. Gestational diabetes mellitus: Is it a clinical entity? *Diabetes Rev, 3,* 605.)

leads to rapid insulin secretion and rebound hypoglycemia after an intravenous glucose bolus in the newborn.[116]

Large-for-Gestational-Age (LGA) Infants. LGA infants (weight greater than 90th percentile or greater than 2 standard deviations for their gestational age) who are not offspring of diabetic women are also at higher risk for developing hypoglycemia and hyperinsulinemia.[107,116] The exact mechanism is unclear but may be related to increased insulin sensitivity or due to borderline maternal glucose tolerance.[71,107,116]

The Infant with Asphyxia

After intrauterine stress, levels of IGF-I are low with increased insulin-like growth factor binding protein-1 and interleukin-6. This leads to decreases in peripheral glucose consumption, conserving glucose for the central nervous system.[40] Hypoxia and asphyxia alter glucose production and utilization with an increase in glycogenolysis to meet the increased metabolic and energy demands. Because oxygen availability is compromised, the infant switches from aerobic to anaerobic glycolysis. Anaerobic metabolism is less efficient than aerobic metabolism, producing a net increase of only two molecules of adenosine triphosphate (ATP) per molecule of glucose oxidized (versus 36 molecules of ATP per glucose molecule under aerobic conditions). These changes rapidly deplete glucose (glycogen) reserves, with decreased energy production that may be inadequate to maintain normal cell biologic processes and lead to accumulation of lactic acid.[25] Hypoxic-ischemic damage to the liver may further impair glucose production and delay the postnatal increase in gluconeogenesis. These infants may also develop a transient hyperinsulinemia.[25,93]

Because the fetus normally produces large amounts of lactate, intermediary pathways to metabolize lactate are relatively mature and efficient in the fetus and the newborn. As a result, metabolic acidosis with birth and asphyxia—if it is not severe enough to overwhelm these pathways or associated with postnatal alterations in oxygenation—is often reversed without administration of sodium bicarbonate.

The ability of the infant to mobilize fat stores may be impaired in hypoxia. During hypoxia, release of catecholamines and fatty acids is impaired and oxidation of fats is inhibited. These changes impair the ability of the infant to generate the energy necessary for normal cell functions and to meet the increased demands of the hypoxic state. The infant of a diabetic woman may be further compromised, because although this infant has adequate (or excessive) fat stores, the concomitant hyperinsulinemia and reduced glucagon secretion result in inadequate lipolysis.

Neonatal Hyperglycemia

Neonatal hyperglycemia is a plasma glucose level greater than 180 mg/dL.[71] Hyperglycemia occurs less frequently than hypoglycemia but has the potential for significant alterations in neurodevelopmental outcome.[22,35,71,77] Hyperglycemia is seen predominantly in preterm infants, especially those weighing less than 1000 g and receiving parenteral glucose infusions.[25,35] Hyperglycemia is negatively correlated with birth weight and positively correlated with the rate of glucose infusion. Markedly increased blood glucose levels can lead to osmotic changes and fluid shifts within the CNS (with a risk of intraventricular hemorrhage) and to glycosuria (with increased fluid and electrolyte losses and subsequent dehydration).

Hyperglycemia in low–birth weight infants "is most likely related to the secretion of glucose counter regulatory hormones as a result of stress, or to the release of cytokines in infected infants."[71] Other mechanisms that have been suggested for neonatal hyperglycemia include an inability of the immature infant to suppress endogenous glucose production while receiving a glucose infusion.[25,35] This inability may be due to a decrease in expression of GLUT-2 on hepatocytes, an increased ratio of GLUT-1/GLUT-2 transporters, decreased sensitivity and response to glucose and insulin with hyperglycemia, and decreased ability of the pancreatic β cells to adequately increase insulin in response to increased glucose.[35,98] Stressed infants seem to be at particular risk for hyperglycemia because of the simultaneous increase in catecholamine release (as a stress response), which further increases glucose levels by inhibiting insulin release and glucose utilization. Other infants at risk for hyperglycemia include infants treated with methylxanthines for apnea or with lipid infusions given at rates greater than 0.25 g/kg/hr, infants with sepsis or after surgery, and term newborns with severe growth restriction who develop transient neonatal diabetes. Chronic glucose deficiency in the growth restricted fetus leads to fewer pancreatic β cells with a decreased ability to secrete insulin. As a result these infant may develop hepatic insulin resistance with increased PEP-CK and increased hepatic glucose production rate, which can lead to a persistent hyperglycemia.[116] Hyperglycemia can also occur, rarely, in infants with very early onset diabetes mellitus.[110]

MATURATIONAL CHANGES DURING INFANCY AND CHILDHOOD

Energy and calorie requirements per unit of body weight remain higher in children than in adults because of their higher metabolic rate and growth needs. The relative requirement for carbohydrates is similar for children and adults. For infants, generally not more than 40% of the total calories should be carbohydrates; for children and adults, this value is 40% to 60%.[92] Cerebral glucose utilization is increased until childhood.

The fasting response pattern is similar in infants and children as in adults; however, it proceeds more rapidly due to the greater brain mass–to–body weight ratio and increased glucose utilization rates. Therefore infants and young children develop fasting hyperketonemia more rapidly (within 24 hours) than adults (36 to 48 hours).[122]

IGF-I levels along with insulin continue as important growth regulators during infancy and have an inverse relationship with body weight.[106] Catch-up growth is associated with IGF-I elevations during early childhood.[106] Growth hormone receptors increase in the first 2 years with a gradual transition to growth hormone regulation of growth.[106]

Serum amino acid levels decrease and urinary excretion increases until early childhood. Total body protein increases and reaches adult proportions (3%) by 4 years. Retention of nitrogen decreases during this time to adult values (11 mg/kg/day).[92] Diet alters the fatty acid composition of adipose tissue and possibly the composition of structural lipids during periods of rapid weight gain in the first year of life. This may affect the functional ability of tissues and structures.

SUMMARY

Growth "is an accretion of materials brought together in a synergism involving anabolism and catabolism."[82] Growth involves increases in cell size and in the complexity of cells, tissues, and organs. Alterations in growth during the perinatal period arise from maternal, fetal, or placental factors that alter the availability, accretion, or use of substrates or nutrients. These events are influenced by metabolic processes involved in carbohydrate, protein, and lipid metabolism. When this occurs the fetus or neonate may be unable to adapt to environmental stress and is at increased risk for morbidity and mortality.[82] Implications for clinical practice are summarized in Table 16-6.

Table 16-6 Recommendations for Clinical Practice Related to Changes in Carbohydrate, Protein, and Fat Metabolism in Neonates

Know the usual changes in carbohydrate, protein, and fat metabolism during the fetal and neonatal periods (pp. 573-581).
Monitor neonates for alterations in metabolic processes (pp. 578-582).
Monitor newborn glucose status during transition and in the early neonatal period (pp. 578-580 and Table 16-4).
Initiate early enteral feeding as appropriate (pp. 578-580 and Table 16-4).
Monitor neonates for signs of excessive and inadequate intake of carbohydrates, protein, and fat (pp. 578-582).
Recognize infants at risk for hypoglycemia (pp. 582-584 and Table 16-5).
Know the clinical signs of hypoglycemia (p. 582).
Assess and monitor infants at risk for neonatal hypoglycemia (p. 584 and Table 16-5).
Recognize infants at risk for hyperglycemia (p. 584).
Assess and monitor infants at risk for hyperglycemia (p. 584).
Monitor infants at risk for hyperglycemia for alterations in fluid and electrolyte balance (p. 584).
Recognize and monitor for problems for which the infant of a diabetic mother is at increased risk (pp. 572, 583-584 and Figure 16-11).

References

1. Aberg, A., et al. (2001). Congenital malformations among infants whose mothers had gestational or preexisting diabetes. *Early Hum Dev, 61,* 85.
2. Albareda, M., et al. (2005). Metabolic syndrome at follow-up in women with and without gestational diabetes mellitus in index pregnancy. *Metabolism, 54,* 1115.
3. American Diabetes Association. (2006). Diagnosis and classification of diabetes mellitus. *Diabetes Care, 29,* S43.
4. Atanassova, P., & Popova, L. (2000). Leptin expression during the differentiation of subcutaneous adipose cells of human embryos in situ. *Cells Tissues Organs, 166,* 15.
5. Aynsley-Green, A., & Hawdon, J.M. (1997). Hypoglycemia in the neonate: Current controversies. *Acta Paediatr Jpn, 39,* S12.
6. Baird, J.D. (1986). Some aspects of the metabolic and hormonal adaptation to pregnancy. *Acta Endocrinol, 112,* 11.
7. Baksu, A., et al. (2005). Serum leptin levels in preeclamptic pregnant women: Relationship to thyroid-stimulating hormone, body mass index, and proteinuria. *Am J Perinatol, 22,* 161.
8. Barta, E., & Drugan, A. (2010). Glucose transport from mother to fetus—A theoretical study. *J Theor Biol, 263,* 295.
9. Battaglia, F.C., & Thureen, P.J. (1997). Nutrition of the fetus and premature infant. *Nutrition, 13,* 903.
10. Beardsall, K. (2010). Measurement of glucose levels in the newborn. *Early Human Dev, 86,* 263.
11. Beltrand, J., Meas, T., & Levy-Marchal, C. (2010). Pathophysiology of insulin resistance in small for gestational age subjects: A role for adipose tissue? *Endocr Dev, 19,* 73.
12. Boden, G. (1996). Fuel metabolism in pregnancy and in gestational diabetes mellitus. *Obstet Gynecol Clin North Am, 23,* 1.
13. Boluyt, N., van Kempen, A., & Offringa, M. (2006). Neurodevelopment after neonatal hypoglycemia: A systematic review and design of an optimal future study. *Pediatrics, 117,* 2231.
14. Boyne, M.S., et al. (2003). The relationship among circulating insulin-like growth factor (IGF)-I, IGF-binding proteins-1 and -2, and birth anthropometry: A prospective study. *J Clin Endocrinol Metab, 88,* 1687.
15. Briana, D.D., & Malamitsi-Puchner, A. (2010). The role of adipocytokines in fetal growth. *Ann N Y Acad Sci, 1205,* 82.
16. Butte, N.F. (2000). Carbohydrate and lipid metabolism in pregnancy: Normal compared with gestational diabetes mellitus. *Am J Clin Nutr, 71,* 1256S.
17. Butte, N.F., et al. (2004). Energy requirements during pregnancy based on total energy expenditure and energy deposition. *Am J Clin Nutr, 79,* 1078.
18. Calkins, K., & Devaskar, S.U. (2011). Fetal origins of adult disease. *Curr Probl Pediatr Adolesc Health Care, 41,* 158.
19. Cetin, I., Berti, C., & Calabrese, S. (2010). Role of micronutrients in the periconceptional period. *Hum Reprod Update, 16,* 80.
20. Christou, H., et al. (2001). Cord blood leptin and insulin-like growth factor levels are independent predictors of fetal growth. *J Clin Endocrinol Metab, 86,* 935.
21. Committee on Fetus and Newborn, & Adamkin, D.H. (2011). Postnatal glucose homeostasis in late-preterm and term infants. *Pediatrics, 127,* 575.

22. Cornblath, M., & Ichord, R. (2000). Hypoglycemia in the neonate. *Semin Perinatol, 24,* 136.
23. Cornblath, M., et al. (1990). Hypoglycemia in infancy: The need for a rational definition. *Pediatrics, 85,* 834.
24. Cornblath, M., et al. (2000). Controversies regarding definition of neonatal hypoglycemia: Suggested operational thresholds. *Pediatrics, 105,* 1141.
25. Cowett, R.M., & Farrag, H.M. (2004). Selected principles of perinatal-neonatal glucose metabolism. *Semin Neonatol, 9,* 37.
26. Crowther, C.A., et al. (2005). Australian Carbohydrate Intolerance Study in Pregnant Women (ACHOIS) Trial Group. Effect of treatment of gestational diabetes mellitus on pregnancy outcomes. *N Engl J Med, 352,* 2477.
27. Dennedy, M.C., & Dunne, F. (2010). The maternal and fetal impacts of obesity and gestational diabetes on pregnancy outcome. *Best Pract Res Clin Endocrinol Metab, 24,* 573.
28. Desai, M., & Ross, M.G. (2011). Fetal programming of adipose tissue: Effects of intrauterine growth restriction and maternal obesity/high-fat diet. *Semin Reprod Med, 29,* 237.
29. Devreker, F., & Englert, Y. (2000). In vitro development and metabolism in the human embryo up to the blastocyst stage. *Eur J Obstet Gynecol Reprod Biol, 92,* 51.
30. Di Simone, N., et al. (2009). Resistin modulates glucose uptake and glucose transporter-1 (GLUT-1) expression in trophoblast cells. *J Cell Mol Med, 13,* 388.
31. Duggleby, S.L., & Jackson, A.A. (2002). Protein, amino acid and nitrogen metabolism during pregnancy: How might the mother meet the needs of her fetus? *Curr Opin Clin Nutr Metab Care, 5,* 503.
32. Duttaroy, A.K. (2009). Transport of fatty acids across the human placenta: A review. *Prog Lipid Res, 48,* 52.
33. Dyer, J.S., & Rosenfeld, C.R. (2011). Metabolic imprinting by prenatal, perinatal and postnatal overnutrition: A review. *Semin Reprod Med, 29,* 266.
34. Engstrom, E., et al. (2005). The role of maternal factors, postnatal nutrition, weight gain, and gender in regulation of serum IGF-I among preterm infants. *Pediatr Res, 57,* 605.
35. Farrag, H.M., & Cowett, R.M. (2000). Glucose homeostasis in the micropremie. *Clin Perinatol, 27,* 1.
36. Fernandez-Twinn, D.S., & Ozanne, S.E. (2010). Early life nutrition and metabolic programming. *Ann N Y Acad Sci, 1212,* 78.
37. Gleicher, N., et al. (1998). *Principles of medical therapy in pregnancy* (3rd ed.). New York: McGraw-Hill.
38. Gluckman, P.D. (1997). Endocrine and nutritional regulation of prenatal growth. *Acta Paediatr Suppl, 423,* 153.
39. Godfrey, K.M., Inskip, H.M., & Hanson, M.A. (2011). The long term effects of prenatal development on growth and metabolism. *Semin Reprod Med, 29,* 257.
40. Gustafsson, J. (2009). Neonatal energy substrate production. *Indian J Med Res, 130,* 618.
41. Hadar, E., & Hod, M. (2010). Establishing consensus criteria for the diagnosis of diabetes in pregnancy following the HAPO study. *Ann N Y Acad Sci, 1205,* 88.
42. Hadden, D.R., & McLaughlin, C. (2009). Normal and abnormal maternal metabolism during pregnancy. *Semin Fetal Neonatal Med, 14,* 66.
43. Handwerger, S., & Freemark, M. (2000). The roles of placental growth hormone and placental lactogen in the regulation of human fetal growth and development. *J Pediatr Endocrinol Metab, 13,* 343.
44. Hanebutt, F.L., et al. (2008). Long-chain polyunsaturated fatty acid (LC-PUFA) transfer across the placenta. *Clin Nutr, 27,* 685.
45. HAPO Study Cooperative Research Group (2008). Hyperglycemia and adverse pregnancy outcomes. *N Engl J Med, 358,* 1991.
46. HAPO Study Cooperative Research Group (2009). Hyperglycemia and Adverse Pregnancy Outcome (HAPO) Study: Associations with neonatal anthropometrics. *Diabetes, 58,* 453.
47. Hare, J.W. (1989). *Diabetes complicating pregnancy: The Joslin Clinic method.* New York: Alan R. Liss.
48. Harris, D.L., et al. (2010). Continuous glucose monitoring of newborn babies at risk of hypoglycemia. *J Pediatric, 157,* 198.
49. Hauguel-de Mouzon, S., Lepercq, J., & Catalano, P. (2006). The known and unknown of leptin in pregnancy. *Am J Obstet Gynecol, 194,* 1537.
50. Hawdon, J.M. (1999). Hypoglycemia and the neonatal brain. *Eur J Pediatr, 158,* S9.
51. Hay, W.W., Jr. (2006). Recent observations on the regulation of fetal metabolism by glucose. *J Physiol, 572,* 17.
52. Hay, W.W., Jr., et al. (2009). Knowledge gaps and research needs for understanding and treating neonatal hypoglycemia: Workshop report from Eunice Kennedy Shriver National Institute of Child Health and Human Development. *J Pediatr, 155,* 612.
53. Hay, W.W., Jr., & Rozance, P.J. (2010). Continuous glucose monitoring for diagnosis and treatment of neonatal hypoglycemia. *J Pediatr, 157,* 180.
54. Hay, W.W., Jr., et al.. (2012). Fetal requirements and placental transfer of nitrogenous compounds. In R.A. Polin, W.W. Fox, & S.H. Abman (Eds.), *Fetal and neonatal physiology* (4th ed.). Philadelphia: Saunders.
55. Henson, M.C., & Castracane, V.D. (2006). Leptin in pregnancy: An update. *Biol Reprod, 74,* 218.
56. Herrera, E. (2000). Lipid metabolism in the fetus and the newborn. *Diabetes Metab Res Rev, 16,* 202.
57. Herrera, E. (2000). Metabolic adaptations in pregnancy and their implications for the availability of substrates to the fetus. *Eur J Clin Nutr, 54,* S47.
58. Herrera, E., & Ortega-Senovilla, H. (2010). Disturbances in lipid metabolism in diabetic pregnancy—Are these the cause of the problem? *Best Pract Res Clin Endocrinol Metab, 24,* 515.
59. Herrera, E., & Lasuncion, M.A. (2012). Maternal-fetal transfer of lipid metabolites. In R.A. Polin, W.W. Fox, & S.H. Abman (Eds.), *Fetal and neonatal physiology* (4th ed.). Philadelphia: Saunders.
60. Hume, R., et al. (2005). Glucose homeostasis in the newborn. *Early Hum Dev, 81,* 95.
61. Illsley, N.P. (2000). Glucose transporters in the human placenta. *Placenta, 21,* 14.
62. Illsley, N.P. (2000). Placental glucose transport in diabetic pregnancy. *Clin Obstet Gynecol, 43,* 116.
63. Innis, S.M. (2005). Essential fatty acid transfer and fetal development, *Placenta, 26,* S70.
64. International Association of Diabetes and Pregnancy Study Groups (2010). International Association of Diabetes and Pregnancy Study Groups recommendations on the diagnosis and classification of hyperglycemia in pregnancy. *Diabetes Care, 33,* 676.
65. Jain, V. , Chen, M. & Menon, R.K. (2012). Disorders of carbohydrate metabolism. In C.A. Gleason & S. Devaskar (Eds.). *Avery's Diseases of the newborn* (9th ed.). Philadelphia: Saunders.
66. Jaksic, J., et al. (2001). Effect of insulin and insulin-like growth factor I on fetal macrosomia in healthy women. *Coll Antropol, 25,* 535.
67. Jansson, T., & Powell, T.L. (2000). Placental nutrient transfer and fetal growth. *Nutrition, 16,* 500.
68. Jansson, T., Myatt, L., & Powell, T.L. (2009). The role of trophoblast nutrient and ion transporters in the development of pregnancy complications and adult disease. *Curr Vasc Pharmacol, 7,* 521.
69. Javaid, M.K., et al. (2005). Umbilical cord leptin predicts neonatal bone mass. *Calcif Tissue Int, 76,* 341.
70. Jovanovic, L., & Nakai, Y. (2006). Successful pregnancy in women with type 1 diabetes: From preconception through postpartum care. *Endocrinol Metab Clin North Am, 35,* 79.
71. Kalhan, S.C., & Devaskar, S.U. (2011). Disorders of carbohydrate metabolism. In R.J. Martin, A.A. Fanaroff, & M.C. Walsh (Eds.), *Fanaroff & Martin's Neonatal-perinatal medicine: Diseases of the fetus and infant* (9th ed.). St. Louis: Mosby.
72. Kalhan, S.C. (2000). Protein metabolism in pregnancy. *Am J Clin Nutr, 71,* 1249S.

73. Kalhan, S.C., & Parimi, P.S. (2012). Metabolism of glucose and methods of investigation in the fetus and newborn. In R.A. Polin, W.W. Fox, & S.H. Abman (Eds.), *Fetal and neonatal physiology* (4th ed.). Philadelphia: Saunders.
74. Kanaka-Gantenbein, C. (2010). Fetal origins of adult diabetes. *Ann N Y Acad Sci, 1205,* 99.
75. Kapoor, N. (2007). Diabetes in pregnancy: A review of current evidence. *Curr Opin Obstet Gynecol, 19,* 586.
76. Kashyap, S.H., & Putet, G. (2012). Lipids as an energy source for the premature and full term neonate. In R.A. Polin, W.W. Fox, & S.H. Abman (Eds.), *Fetal and neonatal physiology* (4th ed.). Philadelphia: Saunders.
77. Katz, L.L., & Stanley, C.A. (2005). Disorders of glucose and other sugars. In A.R. Spitzer (Ed.), *Intensive care of the fetus and neonate* (2nd ed.). St. Louis: Mosby.
78. Kenshole, A.B. (2004). Diabetes and pregnancy. In G.N. Burrow, T.P. Duffy, & J.A. Copel (Eds.), *Medical complications during pregnancy* (6th ed.). Philadelphia: Saunders.
79. King, J.C., et al. (1994). Energy metabolism during pregnancy: Influence of maternal energy status. *Am J Clin Nutr, 59,* 439S.
80. King, J.C. (2000). Physiology of pregnancy and nutrient metabolism. *Am J Clin Nutr, 71,* 1218S.
81. Kratzscm J.Y., et al. (2000). Leptin and pregnancy outcome. *Curr Opin Obstet Gynecol, 12,* 501.
82. Kretchmer, N., Schumacher, L.B., & Silliman, K. (1989). Biological factors affecting intrauterine growth. *Semin Perinatol, 13,* 169.
83. Lage, M., et al. (1999). Serum leptin levels in women throughout pregnancy and the postpartum period and in women suffering spontaneous abortion. *Clin Endocrinol, 50,* 211.
84. Laivuori, H., et al. (2000). Leptin during and after pre-eclamptic or normal pregnancy: its relation to serum insulin and insulin sensitivity. *Metabolism, 49,* 259.
85. Landon, M.B., et al. (2009). A multicenter, randomized trial of treatment for mild gestational diabetes. *N Engl J Med, 361,* 1339.
86. Lappas, M., et al. (2005). Release and regulation of leptin, resistin and adiponectin from human placenta, fetal membranes, and maternal adipose tissue and skeletal muscle from normal and gestational diabetes mellitus-complicated pregnancies. *J Endocrinol, 186,* 457.
87. Leary, J., Pettitt, D.J., & Jovanovic, L. (2010). Gestational diabetes guidelines in a HAPO world. *Best Pract Res Clin Endocrinol Metab, 24,* 673.
88. Lesser, K.B., & Carpenter, M.W. (1994). Metabolic changes associated with normal pregnancy and pregnancy complicated by diabetes mellitus. *Semin Perinatol, 18,* 399.
89. Levy-Marchal, C., Jaquet, D., & Czernichow, P. (2004). Long-term metabolic consequences of being born small for gestational age. *Semin Neonatol, 9,* 67.
90. Lindsay, R.S., et al. (2004). The relation of insulin, leptin and IGF-1 to birthweight in offspring of women with type 1 diabetes. *Clin Endocrinol (Oxf), 61,* 353.
91. Lof, M., et al. (2005). Changes in basal metabolic rate during pregnancy in relation to changes in body weight and composition, cardiac output, insulin-like growth factor I, and thyroid hormones and in relation to fetal growth. *Am J Clin Nutr, 81,* 678.
92. Lowrey, G. (1986). *Growth and development of children.* Chicago: Year Book.
93. Lteif, A.N., & Schwenk, W.F. (1999). Hypoglycemia in infants and children. *Endocrinol Metab Clin North Am, 28,* 619.
94. Mericq, V. (2006). Prematurity and insulin sensitivity. *Horm Res, 65,* 131.
95. Metzger, B.E., et al. (2007). Summary and recommendations of the fifth international workshop-conference on gestational diabetes mellitus. *Diabetes Care, 30,* S251.
96. Metzger, B.E. (2003).The Freinkel legacy. In M. Hod, et al. (Eds.), *Textbook of diabetes and pregnancy.* London: Martin Dunitz.
97. Metzger, B.E., et al. (2010). Hyperglycemia and adverse pregnancy outcome study: Neonatal glycemia, *Pediatrics, 126,* e1545.
98. Moore, T.R., & Catalano, P. (2009). Diabetes and pregnancy. In R.K. Creasy, et al. (Eds.), *Creasy & Resnik's Maternal-fetal medicine: Principles and practice* (6th ed.). Philadelphia: Saunders.
99. Mott, G.E. (2012). Lipoprotein metabolism and nutritional programming in the fetus and neonate. In R.A. Polin, W.W. Fox, & S.H. Abman (Eds.), *Fetal and neonatal physiology* (4th ed.). Philadelphia: Saunders.
100. Nelson, S.M., Matthews, P., & Poston, L. (2009). Maternal metabolism and obesity: Modifiable determinants of pregnancy outcome. *Hum Repro Update, 16,* 1.
101. Ogata, E.S. (2012). Carbohydrate metabolism during pregnancy. In R.A. Polin, W.W. Fox, & S.H. Abman (Eds.), *Fetal and neonatal physiology* (4th ed.). Philadelphia: Saunders.
102. Ong, K., et al. (2002). Circulating IGF-I levels in childhood are related to both current body composition and early postnatal growth rate. *J Clin Endocrinol Metab, 87,* 1041.
103. Ortega-Senovilla, H., et al. (2009). Gestational diabetes mellitus upsets the proportion of fatty acids in umbilical arterial but not venous plasma. *Diabet Care,* 32, 120.
104. Pampfer, S. (2000). Peri-implantation embryopathy induced by maternal diabetes. *J Reprod Fertil Suppl, 55,* 129.
105. Persson, B. (2009). Neonatal glucose metabolism in offspring of mothers with varying degrees of hyperglycemia during pregnancy. *Semin Fetal Neonatal Med, 14,* 106.
106. Phillips, A.F. (2012). Oxygen consumption and general carbohydrate metabolism of the fetus. In R.A. Polin, W.W. Fox, & S.H. Abman (Eds.), *Fetal and neonatal physiology* (4th ed.). Philadelphia: Saunders.
107. Poppitt, S.D., et al. (1993). Evidence of energy-sparing in Gambian women during pregnancy: A longitudinal study using whole-body calorimetry. *Am J Clin Nutr, 57,* 353.
108. Poston, L. (2010). Developmental programming and diabetes—The human experience and insight from animal models. *Best Pract Res Clin Endocrinol Metab, 24,* 541.
109. Prentice, A.M., & Goldberg, G.R. (2000). Energy adaptations in human pregnancy: Limits and long-term consequences, *J Clin Nutr, 71,* 1226S.
110. Pridjian, G., & Benjamin, T.D. (2010). Update on gestational diabetes. *Obstet Gynecol Clin North Am, 37,* 255.
111. Ray, J.G., O'Brien, T.E., & Chan, W.S. (2001). Preconception care and the risk of congenital anomalies in the offspring of women with diabetes mellitus: A meta-analysis. *QJM, 94,* 435.
112. Retnakaran, R., et al. (2004). Reduced adiponectin concentration in women with gestational diabetes: A potential factor in progression to type 2 diabetes. *Diabetes Care, 27,* 799.
113. Rozance, P.J., & Hay, W.W., Jr. (2006). Hypoglycemia in newborn infants: Features associated with adverse outcomes. *Biol Neonate, 90,* 74.
114. Rozance, P.J., & Hay, W.W. Jr. (2010). Describing hypoglycemia—definition or operational threshold? *Early Hum Dev, 86,* 275.
115. Sibley, C.P., et al. (2010). Review: Adaptation in placental nutrient supply to meet fetal growth demand: Implications for programming. *Placenta, 31,* S70.
116. Siddiqui, F., & James, D. (2003). Fetal monitoring in type 1 diabetic pregnancies. Review. *Early Hum Dev, 72,* 1.
117. Simmons, R.A. (2012). Cell glucose transport and glucose handling during fetal and neonatal development. In R.A. Polin, W.W. Fox, & S.H. Abman (Eds.), *Fetal and neonatal physiology* (4th ed.). Philadelphia: Saunders.
118. Stanley, C.A., & Hardy, O.T. (2012). Pathophysiology of hypoglycemia. In R.A. Polin, W.W. Fox, & S.H. Abman (Eds.), *Fetal and neonatal physiology* (4th ed.). Philadelphia: Saunders.
119. Sugden, M.C., & Holness, M.J. (1998). Fuel selection: The maternal adaptation to fetal nutrient demand. *Biochem Soc Trans, 26,* 79.

120. Tieu, J., et al. (2010). Oral anti-diabetic agents for women with pre-existing diabetes mellitus/impaired glucose tolerance or previous gestational diabetes mellitus. *Cochrane Database Syst Rev, 10,* CD007724.
121. Tieu, J., et al. (2010). Screening and subsequent management for gestational diabetes for improving maternal and infant health. *Cochrane Database Syst Rev, 7,* CD007222.
122. Touger, L., et al. (2005). Early growth in offspring of diabetic mothers. *Diabetes Care, 28,* 585.
123. Vanverde, J.E., et al. (2012). Accretion of lipid in the fetus and newborn. In R.A. Polin, W.W. Fox, & S.H. Abman (Eds.), *Fetal and neonatal physiology* (4th ed.). Philadelphia: Saunders.
124. Vitoratos, N., et al. (2001). Maternal plasma leptin levels and their relationship to insulin and glucose in gestational-onset diabetes. *Gynecol Obstet Invest, 51,* 17.
125. Waugh, N., et al. (2010). Screening for hyperglycaemia in pregnancy: A rapid update for the National Screening Committee. *Health Technol Assess, 14,* 1.
126. Waugh, N., Pearson, D., & Royle, P. (2010). Screening for hyperglycaemia in pregnancy: Consensus and controversy. *Best Pract Res Clin Endocrinol Metab, 24,* 553.
127. Weindling, M.A. (2009). Offspring of diabetic pregnancy: Short-term outcomes. *Semin Fetal Neonatal Med, 14,* 111.
128. Wells, J.C. (2011). The thrifty phenotype: An adaptation in growth or metabolism? *Am J Hum Biol, 23,* 65.
129. Widmaier, E., Raff, H., & Strang, K.T. (2005). *Vander's Human physiology: The mechanism of body function* (10th ed.). New York: McGraw-Hill.
130. Williamson, D.H., & Thornton, P.S. (2012). Ketone body production and metabolism in the fetus and newborn. In R.A. Polin, W.W. Fox, & S.H. Abman (Eds.), *Fetal and neonatal physiology* (4th ed.). Philadelphia: Saunders.
131. Yamashita, H., Shao, J., & Friedman, J.E. (2000). Physiologic and molecular alteration in carbohydrate metabolism during pregnancy and gestational diabetes mellitus. *Clin Obstet Gynecol, 43,* 87.
132. Yogev, Y., Metzger, B.E., & Hod, M. (2009). Establishing diagnosis of gestational diabetes mellitus: Impact of the hyperglycemia and adverse pregnancy outcome study. *Semin Fetal Neonatal Med, 14,* 94.

CHAPTER 17

Calcium and Phosphorus Metabolism

Calcium and phosphorus are critical in cardiovascular, nervous, homeostatic, and muscular processes and in the function of many hormones and enzyme systems. Maternal calcium metabolism during pregnancy and lactation undergoes a series of hormone-mediated adjustments to enhance transport of this mineral to the fetus without long-term alterations in the maternal skeleton.[35] Calcium serves as a second messenger; this calcium signaling is important in many reproductive processes, including fertilization, implantation and placental development and function.[5]

Calcium, phosphorus, and other minerals are transported across the placenta for fetal bone mineralization and skeletal growth. After birth the neonate loses the placental supply of calcium and must quickly establish homeostasis of this system to avoid metabolic derangements. This chapter discusses alterations in these substances and related hormones during pregnancy and the neonatal period. Calcium and phosphorus homeostasis in nonpregnant individuals is summarized in Box 17-1 on page 590 and in Figure 17-1. The roles of the major calcitropic hormones (parathyroid hormone, calcitonin, and vitamin D) are summarized in Table 17-1.

MATERNAL PHYSIOLOGIC ADAPTATIONS

Calcium and phosphorus metabolism is altered during pregnancy, with an increase in the amount and efficiency of intestinal calcium absorption. During pregnancy, absorption increases to 50%, versus 20% to 25% in nonpregnant individuals.[56,65] The increased absorption is mediated primarily by increased 1,25-dihydroxyvitamin D (1,25-[OH]$_2$D).[62] Calcium accumulation in the fetus by term totals 28 to 30 g.[36,51,59] Most of this accretion (approximately 25 g) occurs in the third trimester and is used for fetal bone formation and mineralization.[56] Maternal calcium metabolism undergoes further changes during lactation to meet the calcium needs of the growing infant. Understanding of changes in maternal calcium metabolism in pregnancy and lactation has grown in recent years with improved assay techniques and recognition of the roles of parathyroid hormone–related peptide (PTHrP) (see Box 17-2 on page 591).[44] PTHrP increases in the first trimester and is critical for placental calcium transport and thought to help protect the maternal skeleton from excess bone loss.[47] PTHrP may also help mediate changes in vitamin D and PTH.[73]

Antepartum Period

Calcium homeostasis during pregnancy is interrelated with changes in extracellular fluid volume, renal function, and fetal needs. The mother meets the fetal requirement for calcium primarily by increasing intestinal calcium absorption. These change are mediated by increased production of 1,25-(OH)$_2$D and PTHrP and under the influence of hormones and growth factors such as estrogens, prolactin (PRL), human placental lactogen (hPL), placental growth factor, and insulin-like growth factor-1.[51,56] These substances increase intestinal absorption of calcium in pregnancy, decrease urinary excretion, alter maternal bone calcium turnover, and stimulate synthesis of both PTHrP and 1,25-(OH)$_2$D.[35,56,65] Changes in calcium and phosphorus homeostasis during pregnancy are summarized in Table 17-2 and Figure 17-2.

Calcium

Maternal total serum calcium levels fall progressively beginning soon after fertilization and decrease by an average of 1 to 1.5 mg/dL (0.25 to 0.38 mmol/L). Calcium reaches its lowest levels at 28 to 32 weeks, followed by a plateau or slight rise to term.[62,85] Serum calcium levels during pregnancy average 9 to 10 mg/dL (2.3 to 2.5 mmol/L)—a decrease of 5% to 6%.[62] The decrease in serum calcium is a relative decrease, in that it is primarily related to and parallels the fall in serum proteins, especially albumin, with a decrease in both total and bound calcium.[36,51,56] Other factors that contribute to alterations in serum calcium include increased plasma volume and hemodilution, increased urinary calcium excretion, and fetal transfer (primarily in the third trimester).[44,62] Ionized calcium (physiologically active form) does not change significantly and is stable or in the low normal range.[35,36,44,51]

Calcium absorption occurs by active transport in the duodenum and proximal jejunum and by passive mechanisms in the distal jejunum and ileum. Intestinal absorption of calcium doubles during pregnancy, with a positive calcium balance noted by as early as 12 weeks' gestation that continues to the third trimester.[18,35,51] The early increase allows the mother to store calcium throughout pregnancy to meet the high fetal

BOX 17-1 Calcium and Phosphorus Homeostasis

Serum calcium is present in three forms: (1) bound to albumin and globulins (40%), (2) complexed to bicarbonate and other buffers (8% to 10%), and (3) physiologically active ionized (50%) calcium. Calcium is also found in extracellular fluid (ECF) and cytoplasm. Calcium is needed for muscle contraction, neurotransmitter secretion, and hormonal secretion.[46] Parathyroid hormone (PTH), vitamin D, and calcitonin are the major hormones involved in calcium homeostasis. Actions of PTH and intestinal absorption of vitamin D are enhanced by magnesium. Hormonal regulation of calcium metabolism is summarized in Figure 17-1.

Calcium and phosphorus are absorbed in the small intestine under the influence of 1,25-dihydroxyvitamin D (1,25-[OH]$_2$D), which stimulates calcium-binding protein carriers. PTH mobilizes calcium and phosphorus in bone by stimulating osteolysis. Active transport of calcium across intestinal cells is vitamin D–dependent and releases calcium and phosphorus into ECF. In the kidneys, 98% of the filtered calcium is reabsorbed, 70% in the proximal tubule, 20% in the distal tubule, and 10% in the ascending loop of Henle. Reabsorption is regulated by PTH and 1,25-(OH)$_2$D.

PTH inhibits proximal tubular reabsorption of phosphate, leading to increased urinary loss and decreased ECF levels. PTH increases distal tubular reabsorption of Ca^{2+} to conserve calcium by decreasing renal excretion. Thus PTH increases the release of both calcium and phosphorus from the bones, increasing ECF levels. PTH alters both osteoblast and osteoclast activity in the bone.[6] Because concentrations of Ca^{2+} and PO_4 in ECF are closely tied to each other, if ECF PO_4 levels increase, further release of calcium from the bones would normally be decreased to keep the total concentration of calcium and phosphorus constant. If the kidneys increase PO_4 excretion, however, extracellular phosphorus decreases and more calcium is released from bone. The net result is increased serum and ECF calcium and decreased phosphorus. Decreased serum PO_4 occurs because the phosphaturic actions of PTH exceed serum phosphate–elevating activities. Release of PTH is regulated by concentrations of serum calcium. Even small changes in serum ionized calcium stimulate PTH release. Calcium reabsorption is also influenced by ionized calcium levels, acid-base balance, and phosphate concentrations.[69] Phosphorus excretion is regulated primarily by PTH, which inhibits renal phosphorus reabsorption. Decreased plasma phosphorus levels stimulate increased 1,25-(OH)$_2$D, which increases plasma calcium and suppresses PTH.[69] Phosphorus is also regulated by phosphatonin peptides such as FGF23 which acts on the bone and kidney.[66]

Vitamin D enhances PTH action to increase calcium release from bone and tubular reabsorption of these minerals (see Figure 17-1). Vitamin D can be produced endogenously in the epidermal layer of skin by ultraviolet light irradiation of 7-dehydrocholesterol to D_3 (cholecalciferol) or ingested as D_2 (ergocalciferol) or D_3. Ingested vitamin D requires bile salts for intestinal absorption and is converted in the liver to serum 25-hydroxyvitamin D (25-[OH]D) (major circulating metabolite). This metabolite is usually transported in the blood bound to vitamin-D binding protein. In the kidneys, 25-(OH)D is hydroxylated to 1,25-(OH)$_2$D$_3$ by 1α-hydroxylase (CYP27B1). This enzyme is found in the proximal tubule and is up-regulated by PTH and down-regulated by fibroblast growth factor.[40] Regulation of vitamin D also occurs through negative feedback from 25-(OH)D levels. 1,25-(OH)$_2$D is also produced in other tissues, including possibly the decidua and placenta during pregnancy, and may play a role in glucose metabolism, skeletal muscle, skin, and cardiovascular and immune system function.[6,9,36,40,45]

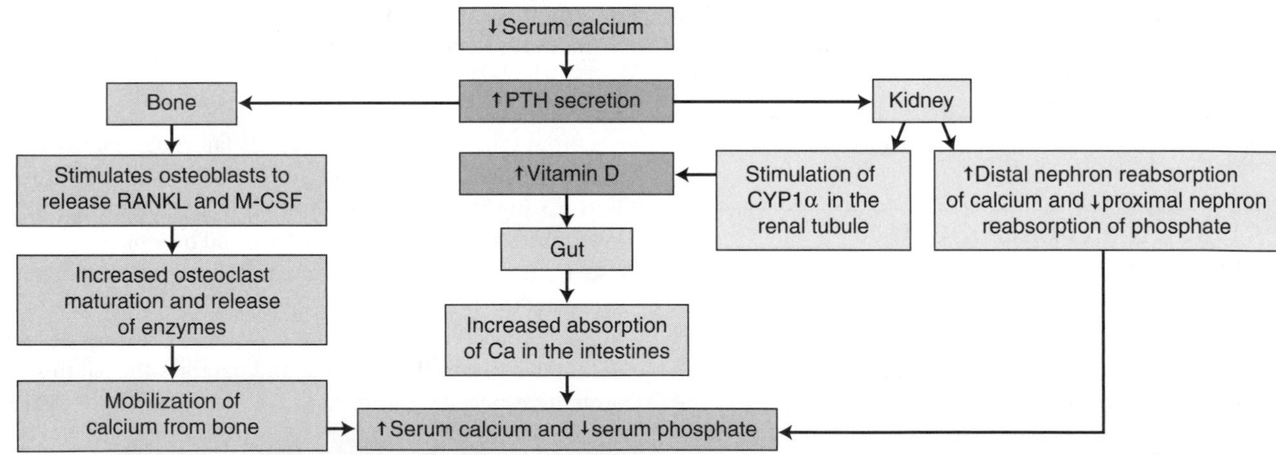

FIGURE 17-1 Normal calcium metabolism regulated by PTH and vitamin D. *CYP1α,* cytochrome P4501α-hydrolase; *M-CSF,* macrophage-colony stimulating factor; *PTH,* parathyroid hormone; *RANKL,* receptor activator of nuclear factor kappa beta (NF-κβ) ligand. (From McCance, K.L., & Huether, S. [2010]. *Pathophysiology: The biological basis for disease in adults & children* [6th edition]. St. Louis: Mosby Elsevier, p. 712.)

demands in the latter part of the third trimester.[44] The rise in calcium absorption parallels the rise in 1,25-(OH)$_2$D, which is the primary mediator of this change. However, since the increased intestinal absorption begins prior to the increase in 1,21,25-(OH)$_2$D, there are likely other as yet unknown mechanisms.[40] Estrogens and other hormones may up-regulate intestinal calcium transporter genes independent of the influence of vitamin D.[80] Prolactin also has a calcitropic role during pregnancy as well as during lactation.[17]

Urinary calcium excretion parallels the rise in intestinal calcium absorption.[35,36] Urinary excretion increases by 12 weeks, with an average increase from the nonpregnant value of

Table 17-1 Hormonal Actions Controlling Calcium and Phosphorus Levels

HORMONE	BONE	INTESTINE	KIDNEY
Parathyroid hormone	Increased calcium release Increased phosphorus release		Increased calcium reabsorption Decreased phosphorus reabsorption
Calcitonin	Decreased calcium release Decreased phosphorus release	May inhibit calcium and phosphorus reabsorption	Increased calcium excretion Increased phosphorus excretion
Vitamin D	Increased calcium release	Increased calcium absorption Increased phosphorus absorption	Increased calcium reabsorption Increased phosphorus reabsorption

BOX 17-2 Roles of Parathyroid Hormone–Related Peptide (or Protein)

Parathyroid hormone–related peptide or protein (PTHrP), first isolated in 1987, is produced from a single gene similar in origin and sequencing to the parathyroid (PTH) gene.[43,81,87] The gene is processed into different circulating fragments or isoforms, each with a different function.[28,81] PTHrP is produced in most tissues of the body and has a broad range of functions. Because few of these functions directly relate to calcium, the name is somewhat of a misnomer. Sources of PTHrP during pregnancy include the breasts, decidua, placenta, fetal membranes, parathyroid gland, and umbilical cord.[44,81]

PTHrP is divided into three peptides that can each produce other peptides, each with differing functions.[44,81,87] The major functions of PTHrP are as follows: (1) stimulation of transepithelial calcium transport, especially in the kidneys, placenta, and breast; (2) smooth muscle (uterus, bladder, stomach, intestines, arterial wall) relaxation; and (3) regulation of cellular proliferation, differentiation, and apoptosis (see Chapter 3).[43,44,81,87] Critical perinatal functions of PTHrP include roles in milk production (see Chapter 5), labor onset (see Chapter 4), fetal maternal calcium gradient, and placental calcium transport.[93] Disruption of the PTHrP gene in the fetus or neonate is lethal.[83]

Table 17-2 Minerals and Hormones Involved in Calcium Homeostasis

MINERAL/ HORMONES	MOTHER	FETUS	NEWBORN
Total calcium*	Low	High	Falls‡
Ionized calcium*	Low normal	High	Falls
Magnesium*	Low normal	High normal	Falls
Phosphorus*	Low	High	Rises‡
Parathyroid hormone	Low	Low	Rises
Calcitonin	Normal/High	High	Falls
25(OH)D*	Variable	Variable	Variable
1,25(OH)$_2$D	High	Low	Rises
Parathyroid hormone–related protein	High†	High	

From Nader, S. (2004). Other endocrine disorders of pregnancy. In R.K. Creasy, R. Resnik, & J.D. Iams (Eds.), *Maternal-fetal medicine: Principles and practice* (5th ed.). Philadelphia: Saunders.
* Placental transfer.
† Of fetal origin.
‡ Toward nonpregnant adult values.

160 to 240 mg/dL (40 to 60 mmol/L) in the third trimester.[56,62] This change is due to up-regulation of 1α-hydroxylase (enzyme involved in 1,25-[OH]$_2$D synthesis) activity by PTHrP, estrogens, prolactin, and human placental lactogen as well as the increased glomerular filtration rate, and occurs even when the maternal diet is calcium deficient.[18,65] After 36 weeks, urinary calcium excretion decreases by about 35%, increasing calcium availability by approximately 50 mg/day. Because fetal needs at this point are approximately 350 mg/day, however, other maternal calcium sources (i.e., dietary sources or the maternal skeleton) are essential.[62]

Phosphorus and Magnesium

Serum inorganic phosphate levels are generally stable during pregnancy, as is renal tubular reabsorption of this mineral.[35,44] Magnesium is at or below the lower reference range limit. These changes are related to hemodilution and decreased serum albumin.

Parathyroid Hormone

PTH levels fall to low-normal in the first trimester and may become undetectable in women with adequate calcium and vitamin D intake, and increase to mid-normal ranges by term in these women.[18,36,44] Newer assays suggest PTH levels decrease to 10% to 30% of prepregnant values before increasing to term.[51] The initial decrease is due to the increased 1,25-(OH)$_2$D in response to increased PTHrP, which may contribute to changes in parathyroid function during pregnancy.[6,27,35,36,51,87]

Vitamin D

Both free and bound levels of 1,25-(OH)$_2$D rise early in pregnancy, double by 10 to 12 weeks' gestation, and remain high to term.[6,35,36,44,51,65] Maternal serum levels of 1,25-(OH)$_2$D are 50% to 100% higher by the second trimester and up to 100% higher in the third trimester.[40] Vitamin D–binding protein

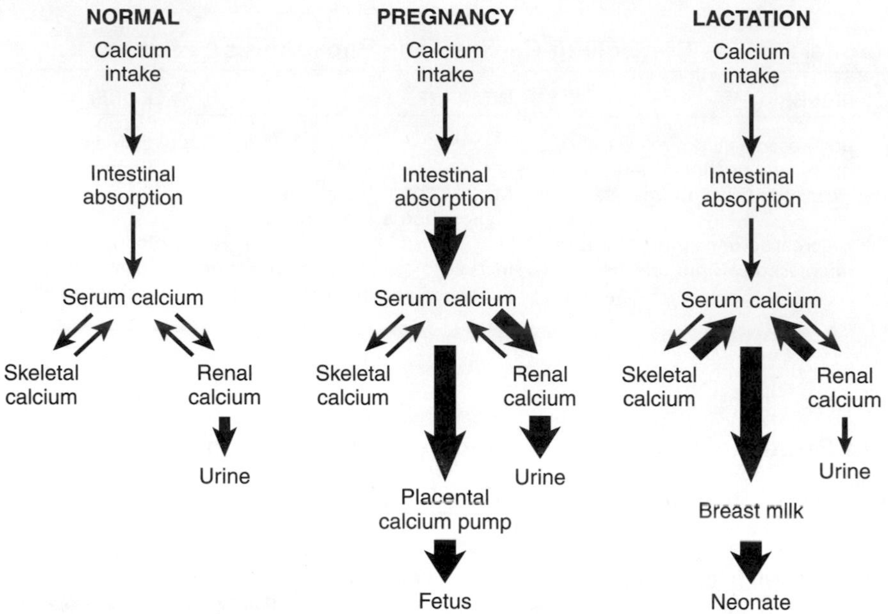

FIGURE 17-2 Adaptive processes of calcium homeostasis in human pregnancy and lactation as compared with the normal nonpregnant state. The thickness of the arrows indicates the relative increase or decrease with respect to the normal, nonpregnancy state. (From Kovacs, C.S., & Kronberg, H.M. [1997]. Maternal-fetal calcium and bone metabolism during pregnancy, puerperium and lactation. *Endocrin Rev, 18,* 859.)

also increases, possibly due to the increased estrogen.[6,61] Changes in 1,25-$(OH)_2$D are not mediated by PTH, because levels of this hormone are low-normal during the first trimester, but are under the influence of estrogens, PRL, hPL, and especially PTHrP, which increases levels of the enzyme 1α-hydroxylase needed for production of 1,25-$(OH)_2$D and suppresses maternal PTH.[6,18,40,51] The increased 1,25-$(OH)_2$D comes primarily from increased production by the maternal kidney, with some from the decidua and fetoplacental unit.[6,35,36,40,44,65,87] 1,25-$(OH)_2$D opens voltage-dependent calcium channels in intestinal cells to increase calcium absorption.[51] Thus the doubling of 1,25-$(OH)_2$D is paralleled by a twofold increase in intestinal calcium absorption. Serum 25-hydroxyvitamin D (25-[OH]D) levels (stored form) do not change significantly during pregnancy. The increase in 1,25-$(OH)_2$D after 34 to 36 weeks has been associated with an increase in a vitamin D–binding protein and bound vitamin D. Thus intestinal absorption of vitamin D is enhanced throughout gestation. Renal clearance of 1,25-$(OH)_2$D does not change during pregnancy.[6]

Calcitonin

Calcitonin levels are generally reported to be normal to high during pregnancy, particularly in the latter half, with about 20% of women having values outside the normal range.[35,51] During pregnancy calcitonin is synthesized by the breasts and placenta in addition to the usual synthesis by the C cells of the thyroid gland. The increase in calcitonin with advancing pregnancy may stimulate the proximal renal tubule to increase 1,25-$(OH)_2$D production.[27] Increased calcitonin inhibits calcium and phosphorus release from the bones, counteracting the action of PTH (see Table 17-1). This may help prevent excessive reabsorption of bone calcium and conserve the maternal skeleton while simultaneously permitting the intestinal and renal actions of PTH and 1,25-$(OH)_2$D to provide the additional calcium needed by the fetus.

Changes in Bone Formation and Density

Uncoupling of bone reabsorption and formation is seen during pregnancy, with increased reabsorption during the first two trimesters and increased formation in the third trimester.[51] For example, markers of bone reabsorption are reported to increase through 28 weeks' gestation, whereas bone formation markers remain stable to 28 weeks and then increase to term.[18,36,51] Maternal bone formation increases early in pregnancy with increased storage of calcium in maternal bones. Maternal bone growth is associated with increases in bone formation and reabsorption markers such as bone alkaline phosphatase and procollagen peptides in the blood.[53,56,65] Osteocalcin, which normally increases with bone formation, is lower in pregnancy, although some increase is noted in late pregnancy. This may be due to increased placental calcium uptake.[44,87] Bone turnover increases in the third trimester at the time of peak calcium transfer to the fetus. During this time, maternal bone stores are mobilized to meet fetal demands.[35,62] However, the fetal calcium accumulation of 28 to 30 g represents only a small proportion of maternal skeletal stores. The changes in maternal bone are transient.[31,56]

Studies of bone mineral density during pregnancy have been inconsistent with small sample sizes and other methodological problems, including time of follow-up and other confounding factors.[18,22,30,31,49,53] However, most indicate that bone mineral density decreases by 2% to 5% during pregnancy and lactation, especially in the trabecular bone sites (lumbar spine and hips).[11,18,40,53,55] This is balanced by increases in the periosteal and endosteal surfaces of cortical bones (arms, legs).[53,56,65,86] Individual variations are seen with an increased risk of loss with frequent pregnancies, short time between pregnancies, adolescent women, lower calcium intake during pregnancy, multiple gestation, and heparin use.[56,65] There do not appear to be any long-term effects of maternal skeletal mass or bone density changes during pregnancy, and bone mineral density has been found to be similar in postmenopausal women who have or have not been pregnant.[31,56] A decrease in hip fractures has been reported in several studies in women who have had children, perhaps because pregnancy-associated changes in calcium and phosphorus metabolism may improve mechanical resistance of the upper femur.[56,57,61].

Intrapartum Period

Calcium is essential for activation of myosin light chain kinase in smooth muscle and thus myometrial contraction. Without calcium, much of which comes from extracellular sources, myometrial contraction does not occur. PTHrP levels in the myometrium and amnion decrease at the onset of labor. The role of calcium in uterine contraction is discussed in Chapter 4.

Postpartum Period

Serum calcium, PTH, and calcitonin gradually return to prepregnant values by 6 weeks postpartum in nonlactating women.[36,62] Resumption of menses is associated with increases in calcium absorption, PTH, and, in most studies, 1,25-$(OH)_2D$.[65] In lactating women, changes in calcium metabolism continue in order for the mother to provide adequate calcium for infant growth and development.[65] Lactation is a greater challenge to calcium homeostasis than pregnancy. During lactation the woman must provide 280 to 400 mg/day of calcium.[44,56] Exclusive breastfeeding for 6 months leads to four times the calcium loss than in pregnancy.[36] In the lactating women, serum calcium levels are slightly decreased with a slight increase in ionized calcium (although still within normal limits), while phosphorus, PTH, PTHrP, and 1,25-$(OH)_2D$ levels are all increased. PTH levels are low normal or slightly lower if the woman has adequate calcium and vitamin D intake.[36]

PTHrP, primarily from mammary tissue, increases and plays an important role in controlling breast calcium content.[6,32,44,51,56] PTHrP is important in regulating movement of calcium and phosphorus from maternal bone to breast milk, renal tubular calcium reabsorption, and suppressing PTH.[51] Suckling and prolactin increase PTHrP, which in conjunction with low estradiol levels, up-regulates bone reabsorption of calcium.[36] PTHrP levels may show a pulsate pattern in response to suckling. Intestinal calcium absorption is not increased in lactation as it was during pregnancy. However, renal calcium excretion is reduced, conserving calcium for milk production.[44,51] Thus the calcium demands of lactation are met primarily through reabsorption of maternal skeletal calcium, probably mediated primarily by PTHrP, and reduction in renal excretion of calcium.[36] Changes in calcium metabolism during lactation are summarized in Figure 17-2.

Markers of bone turnover are increased in early lactation but decrease after 6 to 12 months, even with continuation of lactation.[65] Maternal bone density decreases during lactation, with up to 7% of the maternal bone mass lost by 9 months' lactation.[39] These changes are most prominent in the trabecular bones of the axial skeleton and hip (e.g., pregnancy and lactation are associated with a 2% to 10% loss of bone mass in the spine and hip), in the first six months of lactation, with wide individual variation.[3,18,51,56,65] Calcium losses do not continue beyond 6 months even with continued lactation.[51] Calcium supplementation during lactation does not prevent these losses.[18] These are reversible changes with no long-term adverse effects in most women as the maternal skeleton recovers the calcium within 3 to 6 months of weaning (with a regain of bone mineral density of 0.5% to 2% per month).[18,36,56,65] Very rarely bone reabsorption may be excessive, with fractures and a clinical diagnosis of osteoporosis.[35,44,65]

Changes in the maternal skeleton are reversed in the later stages of lactation and with weaning. Markers of bone reabsorption increase in the first 5 to 12 months of lactation and then decrease.[65] During weaning, there is decreased suckling and milk volume and increase in estradiol levels. PTHrP levels decrease.[56] After weaning, PTHrP and PTH levels are elevated, intestinal absorption increases, and urinary calcium losses decrease.[44,65] These changes may help the woman regain her stores. By 3 to 5 months after lactation, bone mineral status is similar or higher in lactating women than in nonlactating women, regardless of the length of lactation.[65] Increases in PTH and 1,25-$(OH)_2D$ after weaning help restore the maternal skeleton.[65] Lactation physiology is discussed further in Chapter 5.

CLINICAL IMPLICATIONS FOR THE PREGNANT WOMAN AND HER FETUS

Changes in calcium and phosphorus metabolism are essential to provide adequate substrate for fetal growth and development and to simultaneously ensure maternal homeostasis. To support these changes, maternal calcium and phosphorus intake must increase during pregnancy and lactation. This section considers these needs as well as implications of alterations in calcium, phosphorus, and magnesium in relation to leg cramps and selected disorders complicating pregnancy.

Maternal Nutritional Needs

During pregnancy an additional 400 mg/day of both calcium and phosphorus is recommended, especially during the second and third trimesters. This results in a total calcium intake of 1200 mg/day in the pregnant woman (or 1600 mg/day in the pregnant adolescent).[44] The effect of supplemental calcium intake on bone density during pregnancy is unclear, since changes in bone metabolism occur even with increased calcium intakes.[65,83] There is no consistent correlation between dietary calcium intake or 1,25-$(OH)_2D$ bioavailability and intestinal calcium absorption. Hoskings notes that because the fetal skeleton contains only 28 to 30 g of calcium (far less than the average 1000 g of calcium in the adult skeleton), it is unlikely that fetal calcium needs cause clinical bone disease in the mother, but these needs may exacerbate the effects of existing low peak bone mass.[27]

Most studies have not shown significant increase in maternal bone mineral density with use of calcium supplements, although neonatal bone mineral density may be improved.[36,51,75,77] However, women with low calcium intakes (less than 600 mg/day), adolescents, or women with multiple pregnancy may benefit from increased calcium intake or supplementation during pregnancy.[1,37,56,65] Calcium supplementation during pregnancy has been associated with a reduced risk of preeclampsia (see Maternal Calcium Metabolism and Pregnancy Complications), increased birth weight, decreased risk of preterm delivery, decreased fetal lead exposure (calcium decreases circulating lead in the mother), and lower infant blood pressures.[6,26,77,82] Calcium and phosphorus needs during lactation are discussed further in Chapter 5.

Vitamin D intake is critical in maintaining calcium homeostasis. Vitamin D intakes of 400 international units (10 mcg) per day are recommended in pregnancy, although some question whether these values are too low.[6] Vitamin D helps ameliorate fluctuations in the calcium-to-phosphorus ratio and enhances calcium absorption. Five percent to 29% of pregnant women in the United States may have an inadequate vitamin D status.[15] Alterations in calcium and bone metabolism, including increased risk of maternal osteomalacia and neonatal hypocalcemia, tend to occur primarily in women who have diets that are low in both calcium and vitamin D.[44] Supplementation is recommended for women with low levels prior to pregnancy, low dietary intakes, and minimal sunlight exposure, although studies of the efficacy of supplementation are limited.[36,40,50,58] Low intake of vitamin D during pregnancy has been associated with preeclampsia, gestational diabetes, increased cesarean section, bacterial vaginosis, preterm delivery, and lower weight gain and altered fetal mineral accretion, although some data for these effects are contradictory.[2,6,12,15,36,38,40,82]

Milk is an excellent source of calcium, vitamin D, and phosphorus. Alternatives for women who are lactose intolerant include cheese, yogurt, lactose-free milks, sardines, whole or enriched grains, and green leafy vegetables. Some substances alter calcium absorption. For example, lactose increases calcium absorption, possibly by decreasing luminal pH or through chelate formation. Excessive fats, phosphate, phytates (found in many vegetables), or oxalates interfere with calcium absorption by forming insoluble calcium salts within the intestinal lumen. High sodium concentrations may also decrease calcium absorption by interfering with active transport mechanisms.

Adequate intake of phosphorus is as important as that of calcium because these two minerals exist in a constant of solubility in the blood (see Box 17-1 on page 590). Excess dietary phosphorus binds calcium in the intestine, limiting absorption; excess blood phosphorus leads to increased urinary excretion of calcium. Therefore it is essential for the diet of pregnant and lactating women to be balanced in regard to these substances. Foods such as processed meats, snack foods, and cola drinks have high phosphorus but low calcium levels.

Leg Cramps

Sudden tonic or clonic contraction of the gastrocnemius muscles and occasionally the thigh and gluteal muscles is experienced by 25% to 50% of all pregnant women.[25,63,79] These cramps are felt most frequently at night or on awakening and are most common after 24 weeks' gestation.[89] Leg cramps are also more common in sedentary versus active pregnant women.

Cramps may be associated with a lower threshold for increased neuromuscular irritability due to decreased serum ionized calcium levels combined with increased serum inorganic phosphate levels, along with the hormonal and biochemical alterations of pregnancy.[62,63] Systemic relaxin may decrease calcium movement into muscle, increasing the risk of leg cramps.[63] The incidence of leg cramps is not correlated with ionized calcium levels. Muscular irritability in pregnancy also arises from the lowered calcium levels and mild alkalosis caused by changes in the respiratory system (see Chapter 10).[63] Interventions have included reducing milk intake (although milk is rich in calcium, it also contains large amounts of phosphate); supplementation with magnesium lactate or citrate; or use of aluminum hydroxide antacids to promote formation of insoluble aluminum phosphate salts in the gut, thus reducing absorption of phosphorus.[62] Young and Jewell found the best evidence for treatment with magnesium lactate or citrate.[89] Calcium supplements have often been used although data to support their efficacy are weak.[25,89] Thus the specific basis for leg cramps in pregnant women and the most effective interventions remain unclear.

Maternal Calcium Metabolism and Pregnancy Complications

Women with acute and chronic hypertension during pregnancy tend to have lower serum calcium and higher magnesium levels.[35,51] Decreased calcium increases vascular resistance.[64] The incidence of preeclampsia has been reported to vary inversely with calcium intake, primarily in women at high risk for low calcium intake.[26] A recent meta-analysis of 12 studies of calcium supplementation and preeclampsia found that the risk for preeclampsia decreased by 50% (range 31% to 67% reduction) and concluded that the "reduction in preeclampsia, and in maternal death or severe morbidity, support the use of calcium supplementation, particularly for those with low dietary intake.[26] Calcium supplementation during pregnancy was also found in this meta-analysis to reduce the risk of preterm birth; another more recent meta-analysis also found a significant protective benefit of calcium supplementation in the prevention of preeclampsia, but found no additional benefit in preventing preterm birth or low birthweight.[16,26]

Women on long-term heparin therapy for thromboembolism during pregnancy may occasionally develop heparin-induced osteopenia. Heparin inhibits 1α-hydroxylation of 25-(OH)D, decreasing levels of 1,25-$(OH)_2$D; altering calcium homeostasis; and increasing bone calcium absorption.[44,51] Calcium status should be monitored carefully in women receiving this therapy.

Disorders of the parathyroid glands are rare. The diagnosis of primary hyperparathyroidism may be obscured by pregnancy changes in calcium metabolism. Pregnancy may provide some protection to women with this disorder, with 39% to 80% becoming asymptomatic during pregnancy. This is often followed by an acute exacerbation postpartum. Moderate to severe forms of this disorder may lead to maternal hypercalcemia with fetal parathyroid suppression and hypocalcemia and risk for neonatal tetany.[35,44,51,64] In women with hypoparathyroidism the normal replacement dose of vitamin D may need to be increased due to the increased vitamin D–binding hormone in pregnancy.[35,44,51,64]

Osteoporosis is a rare complication of pregnancy and seems to be associated with various factors—such as chronic heparin, anticonvulsant, or steroid use, low bone mineral density prepregnancy, skeletal abnormalities, or excessive reabsorption secondary to chronic inadequate calcium intake, low 1,25-$(OH)_2$D stores, or excessive parathyroid hormone–related peptide (PTHrP)—rather than pregnancy-induced alteration in calcium metabolism.[18,35,44] Similarly the also rare pregnancy-associated osteoporosis of the hip is thought to be unrelated to alterations in mineral balance in pregnancy.[14,35] This condition, seen primarily in primigravida lactating women with small body builds, is self-limiting and usually resolves by 6 to 12 months postpartum.[31]

Maternal-Fetal Interactions

Maternal-placental-fetal calcium metabolism is interrelated. As noted earlier, fetal calcium accumulation is mediated by increased maternal absorption of calcium. Calcium is actively transported across the placenta, mediated primarily by PTHrP to maintain a 1:1.4 maternal to fetal calcium gradient.[28,35,62,69,87] Calcium transport increases from 50 mg/day (20 weeks) to greater than 150 mg/day (mean 200-300 mg/day) at term.[5,17,31,35,36,46] About 80% of fetal mineral accretion occurs after 25 weeks, with peak accretion occurring from 34 to 38 weeks' gestation coinciding with bone development.[18,29,33,34] Total fetal calcium accretion increases during pregnancy from 100 mg (4 months) and averages 25 to 30 g (generally 28-30) at term.[36,51,59,64,69] Fetal serum calcium (10 to 11 mg/dL [2.5 to 2.8 mmol/L]) is about 1 mg/dL (0.25 mmol/L) above maternal values.[44] The higher fetal values are primarily due to increased ionized calcium.

Fetal calcium accretion and active transport across the placenta are independent of maternal calcium levels and stores. Calcium movement across the placenta involves three phases: (1) passive bidirectional movement across the maternal-facing microvillous trophoblast membrane into the syncytiotrophoblast cytosol; (2) binding of calcium to calcium-binding proteins such as calmodulin for transport through the syncytiotrophoblast cytosol (binding buffers the calcium so that it does not disrupt cellular processes in the trophoblast); and (3) active transport across the fetal-facing basolateral trophoblast membrane into fetal circulation via several calcium channels and transporters.[5,7,27,29] Placental transport of both calcium and phosphorus also involves insulin–like growth factor-1, which also stimulates 1,25-$(OH)_2$D synthesis.[69]

PTHrP (see Box 17-2 page 591) regulates control of calcium transport across the placenta.[28] PTHrP is the major factor in maintaining the fetal calcium level higher than maternal levels. PTHrP is also important for bone development.[36] PTHrP is produced by the fetal parathyroid glands, skeletal growth plate, umbilical cord, amnion, chorion, and placenta.[27,87] PTHrP levels are higher in the fetus than in adults.[87] Fetal calcium levels are set at a specific level and appear to be maintained at that level regardless of maternal calcium level, even with maternal hypocalcemia.[35] Although fetal calcium levels are maintained primarily by PTHrP-mediated placental calcium transport, movement of calcium in and out of fetal bone, fetal renal tubular reabsorption and excretion of calcium, and swallowing of amniotic fluid also have a role in maintaining fetal homeostasis.[35] Lack of adequate PTHrP and PTH can lead to fetal growth restriction since both substances are critical for skeletal mineral accretion.[69]

The fetus accumulates 16 g of phosphorus, primarily in the third trimester, and 0.75 g of magnesium (with a peak of 60-75 mg/kg/day in the third trimester).[46,69,70] Most of the fetal phosphorus is used for bone mineralization.[69] Fetal phosphorus and magnesium levels are higher than maternal levels; these minerals are actively transported across the placenta.[39,62,69,72] Magnesium is transported to the fetus in increasing amounts after the fifth month.[20] Fetal magnesium levels depend on adequate placental function and maternal stores. Placental insufficiency and inadequate nutritional intake increase the risk of neonatal hypomagnesemia. Transplacental passage of magnesium is influenced by maternal level; for example, administration of large amounts of magnesium sulfate to the mother leads to elevated magnesium in both mother and fetus.[23]

Fetal mineral homeostasis is not heavily dependent on vitamin D.[46] Placental transport of 1,25-$(OH)_2D$ is low and the fetus is a main source of this substance.[4,40,62,75] The placenta also synthesizes 1,25-$(OH)_2D$ and contains 1,25-$(OH)_2D$ receptors and key enzymes such as 1-hydroxylase needed for vitamin D metabolism.[4] The fetus is dependent upon maternal 25-(OH)D, which is readily transported across the placenta, because fetal hepatic enzyme processes are limited. The 25-(OH)D is 1α-hydroxylated to 1,25-$(OH)_2D$ in the fetal kidneys.[35,44] Maternal vitamin D deficiency is associated with an increased incidence and severity of neonatal hypocalcemia. PTH and calcitonin do not appear to cross the placenta.[44,62,75] Vitamin D is an important factor in the regulation of cellular differentiation and apoptosis.[41] Insufficient vitamin D during gestation can affect development of the fetal skeleton, immune system, and brain and may alter fetal programming, increasing the risk of adult-onset disorders.[41] Maternal vitamin D deficiency during pregnancy has been associated with neonatal hypocalcemia, impaired growth, and later problems in offspring including skeletal problems, type 1 diabetes, altered immunotolerance, risk of autoimmune disease, food allergies, and altered programming of long bone development.[6,13,36,40,41,42,71,82]

SUMMARY

Calcium and phosphorus are essential minerals for many body processes and growth. Alterations in metabolic processes related to these elements during pregnancy can alter maternal, fetal, and infant health status. Health can be promoted by careful assessment and monitoring of maternal and fetal status and initiation of appropriate interventions. Recommendations for clinical practice related to calcium and phosphorus metabolism during pregnancy are summarized in Table 17-3.

DEVELOPMENT OF CALCIUM AND PHOSPHORUS METABOLISM IN THE FETUS

Anatomic Development

Calcium and phosphorus metabolism is regulated by a variety of hormones, including parathyroid hormone (PTH), vitamin D, and calcitonin. This section reviews development of the parathyroid glands; development of the thyroid glands (site of calcitonin synthesis) is discussed in Chapter 19. Because calcium and phosphorus are critical for bone mineralization processes, skeletal growth is also considered.

Parathyroid Glands

Many structures of the head and neck—the maxillary process, mandibular arch, several muscles of the jaw, hyoid and ear bones, thyroid, and cricoid cartilage—develop from the branchial or pharyngeal arches. These are bars of mesenchymal tissue separated by pharyngeal clefts. The pharyngeal pouches are outpouchings along the lateral walls of the pharyngeal gut. Structures that develop from these pouches include the palatine tonsils, thymus, primitive tympanic cavity, and (from the third and fourth pouches) the parathyroid glands (Figure 17-3).[48]

The third and fourth pharyngeal pouches develop bulbar and ventral portions. The inferior parathyroid glands differentiate from the dorsal bulbar portion of the third pharyngeal pouch during the sixth week. The ventral portion of this pouch forms the thymus. The parathyroid glands initially migrate caudally and medially with the thymus, later separating and attaching to the inferior portion of the dorsal surface of the descending thyroid gland (see Chapter 19). The superior parathyroid glands develop from the dorsal bulbar portion of the fourth pharyngeal pouch by the sixth week and attach to the superior portion of the dorsal side of the caudally migrating thyroid gland (see Figure 17-3).[48] Parathyroid glands are active by 12 weeks, but function is suppressed by the high serum calcium concentrations in the fetus.[23,51,69]

Table 17-3 Recommendations for Clinical Practice Related to Changes in Calcium and Phosphorus Metabolism in Pregnant Women

Recognize the usual changes in calcium and phosphorus metabolism during pregnancy (pp. 589-592, Figure 17-2, and Table 17-2).
Assess and monitor maternal nutrition in terms of calcium, phosphorus, and vitamin D intake (p. 594).
Counsel women regarding calcium, phosphorus, and vitamin D requirements to meet maternal and fetal needs during pregnancy (pp. 594-596).
Monitor fetal growth (pp. 595-596).
Know usual parameters for serum calcium during pregnancy (p. 589).
Evaluate diet of women complaining of leg cramps (p. 594).
Counsel women regarding leg cramps and appropriate interventions (p. 594).
Recognize usual changes in calcium and phosphorus metabolism during lactation (p. 593, Figure 17-2).
Assess and monitor nutrition during lactation in terms of calcium, phosphorus, and vitamin D intake (p. 593).
Counsel women regarding calcium, phosphorus, and vitamin D requirements to meet maternal needs during lactation (pp. 593-594 and Chapter 5).
Counsel women with pregnancy complications regarding calcium intake during pregnancy (pp. 594-595).

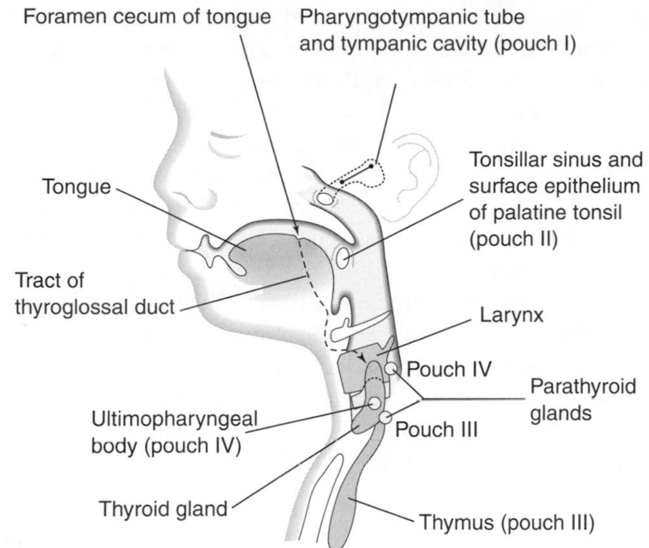

FIGURE 17-3 Schematic sagittal section of the head and neck of a 20-week fetus showing the adult derivatives of the pharyngeal pouches and descent of the thyroid gland. (From Moore, K. [1998]. *The developing human* [6th ed.]. Philadelphia: Saunders.)

Skeletal Development and Growth

Skeletal growth occurs in two phases. During fetal life a cartilage anlage (primordium) is formed that is later replaced by bone. Bone formation also occurs by differentiation of mesenchyme directly into bone cells. Later linear growth depends on cartilaginous growth in the endochondral ossification centers at the epiphyses; appositional growth of the skeleton depends on the laying down of new bone by bone-forming cells with subsequent remodeling (reabsorption of existing bone followed by formation of new bone). Bone formation and remodeling are a cyclic process that occurs continuously throughout life. During growth, bone formation is greater than remodeling. Once maximal growth is achieved, the skeletal mass is stable for 10 to 15 years, and remodeling and bone formation occur at the same rate. With aging, remodeling is greater than bone formation, with a gradual loss of bone mass. Excessive differences between bone formation and remodeling can lead to osteoporosis and compromised skeletal integrity. Stress, such as subjecting bone to heavy loads, or stress that occurs with strenuous exercise, stimulates osteoblastic deposition of new bone, leading to thickening of bones.[24,67]

Skeletal development begins in early embryonic life (apparent by the eighth week) and continues well into postnatal life.[51] Bone consists primarily of organic matrix and bone salts. Compact bone is 30% organic matrix and 70% bone salts; newer bone has a more organic matrix. The organic matrix is composed primarily of collagen fibers that give the bone its tensile strength. The rest of the matrix is ground substance, consisting of extracellular fluid and proteoglycans, which may assist in controlling deposition of calcium salts. Crystalline bone salts (hydroxyapatites) give bone compressional strength and consist primarily of calcium and phosphorus with small deposits of sodium, potassium, magnesium, and carbonate salts.[24,67]

Bone is formed by either intramembranous or endochondral ossification. Intramembranous ossification is the process involved in formation of bones such as the skull, mandible, and maxilla.[67,69] With intramembranous ossification, the fibrous mesenchyme condenses to form a collagenous membrane in which some cells differentiate into osteoblasts. Osteoblasts produce a collagenous material and ground substance to fill the extracellular spaces. The collagen polymerizes to form collagen fibers and the tissue becomes osteoid and similar to cartilage.[67,69] Osteoblasts later secrete alkaline phosphatase, which leads to deposition of calcium salts in the form of calcium hydroxyapatite crystals, with gradual conversion of the osteoid to bone. Some osteoblasts are trapped within lacunae in the bone matrix and develop into osteocytes. The bone matrix grows in all directions as spicules and ossification centers are established.

The osteoblasts deposit spongy bone first, followed by plates of compact bone (periosteal ossification). Spongy bones are filled with fibrous and cellular mesenchymal derivatives that later differentiate into elements characteristic of red bone marrow (reticular tissue, fat cells, sinusoids, and developing blood cells). Bone growth is accompanied by remodeling in which much of the original matrix is reabsorbed by osteoclasts simultaneously with formation of new bone by osteoblasts. During this process the osteoclasts project villi that secrete proteolytic enzymes to dissolve the organic matrix and citric, lactic, and other acids that cause solution of bone salts.[24]

The long bones of the appendicular and axial skeleton form by endochondral ossification in which the condensed mesenchymal cells give rise to hyaline cartilage models that are shaped like the eventual bone. This cartilage is eroded locally and destroyed as bone is formed. Endochondral ossification involves the progressive destruction of cartilage, deposition of calcium salts, and formation of a central area of spongy bone (that will later develop a red marrow matrix) surrounded by compact bone. This process begins in the middle of the bone shaft and progresses toward the epiphysis. At birth the long bones consist of central ossification centers and bony shafts with cartilaginous ends. Secondary areas of ossification later appear in the epiphyses.[48,67]

Bone growth and mineralization are mediated by a variety of regulating hormones and growth factors including calcitropic hormones (e.g., PTH, vitamin D, calcitonin); parathyroid hormone–related peptide (PTHrP); systemic growth-regulating hormones (e.g., growth hormone, insulin, glucocorticoids, thyroid hormones, sex steroids); circulating growth factors (e.g., somatomedin, insulin-like growth factor [IGF], epidermal growth factor, platelet-derived growth factor, fibroblast growth factor); and local factors (e.g., osteoclast activity factor, cartilage-derived growth factor).[67,69,72] In addition, maternal diet (especially vitamin D), physical activity, and smoking during pregnancy may also influence fetal bone mineral acquisition.[19]

Functional Development

Fetal mineral requirements are met by transport of calcium, phosphorus, magnesium, and other minerals across the placenta (see Maternal-Fetal Interactions). Eighty percent of calcium and phosphorus accretion occurs in the third trimester.[72] From 25 weeks' gestation to term, bone mineralization increases fourfold and fetal calcium acquisition ranges from 92 to 119 mg/kg/day or higher (up to 350 mg/day or a mean of 200 mg/day at term) and phosphorous from 2.51 to 3.44 mg/kg/day (Figure 17-4).[33,35] In contrast, calcium accretion immediately after birth increases from 15 mg/kg on day 1 to 45 mg/kg on day 3.[20] Phosphate levels peak at midgestation (15 mg/dL [4.8 mmol/L]) and then decrease to 5.5 to 7 mg/dL (1.8 to 2.3 mmol/L) by term.

1,25-$(OH)_2$D and PTH levels are low in the fetus and probably have a limited role in fetal calcium physiology.[35,46] The parathyroid gland contains PTH by 10 to 12 weeks and actively secretes PTH by 25 to 26 weeks in response to decreased extracellular fluid calcium.[6,48] The fetal parathyroid is less responsive to decreased serum calcium, perhaps because of suppression of the parathyroid by the relative fetal hypercalcemia or placental PTH production.[6,28,62] The predominant hormone regulating fetal calcium homeostasis is PTHrP (see Box 17-2 on page 591) rather than PTH as occurs after birth and in adults, although PTHrP and PTH act synergystically.[27,69]

Cord concentrations of vitamin D metabolites are only about 20% of maternal levels.[6,36] 25-(OH)D is transferred from the mother since fetal liver processes for vitamin D metabolism are limited.[35] Renal 1α-hydroxylation to form 1,25-$(OH)_2$D occurs in the fetal kidneys, placenta, and decidua.[46] The fetus needs to store vitamin D to cope with the relatively high calcium requirements of the early postbirth period. Vitamin D deficiency during fetal development can alter bone growth and development as well as other areas of development in the infant and child and has implications for the development of other disorders.[1,46] These implications and fetal vitamin D synthesis are described further in Maternal-Fetal Interactions on pp. 595-596.

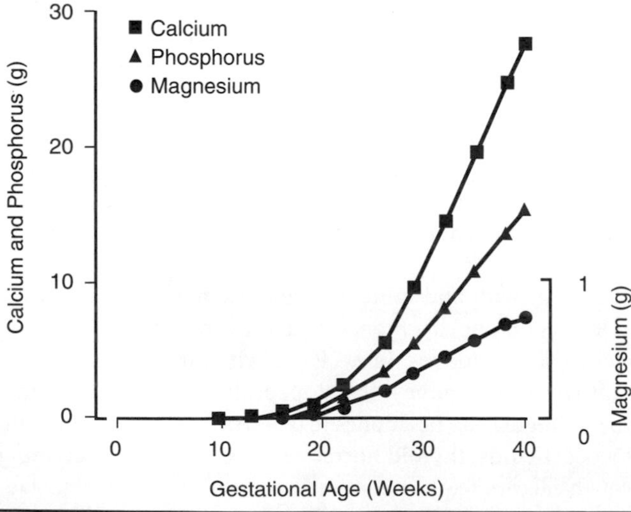

FIGURE 17-4 Calcium, phosphorus, and magnesium accretion in the human fetus from 16 to 40 weeks' gestation. (From Greer, F.R. [2005]. Disorders of calcium homeostasis. In A.R. Spitzer [Ed.], *Intensive care of the fetus and neonate* [2nd ed.]. Philadelphia: Mosby.)

Calcitonin-containing cells appear in the thyroid at about 14 weeks' gestation and secrete immunoreactive calcitonin from 28 weeks.[46] Calcitonin levels are high in the fetus, with increasing concentrations during the third trimester. The role of calcitonin in the fetus is unclear; however, animal evidence suggests that calcitonin does not have a major role in fetal bone metabolism.[35,46]

NEONATAL PHYSIOLOGY

The newborn is relatively hypercalcemic and hyperphosphatemic when compared with the mother. The infant must quickly move from the intrauterine dependence on maternal calcium sources and placental hormones to independent extrauterine control of calcium and phosphorus metabolism and homeostasis with reliance on oral intake and bone stores. Failure to do so may lead to hypocalcemia or other metabolic abnormalities. Calcium and phosphorus homeostasis is summarized in Box 17-1 on page 590 and in Figure 17-1. The roles of the major calcitropic hormones (parathyroid hormone, calcitonin, and vitamin D) are summarized in Table 17-1.

Transitional Events

At birth, maternal supplies of calcium and other minerals are no longer available to the infant. Within 24-48 hours of birth, the infant moves from the hypercalcemic, peptide PTHrP-dominated calcium metabolism to a parathyroid hormone (PTH) and 1,25-$(OH)_2$D environment. In this environment, the infant must mobilize bone calcium and increase intestinal absorption to maintain serum calcium levels.[35] Total and ionized calcium levels are higher in cord blood than in maternal serum; PTH is decreased, but PTHrP is increased.[21,23,35,62,70] Cord blood magnesium levels are slightly increased and related to maternal levels, whereas phosphorus levels are low.[21,69] Cord blood levels of calcitonin are reported to be 68% to 108% of maternal levels and correlate with maternal levels.[23]

Maternal serum 25-(OH)D levels at term correlate with cord blood levels, although cord blood values are about 20% lower; 1,25-$(OH)_2$D levels are about half maternal values.[6,46] At birth serum osteocalcin levels are two to three times higher than in adults. This reflects the rapid rate of fetal bone formation in the last weeks of pregnancy. Osteocalcin is a noncollagenous bone-specific protein that is released into the blood in proportion to the amount of bone formation. Levels increase from birth to 1 to 5 days and then decrease.

Markers of bone formation decrease and markers of bone reabsorption increase for a few days after birth due to the transition to dependence on intestinal mineral absorption and the relatively low intake immediately after birth. After that time, both types of markers increase over the next few weeks.[18]

Calcium

The relative hypercalcemia at birth is followed by a physiologic hypocalcemia as both total and ionized calcium fall to levels lower than those found in older infants and about 1 mg/dL (0.25 mmol/L) lower than birth values.[23,46,62] There is a rapid decrease in ionized calcium, especially in the first 4 to 6 hours after birth, reaching a nadir of 4.4 to 5.4 mg/dL (1.1 to 1.4 mmol/L) by 16 to 24 hours.[35,37,46,54] Calcium levels generally stabilize in the next 24 to 48 hours and then increase along with increases in PTH and 1,25-$(OH)_2$D.[23,35] The fall in calcium is thought to be due to parathyroid suppression in late gestation (from elevated fetal calcium levels), loss of placental transport of calcium, and an increased PTH response.[35,46] This nadir is more pronounced in infants who are preterm or born to mothers with diabetes or vitamin D deficiency.[36] In term infants, total calcium values average 8 to 9 mg/dL (2 to 2.2 mmol/L), with a range of 8 to 11 mg/dL (2 to 2.8 mmol/L), and are slightly lower in preterm infants. Ionized calcium levels are 4 to 4.6 mg/dL (1 to 1.5 mmol/L).[28,69] Calcium levels at birth correlate inversely with gestational age.[33,62,69] The length and degree of the postbirth physiologic hypocalcemia are also correlated inversely with gestational age.[23,69] In very low–birth weight (VLBW) infants this hypocalcemia may persist despite increasing levels of PTH and 1,25-$(OH)_2$D.[23,36]

Intestinal absorption of calcium is correlated with both gestational and postbirth age, but the major factor in determining absorption is postnatal age.[23] Immature intestinal function and decreased intake may limit calcium absorption. Much of the intestinal transport is primarily passive (via paracellular transport) in preterm infants since transcellular active transport, which is vitamin D dependent, is not yet mature.[69] Renal calcium excretion is relatively efficient in both term and preterm infants, although increased renal sodium losses in VLBW infants may also increase calcium loss.[23,69] Renal calcium excretion increases with gestational and postbirth age, ranging from 60 to 88 mg/day during the first 2 weeks to 180 mg/day by 3 to 12 weeks in the term infant and from less than 8 to 80 mg/day to 120 mg/day by 2 weeks of age in the preterm infant.[20]

Phosphorus

Phosphorus levels may decrease slightly during the first 1 to 2 days after birth but remain higher than those of adults.[62] Renal excretion of phosphorus is delayed because of a decreased glomerular filtration rate and increased tubular reabsorption of phosphorus. Increased energy demands during birth with conversion of adenosine triphosphate (ATP) to adenosine diphosphate (ADP) lead to additional phosphorus release. Delayed feeding further elevates phosphorus levels because of tissue catabolism. Phosphorus levels are lower in small-for-gestational-age (SGA) infants and correlate with the degree of growth restriction. Levels are higher in formula-fed than breastfed infants and inversely related to serum calcium concentrations.[69] The fractional excretion of phosphorus is increased in preterm infants, increasing the risk of phosphate deficiency.[69]

Parathyroid Hormone

As serum calcium levels decrease over the first few days after birth, PTH levels gradually increase by about 24 to 48 hours.[37] Levels are higher in hypocalcemic preterm infants.[23] Preterm infants may have a transient pseudohypoparathyroidism for the first 72 hours secondary to immature bone and renal responses to PTH.[23] By 3 to 4 days of age, the preterm infant's parathyroid gland generally responds effectively to calcium. The infant of a diabetic mother may also have impaired PTH production initially; infants following perinatal hypoxic ischemic events may have a decreased PTH response to low calcium.[69] PTH levels do not appear to change with oral administration of calcium supplements, but intravenous bolus administration of calcium can suppress parathyroid function.[23] PTHrP decreases rapidly after birth to the low levels normally seen in adults. Its role in neonatal calcium homeostasis is unclear, but PTH is the major calcitropic hormone by 48 hours of age.[35] The response of the neonatal kidneys to PTH is not well understood, although both term and preterm infants do respond to exogenous PTH.[28] The amount of calcium excreted by the kidneys increases over the first 2 weeks after birth, perhaps mediated by the increasing glomerular filtration rate (see Chapter 11).[28]

Vitamin D

Plasma concentrations of 25-(OH)D are lower than and correlate with maternal serum values and remain stable in both term and preterm infants in the first week.[23] Term infants are able to effectively metabolize vitamin D in the liver and kidneys. The kidneys can convert 25-(OH)D to 1,25-$(OH)_2$D by 28 to 32 weeks' gestational age. However, vitamin D metabolism remains limited in the preterm infant because 25-hydroxylation by the liver does not occur at significant rates until 36 to 38 weeks' gestation.[75] In VLBW infants born at less than 28 weeks gestation the vitamin D activation pathway may remain immature.[69] Absorption of exogenous vitamin D may also be limited because of immature fat absorption. Serum 1,25-$(OH)_2$D levels increase during the first 48 hours, probably because of decreased serum calcium or increased PTH, and elevated levels persist for the first week.[56] The increase parallels the decrease in serum calcium and increase in PTH in both term and preterm infants.[23] This helps maintain calcium levels within physiologic limits by stimulating bone and intestinal reabsorption.[23,35] In preterm infants, levels may remain higher for up to 7 to 9 weeks, reflecting rapid prenatal growth.[23]

Calcitonin

Calcitonin levels may be normal or slightly elevated at birth, followed by a surge that is reported to peak anywhere from two- to 10-fold over cord blood levels by 24 to 48 hours of age.[69] Levels then plateau and decrease to childhood levels by 1 month.[23,52] Calcitonin levels are inversely correlated with gestational age.[52] Increased calcitonin may protect the infant from excessive bone reabsorption and promote mineralization during a period of active bone growth in the face of increased PTH and 1,25-$(OH)_2D$. High calcitonin levels may contribute to the lower serum calcium levels and increased risk of hypocalcemia seen in preterm infants. Calcitonin levels remain high in preterm infants for a longer period of time, slowly decreasing over the first 2 to 3 months to reach normal levels by about 40 weeks' postmenstural age.[52]

Magnesium

Serum magnesium levels increase initially after birth and then fall to levels similar to those in adults (range, 1.5 to 2.8 mg/dL [0.6 to 1.2 mmol/L]) by 2 weeks. Urinary excretion of magnesium may be low for the first few days after birth.

CLINICAL IMPLICATIONS FOR NEONATAL CARE

Bone mineralization and synthesis of new tissues continue after birth and are dependent on adequate substrate. Alterations in calcium and phosphorus metabolism in the neonatal period have implications for nutritional needs of term and preterm infants and are critical in ensuring adequate postnatal growth and development. In addition, these alterations may increase the risk for disorders such as hypocalcemia. This section examines postnatal nutritional needs related to calcium and phosphorus metabolism and the demands of bone mineralization and the basis for common disorders.

A calcium-to-phosphorus ratio of 1.7:1 to 2.0:1 is thought to be ideal for human infants.[20,69] The ratio of calcium to phosphorus can have a significant impact on mineral homeostasis. Hyperphosphatemia may lead to hypocalcemia by blunting the responsiveness of the bone to parathyroid hormone (PTH) and vitamin D. Conversely, low serum phosphorus levels can lead to reduction of calcium entry into bone, bone demineralization, and hypercalcemia.[20] Infant formulas have higher phosphorus and lower ionized calcium concentrations than human milk. However, currently most commercial formulas have ratios that more closely approximate those of human milk.[69,75] Although of calcium are lower in human milk than in cow's milk formulas; the ratio of calcium to phosphorus promotes calcium-phosphorus homeostasis. The efficiency of intestinal calcium absorption increases up to twofold with human milk feedings. The American Academy of Pediatrics recommends that exclusively breastfed infants receive 400 international units of vitamin D daily (10 μg/day) beginning soon after birth, although compliance with this recommendation is low.[60,84] Calcium and phosphorus levels of human milk are not adequate initially for VLBW infants, and supplementation is recommended (see Chapter 12).[78]

Calcium Intake in Preterm Infants

Preterm infants may have difficulty maintaining an adequate calcium intake because of increased growth needs and a low intake. Calcium needs are increased in VLBW infants since they have missed the third trimester when much of the fetal calcium accretion occurs.[72] In addition medications such as phenytoin, phenobarbital, and glucocorticoids can decrease intestinal calcium absorption.[69] Calcium levels in mature breast milk and standard formulas are significantly below daily intrauterine calcium accretion rates in the third trimester.[72] As a result, bone mineralization is reduced in infants fed these feedings. Preterm infants fed breast milk do have increased calcium absorption (60% to 70% versus 35% to 60% with formulas).[23,67] Initially, extremely low–birth weight (ELBW) infants will need parenteral nutrition to supply calcium and phosphorus, although this often does not match intrauterine accretion rates.[23,67] Increased levels of calcium and phosphorus can be delivered with formulations containing calcium glycerophosphate and monobasic phosphate (up to 86 mg/dL [21.5 mmol/L] of calcium and 46 mg/dL [14.9 mmol/L] of phosphorus). Fortification of human milk can increase calcium retention up to 60 mg/kg/day, and if the fortifier contains calcium glycerophosphate, up to 90 mg/kg/day.[67] If supplementation is used for preterm infants fed human milk, calcium-to-phosphorus ratios of 1.7:1 are recommended to maximize intake and retention.[67,69] Ratios should not be greater than 2:1 to prevent hyperphosphatemia. Preterm formulas come closer to duplicating intrauterine calcium accretion rates during the last weeks of the third trimester (120 to 150 mg/kg/day), but have a lower bioavailability of calcium than human milk.[23,33,68,69] Vitamin D levels are increased in these formulas to enhance intestinal calcium absorption. Medium-chain triglycerides (MCTs) are also added to increase fat absorption and thus absorption of vitamin D and calcium.

Bone Mineralization

After birth the neonatal skeleton continues to accrete calcium at a rate of approximately 150 mg/kg/day.[35,37] To accomplish this, the infant must have adequate vitamin D and intestinal absorption of calcium. This may be difficult to achieve in VLBW and ELBW infants. Rigo and colleagues note that the goal for VLBW infants is postnatal growth similar to the intrauterine rate, with a slightly higher rate in ELBW infants.[67] To reach this goal, these infants need not only adequate supplies of calcium, phosphorus, and other minerals, but also protein and energy for formation of the collagen matrix.[67,69] VLBW infants have decreased postnatal bone mineralization and a significant delay in completing bone development in comparison with intrauterine rates.[10] Prolonged (greater than 5 days) maternal magnesium sulfate administration has been reported to alter neonatal bone mineralization.[88]

Preterm infants are at risk for both rickets and osteopenia (reduction of bone mass with demineralization of the bone with or without signs of rickets). By term-corrected age, VLBW infants are still of lower weight and length than term infants with linear growth restriction and lower bone mineral mass and density seen in up to 22% of AGA preterm infants.[8,37] Land and Schoenau suggest that one reason for this difference is that the fetus in utero experiences higher mechanical resistance to extremity movement than occurs after birth. Thus the preterm infant's movements occur against lower resistance, which provides less stimulation for development.[37] Significant bone mineralization problems, ranging from osteopenia to rickets, are seen in more than 30% of ELBW infants.[33,67] Mineralization may also be delayed in SGA infants. Longitudinal follow-up is important after discharge to promote catch-up growth and optimal bone mineralization.[67] Factors leading to inadequate bone mineralization are illustrated in Figure 17-5.

Alterations in Neonatal Calcium Homeostasis

Neonatal Hypocalcemia

The serum calcium level below which an infant is considered to be hypocalcemic varies in the literature from 7 to 8 mg/dL (1.75 to 2 mmol/L).[33,62,69,70] Most sources use a lower limit of 7 mg/dL (1.75 mmol/L) in preterm and 7.8 to 8 mg/dL (1.95 to 2 mmol/L) in term infants.[23,33] Ideally determination of hypocalcemia should be based on the ionized calcium fraction (less than 4.4 mg/dL [1.1 mmol/L]) because this is the biologically active form.[8,20,23,33] In preterm infants the relationship between total and ionized calcium is atypical, so infants may have a greater decrease in total serum calcium than in ionized calcium.[28]

Hypoproteinemia or acid-base changes can alter calcium levels. Serum calcium is either ionized (physiologically active form) or undissociated and bound to protein or complexed to anions. Because these two forms of serum calcium are in equilibrium, hypoproteinemia lowers serum calcium levels. This equilibrium is influenced by acid-base status. Acidosis increases the movement of calcium from bone and decreases the amount of protein-bound calcium. As a result, levels of ionized calcium increase. Opposite effects are seen during alkalosis.[20]

Infants at greatest risk for hypocalcemia are preterm infants, those born to diabetic mothers, and those born after perinatal hypoxic-ischemic events. Possible pathogenic mechanisms are discussed below and are summarized in Table 17-4. Hypocalcemia due to decreased ionized calcium may occur after exchange transfusion, with renal dysfunction, after furosemide therapy, or with magnesium deficiency. Hypocalcemia with a decrease in ionized calcium but without a decrease in total calcium can occur with alkalosis, after exchange transfusion with citrated blood, or with elevated serum free fatty acids after lipid infusion.[20] Alkalosis leads to a decreased affinity of albumin for calcium and thus less ionized calcium. A rapid shift in the amounts of ionized versus albumin-bound calcium can lead to significant hypocalcemia.[69] Hypocalcemia in infants with fetal growth restriction is usually associated with prematurity or perinatal hypoxic-ischemic events.[33]

The usual physiologic course of neonatal hypocalcemia involves a decrease in serum calcium to a nadir at 24 to 48 hours of age in term infants and slightly earlier in preterm infants. This is associated with a concomitant increase in phosphorus

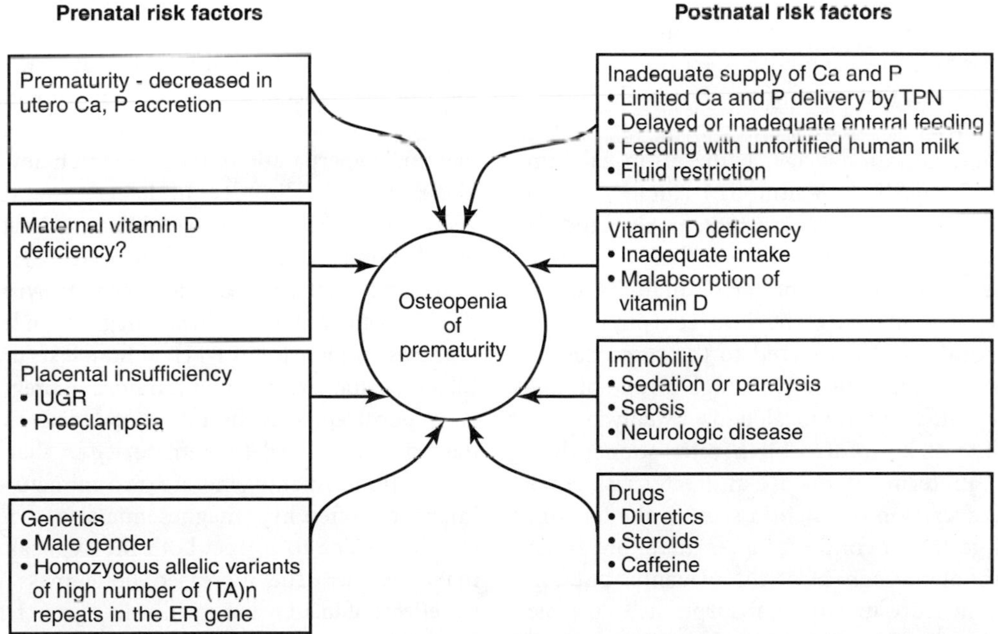

FIGURE 17-5 Prenatal and postnatal risk factors for development of osteopenia of prematurity. *Ca*, calcium; *P*, phosphorus; *IUGR*, intrauterine growth restriction; *TPN*, total parenteral nutrition; *(TA)n*, thymine adenine repeat; *ER*, estrogen receptor. (From Rigo, J., Mohamed, M., & Decurtis, M. [2011]. Disorders of calcium, phosphorus and magnesium metabolism. In R.J. Martin, A.A. Fanaroff, & M.C. Walsh [Eds.], *Fanaroff & Martin's Neonatal-perinatal medicine: Diseases of the fetus and infant* [9th ed.]. St. Louis: Mosby Elsevier.)

Table 17-4 Possible Pathogenic Mechanisms in Early Neonatal Hypocalcemia

CLINICAL PARAMETERS	POSSIBLE PATHOGENIC MECHANISMS
Prematurity	Decreased calcium and phosphorus intake Decreased parathyroid hormone responsiveness altering ability to move calcium out of bone Increased calcitonin Immature absorption Immature renal function with decreased phosphorus excretion Decreased vitamin D intake and absorption Interference with calcium metabolism by acidosis Increased needs
Infant of a diabetic mother	Prematurity (see above) Transient hypoparathyroidism due to fetal parathyroid suppression by maternal hyperparathyroidism
Perinatal hypoxia-ischemia	Increased tissue breakdown with phosphorus release Effects of pH and bicarbonate on protein binding of calcium and levels of ionized calcium Impaired parathyroid function Increased calcitonin

levels. Magnesium levels may be normal or low. Infants can be asymptomatic or symptomatic. Symptoms may include tremors, twitching, hyperexcitability, irritability, high-pitched cry, laryngospasm, tachycardia, apnea, and (rarely) seizures. Early and late forms of hypocalcemia are seen.

Hypocalcemia in the Preterm Infant. Hypocalcemia is seen frequently in preterm infants, and is inversely related to birth weight and gestational age, with serum calcium levels lower than 7 mg/dL (1.8 mmol/L) (total) or 3 to 3.5 mg/dL (0.75 to 0.88 mmol/L) (ionized) reported in 30% to 40% of preterm infants and up to half of VLBW infants.[33,69,70] The hypocalcemic preterm infant is often asymptomatic, possibly because the ionized (physiologically active) calcium is not decreased to the same degree as the total serum calcium resulting in a higher ratio of ionized to total calcium.[70] The hypocalcemia usually occurs within the first 24 to 48 hours after birth, often sooner than in term infants.[28] Preterm infants are at greater risk since the rapid skeletal accretion of calcium seen in the fetus in the last weeks of gestation continues after birth, but in an environment without the benefit of the placental calcium pump and with immature intestinal absorption.[35] Possible causes of hypocalcemia in preterm infants include lack of available calcium with decreased early intake, insufficient PTH release, and thus decreased PTH availability to move calcium out of the bones (although some recent studies do not support immaturity in parathyroid function in these infants), immature absorption, interference with calcium metabolism by acidosis, increased calcitonin levels, decreased vitamin D intake and absorption, and 1,25-$(OH)_2D$ in VLBW infants.[20,23,33,69,70]

Preterm infants may have an imbalance between calcium needs and PTH production, with increased calcium needs due to growth and a decreased supply as well as inadequate PTH response by the renal tubular cells.[69] Increased renal sodium losses in VLBW infants may aggravate calcium loss.[69]

The preterm infant has a marked elevation of calcitonin at 2 to 5 hours that reaches a plateau at 12 to 24 hours; this may also contribute to the risk of hypocalcemia.[69] Serum calcium values are negatively correlated with calcitonin at 12 to 24 hours of age, possibly impeding resolution of the hypocalcemia. Alterations in vitamin D metabolism or availability may also impede resolution. Hyperphosphatemia has also been observed, along with an occasional transient decrease in magnesium at 24 to 48 hours.[33] The decrease in magnesium can be prevented by calcium, suggesting that hypomagnesemia is a consequence and not a cause of this hypocalcemia.[33]

Hypocalcemia in the Infant of a Diabetic Mother. Hypocalcemia occurs in about 50% of infants of insulin-dependent diabetic women, with an increased incidence also reported in infants of women with gestational diabetes.[33,69] A lower incidence is seen in infants of women with tight maternal glycemic control during pregnancy. This form of hypocalcemia tends to appear within the first 24 hours of age and to be more severe and last longer than the hypocalcemia seen in preterm infants. The decrease in calcium level is directly correlated with the severity of the maternal diabetes.[69]

Cord blood of these infants contains decreased levels of PTH and of both total and ionic calcium. The cause of this form of hypocalcemia may be related to suppression of the fetal parathyroid by maternal hypomagnesemia and a relative maternal hyperparathyroidism seen in many diabetic women. These metabolic disorders in diabetic women are believed to be caused by increased urinary losses and may lead to chronic fetal hypomagnesemia and decreased PTH secretion.[20] This results in a transient neonatal hypoparathyroidism. The pregnant diabetic woman has lower magnesium levels and a failure of the usual increase in PTH, although serum total and ionic calcium values are often within normal pregnancy limits.

Hypocalcemia in the infant of a diabetic mother (IDM) may also be related to immaturity in that it is seen more frequently in infants who are also immature. Because these infants are often hypomagnesemic also, magnesium therapy may be needed to correct both the hypocalcemia and hypomagnesemia.[62] The increased bone mass is secondary to the effects of insulin and insulin-like growth factor-1 on bone formation. Because the increased bone mass increases calcium needs, this may also be a factor in the neonatal hypocalcemia in these infants.

Hypocalcemia and Perinatal hypoxic-ischemic events. With these events, tissue breakdown increases with release of phosphorus as well as accelerated conversion of ATP to ADP (to meet the increased energy demands), with subsequent phosphorus release. Administration of bicarbonate or hyperventilation with mechanical ventilators both increase pH, which alters protein binding and decreases ionized calcium.[23] Alkalosis from bicarbonate therapy reduces the flux of calcium from bone and reduces serum ionized calcium.[20] These events are also associated with an impairment of parathyroid function, increased calcitonin levels, and altered serum magnesium and phosphorus.[69]

Late Neonatal Hypocalcemia. Late hypocalcemia is seen infrequently, but is more frequent in term than preterm infants and usually seen at 5-10 days.[69] Late neonatal hypocalcemia may be due to decreased renal responses to PTH so that the kidneys reabsorb more phosphorus, which leads to a reduction in serum calcium levels, and may be exacerbated by the lower glomerular filtration rates in the neonate. This problem used to be seen primarily in formula-fed term infants with increased phosphate intake, but is uncommon with current formulas (although formulas continue to have higher phosphorus levels than breast milk).[69] Other less frequent causes are malabsorption of calcium, hypomagnesemia, and hypoparathyroidism. Late hypocalcemia may be asymptomatic but is associated with tetany. Symptoms range from mild tremors to seizures.

These infants demonstrate hypoparathyroidism in the face of decreased serum calcium and a reduction in efficient parathyroid activity that extends the usual postnatal decrease in calcium beyond 72 hours. The cause of persistent hypoparathyroidism is unknown. These changes may be aggravated by other factors such as vitamin D deficiency or high phosphorus loads from cow's milk formulas.[33] Late hypocalcemia was seen more often in the past, when higher phosphate formulas were more common. The disorder is uncommon with current formulas and essentially nonexistent in breastfed infants. Late hypocalcemia is occasionally seen in preterm infants secondary to immature renal function, transient parathyroid dysfunction, or altered responsiveness to 1,25-$(OH)_2D$.

Neonatal Hypercalcemia

Hypercalcemia is rare in the neonate and is generally defined as a serum calcium level over 11.0 mg/dL (2.75 mmol/L), or ionized calcium over 5.4 mg/dL (1.35 mmol/L).[69] Infants may be asymptomatic, especially if calcium is in the 11 to 13 mg/dL (2.8 to 3.3 mmol/L) range, or symptomatic (hypotonia, poor feeding, lethargy, vomiting, seizures, polyuria, and hypertension). Neurologic manifestations arise from the effects of calcium on nerve cells and cerebral ischemia.[28] Polyuria is due to interference with the action of arginine vasopressin on the collecting ducts and can lead to dehydration. Hypertension is related to the vasoconstrictive effects of calcium and subsequent increased activity of the renin-angiotensin system. Hypercalcemia may be idiopathic, iatrogenic, or due to hypervitaminosis (vitamin A or D) or underlying metabolic or genetic disorders.

Alterations in Neonatal Magnesium Homeostasis

Hypomagnesemia in the neonate (less than 1.6 mg/dL [0.66 mmol/L]) occurs most often in infants who are SGA, preterm, or born to insulin-dependent diabetic women.[69] Clinical signs are often not seen until levels are less than 1.2 mg/dL (less than 0.49 mmol/L). Less frequent causes of neonatal hypomagnesemia include decreased intake due to malabsorption or short-bowel syndrome, increased losses with frequent exchange transfusions or loop diuretic use or aminoglycosides, maternal hyperparathyroidism, neonatal hypoparathyroidism, and hyperphosphatemia from cow's milk formula.[23] Occasionally tissue hypomagnesemia may be present with normal serum magnesium levels.[33] Hypocalcemia and hypomagnesemia often occur simultaneously and symptoms are similar. Magnesium plays an important role in bone-serum calcium homeostasis and intestinal absorption of calcium (see Box 17-1 on p. 590). Decreased magnesium inhibits PTH secretion and response, with subsequent reduction in calcium levels.[69] Transient hypomagnesemia due to magnesium depletion is sometimes seen with use of loop diuretics, aminoglycosides, amphotericin B, or in infants with renal problems.[69]

Hypermagnesemia (greater than 2.8 mg/dL [1.15 mmol/L]) is most often associated with administration of magnesium sulfate to the mother for treatment of preeclampsia or preterm labor prevention.[69] This can lead to elevated neonatal magnesium levels during the first 48 hours and respiratory depression, hypotonia, flaccidity, ileus, and poor feeding (magnesium has a curare-like effect). These infants have lower calcium levels, although they are not necessarily hypocalcemic. Hypermagnesemia may be treated with calcium, which increases magnesium excretion.[23]

Neonatal Osteopenia and Rickets

Preterm infants, especially those ≤1500-g birth weight, are at increased risk of metabolic bone disease including osteopenia, rickets, and fractures.[10,37,47,74] Osteopenia is a reduction in the bone of the skeleton often accompanied by osteomalacia (failure of mineralization of newly formed osteoid leading to hypomineralization of the bone matrix); rickets involves specific histologic, radiographic, and physical findings with accumulation of unmineralized osteoid, which interrupts bone growth plate mineralization.[23,37,47] In preterm infants, osteopenia develops from inadequate mineral stores exacerbated by the mineral demands of extrauterine life and inadequate intake of calcium or phosphorus over an extended period of time during which the infant is growing rapidly.[47] The cause is often multifactorial, including lower calcium and phosphorus stores, lower intake, prolonged use of total parenteral nutrition, especially calcium and phosphorus levels are low, and exposure to medications such as diuretics, anticonvulsants corticosteroids, and methylxanthines, and diuretics may contribute to metabolic bone disease in preterm infants.[37,47,74,75] Factors predisposing to osteopenia in preterm infants are summarized in Figure 17-5.

Another factor may be the absence of bone loading in preterm infants who are hospitalized for prolonged periods.[23,54] Bone loading normally occurs with passive and active exercise. Increased bone loading promotes bone formation; decreased bone loading leads to bone reabsorption.[23] Most preterm infants with osteopenia have normal 25-(OH) D and 1,25-$(OH)_2D$ levels.[23] Altered bone mineralization may continue into the preschool period and beyond and is associated with decreased linear growth.[47,75,76]

Rickets occurs because of a deficiency of calcium or phosphorus in extracellular fluid, usually associated with inadequate vitamin D, which ensures adequate intestinal absorption of these minerals (see Figure 17-5). This results in increased secretion of PTH, which stimulates osteoclastic breakdown and absorption of bone. Additional calcium is then available to maintain serum levels and prevent hypocalcemia. After a time the bone weakens and becomes stressed. Osteoblast activity is stimulated to replace the absorbed bone, leading to production of large amounts of osteoid (organic bone matrix) that never becomes completely calcified because of lack of calcium and phosphorus. Infants on total parenteral nutrition, with chronic health problems such as bronchopulmonary dysplasia, or on long-term diuretic therapy, have higher mineral requirements and are at greater risk for developing rickets. Acidosis increases urinary calcium losses and interferes with synthesis of 1,25-$(OH)_2D$. Rickets has been reported in breastfed infants, but in most cases appears to be related more to lack of ultraviolet (sunlight) exposure of the mother than nutritional deficiencies per se. The greatest risks to the infant seem to occur if the mother's diet is chronically deficient in vitamin D and she also does not get enough sun exposure (see Maternal-Fetal Interactions).[46,47,75]

MATURATIONAL CHANGES DURING INFANCY AND CHILDHOOD

Age-related changes in calcium and phosphorus and their regulating hormones reflect needs of the infant and child to maintain calcium stability while providing for skeletal growth. Measures of bone turnover increase in the first few weeks, then stabilize from 4 to 10 weeks, and decrease after 10 weeks.[10] Phosphorus levels decrease during the first year to 5 mg/dL (2.1 mmol/L) at 1-2 years, 4.4 mg/dL (1.8 mmol/L) by mid-childhood, and 3.5 mg/dL (1.5 mmol/L) by late adolescence.[69] Reference ranges for serum calcium and phosphorus and urinary calcium excretion from birth to adolescence have been published.[46] With increasing exposure to ultraviolet light, 25-(OH)D levels increase during this same period. Levels of 1,25-$(OH)_2D$ are higher than adult values for the first year. Levels of this biologically active metabolite may remain even higher in preterm infants for up to 3 months, perhaps to compensate for immature calcium absorption.[23] Levels of 1,25-$(OH)_2D$ tend to be elevated during periods of growth. Serum magnesium levels tend to remain slightly higher than adult values in infants and young children.[33]

From 3 weeks to 6 months, serum calcium values in exclusively breastfed infants gradually increase, leading to a transient physiologic hypercalcemia.[33] This increase may be related to decreased phosphorus intake due to the lower levels of phosphorus in human milk.[75] Serum calcium levels do not change significantly in formula-fed infants from birth to 18 months. Serum calcium levels gradually decrease from 6 to 20 years. Intestinal absorption of calcium tends to be passive until after weaning. Absorption is mediated by high lactose levels that increase absorptive efficiency.[27] Infants on standard formulas experience a progressive fall in serum parathyroid hormone (PTH) that reaches a nadir at about 3 months, at which time bone mineralization increases. This is analogous to the lowered PTH levels seen in utero and may promote extrauterine bone development. By 2 to 4 months, the renal response to exogenous PTH is similar to that seen in adults.[27] Phosphate renal reabsorption decreases after weaning.[69]

Skeletal bone mass, size, shape, and properties continue to change throughout childhood and early adolescence and are affected by both genetic and environmental factors (such as diet, lifestyle, illness).[18] During prepuberty, bone growth and mineralization are more rapid in the appendicular versus axial skeleton. Puberty stimulates rapid axial skeletal growth, which slows in later adolescence.[18] The prepuberty period is characterized by a relative undermineralization that increases the risk of fractures. This is due to a lag of about 8 months between peak height velocity and peak mineral accrual.[18]

With the increased secretion of estrogens and other steroid hormones at menarche, skeletal mineral acquisition increases, stimulating longitudinal and radial skeletal growth for approximately 10 years, as well as increases in volumetric density.[19] The first 4 years after menarche are characterized by a rapid increase in bone mineral density, followed by a slower increase in late adolescence and early adulthood.[18] In women, peak bone mineral density is reached at 25-35 years (one third of this is achieved in the first 4 years after menarche).[18]

SUMMARY

Calcium and phosphorus are essential minerals for many body processes and normal growth and development. Alterations in metabolic processes related to these elements can significantly alter the infant's health status. Many of these problems can be prevented and normal growth and development promoted by careful assessment and monitoring of neonatal nutritional status and initiation of appropriate interventions. Recommendations for clinical practice related to calcium and phosphorus metabolism are summarized in Table 17-5.

Table 17-5 Recommendations for Clinical Practice Related to Calcium and Phosphorus Metabolism in Neonates

Know the usual changes in calcium, phosphorus, and magnesium metabolism during the neonatal period (pp. 598-600).
Monitor newborn calcium, phosphorus, and magnesium status during transition and in the early neonatal period (pp. 598-600).
Recognize factors that influence bone mineralization and growth (pp. 595-596, 597, 600-601).
Initiate early enteral feeding as appropriate (p. 600).
Monitor the nutritional intake of calcium, phosphorus, and vitamin D in infants (p. 600).
Monitor neonates for signs of excessive and inadequate intake of calcium, phosphorus, and magnesium (pp. 600-604).
Recognize infants at risk for hypocalcemia (pp. 601-603 and Table 17-4).
Know clinical signs of hypocalcemia (pp. 601-602).
Assess and monitor infants at risk for hypocalcemia (pp. 601-603).
Recognize infants at risk for hypomagnesemia and hypermagnesemia (p. 603).
Know the clinical signs of hypomagnesemia and hypermagnesemia (p. 603).
Assess and monitor infants at risk for hypomagnesemia and hypermagnesemia (p. 603).
Recognize and monitor infants at risk for late neonatal hypocalcemia (p. 603).
Recognize and monitor infants at risk for osteopenia and neonatal rickets (pp. 603-604).

References

1. Abrams, S.A. (2007). In utero physiology: Role in nutrient delivery and fetal development for calcium, phosphorus, and vitamin D. *Am J Clin Nutr, 85*, 604S.
2. Adamova, Z., Ozkan, S., & Khalil, R.A. (2009). Vascular and cellular calcium in normal and hypertensive pregnancy. *Curr Clin Pharmacol, 4*, 172.
3. Affinito, P., et al. (1996). Changes in bone mineral density and calcium metabolism in breast-feeding women: A one-year follow-up study. *J Clin Endocrinol Metab, 81*, 2314.
4. Avila, E., et al. (2007). Regulation of vitamin D hydroxylases gene expression by 1,25-dihydroxyvitamin D3 and cyclic AMP in cultured human syncytiotrophoblasts. *J Steroid Biochem Mol Biol, 103*, 90.
5. Baczyk, D., Kingdom, J.C., & Uhlén, P. (2011). Calcium signaling in the placenta. *Cell Calcium, 4*, 350.
6. Barrett, H., & McElduff, A. (2010). Vitamin D and pregnancy: An old problem revisited. *Best Pract Res Clin Endocrinol Metab, 24*, 527.
7. Belkacemi, L., et al. (2005). Calcium channels, transporters and exchangers in placenta: A review. *Cell Calcium, 37*, 1.
8. Berry, M.A., Abrahamowicz, M., & Usher, R.H. (1997). Factors associated with the growth of extremely premature infants during initial hospitalization. *Pediatrics, 100*, 640.
9. Bikle, D. (2009). Nonclassic actions of vitamin D. *JCEM, 94*, 26.
10. Bishop, N. (2005). Metabolic bone disease. In J.M. Rennie (Ed.), *Robertson's textbook of neonatology* (4th ed.). London: Churchill Livingstone.
11. Black, A.J., et al. (2000). A detailed assessment of alteration in bone turnover, calcium homeostasis and bone density in normal pregnancy. *J Bone Miner Res, 15*, 557.
12. Bodnar, L.M., et al. (2007). Maternal vitamin D deficiency increases the risk of preeclampsia. *JCEM, 92*, 3517.
13. Bodnar, L.M., et al. (2010). Maternal serum 25-hydroxyvitamin D concentrations are associated with small-for-gestational-age births in white women. *J Nutr, 140*, 999.
14. Boissonnault, W.G., & Boissonnault, J.S. (2001). Transient osteoporosis of the hip associated with pregnancy. *J Orth Sports Phys Ther, 31*, 359.
15. Brannon, P.M., & Picciano, M.F. (2011). Vitamin D in pregnancy and lactation in humans. *Annu Rev Nutr, 21*, 89.
16. Buppasiri, P., et al. (2011). Calcium supplementation (other than for preventing or treating hypertension) for improving pregnancy and infant outcomes. *Cochrane Database Syst Rev, 10*, CD007079.
17. Charoenphandhu, N., Wongdee, K., & Krishnamra, N. (2010). Is prolactin the cardinal calciotropic maternal hormone? *Trends Endocrinol Metab, 21*, 395.
18. Clarke, B.L., & Khosla, S. (2010). Female reproductive system and bone. *Arch Biochem Biophys, 503*, 118.
19. Cooper, C., et al. (2008). Growth and bone development. *Nestle Nutr Workshop Ser Pediatr Program, 61*, 53.
20. Cruz, M.L., & Tsang, R.C. (1991). Disorders of calcium and magnesium homeostasis. In T.F. Yeh (Ed.), *Neonatal therapeutics* (2nd ed.). St. Louis: Mosby.
21. Elizabeth, K.E., Krishnan, V., & Vijayakumar, T. (2008). Umbilical cord blood nutrients in low birth weight babies in relation to birth weight and gestation age. *Indian J Med Res, 128*, 128.
22. Ensom, M.H., Liu, P.Y., & Stephenson, M.D. (2002). Effect of pregnancy on bone mineral density in healthy women. *Obstet Gynecol Surv, 57*, 99.
23. Greer, F.R. (2005). Disorders of calcium homeostasis. In A.R. Spitzer (Ed.), *Intensive care of the fetus and neonate* (2nd ed.). St. Louis: Mosby.
24. Guyton, A.C., & Hall, J.E. (2010). *Textbook of medical physiology* (12th ed.). Philadelphia: Saunders.
25. Hensley, J. (2009). Leg cramps and restless legs syndrome during pregnancy. *J Midwifery Womens Health, 54*, 211.
26. Hofmeyr, G.J., et al. (2010). Calcium supplementation during pregnancy for preventing hypertensive disorders and related problems. *Cochrane Database Syst Rev, 8*, CD001059.
27. Hoskings, D.J. (1996). Calcium homeostasis in pregnancy. *Clin Endocrinol (Oxf), 45*, 1.
28. Hsu, S.C., & Levine, M.A. (2004). Perinatal calcium metabolism: Physiology and pathophysiology. *Semin Neonatol, 9*, 23.
29. Husain, S.M., Mughal, M.Z., & Tsang, R.C. (2012). Calcium, phosphorus and magnesium transport across the placenta. In R.A. Polin, W.W. Fox, & S.H. Abman (Eds.), *Fetal and neonatal physiology* (4th ed.). Philadelphia: Saunders.
30. Karlsson, C., Obrant, K.J., & Karlsson, M. (2001). Pregnancy and lactation confer reversible bone loss in humans. *Osteoporos Int, 12*, 828.
31. Karlsson, M.K., Ahlborg, H.G., & Karlsson, C. (2005). Female reproductive history and the skeleton—A review. *BJOG, 112*, 851.
32. Kent, J.C., et al. (2009). Why calcium in breastmilk is independent of maternal dietary calcium and vitamin D. *Breastfeeding Review, 17*, 5.
33. Koo, W.K., & Tsang, R.C. (2005). Calcium and magnesium homeostasis. In M.G. MacDonald, M.M.K. Seshia, & M.D. Mullett (Eds.), *Avery's Neonatology: Pathophysiology and management of the newborn* (6th ed.). Philadelphia: Lippincott Williams & Wilkins.
34. Koo, W.W.K., & Warren, L. (2003). Calcium and bone health. *Neonatal Netw, 22*, 23.
35. Kovacs, C.K., & Fuleihan, G.E.H. (2006). Calcium and bone disorders during pregnancy and lactation. *Endocrinol Metab Clin North Am, 35*, 21.
36. Kovacs, C.S. (2008). Vitamin D in pregnancy and lactation: Maternal, fetal, and

neonatal outcomes from human and animal studies, *Am J Clin Nutr, 88*, 520S.
37. Land, C., & Schoenau, E. (2008). Fetal and postnatal bone development: Reviewing the role of mechanical stimuli and nutrition. *Best Pract Res Clin Endocrinol Metab, 22*, 107.
38. Lapillonne, A. (2010). Vitamin D deficiency during pregnancy may impair maternal and fetal outcomes. *Med Hypotheses, 74*, 71.
39. Laskey, M.A., & Prentice, A. (1999). Bone mineral changes during and after lactation. *Obstet Gynecol, 94*, 608.
40. Lewis, S., et al. (2010). Vitamin D deficiency and pregnancy: From preconception to birth. *Mol Nutr Food Res, 54*, 1092.
41. Liu, N.Q., & Hewison, M. (2011). Vitamin D, the placenta and pregnancy. *Arch Biochem Biophys*. In press, doi: 10.1016/j.abb.2011.11.018. [Epub ahead of print.]
42. Lucas, R.M., et al. (2008). Future health implications of prenatal and early-life vitamin D status. *Nutr Rev, 66*, 710.
43. Maioli, E., Fortino, V., & Pacini, A. (2004). Parathyroid hormone-related protein in preeclampsia: A linkage between maternal and fetal failures. *Biol Reprod, 71*, 1779.
44. Masiukiewicz, U.S., & Insogna, K.L. (2004). Calcium and disorders of calcium metabolism during pregnancy and lactation. In G.N. Burrows, T.P. Duffy, & J.A. Copel (Eds.), *Medical complications during pregnancy* (6th ed.). Philadelphia: Saunders.
45. Misra, M., et al. (2008). Drug and Therapeutics Committee of the Lawson Wilkins Pediatric Endocrine Society. Vitamin D deficiency in children and its management: Review of current knowledge and recommendations. *Pediatrics, 122*, 398.
46. Mitchell, D.M., & Jüppner, H. (2010). Regulation of calcium homeostasis and bone metabolism in the fetus and neonate. *Curr Opin Endocrinol Diabetes Obes, 17*, 25.
47. Mitchell, S.M., et al. (2009). High frequencies of elevated alkaline phosphatase activity and rickets exist in extremely low birth weight infants despite current nutritional support. *BMC Pediatr, 9*, 47.
48. Moore, K.L., Persaud, T.V.N, & Torchia, M.G. (2011). *The developing human: Clinically oriented embryology* (9th ed.). Philadelphia: Saunders.
49. More, C., et al. (2001). The effects of pregnancy and lactation on bone mineral density. *Osteoporos Int, 12*, 732.
50. Mulligan, M.L., et al. (2009). Implications of vitamin D deficiency in pregnancy and lactation. *Am J Obst Gynecol, 202*, 429.
51. Nader, S. (2009). Other endocrine disorders of pregnancy. In R.K. Creasy, et al. (Eds.), *Creasy & Resnik's Maternal-fetal medicine: Principles and practice* (6th ed.). Philadelphia: Saunders.
52. Namgung, R., & Tsang, R. (2012). Neonatal calcium, phosphorus and magnesium homeostasis. In R.A. Polin, W.W. Fox, & S.H. Abman (Eds.), *Fetal and neonatal physiology* (4th ed.). Philadelphia: Saunders.
53. Naylor, K.E., et al. (2000). The effect of pregnancy on bone density and bone turnover. *J Bone Miner Res, 15*, 129.
54. Nemet, D., et al. (2002). Evidence for exercise-induced bone formation in preterm infants. *Int J Sports Med, 23*, 82.
55. Olausson, H., et al. (2008). Changes in bone mineral status and bone size during pregnancy and the influences of body weight and calcium intake. *Am J Clin Nutr, 88*, 1032.
56. Oliveri, B., et al. (2004). Mineral and bone mass changes during pregnancy and lactation. *Nutrition, 20*, 235.
57. Paton, L.M., et al. (2003). Pregnancy and lactation have no long term deleterious effect on measures of bone mineral in healthy women: A twin study. *Am J Clin Nutr, 77*, 707.
58. Pawley, N., & Bishop, N.J. (2004). Prenatal and infant predictors of bone health: The influence of vitamin D. *Am J Clin Nutr, 80*, 1748S.
59. Perez-Lopez, F.R. (2007). Vitamin D: The secosteroid hormone and human reproduction. *Gynecol Endocrinol, 23*, 13.
60. Perrine, C.G., et al. (2010). Adherence to vitamin D recommendations among U.S. infants. *Pediatrics, 125*, 627.
61. Petersen, H.C., et al. (2002). Reproduction life history and hip fractures. *Ann Epidemiol, 12*, 257.
62. Pitkin, R.M. (1985). Calcium metabolism in pregnancy and the perinatal period: A review. *Am J Obstet Gynecol, 151*, 99.
63. Ponnapula, P., & Boberg, J. (2010). Lower extremity changes experienced during pregnancy. *J Foot Ankle Surg, 49*, 452.
64. Power, M.L., Heaney, R.P., & Kalkwarf, H.J. (1999). The role of calcium in health and disease. *Am J Obstet Gynecol, 181*, 1560.
65. Prentice, A. (2003). Micronutrients and the bone mineral content of the mother, fetus and newborn, *J Nutr, 133*, 1693S.
66. Quarles, L.D. (2009). Endocrine functions of bone in mineral metabolism regulation. *J Clin Invest, 118*, 3820.
67. Rigo, J., DeCurtis, M., Pieltain, C., et al. (2000). Bone mineralization in the micropremie. *Clin Perinatol, 27*, 147.
68. Rigo, J., et al. (2006). Nutritional needs of premature infants: Current issues, *J Pediatr, 149*, s80.
69. Rigo, J., Mohamed, M., & Decurtis, M. (2011). Disorders of calcium, phosphorus and magnesium metabolism. In R.J. Martin, A.A. Fanaroff, & M.C. Walsh (Eds.), *Fanaroff & Martin's Neonatal-perinatal medicine: Diseases of the fetus and infant* (9th ed.). St. Louis: Mosby.
70. Rubin, L.P. (2012). Disorders of calcium and phosphorus metabolism. In C.A. Gleason & S. Devaskar (Eds.), *Avery's Diseases of the newborn* (9th ed.). Philadelphia: Saunders.
71. Scholl, T.O., & Chen, X. (2009). Vitamin D intake during pregnancy: Association with maternal characteristics and infant birth weight. *Early Hum Dev, 85*, 231.
72. Shah, M.D., & Shah, S.R. (2009). Nutrient deficiencies in the premature infant. *Pediatr Clin North Am, 56*, 1069.
73. Simmonds, C.S., et al. (2010). Parathyroid hormone regulates fetal-placental mineral homeostasis. *J Bone Miner Res, 25*, 594.
74. So, K.W., & Ng, P.C. (2005). Treatment and prevention of neonatal osteopenia. *Curr Paediatr, 15*, 106.
75. Specker, B. (2004). Nutrition influences bone development from infancy through toddler years. *J Nutr, 134*, 691S.
76. Specter, B.L., et al. (2001). Total body bone mineral content and tibial cortical bone measures in preschool children. *J Bone Miner Res, 16*, 2298.
77. Thomas, M., & Weisman, S.M. (2006). Calcium supplementation during pregnancy and lactation: Effects on the mother and fetus. *Am J Obstet Gynecol, 194*, 937.
78. Thomson, K., et al. (2004). Postnatal evaluation of vitamin D and bone health in women who were vitamin D-deficient in pregnancy, and in their infants. *Med J Aust, 181*, 486.
79. Valbo, A., & Bohmer, T. (1999). Leg cramps in pregnancy—How common are they? [English abstract], *Tidsskr Nor Laegeforen, 119*, 1589.
80. Van Cromphaut, S.J., et al. (2003). Intestinal calcium transporter genes are upregulated by estrogens and the reproductive cycle through vitamin D receptor-independent mechanisms. *J Bone Miner Res, 18*, 1725.
81. VanHouten, J., et al. (2004). The calcium-sensing receptor regulates mammary gland parathyroid hormone-related protein production and calcium transport. *J Clin Invest, 113*, 598.
82. Viljakainen, H.T., et al. (2010). Maternal vitamin D status determines bone variables in the newborn. *J Clin Endocrinol Metab, 95*, 1749.
83. Villar, J., & Belizan, J. (2000). Same nutrient, different hypotheses: Disparities in trial of calcium supplementation during pregnancy, *Am J Clin Nutr, 71*, 1375S.
84. Wagner, C.L., & Greer, F.R. (2008). American Academy of Pediatrics Section on Breastfeeding: Committee on Nutrition: Prevention of rickets and vitamin D deficiency in infants, children, and adolescents. *Pediatrics, 122*, 1142.
85. Widmaier, E., Raff, H., & Strang, K.T. (2005). *Vander's Human physiology: The mechanism of body function* (10th ed.). New York: McGraw-Hill.
86. Wisser, J., et al. (2005). Changes in bone density and metabolism in pregnancy. *Acta Obstet Gynecol Scand, 84*, 349.
87. Wysolmerski, J.J., & Stewart, A.F. (1998). The physiology of parathyroid hormone-related protein: An emerging role as a developmental factor. *Ann Rev Physiol, 60*, 431.
88. Yokoyama, K., et al. (2010). Prolonged maternal magnesium administration and bone metabolism in neonates. *Early Hum Dev, 86*, 187.
89. Young, G.L., & Jewell, D. (2002). Interventions for leg cramps in pregnancy. *Cochrane Database Syst Rev, 1*, CD000121.

CHAPTER 18

Bilirubin Metabolism

Physiologic jaundice is a common problem in term and preterm infants during the first week after birth. For most of these infants, this phenomenon is mild and resolves without treatment. A small group of infants develop neonatal hyperbilirubinemia, which may be an exaggeration of normal physiologic processes or may herald underlying disorders such as hemolytic disease of the newborn or sepsis. When any infant develops significant hyperbilirubinemia, concerns arise about possible sequelae in the form of bilirubin encephalopathy. This chapter focuses on bilirubin metabolism in the fetus and neonate along with issues related to neonatal hyperbilirubinemia and its management. Maternal adaptations are discussed only briefly, because bilirubin metabolism is not normally significantly altered in pregnancy. Bilirubin synthesis, transport, and metabolism are summarized in Figure 18-1 and in Box 18-1 on page 609.

MATERNAL PHYSIOLOGIC ADAPTATIONS

Alterations in liver and hepatic function during pregnancy are described in Chapter 12. Bilirubin metabolism is not significantly altered in the pregnant woman, with bilirubin levels generally reported to be similar or slightly lower than those in nonpregnant women; i.e., values of 0.3 to 1 mg/dL (5.3 to 17.1 μmol/L) for total bilirubin and an upper limit of 0.2 mg/dL (3.4 μmol/L) for direct bilirubin.[102] However, others report that both total and free bilirubin levels are slightly lower across all three trimesters and direct is lower in the second and third trimesters, due to hemodilution and decreased albumin.[9,52] This discrepancy may be because of differences in the reference ranges used. Reference ranges for liver function tests during pregnancy have been proposed, with the upper limit of normal values lower than previous values for both pregnant and nonpregnant women of childbearing age.[9,40,52] Activity of phase II enzymes involved in bilirubin metabolism is increased in pregnant women.[82] Elevated serum bilirubin levels in pregnancy warrant further evaluation for liver or hematologic dysfunction.[72,102,133]

CLINICAL IMPLICATIONS FOR THE PREGNANT WOMAN AND HER FETUS

A major difference between fetal and adult handling of bilirubin is that the fetus uses the placenta rather than its own intestines as the major elimination pathway. Most of the bilirubin produced by the fetus remains in the indirect state, a form that can be readily cleared by the placenta. The indirect fetal bilirubin eliminated across the placenta is conjugated and excreted by the maternal liver. Even with severe hemolysis, infants are rarely born jaundiced because the placenta efficiently clears excess fetal indirect bilirubin.[59] However, these infants may have an accumulation of direct bilirubin and are often severely anemic due to the ongoing hemolysis. The maternal system efficiently handles the fetal bilirubin load and has sufficient reserve so maternal hyperbilirubinemia secondary to fetal hemolysis is rare.[102] Immunologic aspects of hemolytic disorders secondary to blood group incompatibility are discussed in Chapter 13.

Maternal Hyperbilirubinemia

Elevated total and direct serum bilirubin levels during pregnancy may occur with viral hepatitis, hyperemesis gravidarum (usually less than 5 mg/dL [85.5 μmol/L]), intrahepatic cholestasis of pregnancy (usually less than 4 to 5 mg/dL [68.4 to 85.8 μmol/L]), preeclampsia/eclampsia (often normal but if increased levels are generally less than 5 mg/dL [85.5 μmol/L]), acute fatty liver of pregnancy (usually less than 10 mg/dL [171 μmol/L]), cholelithiasis, and hepatic rupture.[52,102] The most common cause of jaundice in the first two trimesters of pregnancy is viral hepatitis.[102] Other causes of jaundice in early pregnancy include drug-induced hepatotoxicity, septicemia, or cholelithiasis, with biliary tract disease becoming more prominent in the second trimester.[99] Causes of jaundice in the third trimester include intrahepatic cholestasis of pregnancy (see Table 14-2), viral hepatitis, gallstone disease, HELLP syndrome (characterized by hemolysis [H], elevated liver enzymes [EL], and a low platelet [LP] count), acute fatty liver of pregnancy, and disseminated herpes. Postpartum jaundice is most often a result of septicemia, drug use, viral hepatitis, or cholelithiasis.[52,72] Liver function and hepatic disorders during pregnancy are discussed further in Chapter 12.

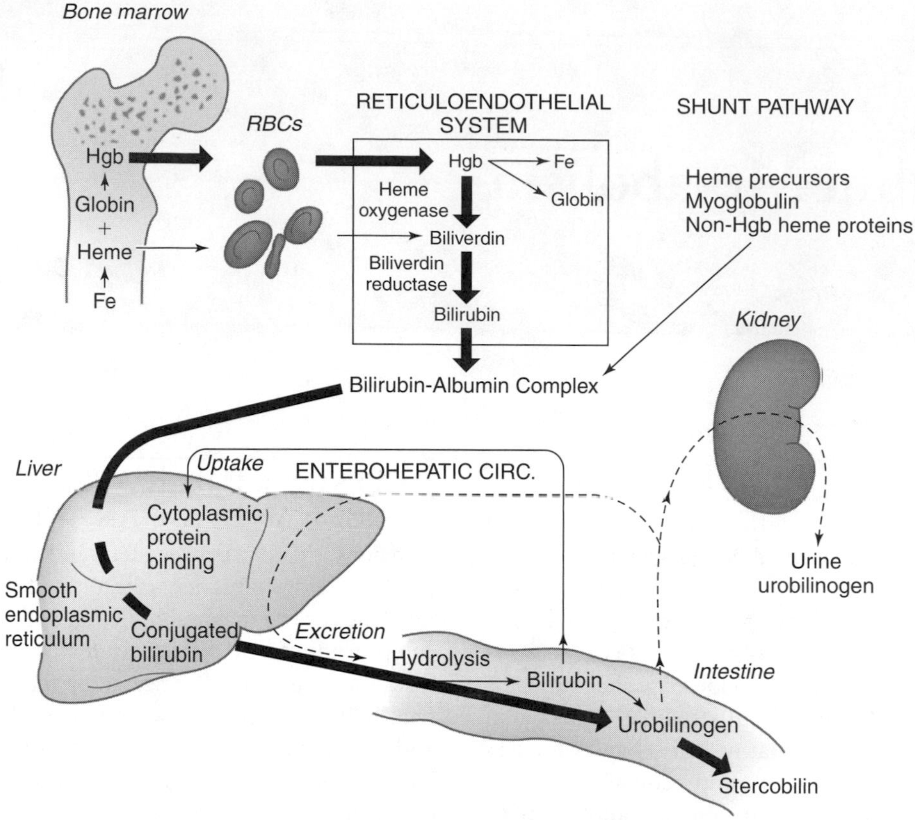

FIGURE 18-1 Bilirubin synthesis, transport, and metabolism. (From Gartner, L.M., & Hollander, M. [1972]. Disorders of bilirubin metabolism. In N.S. Assali [Ed.], *Pathophysiology of gestation* [Vol. 2]. New York: Academic Press.)

The effects of excessive maternal bilirubin production on the fetus depend on whether the woman has direct or indirect hyperbilirubinemia. Direct (conjugated) bilirubin is not transferred across the placenta in either direction.[71,102] Therefore the fetus of a woman with direct hyperbilirubinemia and jaundice secondary to hepatitis or other functional liver disorders does not have an elevated direct bilirubin level. Indirect (unconjugated) bilirubin has been reported to be transferred across the placenta from mother to fetus (as well as the usual transfer from fetus to mother) and prolonged exposure to elevated levels may increase the risk of neurologic complications in the infant.[74,102] HELLP syndrome is associated with an increase in indirect bilirubin, although levels in the mother are usually less than 5 mg/dL (85.5 μmol/L) and the mother usually does not appear jaundiced.[102] Neonatal hyperbilirubinemia is seen in about half of the infants in pregnancies complicated by this syndrome. Isolated indirect hyperbilirubinemia is rare in adults; however, several cases of elevated indirect bilirubin levels in cord blood have been reported in infants of women with end-stage cirrhosis.[102] It is unclear whether this increase results from maternal-to-fetal transfer or whether the elevated maternal bilirubin levels prevented the normal fetal-to-maternal transfer of indirect bilirubin. Intrahepatic cholestasis of pregnancy can alter the removal of bile acids and bilirubin from the fetus across the placenta. If this occurs, these substances may accumulate in the maternal liver and eventually in the placenta and fetal liver.[8,71,82]

DEVELOPMENT OF BILIRUBIN METABOLISM IN THE FETUS

In early pregnancy, the fetus begins producing bile acids and bile pigments (the most prominent being biliverdin and bilirubin). Elimination of these cholephilic organic anions requires a complex interplay of the mother, placenta, and fetus.[71,82] The placenta contains detoxifying enzymes and organic anion carrier transport systems, which facilitate this removal and prevent fetal accumulation of these potentially harmful substances.[71,82] For example, expression and activity of phase II enzymes are increased in the placenta.[82] As a result, bile acids and bilirubin levels remain low in the fetus.[71] Biliverdin crosses the placenta poorly; thus conversion to bilirubin facilitates carrier-mediated transport across the placenta.[71] The early production of bile acids may have a role in development that is as yet incompletely understood, since bile acids act as signaling molecules with both endocrine and paracrine functions.[62] Most fetal bilirubin remains in an unconjugated state.[22,71] This is facilitated by immaturity of the liver and intestine, decreased hepatic blood flow as a result of shunting of

BOX 18-1 Bilirubin Synthesis, Transport, Metabolism, and Excretion

Bilirubin is a chain of four pyrrole rings with carbon bridges that is an end product of hemoglobin catabolism. Hemoglobin is broken down into a heme iron–porphyrin complex and globin in the reticuloendothelial system (see Figure 18-1). Heme is degraded by a series of oxidation-reduction reactions releasing ferrous iron (Fe^{++}) and carbon monoxide (CO) to form biliverdin under the influence of heme oxygenase (HO). HO is a membrane-bound isoenzyme with several forms and is found primarily in the spleen, liver, and bone marrow, although it is also found in the lungs, vascular endothelium, and nervous system.[22,118] HO is the rate-limiting step in bilirubin production.[24,118] The iron is stored and reused. The CO is excreted via the lungs. Bilirubin, iron, and CO are formed in equimolar proportions, so CO production has been used an index of bilirubin production.[24,118] About 80% of the CO produced by the newborn comes from bilirubin.[24,118] Biliverdin is a water-soluble, nontoxic, blue-green pigment that is catabolized to indirect (unconjugated) bilirubin (4Z-15Z-bilirubin-IXa) by action of nicotinamide adenine dinucleotide phosphate (NADPH)–dependent biliverdin reductase.[118] Most of the heme comes from catabolism of senescent red blood cells (RBCs) and ineffective erythropoiesis (each gram of hemoglobin produces 34 mg of unconjugated bilirubin).[59] Bilirubin also comes from catabolism of nonhemoglobin heme proteins and free heme in the liver. Indirect bilirubin is orange-yellow, fat-soluble, and not readily excreted in bile or urine. Indirect bilirubin is transported in plasma—bound to albumin (1 g albumin binds 7 to 8 mg of unconjugated bilirubin) with a small amount of free bilirubin—to the liver for metabolism and excretion.[59] The albumin-bilirubin complex is rapidly reversible.[85] Direct (conjugated) bilirubin is a water-soluble complex that has been metabolized by the liver to form bilirubin monoglucuronides or diglucuronides (see Figure 18-1).

Bilirubin is dissociated from albumin and transported into the hepatocyte via carrier-mediated diffusion or mediated by organic anion transporters.[59] Intracellular carrier proteins that bind organic anion move bilirubin from the hepatocyte plasma membrane to the liver's smooth endoplasmic reticulum. A cytosolic form of glutathione *S*-transferase, ligandin, is the major intracellular carrier protein for bilirubin.[22,59,74] Indirect bilirubin is conjugated in the smooth endoplasmic reticulum of the liver to form polar (water soluble) bilirubin monoglucuronide or diglucuronide. The major conjugation pathway involves action of the microsomal enzyme uridine diphosphate-glucuronosyltransferase (UGT). There are multiple isoforms of this liver enzyme, including a bilirubin-specific isoform (UGT1A1) coded by genes on chromosome 2. Mutations in this gene lead to diseases such as Gilbert syndrome and Crigler-Najjar syndrome, which are characterized by an indirect hyperbilirubinemia.[129] Other isoforms are involved in conjugation of various drugs and hormones. Polymorphisms in this gene can increase the risk of hyperbilirubinemia in newborns by altering enzyme activity and decreasing production of conjugated bilirubin production or delaying bilirubin clearance.[129]

Conjugation of each bilirubin molecule involves an enzymatic combination with sugars and glucuronic acid to produce bilirubin monoglycerides and diglycerides.[74] In children and adults, about two thirds of the monoglucuronides are conjugated to form diglucuronides. In neonates, most of the conjugated bilirubin is monoglucuronide. The glucuronyl-conjugating system is dependent on adequate supplies of glucose and oxygen for proper functioning. Most conjugated bilirubin is transported into the intestines in bile and is excreted in feces. A small amount is reabsorbed in the colon and subsequently excreted in urine (increases with elevated serum direct bilirubin levels).[44,59,105] The excretion of bilirubin into the biliary tree is by carrier-mediated active transport. These carriers may become saturated at high bilirubin levels.[24] This is a rate-limiting step in clearance of bilirubin from the blood. If these carriers become saturated (as occurs with hepatocellular disorders such as hepatitis), direct hyperbilirubinemia develops.[17,18,59,74] Some direct bilirubin is also found in circulation bound to albumin to form δ bilirubin. δ bilirubin is not seen in the first 2 weeks.[59] Direct or conjugated bilirubin is relatively unstable in the circulation so that the mono- and diglucuronide isomers that make up its structure can be rearranged to form other isomers reducing accuracy of direct bilirubin measurements.[85]

In the intestines, conjugated bilirubin is further catabolized by intestinal bacteria into urobilins. Urobilinogen is oxidized by intestinal bacteria to stercobilin, which is excreted in stool. Stercobilin has a characteristic brown-orange color that contributes to the color of feces. Direct bilirubin is unstable and can be hydrolyzed by the relatively alkaline environment of the duodenum and jejunum, by intestinal brush border enzymes such as β-glucuronidase, and by intestinal bacteria back into glucuronic acid and unconjugated (indirect) bilirubin. β-glucuronidase is found in high concentrations in both term and preterm newborns.[59] Some urobilinogen is also deconjugated in the small intestine by β-glucuronidase, absorbed across the intestinal mucosa, and returned to the circulation and portal venous system through enterohepatic circulation (see Figure 18-1). Recirculated bilirubin eventually is reconjugated by the liver.[17,18,51,59,74]

some placental blood away from the fetal liver by the ductus venosus, and increased recirculation of bilirubin by the enterohepatic shunt (see Figure 18-1 and Box 18-1). Bilirubin production from biliverdin before liver maturation may play a role in protecting the fetus from oxidative stress and in inducing expression of antioxidant systems.[71,108]

Hepatic uptake is reduced by very low levels of the intracellular carrier protein ligandin.[74] Conjugation of indirect bilirubin by the fetal liver is reduced because of immaturity of a hepatic microsomal enzyme 1A1 isoform of uridine diphosphate-glucuronosyltransferase (UGT) and other liver enzyme systems, and decreased hepatocyte uptake and excretion of bilirubin. UGT1A1 can be detected by 16 weeks' gestation.[61] Activity of this enzyme remains low in the fetus and is 0.1% of adult activity at 17 to 30 weeks, increasing to 1% by term.[61,74,129]

Elevated concentrations of β-glucuronidase in the fetal small intestine lead to increased deconjugation of direct bilirubin with recirculation to the blood for removal by the placenta. Limited intestinal motility also promotes intestinal reabsorption of bilirubin by lengthening the time available for β-glucuronidase to act. Fetal total bilirubin levels are slightly higher than maternal values (averaging 1.5 ± 0.3 mg/L [25.6 ± 5.1 μmol/L]), which may facilitate diffusion across the placenta.[101] The fetus demonstrates little hepatobiliary elimination of bilirubin. Unconjugated bilirubin levels are also greater in the fetus than the mother.[71] Bilirubin and its conjugates can be detected in fetal bile by 22 to 24 weeks' gestation.[41] Fetal total and direct bilirubin increases with increasing gestational age, probably due to increasing numbers of red blood cells (RBCs) that then undergo physiologic hemolysis. Bilirubin production increases about 150% per unit of body weight in late gestation as RBCs formed earlier in gestation undergo normal degradation.

Indirect bilirubin can be found in the amniotic fluid beginning at about 12 weeks' gestation.[59] Amniotic fluid bilirubin levels initially rise, plateau between 16 and 25 weeks, and then decrease, essentially disappearing by about 36 weeks.[59,101] This pattern has been plotted on graphs used to monitor and manage the fetus in pregnancies complicated by Rh sensitization and other blood group incompatibilities. The increased bilirubin reflects increased RBC destruction by maternal antibodies (see Chapter 13).

The mechanisms by which bilirubin reaches amniotic fluid are uncertain.[59] The fetal kidney excretes small amounts of organic anions into amniotic fluid.[22] Bilirubin may be transferred directly across placental tissue from the mother or across the amnion or umbilical cord from fetal blood vessels.[59,61] The lipid-soluble indirect bilirubin may enter the amniotic fluid dissolved in phospholipids from tracheobronchial secretions.[59] Failure of amniotic fluid bilirubin levels to decrease during gestation is associated with hemolytic disease or disorders that interfere with the normal production and turnover of amniotic fluid (see Chapter 3), such as high intestinal obstruction or anencephaly with decreased fetal swallowing.

Heme oxygenase, an enzyme involved in bilirubin production, is found in the placenta. Heme oxygenase catabolizes heme into carbon monoxide and biliverdin, which is subsequently catabolized to bilirubin (see Figure 18-1 and Box 18-1). Carbon monoxide is a potent vasodilator and bilirubin a potent antioxidant (see Benefits of Bilirubin). Thus, these substances may have a local role in control of placental vascular tone and protection of fetal-placental endothelium and syncytiotrophoblast from oxidative injury.[24,115,118]

NEONATAL PHYSIOLOGY

Before birth, bilirubin clearance is handled efficiently by the placenta and mother. After birth, the liver of the newborn must assume full responsibility for bilirubin metabolism. Immaturity of liver and intestinal processes for metabolism, conjugation, and excretion can result in physiologic jaundice and interact with other factors to increase the risk of neonatal hyperbilirubinemia.

Transitional Events

Cord blood bilirubin levels are normally less than 2 mg/dL (34.2 μmol/L) and range from 1.4 to 1.9 mg/dL (23.9 to 32.5 μmol/L).[74] With clamping of the umbilical cord, blood flow and pressure in the venous circulation decrease, the ductus venosus constricts, and flow of relatively desaturated blood to the liver increases. Persistent or fluctuating patency of the ductus venosus, which occurs in some immature or ill infants, results in shunting of portal blood past the liver sinusoidal circulation (reducing the amount of blood perfusing the liver) and may interfere with normal clearance of bilirubin from the plasma.[84]

At birth the meconium in the intestines may contain 100 to 200 mg of bilirubin.[41] About half of this is deconjugated bilirubin and equals 5 to 10 times the daily bilirubin production rate from heme catabolism in the term neonate. Meconium passage usually occurs within 6 to 12 hours (69% of infants); it occurs in 94% of term infants by 24 hours of age (see Chapter 12). Any delay in passage of meconium through the intestinal tract increases the likelihood that conjugated bilirubin will be deconjugated (see Box 18-1 on page 609) and returned to the circulation.

Benefits of Bilirubin

The by-products of heme degradation (CO, iron, and bilirubin) have both toxic and beneficial effects.[24,118] Unconjugated bilirubin can diffuse into any cell. While high levels of bilirubin are toxic, at low levels, bilirubin acts as a potent intracellular antioxidant by binding to membranes to prevent their peroxidation and scavenging reactive oxygen species.[10,24,45,59,71,74,85,108,109] Levels of bilirubin correlate with total blood oxidative capacity in the newborn.[108] Highly reactive metabolites of oxygen (free radicals) are a by-product of oxidative phosphorylation. Cellular enzymes normally scavenge for and destroy these radicals before they can interfere with cell metabolic functions and destroy cell lipid membranes. Bilirubin accumulation after birth may augment other antioxidant systems and help protect the fetus in moving from the lower oxygenation of the intrauterine environment to the oxygen-rich extrauterine environment.[21,71,74,108] Infants with neonatal disorders associated with free radical production (e.g., respiratory distress syndrome, intraventricular hemorrhage, necrotizing enterocolitis, and retinopathy of prematurity) have been found to have lower serum bilirubin levels than those of similar gestational ages with non-oxidative disorders, which is suggestive that bilirubin is being used to cope with oxidative stress.[108] Bilirubin may also have a protective role against cardiovascular disease in adults.[71]

Bilirubin Production in the Neonate

The usual destruction of circulating red blood cells (RBCs) accounts for about 75% of the bilirubin produced in the healthy term newborn. Catabolism of nonhemoglobin heme, ineffective erythropoiesis, and enterohepatic recirculation (enterohepatic shunt) account for 20% of the bilirubin produced in the term and 30% in the preterm infant.[74] In newborns the amount of nonhemoglobin heme is increased by heme from the large pool of hematopoietic tissue that ceases to function after birth.[59] Bilirubin produced by catabolism of nonhemoglobin heme and immature RBCs is sometimes referred to as *early* bilirubin.

The newborn produces up to 8 to 10 mg/kg/day of bilirubin (more than twice as much as adults).[74] Bilirubin production is inversely correlated with gestational age and remains higher (per kilogram) for 3 to 6 weeks.[59] Increased bilirubin production in the newborn is due to a greater circulating RBC volume per kilogram (and subsequent breakdown of senescent cells), decreased RBC life span (80 to 100 days in term, 60 to 80 days in preterm, and 35 to 50 days in extremely low–birth weight [ELBW] infants, versus 120 days in adults), increased numbers of immature or fragile cells, and an increase in early bilirubin.[51,74]

Levels of unbound bilirubin are also higher in the newborn, and more so in the preterm infant, because of lower albumin concentrations, decreased albumin-binding capacity, and decreased affinity of albumin for bilirubin.[4,23,21,59] This may be due to a maturational defect in albumin structure, or endogenous metabolic products produced during periods of stress or abnormal metabolism may block or interfere with albumin-binding sites.[22] Bilirubin processing (conjugation) by the liver and excretion are also altered in the newborn (see Causes of Physiologic Jaundice).

Physiologic Jaundice

Physiologic jaundice in the newborn is seen in 50% to 60% of term infants and up to 80% of preterm infants during the first days after birth.[59,74] Visible jaundice in neonates usually appears as the bilirubin levels reach 5 to 6 mg/dL (85.5 to 103 μmol/L).[59] Almost all term infants develop bilirubin levels over 2 mg/dL (34.2 μmol/L) in the first week and two thirds or more develop clinical jaundice.[71] Neonatal jaundice accounts for 75% of hospital readmissions in the first week after birth.[86]

Patterns of Physiologic Jaundice

The usual pattern of bilirubin change is a two-phase process.[38,39,59] These general phases are seen in term and preterm infants and in breastfed and formula-fed infants, although characteristics of the phases vary depending on gestation, ethnicity and method of feeding. Phase I is primarily secondary to the reduced hepatic UGT1A1 activity and phase II to low levels of ligandin binding.[51] During phase I in white and African-American term infants, total bilirubin levels peak at 48 to 120 hours (most infants peak at 72 to 96 hours) at 5 to 6 mg/dL (86 to 103 μmol/L) and then decrease to less than 3 mg/dL (51 μmol/L) by day 5.[59] Infant of East Asian ethnicity usually peak slightly later (72 to 120 hours) at 10 to 14 mg/dL (171 to 239 μmol/L), and fall to less than 3 mg/dL (51 μmol/L) by 7 to 10 days.[59] All groups gradually fall to adult values of less than 2 mg/dL (34 μmol/L) over the first 1 to 2 weeks (phase II).

The reason for the increased bilirubin levels in infants of East Asian ethnicity is not known, although there is some evidence to suggest that their rate of bilirubin synthesis may be slightly elevated.[59] These infants are also more likely to have glucose-6-phosphate dehydrogenase (G6PD) deficiency. In addition, genomic polymorphisms (variations in gene sequencing) in the genes involved in bilirubin production and conjugation are seen with greater frequency.[59,129] Polymorphisms in these genes increase the risk of hyperbilirubinemia and are seen in other infants as well. For example, alterations in UGT1A1, which is involved in bilirubin conjugation, and soluble carrier organic anion transporter polypeptide (SLCO1B1), which is involved in uptake of unconjugated bilirubin by the hepatocyte, alone or in conjunction with environmental influences can alter bilirubin clearance and increase the risk of hyperbilirubinemia.[129]

Patterns of physiologic jaundice in term breastfed infants are similar to phases in term formula-fed infants, except that the peak is higher (may be up to 7 to 14 mg/dL [119.7 to 239.4 μmol/L]) and later and phases I and II are longer. This difference is due in part to a delay in UGT1A1 maturation. In these infants, bilirubin levels generally decrease over 2 to 4 weeks, although it may take up to 6 weeks.[51,59,74]

Preterm infants also have two phases with a higher peak and longer phase I and II. The mean peak total bilirubin is 10 to 12 mg/dL (171 to 205 μmol/L) by day 5.[59] These patterns are only seen if early prophylactic phototherapy is not used. The greater the immaturity of the infant, the greater the alterations in phases and the risk of hyperbilirubinemia. Maisels suggests that the term *physiologic jaundice* has little usefulness with preterm and especially very low–birth weight (VLBW) infants since these infants are treated with phototherapy even at physiologic levels.[74]

Causes of Physiologic Jaundice

Physiologic jaundice is not caused by a single factor, but rather reflects a combination of factors related to the newborn's physiologic maturity (Table 18-1 and Figure 18-2). The increased levels of circulating indirect bilirubin in the newborn are due to the combination of increased bilirubin availability and decreased clearance. Phase I bilirubin elevations are primarily due to a sixfold increase in bilirubin load, decreased bilirubin-specific hepatic UGT1A1 activity, and increased enterohepatic shunting.[59] Phase II elevations are primarily due to the continuing high bilirubin load from increased reabsorption of bilirubin by the enterohepatic shunt (see Figure 18-1), increased bilirubin production, and

Table 18-1 Factors Associated with the Development of Physiologic Jaundice

BASIS	CAUSES
Increased bilirubin availability	
Increased bilirubin production	Increased red blood cells (RBCs) Decreased RBC lifespan Increased early bilirubin
Increased recirculation via enterohepatic shunting	Increased β-glucuronidase activity Absent bacterial flora Delayed passage of meconium
Decreased clearance of bilirubin:	
Decreased clearance from plasma	Deficiency of carrier proteins
Decreased hepatic metabolism	Decreased uridine diphosphate-glucurosyltransferase (UDPGT1A1) activity

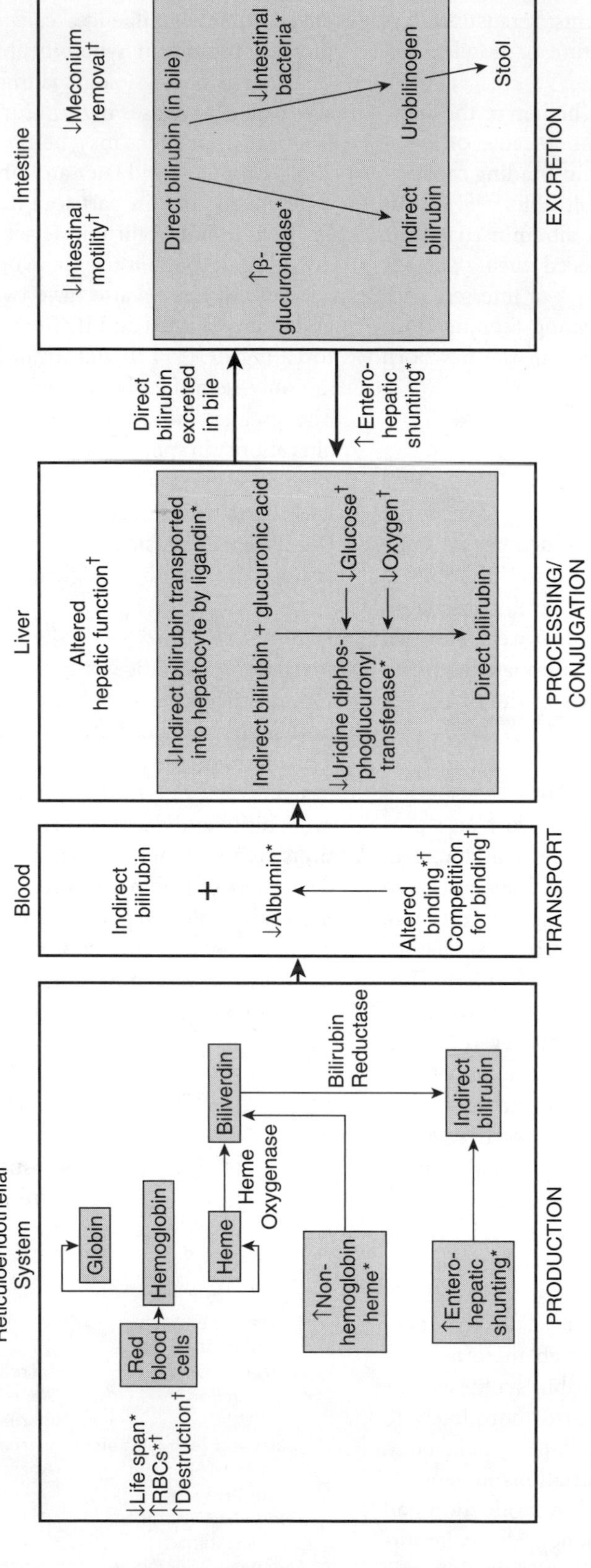

FIGURE 18-2 Basis for increased bilirubin levels in the newborn.

decreased hepatic uptake of bilirubin.[39] Table 18-2 lists other factors associated with the development of increased bilirubin levels in newborns.

Increased bilirubin availability results from greater bilirubin production (with more RBCs per kilogram), decreased RBC life span, and greater early bilirubin. Active recirculation of bilirubin by the enterohepatic shunt also raises serum indirect bilirubin levels (see Figure 18-1 and Box 18-1 on page 609). Increased recirculation of bilirubin is promoted by reduced bacterial flora (which normally further metabolizes direct bilirubin for excretion in feces), high levels of β-glucuronidase activity (which deconjugates direct bilirubin back into indirect bilirubin), and decreased intestinal motility. Concentrations of β-glucuronidase, an intestinal brush border enzyme, are 10 times higher in newborns than in adults, in whom little bilirubin is normally reabsorbed from the small intestine.[51]

The longer direct bilirubin remains in the small intestine, the greater the likelihood it will be deconjugated. Thus infants who are fed earlier (before 4 hours of age versus after 24 hours) or fed more frequently, and infants with meconium staining or early passage of meconium tend to have a lower incidence of physiologic jaundice.[17,38] Formula-fed infants tend to excrete more bilirubin in their meconium during the first 3 days after birth than breastfed infants. Among breastfed infants, bilirubin levels tend to be lower in those who defecate more frequently.[28] Infants with delayed passage of meconium, meconium ileus, or intestinal obstructions are more likely to develop physiologic jaundice. Recirculated bilirubin puts an additional load on an already stressed and functionally immature liver.

Clearance of bilirubin from the plasma and metabolism by the liver are impaired in the newborn because of deficient ligandin (the main hepatocyte intracellular bilirubin-binding protein), reduced UGT1A1 activity, and diminished excretion by a liver overloaded with bilirubin. Levels of ligandin reach adult values by 5 days of age.[51,71]

UGT1A1 activity is 0.1% at 17 to 30 weeks, gestation and remains minimal (less than 1% of adult activity) from 30 to 40 weeks and during the first 24 hours after birth.[74,129] Activity of this enzyme increases rapidly after the first 24 hours, due to a gradual up-regulation of UGT1A1 activity. This up-regulation is seen across all gestational ages.[129] Activity is lower in preterm than term infants; however, increases in activity after birth are related more to postbirth age than to gestational age. The increase in bilirubin levels in the newborn infant help induce UGT1A1 activity and bilirubin conjugation in the liver after birth.[21] UGT1A1 activity does not reach adult levels for 6 to 14 weeks.[59,61,74,129] The major bilirubin conjugate formed in the newborn infant is monoglucuronide rather than diglucuronide, as in older individuals (see Box 18-1 on page 609). Monoglucuronide is more easily hydrolyzed to indirect bilirubin than diglucuronide, and only indirect bilirubin is reabsorbed across the intestinal mucosa via enterohepatic shunting.[39]

Hypoglycemia or hypoxemia may interfere with bilirubin conjugation. Decreased liver perfusion due to persistent patency of the ductus venosus may also impede clearance of bilirubin from plasma, particularly in preterm infants.[74] Hypoxemia further reduces blood flow to the liver and alters hepatocyte function. The ability of the newborn's liver to excrete conjugated bilirubin may also be decreased. This may be critical in disorders with large bilirubin loads (e.g., severe erythroblastosis fetalis) and leads to the direct hyperbilirubinemia seen in these infants.[59,74]

The preterm infant is more likely to develop physiologic jaundice and hyperbilirubinemia than the term infant. All of the factors previously described that contribute to physiologic jaundice in the term infant are more prominent in the preterm infant and are magnified with decreasing gestational age. For example, RBC life span is related to gestational age and may be only 35 to 50 days in the ELBW infant.

Table 18-2 Causes of Neonatal Indirect Hyperbilirubinemia

BASIS	CAUSES
INCREASED PRODUCTION OF BILIRUBIN	
Increased hemoglobin destruction	Fetomaternal blood group incompatibility (Rh, ABO) Congenital red blood cell abnormalities Congenital enzyme deficiencies (glucose-6-phosphate dehydrogenase deficiency, galactosemia) Enclosed hemorrhage (e.g., cephalohematoma, bruising) Sepsis
Increased amount of hemoglobin	Polycythemia (maternal-fetal or twin-twin transfusion, small for gestational age) Delayed cord clamping
Increased enterohepatic circulation	Delayed passage of meconium, meconium ileus, or plug Fasting or delayed initiation of feeding Intestinal atresia or stenosis
ALTERED HEPATIC CLEARANCE OF BILIRUBIN	
Alteration in UDT1A1 production or activity	Immaturity Metabolic/endocrine disorders (e.g., Crigler-Najjar disease, hypothyroidism, disorders of amino acid metabolism)
Alteration in hepatic function and perfusion (and thus conjugating ability)	Asphyxia, hypoxia, hypothermia, hypoglycemia Sepsis (also causes inflammation) Drugs and hormones (e.g., novobiocin, pregnanediol)
Hepatic obstruction (associated with direct hyperbilirubinemia)	Congenital anomalies (biliary atresia, cystic fibrosis) Biliary stasis (hepatitis, sepsis) Excessive bilirubin load (often seen with severe hemolysis)

G6PD, Glucose-6-phosphate dehydrogenase; *SGA*, small for gestational age.

The lower serum albumin levels in the ELBW infant may limit extracellular binding and transport of bilirubin when concentrations are high.[21] These infants often have delayed feeding, with a low caloric intake initially and slower intestinal transit time. Feeding provides a substrate for intestinal flow and bacterial colonization. A major factor contributing to the increased risk in the preterm infant is decreased UGT1A1 activity. Postnatal maturation of UGT1A1 and ligandin and canalicular transportation pathways for bile may be slower in ELBW infants.[21]

CLINICAL IMPLICATIONS FOR NEONATAL CARE

Alteration in bilirubin metabolism is a relatively common event during the first week after birth. Neonatal jaundice results from either physiologic or pathologic causes. Physiologic jaundice is a normal process in the first days after birth and is due to normal physiologic adaptations. Physiologic jaundice is seen in 50% to 60% of term infants and up to 80% of preterm infants. Pathologic jaundice is due to pathologic factors, such as Rh or ABO incompatibility, polycythemia, glucose-6-phosphate dehydrogenase (G6PD) deficiency, intestinal obstruction, sepsis, and other factors that alter normal bilirubin metabolism. Neonatal jaundice reflects an increase in bilirubin. At times these increases may reach levels that characterize hyperbilirubinemia. Readmission rates for treatment of jaundice have increased twofold to threefold in recent years and are higher in late preterm infants (born between 35 and 36 6/7 weeks' gestation).[14,22,74] In addition, although still rare, bilirubin encephalopathy and kernicterus continues to occur with breastfed and late preterm infants at higher risk.[22,42,53] This section addresses these issues and discusses the basis for phototherapy and other methods of managing hyperbilirubinemia. Guidelines for the management of neonatal hyperbilirubinemia are available from professional groups in several countries, including the American Academy of Pediatrics, the Canadian Pediatric Society, the United Kingdom's National Institute for Health and Clinical Excellence, and others.[7,19,29]

Neonatal Hyperbilirubinemia

Hyperbilirubinemia can be due to physiologic or pathologic causes or may be due to a combination of physiologic and pathologic causes. The risk of this disorder is increased in breastfed, late preterm, and preterm infants. Neonatal hyperbilirubinemia is of concern because it may be a sign of an underlying pathologic problem, such as hemolysis or sepsis, and because of its association with bilirubin encephalopathy and kernicterus.[16]

Neonatal hyperbilirubinemia is due to increased production or decreased hepatic clearance of bilirubin (see Table 18-2 and Figure 18-2). Significant hyperbilirubinemia within the first 36 hours after birth is usually due to increased production (primarily from hemolysis), because hepatic clearance is rarely altered enough during this period to produce bilirubin values greater than 10 mg/dL (171 μmol/L).[59,74] An increase in the hemoglobin destruction rate by 1% leads to a fourfold increase in the bilirubin production rate.

According to the American Academy of Pediatrics (AAP), the major risk factors for developing severe hyperbilirubinemia in late preterm and term infants are total serum bilirubin (TSB) or transcutaneous bilirubin (TcB) level in the high-risk zone on the bilirubin nomogram,[7] jaundice in the first 24 hours postbirth, blood group incompatibility with a positive direct Coombs test, other known hemolytic disease (e.g., G6PD deficiency), gestational age of 35 to 36 weeks, previous sibling who received phototherapy, cephalohematoma or significant bruising, East Asian ethnicity, and exclusive breastfeeding, particularly in infants with difficulties with nursing and excessive infant weight loss.[7] Any infant born prematurely is also at greater risk for hyperbilirubinemia, with the risk increasing with decreasing gestational age and the factors listed previously.

There is no consistent definition for neonatal hyperbilirubinemia; what is considered to be in that range varies with population characteristics and postbirth age. One definition is "an elevation of plasma bilirubin two standard deviations or greater than the expected mean values for the infant's age" or greater than 90th percentile values on the bilirubin nomogram.[7,22] Kaplan et al. define *unconjugated (indirect) hyperbilirubinemia* in the newborn as bilirubin levels greater than 20 mg/dL (34 μmol/L) and *conjugated (direct) hyperbilirubinemia* as bilirubin levels greater than 1.5 mg/dL (26 μmol/L).[59] With more diverse populations and increases in breastfeeding, total serum bilirubin (TSB) levels are higher than have been previously reported, and may approach values of 15 to 18 mg/dL (256.5 to 307.8 μmol/L).[22,56,74] Bhutani et al. calculated that about 1:10 infants will have TSB levels equal to or greater than 17 mg/dL (290.7 μmol/L); 1:70 will have levels equal to or greater than 20 mg/dL (342 μmol/L); 1:700 will have levels equal to or greater than 25 mg/dL (425 μmol/L); and 1:10,000 will have levels equal to or greater than 30 mg/dL (513 μmol/L).[14] Jaundice within the first 24 hours after birth; increases of more than 0.25 mg/dL/hr (4.3 μmol/L/hr), which is equivalent to greater than 6 mg/dL/day; and jaundice associated with other abnormal findings such as feeding problems, G6PD deficiency, irritability, hepatosplenomegaly, acidosis, or metabolic abnormalities are also of concern.[7,55,56,59] Infants with G6PD deficiency are at high risk for both hyperbilirubinemia and kernicterus. G6PD deficiency is an inherited X-linked metabolic disorder that is one of the most common genetic diseases in the world. G6PD is an enzyme that normally protects the RBC and other cells from oxidative injury and hemolysis.[55,116]

Investigators have attempted to predict the risk of later significant hyperbilirubinemia in healthy term infants before early hospital discharge.[5,7,12,110,124] For example, Alpay reported that a serum bilirubin level of 6 mg/dL (102.6 μmol/L) or greater in the first 24 hours after birth predicted nearly all healthy term infants who later developed significant hyperbilirubinemia and all who required phototherapy for bilirubin levels greater than 20 mg/dL (342 μmol/L).[5] Bhutani and colleagues developed an hour-specific nomogram by plotting total serum bilirubin levels with age in hours to identify infants at high, intermediate, and low risk of later requiring phototherapy.[12] They reported that no infant who fell into the low-risk area of the graph later required phototherapy. This nomogram has been incorporated into the revised AAP guidelines for management of hyperbilirubinemia in newborns of 35 weeks' gestational age and older.[7] In a comparison of the predictive value of predischarge bilirubin measurement with this nomogram and clinical risk factor assessment, Keren and colleagues reported that the predischarge bilirubin measurement was more accurate in identifying infants at risk for severe hyperbilirubinemia (TSB greater than 95th percentile) and generated a wider risk stratification.[63] Several investigators have noted that the factors most predictive of readmission for phototherapy are infants with a peak transcutaneous bilirubin greater than 75th percentile (or high-intermediate to high zone) on the nomogram, exclusive breastfeeding, and less than 38 weeks' gestation.[64,80] Concerns have been raised about methodological flaws in the development of the nomogram and the risks of false positives and, particularly, false negatives.[33]

Direct Hyperbilirubinemia

Direct or conjugated hyperbilirubinemia (obstructive jaundice), which is common in adults with jaundice, is rare in the neonate. A direct bilirubin greater than 1 mg/dL (17.1 μmol/L) with TSB levels ≤5 mg/dL (85.5 μmol/L), or TSB levels greater than 5 mg/dL (85.5 μmol/L) with the direct bilirubin equal to 20% of the TSB, are abnormal.[7] Elevations of direct bilirubin involve cholestasis and are associated with alterations in hepatic function and interference with excretion of bilirubin into bile or obstruction of bile flow in the biliary tree. In neonates this can occur with hepatitis, severe erythroblastosis, sepsis, biliary atresia, and inborn errors of metabolism, (including galactosemia, α1-antitrypsin deficiency, tyrosinemia, and cystic fibrosis), prolonged parenteral alimentation.

Breastfeeding and Neonatal Jaundice

The increased incidence of hyperbilirubinemia in the United States over the past 25 years has been attributed primarily to the increase in breastfeeding. The majority of infants with hyperbilirubinemia for which no specific cause can be found are breastfed.[86] Two forms or phases of neonatal jaundice are described in breastfed infants: the more common early (breastfeeding-associated) jaundice, and late (breast milk) jaundice. However, these forms overlap and may not be readily distinguishable from each other.[40,42,51,59,74]

The early-onset form, often referred to as *breastfeeding-associated jaundice,* is believed to be related primarily to the process of feeding.[38,42] The major factor leading to breastfeeding-associated jaundice is increased enterohepatic shunting due to lower fluid and caloric intake, less frequent feedings, stooling patterns, increased β-glucuronidase activity, and decreased formation of urobilins.[42,74,81] Decreased caloric intake results in increased fat breakdown for energy and fatty acid production that increases intestinal fat absorption and may indirectly interfere with UGT1A1 and ligandin.[74] When fatty acids reach the liver, they may inhibit UGT1A1 activity or saturate the hepatic protein carrier system.[27] The increased absorption of fat from breast milk may also increase intestinal bilirubin absorption. Breastfed infants produce lower weight individual stools, have a lower initial stool output, and have stools that contain less bilirubin than formula-fed infants.[74] Greater weight loss after birth and less stooling are associated with higher bilirubin production. These infants also have slower urobilinogen formation, possibly due to different intestinal colonization patterns after birth (see Chapter 13). Breastfed infants excrete less bilirubin in stools than formula-fed infants because more conjugated direct bilirubin is changed back to indirect bilirubin by β-glucuronidase, which has greater activity in breastfed infants.[28,42,43] Breastfeeding-associated jaundice is not associated with increased new bilirubin production or abnormal hepatic uptake or conjugation of bilirubin, suggesting that the most likely mechanism is increased enterohepatic shunting.[39]

Breastfed infants also develop a later onset, prolonged hyperbilirubinemia. The late-onset form is less common and is believed to be related primarily to attributes of breast milk that interfere with normal conjugation and excretion.[39,59] Many of these infants also have a history of the early-onset form of jaundice. Late-onset jaundice is characterized by increasing bilirubin levels after 3 to 5 days, peaking at 5 to 10 mg/dL (86-171 μmol/L) by 2 weeks, followed by a slow decrease in bilirubin values to normal limits over the next 3 to 12 weeks.[38,59] These infants do not have any signs of hemolysis or abnormal liver function.

The cause of late-onset jaundice in breastfed infants is unknown but has been attributed to the presence of specific factors in breast milk that appear to be minimal or absent in colostrum but appear in transitional and mature milk.[39] Although the specific factor or factors have not been identified, these may include the following: 3α-20β-pregnanediol (which may interfere with UGT1A1 activity or release of conjugated bilirubin from the hepatocyte); increased lipoprotein lipase activity with subsequent release of free fatty acids in the intestines; inhibition of conjugation by the increased amounts of unsaturated fatty acids found in breast milk; or β-glucuronidase or other factors in breast milk that may increase enterohepatic shunting.[39,41,59,74]

Prevention of Hyperbilirubinemia in Breastfed Infants

Hyperbilirubinemia in breastfed infants may be reduced by preventive interventions. Encouraging feeding soon after delivery will increase intestinal activity and begin establishing gut flora. Frequent feeding stimulates intestinal activity and meconium removal (less bilirubin for enzymes to convert back to the indirect form), and reduces enterohepatic shunting, and stimulates maternal milk production.[7,16,59] Infants fed in the first 1 to 3 hours after birth pass meconium sooner than infants fed after 4 hours.[17] Feeding stimulates the gastrocolonic reflex, increases intestinal motility, and stimulates meconium passage (colostrum acts as a laxative). This removes conjugated bilirubin from the small intestine, thus reducing the likelihood that this bilirubin will be recirculated by the enterohepatic shunt.

A critical factor in reducing the risk of jaundice in breastfed infants seems to be enhancing breast milk intake.[7,37,38,42,59] Bilirubin levels in these infants tend to correlate negatively with breast milk intake; that is, as intake decreases, bilirubin levels tend to rise. Supplements should be avoided as they can interfere with establishment of breastfeeding.[7] If supplementation is required for medical reasons, supplementation with formula provides more calories. Supplementation of breastfeeding with water or dextrose water does not lower bilirubin levels in healthy breastfeeding infants. Supplemental feedings with dextrose water have been found to decrease breast milk intake, increase bilirubin levels, and possibly increase the risk of hyponatremia.[26,69] Dextrose water supplementation may satiate the infant but lead to inadequate caloric intake; caloric deprivation increases bilirubin levels.[38] Use of any form of supplementation can alter intake of breast milk and establishment of the mother's milk supply (see Chapter 5). Use of supplementation is associated with a significant decrease in the number of infants still breastfeeding at 3 months.[47]

An inverse relationship between the number of feedings per day and bilirubin levels has been reported.[27,28] Bilirubin levels were lowest in infants who were breastfed more than eight or nine times in 24 hours during the first 3 days after birth.[135] Increasing the frequency of feedings may stimulate gut motility and decrease intestinal absorption of bilirubin.[27] Current AAP recommendations are to breastfeed at least 8 to 10 times per 24 hours initially to ensure adequate milk intake.[7] Signs of inadequate milk intake include delayed meconium passage, fewer bowel movements (less than 3 to 4 stools per day by day 4), decreased urine output (less than 4 to 6 thoroughly wet diapers in 24 hours), and weight loss greater than 7%.[7,39,69]

Initial and continuing support of the mother and other family members is essential to enhance breastfeeding success.[73] The American Academy of Pediatrics (AAP) recommends that all newborns be seen by 72 hours if discharged before 24 hours of age, at 96 hours if discharged at 24 to 49.9 hours of age, and at 120 hours if discharged at 48 to 72 hours of age with earlier and more frequent follow-up for infants at risk for hyperbilirubinemia.[7] Some infants discharged before 48 hours may need multiple follow-up visits at 24 to 72 hours depending on their clinical status.[7] Several studies examining compliance with these recommendations have reported that only about one third of all newborns were seen in a timely manner after hospital discharge.[34,96,100]

Management of Hyperbilirubinemia in Breastfed Infants

Management of hyperbilirubinemia in breastfed infants is often challenging. Multiple issues and concerns, including maternal desire to breastfeed, advantages of breastfeeding to both mother and infant, effects on maternal-infant interaction, parental stress with the potential for bilirubin toxicity, and legal implications related to "safe" bilirubin values must be balanced.[59] This has been further complicated by the continuing reports of kernicterus (although still rare) in breastfed term and late preterm infants.[15,23,56,64,70,73,86,93] In the early 1990s, less aggressive treatment of hyperbilirubinemia in term infants was advocated and reflected in guidelines released by the AAP in 1994. One of the bases for these guidelines was the estimate that the risk of kernicterus in well term infants with bilirubin levels of 20 to 25 mg/dL (342 to 428 μmol/L) was lower than the risks associated with exchange transfusion.[93]

The AAP guidelines recommend that breastfeeding be continued whenever possible, but that supplementation with expressed breast milk or formula be considered if "the infant's intake is inadequate, weight loss is excessive, or the infant seems dehydrated."[7] Amato and colleagues report no difference in the time needed to reduce bilirubin levels with jaundice managed by discontinuing breastfeeding versus the use of phototherapy and continued breastfeeding.[6] Martinez and associates compared four interventions (continue breastfeeding and observe; discontinue breastfeeding and begin formula feeding; discontinue breastfeeding, begin formula feeding, and start phototherapy; and continue breastfeeding and start phototherapy) once bilirubin levels reached 17 mg/dL (291 μmol/L).[83] They found that if an adequate dosage of phototherapy was provided, there was no significant advantage to stopping breastfeeding.[83]

Maisels recommends that any interruption of breastfeeding be avoided, unless the infant develops bilirubin levels above 25 mg/dL (428 μmol/L), and rather to continue frequent breastfeeding (every 2 to 3 hours) while using intensive phototherapy, unless the infant's weight loss from birth is greater than 12% or there is clinical evidence of dehydration.[7,74] Lawrence emphasizes an approach, focusing on prevention and modifying factors (particularly inadequate frequency of feeding) that are associated with early-onset jaundice in breastfed infants (Table 18-3).[69] Any interruption of breastfeeding must be accompanied by parental emotional support and facilitation of breast pumping or manual expression of milk.

Measurement of Serum Bilirubin

Serum bilirubin levels are measured by laboratory and transcutaneous methods. Clinical estimations of serum bilirubin levels by the cephalopedal progression of jaundice are correlated with serum bilirubin concentrations in most but not all studies.[66,67,89] Cephalopedal progression is most useful at low bilirubin levels and is less reliable at levels greater than 12 mg/dL (205 μmol/L).[74] Knudsen suggests that the basis for this progression may be due to conformational changes in the bilirubin-albumin complex and in the binding affinity of bilirubin for albumin.[66,67] Indirect bilirubin leaving the reticuloendothelial system, where it is produced, binds to albumin. Initially binding affinity is lower with less effective

Table 18-3 Management Outline for Early Jaundice While Breastfeeding

1. Monitor all infants for initial stooling. Consider stimulating stooling if no stool in 24 hours.
2. Initiate breastfeeding early and frequently. Frequent short feedings are more effective than infrequent prolonged feeding, although total time may be the same.
3. Discourage water, dextrose water, or formula substitutes.
4. Monitor weight, voidings, stooling in association with breastfeeding pattern.
5. When bilirubin level approaches 15 mg/dL (256.5 μmol/L), augment feedings, stimulate breast milk production with pumping, and use phototherapy per the American Academy of Pediatrics guidelines.[7]

Modified from Lawrence, R.A., & Lawrence, R.M. (2005). *Breastfeeding: A guide for the medical profession* (6th ed.). Philadelphia: Mosby.
AAP, American Academy of Pediatrics.

binding, so bilirubin is more likely to be deposited in this area (i.e., in more proximal tissues). By the time bilirubin reaches more distal areas, it is more tightly bound and less likely to be deposited in the peripheral tissues unless bilirubin levels are high (overwhelming the available albumin-binding capacity).[66,67] Several studies suggest that visual assessment may be useful for deciding about which infants need a transcutaneous bilirubin assessment.[20,58,65,76,103] These assessments are not predictive of who will develop severe hyperbilirubinemia.[64] Thus laboratory assessments are also necessary.[56]

Laboratory methods involve measurement of total and direct bilirubin and calculation of indirect values. Total serum bilirubin (TSB) is the gold standard for assessment of neonatal jaundice.[70] Peak total bilirubin concentrations are poorly associated with development of bilirubin toxicity.[3] Plasma unbound bilirubin is a better predictor of abnormal outcomes, but more difficult to measure.[2,3,132]

Transcutaneous bilirubinometry is an alternative method that is most appropriate for screening and monitoring healthy term infants with physiologic jaundice because it avoids repeated heel sticks. These devices work by either calculating changes in light optical density between reflected light sources or measuring the amount of light reflected from light transmitted into the skin.[70] TcB is linearly related to laboratory measurements of TSB, especially in infants of more than 30 weeks' gestation.[7,13,20,32,50,70,74,121] TcB levels have been reported to also correlate with TSB in preterm infants but more study is needed.[107] Newer TcB instruments have a correlation that is within 2 to 3 mg/dL (34.2 to 51.3 μmol/L) of TSB if the TSB is less than 15 mg/dL (356.5 μmol/L).[56,59] This correlation is poorer once infants are under phototherapy. Other studies report that TcB levels significantly underestimate TSB in both term and late preterm infants, especially at higher bilirubin levels.[35,36,48,54,60,75] Measurement of TcB at the sternum has been reported to more closely approximate TSB than forehead measurements.[95] If therapy is being considered, a TSB should be obtained.[79] Universal bilirubin screening has been recommended by some, whereas others have noted the lack of evidence that this will prevent acute bilirubin encephalopathy and concerns about excessive use of phototherapy.[68,79,94,122,123] Implementation of universal screening has been associated with a lower incidence of hyperbilirubinemia, but increased phototherapy use.[122,123]

Serum albumin and bilirubin/albumin levels may also be measured in addition to the TSB and may be useful as additional data in those infants at risk for an exchange transfusion.[7] Lower albumin levels or low albumin binding of bilirubin suggests that these infants may be at increased risk for deposition of bilirubin in the brain. However, the bilirubin/albumin ratio does not correlate well with unbound bilirubin and significant differences can occur between newborns.[7] End-tidal carbon monoxide (CO) monitors have been evaluated to assess excessive bilirubin production due to hemolysis.[24,59,116,117,118] The breakdown of heme by heme oxygenase produces biliverdin and CO. CO binds to RBCs and is circulated to the lungs where the CO detaches and is exhaled. The amount of CO exhaled can be measured. These monitors have a low positive but strong negative predictive value, so they are not often used clinically.[56]

Management of Neonatal Hyperbilirubinemia

Various techniques have been used to manage neonates with indirect hyperbilirubinemia. Strategies have included prevention, use of pharmacologic agents, exchange transfusion, and phototherapy. Prevention has focused on early initiation of feedings and frequent breastfeeding to decrease enterohepatic shunting, promote establishment of normal bacterial flora, and stimulate intestinal activity. Specific pharmacologic agents have been used to prevent hyperbilirubinemia or reduce bilirubin levels.

Pharmacologic Agents

Pharmacologic agents have been used in the management of hyperbilirubinemia to stimulate the induction of hepatic enzymes and carrier proteins, to interfere with heme degradation, or to bind bilirubin in the intestines to decrease enterohepatic reabsorption. Inert nonabsorbable substances such as charcoal and agar have been tried for the latter purpose with equivocal results and are not recommended.[74] Intravenous immunoglobulin has been used with infants with severe Rh and ABO incompatibility to suppress isoimmune hemolysis and decrease the number of exchange transfusions.[7,51] Phenobarbital has also been used, although generally only with some rare forms of congenital hyperbilirubinemia.[59] Phenobarbital stimulates activity and concentrations of UGT1A1 and ligandin and may increase the number of bilirubin-binding sites.[74] β-glucuronidase inhibitors, such as L-aspartic acid and enzymatically hydrolyzed casein, and other nonabsorbable substances that bind bilirubin in the intestines (and thus possibly reduce enterohepatic shunting) have also been examined with further investigation needed.[43,59] Kaplan suggests that frequent breastfeeding may be as effective as these interventions.[59]

Prevention of hyperbilirubinemia with the use of synthetic metalloprotoporphyrins has also been investigated.[51,118,119,134] These substances are synthetic heme analogues. Protoporphyrin has been shown to be an effective competitive inhibitor of heme oxygenase, the enzyme necessary for catabolism of heme to biliverdin (see Figure 18-1), and the rate-limiting step in the formation of bilirubin. With use of these substances, the heme that is prevented from being catabolized does not accumulate but is excreted intact in bile.[51] In studies with both term and preterm infants, and in infants with and without hemolytic diseases, tin-protoporphyrin (Sn-PP) and tin-mesoporphyrin (Sn-MP) have decreased serum bilirubin levels and the need for phototherapy.[24,30,51,118,119,134] Use of phototherapy after the administration of Sn-PP has been associated with phototoxic erythema. Sn-MP is a less toxic variant, especially when used in conjunction with phototherapy. Studies continue with use of Sn-MP and other metalloprotoporphyrins such as chromium mesoporphyrin and zinc deuteropophyrin.[24,59,134] Long-term outcomes have not been established.

Exchange Transfusion

Exchange transfusions are used in the management of indirect hyperbilirubinemia and hemolytic disease of the newborn. An exchange transfusion removes antibody-coated blood cells and bilirubin and helps to correct the anemia associated with hemolytic disease. A two-volume exchange replaces 85% of the circulating red blood cell (RBC) volume and reduces the bilirubin by approximately 50%. Post exchange, bilirubin rebounds by up to 60% of pre-exchange values as bilirubin diffuses into the vascular space from extravascular tissues. The frequency of exchange transfusions has been significantly reduced with the availability of Rho(D) immune globulin (see Chapter 13) and phototherapy.

Phototherapy

Phototherapy was first introduced in 1958 and has been used extensively and effectively in treating neonatal indirect hyperbilirubinemia since the late 1960s.[25] Multiple studies have documented the effectiveness of phototherapy in preventing and treating neonatal hyperbilirubinemia.[74,77,91] Protocols are available to guide initiation of phototherapy in healthy term and late preterm infants (greater than or equal to 35 weeks' gestational age) and in preterm infants.[7,19,29,59,74]

Physics of Phototherapy. Absorbance of light by bilirubin is strongest in the blue light spectrum at about 460-nm wavelength.[104] Absorption of a photon of light excites the bilirubin molecule due to the accumulation of excess energy. In order to lose this excess energy, the bilirubin molecule can reemit the light photon (rare), use the excess energy to produce heat (accounts for about 80% of the excess energy), or the energy can alter the bilirubin molecule (about 20% of the excess energy) by photochemical reactions.[22] These photochemical reactions are photoisomerization and photo-oxidization. Indirect bilirubin is composed of four pyrrole rings. Photoisomerization involves conversion of poorly soluble indirect bilirubin into water-soluble reversible configurational (rearrangement of chemical groups in the molecule by temporarily disrupting the chemical bonds between carbon atoms in the molecule, resulting in a 180-degree rotation of the pyrrole rings) or irreversible structural (rearrangement of the atoms) photoisomers (i.e., photobilirubin, lumirubin).[51,59,104,125] The photoisomers can be excreted into bile without conjugation. Since these photoisomers are polar and need transporters to reach neurons, Hansen suggested that they are less likely to cross the blood-brain barrier than unconjugated bilirubin.[104] Formation of configurational isomers is rapid (nanoseconds), but these isomers are excreted slowly in bile, with a serum half-life of 12 to 21 hours.[51,85,90,105] By 6 to 12 hours after phototherapy has been initiated, 20% of TSB has been converted to configurational isomers.[105] These isomers are unstable and may be changed back into unconjugated bilirubin in the intestines and recirculated via enterohepatic shunting.

Lumirubin, a structural nonreversible isomer, is formed at a slower rate but is excreted in bile more rapidly with a serum half-life of 2 hours. Lumirubin is the major pathway through which bilirubin is eliminated during phototherapy. Lumirubin accounts for 2% to 6% of the TSB under steady-state conditions during phototherapy.[51,104,105,125] There is a dose-response relationship between lumirubin formation and phototherapy irradiance.[51] Formation of lumirubin is irreversible; it is excreted in bile or, to a lesser extent, in urine. Excretion of these isomers increases bile flow, which may stimulate intestinal activity and more rapid removal of bilirubin. As a result, phototherapy is often more effective in infants being fed and less effective in infants who are not being fed or infants with bowel obstruction.

Photo-oxidization has a minor role in elimination of bilirubin with phototherapy.[59,105] In this process the bilirubin molecule absorbs light energy from the phototherapy lights. Some of this energy is transferred to oxygen, leading to the formation of a highly reactive oxygen molecule (singlet oxygen). This molecule aids in oxidation and breakdown of bilirubin into water-soluble breakdown products (e.g., monopyrroles, dipyrroles) that are excreted primarily in urine. Decomposition of bilirubin under phototherapy occurs in the superficial capillaries of the and in interstitial spaces.

Side Effects of Phototherapy. Although many concerns have been raised about the safety of phototherapy and possible short-term and long-term effects, significant side effects are rare. Concerns focus on complications of photoisomerization and photo-oxidization; long-term concerns focus on irradiation damage, retinal damage (eye protection is always needed), and neurodevelopmental issues.[7,59] Investigations have generally failed to demonstrate any significant long-term problems with phototherapy usage in human infants and side effects are usually transient.[7,50,59] Transient effects include thermal and metabolic changes, hemodynamic changes, increased insensible water loss (IWL) and stool water loss, altered physiologic function and weight gain, skin and ocular effects, behavioral alterations, and hormonal changes (Table 18-4).[1,43,50,74] IWL loss may increase up to 25%, increasing the needs for fluids and monitoring. IWL is less with light-emitting diode (LED) units and slightly less with fiberoptic blankets.[59] Some infants with an elevated direct bilirubin and cholestasis develop bronze baby syndrome, which is characterized by a dark gray-brown discoloration of the skin, serum, and urine. This syndrome may be due to retention of bile pigments with accumulation of porphyrins and other metabolites secondary to impaired bile excretion due to cholestasis.[7,59]

Psychobehavioral concerns associated with the use of phototherapy include the potential effect of isolation and the lack of usual sensory experiences, behavioral and activity changes (including lethargy, irritability, and altered feeding behavior), and alterations in state organization and biologic rhythms as well as effects of parental stress (see Table 18-4). These concerns may influence parental perceptions of their infant and early parent-infant interactions.

Methods of Providing Phototherapy. Phototherapy can be provided using a bank of fluorescent lights, tungsten-halogen or quartz halide spotlights, high-intensity blue gallium nitride light-emitting diodes (LEDs), and fiberoptic blankets. Plexiglas covering lights protects against ultraviolet irradiation.[59] A bassinet system is also available that provides simultaneous phototherapy above and below the infant. Bilirubin blankets are woven fiberoptic pads. Halogen light beams are transmitted through a cord of fiberoptic filaments to a flexible pad that is placed beneath or wrapped around the infant. These pads remain at room temperature and deliver light within the 425- to 475-nm wavelength. In most studies, the fiberoptic pads have been shown to be somewhat less effective than single conventional phototherapy (in both term and preterm infants) in reducing bilirubin levels in infants with mild to moderate hyperbilirubinemia but more effective than no treatment.[59,74,87,125] A disadvantage of these pads is lower spectral power due to small surface area, making them less useful in treating infants with severe hyperbilirubinemia, unless used in conjunction with overhead bililights to provide intensive phototherapy. Tungsten-halogen spotlights cover a smaller infant surface area; therefore they also provide less spectral power than fluorescent bank lights.[74] High-intensity blue gallium nitride LEDs produce less ultraviolet light, infrared radiation, and heat, and the amount of blue-green light can be customized.[59,116,126] Because these units generate little heat, the unit can be placed a shorter distance from the infant to deliver high irradiances, thus enhancing lumirubin formation.[59,111,116,126]

An issue in caring for infants under phototherapy is whether to turn off the "lights" or remove the infant from under them during feeding and other caregiving. The benefits to both the infant and the parents of removing the eye shields and holding the infant during feeding seem to outweigh concerns regarding the effectiveness of bilirubin reduction in most situations.[7] The most rapid catabolism of bilirubin appears to take place within the first few hours after the start of each phototherapy period. It takes bilirubin about 3 hours to return to the skin after removal of photoisomers.[51] Thus for infants with mild to moderate hyperbilirubinemia, the irradiance, area of skin exposed, and initial effects of phototherapy on bilirubin in the skin seem to have more influence than whether the infant is removed for short periods of feeding or holding.[22,74] A significant post-phototherapy bilirubin rebound has been reported in infants who are preterm, have a positive direct Coombs test, or are under phototherapy for less than 72 hours.[57] Alternating positions from supine to prone while under phototherapy has not been reported to affect the pattern of decreased TSB.[31]

Effective phototherapy requires sufficient illumination over an adequate area of exposed skin at a sufficiently short distance to produce the desired effect of light on bilirubin molecules.[7,59] Therefore, the effectiveness of phototherapy depends on factors such as the spectrum of light delivered by the phototherapy unit, intensity of the energy output (power output) or irradiance, peak wavelength of the light delivered, and the surface area of the infant exposed to the light.[74,104] The surface area of exposure can be increased with the use of intensive phototherapy.

Irradiance is the radiant power of light on a surface per unit of surface area ($\mu W/cm^2/nm$). Irradiance is directly related to the distance of the light source from the infant.[74] Spectral irradiance—the irradiance of the light source (radiant power per unit area) within the therapeutic wavelength of maximum light absorbance by the bilirubin molecule (425 to 550 nm), not the intensity (i.e., illumination or brightness)—determines effectiveness.[74] Maximal absorbance of albumin-bound bilirubin is about 460-nm wavelength and 440-nm wavelength for unbound bilirubin.[59] The intensity of the light is inversely related to the distance between the light source and the skin surface.[7,86] There is a significant linear relationship between the spectral irradiance received by the infant and the decrease in serum bilirubin levels over a 24-hour period.[7,46,74]

Phototherapy units vary in effectiveness, and light emission may decrease over time. Irradiance levels can be monitored with a radiometer using the instructions in equipment manuals or unit protocol. The radiometer has a wide bandwidth so that the effective irradiance of the phototherapy unit (as amount of blue light) can be measured. Measurement is in $\mu W/cm^2/nm$ and evaluates the spectral irradiance. A spectral irradiance of 6 $\mu W/cm^2/nm$ in the 425- to 475-nm waveband is sufficient for production of configurational isomers; however, for production of the structural isomer lumirubin, a higher spectral irradiance of 8 to 10 $\mu W/cm^2/nm$ is required.[7,22] A spectral radiance of 10 $\mu W/cm^2/nm$ should reduce the TSB 20% to 50% during the first 24 hours of therapy.[104] Intensive phototherapy requires a spectral irradiance of greater than 30 $\mu W/cm^2/nm$.[7,59] In comparing different devices, spectral

Table 18-4 Side Effects of Phototherapy

SIDE EFFECT	SPECIFIC CHANGES	IMPLICATIONS
Thermal and other metabolic changes	Increased environmental and body temperature Increased oxygen consumption Increased respiratory rate Increased skin blood flow	Influenced by maturity, caloric intake (energy to respond to thermal changes), adequacy of heat dissipation from phototherapy unit, distance of unit from infant and incubator hood (related to space for air flow and radiant heat loss), use of servocontrol
Cardiovascular changes	Transient changes in cardiac output and decrease in left ventricular output	Reopening of ductus arteriosus, possibly due to photorelaxation; usually not hemodynamically significant Hemodynamic changes are seen primarily in the first 12 hours of phototherapy use; after that, return to previous levels or higher
Fluid status	Increased peripheral blood flow	Increases fluid loss May alter uptake of intramuscular medications
	Increased insensible water loss	Due to increases in evaporative water loss, metabolic rate, and possibly respiratory rate Influenced by environment (e.g., air flow, humidity, temperature); characteristics of phototherapy unit (e.g., heat dissipation, distance from infant); ambient temperature alteration; infant alterations in skin and core temperature, heart rate, respiratory rate, metabolic rate, caloric intake; type of bed (increased with radiant warmer and incubator)
Gastrointestinal function	Increased number, frequency of stools	May be related to increased bile flow, which stimulates gastrointestinal activity
	Watery, greenish brown stools	Increases stool water loss
	Decreased time for intestinal transit	Increases stool water loss and risk of dehydration
	Decreased absorption; retention of nitrogen, water, electrolytes	Transient alterations in fluids and electrolytes
	Altered lactose activity, riboflavin	Temporary lactose intolerance with decreased lactase at epithelial brush border and increased frequency and water content of stools
Altered activity	Lethargy or irritability Decreased eagerness to feed	May impact parent-infant interaction May alter fluid and caloric intake
Altered weight gain	Decreased initially but generally catches up in 2 to 4 weeks	Due to poor feeding and increased gastrointestinal losses
Ocular effects	Not documented in humans, but continued concerns about effects of light versus effect of eye patches	Lack of appropriate sensory input and stimulation Eye patches may increase risk of infection, corneal abrasion, and increased intracranial pressure if they are too tight
Skin changes	Tanning	Due to induction of melanin synthesis or dispersion by ultraviolet light
	Rashes	Due to injury to skin mast cells with release of histamine; erythema from ultraviolet light
	Burns	From excessive exposure to short-wave emissions from fluorescent light
	Bronze baby syndrome	Due to interaction of phototherapy and cholestasis jaundice, producing a brown pigment (bilifuscin) that stains the skin; reversible change which may take months to resolve
Endocrine changes	Alterations in serum gonadotropins (increased luteinizing hormone and follicle-stimulating hormone)	Significance unclear
Hematologic changes	Increased rate of platelet turnover	May be a problem in infants with low platelets and sepsis
	Injury to circulating red blood cells with decreased potassium and increased adenosine triphosphate activity	May lead to hemolysis, increased energy needs
Psychobehavioral concerns	Isolation or lack of usual sensory experiences, including visual deprivation	Impact can be mediated by provision of appropriate nursing care
	Alteration in state organization and neurobehavioral organization	May interfere with parent-infant interaction and increase parental stress May also affect circadian rhythms (unclear)

power may be a more useful measure since it measures the average spectral irradiance across the skin surface area of the infant.[74]

For phototherapy to be effective, light photons must penetrate the skin and be absorbed by bilirubin molecules. Only certain wavelengths are absorbed by bilirubin; longer waves penetrate deeper into the skin. Light wavelengths in the blue-green spectrum (425 to 550 nm) are most effective in reducing bilirubin levels. Daylight white, blue, green, and special blue (super blue) fluorescent bulbs have been used in conventional phototherapy devices. Special blue (narrow spectrum) bulbs are the most effective because they provide more irradiance at 450 nm (maximal blue wavelength absorbance).[74] Green light favors formation of lumirubin, and its longer waves penetrate farther into the skin.[51,86] Blue-green lights found in LED devices may thus be advantageous.[111]

Intensive phototherapy is used for infants with severe hyperbilirubinemia to produce irradiance in the 430- to 490-nm wavelength with an irradiance of greater than 30 μW/cm²/nm.[7] By using multiple (fluorescent or halogen) phototherapy units or combining overhead phototherapy with fiberoptic blankets or using special blue lights on an uninterrupted schedule, over as much of the infant's body as possible, the intensity and thus effectiveness of phototherapy can be increased.[59,74] Simultaneous use of overhead phototherapy and fiberoptic blankets increases the surface area exposed to light and spectral irradiance, which can also increase effectiveness. As compared to single phototherapy, double phototherapy has been reported to be twice as effective in preterm infants and 50% more effective in term infants.[106,120] Although use of special blue fluorescent bulbs is most effective in reducing bilirubin levels, these lights can interfere with skin color assessment and are associated with reports of nausea and dizziness in caregivers.[59] Exposure can be increased by using a reflective surface (such as a white sheet) around the incubator or bassinet or two to three fiberoptic blankets to cover more surface area.[59,74] The spectral irradiance can also be increased by placing the lights at the minimum safe distance from the infant's surface.[59] Care must be taken to keep all phototherapy lights, halogen lights in particular, at the manufacturer's recommended distance from the infant's skin, because these lights can cause burns if too close.[51,74]

Competition for Albumin Binding

Most indirect bilirubin is transported in plasma bound to albumin (1 g albumin binds 8.5 to 10 mg of bilirubin). Two terms used to describe albumin binding are *capacity* and *affinity*. Each molecule of albumin has a certain number of binding sites available (the binding capacity). The tightness by which bilirubin is bound to sites available for binding is the affinity. Avidity increases with increasing plasma albumin concentration as well as the ability of the albumin to bind bilirubin.[3]

In adults, each molecule of albumin can bind at least two molecules of bilirubin, with the first molecule bound more tightly.[59] Binding sites may be primary (tight or high affinity) or secondary (weak affinity). Each albumin molecule has one primary binding site and one or more secondary sites. If the primary site is saturated, there is a rapid increase in loosely bound or free bilirubin.[74] Albumin-binding capacity is lower in the neonate due to lower albumin levels and decreased albumin-binding capacities.[4,59] Albumin-binding capacity increases with both gestational and postnatal age and is impaired in sick infants.[11,130] Unbound bilirubin can leave the vascular system and enter the skin, brain, and other organs. Albumin-bound bilirubin does not enter the brain.[104] The unbound fragment of bilirubin is thought to be more closely associated with bilirubin levels in the central nervous system and risk of bilirubin encephalopathy than TSB.[2,59,131] An infant with a greater binding capacity may have a greater TSB, but lower risk of toxicity since more of the bilirubin is bound to albumin.[3] Various techniques have been developed to measure albumin binding of bilirubin, but to date none of them has been acceptable for widespread clinical management in terms of either application or interpretation.[2,22,59,74,85]

Many substances can influence bilirubin binding to albumin.[11] Competing substances easily displace bilirubin bound to secondary sites. Drugs such as sulfisoxazole and other sulfonamides, salicylate, chlorothiazide, ceftriaxone, rifampicin, indomethacin, certain x-ray contrast substances, and sodium benzoate (a preservative once used in some multiple-injection vials) may displace bilirubin.[22,51,59] Combinations of drugs may exacerbate these effects. Bilirubin also displaces some drugs (including ampicillin, phenobarbital, and phenytoin) from albumin (see Chapter 7).

Albumin binding of bilirubin can be altered by pathologic events. Plasma free fatty acids compete with bilirubin for albumin-binding sites.[51] Hypothermia increases metabolism and catabolism of fatty acids, which may displace bilirubin from albumin. However, the risk is minimal if molar concentrations of free fatty acids to albumin are less than 4:1.[51] Fatty acids are also elevated with sepsis and hypoxemia.[59,130] Although concerns have been raised about risks with the use of emulsified lipid solutions (e.g., Intralipid) in neonates, dosages of 2 to 3 g/kg every 15 hours produce fatty acid to albumin ratios of only 0.1 to 1.8.[74] The amount of unbound indirect bilirubin may also be increased if there is more bilirubin than available albumin because of excess production of bilirubin or decreased albumin (e.g., with malnourishment). Serum pH per se may not alter binding but may influence deposition of unbound bilirubin in the central nervous system.[74,104] Thus there may be an advantage to monitoring bilirubin to albumin ratios as well as TSB levels in determining the need for exchange transfusions.[7]

Bilirubin Encephalopathy and Kernicterus

Development of bilirubin encephalopathy and kernicterus is a concern for any infant with elevated bilirubin levels. These complications, although rare, still occur.[3,23,78,81] Early discharge, breastfeeding, and lack of adequate early follow-up may increase the risk.[3,23,78,81] Other infants at higher risk are late preterm infants, other preterm infants, male infants, and infants with low albumin levels and other factors that alter the blood-brain barrier, such as asphyxia, hypoxia, infection, and hypothermia.[7,22,78,79,97,125] Although the terms *acute bilirubin encephalopathy* and *kernicterus* are sometimes used interchangeably, acute bilirubin encephalopathy usually refers to early, acute clinical central nervous system symptoms of bilirubin toxicity, whereas kernicterus (or chronic bilirubin encephalopathy) refers to the chronic, permanent changes to the brain secondary to deposition of bilirubin in brain cells, with yellow staining and neuronal necrosis.[51,53,56,73,78,113] Another term used is *bilirubin-induced neurologic dysfunction* (BIND).[112,113] The risk of neurotoxicity is related to the amount of unbound bilirubin, blood pH, duration of exposure, and albumin-binding capacity; co-morbidities such as infection, hemolysis, and hypoxic-ischemic injury may increase the risk.[7,50,79,112,117]

Early signs of acute bilirubin encephalopathy, which is reversible in early stages, include progressive lethargy, poor feeding, vomiting, temperature instability, hypotonia, alternating hypotonia and hypertonia of the extensor muscles, and a high-pitched cry.[85,113,114] Many infants, especially VLBW infants, are asymptomatic in the neonatal period.[113] Signs of kernicterus include ataxia, opisthotonos, extrapyramidal disturbances, dental enamel hypoplasia of the primary teeth, deafness, seizures, and developmental and motor abnormalities. The neurotoxic effects of bilirubin are exacerbated by other pathologic conditions such as hypoxia, asphyxia, and hypercapnia.[51,55,74,113,114]

Bilirubin has a high affinity for phospholipids in cell membranes.[22] Although the specific effects of bilirubin on the brain are still unclear, acidic forms of bilirubin act as mitochondrial poisons that uncouple oxidative phosphorylation in the mitochondria, interfering with cellular respiration, blocking adenosine triphosphate (ATP) production, inhibiting cellular enzymes, and altering cerebral glucose metabolism, water and electrolyte transport, and protein synthesis, and damaging or interfering with DNA.[22,51,55,59,74,104,113] Some bilirubin may be produced in the brain and interference with its transport out of the brain (by alterations in the blood-brain barrier) may increase the risk of kernicterus.[59] Areas of the brain most often affected include the basal ganglia, brainstem auditory pathways, and oculomotor nuclei. The reason for the increased risk in these area may be related to increased blood flow and metabolic activity in these areas.[51] Some infants also have extraneural lesions, primarily in the renal tubular cells, lungs, adrenal glands, or gastrointestinal system.[59,74] Bilirubin toxicity may be prevented in individual cells by specific transporter proteins that maintain intracellular bilirubin levels at nontoxic levels.[92] Genetic differences in the expression and function of these proteins might lead to differences in susceptibility to the effects of unbound bilirubin and risk of kernicterus.[127,129]

In order for bilirubin to pass into neural tissue, it must cross the blood-brain barrier.[18] The blood-brain barrier has tight junctions between endothelial cells of the cerebral blood vessels. These junctions are permeable to lipid-soluble substances but usually are impermeable to water-soluble substances, proteins, and other large molecules (see Chapter 15).[51] Unbound (free) indirect bilirubin crosses the blood-brain barrier in both directions, although its passage is slowed by this barrier. Factors that influence the passage of bilirubin include the amount of free bilirubin, blood flow, the bilirubin-albumin dissociation rate, transit time in the capillary bed, permeability and surface area of the capillary epithelium, and perhaps energy-dependent and multidrug-resistant transporters such as P-glycoprotein.[131] Because indirect bilirubin is fat soluble, at high levels it accumulates in the brain, especially in the basal ganglia and in other areas with a high lipid content. The intact blood-brain barrier is normally impermeable to albumin-bound bilirubin.[56] However, if the blood-brain barrier is damaged, reversible alterations ("openings") in the blood-brain barrier (caused by infection, dehydration, hyperosmolality, severe respiratory acidosis, hypoxemia, or other injury) allow entry of albumin-bound bilirubin as well as increased movement of unbound bilirubin.[22,56,74,131]

The critical level of bilirubin beyond which brain damage occurs is not certain.[55] In addition, the role of small elevations of TSB in neurologic damage in the preterm infant is uncertain.[88] Most healthy term infants with kernicterus in the recent resurgence have had bilirubin levels greater than 30 mg/dL (513 μmol/L).[74] Ip and colleagues examined reports of outcomes of infants with kernicterus over 30 years and concluded that "kernicterus, although infrequent, has at least 10% mortality and at least 70% long-term morbidity. It is evident that the preponderance of cases of kernicterus occurred in infants with bilirubin levels higher than 20 mg/dL (342 μmol/L)."[50]

Reanalysis of data from the Collaborative Perinatal Project as well as follow-up studies of bilirubin in healthy term infants shows no consistent association between bilirubin levels, hearing loss, and neurologic abnormalities.[50,74,92,98] Most infants with hyperbilirubinemia do not develop neurodevelopment problems.[49] Low bilirubin values are not safe for all infants, because pathologic changes associated with bilirubin encephalopathy have been clearly demonstrated on autopsy at much lower values.[74,130] Factors associated with greater risk for developing kernicterus at lower bilirubin levels are prematurity, respiratory distress syndrome, G6PD deficiency, hypoxia, and acidosis.[7,21,22,79] However, there has not been a consistent pattern of hazardous bilirubin levels related to birth weight or gestational age with low-bilirubin-level kernicterus nor have serum bilirubin concentrations or treatment been significant independent variables affecting long-term neurodevelopmental outcome.[21,88,130] As a group, peak bilirubin levels in VLBW infants (less than 1500 g), are associated with an increased risk of hearing loss, altered psychomotor development, and possibly neurodevelopmental problems, although these findings are confounded by many co-morbidities in this group of infants.[74,88,128,130]

MATURATIONAL CHANGES DURING INFANCY AND CHILDHOOD

The bilirubin load tends to remain higher in infants for 3 to 6 weeks after birth. In older children and adults, visible jaundice may be noticed at bilirubin levels as low as 2 mg/dL (34.2 μmol/L). Bilirubin-specific UGT1A1) activity increases to adult values by 3 months of age.[59] Plasma levels of indirect bilirubin reach adult values by 2 to 4 weeks postbirth in most healthy infants.[22] δ-bilirubin, absent in the first two weeks, is seen in older neonates and children and is increased in children with congenital hyperbilirubinemia associated with liver problems.[59]

SUMMARY

Alterations in bilirubin metabolism that occur with birth result in one of the more frequent problems seen in the neonate: physiologic jaundice. These changes also interact with pathologic factors in the development of hyperbilirubinemia. Hyperbilirubinemia is of concern because it may be a sign of underlying pathologic processes, such as hemolysis or sepsis, and may lead to adverse consequences—namely, kernicterus. Therefore it is essential for caregivers to appreciate the processes involved in bilirubin metabolism and its maturation, to understand the basis for physiologic jaundice and hyperbilirubinemia, and to recognize infants at risk for these disorders. Clinical recommendations are summarized in Table 18-5.

Table 18-5 Recommendations for Clinical Practice Related to Bilirubin Metabolism in Neonates

Know the usual cord blood values for serum bilirubin (p. 610).
Know the usual patterns for serum bilirubin in term and preterm neonates, as well as breastfed infants (p. 611).
Recognize infants at risk for physiologic jaundice (pp. 611, 613-614, Figure 18-2, and Table 18-1).
Monitor fluid intake and stooling patterns (pp. 613, 615-616).
Assess and monitor infants at risk for physiologic jaundice (pp. 611, 613-614).
Recognize infants at risk for hyperbilirubinemia (pp. 614-615 and Table 18-2).
Know the substances and pathophysiologic events that may compete with bilirubin for albumin-binding sites and monitor status of exposed infants (p. 621).
Counsel and support the family of a jaundiced infant (p. 619 and Table 18-4).
Monitor breastfed infants for early and late hyperbilirubinemia (pp. 615-616).
Institute interventions to prevent early-onset jaundice in breastfed infants (pp. 615-616 and Table 18-3).
Counsel and support parents of a jaundiced breastfed infant (pp. 615-616).
Teach parents to monitor for hyperbilirubinemia and importance of health care following early hospital discharge (pp. 615-616, 621-622).
Plan with parents of term infants for follow-up care with the primary care provider after discharge (pp. 614-616).
Assess and monitor infants at risk for hyperbilirubinemia (pp. 614-615, 621-622 and Table 18-2).
Know the methods of monitoring serum bilirubin levels and factors that can alter accuracy of measurement (pp. 616-617).
Monitor infants during and after exchange transfusion for alterations in fluid, electrolyte, and acid-base status (p. 618).
Recognize and monitor for physiologic and psychobehavioral side effects associated with phototherapy (pp. 618-619 and Table 18-4).
Provide a safe environment for the infant under phototherapy (pp. 618-621 and Table 18-4).
Recognize infants at risk for bilirubin encephalopathy and kernicterus (pp. 621-622).
Monitor for signs of bilirubin encephalopathy and kernicterus (pp. 621-622).

References

1. Abrol, P., & Sankarasubramanian, R. (1998). Effect of phototherapy on behavior of jaundiced neonates. *Indian J Pediatr, 65,* 603.
2. Ahlfors, C.E., et al. (2009). Unbound (free) bilirubin (Bf): Improving the paradigm for evaluating neonatal jaundice. *Clin Chem, 55,* 1288.
3. Ahlfors, C.E. (2010). Predicting bilirubin neurotoxicity in jaundiced newborns. *Curr Opin Pediatr, 22,* 129.
4. Ahlfors, C.E., & Parker, A.E. (2010). Bilirubin binding contributes to the increase in total bilirubin concentration in newborns with jaundice. *Pediatrics, 126,* e639.
5. Alpay, F. (2000). The value of first-day bilirubin measurement in predicting the development of significant hyperbilirubinemia in healthy term newborns, *Pediatrics, 106,* E6.
6. Amato, M., Howald, H., & van Murah, G. (1985). Interruption of breastfeeding versus phototherapy as treatment of hyperbilirubinemia in full term infants. *Helv Paediatr Acta, 40,* 127.
7. American Academy of Pediatrics, Subcommittee on Hyperbilirubinemia. (2004). Management of hyperbilirubinemia in the newborn infant 35 or more weeks of gestation. *Pediatrics, 114,* 297.
8. Arrese, M., et al. (2008). Molecular pathogenesis of intrahepatic cholestasis of pregnancy. *Expert Rev Mol Med, 10,* e9.
9. Bacq, Y., et al. (1996). Liver function tests in normal pregnancy: A prospective study of 103 pregnant women and 103 matched controls. *Hepatology, 23,* 1030.
10. Belanger, S., Lavoie, J.C., & Chessex, P. (1997). Influence of bilirubin on the antioxidant capacity of plasma of newborn infants. *Biol Neonate, 71,* 233.
11. Bender, G.J., Cashore, W.J., & Oh, W. (2007). Ontogeny of bilirubin-binding capacity and the effect of clinical status in premature infants born at less than 1300 grams. *Pediatrics, 120,* 1067.
12. Bhutani, V.K., Johnson, L., & Silvieri, E.M. (1999). Predictive ability of a predischarge hour-specific serum bilirubin for subsequent significant hyperbilirubinemia in healthy term and near-term newborns. *Pediatrics, 103,* 6.
13. Bhutani, V.K., et al. (2000). Noninvasive measurement of total serum bilirubin in a multiracial predischarge newborn population to assess risk of severe hyperbilirubinemia. *Pediatrics, 106,* E17.
14. Bhutani, V.K., et al. (2004). Kernicterus: Epidemiological strategies for its prevention through systems-based approaches. *J Perinatol, 24,* 650.

15. Bhutani, V.K., & Johnson, L.H. (2006). Kernicterus in preterm infants cared for as term healthy infants. *Semin Perinatol, 30,* 89.
16. Blackburn, S. (1995). Hyperbilirubinemia and neonatal jaundice. *Neonatal Netw, 14,* 15.
17. Boyer, D.B., & Vidyasagar, D. (1987). Serum indirect bilirubin levels and meconium passage in early fed normal newborns. *Nurs Res, 36,* 174.
18. Bratlid, D. (1990). How bilirubin gets into the brain. *Clin Perinatol, 17,* 449.
19. Canadian Paediatric Society, Fetus and Newborn Committee. (2007). Guidelines for detection, management and prevention of hyperbilirubinemia in term and late preterm newborn infants (35 or more weeks' gestation), *Paediatr Child Health, 12,* 1B.
20. Carceller-Blanchard, A., Cousineau, J., & Delvin, E.E. (2009). Point of care testing: Transcutaneous bilirubinometry in neonates. *Clin Biochem, 42,* 143.
21. Cashore, W.J. (2000). Bilirubin and jaundice in the micropremie. *Clin Perinatol, 27,* 171.
22. Cashore, W.J. (2012). Neonatal bilirubin metabolism. In R.A. Polin, W.W. Fox, & S.H. Abman (Eds.), *Fetal and neonatal physiology* (4th ed.). Philadelphia: Saunders.
23. Centers for Disease Control and Prevention. (2001). Kernicterus in full-term infants—United States, 1994-1998. *JAMA, 18,* 299.
24. Cohen, R.S., Wong, R.J., & Stevenson, D.K. (2010). Understanding neonatal jaundice: A perspective on causation. *Pediatr Neonatol, 51,* 143.
25. Cremer, R.J., Perryman, P.W., & Richards, D.H. (1958). Influence of light on the hyperbilirubinemia of infants. *Lancet, 1,* 1094.
26. De Carvalho, M., Holl, M., & Harvey, D. (1981). Effects of water supplementation on physiological jaundice in breastfed babies. *Am J Dis Child, 56,* 568.
27. De Carvalho, M., Klaus, M., & Merkatz, R.B. (1982). Frequency of breast-feeding and serum bilirubin concentration. *Am J Dis Child, 136,* 737.
28. De Carvalho, M., Robertson, S., & Klaus, M. (1985). Fecal bilirubin excretion and serum bilirubin concentrations in breast-fed and bottle-fed infants. *J Pediatr, 107,* 786.
29. De Luca, D. (2010). NICE guidelines on neonatal jaundice: At risk of being too nice. *Lancet, 376,* 771.
30. Dennery, P.A. (2005). Metalloporphyrins for the treatment of neonatal jaundice. *Curr Opin Pediatr, 17,* 167.
31. Donneborg, M.L., Knudsen, K.B., & Ebbesen, F. (2010). Effect of infants' position on serum bilirubin level during conventional phototherapy. *Acta Paediatr, 99,* 1131.
32. Engle, W.D., et al. (2005). Evaluation of a transcutaneous jaundice meter following hospital discharge in term and near-term neonates. *J Perinatol, 25,* 486.
33. Fay, D.L., Schellhase, K.G., & Suresh, G.K. (2009). Bilirubin screening for normal newborns: A critique of the hour-specific bilirubin nomogram. *Pediatrics, 124,* 1203.
34. Feldman-Winter, L.B., et al. (2008). Pediatricians and the promotion and support of breastfeeding. *Arch Pediatr Adolesc Med, 162,* 1142.
35. Fouzas, S., et al. (2010). Transcutaneous bilirubin levels in late preterm neonates. *Pediatrics, 157,* 762.
36. Fouzas, S., et al. (2010). Transcutaneous bilirubin levels for the first 120 postnatal hours in healthy neonates. *Pediatrics, 125,* e52.
37. Gartner, L.M. (1998). Practice patterns in neonatal hyperbilirubinemia. *Pediatrics, 101,* 25.
38. Gartner, L.M. (1994). On the question of the relationship between breastfeeding and jaundice in the first five days of life. *Semin Perinatol, 18,* 502.
39. Gartner, L.M., & Lee, K.S. (1999). Jaundice in the breastfed infant. *Clin Perinatol, 26,* 431.
40. Girling, J.C., Dow, E., & Smith, J.H. (1997). Liver function tests in pre-eclampsia: Importance of comparison with a reference range derived for normal pregnancy. *Br J Obstet Gynaecol, 104,* 246.
41. Gourley, G.R. (1998). Pathophysiology of breast-milk jaundice. In R.A. Polin & W.W. Fox (Eds.), *Fetal and neonatal physiology* (2nd ed.). Philadelphia: Saunders.
42. Gourley, G.R. (2002). Breast-feeding, neonatal jaundice and kernicterus. *Semin Neonatol, 7,* 135.
43. Gourley, G.R., et al. (2005). A controlled, randomized, double-blind trial of prophylaxis against jaundice among breastfed newborns. *Pediatrics, 116,* 385.
44. Guyton, A.C., & Hall, J.E. (2010). *Textbook of medical physiology* (12th ed.). Philadelphia: Saunders.
45. Hammerman, C., et al. (1997). Antioxidant potential of bilirubin in the premature infant, *Pediatr Res, 41,* 157A.
46. Hart, G., & Cameron, R. (2005). The importance of irradiance and area in neonatal phototherapy, *Arch Dis Child Fetal Neonatal Ed, 90,* F437.
47. Herrera, H.A. (1984). Supplemented versus unsupplemented breastfeeding. *Perinatol Neonatol, 8,* 70.
48. Holland, L., & Blick, K. (2009). Implementing and validating transcutaneous bilirubinometry for neonates. *Am J Clin Pathol, 132,* 555.
49. Holtzman, N.A. (2004). Management of hyperbilirubinemia: Quality of evidence and cost. *Pediatrics, 114,* 1086.
50. Ip., S., et al. (2004). An evidence-based review of important issues concerning neonatal hyperbilirubinemia, *Pediatrics, 114,* e130.
51. Ives, N.K. (2005). Neonatal jaundice. In I.M. Rennie (Ed.), *Textbook of neonatology* (4th ed.). Edinburgh: Churchill Livingstone.
52. Jamjute, P., et al. (2009). Liver function test and pregnancy. *J Matern Fetal Neonatal Med, 22,* 274.
53. Joint Commission on Accreditation of Healthcare Organizations (JCAHO). (2001). Kernicterus threatens healthy newborns. *Sentinel Event Alert, 18,* 1.
54. Kamath, B.D., Thilo, E.H., & Hernandez, J.A. (2011). Jaundice. In S.L. Gardner et al. (Eds.), *Merenstein & Gardner's Handbook of neonatal intensive care* (7th ed.). St. Louis: Mosby.
55. Kaplan, M., & Hammerman, C. (2004). Glucose-6-phosphate dehydrogenase deficiency: A hidden risk for kernicterus. *Semin Perinatol, 28,* 356.
56. Kaplan, M., & Hammerman, C. (2005). Understanding severe hyperbilirubinemia and preventing kernicterus: Adjuncts in the interpretation of neonatal serum bilirubin. *Clin Chim Acta, 356,* 9.
57. Kaplan, M., et al. (2006). Post-phototherapy neonatal bilirubin rebound: A potential cause of significant hyperbilirubinaemia. *Arch Dis Child, 91,* 31.
58. Kaplan, M., et al. (2008). Visual screening versus transcutaneous bilirubinometry for predischarge jaundice assessment. *Acta Paediatr, 97,* 759.
59. Kaplan, M., et al. (2011). Neonatal jaundice and liver disease. In R.J. Martin, A.A. Fanaroff, & M.C. Walsh (Eds.), *Neonatal-perinatal medicine: Diseases of the fetus and infant* (9th ed.). St. Louis: Mosby.
60. Karon, B.S., et al. (2010). BiliChek transcutaneous bilirubin meter overestimates serum bilirubin as measured by the Doumas reference method. *Clin Biochem, 43,* 1009.
61. Kawade, N., & Onishi, S. (1981). The prenatal and postnatal development of UGT-glucuronyl transferase activity towards bilirubin and the effect of premature birth on this activity in the human liver. *Biochem J, 196,* 257.
62. Keitel, V., Kubitz, R., & Haussinger, D. (2008). Endocrine and paracrine role of bile acids. *World J Gastroenterol, 14,* 5620.
63. Keren, R., et al. (2005). Identifying newborns at risk of significant hyperbilirubinaemia: A comparison of two recommended approaches. *Arch Dis Child, 90,* 415.
64. Keren, R., et al. (2008). A comparison of alternative risk-assessment strategies for predicting significant neonatal hyperbilirubinemia in term and near-term infants. *Pediatrics, 121,* e170.
65. Keren, R., et al. (2009). Visual assessment of jaundice in term and late preterm infants, *Arch Dis Child Fetal Neonatal Ed, 94,* F317.
66. Knudsen, A. (1990). The cephalocaudal progression of jaundice in newborns in relation of transfer of bilirubin from plasma to skin. *Early Hum Dev, 22,* 23.
67. Knudsen, A. (1991). The influence of the reserve albumin concentration and pH on the cephalocaudal progression of jaundice in newborns. *Early Hum Dev, 25,* 37.
68. Kuzniewicz, M.W., et al. (2009). Impact of universal bilirubin screening on severe hyperbilirubinemia and phototherapy use. *Pediatrics, 124,* 1031.
69. Lawrence, R.A. (2011). *Breastfeeding: A guide for the medical profession (7th ed.).* Philadelphia: Saunders.

70. Lease, M., & Whalen, B. (2010). Assessing jaundice in infants of 35-week gestation and greater. *Curr Opin Pediatr, 22,* 352.
71. Macias, R.I., Marin, J.J., & Serrano, M.A. (2009). Excretion of biliary compounds during intrauterine life. *World J Gastroenterol, 15,* 817.
72. Mackillop, L., & Williamson, C. (2010). Liver disease in pregnancy. *Postgrad Med J, 86,* 160.
73. Maisels, M.J., & Newman, T.B. (1998). Jaundice in full-term and near-term babies who leave the hospital within 36 hours. The pediatrician's nemesis. *Clin Perinatol, 25,* 295.
74. Maisels, M.J. (2005). Jaundice. In M.G. MacDonald, M.M.K. Seshia, & M.D. Mullett (Eds.), *Avery's Neonatology: Pathophysiology and management of the newborn* (6th ed.). Philadelphia: Lippincott Williams & Wilkins.
75. Maisels, M.J. (2006). Transcutaneous bilirubinometry. *NeoReviews, 7,* e217.
76. Maisels, M.J., & Kring, E. (2006). Transcutaneous bilirubin levels in the first 96 hours in a normal newborn population of ≥ 35 weeks' gestation. *Pediatrics, 117,* 1169.
77. Maisels, M.J., & McDonagh, A.F. (2008). Phototherapy for neonatal jaundice. *N Engl J Med, 358,* 920.
78. Maisels, M.J. (2009). Neonatal hyperbilirubinemia and kernicterus—not gone but sometimes forgotten. *Early Hum Dev, 85,* 727.
79. Maisels, M.J., et al. (2009). Hyperbilirubinemia in the newborn infant ≥35 weeks' gestation: An update with clarifications. *Pediatrics, 124,* 1193.
80. Maisels, M.J., et al. (2009). Routine transcutaneous bilirubin measurements combined with clinical risk factors improve the prediction of subsequent hyperbilirubinemia. *J Perinatol, 29,* 612.
81. Maisels, M.J. (2010). Screening and early postnatal management strategies to prevent hazardous hyperbilirubinemia in newborns of 35 or more weeks of gestation. *Semin Fetal Neonatal Med, 15,* 129.
82. Marin, J.J., et al. (2008). Molecular bases of the fetal liver-placenta-maternal liver excretory pathway for cholephilic compounds. *Liver Int, 28,* 435.
83. Martinez, J.C., et al. (1993). Hyperbilirubinemia in the breast-fed newborn: A controlled trial of four interventions. *Pediatrics, 91,* 470.
84. McDonagh, A.F. (1990). Is bilirubin good for you? *Clin Perinatol, 17,* 359.
85. McDonagh, A.F. (2010). Controversies in bilirubin biochemistry and their clinical relevance. *Semin Fetal Neonatal Med, 15,* 141.
86. Melton, K., & Akinbi, H.T. (1999). Neonatal jaundice: Strategies to reduce bilirubin-induced complications. *Postgrad Med, 106,* 167.
87. Mills, J.F., & Tudehope, D. (2001). Fiberoptic phototherapy for neonatal jaundice. *Cochrane Database Syst Rev, 1,* CD002060.
88. Morris, B.H., et al. (2008). Aggressive vs. conservative phototherapy for infants with extremely low birth weight. *N Engl J Med, 359,* 1885.
89. Moyer, V.A., Ahn, C., & Sneed, S. (2000). Accuracy of clinical judgment in neonatal jaundice. *Arch Pediatr Adolesc Med, 154,* 301.
90. Mreihil, K., et al. (2010). Early isomerization of bilirubin in phototherapy of neonatal jaundice. *Pediatr Res, 67,* 656.
91. National Institute of Child Health and Human Development. (1985). Randomized controlled trial of phototherapy for neonatal hyperbilirubinemia. *Pediatrics, 75,* 365.
92. Newman, T.B., & Klebanoff, M.A. (1993). Neonatal hyperbilirubinemia and long-term outcome: Another look at the Collaborative Perinatal Project. *Pediatrics, 92,* 651.
93. Newman, T.B., & Maisels, M.J. (2000). Less aggressive treatment of neonatal jaundice and reports of kernicterus: Lessons about practice guidelines. *Pediatrics, 105,* 242.
94. Newman, T.B. (2009). Universal bilirubin screening, guidelines, and evidence. *Pediatrics, 124,* 1199.
95. Newman, T.B. (2009). Data suggest visual assessment of jaundice in newborns is helpful. *J Pediatr, 154,* 466.
96. Newman, T.B., et al. (2009). Numbers needed to treat with phototherapy according to American Academy of Pediatrics guidelines. *Pediatrics, 123,* 1352.
97. Oh, W., et al. (2003). Association between peak serum bilirubin and neurodevelopmental outcomes in extremely low birth weight infants. *Pediatrics, 112,* 773.
98. Palmer, R.H., et al. (2004). National Institute of Child Health and Human Development NICHD) conference on kernicterus: A population perspective on prevention of kernicterus. *J Perinatol, 24,* 723.
99. Pathak, B., Sheibani, L., & Lee, R.H. (2010). Cholestasis of pregnancy. *Obstet Gynecol Clin North Am, 37,* 269.
100. Profit, J., et al. (2009). Delayed pediatric office follow-up of newborns after birth hospitalization. *Pediatrics, 124,* 548.
101. Ramsay, M.M., et al. (2000). *Normal values in pregnancy* (2nd ed.). Philadelphia: Saunders.
102. Riely, C.A., & Fallon, H.J. (2004). Liver diseases. In G.N. Burrow, T.P. Duffy, & J.A. Copel (Eds.), *Medical complications during pregnancy* (5th ed.). Philadelphia: Saunders.
103. Riskin, A., et al. (2008). Is visual assessment of jaundice reliable as a screening tool to detect significant neonatal hyperbilirubinemia? *J Pediatr, 152,* 782.
104. Ruud Hansen, T.W. (2010). Phototherapy for neonatal jaundice—therapeutic effects on more than one level? *Semin Perinatol, 34,* 231.
105. Ruud-Hansen, T.W. (2012). Mechanisms of action of phototherapy. In R.A. Polin, W.W. Fox, & S.H. Abman (Eds.), *Fetal and neonatal physiology* (4th ed.). Philadelphia: Saunders.
106. Sarici S., et al. (2000). Double versus single phototherapy in term newborns with significant hyperbilirubinemia. *J Trop Pediatr, 46,* 36.
107. Schmidt, E.T., et al. (2009). Evaluation of transcutaneous bilirubinometry in preterm neonates. *J Perinatol, 29,* 564.
108. Sedlak, T.W., & Snyder, S.H. (2004). Bilirubin benefits: Cellular protection by a biliverdin reductase antioxidant cycle. *Pediatrics, 113,* 1776.
109. Sedlak, T.W., et al. (2009). Bilirubin and glutathione have complementary antioxidant and cytoprotective roles. *Proc Natl Acad Sci U S A, 106,* 5171.
110. Seidman, D.S., et al. (1999). Predicting the risk of jaundice in full-term healthy newborns: A prospective population-based study. *J Perinatol, 19,* 564.
111. Seidman, D.S., et al. (2000). A new blue light-emitting phototherapy device: A prospective randomized controlled study. *J Pediatr, 136,* 771.
112. Shapiro, S.M. (2005). Definition of the clinical spectrum of kernicterus and bilirubin-induced neurologic dysfunction (BIND). *J Perinatol, 25,* 54.
113. Shapiro, S.M. (2010). Chronic bilirubin encephalopathy: Diagnosis and outcome. *Semin Fetal Neonatal Med, 15,* 157.
114. Smitherman, H., Stark, A., & Bhutani, V. (2006). Early recognition of neonatal hyperbilirubinemia and its emergent management. *Semin Fetal Neonatal Med, 11,* 214.
115. Soares, M., & Bach, F. (2009). Heme oxygenase-1: From biology to therapeutic potential. *Trends Mol Med, 15,* 50.
116. Steffensrud, S. (2004). Hyperbilirubinemia in term and near-term infants: Kernicterus on the rise? *Newborn Infant Nurs Rev, 4,* 191.
117. Stevenson, D.K., et al. (2004). NICHD Conference on kernicterus: Research on prevention of bilirubin-induced brain injury and kernicterus: Bench-to-bedside—diagnostic methods and prevention and treatment strategies. *J Perinatol, 24,* 521.
118. Stevenson, D.K., & Wong, R.J. (2010). Metalloporphyrins in the management of neonatal hyperbilirubinemia. *Semin Fetal Neonatal Med, 15,* 164.
119. Suresh, G.K., Martin, C.L., & Soll, R.F. (2003). Metalloporphyrins for treatment of unconjugated hyperbilirubinemia in neonates. *Cochrane Database Syst Rev, 2,* CD004207.
120. Tan, K.L. (1997). Efficacy of bi-directional fiber-optic phototherapy for neonatal hyperbilirubinemia. *Pediatrics, 99,* 5.
121. Thayyil, S., & Marriott, L. (2005). Can transcutaneous bilirubinometry reduce the need for serum bilirubin estimations in term and near term infants? *Arch Dis Child, 90,* 1311.
122. Trikalinos, T., et al. (2009). Systematic review of screening for bilirubin encephalopathy in neonates. *Pediatrics, 124,* 1162.
123. U.S. Preventive Services Task Force. (2010). Screening of infants for hyperbilirubinemia to prevent chronic bilirubin encephalopathy: Recommendation statement. *Am Fam Physician, 82,* 408.

124. Varvarigou, A., et al. (2009). Transcutaneous bilirubin nomogram for prediction of significant neonatal hyperbilirubinemia. *Pediatrics, 124,* 1052.
125. Vitek, L., & Ostrow, J.D. (2009). Bilirubin chemistry and metabolism: Harmful and protective aspects. *Curr Pharm Des, 15,* 2869.
126. Vreman, H.J., et al. (2008). Standardized bench method for evaluating the efficacy of phototherapy devices. *Acta Paediatr, 97,* 308.
127. Watchko, J.F., Daod, M.J., & Biniwale, M. (2002). Understanding neonatal hyperbilirubinaemia in the era of genomics. *Semin Neonatol, 7,* 143.
128. Watchko, J.F., & Maisels, M.J. (2003). Jaundice in low birthweight infants: Pathobiology and outcome, *Arch Dis Child Fetal Neonatal Ed, 88,* F455.
129. Watchko, J.F., & Lin, Z. (2010). Exploring the genetic architecture of neonatal hyperbilirubinemia. *Semin Fetal Neonatal Med, 15,* 169.
130. Watchko, J.F., & Maisels, M.J. (2010). Enduring controversies in the management of hyperbilirubinemia in preterm neonates. *Semin Fetal Neonatal Med, 15,* 136.
131. Wennberg, R.P., et al. (2006). Toward understanding kernicterus: A challenge to improve the management of jaundiced newborns. *Pediatrics, 117,* 474.
132. Wennberg, R.P., Ahlfors, C.E., & Aravkin, A.Y. (2009). Intervention guidelines for neonatal hyperbilirubinemia: An evidence based quagmire. *Curr Pharm Des, 15,* 2939.
133. Williamson, C., & Mackillop, L. (2009). Diseases of the liver, biliary system, and pancreas. In R.K. Creasy et al. (Eds.), *Creasy and Resnik's Maternal-fetal medicine: Principles and practice* (6th ed.). Philadelphia: Saunders.
134. Wong, R.J., et al. (2007). Tin mesoporphyrin for the prevention of severe neonatal hyperbilirubinemia. *NeoReviews, 8,* e77.
135. Yamauchi, Y., & Yamanouchi, H. (1990). Breast-feeding frequency during the first 24 hours after birth in full-term neonates. *Pediatrics, 86,* 171.

CHAPTER 19

Pituitary, Adrenal, and Thyroid Function

Pituitary, adrenal, and thyroid function and the hypothalamic-pituitary-adrenal (HPA) and hypothalamic-pituitary-thyroid (HPT) axes are critical for normal function and adaptation during pregnancy, growth, and development of the fetus, and adaptation of the newborn to the extrauterine environment. HPA axis function in the mother and fetus are closely interrelated with placental function. The hormones of the HPA and HPT axes (see Figure 2-7) are necessary for many body functions, for development of the central nervous system (CNS) and other growth processes, and for reproductive function. Disorders of these systems are associated with infertility, alterations in normal changes at puberty, and complications of pregnancy. Concentrations of HPA and HPT axis hormones are altered in pregnant women and neonates. In the neonate marked changes in adrenal and thyroid function occur with birth. This chapter examines changes in the glands and hormones of the HPA and HPT axes during pregnancy; development of neuroendocrine function in the fetus and neonate; and implications for the mother, fetus, and neonate.

MATERNAL PHYSIOLOGIC ADAPTATIONS

Pregnancy is associated with significant alterations in the morphology of the pituitary, adrenal, and thyroid glands. Concentrations of adrenocorticotropin (ACTH), corticotropin-releasing hormone (CRH), growth hormone (GH), cortisol, thyroid hormones (thyroxine [T_4] and triiodothyronine [T_3]), and thyroxine-binding globulin (TBG) are altered during pregnancy. Placental hormones, particularly estrogen, human chorionic gonadotropin (hCG), placental growth hormone, and placental CRH, and alterations in liver and kidney function influence these changes.

Antepartum Period

Hypothalamic-Pituitary-Adrenal Axis

Marked changes occur in the hypothalamic-pituitary-adrenal (HPA) axis during pregnancy, resulting in a state of increased HPA function.[77,113] (See Figure 2-7 for an illustration of the HPA axis.) These changes are mediated primarily by placental hormones, including placental ACTH, GH, and CRH. Maternal hypothalamic-pituitary function is discussed further in Chapter 2 in conjunction with the hypothalamic-pituitary-ovarian axis. Changes in the hypothalamus and pituitary during pregnancy are summarized in Box 19-1 on page 628.

Anterior Pituitary Function. The anterior pituitary is composed of six cell types, each of which produces different hormones. These types of cells and their major hormones include lactotroph (prolactin), corticotroph (pro-opiomelanocortin [POMC] and its derivatives including ACTH, β-endorphin, and β-lipotropin), somatotroph (GH), gonadotroph (follicle-stimulating hormone [FSH] and luteinizing hormone [LH]), and cells producing thyroid-stimulating hormone (TSH) (thyrotropin). The anterior pituitary gland increases in size and weight (from an average of 660 mg in the nonpregnant woman to 760 mg or greater during pregnancy) due to an estrogen-induced increase in the lactotroph cells.[32,35,86,93,97,151] The anterior pituitary also develops a more convex, dome-shaped surface, which may cause it to bulge upward in some women, compressing the optic chiasma.[32] For these women, this can result in a transient hemianopia. Changes in pituitary function during pregnancy are summarized in Box 19-1 on page 628.

In the nonpregnant woman, the prolactin-producing lactotroph cells make up approximately 20% of the anterior pituitary; this increases to around 60% during pregnancy.[151] Prolactin isoforms increase during pregnancy, with the non-glycosylated forms exceeding the N-linked glycosylated form that is most common in nonpregnant women.[32,151] The nonglycosylated form may be more bioactive and function to prepare the breast for lactation (see Chapter 5). Prolactin increases 10-fold during pregnancy to peak at delivery at 140 ng/mL (6068 pmol/L).[32,35,74,97] Most of the increase in maternal prolactin is from the maternal anterior pituitary, although prolactin is also produced by the maternal decidua. Decidual prolactin is found primarily in amniotic fluid; little enters the maternal circulation. Prolactin levels in the amniotic fluid peak in the second trimester at 6000 ng/mL (260,886 pmol/L).[32,35,151]

Corticotroph cells do not change in size during pregnancy.[151] However, ACTH secretion and plasma ACTH levels increase progressively, peaking during the intrapartum period (Figure 19-1), from approximately 10 pg/mL (2.2 pmol/L) in

BOX 19-1 Physiologic Changes in the Hypothalamic-Pituitary Axis during Pregnancy

Lactotroph hypertrophy and hyperplasia
Progressive increase in serum prolactin
Doubling or more of anterior pituitary volume
Decline in gonadotropins, luteinizing hormone, and follicle-stimulating hormone
Decline in pituitary growth hormones
Production of a placental variant of growth hormone
Increase in corticotropin-releasing hormone (CRH), mainly of placental origin
Placental corticotropin stimulating hormone activates maternal and fetal pituitary gland
Increased ACTH and cortisol
Increase in cortisol stimulates placental CRH and leads to hypercortisolism
Decline in thyroid-stimulating hormone in first trimester because of the thyrotropic effect of human chorionic gonadotropin
Decline in plasma osmolality by 5 to 10 mOsm/kg as a result of resetting of osmoreceptors for vasopressin release
Decline in osmotic threshold for thirst
Increase in metabolic clearance of vasopressin as a result of a placental vasopressinase

From Nader, S. (2004). Thyroid disease and other endocrine disorders in pregnancy. *Obstet Gynecol Clin North Am, 31,* 258.
ACTH, Adrenocorticotropic hormone; *CRH,* corticotropin stimulating hormone.

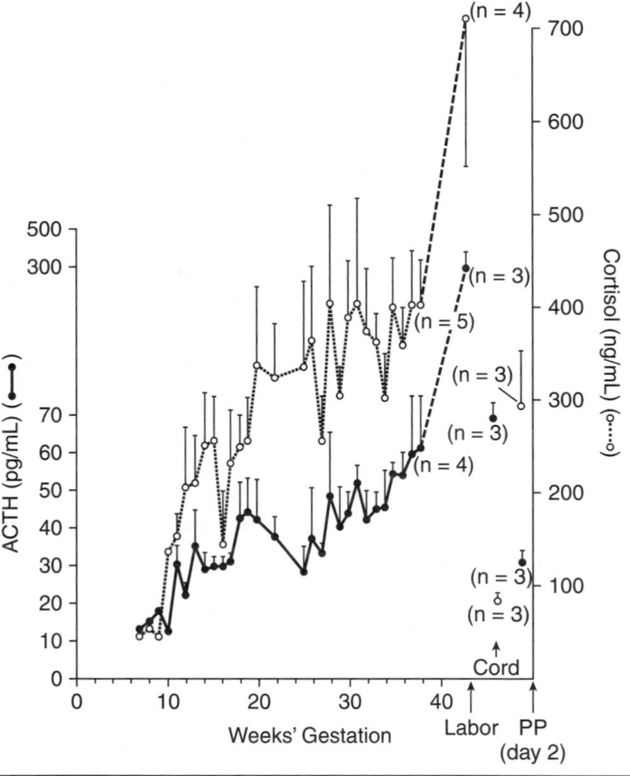

FIGURE 19-1 ACTH and cortisol concentration in maternal circulation throughout gestation. (From Carr, B.R., et al. [1981]. Maternal plasma adrenocorticotropin [ACTH] and cortisol relationships throughout human pregnancy. *Am J Obstet Gynecol, 139,* 416.)

nonpregnant women to 50 pg/mL (11 pmol/L) at term.[32,35,97,151] ACTH secretion is stimulated by CRH and, in turn, stimulates release of cortisol by the adrenal gland. Changes in ACTH parallel the increase in free and total cortisol (see Figure 19-1).[35,86] During pregnancy, the adrenal gland is more responsive to ACTH with a blunted HPA axis response to exogenous glucocorticoids.[77] There is a two- to fourfold increase in ACTH from the first to third trimesters, in spite of the increased bound and free plasma cortisol.[97] The increase in ACTH in the face of increased cortisol suggests a change in the set point for cortisol release that alters the ACTH-cortisol feedback loop.[44,97] ACTH maintains its diurnal variation during pregnancy, although this cycling may be blunted.[35,43,77,86,97] Placental ACTH increases in the second and third trimesters and it is unclear how much of increased maternal serum ACTH comes from the maternal anterior pituitary versus the placenta.[93] The effects of ACTH on the adrenal gland and changes in cortisol during pregnancy are described further under Adrenal Function.

The increased ACTH secretion during pregnancy is thought to be due primarily to increased placental (and some decidual and fetal membrane) CRH, rather than maternal hypothalamic CRH (Figure 19-2, *B*).[32,35,77,86,151,159] Other factors that may contribute to this increase are the decreased pituitary gland sensitivity to cortisol feedback, enhanced pituitary responsiveness to corticotropin-releasing factors such as vasopressin, and CRH.[77,159] Maternal serum CRH increases markedly beginning by 8 to 10 weeks and rises from prepregnant values of 10 to 100 pg/mL (47.6 to 476 pmol/L) to 300 to 1000 pg/mL (1429 to 4762 pmol/L) by the third trimester.[86,151,159] CRH-binding protein (CRH-BP) decreases the bioactivity of CRH throughout most of gestation. CRH-BP levels are similar to nonpregnant levels until the third trimester and then fall by two thirds during the last 6 weeks in preparation for birth. CRH has multiple roles in establishing and maintaining pregnancy and is produced by placental and uterine tissues in addition to the hypothalamus.[159] CRH plays an important role in the onset of parturition; increased CRH prior to term plays a role in preterm labor onset (see Chapter 4).[159]

Somatotroph and gonadotroph cells of the anterior pituitary decrease during pregnancy.[6] Hypothalamic gonadotropin-releasing hormone (GnRH) is suppressed in pregnancy by the elevated CRH, β-endorphins, and cortisol, with a blunted response of the pituitary to GnRH and low LH and FSH levels by 6 to 7 weeks.[159] By midpregnancy, LH and FSH levels are undetectable.[32,35,97,151] Gonadotropin function is described in Chapter 2. β-endorphins during pregnancy and the intrapartum period are described in Chapter 15.

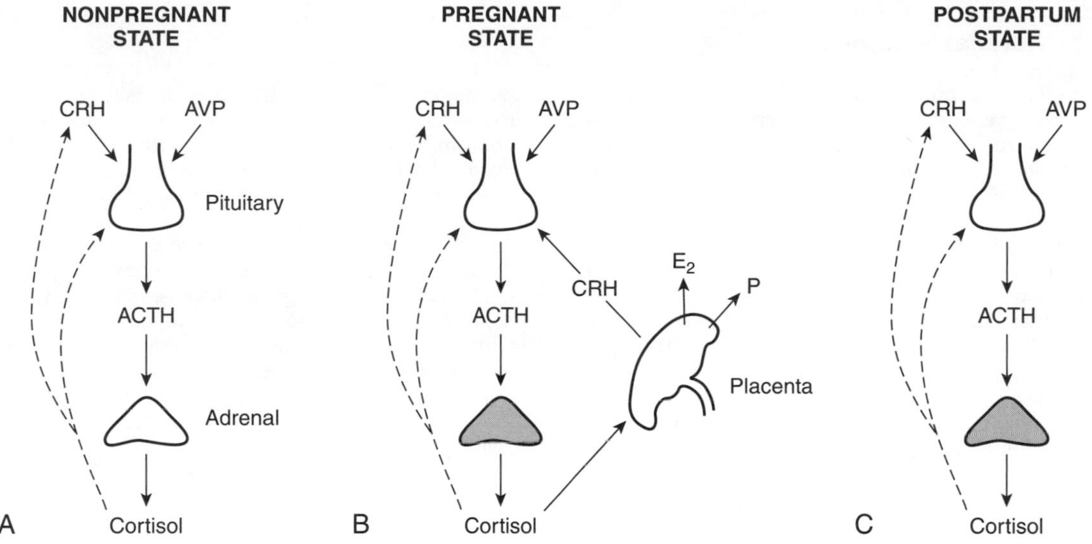

FIGURE 19-2 Schematic representation of the hypothalamic-pituitary-adrenal (HPA) axis in the nonpregnant, pregnant, and postpartum woman. *CRH*, Corticotropin releasing hormone; *AVP*, arginine vasopressin; *ACTH*, adrenocorticotropin; E_2, estradiol; *P*, progesterone. Shaded areas represent relative hypertrophy of the adrenals. (From Mastorakos, G., & Ilias, I. [2000]. Maternal hypothalamic-adrenal axis in pregnancy and the postpartum period: Postpartum-related disorders. *Ann N Y Acad Sci, 900,* 100.)

Pituitary GH (GH-N) decreases after the first trimester as placental GH (GH-V) increases.[35,93,97] GH-V is a GH variant that stimulates bone growth and regulates maternal insulin-like growth factor-I (IGF-I), which in turn alters maternal metabolism, stimulating gluconeogenesis and lipolysis.[93] GH-V is secreted continuously, as opposed to the pulsatile secretion characteristic of GH-N.[5] GH-N is the main maternal GH until 15 to 20 weeks; then it decreases and becomes undetectable by term. GH-V increases progressively from 15 to 20 weeks until term.[97] GH-V stimulates IGF-I, with negative feedback suppression of maternal GH-N.[5,32]

Posterior Pituitary Function. The major posterior pituitary hormones are arginine vasopressin (AVP) and oxytocin. Posterior pituitary function changes are associated with osmoregulatory changes and parturition. AVP levels are within normal ranges during pregnancy; however, the threshold at which AVP is secreted is reset so that AVP is secreted at a lower plasma osmolality during pregnancy (see Chapter 11) with a decline in plasma osmolality by 5 to 10 mOsm/kg below the nonpregnant mean of 285 mOsm/kg.[97,98] AVP also modulates ACTH release.[43] Oxytocin levels progressively increase during pregnancy, with further increase at term (see Chapter 4) and with lactation (see Chapter 5).[35,97]

Adrenal Function. Pregnancy is characterized by a transient hypercortisolism that begins by at least 12 weeks (see Figure 19-1).[59,86] Both total serum cortisol (the primary glucocorticoid) and free cortisol increase, with total cortisol peaking at levels three- to eightfold times higher by term.[97,127] Salivary cortisol increases twofold by 25 weeks and then plateaus to term.[21] The pregnant woman does not demonstrate signs of hypercortisolism because the free cortisol fraction is still within normal range.[21] Urinary cortisol increases at least 180% by term.[97] The diurnal secretion of cortisol—with higher levels in the morning versus evening—is blunted but maintained.[77,86,97] Physiologic responses to stress are maintained during pregnancy, but appear to be blunted.[21,159]

The increase in plasma cortisol parallels the increase in ACTH (see Figure 19-1). The increase in total cortisol is primarily due to an estrogen-stimulated increase in cortisol-binding globulin (CBG) that increases to two- to threefold during pregnancy.[97] Increased CBG reduces liver catabolism and clearance of cortisol, yielding a twofold increase in cortisol half-life.[86] The increase in free cortisol is also due in part to displacement of cortisol from CBG by progesterone.[35]

The adrenal gland becomes hypertrophic as the zona fasciculata (site of glucocorticoid production) widens, with no changes in the size of the zona glomerulosa or reticularis (see Box 19-2 on page 630).[35] Levels of aldosterone (the primary mineralocorticoid) also are markedly increased in pregnancy (see Chapter 11). Synthesis of androgens and dehydroepiandrosterone sulfate (DHEA-S) by the zona reticularis also increases, but less so than the glucocorticoids and mineralocorticoids. An increase in sex hormone binding globulin during pregnancy increases total and protein bound testosterone levels. Levels of free testosterone are low to normal to 28 weeks and then increase along with levels of androstenedione.[97] Maternal serum DHEA-S levels remain low due to placental uptake and metabolism.[44]

Hypothalamic-Pituitary-Thyroid Axis

Marked changes are also seen in the HPT axis during pregnancy. These changes occur primarily in the first half of gestation so that the woman achieves a new steady state in HPT function by midgestation that is maintained until

BOX 19-2 Adrenal Hormones

The adrenal gland is composed of the outer adrenal cortex and the inner adrenal medulla. The mature adrenal cortex is divided into three zones: zona fasciculata, zona glomerulosa, and zona reticularis. Although the adrenal cortex produces more than 50 steroid hormones, the major hormones are cortisol and aldosterone. The zona fasciculata is the site of glucocorticoid/cortisol production, which is regulated by corticotropin-releasing hormone (CRH) from the hypothalamus and adrenocorticotropin (ACTH) from the pituitary gland (see Fig. 19-2, *A*). ACTH is derived from pro-opiomelanocortin (POMC) precursors. Placental cortisol inhibits ACTH release and POMC synthesis. ACTH binds to membrane receptors on cells of the adrenal gland, activating adenylate cyclase. This increases movement of cholesterol, a precursor for pregnenolone, into the cells. Pregnenolone is metabolized in the smooth endoplasmic reticulum to cortisol, the main glucocorticoid. Glucocorticoids, primarily cortisol, are involved in the regulation of fluid and electrolyte balance, metabolism, vascular permeability, endothelial integrity, and blood glucose; maintenance of hemodynamic stability; increase with stress; and suppress immune functions.[27] The zona glomerulosa produces mineralocorticoids, the major one being aldosterone. Mineralocorticoids regulate fluid and electrolyte balance (see Chapter 11). The zona reticularis produces androgens that are important for sexual differentiation (see Chapter 1), although the major source of androgens is the gonads (see Chapter 2). A major androgen is androstenedione, which is converted to testosterone, estrone, and estriol in peripheral tissues.[97] The adrenal medulla is the source of epinephrine and norepinephrine, which are also involved in stress responses and cardiovascular function.

delivery.[62,71] The net result of changes in thyroid function during pregnancy is to increase the availability of thyroid hormones by 40% to 100%.[142] Morreale de Escobar et al. summarized the major changes in thyroid function during pregnancy: (1) Increased estrogen leads to a two- to threefold increase in thyroid-binding globulin production by the liver. This decreases levels of free thyroid hormone and stimulates the hypothalamic-pituitary-thyroid (HPT) axis; (2) increased human chorionic gonadotropin (hCG), which has a structure similar to thyroid-stimulating hormone (TSH), stimulates increased T_3 and T_4. This leads to negative feedback to the pituitary gland and a decrease in TSH (especially during weeks 8 to 14 when hCG is peaking); (3) peripheral metabolism of thyroid hormones increases in the second and third trimesters due to increased production of type II and III monodeiodinases (see Box 19-3 below) by the placenta.[95]

Adaptations during pregnancy related to thyroid physiology mimic hyperthyroidism. The pregnant woman can be described as being in a state of euthyroid hyperthyroxinemia, however, since thyroid function per se does not change during pregnancy.[95] Thyroid hormone changes are important in supporting the altered carbohydrate, protein, and lipid metabolism of pregnancy and changes in basal

BOX 19-3 Thyroid Function

The thyroid gland consists of multiple colloid-filled follicles that serve as a storage site for thyroid hormone (see Figure 19-3). The major component of the colloid is thyroglobulin. Thyroid cellular functions include iodine transport and thyroxine (T_4) and triiodothyronine (T_3) formation and release into the blood. T_4 acts as a prohormone for T_3 and by itself has little intrinsic metabolic activity.[131] Iodide is actively transported into the thyroid cell, where it is stored and oxidized. Oxidized iodide is bound to tyrosine to form monoiodotyrosines (MIT) and diiodotyrosines (DIT). T_3 is composed of 1 MIT and 1 DIT; T_4 is formed from 2 DIT. These substances are held within the thyroglobulin and used to form T_4 and T_3. T_4 and T_3 are stored in the thyroid, bound to thyroglobulin. Under the influence of thyroid-stimulating hormone (TSH), T_4 and a small amount of T_3 are cleaved from thyroglobulin and secreted. In peripheral tissue, T_4 is deiodinated to T_3 (80% of T_3 in tissues is derived from this process).[131] The iodine released by this process is reconcentrated by the thyroid or excreted by the kidneys. T_4 can also be metabolized to reverse T_3 (rT_3), which is an inactive compound. T_3 and rT_3 are in a reciprocal relationship. Nearly all of the thyroid hormones circulate in plasma bound to proteins, including thyroxine-binding globulin (TBG) (the major carrier), transthyretin (TTR), or albumin. Changing levels of TBG, such as occurs during pregnancy, alter serum thyroxine levels without changing thyroid status. The small amount of free T_3 in the blood forms the most physiologically active fraction.

Three types of the monodeiodinase (MDI) enzymes catabolize thyroid hormones: (1) MDI-I (found in the liver, kidney, thyroid, and pituitary); (2) MDI-II (found in the brain, pituitary, brown adipose tissue, keratinocytes, and placenta; and (3) MDI-III (found in the placenta, brain, and epidermis). MDI-I and MDI-II act on the outer ring of the iodothyronine molecule; MDI-III acts primarily on the inner ring. MDI action on the inner rings catabolizes T_4 to the inactive rT_4 or T_3 to the inactive T_2. MDI action on the outer ring converts T_4 to T_3.

Thyroid hormones bind to nuclear thyroid hormone protein receptors in cells, which have a 10-fold greater affinity for T_3 than for T_4, that regulate gene transcription resulting in the production of proteins that affect a variety of metabolic and other proces ses.[29,99,131] Thyroid hormones are involved in the regulation of protein and lipid metabolism, glucose absorption and utilization, increasing the rate of cellular oxidation, heat production, fluid balance, calcium and vitamin D homeostasis, and liver functions.[131] Thyroid hormones are also critical for maturation of the retina, cochlea, and brain, including neural differentiation and migration (see Chapter 15).[131]

From references 29, 47, 99, 131.

metabolic rate (see Chapter 16).[79] The factors primarily responsible for changes in HPT axis function during pregnancy are the elevated hCG and thyroid-binding globulin (TBG) levels and the increased urinary iodide excretion that lowers maternal plasma iodine.[40,43] Box 19-3 on page 630, Box 19-4 below and Figure 19-3 review thyroid hormone production and regulation. Figure 19-4 illustrates regulation of maternal thyroid hormone function during pregnancy.

Thyroid hormones are transported in the blood bound to binding proteins, such as TBG, albumin, and transthyretin (TTR; formerly called thyroxine-binding prealbumin). In the nonpregnant individual, about two thirds of the T_4 is bound to TBG, increasing to 75% or greater during pregnancy.[34,43] Under the influence of estrogen, hepatic synthesis and sialylation of TBG increase twofold to threefold beginning within a few weeks after fertilization and plateau from midgestation to delivery.[34,71,99,100,144] Increased sialylation increases the half-life of TBG. The ability of TBG to bind thyroxine doubles during this period; TTR, also influenced by estrogen, decreases.[43] These changes increase serum TBG levels, decrease the percent of T_4 bound to TTR and increase total T_4 and T_3.[100] The increased TBG is accompanied by 10% to 15% decrease in free T_4 and free T_3 if iodine is sufficient; if iodine is inadequate, T_4 levels increase.[99]

A transient increase in free T_4 is reported in the first trimester, related to the increase in hCG, with a decrease in the second and third trimesters.[71,72] Variations in findings are most often due to differences in the iodine status of the populations studied and measurement techniques.[73] Free T_3 changes parallel those of free T_4.[72] Concentrations of free T_3 and free T_4, although low, remain within normal physiologic limits.[72,99] The basis for these changes is thought to be primarily related to the interaction of estrogen, TSH, and thyroid-binding proteins.[72]

BOX 19-4 Regulation of Thyroid Hormone Secretion

Thyroid-stimulating hormone (TSH) acts through receptors on the thyroid cell membrane to activate adenyl cyclase. This stimulates formation of cyclic adenosine monophosphate (cAMP), which activates cellular systems to increase iodide uptake and thyroid hormone production and synthesis. TSH secretion is stimulated by thyrotropin-releasing hormone (TRH). TRH is secreted primarily by paraventricular nuclei of the hypothalamus and is released into the hypothalamic-pituitary portal system. TRH binds to receptors on the plasma membrane of thyrotropic cells within the anterior pituitary to activate synthesis and secretion of TSH. Secretion of thyroid hormones decreases the responsiveness of the pituitary to TRH. Secretion of TSH is also influenced by circulating levels of free thyroid hormone and intrapituitary triiodothyronine (T_3) levels via negative feedback to the pituitary gland; that is, increased free thyroid hormone levels decrease secretion of TSH by the pituitary and vice versa. Circulating thyroxine (T_4) regulates TSH primarily through intrapituitary deiodination of T_4 to T_3. The pituitary-thyroid axis is controlled in turn by the hypothalamus and TRH. TSH is inhibited by excess circulating thyroid hormone.

From references 29, 47, 99, 131.

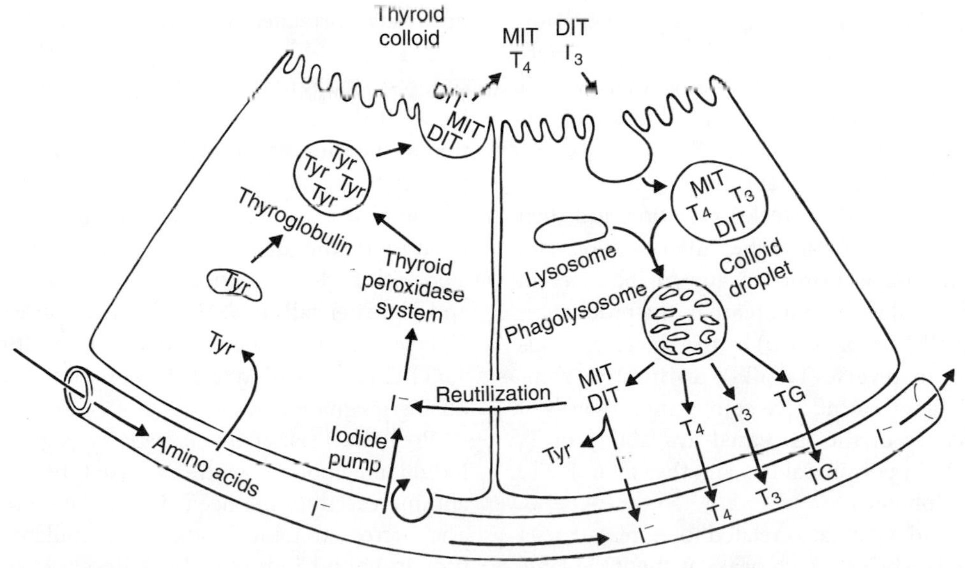

FIGURE 19-3 Thyroid hormone synthesis. *DIT*, Diiodotyrosine; *MIT*, monoiodotyrosine, thyroglobulin; *Tyr*, tyrosine. (From Lane, A.H., & Wilson, T.A. [2005]. Neonatal thyroid disorders. In A.R. Spitzer [Ed.], *Intensive care of the fetus & neonate* [2nd ed.]. St. Louis: Mosby, p. 1141.)

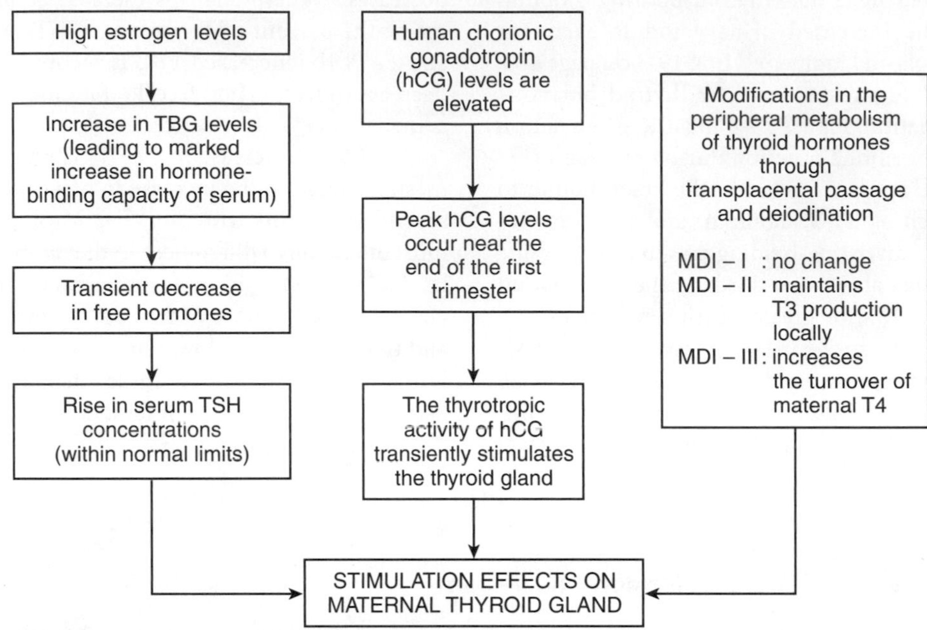

FIGURE 19-4 Regulation of maternal thyroid function in normal pregnancy. Three series of separate events exert stimulatory effects on maternal thyroid function. The first event is linked to the progressive rise in thyroid binding (TBG) levels during the first trimester; the second event takes place transiently near the end of the first trimester and is related to the thyrotropic action of peak human chorionic gonadotropin (hCG) concentrations; the third event takes place mainly during the second half of gestation and is related to modifications in peripheral metabolism of maternal thyroid hormones, mainly at the placental level. *TSH*, Thyroid stimulating hormone; *MDI*, monodeiodinase. (From Glinoer, D. [1999]. Thyroid regulation and disease in pregnancy. In M.I. Surks [Ed.], *Atlas of clinical endocrinology-thyroid disease* [volume I]. Philadelphia: Blackwell Science, p. 161.)

Resin T_3 uptake (RT_3U) decreases during pregnancy. RT_3U measures TBG-binding capacity by quantifying the number of unbound sites, and approximates the amount of free T_4. Although T_4-binding sites and binding capacity increase in pregnancy, the number of binding sites exceeds the available T_4. The increased number of unbound sites is reflected by decreased RT_3U.

In contrast to changes in free T_3 and free T_4, total T_3 and T_4 increase, peaking at 10 to 15 weeks' gestation and then plateauing at levels 40% to 100% higher than nonpregnant values.[142,144] This increase is primarily due to increases in TBG and hCG, and possibly to an increase in the production of MDI-III (see Box 19-3 on page 630) by the placenta.[71] This enzyme converts T_4 to reverse T_3 (rT_3), an inactive compound, and T_3 to T_2, another inactive compound.[98] Levels of T_3 are elevated because of the increased availability of T_4 for deiodination to T_3 in peripheral tissue rather than due to increased T_3 production per se.

The increased T_3 and T_4 are also related to increased TSH bioactivity stimulated by hCG, which peaks at about the same time.[58] hCG has a mild TSH-like activity that increases secretion of T_4.[34,100] hCG is a partial inhibitor of the pituitary gland and has β subunits similar to TSH (as well as luteinizing and follicle-stimulating hormone). Thus hCG has thyrotropic activity and can activate TSH receptors.[34,100] Serum hCG is positively correlated with free T_4 and inversely correlated with TSH levels in early pregnancy.[40,73] Elevated T_3 and T_4 suppress endogenous TSH secretion by the anterior pituitary.[98] TSH decreases transiently from 8 to 14 weeks' gestation at the time of the hCG peak, progressively returning to prepregnancy levels by term.[34,100,151] Occasionally some otherwise healthy pregnant women will experience a transient hyperthyroxinemia (generally without clinical signs) associated with higher than usual hCG levels in the first trimester and a greater fall in TSH.[43,72,99] The increase in total T_3 and T_4 is less than the increase in TBG, resulting in a decreased T_4/TBG ratio, leading to a state of relative hypothyroxinemia during pregnancy.

Pregnancy is characterized by significant changes in iodide metabolism with increased renal iodide clearance and increased iodine needed to make thyroid hormones.[38,71] The increased total T_4 and T_3 stimulate increased serum protein-bound iodine (PBI).[38] Because circulating levels of free thyroid hormone are not significantly altered, increased PBI does not reflect maternal hyperthyroidism. Thyroid iodine uptake increases because of a decrease in the total body iodine pool. This pool is altered because of increased renal iodide loss secondary to the increased renal blood flow and glomerular filtration rate (see Chapter 11) and placental transfer of iodine to the fetus.[43,71,99,144]

The thyroid compensates for the increased loss of iodine by hyperplasia and increased plasma iodine clearance, reducing plasma iodine levels.[88,99] Iodine is stored in the colloid of the thyroid gland follicles (see Figure 19-3). With TSH stimulation, thyroglobulin is catabolized to form T_4 and T_3.[99] Serum thyroglobulin increases in the first trimester but is most marked in later pregnancy. This increase is associated with an increase in thyroid volume, especially in areas of low iodine intake.[43,72,99] The degree of hyperplasia is related to the degree of imbalance between iodine needs versus iodine intake and stores (see Iodine Needs during Pregnancy).[72] Mild thyroid hyperplasia (10% to 15% increase), due primarily to increased vascularity, is seen in areas such as North America, where diets are generally thought to be iodine sufficient.[38,99,100] Therefore moderate to marked thyroid enlargement in these women cannot be considered normal and requires further evaluation. Women who live in iodine-poor areas have an increase in thyroid volume of 15% to 30% during pregnancy.[38,99] Goiter is generally not a risk if iodine levels are greater than 0.08 mcg/dL (0.006 μmol/L); in North America, levels average 0.3 mcg/dL (0.023 μmol/L). Goiter is a significant risk in areas with low iodine intake.

Intrapartum Period

The HPA and HPT axes undergo further alterations during the intrapartum period. CRH appears to be a trigger in the initiation of labor, and activation of the HPA axis may serve as a "biologic clock" timing the length of gestation.[99] Maternal plasma CRH, ACTH, β-endorphin, and cortisol levels increase up to sevenfold with labor onset and during labor (see Chapter 4).[20,35,77,86,93,172] ACTH reaches its highest level, increasing from 50 pg/mL (11 pmol/L) at term to 300 pg/mL (66 pmol/L) in labor (see Figure 19-1).[32,77,151] Further increases in ACTH and cortisol are seen in women with poor progress in labor.[31] Low β-endorphin levels at term have been associated with an increased need for pain medication during labor, although a causal relationship is unclear.[20]

Levels of total and free T_3 increase during labor. This change probably reflects the energy demands of labor on the maternal system. T_3 and T_4 have similar functions, but T_3 is three to five times more active. T_3 and T_4 increase intracellular enzymes (increased cellular metabolism), the number and activity of mitochondria (to provide energy for cellular enzyme systems), and Na-K adenosine triphosphatase (ATPase) (because of the increased energy use for myometrial contractions).[47]

Postpartum Period

The alterations in the HPA (see Figure 19-2, *C*) and HPT axes during pregnancy are reversed during the postpartum period. CRH levels drop rapidly with removal of the placenta and placental CRH.[151] Maternal ACTH and cortisol levels decrease rapidly in the immediate postpartum period and reach nonpregnant values by 1 to 4 days postpartum.[35,77,86] The HPA axis is depressed with a reduction in hypothalamic CRH for 3 to 6 weeks, returning to normal levels by 12 weeks.[86] This depression of the HPA axis may play a role in postpartum mood disorders or in exacerbation of autoimmune disorders in the postpartum period.[1,62] Although ACTH secretion may be suppressed, total serum cortisol is within normal limits, probably secondary to a mild hypertrophy of the adrenal cortex.[86] Hyperplasia of the lactotrophs of the anterior pituitary gland peaks in the first 3 days postpartum. This tissue decreases in size by 1 month in nonlactating and more slowly in lactating women, but never returns to nulliparous size.[32,93,97] Prolactin falls at delivery and returns to nonpregnant values by 3 months; in breastfeeding women, prolactin increases after delivery.[32,35,151] β-endorphins decrease by 24 hours after birth and are higher in colostrum than in maternal plasma.[173] Serum growth hormone levels may remain elevated for several months.[32] Postpartum changes in prolactin, FSH, and LH are described in Chapter 5.

After delivery with removal of the placenta and reduction in estrogen, hepatic synthesis of TBG decreases, as does the renal excretion of iodine. As a result, the metabolic alterations in thyroid processes gradually reverse over 4 to 6 weeks, although they may persist for up to 6 to 12 weeks.[43,144] Thyroid-releasing hormone (TRH) is a (minor) stimulus of prolactin release and has been used to induce relactation.[70] Free T_4 may be low and TSH elevated in the first 3 to 4 days, which may confound assessment of thyroid function.[65] Transient disorders in thyroid function are seen in some postpartum women (see Postpartum Thyroid Disorders).

Thyroid hormones are secreted in breast milk. Levels are low initially and then rise. Breast milk T_4 and T_3 have been reported to delay the development of hypothyroidism in some infants with this disorder.[131]

CLINICAL IMPLICATIONS FOR THE PREGNANT WOMAN AND HER FETUS

Changes in the hypothalamic-pituitary-adrenal (HPA) and hypothalamic-pituitary-thyroid (HPT) axes are critical for maintenance of pregnancy. In addition, the maternal and fetal HPA axes and the interrelationship between maternal and fetal-placental function are essential for initiation of labor (see Chapter 4). Alterations in the HPA axis with infection or stress may lead to preterm labor. These risks are discussed further in Chapter 4. Thyroid disorders are more common in women and are not uncommon in pregnant women, being the second most common endocrine disorder (after diabetes mellitus) seen during pregnancy. Disorders of the adrenal and pituitary gland, such as prolactinomas, which may increase in size during pregnancy due the stimulating effects of elevated prolactin levels, and Cushing disease, are uncommon.[78,93,97,98] Cushing disease tends to be exacerbated during pregnancy with remission postpartum and is more often due to adrenal lesions than excess adrenocorticotropin

(ACTH).[78] Diagnosis of thyroid dysfunction during pregnancy may be more difficult in that symptoms of thyroid disorders often mimic some of the usual physiologic changes of pregnancy, and radioactive iodine tests cannot be used because of fetal risks. Implications of alterations in thyroid function and changes in laboratory tests during pregnancy are discussed in this section, along with disorders of thyroid function unique to the postpartum period.

Iodine Needs during Pregnancy

Adequate iodine stores and nutrition are essential for normal function of the maternal and fetal thyroid.[23,36,39] Iodine needs increase during pregnancy due to increased renal loss and increased placental—and thus fetal—uptake.[30,36,131] Dietary iodine is converted to iodide; 20% of this is absorbed by the thyroid gland, the rest is cleared by the kidney. During pregnancy renal iodide clearance doubles due to the increased renal blood flow and glomerular filtration rate (see Chapter 11).[99] The World Health Organization recommends an iodine intake of 250 μg/day during pregnancy and lactation; others recommend 200 or up to 300 μg/day.[30,76,88,131,174,175] Iodine needs can be met by iodine in prenatal vitamins and use of iodinated salt.[43] Mean urinary iodine excretion, used to assess iodine deficiency, is insufficient if less than 150 μg/L during pregnancy or less than 100 μg/L during lactation.[30]

Iodine deficiency is lowest in North America, higher in Europe, with Southeast Asia accounting for nearly one fourth of the worldwide population with insufficient iodine uptake.[88] Iodine stores are low in developing countries and have been falling in many developed countries, for example, 50% to 65% of women in western and central Europe were found to be iodine deficient (versus 11% of women in the United States).[36,175] Recent reports suggest a decline in iodine sufficiency in childbearing women in the United States.[15] Women who enter pregnancy in an iodine-deficient state fall even further behind so that iodine deficiency in the first trimester tends to become more severe in later pregnancy.[71,73] Iodine deficiency is the most frequent cause worldwide of preventable mental retardation and often the damage is done by the time of birth.[88,175] Iodine deficiency is also associated with an increased risk of spontaneous abortion and stillbirths.[88,175] Even in iodine-sufficient areas, there has been increasing concern that iodine deficiency may increase the risk of later neurodevelopmental impairment of offspring in women with marked subclinical thyroid dysfunction.[72] Various professional groups have differing recommendations regarding whether all pregnant women should be routinely screened to identify subclinical hypothyroidism.[1,2,9,14,30,62,167]

Thyroid Function Tests during Pregnancy

Changes in TBG and thyroid hormones during pregnancy alter parameters for many tests used to assess thyroid status. These alterations, which vary with trimester, must be considered when evaluating thyroid function in pregnant and postpartum women. Free T_3 and T_4 assays, rather than total values, are generally preferred because of the increased thyroxine-binding globulin (TBG).[30] Glinoer and Spencer indicate that serum TSH assay "is the most sensitive index to reliably detect thyroid function abnormalities" during pregnancy.[40] Reference ranges for thyroid function tests during pregnancy have been described in several studies, with variations by trimester of testing, number of fetuses, and testing method.[30] Table 19-1 summarizes the changes in thyroid function during pregnancy that lead to alterations in these tests. As noted in the previous section, recommendations for routine thyroid screening during pregnancy vary among different professional groups worldwide.[1,2,9,14,30,62,167]

Antithyroid peroxidase enzymes have been reported in 10% to 14% of women at 14 weeks' gestation and may increase the risk of gestational thyroid dysfunction and

Table 19-1 Thyroid Function Tests during Pregnancy

PHYSIOLOGIC CHANGES	RESULTING CHANGE IN THYROID ACTIVITY
↑ Serum estrogens ↑ Serum TBG	↑ Serum TBG ↑ Demand for T_4 and T_3 ↑ In total T_4 and T_3
↑ hCG	↓ TSH in first trimester (in reference range unless hCG is >50,000 IU/L) ↑ Free T4 in first trimester (still within normal reference range unless hCG is >50,000 IU/L)
↑ Iodine (I) clearance	↑ In dietary requirement for iodine ↓ In thyroid hormone production in iodine-deficient areas ↑ Goiter in iodine-deficient areas
↑ Type III deiodinase	↑ T_4 and T_3 degradation ↑ Demand for T_4 and T_3
↑ Demand for T_4 and T_3	↑ Serum thyroglobulin ↑ Thyroid volume ↑ Goiter in iodine-deficient areas

Modified from Brent, G.A. (1997). Maternal thyroid function: Interpretation of thyroid function test in pregnancy. *Clin Obstet Gynecol, 40,* 3, by Fantz, C.R., et al. (1999). Thyroid function during pregnancy. *Clin Chem, 45,* 2250.

hCG, Human chorionic gonadotropin; T_3, triiodothyronine; T_4, thyroxine; *TBG,* thyroxine-binding globulin; *TSH,* thyroid-stimulating hormone.

postpartum thyroiditis.[72] Most women are euthyroid but some have increased thyroid-stimulating hormone (TSH) or decreased free T_4 or both.[72]

Thyroid Function and Nausea and Vomiting in Pregnancy

Nausea and vomiting in pregnancy (NVP) has been linked to alterations in T_4, TSH, and human chorionic gonadotropin (hCG) (which has TSH-like activity). hCG stimulates receptors for both TSH (increases T_4) and hCG (increases estriol and possibly NVP). NVP severity has been correlated with increased free T_4 and decreased TSH, with values returning to normal pregnant ranges as the nausea and vomiting resolve.[71] These findings may lead to or be a consequence of emesis during early pregnancy. NVP is discussed further in Chapter 12.

Hyperemesis gravidarum in women without any history or evidence of thyroid dysfunction has also been associated with increased free T_4 and decreased TSH. These findings, seen in about 60% of women with hyperemesis, are similar to those of the euthyroid sick syndrome seen with severe illness.[73] T_4 levels in women with hyperemesis return to usual values in 1 to 4 weeks after resolution with or without treatment with antithyroid drugs.[1,43,72,98]

The Pregnant Woman with Hyperthyroidism

A transient hyperthyroidism is seen in 10% to 20% of otherwise healthy pregnant women during the first trimester; this may be associated with increased hCG levels, multiple gestation, or NVP.[34,36] This transient form of subclinical hyperthyroidism is characterized by normal free T_4 and decreased TSH.

Another form of transient clinical hyperthyroidism, characterized by increased free T_4 and decreased TSH, is seen less frequently and may be associated with multiple gestation, hyperemesis gravidarum, and gestational trophoblast disorders with markedly increased hCG production.[34,62,72] Trophoblast disorders such as a molar pregnancy occasionally cause biochemical and, in some women (5% to 64%), clinical findings of hyperthyroidism because of the high levels of hCG secreted by the trophoblastic mass.[100]

Chronic hyperthyroidism occurs in 0.05% to 0.2% of pregnant women.[99] The diagnosis of hyperthyroidism during pregnancy may be difficult in that many of the signs and symptoms associated with this disorder are often seen normally during pregnancy. Findings common to hyperthyroidism and certain stages of pregnancy include fatigue, heat intolerance, warm skin, emotional lability, insomnia, increased appetite, sweating, breathlessness, ankle edema, palpitations, and increased pulse pressure.[30,34,43,72,99,100] Failure to gain weight with a good appetite and persistent tachycardia (greater than 100 beats/min) are most suggestive of hyperthyroidism in pregnancy.[43] Increased free T_3 and total T_4 (greater than 15 mcg/dL [193 nmol/L]) and increased or high-normal RT_3U are seen with hyperthyroidism. Alterations in thyroid function tests during pregnancy (see Table 19-1) must be considered when interpreting test results. For example, because RT_3U is decreased in pregnancy, values in the nonpregnant range suggest hyperthyroidism. TSH levels less than 0.05 μU/L (mIU/mL) and increased free T_4 levels greater than 11.6 mcg/dL (149 pmol/L) are diagnostic.[99]

Hyperthyroidism in pregnant women in North America is usually due to either an autoimmune disorder or an unknown cause; it is rarely due to goiter. The risk of goiter during pregnancy is attributed to increased avidity of the thyroid for iodine in response to increased renal loss and placental transport. In most women these losses are compensated for by a higher dietary iodine intake.

Hyperthyroidism in pregnant women is almost always (85% to 95%) due to Graves' disease.[34,72,73,81] Graves' disease is an autoimmune disorder in which thyroid-stimulating immunoglobulins (TSIs), such as TSH receptor antibody (TRAb), attach to and activate TSH receptors on the thyroid follicular cells. This leads to increased production of thyroid hormones and the clinical finding of hyperthyroidism.

Women with mild hyperthyroidism generally do well during pregnancy because increased serum TBG offsets the increased secretion of thyroid hormones. In women with Graves' disease, their disorder may be aggravated in the first trimester (due to the increased hCG) and then improve during the third trimester, with remission and occasionally complete resolution.[30,165] This improvement is related to suppression of the maternal immune system responses (see Chapter 13) by fetal cytokines with lower TSI levels and decreased thyroid hormone production. Relapse or exacerbation generally occurs postpartum, usually within several weeks of delivery, as immune system alterations and production of TBG return to prepregnancy levels.[100,165]

Pregnant women with hyperthyroidism usually require a caloric intake that is higher than that generally recommended during pregnancy to compensate for their increased metabolic rate. These women are also at risk for fluid loss and dehydration as a result of the diarrhea and tachycardia that often accompany hyperthyroidism.[99] Women with hyperthyroidism, particularly if this disorder is poorly controlled, are at increased risk for placental abruption, miscarriage, preterm labor, fetal growth restriction, congestive heart failure, and thyroid storm.[30,34,36,69,72,119] Their infants can develop transient hyperthyroidism from transplacental passage of TSIs or hypothyroidism secondary to the effects of maternal antithyroid drugs.[36,119] Hyperthyroidism also alters sex steroid metabolism, sperm motility, and fertility.[61,131]

Transplacental passage of TSIs, especially TRAbs, leads to a transient neonatal hyperthyroidism in about 1% to 5% of infants of mothers with Graves' disease (see Chapter 13).[1,30,33,116] The risk is present even if the woman is euthyroid in pregnancy or has had thyroid ablation via surgery or radiation before pregnancy because TSIs are still present.[82,100] The fetal risk increases after 20 weeks when fetal TSH receptors become responsive to TSH.[81] TSH-binding inhibitory immunoglobulins may also cross the placenta, causing a transient neonatal hypothyroidism.[131]

Hyperthyroidism is treated with antithyroid drugs (thioamides), surgical removal, or thyroid ablation with ^{131}I. The most common thioamides are propylthiouracil (PTU) and methimazole (Tapazole or carbimazole, which is metabolized to methimazole). Thioamides cross the placenta and can block synthesis of thyroid hormones by the fetus.[119] The lower hormone levels stimulate increased TSH production, which can lead to goiter and tracheal obstruction. Infants of mothers treated with thioamides may have decreased T_4 and increased TSH levels after birth. These values are generally within normal neonatal limits by 4 to 5 days of age. PTU is recommended as the first-line drug during pregnancy.[1,34,36,69] Although methimazole (MMI) has the advantage of less frequent dosing and fewer tablets per dose, MMI is associated with a risk of fetal scalp defects (cutis aplasia) and possibly esophageal and choanal atresia.[30,36,73,100,152] Pharmacologic effects must be monitored carefully, particularly during the third trimester in women with Graves' disease, when remission can lead to decreased thyroid hormone production and a transient decrease in required drug dosage by 32 to 36 weeks.[99] In some women, the drug can be transiently discontinued in late pregnancy.[165]

Pregnant women may also develop a transient subacute thyroiditis that often occurs in association with viral infections. The inflammation and destruction of thyroid tissue lead to release of stored thyroid hormone into serum and a transient hyperthyroxinemia. As the disorder resolves, the woman may develop hypothyroidism because the released thyroid hormones are used up before the thyroid gland can produce an adequate new supply. If treatment is initiated, β-blockers such as propranolol are required rather than antithyroid drugs that block thyroid hormone production, because with subacute thyroiditis the thyroid is not making hormones.[43,72] Propranolol is generally not indicated for long-term treatment of pregnant women with hyperthyroidism. This drug crosses the placenta and has been associated with fetal growth restriction and impaired responses to anoxia and neonatal hypoglycemia and bradycardia.

The Pregnant Woman with Hypothyroidism

Hypothyroidism in iodine-sufficient pregnant women is usually secondary to autoimmune disorders (after surgical removal or ablation of the thyroid with radioactive ^{131}I for Graves' disease and idiopathic myxedema) or Hashimoto thyroiditis.[30,62] Worldwide, iodine deficiency is the most common cause of hypothyroidism and can lead to cretinism (mental retardation, deafness, other neurologic symptoms in the infant).[36,48,62,100] Iodine deficiency leads to hypothyroxinemia, thyroid stimulation from thyroid-releasing hormone (TRH) and TSH feedback loops, and development of goiter.[71] Women with untreated hypothyroidism have a high incidence of infertility and spontaneous abortion.[30,34,43,73,124]

The diagnosis of hypothyroidism during pregnancy may be missed because some of the signs and symptoms associated with this disorder—fatigue, weight gain, muscle cramps, constipation, and amenorrhea—are also seen normally during pregnancy.[30,43,99] The increase in TBG in pregnancy may mask the decrease in thyroid hormones; however, levels are usually still low for pregnant norms. In addition, free T_4 is low and TSH is elevated.[72]

Pregnancy in women with primary hypothyroidism or autoimmune thyroiditis may be complicated by an increased risk of fetal loss or prolonged pregnancy, possibly due to compromised placental blood flow or the inability of the thyroid gland to meet the metabolic demands of pregnancy. These women are also at greater risk for preterm delivery, preeclampsia, and cesarean section.[30,34,36,62,92,107,148] Weight gain patterns must be carefully monitored in the woman with hypothyroidism. These women may also have difficulty with fatigue and constipation during pregnancy.

Thyroid hormone replacement doses usually need to be increased as a result of the increased TBG and T_4 demand.[3,49,72,100,145,158] For example, levothyroxine may need to be increased 25% to 40% to maintain normal serum TSH levels.[3,34,73] Increased requirements may occur as early as the fifth week of gestation and are influenced by maternal estrogen levels, pregestation TSH levels, maternal volume of distribution, parity, and etiology of the hypothyroidism.[3,4,34,80] Postpartum levothyroxine levels usually decrease to prepregnancy levels, but some women continue to have a greater requirement.[30,34]

Although overt hypothyroidism is associated with neurodevelopmental problems in offspring, the role of subclinical hypothyroidism is less clear.[1,48,88,101,170] Subclinical hypothyroidism (elevated TSH but normal free T_4) occurs in 2% to 5% of pregnancies and increases the risk of prematurity, abruption, and impaired neurologic outcome in infants.[1,30,48,72,88] The risk of later neurologic problems in offspring is thought to be greatest with untreated or subclinical hypothyroidism in the first 10 to 12 weeks of gestation because the fetus is completely dependent on maternal thyroid hormone for brain development during this time.[115] However, the role of subclinical hypothyroidism in infants' later development is still an area of debate, due to inadequate data on the causal relationship between subclinical hypothyroidism and lower IQ levels.[30,48,114] Routine screening is recommended for all pregnant women or for all who are high risk for this disorder by some, but not all professional organizations[1,2,9,14,62,167]

Postpartum Thyroid Disorders

The postpartum period is associated with transient thyroid disorders. Physiologic alterations and experiences of pregnancy can mask clinical findings of hypothyroidism or hyperthyroidism. As a result, these disorders may first become apparent in the postpartum period. Although less common than these transient disorders, postpartum women are also at increased risk of developing Graves' disease, especially women older than 35 years of age.[10]

Postpartum thyroid disorder (PPTD) is a transient disorder seen in 6% to 9% of postpartum women.[62] The incidence of PPTD is 33% to 50% in women with thyroid peroxidase antibodies in early pregnancy (versus 0.5% in those without these antibodies).[62,72] PPTD is also more prevalent in women with type 1 diabetes.[62] Classic PPTD accounts for about 28% of these cases and generally appears in the first 6 months (usually by 6 to 8 weeks after delivery). PPTD (Figure 19-5) is generally characterized by weeks or months (average, 2 to 4 months, but can be up to 6 months) of mild hyperthyroidism, followed by weeks or months (up to a year) of hypothyroidism, and finally a return to normal thyroid function in most women—usually by 12 months postpartum.[1,43,62,72,100] Others present with only hypothyroidism or hyperthyroidism.

The exact cause of PPTD is unclear but it appears to be an autoimmune disorder with increased susceptibility in the postpartum woman as her immune system rapidly changes from Th2 to Th1 T-lymphocyte dominance (see Chapter 13).[1,72] The initial hyperthyroid phase is characterized by thyroid cell destruction with excessive release of thyroid hormone. PPTD may reflect postpartum exacerbation of a subclinical autoimmune disorder that, with release of pregnancy-induced immunosuppression, leads to rebound of immune components with excessive production of thyroid autoantibodies.[43,62] The subsequent hypothyroid phase is due to decreased thyroid hormones from excessive loss of thyroid cells during the first phase. As the thyroid cells regrow, normal function returns.

Up to 30% to 50% of women with PPTD remain hypothyroid or develop permanent hypothyroidism within 5 to 15 years.[1,62] Biochemical abnormalities include elevated free T_4, suppression of TSH, presence of microsomal antibodies, and a low ^{131}I uptake.[72] PPTD may be misdiagnosed as postpartum depression and often recurs with subsequent deliveries.[30,72] Transient hypothyroidism is also seen occasionally during the postpartum period. Findings include fatigue, weight gain, low free T_4 and elevated TSH levels, and elevated antimicrosomal and antithyroglobulin antibody titers.

Breastfeeding in Women with Thyroid Disorders

Breastfeeding is not contraindicated in women with hypothyroidism, because thyroid hormones cross in only small amounts and the infant should receive a dose no higher than that from a euthyroid woman.[58,70] Breastfeeding in women with hyperthyroidism may be a concern because of passage of antithyroid medications in breast milk.[90] However, PTU is excreted in breast milk in relatively small amounts (0.025% to 0.077% of the maternal dose).[70] Most sources suggest that breastfeeding is not routinely contraindicated in women on PTU who are carefully monitored, but that each woman needs to weigh the risks and benefits and the infant must be carefully monitored. Propranolol and thiouracil cross in significant amounts and are generally contraindicated in breastfeeding women.[70]

The mammary glands actively take up, concentrate, and secrete iodine in breast milk. Thus breastfeeding is interrupted if the woman requires thyroid uptake studies or scans involving use of ^{123}I or ^{131}I. If radioactive iodine is needed, ^{123}I is preferred over ^{131}I, since breastfeeding generally needs to be stopped for only about 48 hours with ^{123}I versus for a prolonged period of time with ^{131}I.[43]

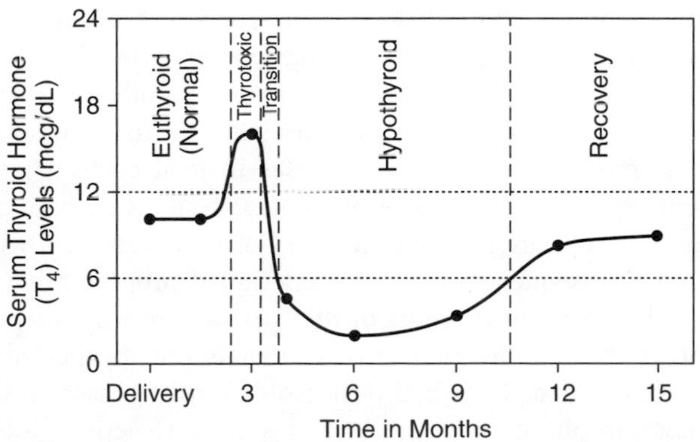

FIGURE 19-5 Thyroid function during postpartum thyroiditis. *T_4*, Thyroxine. (From Smallridge, R.C., et al. [1988]. Postpartum thyroiditis. *The Bridge*, 3, 3. Newsletter of the Thyroid Foundation of America, Inc.)

Use of Radioiodine and Iodides

Iodine is actively transported across the placenta and taken up by the fetal thyroid (Figure 19-6). Avidity of the fetal thyroid for iodine is 20 to 50 times greater than that of the

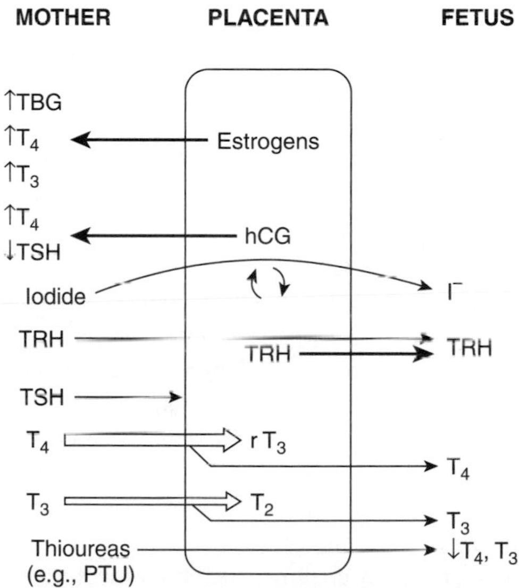

FIGURE 19-6 Placental role in maternal and fetal thyroid function. Heavy arrows indicate placental production of estrogens and human chorionic gonadotropin (hCG), which predominantly moves into maternal blood, and of thyroid-releasing hormone (TRH), which moves primarily into fetal blood. Iodide is actively transported from mother to fetus. The placenta is impermeable to thyroid-stimulating hormone (TSH) in either direction. Transfer of thyroxine (T_4) and triiodothyronine (T_3) is controlled by placental type III iodothyronine deiodinase, which convert T_4 to rT_3 and T_3 to T_2 (rT_3 and T_2 are inactive compounds). Thyroid hormones from the mother cross the placenta throughout gestation and are critical for fetal development. The relatively free transport of antithyroid drugs (propylthiouracil [PTU] and methimazole) can inhibit fetal thyroid hormone production. (From Fisher, D.A., & Polk, D.H. [1994]. The ontogenesis of thyroid function and actions. In D. Tulchinsky & A.B. Little [Eds.], *Maternal-fetal endocrinology* [2nd ed.]. Philadelphia: Saunders.)

mother.[43] Administration of any form of iodine to pregnant women results in significantly higher concentrations per weight in fetal tissues and can lead to development of a goiter, especially after 12 weeks' gestation, when the fetal thyroid begins to concentrate iodine.[53] Fetal risks of radioactive substances include thyroid damage, microcephaly, growth restriction, mental retardation, later malignancy, and death. As a result, radioiodine is contraindicated during pregnancy. Radioiodine also alters spermatogenesis, so a waiting period is recommended in males between therapy and fertilization.

All women should have a pregnancy test before radioactive iodine studies. If these studies are done with ^{123}I in a woman who is later found to be pregnant, however, the risks are minimal since the dose of ^{123}I used is generally low. The use of ^{131}I for definitive diagnosis and therapy of Graves' disease is associated with increased pregnancy loss and potential damage to the fetal thyroid; thus this agent is avoided during pregnancy.[34]

The use of nonradioactive iodides has also been reported to increase the risk of fetal goiter, risk of tracheal obstruction, and hypothyroidism. Iodides are found in Betadine-containing vaginal suppositories and douches, saturated solution of potassium iodide (SSKI), iodinated medications for asthmatics, and some contrast materials.[43,131] The incidence of drug-induced fetal goiter is 1 in 10,000 and is seen primarily with daily iodide doses over 12 mcg.

Maternal-Fetal Endocrine Relationships

Maternal, fetal, and placental HPA functions are closely interrelated. The placenta produces significant amounts of some hypothalamic and pituitary hormones such as corticotropin-releasing hormone (CRH) and growth hormone (GH). The fetus and placenta, via CRH production, influence the timing of parturition (see Chapter 4). Large quantities of steroids are produced by interaction of the mother, placenta, and fetus. Some of these substances are dependent upon the viability and well-being of the fetus and placenta, whereas others, such as progesterone, do not require the fetus to be viable for production to continue. Steroid-producing cells appear early in placental development. They can be seen first in the trophoblast tissue of the placenta; however, the syncytiotrophoblast lacks several of the key enzymes necessary for steroid metabolism. Therefore the placenta is an incomplete steroidogenic tissue and must receive precursors from exogenous sources (i.e., the fetus or maternal system) (see Chapter 3).

During early gestation, maternal cortisol crossing the placenta provides negative feedback to the fetal HPA axis. This suppresses fetal cortisol production. Later in pregnancy, as placental metabolic activity matures, less maternal cortisol reaches the fetus as much of this cortisol is converted to inactive cortisone in the placenta. In late pregnancy, there is less negative feedback to the fetal HPA axis and increased fetal cortisol production. Placental CRH, which increases during gestation, has a stimulatory effect on the fetal HPA axis and is stimulated by cortisol.[162]

The fetal HPT axis develops relatively independently of maternal influences.[28,45] Maternal TRH does cross the placenta but does not seem to have a major influence on fetal pituitary or thyroid function, probably because maternal TRH levels are low and much of the maternal TRH is degraded in the placenta.[29,100] TSH does not cross the placenta.[131] Administration of thyroid hormone to the mother does not significantly increase fetal hormone levels.[28]

Maternal T_4 crosses the placenta to the fetus and is critical for normal development of the central nervous system and other organ systems, especially in the first trimester before the fetal thyroid is functional when the mother is the only source of T_4 (see Role of Maternal Thyroid Hormones).[28,29,43,71,95,99,144] Transfer continues throughout pregnancy but is decreased in later pregnancy due to increased placental deiodination of T_4 (to inactive rT_3) and T_3 (to T_2) by MDI-III.[29,131] Inadequate maternal iodine may decrease transfer of maternal T_4 to the fetus.[76,84,88,175] Increased T_4 transfer has been reported in late gestation with fetuses with severe congenital hypothyroidism.[28] Athyroid fetuses have T_4 levels that are 25% to 50% of normal.[131] The fetus is also dependent on the mother for iodides—either via direct transfer or breakdown of maternal T_4 by the placenta (see Figure 19-6).[28] The placenta is permeable to commonly used antithyroid drugs (PTU and methimazole), β-blockers (propranolol), and iodine.[131] Placental permeability to TSIs can lead to development of transient neonatal hyperthyroidism in infants of women with Graves' disease (see The Pregnant Woman with Hyperthyroidism and Chapter 13).

Maternal Stress Responses and Fetal Endocrine Programming

Even though both ACTH and cortisol are elevated during pregnancy, physiologic responses (e.g., blood pressure, heart rate, and cortisol reactivity) to stress, although maintained, appear to be blunted in the pregnant woman.[13,21,25] However, data are limited and wide individual differences have been reported. This blunting may be due to glucocorticoid negative feedback, possibly nitric oxide, urocortins, β-endorphins, and other endogenous opioids.[13]

Fetal programming refers to the effects of the fetal environment on susceptibility to later disorders. For example, the nutritional/hormonal status during fetal/early postbirth life can alter organ development including the hypothalamus and other endocrine structures. Increases in cortisol with stress in the mother can lead to increases in fetal cortisol. This is important because before birth, fetal systems such as the fetal HPA axis are programmed for postnatal function, with adverse consequences for later function if programming is altered.[13,159] Normally most of the cortisol reaching the placenta is broken down into inert metabolites by placental enzymes, such as 11-β-hydroxysteroid dehydrogenase, in the syncytiotrophoblast. These enzymes convert active glucocorticoids, such as cortisol and corticosterone, to inactive metabolites.[77] As a result, fetal circulating cortisol levels are maintained lower than maternal levels.

Wide individual differences have been reported in both maternal stress reactivity and in the activity and sensitivity of these placental enzymes.[21,25] There is increasing evidence in both human and animal studies of the effects of prenatal stress on offspring, including prematurity, low birth weight, delivery complications, and impaired prenatal and postnatal growth and development.[18,21,41,109,159,161,166] For example, the risk of early pregnancy loss with maternal stress may be mediated by alterations in glucocorticoids, progesterone/prolactin, and the immune system, leading to alterations in the early pregnancy cytokine environmental balance (see Chapter 13) needed for implantation and early pregnancy maintenance.[13] Early stress may also induce epigenetic changes in gene expression that increase the risk of later metabolic, vascular, and neurodevelopmental disorders in offspring.[18,89,159] Prolonged exposure to maternal stress mediators may permanently reset the HPA axis and increase the risk of adult-onset disorders such as type 2 diabetes, hypertension, obesity, coronary artery disease, end-stage renal disease, and depression.[13,150,159,162]

The specific mechanisms by which maternal stress affects the fetus are unclear, but probably involve changes in the fetal HPA axis from maternal increases in sympathetic nervous system and HPA activity and perhaps changes in the limbic system with stress.[24] Glucocorticoids are thought to have a major role in fetal tissue programming because excess levels can inhibit growth; alter expression of receptors, enzymes, ion channels, and transporters; and alter growth factors, structural proteins, binding proteins, and signaling pathways.[113] Possible mechanisms include (1) stress-induced increase in maternal cortisol results in increased fetal cortisol and changes in the feedback regulation of the fetal HPA axis; (2) hormones from the maternal HPA axis stimulate the placenta to increase CRH, which alters brain glucocorticoid receptor development and function in the fetus; and (3) increased cortisol and catecholamines seen with stress may alter uteroplacental blood flow, leading to poorer fetal growth, prematurity, and other complications.[21,56,113,159,166] Figure 19-7 illustrates a proposed model of factors contributing to indirect and direct effects of stress on the fetus. Fetal programming is discussed further in Chapters 12 and 16.

SUMMARY

Changes in the hypothalamic-pituitary-adrenal (HPA) axis during pregnancy enhance maternal adaptations and availability of nutrients to the fetus. Maternal HPA function is interrelated with placental function, because the placenta produces hypothalamic and pituitary hormones such as corticotropin-releasing hormone (CRH) and growth hormone (GH). Placental CRH plays a major role in initiation of parturition (see Chapter 4). Changes in HPA and hypothalamic-pituitary-thyroid (HPT) function can alter reproductive processes. The pregnant woman is in a state of euthyroid hyperthyroxinemia and transient hypercortisolism, although control set points are reset so the woman responds to stress in a manner that is similar to that of nonpregnant individuals. As a result, values for some endocrine function tests are altered. These changes must be considered when evaluating neuroendocrine function during pregnancy. Thyroid disorders are not uncommon in pregnant women. Knowledge of the effects of these disorders and their treatment is important to optimize fetal and neonatal outcome. Clinical recommendations related to thyroid function during pregnancy are summarized in Table 19-2.

DEVELOPMENT OF HYPOTHALAMIC, PITUITARY, ADRENAL, AND THYROID FUNCTION IN THE FETUS

Maturation of thyroid and adrenal function is interrelated with that of the hypothalamic and pituitary glands and the hypothalamic-pituitary-adrenal (HPA) and hypothalamic-pituitary-thyroid (HPT) axes. This process can be divided into three overlapping phases: embryogenesis (phase I), hypothalamic maturation (phase II), and maturation of thyroid and adrenal system function (phase III).[29] During the first phase (10 to 12 weeks), the adrenal and thyroid glands develop morphologically. Hypothalamic function matures during phase II (from 4 to 5 until 35 to 40 weeks). Thyroid-releasing hormone (TRH), gonadotropin-releasing hormone (GnRH), and somatostatin are detected in the hypothalamus by 10 to 12 weeks (by radioimmunoassay) and in fetal blood in the third trimester.[42] Phase III lasts from midgestation until term or 1 month after birth if transitional changes are considered. This stage involves increasing maturation and integration of endocrine system function.

Hypothalamus and Pituitary Gland

Anatomic Development

The hypothalamus and anterior pituitary glands develop simultaneously but independently of each other. As a result, growth of the various cell types within the anterior pituitary is not dependent on the presence of the hypothalamus. For example, anencephalic infants do not have a hypothalamus but have thyroid-stimulating hormone (TSH) cells within their rudimentary anterior pituitary gland.

The hypothalamus develops from 6 to 12 weeks from the ventral portion of the diencephalon. Hypothalamic nuclei and supraoptic track fibers develop by 12 to 14 weeks, with maturation of the hypothalamic neurons by 30 to 35 weeks.[28] The anterior pituitary arises from the anterior wall of the Rathke pouch, an upward offshoot of the primitive oral cavity.[45] The posterior pituitary and stalk develop from the infundibulum, a thickening on the floor of the diencephalon.[135] The anterior pituitary can be seen by 4 weeks and is independent of the oral cavity by 12 weeks. During the fifth week, the primitive anterior pituitary becomes connected with the infundibulum.

Cellular differentiation within the anterior pituitary gland begins at 7 to 8 weeks, under the influence of Pit-1 (a transcription regulator) that activates expression of genes encoding growth hormone (GH) and prolactin and differentiation

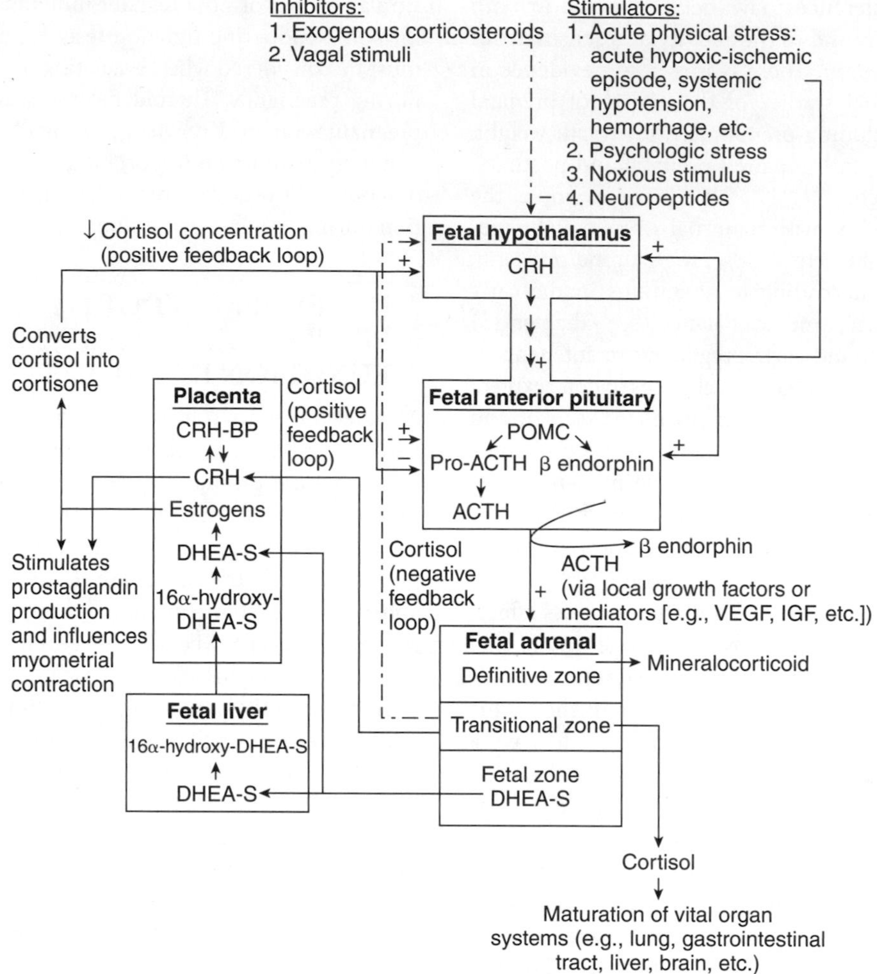

FIGURE 19-7 Schematic model illustrating neuroendocrine interaction between the fetal hypothalamic-pituitary-adrenal axis and the placenta. The solid arrows represent positive stimulatory pathways and the broken arrows represent negative inhibitory pathways. *ACTH,* Adrenocorticotropin; *CRH,* corticotropin-releasing hormone; *CRH-BP,* corticotropin-releasing hormone binding protein; *DHEA-S,* dehydroxy-epiandrosterone sulfate; *IGF,* insulin-like growth factor; *POMC,* pro-opiomelanocortin; *pro-ACTH,* pro-adrenocorticotropin; *VEGF,* vascular endothelial growth factor. (From Ng, P.C. [2000]. The fetal and neonatal hypothalamic-pituitary-adrenal axis. *Arch Dis Child Fetal Neonatal Ed, 82,* F250.)

Table 19-2 Recommendations for Clinical Practice Related to Changes in Pituitary, Adrenal, and Thyroid Function in Pregnant Women

Recognize the usual changes in pituitary and adrenal function during pregnancy (pp. 627-629 and Box 19-1).
Recognize the usual changes in thyroid function during pregnancy (pp. 629-633).
Assess and monitor maternal nutrition in terms of iodine intake (p. 634).
Monitor fetal growth in women with normal and abnormal thyroid function (pp. 635-636, 638).
Know the usual parameters for thyroid function tests during pregnancy (pp. 634-635 and Table 19-1).
Recognize the signs and symptoms of thyroid dysfunction and similarities with certain pregnancy-related findings (pp. 635-636).
Counsel women with hyperthyroidism and hypothyroidism regarding the effects of their disorder on pregnancy and the fetus and of pregnancy on the thyroid disorder (pp. 635-636).
Monitor medication levels and requirements in the pregnant woman with hyperthyroidism (pp. 635-636).
Know the fetal and neonatal risks of maternal iodide and radioactive iodine administration (pp. 637-638).
Avoid the use of iodides and radioactive iodine in pregnant women (pp. 637-638).
Know the fetal and neonatal risks associated with the use of thyroid and antithyroid agents (pp. 635-638).
Recognize and monitor for transient postpartum thyroid disorders (pp. 636-637 and Figure 19-5).
Counsel women with hypothyroidism and hyperthyroidism regarding breastfeeding considerations (p. 637).

of the different anterior pituitary cell types.[45] Thyrotropic cells appear at 12 to 13 weeks. An increase in TSH-secreting cell volume occurs by 23 weeks. Corticotroph cells can be identified by 6 weeks and express adrenocorticotropic hormone (ACTH) by 7 weeks; somatotroph can be seen by 8 weeks. TSH and gonadotropin β subunits are seen by 12 weeks. Lactotroph cells do not produce prolactin until after 24 weeks.[32]

Hypothalamic and Pituitary Function

The HPA axis is essential for regulating intrauterine homeostasis and maturation of the lungs, liver, and central nervous system; in conjunction with the placenta, this axis essential in the timing of parturition (see Chapter 4).[103] The hypothalamus and pituitary gland also play major roles in regulating the principal fetal steroid-secreting glands (adrenal glands and gonads) via a negative feedback mechanism. Figure 19-7 summarizes the HPA axis in the fetus and its interaction with placental function.

The fetal hypothalamus is visible by 7 weeks' gestation.[123] The hypothalamus-pituitary axis is generally complete by 12 to 18 weeks' gestation.[123] The HPA axis is established by 20 weeks and matures throughout the remainder of gestation; integrated HPA function matures postnatally.[29] The hypothalamic pituitary portal system is functional by 10 to 12 weeks and most of the hormones of the HPA axis are present by 10 to 16 weeks' gestation (Table 19-3).[29,90,98] For example, ACTH is seen in pituitary cells by 5 to 8 weeks and is measurable in fetal plasma by 16 weeks.[123] Plasma concentrations of these hormones rise for the first half of gestation. At this time the negative feedback loop comes into operation and the production and release of pituitary hormones become more finely regulated. Corticotropin-releasing hormone (CRH) from the fetus and placenta stimulates ACTH, which controls growth, differentiation, and function of the adrenal cortex in conjunction with growth factors (GFs) and other mediators.[103]

GnRH appears by 18 weeks and increases to 30 weeks.[90] Luteinizing hormone (LH) and follicle-stimulating hormone (FSH) appear in the fetal pituitary gland during the tenth week and reach their peaks at about 20 to 22 weeks' gestation. The concentration of LH is higher than that of FSH, and females have higher levels than males.[90] FSH promotes development of follicles in females; it stimulates growth of seminiferous tubules and initiates spermatogenesis in males. LH increases the synthesis and secretion of testosterone in the male embryo and stimulates steroid synthesis in ovarian cells.

Fetal growth hormone (GH) levels are higher than after birth due to immature inhibitory control and lack of GH receptors on fetal tissues.[42] Increases in cortisol before delivery are thought to induce GH receptors and changes in insulin-like growth factor-I (IGF-1).

Table 19-3 Ontogeny of Human Fetal Hypothalamic and Pituitary Hormones

HORMONE	AGE DETECTED (WEEKS)
HYPOTHALAMIC	
Gonadotropin-releasing hormone	14
Thyrotropin-releasing hormone	10
Somatostatin	14
Dopamine	11
Growth hormone–releasing hormone	18
Corticotropin-releasing hormone	16
PITUITARY	
Prolactin	16.5
Growth hormone	10.5
Adrenocorticotropin	7
Thyroid-stimulating hormone	13
Luteinizing hormone	10.5
Follicle-stimulating hormone	10.5

From Mesiano, S., & Jaffe, R.B. (2004). The endocrinology of human pregnancy and fetal-placental neuroendocrine development. In J.F. Strauss & R.L. Barbieri (Eds.), *Yen and Jaffe's Reproductive endocrinology: Physiology, pathophysiology, and clinical management* (5th ed.). Philadelphia: Saunders.

Adrenal Glands

Anatomic Development

The adrenal cortex arises in the fourth to fifth week from the intermediate mesoderm in the notch between the primitive urogenital ridge and the dorsal mesentery.[19] These cells proliferate and form cords migrating medially and laterally to the cranial end of the mesonephros (primitive transitional renal structures).[90,96] Neural crest cells form a medial mass on the primitive cortex. These cells are surrounded by the cortex cells and differentiate into the adrenal medulla. Later, another wave of cells surrounds the initial cortical cells to form the definitive cortex.[19,135] By 8 weeks, the cortex is organized into the fetal zone, with the definitive zone appearing a week later.[19,90,96] The fetal zone increases in size from 10 to 15 weeks and dominates from 16 to 20 weeks, being similar in size to the fetal kidneys.[19] By 28 to 30 weeks, a transitional zone that is initially similar to the fetal zone appears between the fetal and definitive zones. During the second and third trimesters, the adrenal glands continue to enlarge, with hypertrophy of the fetal zone and hyperplasia of the definitive zone.[19,90] Adrenal growth and zonation are stimulated by fetal ACTH, IGF-II, fibroblast growth factor, and epidermal growth factor.[19]

By midgestation, the fetal zone occupies 85% of the adrenal volume and is highly vascularized.[127,128] The adrenals double in size between 20 and 30 weeks and double again between 30 and 40 weeks as steroidogenic activity increases.[19] At term, the adrenal glands weigh 3 to 4 g and, relative to adult proportions, are 20 to 30 times larger.[19,90,96,127] After birth, the adrenal undergoes extensive remodeling, with a decrease in size and disappearance of the fetal zone.

Adrenal Function

As noted above, the fetal adrenal gland initially consists of two zones: the fetal zone (analogous to the adult zona reticularis) and the definitive zone (becomes the postnatal adrenal neocortex producing aldosterone—see Chapter 11). Later the transitional zone, which gives rise to the glucocorticoid-producing zona fasciculata, develops between the fetal and definitive zones. The fetal zone contains large lipid-containing steroidogenic cells, which are the major source of dehydroepiandrosterone (DHEA) and its sulfate (DHEA-S), which are precursors for production of estrone and estradiol-17β in the placenta. DHEA-S is also the precursor for 16-hydroxydehydroepiandrosterone, which is needed for estriol production by the placenta (see Chapter 3). Cholesterol is the precursor for these steroid hormones and the fetus uses both endogenous cholesterol synthesized from low-density lipoproteins and cholesterol transferred across the placenta.[57,127]

The placenta does not produce these precursors, so is dependent upon the fetal adrenal (primary source) or mother. In fetuses with decreased adrenal function, such as anencephalic fetuses, estriol production by the placenta remains low. Enzymes to synthesize DHEA-S are present by 6 to 8 weeks.[90,123] High levels of 17α-hydroxylase (17-OH or CYP17) and probably 21-hydroxylase (21-OH or CYP21) are seen early in gestation (Figure 19-8). 17-OH and 21-OH are cytochrome P-450 enzymes not expressed by the placenta.[164] Deficiency of 21-OH is the most common cause of congenital adrenal hyperplasia (see p. 651); a lack of 21-OH can result in virilization of the female external genitalia. Because the genital tract differentiates at 7 to 10 weeks (see Chapter 1), this enzyme must be present early in gestation.[19] Levels of 3β-hydroxysteroid dehydrogenase (involved in cortisol production) are low in the fetus.[19] The large size of the adrenal glands allows the fetus to secrete larger amounts of adrenal androgens daily, predominantly DHEA-S, than do adults. The fetus supplies 90% of the DHEA-S to the placenta after 16-hydroxylation by the fetal liver (see Figure 19-7).[127,128]

Cortisol is produced as early as 8 to 12 weeks but in small amounts and primarily from progesterone.[19,90,123] Production of cortisol from cholesterol, the usual precursor in later life, requires 3β hydroxysteroid dehydrogenase (3β HSD) which is not available in early gestation.[162] 3β HSD is not expressed before 23 weeks' gestation, with limited adrenal capacity for synthesis until after 30 weeks.[97,123] Cortisol secretion is present by 20 to 24 weeks' gestation.[29] Fetal cortisol levels gradually increase to term. Cortisol is essential for fetal maturation of the lungs, gut, liver, and central nervous system.[103] Cortisol is also found in amniotic fluid. During labor, fetal cortisol levels double.[96] Most fetal tissues and especially the placenta contain enzymes such as 11β hydroxysteroid dehydrogenase type 2 (11β HSD2) that convert cortisol to inactive cortisone. This serves as a protective mechanism against elevated cortisol in the fetus.

Maternal cortisol enters the placenta. However, since about 85% is deactivated by 11β HSD2, little reaches the fetus.[96,162] Maternal cortisol that does reach the fetus has a negative feedback effect on the fetal HPA axis, suppressing fetal cortisol production. Placental CRH stimulates pituitary ACTH production that in turn stimulates the fetal adrenal to produce cortisol, DHEA, and DHEA-S.[162] In the third trimester, placental 11β HSD2 activity increases with increased conversion of both fetal and maternal cortisol to cortisone. This reduction in active cortisol reaching the fetal

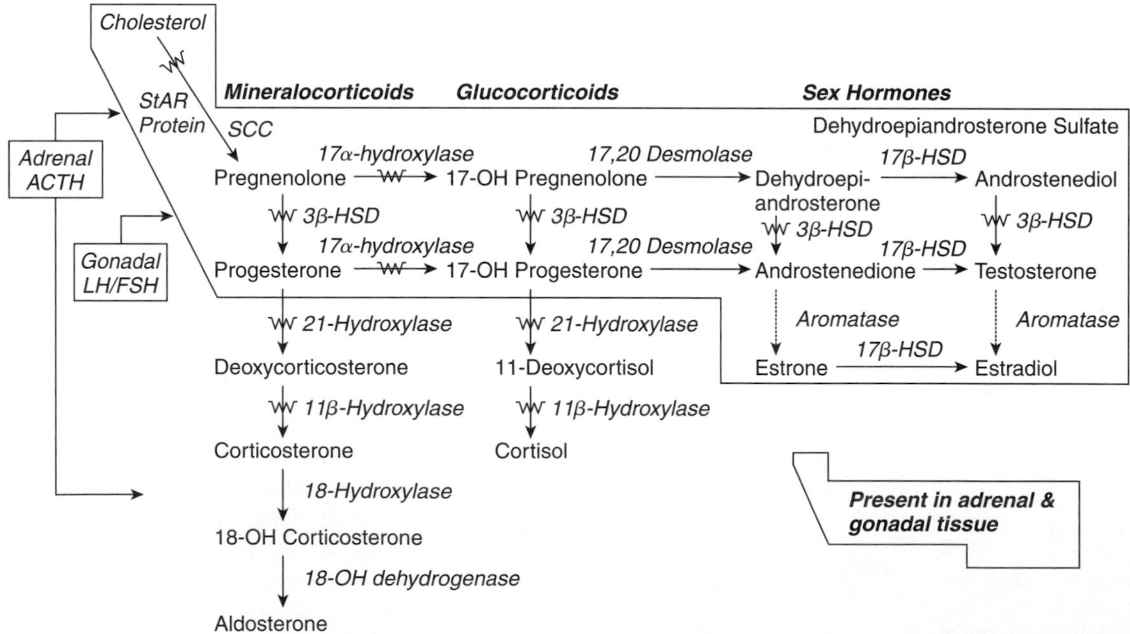

FIGURE 19-8 Adrenal and gonadal steroidogenesis. *Solid line* represents a major pathway; *dotted line* represents a major pathway in ovaries and minor pathway in adrenals; ʌʌ represents one of the potential areas of deficient enzymatic activity causing congenital adrenal hyperplasia; *StAR* represents steroidogenic auto regulatory protein; *SCC* represents cholesterol side chain cleavage enzyme; 3β-HSD represents 3β-hydroxysteroid dehydrogenase; 17β-HSD represents 17β-hydroxysteroid dehydrogenase. (From Pang, S. [1997]. Congenital adrenal hyperplasia. *Endocrinol Metab Clin North Am, 26,* 854.)

hypothalamus and pituitary further reduces negative feedback to the HPA axis that would normally reduce CRH, ACTH, and cortisol levels. This increases adrenal DHEA-S synthesis. DHEA-S production increases estrogen production, which in turn stimulates increased 11β HSD2.[29,103,127,162] CRH plays a major role in regulating fetal adrenal steroidogenesis in late gestation and in labor onset (see Chapter 4).[127] Placental CRH stimulates the fetal HPA axis and is itself stimulated by fetal cortisol (whereas hypothalamic CRH is inhibited by high cortisol levels). Seven to ten weeks prior to birth fetal adrenal cortisol production increases with a decrease in the conversion of cortisol to inactive cortisone, mediated by an increase in 11β HSD activity (stimulated by estrogens).[29] Factors influencing fetal adrenal function are summarized in Table 19-4.

Growth of the adrenal glands is probably not dependent on ACTH, because the anencephalic fetus with low ACTH levels develops adrenal glands, but ACTH is required for adrenal function.[19,128] ACTH may exert its effect via local GFs and other mediators such as fibroblast GF, epidermal GF, transforming growth factor-α (TGF-α), IGF-I, IGF-II, transforming growth factor-β (TGF-β), activin, and inhibin.[19,54,90] ACTH, estrogens, and IGF II stimulate growth of the definitive zone and activation of 3β HSD and P450 17α-hydroxylase, which mediate the increase in fetal cortisol production in late gestation.[29] Fisher summarizes the significance of this increase in fetal cortisol in late gestation in anticipation of transition to extrauterine life: "The increase in fetal circulating cortisol concentration during the final weeks of gestation is associated with a variety of physiologic responses. These include (a) increased conversion of T_4 to T_3 by stimulation of hepatic MDI-I and inhibition of MDI-III leading to an increase in circulating T_3 and decrease in rT_3 levels; (b) increased epinephrine secretion by sympathetic chromaffin tissue (including adrenal medulla) because of augmented phenylethanolamine transferase activity (which converts norepinephrine to epinephrine); (c) augmented synthesis and secretion of surfactant and maturation of surfactant composition; (d) stimulation of maturation of hepatic gluconeogenic enzyme activities; (e) increased β-adrenergic receptor density in a variety of tissues, including lung, heart, and brown adipose tissue; and (f) induction and maturation of a variety of gut enzymes for nutrient absorption and maturation of gut transport processes, motility, and structure."[29,p.390]

Intrauterine stress may activate adrenal cortisol secretion (see Maternal Stress Responses and Fetal Endocrine Programming). This often occurs at the cost of decreased DHEA-S production and thus lowered estriol production. The fetus may be exposed to elevated cortisol passively (due to increased maternal cortisol secondary to maternal stress or lowered placental 11β HSD2 activity) or actively secondary to proinflammatory cytokine secretion.[162] Passive exposure tends to suppress the fetal HPA axis and may increase the risk of low birth weight, prematurity, and other complications as well as alter growth and development and increase risks of adult-onset disorders; active exposure tends to enhance cortisol production after birth.[21,162,166] The fetus also responds to stress after 18 to 19 weeks by increasing β-endorphin (BE) levels.[126,143]

Table 19-4 Factors Affecting Fetal Adrenal Function

FACTOR	EFFECT
Maternal cortisol passively transferred to the fetus suppresses the fetal HPA axis	Increased production during maternal stress Increased transfer during early gestation Increased transfer in the presence of decreased placental 11β-HSD2 activity
Placental 11β-HSD2	Converts maternal cortisol to cortisone Modulates exposure of fetus to maternal cortisol
Placental CRH	Stimulates fetal HPA axis Is in turn stimulated by increased fetal cortisol Increases exponentially prior to delivery
Chorioamnionitis	Pro-inflammatory cytokines stimulate fetal HPA axis
Fetal responses to maternal and placental signaling during development	HPA axis is suppressed by maternal cortisol HPA axis is stimulated by placental CRH or chorioamnionitis

From Watterberg, K.L. (2004). Adrenocortical function and dysfunction in the fetus and neonate. *Semin Neonatol*, 9, 14.
HPA axis, Hypothalamus-pituitary-adrenal axis; *11β-HSD2*, 11β hydroxysteroid dehydrogenase type 2; *CRH*, corticotropin-releasing hormone.

Thyroid Gland

Anatomic Development

The thyroid gland develops during the first 12 weeks of gestation. The thyroid begins as an epithelial thickening at the base of the tongue around 17 days.[131] As the primordial gland migrates down the trachea, it becomes bilobular with a small median isthmus and begins to form follicles.[63] The thyroid initially descends in front of the pharyngeal gut. Later the thyroid descends in front of the hyoid bone and larynx to reach its final position in front of the trachea by 45 to 50 days of gestation.[131] Thyroid gland volume further increases eight- to 10-fold between 30 and 42 weeks' gestation with increasing iodine, thyroglobulin, iodothyronine, and thyroid hormone reserves.[29]

Thyroid Function

TRH synthesis begins in the hypothalamus by 6 to 8 weeks and is found in fetal serum by 9 weeks.[90,100,129,138] TRH is also synthesized by the placenta, fetal pancreas, and gut. Fetal serum TRH levels are high during the first and second trimesters due to these extrahypothalamic sources; hypothalamic

TRH production matures by 35 to 40 weeks along with maturation of the hypothalamic-pituitary portal system.[29,103] TSH can be detected in fetal serum by 10 to 12 weeks.[131] Levels are low until 18 weeks, then increase to 28 weeks, and then plateau and decrease to term.[43,90,131]

By 10 to 12 weeks, the thyroid gland begins to accumulate and concentrate iodine and has begun to synthesize and secrete iodothyronines. T_4 can be detected in fetal serum by 12 weeks, increasing to 2 μg/dL by 20 weeks and 10 μg/dL by term.[30,63,90,100,119,129,131,156] Fetal thyroid function remains at basal levels until midgestation, even though the capacity to secrete these hormones as well as TSH and TRH develops earlier.[28,43,90] As a result, significant amounts of fetal thyroid hormone are not produced before 18 to 20 weeks' gestation.[95,99] TSH, T_4, and free T_4 increase from 15 to 42 weeks.[168] At term, T_4 levels in cord blood are 10% to 20% lower than maternal values; most fetal T_4 is bound to TTR and albumin.[131] Free T_4 concentrations in fetal fluids reflect the interaction between T_4-binding proteins and maternal T_4, which maintains sufficient free T_4 for fetal needs but prevents toxic levels.[95] Thyroxine-binding globulin (TBG) can be detected by 12 weeks and reaches term values by midgestation.[131] Concentrations of iodine increase after 13 to 15 weeks with peak concentrations at 20 to 24 weeks.[72] Changes in fetal thyroid hormones are summarized in Figure 19-9.

Serum T_3 levels remain low until 30 weeks and then increase slightly, but never approach maternal values.[28,100,156] At term, fetal T_3 and free T_3 levels are 30% to 50% of maternal values.[131] T_3 levels remain low because the fetus is unable to convert T_4 to T_3 peripherally due to incomplete enzyme systems. The increase in T_3 after 30 weeks is associated with maturation of these enzymes.[28] Type II and type III monodeiodinases (MDI; see Box 19-3 on page 630) are present by midgestation; MDI-I (which converts T_4 to the highly active T_3) matures later and levels are low during gestation.[29,156] As a result, a greater proportion of T_4 is converted to the inactive rT_3 in the fetus than in the adult.[28,98] Iodothyronines are inactivated by sulfation as well, which also helps to regulate the amount of active thyroid hormone; these analogues are

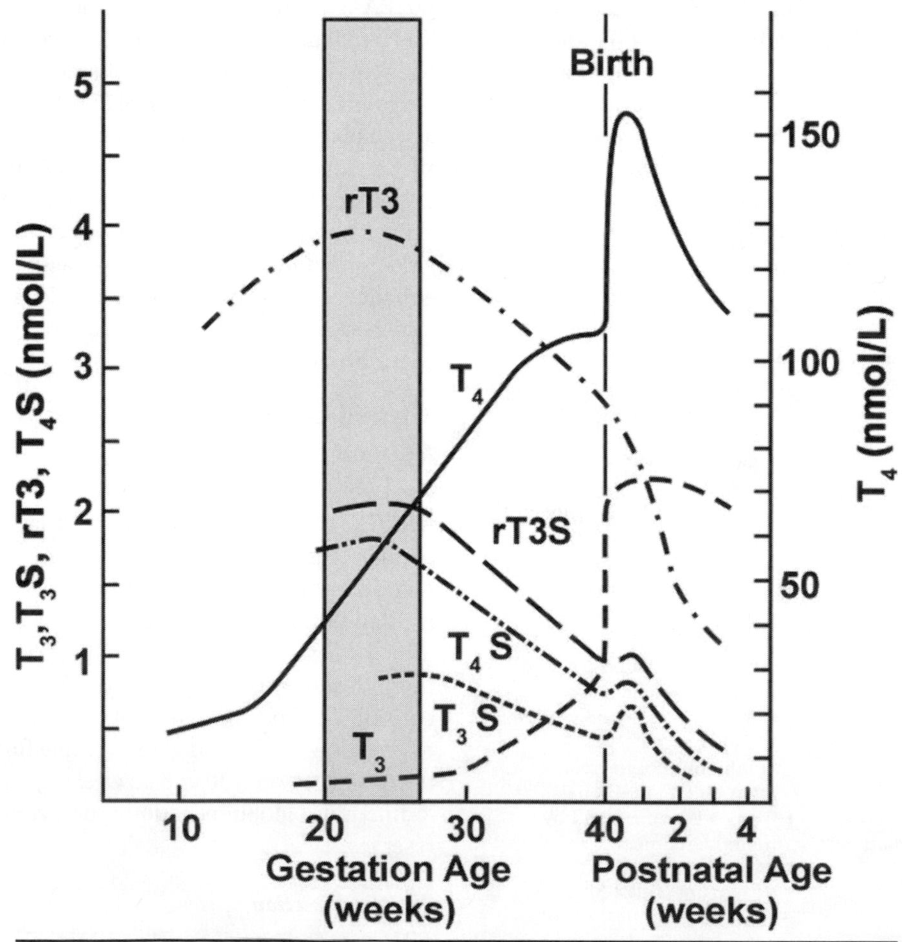

FIGURE 19-9 Maturation of serum iodothyronine concentrations in the human fetus and newborn. T_4 = thyroxine; T_3 = triiodothyronine; rT_3 = reverse T_3. T_4S, T_3S, and rT_3S are sulfated analogues. The neonatal TSH surge peaks at 60 to 70 mU/L. The shaded area highlights levels in the ELBW fetus. (From Fisher, D.A. (2008). Thyroid system immaturities in very low–birth weight premature infants. *Semin Perinatol, 32,* 389.)

also metabolized to the inactive rT_3S.[168] Increased production of sulfated analogues of thyroid hormones are seen in the fetus.[29] In the hypothyroid fetus, MDI-II increases and MDI-I is suppressed so T_4 is shunted to the central nervous system (CNS), where it is converted to T_3 by MDI-II.[29] The control by these monodeiodinases of the levels of active thyroid hormones at different stages of development is an important protective mechanism because too much T_3 could damage cells. Organs such as the brain, which are dependent on T_3 for normal development, have higher levels of enzymes needed to convert T_4 to T_3.[88,98,99]

Serum rT_3 levels rise early in the third trimester and then progressively decrease to term as MDI activity increases.[90,131,156] As noted earlier, the elevated serum rT_3 levels in the fetus are a result of increased MDI-III activity (see also Box 19-3 on page 630).[28] MDI-III is the predominant deiodinase in the fetus and placenta with levels 10 to 15 times greater than in adults.[28,29] This increases conversion of T_4 to the biologically inactive rT_3 (rather than to biologically active T_3) and T_3 to the inactive T_2; this may be a way the fetus counteracts high T_4 levels and maintains metabolic homeostasis.[28,29] Thyroid maturation in the late fetal and early neonatal period is related to progressive increases in hypothalamic TRH secretion, TRH responsiveness by the pituitary (by 26 to 28 weeks, the fetus responds to TRH in a manner similar to that of adults), sensitivity of the thyroid to TSH, and maturation of feedback mechanisms.[28,29] Fetal thyroid function is summarized in Table 19-5.

Role of Maternal Thyroid Hormones

Thyroid hormones are critical for brain development, neuronogenesis, neuron migration, axon and dendrite formation, and organization. Thyroid hormone receptors develop early in the fetal brain, appearing by at least 9 weeks' postmenstrual age, increasing 10-fold by 18 weeks; 25% to 30% of the receptors are occupied by T_3 during this time.[95] Levels of T_3 in the cerebral cortex reach adult values by midgestation.[108] Thyroid hormones are much higher in the brain than fetal serum at each stage of development due to activity of MDI-II and brain MDI-III.[95]

Maternal thyroid hormones are transferred to the fetus in the first trimester, beginning soon after conception and increase rapidly over the next weeks to biologically relevant values that correlate with maternal values.[88,94,95,100] Even during the second and third trimesters when the fetal thyroid is producing hormone, much of the T_4 needed for development and neuroprotection is of maternal origin.[88,94] This has implications for the infant born prematurely, especially very low–birth weight (VLBW) infants, who lose this protection by their early birth.[95] Maternal hypothyroidism is particularly damaging to the fetal brain in the first half of pregnancy when fetal T_4 production is low.[94,129] T_3 generation from T_4 by MDI-II increases in the cerebral cortex until midgestation, reaching values similar to those in the adult brain. Cerebral T_3 levels are dependent on local production in the brain, via MDI-II that converts T_4 to T_3, and are thus not affected by circulating T_3 levels, but by circulating T_4. Therefore if the mother is hypothyroxinemic with low T_4 levels, the fetal brain will have a deficiency of T_3 for normal development, even if circulating T_3 is normal or increased.[94] Maternal iodine deficiency results in altered thyroid function and inadequate thyroid hormone for development; maternal iodine excess can also block thyroid hormone synthesis and secretion.[129]

Table 19-5 Characteristics of Fetal Thyroid Function

- Placental transfer of iodine and maternal T_4
- Extrahypothalamic (placenta, pancreas, gut) production of thyrotropin-releasing hormone by the placenta and selected fetal tissue
- Progressive maturation of T_4 production and T_4 negative feedback control of thyroid-stimulating hormone (thyrotropin) secretion
- Predominant metabolism of T_4 to inactive reverse T_3 and sulfated analogues
- Local monodeiodinase type II mediated T_3 production from T_4 in selected fetal tissues including brain
- Developmentally programmed maturation of thyroid hormone nuclear receptors in individual fetal tissues
- Developmentally programmed maturation of thyroid hormone gene transcription in individual fetal tissues

Adapted from Fisher, D.A. (1999). Hypothyroxinemia in premature infants: Is thyroxine treatment necessary? *Thyroid, 9,* 715.
T_3, Triiodothyronine; *T_4*, thyroxine.

NEONATAL PHYSIOLOGY

Transitional Events

Catecholamines and cortisol surge at birth. Catecholamines, including epinephrine, norepinephrine, and dopamine, increase to levels 20 times greater than those of adults.[29] This increase is greater with vaginal delivery than with cesarean delivery. Levels decrease after the first few hours. The catecholamine surge promotes extrauterine cardiorespiratory adaptation (see Chapters 9 and 10) and is accompanied by a surge in other hormones, including renin, angiotensin II, arginine vasopressin (AVP; see Chapter 11), adrenocorticotropic hormone (ACTH), β-endorphins (BEs), and cortisol (see next section). BEs are increased with fetal distress.[16] Cord blood and maternal BE levels are not correlated.[126] Thyroid hormones are involved in the regulation of thermogenesis, cardiac contractility, and metabolic function during the transition to extrauterine life.[11,122]

Hypothalamic-Pituitary-Adrenal Axis

Remodeling of the adrenal glands after birth occurs via apoptosis of the fetal zone, remodeling of the fetal zone cells, and development of the other zones.[19,90,164] Apoptosis of the fetal zone is mediated by activin and transforming growth factor-β (TGF-β). The size of the adrenals decreases 25% in the first 4 days after birth.[164] Adequate pituitary function is seen in both term and preterm infants.[86]

At birth, the infant's free cortisol levels are about one third or less than maternal levels, possibly related to higher levels of cortisol-binding globulin (CBG) in the mother. A cortisol surge begins in late gestation, increasing during labor and transition to extrauterine life.[29] This surge is blunted in VLBW infants.[29] Cortisol levels double during labor, increase further in the first 1 to 2 hours after birth, and then gradually fall during the first week.[96] There is an inverse relationship between cortisol levels and gestational age. ACTH and cortisol levels are higher in infants delivered vaginally than in those delivered by cesarean birth.[91,134] ACTH and BE levels are elevated in cord blood and decrease significantly by 24 hours and reach adult levels by 4 to 5 days in healthy infants.[75,83,126] After birth the high placental corticotropin releasing hormone (CRH) levels fall. This may lead to a refractory period over the first few days where newborn CRH production by the hypothalamus is transiently suppressed, accompanied by a refractory pituitary gland response. These changes result in a decreased ability to increase ACTH to stimulate the adrenal gland. This transition is tolerated well in healthy infants, but in immature or ill infants may lead to a relative adrenal insufficiency and cardiovascular compromise (see Adrenal Cortex Insufficiency).[27,105,123]

BEs are endogenous opioid-like substances that are derived, along with ACTH and other substances, from a large precursor molecule (pro-opiomelanocortin). BEs increase markedly with birth in both term and preterm infants. The BE increase at birth is greater with perinatal hypoxic-ischemic events or other stress such as forceps delivery and is reported to be inversely related to PO_2.[16,126,149] Other endogenous opioids, such as the enkephalins, are also increased at birth and further increased with hypoxia, acidosis and ischemia.

Both term and preterm infants in the neonatal intensive care unit (NICU) have higher BE levels than healthy term infants. Preterm infants (especially preterm males) have higher BE levels than both healthy term and ill term infants.[75] Elevated BE levels are seen in stressed preterm infants with apnea, but not in nonstressed infants.[83] Release of BE is a component of neonatal respiratory control and is triggered by hypoxia.[83] BE levels are also higher in infants with respiratory distress.[75]

The administration of antenatal corticosteroids (see Chapter 10) leads to a transient suppression of the pituitary and adrenal glands. Long-term effects on hypothalamic-pituitary-adrenal (HPA) function have not been well studied.[87] Even with this suppression, healthy, preterm infants respond to stress with increased cortisol.[103] The ill infant, however, is less able to respond to stress and is more vulnerable to stress-related morbidity (see sections on Neonatal Stress and Adrenal Cortex Insufficiency).

Growth hormone (GH) decreases rapidly after birth as free fatty acids, which block GH release, increase with nonshivering thermogenesis.[42] GH levels are higher in preterm infants than in term infants. Somatostatin levels in preterm infants are higher during the second week but decrease by the third to fourth weeks. Levels are even higher in infants with respiratory distress syndrome.[55]

Prolactin increases in the late fetal and early neonatal periods. Levels are higher in preterm infants than in term infants due to increased sensitivity to thyroid-stimulating hormone (TSH) and estrogens, pituitary insensitivity to dopaminergic inhibition, and reduced renal excretion by the immature kidney (with its lower glomerular filtration rate).[149] Prolactin may have a role in lung maturation and fluid homeostasis with transition. Dopamine levels are twice those of adults and function as a prolactin release–inhibiting factor.[90]

Hypothalamic-Pituitary-Thyroid Axis

The newborn is in a state of physiologic hyperthyroidism because of marked changes in thyroid function at birth (Table 19-6 and Figure 19-9).[121,131] Thyroid-releasing hormone (TRH) and TSH levels increase rapidly after birth, followed by increases in T_4, free T_4, T_3, and free T_3.[124] Exposure of the newborn to the cooler extrauterine environment is believed to stimulate skin thermal receptors, TRH release by the hypothalamus, and TSH release by the pituitary gland.[29] The TSH surge is also stimulated by cutting of the umbilical cord and the catecholamine surge at birth.[29,121] The increase in TSH (and T_4) with cord cutting is limited in extremely low–birth weigh (ELBW) infants.[29] TSH increases from 9 to 10 μU/mL (IU/L) at birth to peak at 60 to 70 mU/L within the first hour after birth.[29] TSH rapidly decreases to 50% of peak values by 2 hours and to 20% by 24 hours, followed by a progressive decrease over the next 2 to 3 days to levels similar to or lower than cord blood values (see Figure 19-9).[28,29,74,90] During the first week, periodic oscillations in serum TSH have been reported, possibly reflecting establishment of a new equilibrium in the negative feedback exerted by thyroid hormone on the anterior pituitary.[135] Although TSH generally falls to adult ranges within 3 to 10 days, TSH may remain somewhat elevated for several months.[129,131]

The TSH surge leads to a rapid threefold to sixfold increase in T_4, and twofold increase in free T_4.[29,168] T_3 and rT_3

Table 19-6 Changes in Thyroid Function Associated with Fetal Transition to Extrauterine Life at Term

Neonatal TSH surge
Increased T_4 and T_3 production
Stimulation of brown adipose tissue thermogenesis
Increased T_4 to T_3 conversion
Permanently increased serum T_3 level
Decreased production of inactive thyroid hormone analogues (rT_3, T_4S, rT_3S, T_2S)
Decreased extrahypothalamic thyrotropin-releasing hormone production
Decreased TSH concentration
Resetting of hypothalamic-pituitary free T_4 set point for control of TSH secretion

From Fisher, D.A. (1999). Hypothyroxinemia in premature infants: Is thyroxine treatment necessary? *Thyroid, 9*, 715.

T_3, Triiodothyronine; *T_4*, thyroxine; *TSH*, thyroid-stimulating hormone (thyrotropin).

levels are correlated with gestational age and birth weight.[129] T_4 levels peak at 24 to 48 hours after birth (see Figure 19-9), and then slowly decrease over the next few weeks.[29,100,129,131,156] Newborn T_4 levels are usually 10% to 20% less than maternal values.[131]

Cord blood T_3 values average 45 to 50 ng/dL (0.69 to 0.77 pmol/L) (30% to 50% of maternal values). The newborn quickly changes from a state of T_3 deficiency to T_3 excess. T_3 levels increase rapidly with birth with a sixfold increase in T_3 secretion and eightfold increase in free T_3.[156] T_3 peaks at 24 to 48 hours at 260 to 300 ng/mL (4 to 4.62 pmol/L) (values exceeding those in adults) in most infants and then gradually fall.[28,29,129,131] The increase in T_3 is due to the TSH surge and increased MDI-I activity (see Box 19-3 on page 630), with increased conversion of T_4 to T_3 and removal of the placenta (with its high levels of MDI-III that convert T_3 to inactive forms).[29,156] The increase in T_3 is also related to cutting the umbilical cord, which increases liver blood flow and conversion of T_3 to T_4.[29] Serum T_3 and T_4 levels gradually fall to values seen in infancy with the first few weeks after birth.[129]

Levels of rT_3 remain high for 3 to 5 days and then gradually decrease to adult values by 1 to 2 months.[131] Thyroxine-binding globulin (TBG) tends to be high because of transplacental passage of estrogens that stimulate its production. TBG-binding capacity in the infant is higher than in the pregnant woman and about 1.5 times that of the adult.[131] Radioactive iodine uptake by the thyroid is higher in the newborn because of increased avidity of the neonatal thyroid for iodine. Iodine concentrations in the thyroid gland at birth are correlated with gestational age with increased 24-hour ^{123}I uptake for the first month and a greater concentration of ^{123}I in infants than adults.[131]

The TSH surge is also seen in preterm and SGA infants, although it may be blunted.[29,168] Thyroid hormones in preterm infants follow patterns similar to those in term infants but may take longer to reach stable values.[43,129,131,175] Thyroid hormone levels are inversely related to gestational age.[29,99,129] Free T_4 and T_3 levels are lower and rT_3 levels higher in preterm infants than in term infants for the first weeks due to persistence of fetal levels of MDI enzymes (see p. 630) and higher sulfated iodothyronine analogues.[29,100,125,156,168] TSH levels and response are generally similar to those in term infants, but TSH may be in the normal adult range.[100] In ELBW infants, TSH response to low T_4 levels is limited.[29] Serum T_4 and T_3 levels may decrease to below birth levels in VLBW preterm infants during the first week to levels two to three times lower than in term infants.[124,129,156] In addition, some ill and VLBW preterm infants develop a characteristic syndrome of transient hyperthyroxinemia with normal or low TSH and low free T_4 levels without other evidence of hypothyroidism (see Transient Alterations in Thyroid Function in Preterm Infants).[29,99,124,129,156,168] T_4 levels are higher in infants of mothers who received a course of antenatal glucosteroids.[85] The preterm infant may take 3 to 8 weeks to reach term levels of these hormones.[156]

CLINICAL IMPLICATIONS FOR NEONATAL CARE

Endocrine adaptation at birth is influenced by gestational age, stresses of delivery, postnatal disease states, and hypoxic-ischemic events.[149] Normal endocrine function is critical for normal growth and development both before and after birth. For example, biochemical maturation of the lungs and surfactant production (see Chapter 10) are dependent on the hypothalamic-pituitary-adrenal (HPA) axis and its hormones, including corticotropin-releasing hormone (CRH) and cortisol, as well as thyroid hormones. Thyroid hormones are needed for lung development and surfactant production, bone growth (including calcium and vitamin D homeostasis), thermogenesis, and central nervous system (CNS) maturation.[11] Within the CNS, these hormones are critical for differentiation of neural stem cells, cerebral neuronogenesis, and regulation of expression of genes involved in neuronal migration, brain dendritic arborization, synaptogenesis, neuronal migration, axon development, and growth (see Chapter 15).[7,11,47,71,144] Effects on bone growth and CNS development continue into early childhood. An intact HPA axis is necessary for the infant to respond appropriately to stress and to prevent maladaptation.

Alterations in HPA and hypothalamic-pituitary-thyroid (HPT) function influence the transition to extrauterine life. For example, thyroid function is closely linked to thermoregulation and production of heat from brown adipose tissue. Alterations in health status from immaturity or acute illness can result in transient adrenal or thyroid dysfunction. Screening for hypothyroidism and congenital adrenal hyperplasia and recognition of hyperthyroidism and hypothyroidism have important ramifications for the infant's future growth and development. This section examines the implications of these events.

Neonatal Stress

Although definitions and depictions of the stress response may vary, all or most propose an integrated biologic response pattern during or after stressor exposure. Activation of endocrine and neurotransmitter systems represents the major mechanisms upon which other aspects of this response are built. Responses to stressors are normally of short duration (acute stress) and are aimed at survival followed by a return to a state of dynamic homeostasis.[118,132] Stress responses that go on for extended periods (chronic stress) can produce long-term changes in stress response systems, leading to decreases in adaptive capacity and increased risk for physical and psychological disorders.[171]

The NICU has the potential for significant stress during a period of critical brain development. There are many sources of stress in the NICU from both internal (e.g., pain, distress, pathologic processes) and external (e.g., physical environment, caregiver interventions, medical or surgical procedures, multiple simultaneous modes of stimulation) demands. Stress and pain (see Chapter 15) interact. Preterm infants may be simultaneously exposed to pain stimuli and other potentially noxious sensations (e.g., handling, light, sound, and temperature changes) that cause further activity in nociceptive pathways and systemic stress responses. An infant's stress tolerance may be reached or exceeded repeatedly, contributing to short- and long-term morbidity. Infants in the NICU experience both acute and chronic stress. Many handling procedures in small and sick infants lead to stress, which if not controlled, may cause cumulative harm.[6]

Baseline responses to stress are set early in life and can influence later responses and adaptation.[13,33,41,109,159] Stress activates the HPA axis with release of catecholamines, CRH, adrenocorticotropin (ACTH), β-endorphins (BEs), and cortisol. Stress responses affect many systems: cardiovascular (increased blood pressure and heart rate), gastrointestinal (increased gut motility and splanchnic vasoconstriction), renal (sodium and water retention), and respiratory (increased oxygen consumption, decreased tidal volume, and functional residual capacity or ventilation-perfusion mismatch). Stress can alter coagulation, immune function, and cytokine production. Stress has profound metabolic consequences; metabolic stability may be more difficult to maintain in the stressed neonate, especially in immature infants.[6] Stress can lead to hyperglycemia or hypoglycemia. Stress increases counterregulatory hormones (e.g., glucagon, ACTH, catecholamines, cortisol) that decrease insulin secretion. Glucagon, fat, and protein are converted to glucose, which—in the face of insulin resistance from the counterregulatory hormones—results in hyperglycemia. In immature infants, this response and the infant's nutrient stores may become exhausted, so over time the infant becomes hypoglycemic.[6]

Term infants, whether healthy or ill, have an intact HPA axis and can identify and respond to stress.[117] Healthy preterm infants older than 28 weeks' gestational age respond to stress with increased cortisol secretion, although at lower levels than in term infants.[117] Healthy term infants have relatively low basal cortisol levels that rapidly increase with stress.[50] Salivary cortisol has been used to examine responses of both term and preterm infants to stressful or soothing events.[46,91,137,146,147]

However, in preterm infants who are ill or younger than 28 weeks' gestational age, the HPA is suppressed during the first few weeks after birth. These VLBW infants seem unable to "recognize" stress and to respond by increasing cortisol secretion.[50] Preterm infants—especially those who are ill or weigh less than 1000 g—have lower basal cortisol levels and are less able to increase cortisol production with stress. In these infants there is an increase in precursors but not in cortisol, suggesting immature activity of enzymes to convert these precursors to cortisol. In very immature infants, this may reflect the persistence of fetal protective responses against higher maternal cortisol levels.[52]

Exposure of VLBW infants to significant early pain and stress has been reported to alter later cortisol response patterns with a "resetting" of the basal arousal system postulated.[46] Early stress in the fetus and neonate may produce permanent changes in neural pathways, increasing the risk of later disorders such as adult psychopathology and hypertension (see Maternal Stress Responses and Fetal Endocrine Programming).[6,13,41,136,159] Maternal stress in the third trimester is associated with increased ACTH and cortisol and increased placental CRH. Because CRH is a primary factor in labor onset, this may lead to preterm labor and decrease the sensitivity of the fetal-neonatal anterior pituitary to CRH, with permanent elevations in cortisol and BEs.[136]

Adrenal Cortex Insufficiency

A transient adrenal cortex insufficiency is seen in some ELBW infants. These infants have poor or limited ability to respond to shock and develop hypotension unresponsive to fluid and pressor management.[26,104,162] In these infants the adrenal cortex may be unable to produce enough cortisol to maintain blood pressure (cortisol is involved in blood pressure regulation).[103] This insufficiency is related to an immature HPA axis with an inadequate pituitary response to CRH stimulation and decreased cortisol production due to immature synthesis of 11β hydroxylase and limited 3β HSD and other enzymes.[27,105,123] Some ELBW infants were reported to have an increase in ACTH and cortisol following CRH administration and increased cortisol after ACTH administration, which are expected responses. However, other ELBW infants in this study, especially those who were ill, had very low serum cortisol levels that remained low even under stimulation.[50] Others have found that only one third to one half of sick preterm infants were able to achieve a normal response to ACTH and CRH stimuation.[51,105,162] Decreased responses to ACTH stimulation have also been reported in small-for-gestational-age (SGA) infants.[12]

Acutely ill preterm infants may have lower cortisol values than healthy preterm infants with low cortisol associated with hypotension, inflammation, bronchopulmonary dysplasia (BPD), and patent ductus arteriosus and an increase in mortality.[8,27,139,162] A multicenter study of prophylactic hydrocortisone to prevent BPD did not improve survival without BPD, although infants who were treated after chorioamnionitis had decreased mortality.[163] However, the study was stopped early due to an increased risk of gastrointestinal perforation in the hydrocortisone-treated group, especially with simultaneous use of hydrocortisone and indomethacin or ibuprofen.[27,163] Term infants following severe perinatal stress may also demonstrate a transient relative adrenal insufficiency with low circulating levels of cortisol.[27,105]

Thyroid Function and Thermoregulation

Thyroid function and neonatal temperature regulation are interrelated (see Chapter 20). T_3 and T_4 increase basal metabolic rate and heat production, whereas T_4 and norepinephrine stimulate metabolism of brown adipose tissue. Occlusion of the umbilical cord activates brown adipose tissue catabolism via a catecholamine surge and withdrawal of placental prostaglandins and adenosine.[28,29] T_4 enhances the effects of catecholamines to increase oxygen consumption (and metabolic rate) and increases brown adipose tissue lipolysis. Within

6 hours of birth, the term neonate can respond to cold stress by increasing his or her metabolic rate 100%; by 6 to 9 days, this increase may be 170%. The preterm infant responds similarly to cold stress, although at a slower rate and lower percentage increase (~40%).[42]

Transient Alterations in Thyroid Function in Preterm Infants

In healthy preterm infants, cord blood T_4 levels range from 5.5 to 6 mcg/dL (72 to 77 nmol/L), increasing to 7 to 9 mcg/dL (90 to 116 nmol/L) by 21 to 28 days and reaching values similar to those of term infants by 4 to 6 weeks or perhaps sooner.[17] As a result, preterm infants are more likely to have below normal values on thyroid screening tests compared with term infants.[131,141,156] Thyroid hormone values after birth are correlated with gestational age. For example, infants of 25 to 27 weeks' gestation have free T_4 levels that are two to three times lower than those of term infants.[29] Maturation of thyroid function in VLBW infants is illustrated in Figure 19-10.

Early loss of placental transfer of maternal T_4, which at that point in gestation may account for 30% of fetal T_4, along with iodine deficiency from inadequate stores and intake, may alter thyroid homeostasis in preterm infants, especially ELBW infants.[7,29,168] As a result some preterm infants develop transient thyroid alterations in the early weeks after birth as T_4 and T_3 levels fall in the first week to values lower than at birth. Other factors in the etiology of these alterations include decreased liver thyroxine-binding globulin (TBG) production, immaturity of the hypothalamic-pituitary-thyroid axis, inadequate nutrition, decreased MDI-I, decreased brown adipose tissue, and immature tissue thyroid systems (Table 19-7).[29,129] Thyroid function tends to return to normal as the infant matures or recovers from the underlying illness, with achievement of stable serum T_4 values by 6 to 7 weeks.[131] Three transient patterns of altered thyroid function have been described in preterm infants: physiologic hypothyroxinemia, transient primary hypothyroidism, and transient secondary/tertiary hypothyroidism.[29,63] These are more likely to occur in VLBW infants who weigh less than 1000 g and infants who are ill or stressed. Ill preterm, such as those with respiratory distress syndrome, patent ductus arteriosus, necrotizing enterocolitis, and prolonged oxygen dependence, may also develop nonthyroidal illness syndrome.[29,168] This disorder is similar to the euthyroid sick syndrome seen in severely ill adults and children.[140]

Table 19-7 Thyroid System Immaturities in the Premature Infant

Loss of maternal T_4
Limited postnatal thermogenesis
Hypothalamic-pituitary immaturity
Limited thyroid gland reserve
Persistent fetal thyroid hormone metabolism
Predisposition to nonthyroidal illness syndrome

From Fisher, D.A. (2008). Thyroid system immaturities in very low birth weight premature infants. *Semin Perinatol, 32,* 391.

Physiologic hypothyroxinemia of prematurity is seen in many preterm infants younger than 35 weeks' gestational age and referred to as *transient hypothyroxinemia of prematurity* (THOP).[29,168] There is a lack of consensus regarding what values define THOP.[168,169] These infants have low T_4 levels with low to normal TBG and thyroid-stimulating hormone (TSH) levels.[29,129,168] This is a transient phenomenon that usually resolves within 2 to 3 weeks, although it may last for 2 to 3 months.[29,63] Thus most preterm infants are hypothyroxinemic. The frequency increases with decreasing gestational age. The mechanism and pattern of this disorder vary with gestational age.[29]

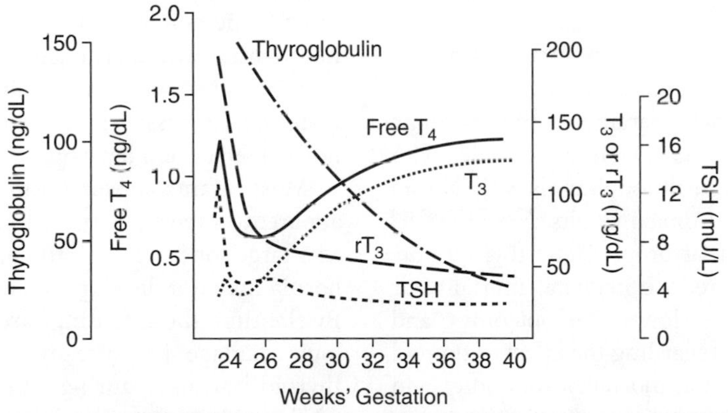

FIGURE 19-10 Maturation of thyroid function parameters in the very low–birth weight (23 to 35 weeks' gestation) premature infant. (Data from van Wassenaer, A.G., et al. [1997]. *Pediatr Res, 42,* 604; and Ares, S., et al. [1997]. *J Clin Endocrinol Metab, 82,* 1704. From Fisher, D.A. [1998]. Thyroid function in premature infants. The hypothyroxinemia of prematurity. *Clin Perinatol, 25,* 1008.)

In infants born at greater than 30 to 32 weeks' gestational age, T_4 and free T_4 increase transiently after birth in conjunction with the TSH surge (which is similar to the pattern seen with term infants) and then decrease. This is followed by a gradual increase in TBG, T_4, free T_4, and T_3, reaching term values by 38 to 42 weeks.[29] These infants probably have immaturity of the thyroid's ability to respond to TSH and ability to convert T_4 to T_3.[29]

In VLBW infants younger than 30 weeks' gestational age, there is a limited TSH surge and increase in T_4, followed by a decrease in T_4 and free T_4 to a nadir at 1 to 2 weeks.[29,156] These infants usually achieve cord blood levels of serum T_4 by 3 to 4 weeks.[29] The greatest fall is seen in the lowest gestation infants.[156] As T_4 decreases, TSH rises, but often remains below 20 μU/L (the cutoff value for hypothyroidism).[156] The etiology of the hypothyroxinemia in these infants is not completely understood but probably due to immaturity of the HPT axis, interruption of transfer of maternal thyroid hormones and iodine across the placenta, iodine deficiency, immaturity of MDI enzymes, decreased TBG and probably an inability to increase iodine uptake and T_4 production with extrauterine adaptation.[7,29,63] Because of immaturity, these infants also have inefficient production of thyroglobulin and a decreased ability to convert T_4 to T_3 due to low levels of liver MDI-I activity (see Box 19-3 on page 630).[29]

Transient primary hypothyroidism is less common.[29] These infants have low T_4 and free T_4, with increased TSH levels during the first 2 to 3 weeks after birth.[63] Thyroglobulin and iodine stores are low, with increased T_4 utilization and demand. The frequency of transient secondary/tertiary hypothyroidism is unknown but may occur in up to 10% of VLBW infants. These infants have low T_4 and free T_4 levels without changes in TSH during the first 1 to 2 weeks after birth.[29] There may be some benefit to treating these infants in that low thyroid hormone may contribute to later neurologic problems, although it is unclear if supplementation improve outcomes.[155,156]

The decision of whether to treat healthy or ill preterm infants with THOP is controversial.[29,63,66,131,155] Exogenous TRH significantly increases serum T_4 and TSH levels. However, most studies of use of T_4 for thyroid hormone replacement do not demonstrate significant differences in the age at which serum T_4 values normalize or in infant growth parameters.[130,155,160] Some observational evidence suggests that THOP is associated with adverse developmental outcomes, although trials with thyroid hormone replacement have had mixed results.[22,29,155,157,168,169] Osborn and Hunt concluded that prophylactic thyroid hormone administration did not reduce neonatal mortality or morbidity or improve neurodevelopmental outcomes, and there was insufficient evidence regarding the effect of thyroid hormone replacement on neonatal mortality, morbidity, and improvement in neurodevelopmental outcomes.[110,111]

Neonatal Hyperthyroidism

Neonatal hyperthyroidism is rare and is usually a transient disorder associated with transplacental passage of maternal thyroid-stimulating immunoglobulins (TSIs) in women with Graves' disease (see Chapter 13). This may occur even in euthyroid women after thyroid removal or ^{131}I thyroid ablation, because TSIs are still present in the woman's system. TSI levels correlate positively with development of neonatal hyperthyroidism; thus maternal screening can identify the infant at risk. An increased fetal heart rate (greater than 160 beats/min) after 22 weeks is of concern.[72] The mother may be treated with antithyroid drugs, if she is not already being treated, to maintain the fetal heart rate around 140. The incidence of neonatal effects is 0.6% to 9.5%.[72] Although this disorder is usually transient, increased mortality has been reported, usually as a result of respiratory obstruction or a difficult delivery due to the enlarged thyroid, or high-output cardiac failure secondary to tachycardia (heart rates greater than 200 beats/min).[72] If the disorder is recognized prior to birth, infants have been treated by giving medications such as propylthiouracil (PTU) to the mother.[120,154]

Clinical findings such as low birth weight, irritability, hunger, tachycardia, diarrhea, sweating, and arrhythmias may be present at birth. T_4 and free T_4 levels are increased, but they are also increased in the normal newborn. If the mother is on antithyroid medication, manifestations may be delayed for 2 to 10 days.[43] These infants have an advanced bone age and occasionally craniosynostosis. Clinical effects, although transient, last for 1 to 5 months (generally 2 to 3 months) or up to 10 months in some infants.[43]

Neonatal Hypothyroidism

The most common cause of congenital hypothyroidism in North America is thyroid dysgenesis, with an incidence of 1 in 3500 to 4000 live births.[76,131] The cause is often unclear. In some infants, the hypothyroidism is due to a single gene defect or familial autoimmune factors. In the majority (85%) of infants, the cause is a nonfamilial embryogenic defect.[67] This may be due to mutations in gene coding transcription factors that are needed for thyroid or pituitary gland morphogenesis and differentiation.[63,67] Females are affected twice as often as males. Hypothyroidism and cretinism secondary to endemic goiter are rare in North America. Infants with intrauterine hypothyroidism may not experience significant impairment of somatic or brain growth before birth, because maternal T_4 crosses the placenta and is catabolized to T_3 for normal fetal brain development.[28]

Most infants appear normal at birth, with clinical signs apparent in fewer than 5% to 30%. Common findings such as a large fontanel, hypotonia, macroglossia, and umbilical hernia may not develop for several weeks or months.[43,74,131] By the time these findings are apparent, significant neurologic damage has already occurred, because inadequate thyroid hormone during fetal life and early infancy alters CNS development. The exact mechanism of injury is not well understood, but the degree of neurologic abnormality correlates with the duration and severity of the hypothyroidism.[43] Even with relatively early diagnosis and treatment after birth, these individuals may have subtle, selective neurologic impairments.[133]

Table 19-8 **Enzyme Deficiencies in Congenital Adrenal Hyperplasia**

DEFICIENT ENZYME	EFFECTS ON HORMONES	EFFECT IN THE NEWBORN
21-Hydroxylase	Inability to synthesize glucocorticoids and aldosterone; increased androgen production in response to increased adrenocorticotropin	Ambiguous genitalia (females), hyponatremia, hyperkalemia, weight loss, acidosis, shock
11-Hydroxylase	Inability to synthesize glucocorticoids; suppression of renin activity	Ambiguous genitalia (females), hypertension, hypernatremia, hypokalemia, alkalosis
3β-Hydrosteroid dehydrogenase	Decreased androgen production; decreased glucocorticoid production	Incomplete genital development (males), mild virilization (females), hypotension, hypoglycemia, hyponatremia, hyperkalemia, acidosis, shock
17α-Hydroxylase	Impaired glucocorticoid and androgen production	Ambiguous genitalia (males), hypernatremia, hypokalemia, hypertension
Lipoid adrenal hyperplasia	Decreased glucocorticoid, mineralocorticoid, and androgen production	Ambiguous genitalia (males), hyponatremia, hyperkalemia, hypoglycemia, acidosis, shock

From Witt, C.L. (1999). Adrenal insufficiency in the term and preterm neonate. *Neonatal Netw, 18,* 25.

Neonatal Screening for Hypothyroidism

Diagnosis and treatment of congenital hypothyroidism before 1 to 3 months of age are associated with an increased likelihood of normal mental development. Therefore routine screening of newborns for hypothyroidism has been implemented in all U.S. states and Canadian provinces as well as in many other countries.[131] Screening involves evaluating T_4 or TSH levels. Infants with congenital hypothyroidism have decreased T_4 levels because of the thyroidal dysgenesis and elevated TSH levels. TSH levels are elevated because the low T_4 level does not provide the usual negative feedback inhibition of the anterior pituitary.[28,64,67] TSH screening is more useful to detect subclinical and primary hypothyroidism; T_4 screening is most useful in detecting central hypothalamic-pituitary hypothyroidism and for infants with a delayed TSH increase.[12,72] Use of TSH as the initial screen has increased in recent years due to increased sensitivity with this test.[76,129] Specimens taken immediately after birth (usually within the first 24 hours) are avoided because of the usual TSH surge. Infants screened before 48 hours of age have a higher rate of intermediate results.[131] Preterm infants are at greater risk of false-positive tests due to their HPT immaturity.[64,141] Infants with a positive screen are further evaluated and those with a positive diagnosis are treated with thyroid hormone replacement therapy to normalize serum T_4 levels.

Congenital Adrenal Hyperplasia

Congenital adrenal hyperplasia (CAH) is the most common cause of ambiguous genitalia and adrenal insufficiency.[127] CAH comprises a group of autosomal recessive genetic disorders, characterized by enzymatic defects in adrenal cortex hormone synthesis (see Figure 2-10), with a frequency of 1 in 15,000 live births in North America.[102] These infants have a defect in cortisol synthesis. Without adequate cortisol negative feedback, ACTH levels are elevated, especially in the last half of gestation. The excess ACTH stimulates the adrenal glands to overproduce precursors for cortisol and leads to adrenal hyperplasia.[96,102,131,153]

CAH is due to a complete or partial block in one of the enzymes involved in synthesis of adrenal cortex hormones (see Figure 19-8). Symptoms vary from mild to severe depending on the enzyme defect. Depending on the enzyme involved and the severity of the enzyme block, some female infants may have ambiguous genitalia due to virilization. Because some of the same enzymes are found in the gonads as the adrenals, both tissues are affected.[96] Prenatal therapy with maternal dexamethasone may prevent or reduce virilization of female genitalia if therapy is begun by 6 to 7 weeks' gestation.[68,97,106,154] This glucocorticoid crosses the placenta, suppressing fetal ACTH secretion (see Chapter 7).[68,97] In infants with partial enzyme defects, results may not be apparent until later in childhood or adolescence.

Table 19-8 summarizes the effects of various enzyme blocks that can lead to CAH. The most common block (90% to 95%) is in the cytochrome P-450 type enzyme 21-hydroxylase (21-OH) located on the short arm of chromosome 6, in which multiple types of mutations and clinical phenotypes are seen.[96,102,127] The 21-OH mutations block conversion of progesterone to precursors needed for production of aldosterone and cortisol (see Figure 19-8), leading to lower levels of these hormones. The excess precursors are instead converted to androgens that therefore increase. CAH is one of the disorders evaluated in newborn screening. Screening is done by measuring plasma levels of 17-hydroxy progesterone, which is elevated in CAH. High rates of false positives to true positives have been reported, especially in stressed preterm and low-birth weight infants.[12] Treatment involves glucocorticoid therapy to suppress ACTH. Aldosterone may be needed if the infant has a salt-wasting form of the disorder (see Table 19-8).

MATURATIONAL CHANGES DURING INFANCY AND CHILDHOOD

HPA maturation continues during infancy and childhood, followed by marked changes at puberty. Involution of the adrenal gland is most prominent in the first month after birth and is complete during the first year of life. By 1 month the adrenal is 50% of the size at birth.[164] Dehydroepiandrosterone sulfate (DHEA-S) rapidly decreases after birth to low levels and then rises again beginning at 5 to 6 years of age, peaking in early adulthood, and then gradually decreasing.[51] Circadian rhythmicity of cortisol secretion is seen by 8 to 12 weeks after birth in term infants.[60]

Within the adrenal gland, the fetal zone involutes after birth and has disappeared by 6 months. The definitive zone (possibly with the transitional zone) develops into the zona glomerulosa and zona fasciculata by 2 years. The final zone, the zona reticularis, develops later becoming fully differentiated by mid-adolescence.[123]

Adrenarche is maturation of the adrenal cortex, with increased production of DHEA, DHEA-S, and other androgens, and development of the zona reticularis. DHEA rises to a maximum around 25 years of age and then declines gradually thereafter.[51] Adrenarche begins in the prepuberty period around 6 to 8 years of age and precedes gonadarche. Steroid hormones increase progressively and are associated with a transient increase in linear growth and bone maturation.[112] Adrenarche increases production of androgens and estrogens needed for puberty changes and occurs several years before the onset of puberty. The exact trigger for this change is unknown. It may be related to a decrease in levels of 3β-hydroxysteroid dehydrogenase (3β HSD) in the zona reticularis and may be influenced by insulin-like growth factor-I.[37,51] Gonadal maturation and changes in the hypothalamic-pituitary-adrenal (HPA) axis with puberty are discussed in Chapter 2.

HPT function gradually changes during infancy and childhood. Thyroid hormones are critical for continued CNS maturation and bone growth. The critical period for thyroid hormone influences on the CNS continues to 6 to 8 months after birth. It has been estimated that infants with significant hypothyroidism lose 3 to 5 IQ points per month if untreated during this period.[28] The ability of the infant to convert T_4 to T_3 matures over the first month. Twenty-four-hour ^{123}I uptake by the thyroid at 1 month is similar to adult values, but concentrations per gram of thyroid tissue are greater since the thyroid gland at this age is only one tenth that of an adult.[131] During childhood, TSH levels tend to remain higher than adult levels. The T_4 turnover rate is higher in infants and children, accounting for the increased requirement of children for thyroid hormone per unit weight.[131] TBG levels gradually fall over the first few years. Thyroid hormones fall to high adult values by 4 to 6 weeks, but they do not reach mean adult values until mid-puberty due to higher TBS levels in children.[131]

SUMMARY

Maturation of the hypothalamic-pituitary-adrenal (HPA) and hypothalamic-pituitary-thyroid (HPT) axes and neuroendocrine function in the fetus and infant is essential for development of the CNS, lungs, bones, and other systems. These functions undergo significant changes during the transition to extrauterine life. In addition, thyroid function is interrelated with thermoregulation and changes dramatically at birth. Newborns normally have a relative hyperthyroidism, but immaturity or illness can lead to transient hypothyroidism. Screening for congenital hypothyroidism and congenital adrenal hyperplasia is a part of newborn metabolic screening. Use of this screening is essential for early identification and reduction of mortality and morbidity in these infants. All neonates should be monitored for stress, and protective interventions should be initiated. Preterm infants—especially those who are ill or younger than 28 weeks' gestational age—are particularly vulnerable to the adverse consequences of stress. Table 19-9 summarizes clinical recommendations related to neonatal pituitary, adrenal, and thyroid function.

Table 19-9 Recommendations for Clinical Practice Related to Pituitary, Adrenal, and Thyroid Function in Neonates

Know the usual changes in pituitary and adrenal function in the fetus and during the neonatal period (pp. 649-643, 645-646, Table 19-4, and Figure 19-7).
Know the usual changes in thyroid function during the neonatal period in term infants (pp. 645-647, Figure 19-9, Table 19-6).
Know the usual changes in thyroid function during the neonatal period in preterm infants (pp. 646-647 and Table 19-7).
Recognize the normal parameters related to thyroid function in term and preterm neonates (pp. 646-647, 648-658).
Recognize and monitor for transient alterations in thyroid function in the preterm infant (pp. 649-650).
Recognize the signs of and monitor for transient hyperthyroidism in infants of mothers with Graves' disease (p. 650).
Recognize the clinical signs of hypothyroidism in infants (p. 650).
Screen newborns for congenital hypothyroidism and congenital adrenal hyperplasia per state newborn screening protocol (pp. 650-651).
Monitor growth and neurologic status in infants with congenital hypothyroidism (p. 650).
Monitor for signs of stress and pain in neonates (pp. 647-648 and Chapter 15).

References

1. Abalovich, M., et al. (2007). Management of thyroid dysfunction during pregnancy and postpartum: An Endocrine Society Clinical Practice Guideline. *J Clin Endocrinol Metab, 92,* S1.
2. ACOG Committee Opinion. (2007). Subclinical hypothyroidism in pregnancy. *Obstetrics & Gynecology, 110,* 959.
3. Alexander, E.K., et al. (2004). Timing and magnitude of increases in levothyroxine requirements during pregnancy in women with hypothyroidism. *N Engl J Med, 351,* 241.
4. Alexander, E.K. (2009). Thyroid function: The complexity of maternal hypothyroidism during pregnancy. *Nat Rev Endocrinol, 5,* 480.
5. Alsat, E., et al. (1997). Human placental growth hormone. *Am J Obstet Gynecol, 177,* 1526.
6. Anand, K.J., & Scalzo, F.M. (2000). Can adverse neonatal experiences alter brain development and subsequent behavior? *Biol Neonate, 77,* 69.
7. Ares, S., Quero, J., & Morreale de Escobar, G. (2008). Iodine balance, iatrogenic excess, and thyroid dysfunction in premature newborns. *Semin Perinatol, 32,* 407.
8. Aucott, S.W. (2010). Stress and severity of illness in very low birth weight infants: What are we measuring? *J Perinatol, 30,* 503.
9. Baskin, H.J., et al. (2002). American Association of Clinical Endocrinologists Medical guidelines for clinical practice for the evaluation and treatment of hyperthyroidism and hypothyroidism. *Endocr Pract, 8,* 457.
10. Benhaim, R.D., & Davies, T.F. (2005). Increased risk of Graves' disease after pregnancy. *Thyroid, 15,* 1287.
11. Blackburn, S. (2009). Maternal-fetal thyroid interactions. *J Perinat Neonatal Nurs, 23,* 312.
12. Bolt, R.J., et al. (2002). Fetal growth and the function of the adrenal cortex in preterm infants. *J Clin Endocrinol Metab, 87,* 1194.
13. Brunton, P.J. (2010). Resetting the dynamic range of hypothalamic-pituitary-adrenal axis stress responses through pregnancy. *J Neuroendocrinol, 22,* 1198.
14. Burman, K.D. (2009). Controversies surrounding pregnancy, maternal thyroid status, and fetal outcome. *Thyroid, 19,* 323.
15. Caldwell, K.L., et al. (2008). Iodine status of the U.S. population, National Health and Nutrition Examination Survey 2003–2004. *Thyroid, 18,* 1207.
16. Cao, L., et al. (1993). Endogenous opioid-like substances in perinatal asphyxia and cerebral injury due to anoxia. *Chin Med J (Engl), 106,* 783.
17. Carrascosa, A., et al. (2004). Thyroid function in seventy-five healthy preterm infants thirty to thirty-five weeks of gestational age: A prospective and longitudinal study during the first year of life. *Thyroid, 14,* 435.
18. Charil, A., et al. (2010). Prenatal stress and brain development. *Brain Res Rev, 65,* 56.
19. Coulter, C.L. (2004). Functional biology of the primate fetal adrenal gland: Advances in technology provide new insight. *Clin Exp Pharmacol Physiol, 31,* 475.
20. Dabo, F., et al. (2010). Plasma levels of beta-endorphin during pregnancy and use of labor analgesia. *Reprod Sci, 17,* 742.
21. de Weerth, C., & Buitelaar, J.K. (2005). Physiological stress reactivity in human pregnancy—A review. *Neurosci Biobehav Rev, 29,* 295.
22. Delahunty, C., et al. (2010). Levels of neonatal thyroid hormone in preterm infants and neurodevelopmental outcome at 5½ years: Millennium cohort study. *J Clin Endocrinol Metab, 95,* 4898.
23. Delange, F. (2007). Iodine requirements during pregnancy, lactation and the neonatal period and indicators of optimal iodine nutrition. *Public Health Nutr, 10,* 1571.
24. DiPietro, J.A., Costigan, K.A., & Gurewitsch, E.D. (2003). Fetal response to induced maternal stress. *Early Hum Dev, 74,* 125.
25. Douglas, A.J. (2005). Central noradrenergic mechanisms underlying acute stress responses of the hypothalamo-pituitary-adrenal axis: Adaptations through pregnancy and lactation. *Stress, 8,* 5.
26. Efird, M.M., et al. (2005). A randomized-controlled trial of prophylactic hydrocortisone supplementation for the prevention of hypotension in extremely low birth weight infants. *J Perinatol, 25,* 119.
27. Fernandez, E.F., & Watterberg, K.L. (2009). Relative adrenal insufficiency in the preterm and term infant. *J Perinatol, 29,* S44.
28. Fisher, D.A. (1997). Fetal thyroid function: Diagnosis and management of fetal thyroid disorders. *Clin Obstet Gynecol, 40,* 16.
29. Fisher, D.A. (2008). Thyroid system immaturities in very low birth weight premature infants. *Semin Perinatol, 32,* 387.
30. Fitzpatrick, D.L., & Russell, M.A. (2010). Diagnosis and management of thyroid disease in pregnancy. *Obstet Gynecol Clin North Am, 37,* 173.
31. Florido, J., et al. (1997). Plasma concentrations of β-endorphin and adrenocorticotropic hormone in women with and without childbirth preparation. *Eur J Obstet Gynecol Reprod Biol, 73,* 121.
32. Foyouzi, N., Frisbaek, Y., & Norwitz, E.R. (2004). Pituitary gland and pregnancy. *Obstet Gynecol Clin North Am, 31,* 873.
33. Fu, J., et al. (2005). Risk factors of primary thyroid dysfunction in early infants born to mothers with autoimmune thyroid disease. *Acta Paediatr, 94,* 1043.
34. Galofre, J.C., & Davies, T.F. (2009). Autoimmune thyroid disease in pregnancy: A review. *J Womens Health (Larchmt), 18,* 1847.
35. Garner, P.R., & Burrow, G.N. (2004). Adrenal and pituitary disorders. In G.N. Burrow, T.P. Duffy, & J.A. Copel (Eds.), *Medical complications during pregnancy* (6th ed.). Philadelphia: Saunders.
36. Gärtner, R. (2009). Thyroid diseases in pregnancy. *Curr Opin Obstet Gynecol, 21,* 501.
37. Gell, J.S., et al. (1998). Adrenarche results from development of a 3beta-hydroxysteroid dehydrogenase-deficient adrenal reticularis. *J Clin Endocrinol Metab, 83,* 3695.
38. Glinoer, D. (2004). The regulation of thyroid function during normal pregnancy: Importance of the iodine nutrition status. *Best Pract Res Clin Endocrinol Metab, 18,* 133.
39. Glinoer, D. (2007). Clinical and biological consequences of iodine deficiency during pregnancy. *Endocr Dev, 10,* 62.
40. Glinoer, D., & Spencer, C.A. (2010). Serum TSH determinations in pregnancy. How, when and why? *Nat Rev Endocrinol, 6,* 526.
41. Glover, V., O'Connor, T.G., & O'Donnell, K. (2010). Prenatal stress and the programming of the HPA axis. *Neurosci Biobehav Rev, 35,* 17.
42. Gluckman, P.D., et al. (1999). The transition from fetus to neonate—An endocrine perspective. *Acta Paediatr Suppl, 88,* 7.
43. Golden, L.H., & Burrow, G.N. (2004). Thyroid diseases. In G.N. Burrow, T.P. Duffy, & J.A. Copel (Eds.), *Medical complications during pregnancy* (6th ed.). Philadelphia: Saunders.
44. Griffing, G.T., & Melby, J.C. (1994). The maternal adrenal cortex. In D. Tuchinsky & A.B. Little (Eds.), *Maternal-fetal endocrinology* (2nd ed.). Philadelphia: Saunders.
45. Grumbach, M., & Gluckman, P.D. (1994). The human fetal hypothalamus and pituitary gland: The maturation of neuroendocrine mechanisms controlling the secretion of fetal pituitary growth hormone, prolactin, gonadotropins, adrenocorticotropin-related peptides, and thyrotropin. In D. Tuchinsky & A.B. Little (Eds.), *Maternal-fetal endocrinology* (2nd ed.). Philadelphia: Saunders.
46. Grunau, R.E., Weinberg, J., & Whitfield, M.F. (2004). Neonatal procedural pain and preterm infant cortisol responses to novelty at 8 months. *Pediatrics, 114,* e77.
47. Guyton, A.C., & Hall, J.E. (2010). *Textbook of medical physiology* (12th ed.). Philadelphia: Saunders Elsevier.
48. Gyamfi, C., Wapner, R.J., & D'Alton, M.E. (2009). Thyroid dysfunction in pregnancy: The basic science and clinical evidence surrounding the controversy in management. *Obstet Gynecol, 113,* 702.
49. Hallengren, B., et al. (2009). Pregnant women on thyroxine substitution are often dysregulated in early pregnancy. *Thyroid, 19,* 391.

50. Hanna, C.E., et al. (1993). Hypothalamic-pituitary adrenal function in the extremely low birth weight infant. *J Clin Endocrinol Metab, 76,* 384.
51. Havelock, J.C., Auchus, R.J., & Rainey, W.E. (2004). The rise in adrenal androgen biosynthesis: Adrenarche. *Semin Reprod Med, 22,* 337.
52. Heckmann, M., et al. (2005). Cortisol production rates in preterm infants in relation to growth and illness: A noninvasive prospective study using gas chromatography-mass spectrometry. *J Clin Endocrinol Metab, 90,* 5737.
53. Hyer, S.L., et al. (2011). Outcome of pregnancy after exposure to radioiodine in utero. *Endocr Pract, 17,* 1.
54. Jaffe, R.B., et al. (1998). The regulation and role of fetal adrenal development in human pregnancy. *Endocr Res, 24,* 191.
55. Jain, L., et al. (1995). Somatostatin in preterm infants: Postnatal changes and response to stress. *Biol Neonate, 68,* 81.
56. Kajantie, E., et al. (2002). Size at birth, gestational age and cortisol secretion in adult life: Foetal programming of both hyper- and hypocortisolism? *Clin Endocrinol (Oxf), 57,* 635.
57. Kallen, G.B. (2004). Steroid hormone synthesis in pregnancy. *Obstet Gynecol Clin North Am, 31,* 795.
58. Karras, S., et al. (2010). Pharmacological treatment of hyperthyroidism during lactation: Review of the literature and novel data. *Pediatr Endocrinol Rev, 8,* 25.
59. Keller-Wood, M., & Wood, C.E. (2001). Pituitary-adrenal physiology during pregnancy. *Endocrinologist, 11,* 159.
60. Kidd, S., et al. (2005). Lack of adult-type salivary cortisol circadian rhythm in hospitalized preterm infants. *Horm Res, 64,* 20.
61. Krassas, G.E., & Pontikides, N. (2004). Male reproductive function in relation with thyroid alterations. *Best Pract Res Clin Endocrinol Metab, 18,* 183.
62. Krassas, G.E., Poppe, K., & Glinoer, D. (2010). Thyroid function and human reproductive health. *Endocr Rev, 31,* 702.
63. Kratzsch, J., & Pulzer, F. (2008). Thyroid gland development and defects. *Best Pract Res Clin Endocrinol Metab, 22,* 57.
64. Kugelman, A., et al. (2009). Pitfalls in screening programs for congenital hypothyroidism in premature newborns. *Am J Perinatol, 26,* 383.
65. Kurioka, H., Takahashi, K., & Miyazaki, K. (2005). Maternal thyroid function during pregnancy and puerperal period. *Endocr J, 52,* 587.
66. La Gamma, E.F., et al. (2009). Phase 1 trial of 4 thyroid hormone regimens for transient hypothyroxinemia in neonates of <28 weeks' gestation. *Pediatrics, 124,* e258.
67. LaFranchi, S. (1999). Congenital hypothyroidism: Etiologies, diagnosis, and management. *Thyroid, 9,* 735.
68. Lajic, S., Nordenström, A., & Hirvikoski, T. (2008). Long-term outcome of prenatal treatment of congenital adrenal hyperplasia. *Endocr Dev, 13,* 82.
69. Laurberg, P., et al. (2009). Management of Graves' hyperthyroidism in pregnancy: Focus on both maternal and foetal thyroid function, and caution against surgical thyroidectomy in pregnancy. *Eur J Endocrinol, 160,* 1.
70. Lawrence, R.A. (2011). *Breastfeeding: A guide for the medical profession* (7th ed.). Philadelphia: Saunders.
71. Lazarus, J.H. (2005). Thyroid disease in pregnancy and childhood. *Minerva Endocrinol, 30,* 71.
72. Lazarus, J.H. (2005). Thyroid disorders associated with pregnancy: Etiology, diagnosis, and management. *Treat Endocrinol, 4,* 31.
73. LeBeau, S.O., & Mandel, S.J. (2006). Thyroid disorders during pregnancy. *Endocrinol Metab Clin North Am, 35,* 117.
74. Lee, M.M., & Moshang, T. (2005). Endocrine disorders of the newborn. In M.G. Macdonald, M.M.K. Sheshia, & M.D. Mullett (Eds.), *Neonatology: Pathophysiology and management of the newborn* (6th ed.). Philadelphia: Lippincott Williams & Wilkins.
75. Leuschen, M.P., et al. (1991). Plasma beta-endorphin in neonates: Effect of prematurity, gender, and respiratory status. *J Clin Endocrinol Metab, 73,* 1062.
76. Li, M., & Eastman, C.J. (2010). Neonatal TSH screening: Is it a sensitive and reliable tool for monitoring iodine status in populations? *Best Pract Res Clin Endocrinol Metab, 24,* 63.
77. Lindsay, J.R., & Nieman, L.K. (2005). The hypothalamic-pituitary-adrenal axis in pregnancy: Challenges in disease detection and treatment. *Endocr Rev, 26,* 775.
78. Lindsay, J.R., & Nieman, L.K. (2006). Adrenal disorders in pregnancy. *Endocrinol Metab Clin North Am, 35,* 1.
79. Lof, M., et al. (2005). Changes in basal metabolic rate during pregnancy in relation to changes in body weight and composition, cardiac output, insulin-like growth factor I, and thyroid hormones and in relation to fetal growth. *Am J Clin Nutr, 81,* 678.
80. Loh, J.A., et al. (2009). The magnitude of increased levothyroxine requirements in hypothyroid pregnant women depends upon the etiology of the hypothyroidism. *Thyroid, 19,* 269.
81. Luton, D., et al. (2005). Management of Graves' disease during pregnancy: The key role of fetal thyroid gland monitoring. *J Clin Endocrinol Metab, 90,* 6093.
82. Luton, D., et al. (2005). Thyroid function during pregnancy in women with past Graves' disease. *BJOG, 112,* 1565.
83. MacDonald, M.G., et al. (1990). Cerebrospinal fluid and plasma beta-endorphin-like immunoreactivity in full-term neonates and in preterm neonates with and without apnea of prematurity. *Dev Pharmacol Ther, 15,* 8.
84. Marco, A., et al. (2010). Patterns of iodine intake and urinary iodine concentrations during pregnancy and blood thyroid-stimulating hormone concentrations in the newborn progeny. *Thyroid, 20,* 1295.
85. Martin, C.R., Van Marter, L.J., & Allred, E.N. (2005). Antenatal glucocorticoids increase early total thyroxine levels in premature infants. *Biol Neonate, 87,* 273.
86. Mastorakos, G., & Ilias, I. (2003). Maternal and fetal hypothalamic-pituitary-adrenal axes during pregnancy and postpartum. *Ann N Y Acad Sci, 997,* 136.
87. Matthews, S.G., et al. (2004). Fetal glucocorticoid exposure and hypothalamo-pituitary-adrenal (HPA) function after birth. *Endocr Res, 30,* 827.
88. Melse-Boonstra, A., & Jaiswal, N. (2010). Iodine deficiency in pregnancy, infancy and childhood and its consequences for brain development. *Best Pract Res Clin Endocrinol Metab, 24,* 29.
89. Merlot, E., Couret, D., & Otten, W. (2008). Prenatal stress, fetal imprinting and immunity. *Brain Behav Immunol, 22,* 42.
90. Mesiano, S. (2009). The endocrinology of human pregnancy and fetoplacental neuroendocrine development. In J.F. Strauss & R. Barbieri (Eds.), *Yen and Jaffe's Reproductive endocrinology: Physiology, pathophysiology, and clinical management* (6th ed.). Philadelphia: Saunders.
91. Miller, N.M., et al. (2005). Stress responses at birth: Determinants of cord arterial cortisol and links with cortisol response in infancy. *BJOG, 112,* 921.
92. Moleti, M., et al. (2009). Gestational thyroid function abnormalities in conditions of mild iodine deficiency: Early screening versus continuous monitoring of maternal thyroid status. *EJE, 160,* 611.
93. Molitch, M.E. (2006). Pituitary disorders during pregnancy. *Endocrinol Metab Clin North Am, 35,* 99.
94. Morreale de Escobar, G., Obregon, M.J., & Escobar del Rey, F. (2004). Maternal thyroid hormones early in pregnancy and fetal brain development. *Best Pract Res Clin Endocrinol Metab, 18,* 225.
95. Morreale de Escobar, G., et al. (2008). The changing role of maternal thyroid hormone in fetal brain development. *Semin Perinatol, 32,* 380.
96. Murphy, B.E.P., & Branchaud, C.L. (1994). The fetal adrenal. In D. Tuchinsky & A.B. Little (Eds.), *Maternal-fetal endocrinology* (2nd ed.). Philadelphia: Saunders.
97. Nader, S. (2004). Other endocrine disorders of pregnancy. In R.K. Creasy, R. Resnik, & J.D. Iams (Eds.), *Maternal-fetal medicine: Principles and practice* (5th ed.). Philadelphia: Saunders.
98. Nader, S. (2004). Thyroid disease and other endocrine disorders in pregnancy. *Obstet Gynecol Clin North Am, 31,* 257.
99. Nader, S. (2004). Thyroid disease and pregnancy. In R.K. Creasy, R. Resnik, & J.D. Iams (Eds.), *Maternal-fetal medicine: Principles and practice* (5th ed.). Philadelphia: Saunders.
100. Neale, D., & Burrow, G. (2004). Thyroid disease in pregnancy. *Obstet Gynecol Clin North Am, 31,* 893.

101. Negro, R., et al. (2010). Universal screening versus case finding for detection and treatment of thyroid hormonal dysfunction during pregnancy. *J Clin Endocrinol Metab, 95,* 1699.
102. New, M.I. (2004). An update of congenital adrenal hyperplasia. *Ann N Y Acad Sci, 1038,* 14.
103. Ng, P.C. (2000). The fetal and neonatal hypothalamic-pituitary-adrenal axis. *Arch Dis Child Fetal Neonatal Ed, 82,* F250.
104. Ng, P.C., et al. (2004). Transient adrenocortical insufficiency of prematurity and systemic hypotension in very low birthweight infants. *Arch Dis Child Fetal Neonatal Ed, 89,* F119.
105. Ng, P.C. (2011). Effect of stress on the hypothalamic-pituitary-adrenal axis in the fetus and newborn. *J Pediatr, 158,* e41.
106. Nimkarn, S., & New, M.I. (2010). Congenital adrenal hyperplasia due to 21-hydroxylase deficiency: A paradigm for prenatal diagnosis and treatment. *Ann N Y Acad Sci, 1192,* 5.
107. Nor Azlin, M.I., et al. (2010). Thyroid autoantibodies and associated complications during pregnancy. *J Obstet Gynaecol, 30,* 675.
108. Obregon, M.J., et al. (2007). Ontogenesis of thyroid function and interactions with maternal function. *Endocr Dev, 10,* 86.
109. O'Donnell, K., O'Connor, T.G., & Glover, V. (2009). Prenatal stress and neurodevelopment of the child: Focus on the HPA axis and role of the placenta. *Dev Neurosci, 31,* 285.
110. Osborn, D.A., & Hunt, R.W. (2007). Postnatal thyroid hormones for preterm infants with transient hypothyroxinaemia. *Cochrane Database Syst Rev* 1, CD005945.
111. Osborn, D.A., & Hunt, R.W. (2007). Prophylactic postnatal thyroid hormones for prevention of morbidity and mortality in preterm infants. *Cochrane Database Syst Rev* 1, CD005948.
112. Parker, L.N. (1991). Adrenarche. *Endocrin Metab Clin North Am, 20,* 71.
113. Parker, V.J., & Douglas, A.J. (2010). Stress in early pregnancy: Maternal neuro-endocrine-immune responses and effects. *J Reprod Immunol, 85,* 86.
114. Pearce, E.N., & Stagnaro-Green, A. (2010). Hypothyroidism in pregnancy: Do guidelines alter practice? *Thyroid, 20,* 241.
115. Pemberton, H.N., Franklyn, J.A., & Kilby, M.D. (2005). Thyroid hormones and fetal brain development. *Minerva Ginecol, 57,* 367.
116. Peter, F. (2005). Thyroid dysfunction in the offspring of mothers with autoimmune thyroid diseases. *Acta Paediatr, 94,* 1008.
117. Peters, K.L. (1998). Neonatal stress reactivity and cortisol. *J Perinat Neonat Nurs, 11,* 45.
118. Pierro, A. (1999). Metabolic response to neonatal surgery. *Curr Opin Pediatr, 11,* 230.
119. Polak, M., et al. (2004). Fetal and neonatal thyroid function in relation to maternal Graves' disease. *Best Pract Res Clin Endocrinol Metab, 18,* 289.
120. Polak, M., & Van Vliet, G. (2010). Therapeutic approach of fetal thyroid disorders. *Horm Res Paediatr, 74,* 1.
121. Polk, D.H., & Fisher, D.A. (2012). Fetal and neonatal thyroid physiology. In R.A. Polin, W.W. Fox, & S.H. Abman (Eds.), *Fetal and neonatal physiology* (4th ed.). Philadelphia: Saunders.
122. Portman, M.A. (2008). Thyroid hormone regulation of perinatal cardiovascular function. *Semin Perinatol, 32,* 419.
123. Quintos, J.B., & Boney, C.M. (2010). Transient adrenal insufficiency in the premature newborn. *Curr Opin Endocrinol Diabetes Obes, 17,* 8.
124. Rabin, C.W., et al. (2004). Incidence of low free T4 values in premature infants as determined by direct equilibrium dialysis. *J Perinatol, 24,* 640.
125. Radetti, G., et al. (2004). Altered thyroid and adrenal function in children born at term and preterm, small for gestational age. *J Clin Endocrinol Metab, 89,* 6320.
126. Radunovic, N., et al. (1992). Beta-endorphin concentrations in fetal blood during the second half of pregnancy. *Am J Obstet Gynecol, 167,* 740.
127. Rainey, W.E., Rehman, K.S., & Carr, B.R. (2004). Fetal and maternal adrenals in human pregnancy. *Obstet Gynecol Clin North Am, 31,* 817.
128. Rainey, W.E., Rehman, K.S., & Carr, B.R. (2004). The human fetal adrenal: Making adrenal androgens for placental estrogens. *Semin Reprod Med, 22,* 327.
129. Raymond, J., & LaFranchi, S.H. (2010). Fetal and neonatal thyroid function: Review and summary of significant new findings. *Curr Opin Endocrinol Diabetes Obes, 17,* 1.
130. Reuss, M.L., et al. (1996). The relation of transient hypothyroxinemia in preterm infants to neurologic development at two years of age. *N Engl J Med, 334,* 821.
131. Rose, S.R. (2004). Thyroid disorders. In A.A. Fanaroff & R.J. Martin (Eds.), *Neonatal-perinatal medicine: Diseases of the fetus and infant* (7th ed.). St. Louis: Mosby.
132. Rosendahl, W., et al. (1995). Surgical stress and neuroendocrine responses in infants and children. *J Pediatr Endocrinol Metab, 8,* 187.
133. Rouet, J.F. (2002). Congenital hypothyroidism: An analysis of persisting defects and associated factors. *Child Neuropsychol, 8,* 150.
134. Ruth, V., et al. (1993). Corticotropin-releasing hormone and cortisol in cord plasma in relation to gestational age, labor and fetal distress. *Am J Perinatol, 10,* 115.
135. Sadler, T.W. (2012). *Langman's Medical embryology* (12th ed.). Philadelphia: Lippincott & Wilkins.
136. Sandman, C.A., et al. (1997). Maternal stress, HPA activity, and fetal/infant outcome. *Ann N Y Acad Sci, 24,* 266.
137. Santiago, L.B., et al. (1996). Longitudinal analysis of the development of salivary cortisol rhythm in infancy. *Clin Endocrinol (Oxf), 44,* 157.
138. Savin, S., et al. (2003). Thyroid hormone synthesis and storage in the thyroid gland of human neonates. *J Ped Endocrinol Metab, 16,* 521.
139. Scott, S.M., & Cimino, D.F. (2004). Evidence for developmental hypopituitarism in ill preterm infants. *J Perinatol, 24,* 429.
140. Shih, J.L., & Agus, M.S. (2009). Thyroid function in the critically ill newborn and child. *Curr Opin Pediatr, 21,* 536.
141. Slaughter, J.L., et al. (2010). The effects of gestational age and birth weight on false-positive newborn-screening rates. *Pediatrics, 126,* 910.
142. Smallridge, R.C., et al. (2005). Thyroid function inside and outside of pregnancy: What do we know and what don't we know? *Thyroid, 15,* 54.
143. Smith, R.P., et al. (2000). Pain and stress in the human fetus. *Eur J Obstet Gynecol Reproduct Biol, 92,* 161.
144. Soldin, O.P., et al. (2004). Trimester-specific changes in maternal thyroid hormone, thyrotropin, and thyroglobulin concentrations during gestation: Trends and associations across trimesters in iodine sufficiency. *Thyroid, 14,* 1084.
145. Soldin, O.P., et al. (2010). Longitudinal comparison of thyroxine pharmacokinetics between pregnant and nonpregnant women: A stable isotope study. *Ther Drug Monit, 32,* 767.
146. Sonir, R.R., et al. (2000). The emergence of salivary cortisol circadian rhythm and its relationship to sleep activity in preterm infants. *Clin Endocrinol, 52,* 423.
147. South, M.M., et al. (2005). The use of non-nutritive sucking to decrease the physiologic pain response during neonatal circumcision: A randomized controlled trial. *Am J Obstet Gynecol, 193,* 537.
148. Stagnaro-Green, A. (2009). Maternal thyroid disease and preterm delivery. *J Clin Endocrinol Metab, 94,* 21.
149. Sulyok, E. (1989). Endocrine factors in the neonatal adaptation. *Acta Physiol Hung, 74,* 329.
150. Swamy, G.K., Ostbye, T., & Skjaerven, R. (2008). Association of preterm birth with long-term survival, reproduction, and next-generation preterm birth. *JAMA, 299,* 1429.
151. Thung, S.F., & Norwtiz, E.R. (2009). Endocrine diseases of pregnancy. In J.F. Strauss & R. Barbieri (Eds.), *Yen and Jaffe's Reproductive endocrinology: Physiology, pathophysiology, and clinical management* (6th ed.). Philadelphia: Saunders.
152. Van Djihe, U.P., et al. (1987). Methimazole, carbimazole, and congenital skin defects. *Ann Int Med, 106,* 60.

153. Van Vliet, G., & Czernichow, P. (2004). Screening for neonatal endocrinopathies: Rationale, methods and results. *Semin Neonatol, 9,* 75.
154. Van Vliet, G., Polak, M., & Ritzén, E.M. (2008). Treating fetal thyroid and adrenal disorders through the mother. *Nat Clin Pract Endocrinol Metab, 4,* 675. Erratum in: *Nat Clin Pract Endocrinol Metab* (2009). *5,* 122.
155. van Wassenaer, A.G., et al. (1997). Effects of thyroxine supplementation on neurologic development in infants born at less than 30 weeks gestation. *N Engl J Med, 336,* 21.
156. van Wassenaer, A.G., & Kok, J.H. (2004). Hypothyroxinaemia and thyroid function after preterm birth. *Semin Neonatol, 9,* 3.
157. van Wassenaer, A.G., & Kok, J.H. (2008). Trials with thyroid hormone in preterm infants: Clinical and neurodevelopmental effects. *Semin Perinatol, 32,* 423.
158. Verga, U., et al. (2009). Adjustment of L-T4 substitutive therapy in pregnant women with subclinical, overt or post-ablative hypothyroidism. *Clin Endocrinol (Oxf), 70,* 798.
159. Vrekoussis, T., et al. (2010). The role of stress in female reproduction and pregnancy: An update. *Ann N Y Acad Sci, 1205,* 69.
160. Vulsma, T., & Kok, J.H. (1996). Prematurity-associated neurological and developmental abnormalities and neonatal thyroid function. *N Engl J Med, 334,* 857.
161. Ward, A.M., et al. (2004). Fetal programming of the hypothalamic-pituitary-adrenal (HPA) axis: Low birth weight and central HPA regulation. *J Clin Endocrinol Metab, 89,* 1227.
162. Watterberg, K.L. (2004). Adrenocortical function and dysfunction in the fetus and neonate. *Semin Neonatol, 9,* 13.
163. Watterberg, K.L., et al. (2004). Prophylaxis of early adrenal insufficiency to prevent bronchopulmonary dysplasia: A multicenter trial. *Pediatrics, 114,* 1649.
164. Watterberg, K.L. (2012). Fetal and neonatal adrenocortical physiology. In R.A. Polin, W.W. Fox, & S.H. Abman (Eds.), *Fetal and neonatal physiology* (4th ed.). Philadelphia: Saunders.
165. Weetman, A.P. (2010). Immunity, thyroid function and pregnancy: Molecular mechanisms. *Nat Rev Endocrinol, 6,* 311.
166. Weinstock, M. (2005). The potential influence of maternal stress hormones on development and mental health of the offspring. *Brain Behav Immun, 19,* 296.
167. Wier, F.A., & Farley, C.L. (2006). Clinical controversies in screening women for thyroid disorders during pregnancy. *J Midwifery Womens Health, 51,* 152.
168. Williams, F., & Hume, R. (2011). The measurement, definition, aetiology and clinical consequences of neonatal transient hypothyroxinaemia. *Ann Clin Biochem, 48,* 7.
169. Williams, F.L., & Hume, R. (2008). Perinatal factors affecting thyroid hormone status in extreme preterm infants. *Semin Perinatol, 32,* 398.
170. Winkner, B.N., et al. (2008). Maternal use of thyroid hormones in pregnancy and neonatal outcome. *Acta Obstet Gynecol, 87,* 617.
171. Yehuda, R., et al. (1993). Long-lasting hormonal alterations to extreme stress in humans: Normative or maladaptive? *Psychosomatic Med, 55,* 287.
172. Yildirim, M., Oktem, M., & Yilmaz, A.O. (2004). Fetal and maternal adrenal steroid levels and labor. *Int J Gynaecol Obstet, 85,* 274.
173. Zanardo, V., et al. (2001). Labor pain effects on colostral milk beta-endorphin concentrations of lactating mothers. *Biol Neonate, 79,* 87.
174. Zimmermann, M.B. (2007). The impact of iodised salt or iodine supplements on iodine status during pregnancy, lactation and infancy. *Public Health Nutr, 10,* 1584.
175. Zimmermann, M.B. (2009). Iodine deficiency in pregnancy and the effects of maternal iodine supplementation on the offspring: A review. *Am J Clin Nutr, 89,* 668S.

CHAPTER 20

Thermoregulation

Thermoregulation is the balance between heat production and heat loss involved in maintaining thermal equilibrium. Heat is produced by the body as a by-product of metabolic processes and muscular activity; thus a major function of the thermoregulatory system is dissipation of this heat.[18] The thermoregulatory system must also respond appropriately to alterations in environmental temperature to preserve thermal equilibrium. Maintenance of thermal stability is particularly critical in the newborn in that exposure to cold environments and lowered body temperatures are closely correlated with survival, especially in very low–birth weight (VLBW) infants. Maternal temperature changes are also important in relation to fetal well-being and the potential adverse consequences of maternal hyperthermia. Regulation of body temperature is summarized in Figure 20-1 and Box 20-1 on page 658.

MATERNAL PHYSIOLOGIC ADAPTATIONS

Hormonal and metabolic alterations during pregnancy result in changes in maternal temperature. These changes are transient and may cause discomfort but are generally not associated with significant physiologic alterations.

Antepartum Period

The amount of heat generated increases 30% to 35% during pregnancy because of the thermogenic effects of progesterone, alterations in maternal metabolism and basal metabolic rate (see Chapter 16), and maternal dissipation of heat generated by the fetus.[30,91] As a result, many pregnant women develop an increased tolerance for cooler weather and decreased tolerance for heat. The additional heat is dissipated by peripheral vasodilation with a fourfold to sevenfold increase in cutaneous blood flow and increased activity of the sweat glands (see Chapter 14). Cutaneous vasodilation leads to skin warmth.

The maternal temperature usually increases by 0.5° C (0.3° F). Both core and skin temperature increase during pregnancy, with a slight decrease reported in late pregnancy. The core temperature peaks by midpregnancy.[85] The decrease in core temperature in late pregnancy may be related to decreases in progesterone and physical activity (which generates heat) during this time. The rise in skin temperature is particularly evident in the hands and feet, probably due to arteriovenous shunting in these areas.[129] In general, heat accumulation may be slower and heat dissipation faster in later pregnancy than before pregnancy or in early pregnancy. The increased plasma volume during pregnancy provides a greater area for heat storage and may enhance heat transfer from the fetus to the mother.[85] The pregnant woman has decreased vasoconstriction in response to cold during pregnancy. This may alter her ability to conserve heat during cold stress.[85]

Body temperature increases with exercise due to heat generated by increased metabolic energy production. Some of this heat is dissipated by increased skin blood flow; the remainder is stored transiently, increasing the core temperature. Changes in temperature with exercise during pregnancy are moderate, as compared with changes in nonpregnant women, suggesting that the enhanced thermoregulatory capacity of the pregnant woman may help protect her against hyperthermia.[85] The increased plasma volume in pregnancy may assist in maintaining uterine and placental blood flow during exercise and in maximizing heat transfer from the fetus and heat dissipation in the mother. Aerobic exercise in water is associated with minimal changes in either core or skin temperature.[85,129] Exercise during pregnancy is discussed further in Chapters 9 and 10.

Intrapartum Period

An increase in body temperature, averaging 1° C (1.7° F), may occur during labor as a result of physical activity with uterine contractions and the release of substances from the fetal-placental unit that may stimulate the maternal hypothalamic thermoregulatory center.[87,91,104] However, Bartholomew and colleagues reported that 95% of 147 women had temperatures between 36.2° C and 37.8° C (97.2° F and 100.0° F) during labor.[11] Diurnal variations were noted with a nadir at midday and peak in the evening.[11]

In some women the increase in temperature during labor is high enough to generate concern that the mother is infected. Although this may sometimes be the case, the most common cause for maternal fever during labor is use of epidural analgesia, not infection.[1,11,134] Women with epidural

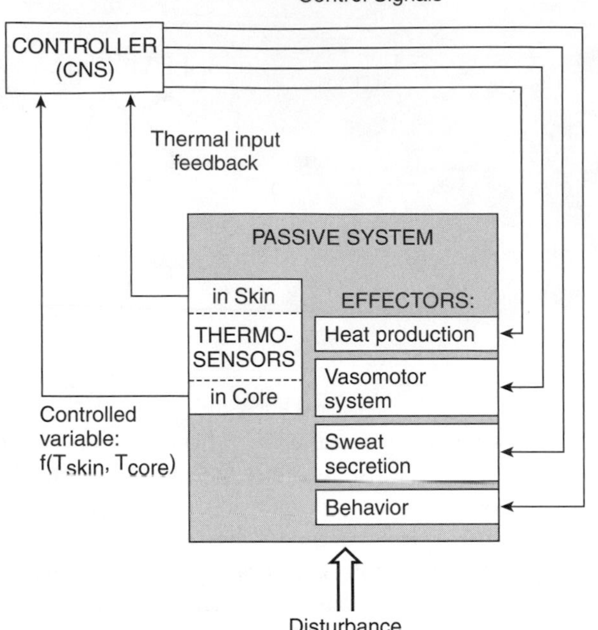

FIGURE 20-1 Regulation of body temperature. The diagram represents the biocybernetic concept of temperature regulation in humans. Temperature is sensed at various sites of the body, and the temperature signals are fed into the central controller *(multiple input system)*. (From Sahni, R., & Schulze, K. [2012]. Temperature control in newborn infants. In R.A. Polin, W.W. Fox, & S.H. Abman [Eds.], *Fetal and neonatal physiology* [4th ed.]. Philadelphia: Saunders.)

BOX 20-1 Body Temperature Regulation

Regulation of temperature depends on the ability to (1) sense temperature changes in the external environment by skin receptors; (2) regulate heat production by increasing or decreasing metabolic rate; (3) conserve or dissipate heat (by sweating or altering skin blood flow); and (4) coordinate sensory input about environmental changes with appropriate body-temperature-regulating responses.[68] Thermoregulation involves a "multiple-input system" controlled by the anterior and posterior portions of the hypothalamus. The anterior hypothalamus is temperature-sensitive and controls heat loss mechanisms. The preoptic and anterior nuclei of the anterior hypothalamus are the sites of the set point or threshold temperature. The set point is a mechanism through which heat production and loss are regulated to maintain the core temperature within a narrow range. The posterior hypothalamus, which is the central controller of responses (heat production or dissipation) to cold or heat stimuli, receives input from central receptors (in deep body structures such as the hypothalamus, abdominal organs and spinal cord) and peripheral receptors (skin, abdomen, spinal cord, hypothalamic preoptic nuclei, internal organs). The peripheral receptors are free nerve endings in the skin that send impulses to the hypothalamus via afferent nerve fibers as well as to the thalamus and cerebral cortex, when there is conscious perception of temperature changes.[64] With cold stress, the thermoregulatory center acts to conserve heat (through cutaneous vasoconstriction and abolition of sweating) or increase heat production (through voluntary skeletal muscle activity, shivering, or nonshivering thermogenesis). This center dissipates heat by activation of sweat glands to increase evaporative loss, peripheral vasodilation, and respiration. Thermal regulation is also influenced by thyroid hormones and the sympathetic nervous system.[112]

analgesia are more likely to develop a fever during labor than women without this form of anesthesia.[50,97,104,134] Epidural anesthesia in nonpregnant individuals is more likely to lead to a decreased rather than increased temperature. The fever seen with epidurals is usually characterized by a slow increase in temperature of approximately 0.07° C/hour, although the temperature may rise to greater than 37.5° C (99.5° F) or 38° C (100.4° F) in some women.[50,104] The basis for the increased temperature in pregnant women during the intrapartum period may be due to decreased heat dissipation (due to a decreased sweating threshold, alterations in ventilation, and altered hypothalamic responses) and an increase in heat production, possibly due to increased shivering.[1,5,104,134,136] The autonomic block with epidural analgesia inhibits peripheral vasoconstriction and sweating in the lower body. The impairment of sweating and behavioral responses may decrease heat loss.[11,91] Maternal fever with epidural anesthesia is associated with an inflammatory state with increased cytokines, especially interleukin-6, but this state is rarely due to infection.[5,97,104,136] Prophylactic administration of acetaminophen has not been found to suppress the fever associated with epidurals.[69,104] Panzer and colleagues reported that women during labor do not show the same relationship between temperature, sweating, and shivering as nonpregnant individuals.[91] In the parturient, shivering was not necessarily triggered by decreased temperature nor was sweating necessarily triggered by increased temperature; the woman might shiver and sweat simultaneously. Temperature increases can lead to an increased maternal heart rate, cardiac output, oxygen consumption, and catecholamine production.[104]

The laboring woman is also at risk for hypothermia during the intrapartum period due to vasodilation (limiting usual vasoconstrictive responses to cold); administration of anesthetics, narcotics, and other pharmacologic agents; blood loss, rapid fluid replacement, especially if cool fluids are used; or other events that increase maternal heat loss (e.g., cold drafts, wet drapes or towels). Prolonged exposure to a cool environment can aggravate heat loss. Hypothermia can result in shivering, hypotension, and hemodynamic and cardiorespiratory instability.[91]

Postpartum Period

Maternal temperature is monitored closely during the postpartum period because elevations may indicate infection or dehydration. A transient postpartum chill or shivering is often experienced about 15 minutes after birth of the infant or delivery of the placenta. The cause of this chill is unknown and various causes have been proposed. This phenomenon may represent muscular exhaustion or result from disequilibrium between the internal and external thermal gradients secondary to muscular exertion during labor and delivery, sudden changes in intraabdominal pressure with emptying of the uterus, or small amniotic fluid emboli. Most women who experience early postpartum shivering are normothermic, suggesting that this phenomenon is nonthermoregulatory in origin.[91] Shivering is seen in about 20% of women who did not receive neuraxial analgesia and more frequently in women after epidural analgesia.[91]

Transient maternal temperature elevations up to 38° C (100.4° F) occur in up to 6.5% of vaginally delivering women during the first 24 hours after delivery. In most women this resolves spontaneously and is secondary to noninfectious causes such as dehydration or to a transient bacterial endometritis.[42] Maternal fever in the postpartum period may be a sign of puerperal infection, mastitis, endometritis, or urinary tract infection, although these infections are usually the cause of fever after 24 hours. Any temperature elevation merits close monitoring, especially with increasingly early discharge.[3,30]

CLINICAL IMPLICATIONS FOR THE PREGNANT WOMAN AND HER FETUS

The fetal ambient environmental temperature is the maternal temperature. Fetal temperature is linked to maternal temperature and the maternal-fetal thermal gradient (see section on Development of Thermoregulation in the Fetus), so that if maternal temperature rises, so will the fetal temperature. Maternal oral temperature has been reported to correlate with intrauterine temperature, with maternal oral temperature lower than intrauterine temperature by 0.8° C (1.3° F) (95% confidence interval, 0.7° C, 1° C [1.28° F, 1.7° F]).[10] In this study a maternal "oral temperature greater than 37.2° C (99.0° F) detected an intrauterine temperature greater than 38° C (100.4° F) with a sensitivity of 81% and a specificity of 96%."[10]

The increase in maternal temperature during pregnancy may cause transient discomfort and alter the woman's heat tolerance. The major concerns related to thermoregulation during pregnancy are the effects of maternal hyperthermia and fever on the fetus.

Maternal Hyperthermia and Fever

Maternal fever has three potential detrimental effects on the fetus: (1) hypoxia secondary to maternal and fetal tachycardia and altered hemodynamics; (2) teratogenesis; and (3) preterm labor from the fever per se, from underlying infection, or from associated hemodynamic alterations.[30] Maternal intrapartum fever due to infection has been linked to a risk of cerebral palsy, cognitive defects, and neonatal seizures and encephalopathy, as well as later disorders such as schizophrenia and autism.[58,80,95,104] Maternal hyperthermia increases maternal oxygen consumption and shifts the oxygen-hemoglobin dissociation curve to the right. Although this latter change increases the oxygen supply to the placenta, fetal oxygen uptake becomes more difficult because of the altered thermal gradient.[57]

Research regarding adverse fetal effects has focused primarily on maternal temperature elevations due to fever secondary to illness, exercise, and the use of saunas or hot tubs. Animal studies show specific effects of maternal hyperthermia, especially when the maternal core temperature increases to 2° C or more above baseline; the longer the temperature elevation is maintained or the higher the temperature, the greater the risk to the fetus.[24] Some of the human studies have been retrospective and suggestive but inconclusive, while other have demonstrated a clear association.[7,23,24,39,85,89,120] A meta-analysis of studies, including both retrospective case-controlled and prospective cohort studies, reported an overall odds ratio of neural tube defects (NTDs) when associated with maternal hyperthermia of 1.92 (95% confidence interval, 1.16, 2.29).[89] Definitions of hyperthermia in the various studies ranged from temperature greater than 37.8° C (greater than 100.4° F) to temperature greater than 38.9° C (greater than 102.0° F). Most of the hyperthermia was due to maternal influenza or other febrile illness. Others have reported a twofold to fourfold increase in the risk for NTD with maternal first trimester hyperthermia for any reason.[120]

Maternal febrile illness is thought to pose the greatest hyperthermic risk; however, susceptibility may be modified by genotype.[20] Elevated maternal temperature secondary to illness-induced fever during early pregnancy has been associated with increased risk of anencephaly and spina bifida (especially around the time of neural tube closure (22 to 28 days), microcephaly, and other central nervous system disorders; alterations in growth; cleft lip; and facial dysmorphogenesis in humans.[10,23,51] In a prospective study, Chambers and colleagues reported a 10-fold increase in NTDs in women who had a temperature of 38.9° C (102° F) or greater lasting for more than 24 hours in the first month of pregnancy.[23] Whether these disorders are primarily due to the elevated temperature, the underlying infection, or a combination of these events has been debated. Most human and animal studies suggest that the increased risk is correlated to the maternal fever and not the viral illness per se.[39,89] Several investigators have reported increased cleft lip and palate, NTDs, and cardiovascular disorders in women with influenza accompanied by high temperature in the first trimester with a reduction in risk with treatment of the fever with antipyretics.[16,120] Reductions in risk have also been reported with folic acid supplementation.[16] Antifever medications and folic acid may reduce the risk of vascular disruption and apoptosis leading to congenital anomalies.[16,39]

Several studies have reported an increase in neural tube defects and oral clefts in infants born to women with an extended heat exposure secondary to sauna or hot tub use in the first trimester, suggesting that an elevated temperature may be the critical factor.[23,24,120] Milunsky and colleagues found that the hot tub exposure, especially in the first two months of pregnancy (and the risk increased with number of exposures during this time), posed a greater risk than sauna use, with no risk from electric blanket use.[88] Prospective studies from Finland of sauna use in pregnancy have not shown an increased risk. However, in these studies, maximal temperature was 38.1° C (100.6° F), below the value of 38.9° C (102° F) thought to be critical.[85]

Table 20-1 Clinical Recommendations Related to Clinical Practice in Pregnant Women

Counsel pregnant women regarding basis for heat intolerance during pregnancy and intervention strategies (p. 657).
Counsel pregnant women to avoid activities that may lead to hyperthermia (pp. 659-660).
Encourage adequate fluid intake before and during exercise (p. 660).
Discourage prolonged exercise especially in a hot, humid environment (p. 660).
Maintain adequate ambient temperature in the delivery area (p. 658).
Protect from cold drafts during delivery (p. 658).
Avoid infusing cold solutions (p. 658).
Avoid contact of maternal skin with wet drapes and towels (p. 658).
Monitor maternal temperature and assess thermoregulatory status during the intrapartum and postpartum periods (pp. 657-659).
Evaluate women with elevated temperatures for signs of infection (pp. 657-659).

Maternal Exercise and Temperature Elevations

Maternal exercise is associated with increased heat production and body temperature increases that may alter the maternal-fetal thermal gradient and fetal heat dissipation. Uterine blood flow decreases during exercise, further altering the ability of the mother to dissipate fetal heat.[57,118] However, most women seem to be able to tolerate moderate intensity exercise without significant changes in core temperature.[118] Low-impact aerobic exercise (to 70% of maximal heart rate) has not been associated with hyperthermia.[72,78] The ability of the mother to dissipate the heat generated by exercise may improve as pregnancy progresses.[85,118] The risks from temperature changes during exercise in late pregnancy are related to decreased uterine blood flow, which can be potentiated by dehydration. Prolonged exercise or exercise in heat (increased ambient heat reduces the thermal gradient between the skin and environment) or high humidity (decreases evaporative heat loss) may result in a higher maternal temperature than exercise in a cool, dry environment or water environment (e.g., aerobic exercise in water).[85,93,129] Physical conditioning before pregnancy can improve thermoregulatory capacity and may decrease the effect of heat stress.[85,93]

SUMMARY

Alterations in thermal status during pregnancy increase the risk of alterations in fetal health and development. Ongoing assessment and monitoring of thermal status in the pregnant woman and neonate and initiation of appropriate interventions to maintain thermal stability can prevent or minimize these risks. Clinical recommendations related to maternal thermoregulation are summarized in Table 20-1.

DEVELOPMENT OF THERMOREGULATION IN THE FETUS

Because fetal temperature is linked to maternal temperature and the maternal-fetal thermal gradient, the fetus cannot control its temperature independently. Under normal resting conditions, the temperature of the fetus is approximately 0.5° C (0.9° F) higher (range, 0.3° C to 1° C [0.5° F to 1.7° F]) than that of the mother, or about 37.6° C to 37.8° C (99.7° F to 100.0° F).[13,14,47,77,87,94,100] About half of this difference is due to placental and uterine heat production.[94] In animal studies, this difference between maternal and fetal temperatures is seen by the time the fetus achieves one third of its body weight, which would be around the beginning of the third trimester in the human fetus.[87] The fetus produces about 5 calories (20.9 J) of heat per every millimeter of oxygen used.[94] Fetal metabolic rate varies to match oxygen availability (adaptive hypometabolism), so that if PO_2 decreases, fetal oxygen consumption also decreases and if fetal PO_2 increases, so does fetal oxygen consumption.[94] Any increase in fetal oxygen consumption increases heat production.[118]

Fetal core and skin temperature and the temperature of amniotic fluid are all similar. The fetal temperature must be higher than the maternal temperature to maintain a gradient to offload heat from the fetus to the mother. Fetal heat dissipation is influenced by fetal and placental metabolic activity, thermal diffusion capacity of heat exchange sites within the placenta, and rates of blood flow in the umbilical cord, placenta, and intervillous spaces.[77,85]

Heat generated by fetal metabolism is dissipated by the amniotic fluid to the uterine wall (conductive pathway) or via umbilical cord and placenta to maternal blood in the intervillous spaces (convective pathway). The majority of heat is transferred via the convective pathway through the placenta via the umbilical circulation, with only 10% to 20% dissipated via amniotic fluid.[47] The large placental surface area, thin membrane barrier, and high blood flow rate enhance thermal exchange. Transfer of heat is facilitated by the maternal-fetal temperature gradient. Therefore if the mother has an elevated temperature (from exercise, illness, or exposure to hot environments such as a sauna), this gradient may be reduced or reversed, leading to an increase in the fetal temperature (see section on Maternal Hyperthermia and Fever).[25] Changes in fetal temperature lag behind maternal changes because amniotic fluid provides some insulation.[57]

Fetal heat production and loss mechanisms are suppressed in utero. Fetal temperature is "heat-clamped" to the maternal system, preventing the fetus from independent thermoregulation before birth.[94] Fetal responses to cooling are minimal and primarily involve shivering-like muscle contractions and endocrine response. Cooling of the fetus does not activate nonshivering thermogenesis (NST). The inability to initiate NST is thought to be linked to placental inhibitors of an uncoupling protein essential for brown adipose tissue (BAT) metabolism that are present in fetal blood. Both BAT and the uncoupling protein (UCP-1) that regulates its metabolism increase from 25 to 26 weeks' gestation to term (see Brown Adipose Tissue Metabolism).[32,56] The placental inhibitors, primarily prostaglandin E_2 and adenosine, are an advantage to the fetus in promoting accumulation of BAT. The rapid decrease in these inhibitors with clamping of the umbilical cord at birth promotes BAT metabolism in the newborn to maintain thermal stability with transition to extrauterine life.[94] Fetal cord occlusion thus leads to an increase in body temperature, although brain temperature tends to remain constant.[32,56,94]

The fetal-maternal temperature gradient is sustained during labor, although it may widen with prolonged labor, during the latent phase or with infection or prolonged rupture of the membranes, or decrease with compression of the umbilical cord (decreasing blood flow from the fetus and thus the ability of the fetus to dissipate heat).[69,94,100] If the maternal temperature rises in labor, as often occurs with epidural analgesia (see Intrapartum Period), the fetal temperature will also increase.[100,104] In the second and third trimesters, increased fetal temperature leads to increased fetal heart rate but not to other thermoregulatory responses. Maternal fever in labor, especially temperature greater than 38° C (100.4° F), in noninfected women has been associated with lower Apgar scores, hypotonia, hypoxia, and an increased need for resuscitation and oxygen at birth.[10,77]

NEONATAL PHYSIOLOGY

Thermoregulation is a critical physiologic function in the neonate that is closely linked to the infant's survival and health status.[62] An understanding of transitional events and neonatal physiologic adaptations is essential for provision of an appropriate environment to maintain thermal stability. Heat losses are greater and more rapid and can easily exceed heat production in both term and preterm neonates if the infants are left unclothed in an environment comfortable for an adult. This is because of the infant's larger surface area–to-body mass ratio, decreased insulating subcutaneous fat, increased skin permeability to water, and small radius of curvature of exchange surfaces.[33] Newborns (even most preterm infants) have a relatively well-developed thermoregulatory capacity. Their major thermoregulatory limitation is a narrow control range that makes them more vulnerable to alterations in the thermal environment.[62]

Transitional Events

With birth the fetus moves from the warm, moist intrauterine environment to the colder, drier extrauterine environment. The infant's temperature falls after birth, triggering cold-induced metabolic responses and heat production.[14,18,103] Because fetal thermoregulation is linked to the mother, thermoregulatory processes are suppressed in the fetus. These processes, especially initiation of nonshivering thermogenesis (NST), must be activated rapidly after birth if the infant is to survive the transition to extrauterine life. Stimulation of cutaneous cold receptors and spinal cord and hypothalamic thermal receptors at birth activates the sympathetic nervous system. This leads to the release of norepinephrine and a twofold to threefold increase in metabolic rate, oxygen consumption, and heat production.[47,94] Occlusion of the umbilical cord, which removes placental factors that suppress NST, increases a brown adipose tissue (BAT)-specific uncoupling protein with a rapid increase in BAT metabolism (see Brown Adipose Tissue Metabolism) and heat production.[94,99] Thermal transition at birth and BAT metabolism are interrelated with changes in thyroid function (see Chapter 19).

Newborns lose heat rapidly after birth, especially through evaporative losses (0.58 kcal/mL [2.4 J/mL] of water loss) from their moist body surface, as well as via convection to cooler room air and radiation to cooler room walls. A newborn's temperature may fall 0.2° C to 1° C/min (0.5° F to 1.7° F/min) if thermal interventions are not initiated.[25,47,62] Rutter estimated that in a cool room, the body temperature of a 1000-g preterm infant falls 1° C (1.7° F) every 5 minutes.[100] Initial temperatures of infants born by cesarean birth are on average 0.3° C (0.5° F) lower than infants born vaginally, perhaps due to slightly lower levels of sympathetic activity, catecholamines, and thyroid activity.[94] Interventions in the delivery room to reduce evaporative and other losses support transition, reduce cold stress, and have been associated with a higher PO_2 at 1 hour of age, lower mortality, and decreased morbidity.[62] Since much of the heat loss immediately after birth is due to evaporative losses, infants should be quickly dried and wrapped in a warm, dry towel and either given to the mother for skin-to-skin contact or placed under a radiant warmer or in a prewarmed incubator.[47,48] A polyethylene bag or wrap can be used with VLBW infants to reduce heat loss after birth (see Methods of Promoting Thermal Stability).[14,29,64] Heat loss in VLBW infants immediately after birth can also be reduced by maintaining adequate ambient temperatures and humidity in the delivery and stabilization room.[122] Bissinger and Annibale recommend 50% humidity and room temperatures of 78° F to 80° F (25.5° C to 26.6° C) for infants less than or equal to 28 weeks' gestation (less than or equal to 1000 g) and greater than or equal to 72° F (22.2° C) with a goal of 75° F (23.8° C) for infants 29 to 32 weeks' gestation (1001-1500 g).[14] Other interventions to reduce evaporative, radiant, conductive, and convective losses are listed in Table 20-2.

Term newborns can increase their metabolic rate by up to 200% to 300%.[18,47] This response is delayed in larger preterm infants, who do not approximate term values until 2 to 3 weeks of age; further delay is seen in VLBW infants.[18,35] VLBW infants may only have a maximal increase in metabolic activity of 25% with cold stress.[25] In extremely low–birth weight

Table 20-2 **Prevention of Heat Loss and Overheating in the Neonate**

MECHANISM	SOURCES OF HEAT LOSS OR OVERHEATING	INTERVENTIONS
Conduction	Cool mattress, blanket, scale, table, x-ray plate, or clothing	Place warm blankets on scales, x-ray plates, and other surfaces in contact with the infant. Warm blankets and clothing before use. Use skin to skin care. Preheat incubators, radiant warmers, and heat shields.
	Heating pads, hot water bottles, chemical bags	Avoid placing infant on any surface or object that is warmer than the infant.
Convection	Cool room, corridors, or outside air	Maintain the room temperature at levels adequate to provide a safe thermal environment for infants according to their gestational ages. Transport the infant in an enclosed, warmed incubator through internal hallways and between external environments (e.g., ambulance to nursery). Open incubator portholes only when necessary and for brief periods. Swaddle with warm blankets (unless under radiant warmer). Use polyethylene bags or wraps with VLBW infants from birth; use transparent plastic across the infant between the radiant warmer side guards; use caps with adequate insulation quality or hooded blankets.
	Convective air flow incubator	Monitor the incubator temperature to avoid temperatures warmer than the infant's body temperature.
	Drafts from air vents, windows, doors, heaters, fans, and air conditioners	Place infants away from air vents, drafts, and other sources of moving air particles. Use side guards on radiant warmers to decrease cross-current air flow across the infant; stretch transparent plastic across the infant between the radiant warmer and side guards.
	Cold oxygen flow (especially near facial thermal receptors)	Warm oxygen and monitor the temperature inside the oxygen hood.
Evaporation	Wet body surface and hair in the delivery room or from bathing	Dry the infant, especially the head, immediately after birth with a warm blanket or towel. Use caps with adequate insulation quality or hooded blankets. Use polyethylene bags or wraps with VLBW infants from birth. Replace wet blankets with dry, warm ones and place in a warm environment. Delay the initial bath until the infant's temperature has stabilized; then give a sponge bath. Bathe the infant in a warm, draft-free environment, place on warmed towels and dry immediately; bathe under a radiant warmer.
	Application of lotions, solutions, wet packs, or soaks to the infant	Prewarm solutions and soaks; maintain warmth during use. Avoid overheating solutions and soaks.
	Water loss from lungs	Warm and humidify oxygen.
	Increased insensible water loss in VLBW or ill infants	Increase incubator humidity levels as needed for VLBW infants.
Radiation	Placement near cold or hot external windows or walls; placement in direct sunlight	Place incubators, cribs, and radiant warmers away from external walls and windows and direct sunlight. Use thermal shades on external windows.
	Cold incubator walls	Use double-walled incubators or heat shields, or cover with plastic film. Prewarm incubators, radiant warmers, and heat shields.
	Heat lamps	Avoid use whenever possible; if used, do not place close to infant skin and monitor temperature every 10 to 15 minutes to avoid burns.

VLBW, Very low–birth weight.

(ELBW) infants, an increase in thermal maturational skills has been reported at 28 weeks' postmenstrual age, possibly due to decreased evaporative losses.[35]

Most healthy infants increase their temperatures by 2 to 3 hours after birth. Thermal stabilization may be affected by timing of the first bath, thermal status at time of bathing, and method of bathing.[19,86,131] VLBW infants are more likely than term infants to have admission temperatures of less than 36° C (96.8° F).[14,69]

Heat Exchange

Heat exchange occurs between the environment and the infant's skin and respiratory tract. Heat transfer involves four mechanisms: evaporation, radiation, conduction, and convection. All four mechanisms operate at the body surface; in the respiratory tract, evaporation and convection are the main mechanisms of heat exchange.[103] The degree of heat exchange depends on these mechanisms as well as other factors such as body surface area, position, body movements, and body shape.[103] Equations are available to calculate heat exchange at the infant's body surface via evaporation, radiation, conduction, and convection as well as heat exchange between the respiratory tract and the environment.[103]

Heat Transfer

Heat transfer involves two interrelated processes: the internal and external gradients. The internal gradient involves transfer of heat from within the body to the surface and relies primarily on blood flow within an extensive capillary and venous plexus. Tissue insulation (subcutaneous fat) and convective movement of heat through blood influence efficiency of heat conduction. Heat conduction can be altered by vasomotor control processes mediated by the sympathetic nervous system that change skin blood flow with peripheral vasoconstriction to conserve heat and vasodilatation to eliminate heat.

Heat transfer through the internal gradient is increased in neonates because of their thinner layer of subcutaneous fat (i.e., less insulation) and a larger surface area–to–body mass ratio, especially in preterm infants. The subcutaneous layer of insulating fat accounts for only 16% of body fat in infants compared with 30% to 35% in adults.[34] The body mass of the neonate is about 5% of adult mass, whereas the surface area is 15%. In term infants, the surface area–to–body mass ratio may be three times, and in preterm infants five times, greater than that of adults.[101] This ratio is even higher in ELBW infants. For example, the surface area–to–body mass ratio of a 500-g infant may be six times greater than that of an adult and twice as great as that of a 1500-g infant.[55]

The external gradient involves transfer of heat from the body surface to the environment. The rate of heat loss is directly proportional to the magnitude of the difference between skin temperature and the environmental temperature and can be expressed as follows: heat loss = h (skin temperature − environmental temperature) × (surface area), where h is the thermal transfer coefficient (the rate at which heat leaves the body surface) and is influenced by body size, tissue conductance, skin blood flow, and vasoactivity.[18,103] Heat loss per unit of body mass is inversely proportional to body size.[18] As noted above, the mechanisms by which heat is transferred from the body surface are conduction, convection, radiation, and evaporation (see Prevention of Excessive Heat Loss or Heat Gain).

Heat transfer by the external gradient is also increased in the neonate because of increased surface area and an increased thermal transfer coefficient.[103] In terms of heat loss, the amount of exposed surface area is most critical; thus an infant who is not in an incubator or radiant warmer will lose less heat if he or she is clothed or swaddled. Factors that increase the thermal transfer coefficient (and thus heat loss), such as decreased skin thickness and altered conductance, are present in the neonate. The threshold for heat production in the newborn is more closely linked to skin temperature than in the adult. As a result, cold responses, especially in preterm infants, are related primarily to skin rather than core temperature changes.[18]

Heat Production and Conservation

Heat production is a result of metabolic processes that generate energy by oxidative metabolism of glucose, fats, and proteins. The amount of metabolic heat produced varies with activity, feeding (calorigenic or specific dynamic action), state (greater heat is produced in awake infants than in sleeping infants and in active versus quiet (deep) sleep), health status, and environmental temperature.[18,26,35] Organs that generate the greatest amount of metabolic energy are the brain, heart, and liver. To maintain a constant body temperature, heat production must equal heat loss from the body surface over a given time. Basal heat production to maintain this stability is generated by body metabolic processes. In the event of cold stress, heat above basal needs can be generated by physical or chemical mechanisms. Because of their surface area–to–body mass ratio (which is an important determinant of heat loss), heat production in infants is low relative to heat loss.[100] In the term infant, heat production at rest (estimated by oxygen consumption) in a thermoneutral environment is similar to that of adults per unit of weight, but approximately half that of the adult per unit of surface area. This is further decreased in preterm infants, who have an even greater surface area–to–body mass ratio and are less likely to spontaneously lie in a flexed position.[100] Prone positioning in low-birth weight (LBW) infants has been reported to increase central and peripheral body temperature in spite of the lower metabolic rates seen in this position.[4] In term infants the maximal heat production increases from 20% to 75% of adult values over the first postbirth week; this change takes longer in preterm infants.[103]

Physical mechanisms to generate include involuntary (shivering) and voluntary muscular activity. Shivering is the most important mechanism for the generation of additional heat in adults. The neonate uses physical methods (shivering and increased muscular activity) to some extent to generate additional heat. Shivering, which is controlled via the somatomotor system, is not as important in the neonate as in the adult, and the shivering threshold is probably at a lower body temperature.[101] Shivering in neonates is primarily seen as a late event associated with decreased spinal cord temperature after prolonged cold exposure. The cervical spinal region is protected from cold stress and preferentially receives heat generated by NST through metabolism of BAT in the intrascapular area. If NST is blocked or the infant is unable to generate adequate heat to compensate for severe or prolonged cold stress, the temperature of the spinal cord eventually decreases.[18]

Infants, primarily term or late preterm infants, produce some heat by increasing muscular activity with restlessness, hyperactivity, or crying. This increases heat production in skeletal muscles with breakdown of glycogen and glucose oxidation.[13,25] Infants may try to conserve heat by postural changes such as flexion that reduce the surface area and heat loss through the internal gradient. The ability to produce heat by physical methods can be markedly reduced or obliterated with the use of anesthetics, muscle relaxants, sedatives, or tight restraints and in infants with brain injury.[18,34,47,103]

Heat can be generated by chemical mechanisms or NST through changes in the metabolic rate and, primarily in neonates, by BAT metabolism. These changes are mediated by the sympathetic nervous system. Both infants and adults can generate heat by increasing their metabolic rate above basal levels. An adult can increase heat production by 10% to 15% by NST; in the neonate, this increase can be 100% or more.[53] NST is mediated by epinephrine in the adult and by norepinephrine in the neonate.[21,119] This results in activation of an adipose tissue lipase and splitting of triglycerides into glycerol and nonesterified fatty acids (NEFA), which are oxidized to produce heat, esterified to form triglycerides, or released into the circulation.[21,115,119] NST is triggered when the mean skin temperature falls to 35° C to 36° C (95° F to 96.8° F).[115]

NST is the major mechanism through which the infant produces heat above basal needs. Increasing the metabolic rate may lead to further problems in immature or compromised neonates, because any increase in metabolic rate increases oxygen consumption. Stressed infants may be unable to provide enough oxygen; oxygen debt with lactic acidosis from anaerobic metabolism and finally exhaustion can result. The ability to generate heat by NST is limited in ELBW infants.[65]

Thermal receptors in the skin are important mediators of the hypothalamic thermal center's response to temperature changes or cold stress. Stimulation of these receptors initially leads to heat-conserving responses with peripheral vasoconstriction.[64] This may result in acrocyanosis in the neonate. In the infant, thermal receptors are most prominent and sensitive over the trigeminal area of the face. For example, cooling the face of an infant who is normothermic causes a rise in metabolic rate. Conversely, warming the facial skin (i.e., use of warmed oxygen in an oxygen hood) when the infant's body is cold may suppress the usual increase in metabolic rate and other heat-generating mechanisms and can be dangerous.[103] A recent study of ELBW found that these infants did not demonstrate peripheral vasoconstriction the first 12 hours after birth even with a low body temperature.[65] Other studies have found minimal or no peripheral vasoconstriction with poor vasomotor control in infants weighing less than 1000 g, increasing their risk of thermoregulatory problems.[65]

Brown Adipose Tissue Metabolism

The neonate relies primarily on BAT metabolism for NST. Large amounts of BAT are found in human and animal newborns, hibernators, and in adult animals after cold acclimatization.[21,34,90] Small amounts of BAT remain in human adults, although it is found primarily in the cervical-supraclavicular area and often interspersed within white adipose tissue.[21,32] Active BAT is seen more frequently in adult females than adult males.[133]

The major function of BAT is heat production. In the newborn, BAT is found in the midscapular region; nape of the neck; around the neck muscles extending under the clavicles into the axillae; in the mediastinum; and around the trachea, esophagus, heart, lungs, liver, and intercostal and mammary arteries; abdominal aorta; kidneys; and adrenal glands. The largest deposits of BAT are around the kidneys and adrenals, with smaller amounts around the great vessels, extending to the neck and from the thoracic cavity to the axillae and clavicles.[34] In children and adults the BAT is less widely dispersed as in the newborn and has a lower lipid content.[32] The total amount of heat produced by BAT metabolism in the neonate is unknown, but it may account for nearly 100% of the infant's needs.

BAT cells begin to differentiate by 25 to 26 weeks' gestation and immature brown adipocytes are seen by at least 29 weeks.[32] BAT increases in the third trimester. BAT stores continue to increase in the early weeks after birth and can double during this time.[32] The term newborn has an estimated 30 g of BAT accounting for approximately 1% of the infant's weight and accounting for one tenth of the adipose tissue in these infants.[32,119] BAT stores are lower in preterm and minimal in VLBW infants.

In appearance and composition, BAT in the infant is markedly different from white adipose tissue (Table 20-3).[18,21,34,90,119] These characteristics promote rapid metabolism, heat production, and heat transfer to the peripheral circulation. The lipolysis rate in BAT is three times higher than in white adipose tissue.[21] The unique structure of BAT gives it the ability to generate more energy than others tissue in the body.

Table 20-3 Characteristics of Brown Adipose Tissue and Their Significance

CHARACTERISTIC	SIGNIFICANCE
Many small fat vacuoles	Large fat-to-cytoplasm ratio, enhancing the rapidity of fat use
Many mitochondria	Production of energy (i.e., adenosine triphosphate [ATP]) for rapid metabolic turnover and heat production
Glycogen stores	Source of glucose for production of ATP and energy
Abundant blood supply	Brings nutrients to cell and transports heat produced to other areas of the body
Abundant sympathetic nerve supply	Metabolism of brown adipose tissue mediated by norepinephrine

Compiled from references 18, 21, 31, 32, 34, 90.

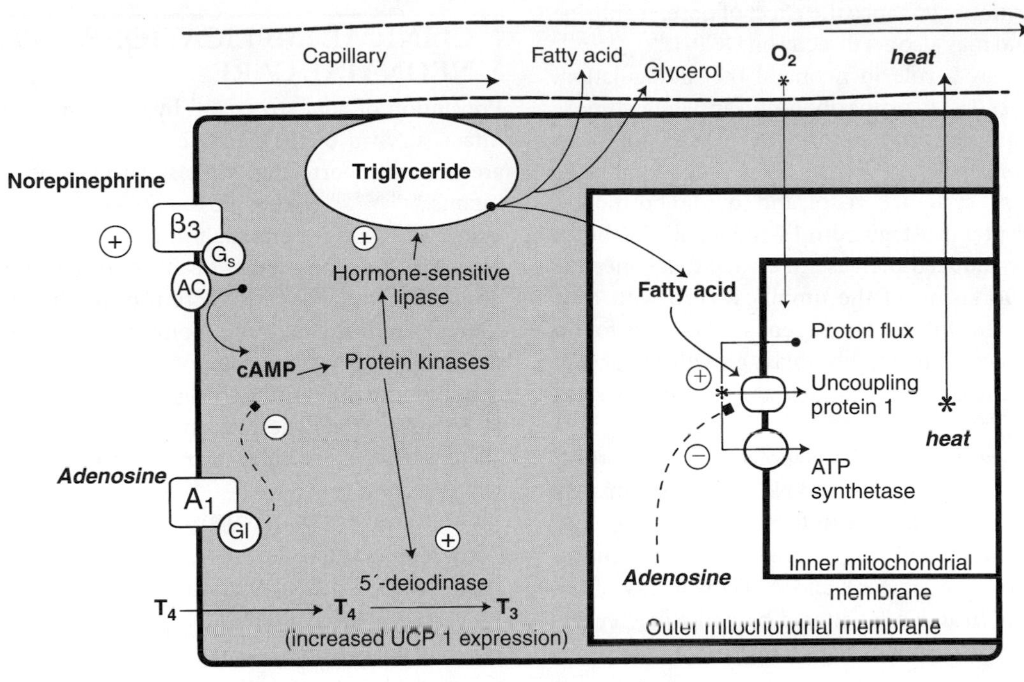

FIGURE 20-2 Metabolic and hormonal controls of brown adipose tissue. Control occurs by regulating blood flow; altering the activity of lipase and 5′ deiodinase and uncoupling protein-1 (UCP-1); and affecting the permeability of the inner mitochondrial membrane to protons. Norepinephrine stimulates thermogenesis through both α_1-receptors and β_3-receptors, but its effects are attenuated in utero. Thyroxine (T_4) is converted to T_3 within the fat cell and increases the expression and activity of the UCP-1. (From Power, G.G., Blood, A.B., & Hunter, C.J. [2004]. Perinatal thermal physiology. In R.A. Polin, W.W. Fox, & S.H. Abman [Eds.], *Fetal and neonatal physiology* [3rd ed.]. Philadelphia: Saunders.)

Heat production within the BAT cell is regulated by uncoupling protein-1 (UCP-1), sometimes called *thermogenin,* located along the inner membrane of brown adipocyte mitochondria (Figure 20-2). UCP-1 permits protons to pass across the mitochondrial membrane without the need to conserve energy. UCP-1 uncouples oxidative phosphorylation and adenosine triphosphate (ATP) synthesis via oxidation of fatty acids. As a result, more energy is used for heat and less is conserved for ATP regeneration.[21,28,82,90,101,113,115] UCP-1 increases from 29.4 ± 3 pmol/mg at 25 weeks' gestation to 62.5 ± 10.2 pmol/mg at 40 weeks with a marked increase seen at 32 weeks' gestation that marks the ability to use NST.[56,64] This gestational age is also the time when levels of enzymes to convert T_4 to T_3 also increase.[56,64] Thus NST is immature in infants of less than 32 weeks' gestation, and especially in ELBW infants, due to low levels of BAT, decreased UCP-1, and decreased thyroid hormones.[64]

UCP-1 is also expressed in the smooth muscle of the uterus, digestive tract, and male reproductive tract, although at much lower levels than in BAT, and may have a role in smooth muscle relaxation.[28] There has been increased interest in the roles of UCP-1 and BAT in recent years since BAT is thought to play a role in energy balance.[28,32,82,96] BAT in adults is associated with low total adipose tissue content and may have a role in weight control. UCP-1 is involved in diet-induced thermogenesis and body weight regulation.[28] Thus there has been increased interest and research recently in BAT related to the prevention and treatment of obesity and age-related disorders.[32,76,82,96,133]

Activation of UCP-1 is controlled by the hypothalamus. The sympathetic nervous system and hormonal mediators control BAT metabolism. Changes in temperature are transmitted from peripheral cutaneous receptors to the posterior hypothalamus (see Figure 20-1). The sympathetic nervous system is stimulated to release norepinephrine within BAT stores and to stimulate catecholamine release from the adrenal medulla.[74,94,112]

Norepinephrine released at the surface of brown adipocytes interacts with α_1-, β_1-, and, primarily, β_3-adrenergic receptors to increase cyclic adenosine monophosphate (cAMP). The cAMP increases lipase activity, allowing rapid hydrolysis of triglycerides and phospholipids within the brown adipocytes. The free fatty acids released activate UCP-1, which further increases heat production.[94] This process is enhanced by triiodothyronine (T_3) and thyroxine (T_4), which up-regulate UCP-1, as well as by cortisol and prolactin.[82,94,113] A thyroid hormone surge occurs with birth (see Chapter 19). The thyroid gland is stimulated by the pituitary release of thyroid-stimulating hormone to produce T_4, which is then converted to T_3. Thyroid hormones enhance the effect of norepinephrine on the BAT cells and may also act directly on UCP-1.[18,34,94,112,113] Leptin may also play a role in neonatal thermoregulation. Leptin (see Chapter 16) is primarily found in white adipose tissue, but small amounts are seen in BAT, increasing from 35 weeks' gestation to term.[21,112] Leptin is regulated by the sympathetic nervous system, cortisol, and thyroid hormones. Before birth, placental prostaglandin E_2 and adenosine block the catecholamine-induced increase in cAMP that is needed to initiate NST. Occlusion of the umbilical cord with cord clamping removes this inhibition. Recent studies have found that signaling molecules of the fibroblast growth factor and bone morphogenetic protein families are also involved in BAT adipogenesis.[32,82]

Production of heat from BAT metabolism involves breakdown of triglycerides into glycerol and NEFAs. Approximately 30% of the NEFAs are oxidized, with formation of energy and metabolic heat. Because oxidation of NEFAs is dependent on the availability of oxygen, glucose, and ATP, the ability of the neonate to generate heat can be altered by pathologic events such as hypoxia, acidosis, and hypoglycemia.

Heat Dissipation and Loss

The neonate can dissipate heat by peripheral vasodilation or by sweating. As the infant's core temperature rises above 37.3° C (99.1° F), cutaneous blood flow and skin thermal conductance increase along with heat loss through the external gradient.[121]

Sweating increases evaporative loss. Each milliliter of water evaporated results in 0.58 cal (2.4 J) of heat loss.[103] Term infants can increase evaporative losses up to 100% but are less effective at sweating than adults. Although the density of sweat glands is six times greater in the neonate, the capacity of these glands is only about one third of adult values.[45] Sweat appears first on the infant's forehead, generally beginning after 35 to 40 minutes of exposure to an ambient temperature above 37° C (98.6° F). By 70 to 75 minutes, evaporative water losses increase four times. In the term small-for-gestational-age (SGA) infant, the onset of sweating is slower (55 to 60 minutes), but evaporative losses increase more rapidly.

Sweating is also altered in infants with central nervous system dysfunction and in preterm infants. Infants of mothers on opiates such as heroin and methadone may have early maturation of sweating.[100] In preterm newborns over 30 weeks' gestation, the onset of sweating is delayed. SGA infants demonstrate thermoregulatory potential similar to that in infants of comparable gestation but are limited by their body size. In preterm infants the maximal rate of sweating is less than that of either term or SGA infants. Sweating is minimal or nonexistent in infants of less than 30 weeks' gestation because of nonfunctional or immature sweat glands.[45,103] However these infants have significant transepidermal water and heat losses due to their immature skin (see Chapter 14).[115,137] These losses are significantly increased in infants cared for in a radiant warmer or receiving phototherapy (see Chapter 18). Neonates also lose heat by radiation, conduction, and convection (discussed in the next section).

CLINICAL IMPLICATIONS FOR NEONATAL CARE

Prevention of cold stress and hypothermia is critical for the intact survival of the neonate. Lowered body temperatures are inversely correlated with survival, especially in VLBW infants.[30,45,62,69,103] Exposure to cool environments and subsequent cold stress often result in physiologic changes that significantly alter the infant's health status, especially in VLBW and ELBW infants. Introduction of the intensive care environment into the delivery room may improve outcomes for these infants.[132] Major components of neonatal care include maintenance of infant thermoregulatory processes, provision of an appropriate thermal environment, and prevention of heat loss, hypothermia, and cold stress.

Neutral Thermal Environment

Body temperature and oxygen consumption are closely related. As the body temperature falls, the amount of oxygen needed for survival increases rapidly. Oxygen consumption is minimal in two thermal regions: the neutral thermal environment (NTE) and with severe hypothermia (Figure 20-3). The NTE (thermoneutrality) is an idealized setting defined as a range of ambient temperatures within which the body temperature is normal, metabolic rate is minimal, and thermoregulation is achieved by basal nonevaporative physical processes alone.[18,25,33] Within the thermal neutral range, the person is in thermal equilibrium with the environment (Figure 20-4). Because all newborns lose fluid through their skin continuously, evaporative loss is always present. Darnell

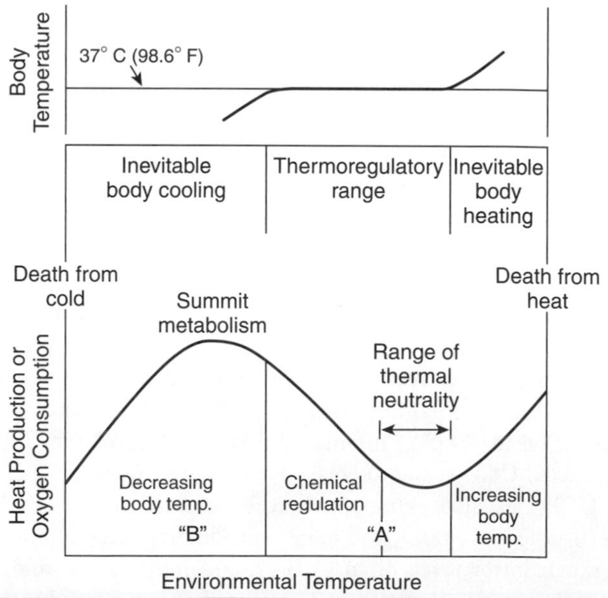

FIGURE 20-3 Effects of environmental temperature on oxygen consumption and body temperature. (From Klaus, M.H., Fanaroff, A.A., & Martin, R.J. [2001]. The physical environment. In M.H. Klaus & A.A. Fanaroff [Eds.], *Care of the high-risk neonate.* [5th ed.]. Philadelphia: Saunders.)

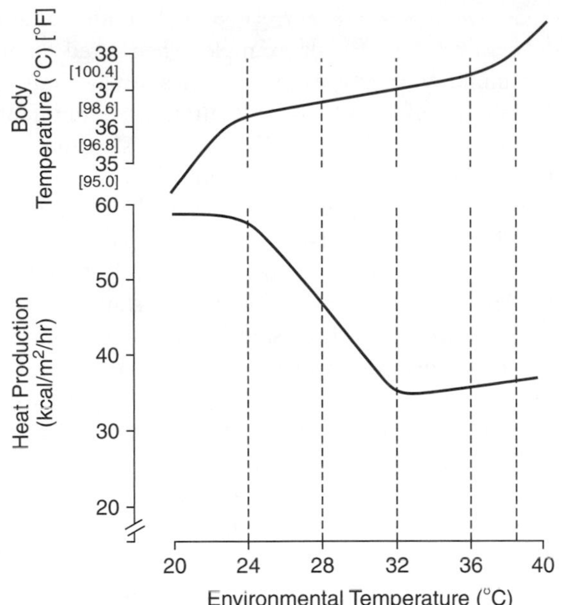

FIGURE 20-4 The effect of environmental temperature on heat production and body temperature of a 1.9-kg infant of 34 weeks' gestation, nursed naked in surroundings of uniform temperature and moderate humidity. Between 32° and 36° C (89.6° F and 93.2° F) heat production is minimal, there is no sweating, and body temperature is normal (neutral thermal range). When the environmental temperature exceeds 36° C (98.6° F), the infant sweats; above 38° C (100.4° F), body temperature rises rapidly. Below 32° C (89.6° F), heat production increases by nonshivering thermogenesis, but below 24° C (75.2° F), heat production has reached its maximum and body temperature rapidly falls. (From Rutter, N. [2005]. Temperature control and its disorders. In J.M. Rennie & N.R.C. Roberton [Eds.], *Roberton's Textbook of neonatology* [4th ed.]. London: Churchill Livingstone.)

proposes the following clinical definition of thermoneutrality for infants: "that environment (usually a range of air temperatures in an incubator or abdominal skin temperature under a radiant warmer) in which the infant, when quiet or asleep, is not required to increase heat production above 'resting' levels to maintain body temperature."[33] Figure 20-3 illustrates the relationships between thermoneutrality, body temperature, and metabolism.

In the thermoneutral state an infant is neither gaining nor losing heat, oxygen consumption is minimal, and the core-to-skin temperature gradient is small. A normal skin or core temperature does not necessarily mean that the infant is in a thermal neutral zone, in that an infant may be maintaining that temperature by increasing metabolic rate and BAT metabolism. Thus body temperature is not a very sensitive indicator of neutral thermal environment stability.[13,25,100] Swaddling or clothing widens the lower range.[100]

Thermoneutrality is generally achieved at environmental temperatures of 25° C to 30° C (77° F to 86° F) in the adult; at 32° C to 33.5° C (89.6° F to 92.3° F) in the unclothed term infant and at 24° C to 27° C (75.2° F to 80.6° F) when clothed; at 34° C to 35° C (93.2° F to 95° F) in the unclothed preterm infant at 30 weeks (1500 g) and at 28° C to 34° C (82.4° F to 93.2° F) when clothed; and at higher temperatures in more immature infants.[18,100,119] Environmental conditions that do not tax an adult may require increased metabolic work by the neonate. The thermoneutral range is narrowest for infants of the lowest birth weights.[100] Guidelines for determining neutral thermal zones for infants of varying ages and weights are available.[62,103] These guidelines were developed for healthy infants at set environmental conditions and must be used in conjunction with evaluation of the temperature of the incubator walls and external environment; humidity; air velocity; posture; clothing; infant weight; health status and activity level; and, especially in the first week, gestational age.[100,103] These guidelines are not appropriate for ELBW infants because these infants require higher neutral temperatures because of increased evaporative losses. The most immature infants may require environmental temperatures equal to or higher than skin and core temperatures.[103]

Preterm infants cared for in environments outside the thermoneutral zone may not grow as well as infants with similar caloric intakes cared for in a thermoneutral environment. VLBW infants may respond to temperatures outside the thermoneutral zone by a change in body temperature unaccompanied by an increase in oxygen consumption. The very high transepidermal water losses in these infants seem to be the major factor in determining their appropriate thermal environment. Use of a neutral thermal environment in the early weeks after birth is associated with smaller feeding and caloric requirements.[62,115]

Prevention of Excessive Heat Loss or Heat Gain

The four mechanisms by which heat is transferred to and from the body surface are conduction, convection, radiation, and evaporation. Examples of each mechanism in the neonate and appropriate interventions are listed in Table 20-2.

Conduction

Conduction involves transfer of heat from the body core to the surface through body tissue and from the body surface to objects in contact with the body (mattress, clothing, and scales). The rate at which heat is transferred is directly proportional to the size of the temperature gradient.[47] Conductive loss can be minimized through insulation such as blankets or clothing or through skin-to-skin contact and is increased by placing the infant on conductive surfaces such as metal.[48] The mattress used in most incubators and radiant warmers has a low conductivity. Room temperature blankets and mattresses can be associated with significant heat loss, especially in the preterm infant, and must be warmed before use.[14,100]

Heat can also be transferred from an object to the infant through conduction. Thus if an infant is placed on a heated pad that is warmer than the infant, hyperthermia or burns can develop. Heat is also conducted to the surrounding stable air (boundary layer) in direct contact with the infant's body. This form of heat loss is minimal unless the air around the infant is moving such that the warmed air is constantly being replaced with cooler air, leading to convective losses.

Convection

With convective losses, heat is dissipated from the interior of the body to the skin surface through the blood, conducted from the body surface to surrounding air (boundary layer), and carried away by diffusion to moving air particles (drafts, colder room or outside air) at the skin surface. Natural (free) or passive convection involves movement of heat molecules into the boundary layer near the skin and then gradually away from the infant.[14,47] Forced convection occurs when a mass of air is physically moving over the infant, conveying heat away from the body.[14,25,47,73] Transfer is dependent on ambient temperature, air flow velocity (usually at velocities of greater than or equal to 0.27 m/sec), and relative humidity (which determines the air's thermal density).[47] In LBW infants, convective losses are increased by the shorter radius of the curvature of the body surface.[121] Heat can be lost by convective means through transfer of warmed inspired air to colder exterior air (or unheated oxygen) through exhalation. During resuscitation, use of cool oxygen (which removes warm carbon dioxide from the lungs) can decrease body temperature.[62] Measurements of air temperature should be made close to the infant's skin surface, because air temperature within an incubator may vary.

Convective losses are increased at higher air-flow velocities.[73,103] This is known as the *wind-chill factor* and may be induced by incubator air circulation. Environments with higher air temperatures and minimal air circulation can reduce convective loss by up to two thirds.[119] Heat can be gained by convection if ambient temperature is higher than the infant's skin temperature. Incubators use this principle to warm infants by circulating warm air around the infant.

Convective heat losses can be minimized by swaddling or using caps on infants in cribs, use of polyethylene bags or wraps with VLBW infants after birth (see Methods of Promoting Thermal Stability), warming oxygen, and placing infants away from drafts or air vents (see Table 20-2).[14,29,64] Warming of oxygen from a face mask is important because of the sensitivity of the thermal receptors in the trigeminal area. If the infant's environment is well heated below the neck but cool around the face, the infant will react as if cold stressed. This can lead to metabolic alterations and hyperthermia.[103] If the infant's face is warmer than the body, apnea may result.

Evaporation

Evaporative heat loss occurs as moisture on the body surface or respiratory tract mucosa vaporizes. These losses depend on air speed and relative humidity. Evaporative loss is the major source of heat loss immediately after delivery, in the first few weeks, and during bathing, accounting for up to 25% of the total heat loss. A wet newborn in the delivery room loses heat and lowers his or her skin temperature at a rate of 0.3° C/min (0.5° F/min) and rectal temperature by 0.1° C/min (0.2° F/min). This change is equivalent to a temperature loss of 3° C (5° F) over 10 minutes.[115]

Evaporative losses are correlated with both gestational age and postbirth age.[103] For example, when cared for in an ambient humidity of 50%, evaporative heat exchange is up to 5 W/m^2 in term infants versus 50 W/m^2 in preterm infants.[103] Transepidermal water loss (TEWL) is up to six times higher per unit of surface area in VLBW infants than in term infants and up to 15 times higher in infants at 25 weeks' gestation.[100,101] TEWL is lower in small-for-gestational-age than appropriate-for-gestational-age infants at similar gestations.[103] In immature infants, higher evaporative loss due to poor skin resistance to water passage from a lack of skin keratinization within the stratum corneum (see Chapter 14) constitutes a significant portion of overall heat loss (Figure 20-5).[14,44,47] The stratum corneum normally provides the greatest resistance to diffusion of water from the skin. In the term newborn the keratin in the stratum corneum creates resistance to water diffusion that is 1000 times greater than the resistance of the dermis.[81] In VLBW infants, evaporative losses in the first days exceed all other sources of heat loss and often exceed heat production.[47,73,115] Preterm infants lose heat via evaporation at a rate of 0.58 kcal/mL (2.4 J/mL).[47] VLBW infants may lose up to 120 mL/kg/day through skin water loss. This represents a loss of up to 72 kcal/kg/day, a significant portion of the infant's total caloric intake.[47,62] Evaporative losses in preterm infants of 26 weeks' gestation or less may be greater than 180 to 200 mL/kg/day.[14,47,103] Evaporative losses decrease with increasing postbirth age.

Evaporative losses in VLBW infants can be reduced by altering the environment. The degree of TEWL depends on the humidity, so infants in environments with greater humidity will lose less water and fewer calories. For example, TEWL at 85% to 95% humidity is approximately 10% that at 50% humidity.[81,103] Evaporative insensible water loss (IWL) increases with activity and tachypnea, under radiant warmers, or with phototherapy (see Chapter 18).[55] Rapid maturation of the skin occurs in the first few weeks after birth in infants of all gestational ages, reducing the degree of TEWL (see

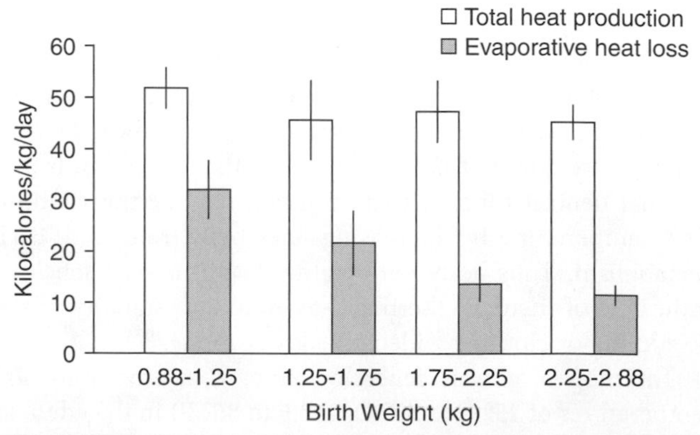

FIGURE 20-5 The relative role of evaporative heat loss at different birth weights. (From Klaus, M.H., Fanaroff, A.A., & Martin, R.J. [1993]. The physical environment. In M.H. Klaus & A.A. Fanaroff [Eds.], *Care of the high-risk neonate* [3rd ed.]. Philadelphia: Saunders.)

Chapter 14). Even at 4 weeks of age, TEWL is still twice as high in preterm versus term infants.[101] The term and older preterm infant can increase evaporative losses via the skin by sweating in response to a warm environment.[100]

Evaporative losses may be minimized by drying infants immediately after delivery or bathing, swaddling them in warm blankets, warming soaks and solutions, and warming and humidifying oxygen (see Table 20-2). Use of polyethylene wrappings, caps, and bags with preterm infants in the delivery room and intensive care nursery can also reduce evaporative losses (see Methods of Promoting Thermal Stability).[22,83,92,103,127,135] Use of topical petroleum emollients to reduce evaporative losses has been associated with an increased risk of bacterial infection and is not recommended.[40,103] Evaporative water losses in infants under radiant warmers can be reduced by stretching a layer of plastic wrap or bubble wrap around the infant or across the infant between the side guards of the radiant warmer, which can reduce IWL up to 75%.[47,100]

In term and preterm infants, the evaporative heat loss is inversely proportional to the partial pressure of water vapor.[63,73] The neutral thermal environment temperature has been calculated to be reduced approximately 0.5° C (0.8° F) for each 1 mm of increase in water vapor pressure.[115] Increasing relative humidity reduces evaporative losses; at a relative humidity of 100%, evaporative loss is nonexistent.[121] Incubator humidity levels may need to be increased to reduce evaporative losses in VLBW infants. These infants may have subnormal temperatures despite incubator temperatures above their body temperatures. The elevated air temperature reduces convective and radiant losses but does little to reduce the extremely high transepidermal evaporative loss in these infants. Vapor pressure increases with higher temperatures, so as long as the infant's skin is warmer than the environment, evaporative losses can occur even with 100% humidity.[103]

Radiation

A major form of heat loss in infants in incubators is radiation. Radiation involves the transfer of radiant energy from the body surface (through absorbance and emission of infrared rays) to surrounding cooler or warmer surfaces (walls, windows, heat lamps, lightbulbs) not in contact with the infant. The rate of transfer depends on the temperature gradient, surface absorption, and geometry (the amount and angle of the infant's surface area facing the object).[47,73,103] Radiant heat losses are independent of ambient temperature, air speed, and other heat loss mechanisms.[119] The infant can also gain heat by radiation, which is the principle of radiant warmers in which the (cooler) infant is placed under the warm radiant heat source.

Regulating incubator temperature only does not prevent heat loss by radiation. Thus infants can get cold in a room containing air warmer than the infant if the walls and windows are cold. Infants in warm incubators can be cold stressed if they radiate body heat to cooler incubator walls or cooler windows and walls or to the cool outside air during transport. The amount of radiant loss is related to the temperatures of the window and walls rather than the temperature of the air in the incubator. Conversely, a baby in a cool incubator can get overheated if the incubator walls or room windows or walls are too hot.[47,62,103] Heat loss by radiation is reduced in double wall versus single wall incubators. Loss of heat by radiation is also influenced by the infant's position and amount of exposed radiating surface area.[25]

Incubators tend to act as greenhouses by trapping heat. The acrylic walls of the incubator are opaque to infrared rays. The walls allow short light waves to enter the incubator and subsequently the infant's body. The infant converts the short waves to heat and reemits them as longer infrared rays. Because these rays cannot escape from the incubator, they heat the incubator and then the infant ("greenhouse effect"). Infants in incubators can become hyperthermic even if they are not subjected to obvious heating and without a change in incubator temperature.[119] Radiant heat losses can be reduced by placing vulnerable infants away from the cooler exterior walls and windows, use of thermal shades, and use of double-walled incubators. Overheating of infants by radiation can be prevented by placing infants away from windows and walls that are warmer than the infant.[47,62,103]

Monitoring Temperature

Neonatal temperature is usually monitored by skin or axillary measurements, and by manual or servocontrol methods. Although rectal temperature provides an approximation of core temperature, it is not used, because of the risks associated with taking rectal temperatures, including trauma, perforation, and cross-contamination with repeated insertions. Axillary temperatures are noninvasive and approximate core temperature. The optimal length of time to obtain an accurate assessment of temperature with axillary measurement using a mercury glass thermometer carefully placed in the axilla is 3 to 5 minutes in most studies.[75,110]

In a cold environment, core temperature may not indicate thermal stability. In a cold-stressed infant, the core temperature may be within normal limits because the infant has successfully compensated by increasing nonshivering thermogenesis. By the time the core temperature falls, the infant may be significantly compromised and difficult to rewarm.[103] Skin temperature measurement is used with preterm and other neonates at risk for thermoregulatory problems. Skin temperature changes provide an early indication of cold or heat stress in that an early mechanism to preserve body heat is peripheral vasoconstriction detected by measuring skin temperature.[62]

Thermocouples or thermistors must be carefully placed because skin temperature can vary widely. The best area for probe placement is not known, although sites usually recommended in textbooks are the skin surface over the liver, between the umbilicus and pubis, or the back in a prone infant. Commonly suggested sites to avoid are over areas of BAT, poorly vasoreactive areas, and excoriated or bruised areas or near transcutaneous gas monitoring transducers.[15] However, there have been few probe placement site studies to determine either the best areas or which areas to avoid. Differences have been reported between various sites used for probe placement, with lower temperatures in sites not exposed to radiant heat.[15,75] Lying on the probe may raise temperature by increasing skin insulation and lead to variable skin temperatures with repositioning.[15]

Disadvantages of skin temperature include accidental displacement of the probe, risk of skin irritation, misleading values with rapid temperature changes, and artifacts altering accuracy of measurement.[3,15,47] Artifacts that can alter readings include inadvertent insulation of the probe and the underlying skin; partial loss of skin contact with the probe; radiant or convective heating or cooling of the probe; increased probe temperature if covered with clothing or blankets or if the infant is lying on the probe (producing falsely high readings); and alteration in evaporative loss in skin covered with probes. This may occur with use of probe covers so that the temperature of the skin under the probe may be different from the skin temperature at other si tes.[3,100,102,103,124] Insulated probes provide different information from exposed probes.[103,124] Insulated probes may result in probe temperatures greater than skin temperatures in either a radiant warmer or incubator and have been reported to alter incubator servocontrol with lower incubator temperatures and a higher skin-to-environment temperature gradient.[100,103,124] Therefore it is important to follow the manufacturer's directions regarding the types of probes and probe covers.

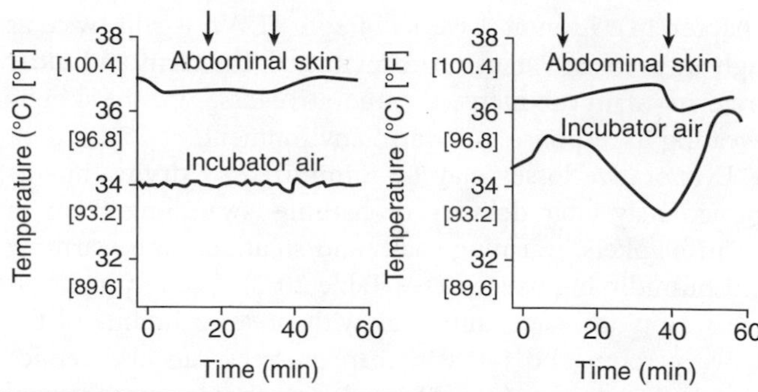

FIGURE 20-6 Fluctuations in incubator and air temperature when used in (a) air mode and (b) servo mode. In air mode, the set temperature (air) is 34° C (93.2° F), and in the servo mode, the set temperature (skin) is 36.3° C (97.3° F). Handling for brief spells of routine nursing care is indicated by the arrows. (From Rutter, N. [2005]. Temperature control and its disorders. In J.M. Rennie [Ed.]. *Roberton's Textbook of neonatology* [4th ed.], London: Churchill Livingstone.)

Servocontrol

Servocontrol methods are used to maintain an infant's temperature within specified ranges. Servocontrol systems regulate both skin and air temperatures. A change in air temperature results in a change in the wall temperature and in heat exchange via convection and radiation.[103] Infant skin servocontrol using proportional control units are standard in current convective incubators.[47] Air and skin servocontrol produce different thermal environments (Figure 20-6).[6,102,124,125] Air servocontrol tends to provide a more stable thermal environment with greater infant temperature variability, whereas skin servocontrol leads to greater variability in air temperature but is more effective in maintaining an NTE.[6,116,124,125] With infant skin servocontrol, the temperature from a skin probe is electronically monitored and used to control heater output decisions in either a convectively heated incubator or radiant warmer. Considerations related to use of skin probes and probe artifacts are discussed in the preceding section. Risks of servocontrol include hyperthermia, if the probe becomes detached or is left in the manual mode, and failure to detect early signs of sepsis because alterations in body temperature are masked.

Servocontrol may be affected by high evaporative water losses. The servocontrol system is based on the assumption that the temperature of the skin under the probe represents that of the surrounding skin; however, attaching the probe to the skin reduces evaporative losses at the site where temperature is being monitored. Thus the servocontrol system may record skin temperatures that are higher than those of the rest of the infant's body and fail to keep the infant warm.[6,47,103] Increasing humidity may reduce these differences. Opening of the portholes may lead to overdamping of the servocontrol system, with undershooting or overshooting of the air temperature for up to 1 hour later.[47] This problem has been reduced with the newer combination convection incubator–radiant warmer devices.

Methods of Promoting Thermal Stability

A major consideration in monitoring thermal status and promoting thermal stability in the neonate involves issues related to the various types of equipment that are currently available. Other methods of supporting thermoregulation are summarized in Table 20-2.

High-risk neonates are generally cared for in convectively heated incubators; open, radiantly heated beds; or hybrid devices. The hybrid devices combine these two methods with an incubator mode in which plastic walls enclose the infants and a radiant warmer mode in which the radiant warmer is turned on and the plastic walls retract. Each of these pieces of equipment and methods has inherent advantages and disadvantages, as do adjuncts to these beds such as humidity and heat shields, thermal blankets, polyethylene skin wraps, and warmed mattresses.[2,14,29,61,70,83,117] There is no consistent evidence supporting either closed, convectively warmed incubators or open, radiant warmers as more effective in reducing morbidity or mortality; each has its advantages and disadvantages, especially for VLBW infants.[43]

Convective Incubators

Convective incubators operate by circulation of warmed air. Air entering the incubator is filtered, providing a barrier against airborne pathogenic organisms from the environment.

Air leaving the incubator is not filtered, so nearby personnel or infants in open warmers and cribs are not protected from airborne organisms in the incubator air. In double-walled incubators, walls are warmed by a layer of warm water or by computer-controlled, electrically conductive plastic panels, thus decreasing heat loss, and reducing radiant losses and oxygen consumption.[62,71]

Up to 60% to 70% of total heat loss in infants cared for in convectively heated incubators is by radiation.[25,121] Because Plexiglas is relatively opaque to radiant waves, infants radiate their body heat primarily to the inner side of the incubator wall. Radiant losses are reduced with double-walled incubators, which place a second layer of Plexiglas between the infant and the outer incubator wall. The infant radiates heat to the inner wall, which is surrounded on both sides by warmed incubator air. Increasing the ambient temperature of the room and placing the infant away from windows or exterior walls can also reduce radiant losses in infants in incubators. Further alterations in radiant losses occur when infants are clothed or incubators are covered with blankets or quilts to reduce light and noise levels. As a result of extremely high transepidermal evaporative losses, VLBW infants may have subnormal temperatures even though incubator temperatures are above their body temperatures and double-walled incubators are used.

A major disadvantage of convective incubators is temperature fluctuations that occur with opening and closing of the portholes or hood. When the portholes are open, the temperature of the air in the incubator falls rapidly and recovers slowly.[137] Laminar flow incubators minimize temperature fluctuations with the opening of portholes. The drop in air temperature when opening the incubator is less in double-walled than single-walled incubators, providing a more stable thermal environment during caregiving. The inner wall in a double-walled incubator acts as a heat reservoir, while in some models warm air is redirected across the front of the incubator when it is opened.[102] The air thermometer or thermistor in an incubator should be near the infant's body and protected from being covered with bedding, clothing, or cool air flow from a resuscitation bag left in the incubator.[25]

Convective losses can also occur in incubators due to either natural convection or forced air convection. Natural convection is the thermal gradient between the skin surface and the surrounding air. Warm air rises from the infant's skin, carrying heat and moisture. This air then cools and falls back to the infant's surface, especially over the curvature of the body. Infants positioned in flexion have less exposed surface area and less heat loss than infants in an extended posture.[25,47] Forced convection usually occurs at air velocities equal to or greater than 0.2 m/sec.[103] Lower air velocities (especially less than 0.1 m/sec) minimize these losses, as can swaddling or clothing and humidity. In incubators currently in use, the primary route of convective loss is through natural convection, because the air velocities near the infant's body are minimal.[47,102]

Air in the incubator is usually humidified by active methods. Active methods use a modular integral or external humidifier, so water vapor is continuously added to the circulating air via vaporization. This method generally uses servocontrol, and the amount of humidity can be individualized. Advantages of active humidification include reduction in infection risk, easier cleaning, and reduced recovery time after incubator doors are opened.[81]

Radiant Warmers

Radiant warmers maintain the infant's temperature using a proportional servocontrol system that maintains skin temperature at a constant level. The optimal skin temperature is not known and may vary from infant to infant.[102] Radiant heat is produced in the infrared spectrum and penetrates below the skin surface, where epidermal cells with a high water content absorb the radiant energy and convert it to heat. This heat is transferred to deeper tissues by conduction and circulating blood. The heat source is usually about 80 to 90 cm from the infant's surface.[47,100]

Radiant warmers are convenient to use, allow direct access to the infant, decrease radiant losses, and eliminate temperature fluctuations with opening of the portholes. Evaporative and convective—and possibly radiant—losses may increase, however, with a risk of dehydration.[13,43,103] Evaporative losses are primarily increased due to the lower humidity and can be reduced by use of plastic wrap or blankets. IWL in infants in radiant warmers is increased 50% to 200%.[53] These losses may counteract the reduction in radiant losses in VLBW infants. Further IWL occurs if infants are simultaneously being treated with phototherapy (see Chapter 18). Although it may be possible to compensate for variations in evaporative and convective heat losses, the increased evaporative water losses are more difficult to manage.[47] Radiant warmers have been associated with an increase in oxygen consumption and metabolic rate, although the increase has not been statistically significant in most trials.[100,115] Other issues in use of radiant warmers include those associated with servocontrol and probe use, discussed earlier.

Convective losses can be reduced by using the sides on the warming bed or by stretching a layer of plastic wrap across the infant between the radiant warmer's side guards or on a special frame. Plastic wrap does not block radiant heat waves as does Plexiglas; thus heat shields made from this material are not recommended for use with radiant warmers.[47,115] Plastic wrap also reduces IWL; plastic shields do not have a similar effect.[47]

Skin-to-Skin Care

At birth, term infants who are dried and covered with a warm blanket and placed skin to skin against their mother or who experience skin-to-skin contact later maintain their temperature as well as infants cared for in standard heating units.[13,46,48] Studies of skin-to-skin (kangaroo) care with stable preterm infants demonstrate that most infants maintain adequate thermal control during this type of holding, especially if the infant is wearing a hat and is covered with a blanket. In some infants, both skin and rectal temperature transiently increase during kangaroo care.[12,17,27,74,102,115] Somewhat less thermal stability has been reported in infants less than 26 weeks' gestation.[17] Others have found no significant differences in skin temperature before, during, and after skin-to-skin care in clinically stable ELBW infants if transfer techniques were standardized to prevent heat loss.[79,130] During kangaroo care, the parent's clothing around the sides and back of the infant forms a "pouch" that provides insulation and reduces non evaporative losses (and possibly evaporative losses).[115] ELBW infants in particular require careful temperature monitoring during kangaroo care to avoid both heat stress and cooling.

Use of Head Coverings, Clothing, Blankets, and Polyethylene Wraps

Clothing and head coverings can provide thermal insulation, reducing radiant and convective losses, and can, depending on the fabric, also reduce evaporative loss.[70,102] In the neonate the head accounts for one fifth of the total body surface area. Brain heat production is estimated to account for 55% of total metabolic heat production in the newborn.[98] Thus the neonate's head is poorly insulated and accounts for a significant proportion of total heat loss. Head coverings are often used to reduce heat loss from this area, and may be especially useful immediately after birth and after a bath when the infant's hair is wet.[103] Head coverings or caps made of stockinette, which is a poor insulator, are relatively ineffective in reducing heat loss.[98] More effective materials include caps made of insulated fabrics, wool, or polyolefin; lined with Gamgee; or insulated with a plastic liner.[98] Head coverings have been found to decrease heat loss after delivery and in neonates cared for in cribs and incubators.[98,123] These coverings are most effective in a cool environment and are less effective in a thermoneutral environment or with use of infant servocontrol.[102] Head coverings and clothing can interfere with radiant heat loss and gain and are not appropriate for infants under radiant warmers. There has been little research on the use of hats with VLBW infants.

Clothing and blankets alter the thermal environment by both widening and lowering the neutral thermal range.[100] Insulation from swaddling with blankets decreases evaporative loss by reducing the amount of exposed surface area and by changing airflow patterns and skin emissivity. In addition, swaddling and nesting maintain flexion, which reduces exposed surface area and thus convective and radiant losses.[47] Swaddled infants in servocontrolled double-walled incubators have been reported to have higher abdominal skin temperatures and require lower incubator temperatures.[111] Swaddling appears to have a greater effect on skin than core temperature. Others have found that nested infants have closer approximation of skin and rectal temperatures.[75]

Polyethylene wraps and bags are recommended for use with preterm infants to reduce heat loss after birth and in the early days postbirth.[22,29,83,92,103,127] These wraps enhance radiant heat gain and reduce evaporative losses, IWL, and TEWL by creating a microenvironment under the wrap.[14,29] Unwrapping the infant disrupts this microenvironment, so it should be minimized.[14]

Neonatal Hypothermia and Cold Stress

Alterations in health status or maturity can compromise the ability of the newborn to efficiently and effectively regulate heat production and respond to cold stress. Infants at risk and the basis for this risk are summarized in Table 20-4.

Signs of hypothermia are often absent or nonspecific in neonates. Clinical findings may include lethargy, restlessness, pallor, cool skin, tachypnea, grunting, poor feeding, or decreased weight gain.[103,119] Hypothermia may be a sign of neonatal sepsis since the newborns have an altered response to pyrogens and as a result may not increase their temperature and run a fever with infection.[13,103] The neonatal response to pyrogens is not well understood.[13] Hypothermia in ELBW infants has been associated with abnormal heart rates (either less than 25th percentile or greater than 75th percentile of the individual infant's baseline heart rate) with a correlation between heart rate and abdominal temperature reported.[66]

"Cold stress occurs when an exposed infant loses more heat than he or she produces."[64] Cold stress can interfere with interpretation of pH, because pH is temperature-dependent.[100] Cold stress may delay transition from fetal to neonatal circulation.[14,64] With severe cold stress the infant may develop peripheral edema and sclerema. The initial temperature decrease is peripheral with stimulation of cutaneous receptors and initiation of NST. If the heat generated by this method is insufficient, the core temperature will drop. ELBW infants are at increased risk of cold stress due to poor vasomotor control with decreased peripheral vasoconstrictive responses, lack of both white and brown adipose tissue, thin skin, increased surface area/weight, and inefficient brown adipose tissue (BAT) metabolism due to decreased BAT, UCP-1, and thyroid hormones.[64]

The hypothermic or cold-stressed neonate tries to compensate by conserving heat and increasing heat production. These compensatory mechanisms can lead to physiologic alterations that may set off a series of adverse metabolic events (Figure 20-7). If uninterrupted, this chain of events can result in hypoxemia, metabolic acidosis, glycogen depletion, hypoglycemia, and altered surfactant production.[52] Physiologic effects of hypothermia and their consequences are summarized in Table 20-5.

Prevention of hypothermia and cold stress is a major component of neonatal health care. Strategies include careful monitoring of all infants, especially those at increased risk for hypothermia; decreasing heat losses by preventing evaporative, convective, conductive, and radiant losses; reducing the frequency and duration of cold exposure; and monitoring both infant and environmental temperatures.

Table 20-4 **Infants at Risk for Problems in Thermoregulation**

INFANT CATEGORY	BASIS FOR RISK
Preterm infants	Decreased subcutaneous fat for insulation Decreased BAT and ability to mobilize norepinephrine and fat Large surface area–to–weight ratio Inadequate caloric intake Inability to effectively increase oxygen consumption Increased open resting posture with less flexion Immature thermal regulatory mechanisms Increased evaporative water losses and higher body water content
Infants with neurologic problems	Alterations in hypothalamic control of body temperature
Infants with endocrine problems	Impairment of BAT metabolism because of inadequate catecholamines, thyroxine, or other hormones
Hypoglycemic infants	Decreased substrate for energy and ATP production in BAT Decreased metabolic response to cold stress
Infants with cardiorespiratory problems	Inability to increase oxygen consumption or minute ventilation further Inability to increase metabolic rate and reduce metabolic response to cold Impairment of BAT metabolism by hypoxia (impaired with PO_2 of 45 to 55 torr; essentially ceases at values below 30 torr)[114] Inadequate caloric intake to meet metabolic demands Increased risk of metabolic acidosis Increased temperature losses through evaporation of water from lungs
Infants with nutritional problems	Inadequate caloric intake to meet increased metabolic demands
Infants with electrolyte imbalances	Alterations in sodium and potassium may lead to sodium pump failure interfering with BAT metabolism
Infants with congenital anomalies (e.g., meningomyelocele, omphalocele, gastroschisis)	Increased surface area for heat loss Increased evaporative losses
Small-for-gestational-age infants	Decreased subcutaneous fat for insulation Increased surface area for weight Higher basal metabolic rate and energy demands
Sedated infants or maternal intrapartal analgesia	Limited physical activity to generate heat Sedation may transiently alter thermal stability

Compiled from references 18,34,47,62,103.
ATP, Adenosine triphosphate; *BAT,* brown adipose tissue.

Use of Hypothermia for Neuroprotection

Mild induced hypothermia has been investigated in recent years as a neuroprotective strategy to reduce secondary reperfusion injuries in infants who are at risk for post-asphyxial hypoxic ischemic encephalopathy.[8,9,36,37,38,54,59,105,106,108,109] The phases of cerebral injury (see Figure 6-4) are described in Chapters 6 and 15. Hypothermia is initiated during the latent stage to prevent or reduce the secondary phase changes. Both selective cooling of the head with mild systemic hypothermia (34° C to 35° C [93.2° F to 95° F]) and whole-body cooling have been studied in several ongoing multinational trials.[8,49,54,106-108] The cooling generally begins within 6 hours after birth and continues for 48 to 72 hours. A recent meta analysis of 13 trials (n = 1440 infants) confirmed beneficial effects in terms of improved survival and outcome with no significant adverse effects up to 18 to 24 months of age, although even with cooling, mortality and morbidity remained high.[106] In this analysis there was a reduction in the combined outcomes of mortality and neurodevelopmental disability and with neurodevelopmental disability in both systemic hypothermia and selective head cooling with decreases in cognitive delay, psychomotor delay, and cerebral palsy also reported in infants with systemic hypothermia.[106] Long-term safety and efficacy have not been established, and the ideal cooling temperatures, method of cooling, and duration of cooling are still unclear.[105]

Hyperthermia in the Neonate

Although discussions regarding alterations in neonatal thermoregulation often focus primarily on hypothermia, the neonate is also at risk for hyperthermia (heat stress). Hyperthermia increases metabolic demands, so even a slight increase in temperature can result in a significant increase in oxygen consumption, especially in preterm infants. Other consequences of hyperthermia include increased heart, respiratory, and metabolic rates; increased IWL; dehydration; peripheral vasodilation with a risk of decreased blood pressure; alteration in weight gain; and the risk of hypoxia and metabolic acidosis.[25,62,103] Neonatal hyperthermia (i.e., temperature above 37.5° C to 37.8° C [99.5° F to 100.0° F]) is primarily due to overheating and less often to hypermetabolism. Hyperthermia also results from dehydration, drugs, or alterations in hypothalamic control mechanisms secondary to birth trauma. Maternal and neonatal fever is associated with maternal epidural anesthesia.[1,47,104,134]

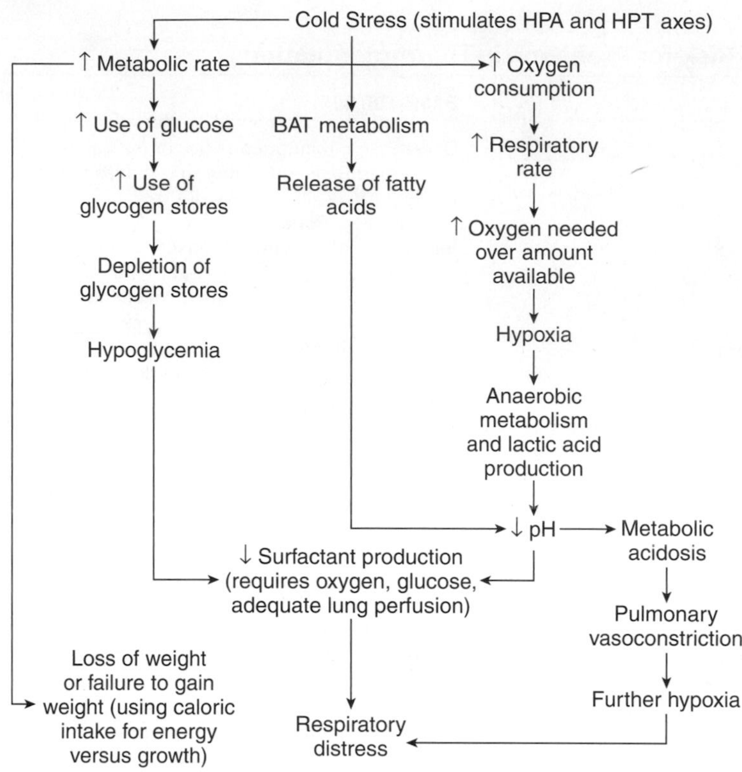

FIGURE 20-7 Physiologic consequences of cold stress. *BAT,* Brown adipose tissue; *HPA,* hypothalamic-pituitary-adrenal; *HPT,* hypothalamic-pituitary-thyroid.

Table 20-5 Consequences of Neonatal Hypothermia

PHYSIOLOGIC EFFECT	PHYSIOLOGIC CONSEQUENCE
Peripheral vasoconstriction	Increased internal (core to skin) gradient and tissue insulation Persistent vasoconstriction can lead to reduced tissue perfusion and metabolism with accumulation of ketone bodies and development of metabolic acidosis
Increased metabolic rate	Increased oxygen consumption by increasing minute ventilation and respiratory rate Risk of hypoxia and respiratory failure in infants unable to increase oxygen intake (e.g., infant with respiratory distress syndrome or other respiratory problems, VLBW)
Increased requirements for oxygen, glucose, and calories	Exhaustion of supplies with subsequent development of hypoglycemia, hypoxia, aggravation of respiratory distress syndrome, or weight loss
Increased production of ketone bodies and accumulation of lactic acid from anaerobic metabolism	Metabolic acidosis with subsequent pulmonary vasoconstriction with further reduction in pulmonary perfusion Risk of hypoxia and altered surfactant synthesis
Norepinephrine release	Increased pulmonary vascular resistance with altered ventilation-perfusion relationships and increased right-to-left shunting through the patent ductus arteriosus Risk of hypoxia and altered surfactant synthesis
Elevation in plasma nonesterified fatty acids	Alteration in glucose–fatty acid relationship with fall in blood glucose Risk of hypoglycemia and altered surfactant synthesis Competition with bilirubin for albumin-binding sites with risk of bilirubin encephalopathy
Dissociation of albumin and bilirubin because of acidosis	Increased indirect (unbound) bilirubin Risk of bilirubin encephalopathy

Compiled from references 18, 34, 47, 62, 103.
VLBW, Very low birth weight.

Overheating because of increased environmental temperatures or radiant gains from exposure to sunlight or heat lamps is associated with peripheral vasodilation, a "flushed" appearance especially prominent in extremities, warm extremities, increased activity, irritability, increased IWL, extended posture, and sweating (in older preterm or term infants). Skin temperatures are higher than core temperatures. Foot temperature is no more than 2° C to 3° C (3.3° F to 5.0° F) cooler than abdominal skin temperature.[100,103] Infants, particularly VLBW infants, are at risk for thermal injury from environmental sources (see Table 20-4).

The neonate is more vulnerable to overheating than are older individuals because the infant has a lower capacity for normothermic heat storage, a larger surface-to-volume ratio, and narrower control range than an adult does.[62] At environmental temperatures above the neutral thermal zone, thermal equilibrium is reestablished by increasing evaporative losses.[18] The adult responds by increasing skin water losses and sweating. The neonate's initial response is to increase respiratory water loss (via tachypnea). Infants more than 30 weeks' gestation can sweat if the environmental temperature exceeds their threshold.[45]

Hyperthermia secondary to hypermetabolism can result from sepsis, cardiac problems, drug withdrawal, or other metabolic alterations. Clinical signs include peripheral vasoconstriction; pale, cool extremities; and a core body temperature that is higher than skin temperature.[13,103] Foot temperature is more than 3° C (5.0° F) cooler than abdominal skin temperature.[100,103] Fever is less commonly seen with infections in neonates due to an immature, weak, or absent response to fever-producing substances such as bacterial endotoxins.[13] Regardless of the cause, hyperthermia can lead to heat stroke, dehydration, and brain damage in the neonate.

MATURATIONAL CHANGES DURING INFANCY AND CHILDHOOD

Nonshivering thermogenesis (NST) is thought to be the major mechanism for thermoregulation in infancy, especially during the first 3 to 6 months.[18,32,76] With increasing age, NST becomes less prominent and the infant begins to rely more on physical methods of heat generation such as activity and shivering.[18] Brown adipose tissue (BAT) is greater in children than adults and plays an important role in thermoregulation until at least 2 years.[32] After that time, BAT in children and adults continues to play a role in energy balance and may have a role in weight control and prevention of obesity.[32,76] After 10 years of age, BAT becomes less widely distributed as more peripherally situated deposits disappear.[32]

Much of the BAT is gradually replaced by white adipose tissue. This change is correlated with the switch in the major thermoregulatory mechanism from NST to shivering.[119] Sweating becomes more efficient as a method of heat dissipation. The threshold body temperature for sweating decreases and maximal sweat production increases.[121] Infants continue to have a decreased hypothalamic response to pyrogens for the first 2 to 3 months.[84]

Differences in thermoregulation may persist in preterm infants after discharge with smaller preterm infants more likely to be underheated at home.[126] Infants increase their temperature more easily with heat exposure and are less able to lose the heat via sweating.[128] By 3 months of age the thermal balance has shifted to favor heat conservation. Mass-to-surface differences and metabolic rate, however, continue to increase so that net heat loss per unit of surface area in a 3-month old is 50% higher than at birth.[60] Children have a greater surface area–to–body mass ratio than adults. "In a warm environment this allows them to rely more on dry heat loss and less on evaporative cooling. However, in extreme conditions, hot or cold, the greater surface area–to–body mass ratio results in a higher rate of heat absorption or heat loss, respectively."[41]

Higher mean temperatures predominate in infants. Average temperatures at 18 months of age are 37.7° C (99.8° F), with marked daily variations seen in some children. Body temperatures gradually decrease from 2 years to puberty, stabilizing at 13 to 14 years of age in girls and 16 to 17 years in boys.[67]

SUMMARY

Thermal stability is one of the most critical processes during the transition to extrauterine life. Thermoregulation is essential for survival and has priority over most other metabolic demands. The infant who does not achieve thermal stability after birth or who is cold stressed in the neonatal period is more likely to experience health problems, poor growth, and increased morbidity and mortality. Ongoing assessment and monitoring of thermal status in the neonate and initiation of appropriate interventions to maintain thermal stability can prevent or minimize these risks. Clinical recommendations related to neonatal thermoregulation are summarized in Table 20-6.

Table 20-6 Recommendations for Clinical Practice Related to Thermoregulation in Neonates

Know the mechanisms of heat production and dissipation in the neonate (pp. 663-669).
Initiate interventions to conserve body heat and reduce neonatal heat loss during transition (pp. 661-662 and Table 20-2).
Recognize the usual values for neonatal temperature (pp. 661-662).
Avoid overheating or cooling the trigeminal area of the neonate's face (pp. 664, 668).
Recognize and monitor for events that increase heat loss by conduction, convection, evaporation, and radiation (pp. 667-669 and Table 20-2).
Institute interventions to reduce heat loss in term and preterm infants by conduction, convection, evaporation, and radiation (pp. 667-669 and Table 20-2).
Provide term and preterm neonates with an appropriate thermal environment (pp. 666-669).
Know the methods for monitoring thermal status and their advantages and limitations (pp. 669-670).
Understand the differences between and implications of core versus skin temperature (pp. 669-670).
Know the advantages and limitations of different types of infant incubators and radiant warmers (pp. 670-671).
Use infant incubators and radiant warmers appropriately to maintain neonatal thermal status and reduce heat loss (pp. 670-671).
Monitor insensible water loss in infants cared for in radiant warmers (p. 671).
Provide opportunities for skin-to-skin care (pp. 671-672).
Use head coverings made of appropriate materials to reduce heat loss in infants in incubators and cribs (p. 672).
Recognize infants at risk for hypothermia and cold stress (p. 672 and Table 20-4).
Monitor neonates for signs of hypothermia and cold stress (p. 672).
Monitor hypothermic or cold-stressed infants for adverse physiologic effects (p. 672, Figure 20-7, and Table 20-5).
Recognize infants at risk for and signs of hyperthermia and thermal injury (pp. 673-674).
Monitor hyperthermic infants for adverse physiologic effects (pp. 673-674).
Use polyethylene wraps or bags with very low birthweight infants (pp. 661, 668-669, 672).

References

1. Alexander, J.M. (2005). Epidural analgesia for labor pain and its relationship to fever. *Clin Perinatol, 32,* 777.
2. Almeida, P.G., et al. (2009). Use of the heated gel mattress and its impact on admission temperature of very low birth-weight infants. *Adv Neonatal Care, 9,* 34.
3. American Academy of Pediatrics and American College of Obstetricians and Gynecologists (2007). *Guidelines for perinatal care* (6th ed.). Elk Grove Village, IL: American Academy of Pediatrics; and Washington, D.C.: American College of Obstetricians and Gynecologists.
4. Ammari, A., et al. (2009). Effects of body position on thermal, cardiorespiratory and metabolic activity in low birth weight infants. *Early Hum Dev, 85,* 497.
5. Anim-Somuah, M., Smyth, R., & Howell, C. (2005). Epidural versus non-epidural or no analgesia in labour. *Cochrane Database Syst Rev 4,* CD000331.
6. Antonucci, R., Porcella, A., & Fanos, V. (2009). The infant incubator in the neonatal intensive care unit: Unresolved issues and future developments. *J Perinat Med, 37,* 587.
7. Au, K.S., Ashley-Koch, A., & Northrup, H. (2010). Epidemiologic and genetic aspects of spina bifida and other neural tube defects. *Dev Disabil Res Rev, 16,* 6.
8. Azzopardi, D., et al. (2008). The TOBY Study: Whole body hypothermia for the treatment of perinatal asphyxia encephalopathy: A randomized controlled trial. *BMC Pediatr, 8,* 17.
9. Azzopardi, D.V., et al. (2009). Moderate hypothermia to treat perinatal asphyxial encephalopathy. *N Engl J Med, 361,* 1349.
10. Banerjee, S., et al. (2004). Maternal temperature monitoring during labor: Concordance and variability among monitoring sites. *Obstet Gynecol, 103,* 287.
11. Bartholomew, M.L., et al. (2002). Maternal temperature variation during parturition. *Obstet Gynecol, 100,* 642.
12. Bauer, K., et al. (1997). Body temperatures and oxygen consumption during skin-to-skin (kangaroo) care in stable preterm infants weighing less than 1500 grams. *J Pediatr, 130,* 240.
13. Baumgart, S. (2008). Iatrogenic hyperthermia and hypothermia in the neonate. *Clin Perinatol, 35,* 183.
14. Bissinger, R.L., & Annibale, D.J. (2010). Thermoregulation in very low-birth-weight infants during the golden hour: Results and implications. *Adv Neonatal Care, 10,* 230. Erratum in: *Adv Neonatal Care 10,* 351.
15. Blackburn, S., et al. (2001). Neonatal nursing thermal care: The effect of position and temperature probe placement. *Neonatal Netw, 20,* 19.
16. Botto, L.D., et al. (2002). Maternal fever, multivitamin use, and selected birth defects: Evidence of interaction? *Epidemiology, 13,* 485.
17. Browne, J.V. (2004). Early relationship environments: Physiology of skin-to-skin contact for parents and their preterm infants. *Clin Perinatol, 31,* 287.
18. Bruck, K. (1978). Heat production and temperature regulation. In U. Stave (Ed.), *Perinatal physiology.* New York: Plenum.
19. Bryanton, J., et al. (2004). Tub bathing versus traditional sponge bathing for the newborn. *J Obstet Gynecol Neonatal Nurs, 33,* 704.
20. Cabrera, R.M., et al. (2004). Investigations into the etiology of neural tube defects. *Birth Defects Res C Embryo Today, 72,* 330.
21. Cannon, B., & Nedergaard, J. (2004). Brown adipose tissue: Function and physiological significance. *Physiol Rev, 84,* 277.
22. Carroll, P.D., et al. (2010). Use of polyethylene bags in extremely low birth weight infant resuscitation for the prevention of hypothermia. *J Reprod Med, 55,* 9.
23. Chambers, C.D., et al. (1998). Maternal fever and birth outcome: A prospective study. *Teratol, 58,* 251.
24. Chambers, C.D. (2006). Risks of hyperthermia associated with hot tub or spa use by pregnant women. *Birth Defects Res A Clin Mol Teratol, 76,* 569.
25. Chandra, S., & Baumgart, S. (2005). Fetal and neonatal thermal regulation. In A.R. Spitzer (Ed.), *Intensive care of the fetus & neonate* (2nd ed.). St. Louis: Mosby.
26. Chardon, K., et al. (2004). Effects of warm and cool thermal conditions on ventilatory responses to hyperoxic test in neonates. *Respir Physiol Neurobiol, 140,* 145.
27. Charpak, N., et al. (1997). Kangaroo mother versus traditional care for newborn infants. A randomized, controlled trial. *Pediatrics, 100,* 682.
28. Cioffi, F., et al. (2009). Uncoupling proteins: A complex journey to function discovery. *Biofactors, 35,* 417.
29. Cramer, K., et al. (2005). Heat loss prevention: A systematic review of occlusive skin wrap for premature neonates. *J Perinatol, 25,* 763.
30. Cunningham, F.G., et al. (2009). *Williams obstetrics* (23rd ed.). New York: McGraw-Hill.

31. Cypess, A.M., et al. (2009). Identification and importance of brown adipose tissue in adult humans. *N Engl J Med, 360,* 1509.
32. Cypess, A.M., & Kahn, C.R. (2010). The role and importance of brown adipose tissue in energy homeostasis. *Curr Opin Pediatr, 22,* 478.
33. Darnell, R.A. (1987). The thermophysiology of the newborn infant. *Med Instrum, 21,* 16.
34. Davis, V. (1980). The structure and function of brown adipose tissue in the neonate. *J Obstet Gynecol Neonatal Nurs, 9,* 368.
35. Dollberg, S., Mimouni, F.B., & Weitraub, V. (2004). Energy expenditure in infants weaned from a convective incubator. *Am J Perinatol, 21,* 253.
36. Drury, P.P., Bennet, L., & Gunn, A.J. (2010). Mechanisms of hypothermic neuroprotection. *Semin Fetal Neonatal Med, 15,* 287.
37. du Plessis, A.J. (2005). Perinatal asphyxia and hypoxic-ischemic brain injury in the full term infant. In A.R. Spitzer (Ed.), *Intensive care of the fetus and neonate* (2nd ed.). St. Louis: Mosby.
38. Edwards, A.D., and Azzopardi, D.V. (2006). Therapeutic hypothermia following perinatal asphyxia. *Arch Dis Child Fetal Neonatal Ed, 91,* F127.
39. Edwards, M.J. (2006). Review: Hyperthermia and fever during pregnancy. *Birth Defects Res A Clin Mol Teratol, 76,* 507.
40. Edwards, W.H., et al. (2004). The effect of prophylactic ointment therapy on nosocomial sepsis rates and skin integrity in infants with birth weights of 501 to 1000 g. *Pediatrics, 113,* 1195.
41. Falk, B. (1998). Effects of thermal stress during rest and exercise in the paediatric population. *Sports Med, 25,* 221.
42. Filker, R., & Monif, G.R.G. (1979). The significance of temperature during the first 24 hours postpartum. *Obstet Gynecol, 53,* 358.
43. Flenady, V.J., & Woodgate, P.G. (2003). Radiant warmers versus incubators for regulating body temperature in newborn infants. *Cochrane Database Syst Rev 2,* CD000435.
44. Fluhr, J.W., et al. (2010). Functional skin adaptation in infancy—almost complete but not fully competent. *Exp Dermatol, 19,* 483.
45. Foster, K.G., Hey, E.N., & Katz, G. (1969). The response of the sweat glands of the newborn baby to thermal stimuli and to intradermal acetylcholine. *J Physiol, 203,* 13.
46. Fransson, A.L., Karlsson, H., & Nilsson, K. (2005). Temperature variation in newborn babies: Importance of physical contact with the mother. *Arch Dis Child Fetal Neonatal Ed, 90,* F500.
47. Friedman, M., & Baumgardt, S. (2005). Thermal regulation. In M.G. Macdonald, M.M.K. Sheshia, & M.D. Mullett (Eds.), *Avery's Neonatology: Pathophysiology and management of the newborn* (6th ed.). Philadelphia: Lippincott Williams & Wilkins.
48. Gardner, S. (1979). The mother as an incubator after delivery. *J Obstet Gynecol Neonatal Nurs, 8,* 174.
49. Gluckman, P.D., et al. (2005). Selective head cooling with mild systemic hypothermia after neonatal encephalopathy: Multicentre randomized trial. *Lancet, 365,* 663.
50. Goetzl, L., et al. (2007). Intrapartum epidural analgesia and maternal temperature regulation. *Obstet Gynecol, 109,* 687.
51. Graham, J.M., Edwards, M.J., & Edwards, M.J. (1998). Teratogen update: Gestational effects of maternal hyperthermia due to febrile illness and resultant patterns of defects in humans. *Teratol, 58,* 209.
52. Gunn, A.J., & Bennet, L. (2012). Responses of the fetus and neonate to hypothermia. In R.A. Polin, W.W. Fox, & S.H. Abman (Eds.), *Fetal and neonatal physiology* (4th ed.). Philadelphia: Saunders.
53. Guyton, A.C., & Hall, J.E. (2010). *Textbook of medical physiology* (12th ed.). Philadelphia: Saunders Elsevier.
54. Higgins, R.D., et al. (2006). Hypothermia and perinatal asphyxia: Executive summary of the National Institute of Child Health and Human Development Workshop. *J Pediatr, 148,* 170.
55. Horns, K. (1994). Physiological and methodological issues: Neonatal insensible water loss. *Neonatal Netw, 13,* 83.
56. Houstek, J., et al. (1993). Type III iodothyronine 5′-deiodinase and uncoupling protein in brown adipose tissue of human newborns. *J Clin Endocrinol Metab, 77,* 382.
57. Huch, R., & Erkkola, R. (1990). Pregnancy and exercise—Exercise and pregnancy. A short review. *Br J Obstet Gynaecol, 97,* 208.
58. Impey, L.W., et al. (2008). The relationship between intrapartum maternal fever and neonatal acidosis as risk factors for neonatal encephalopathy. *Am J Obstet Gynecol, 198,* 49.
59. Jacobs, S., et al. (2003). Cooling for newborns with hypoxic ischaemic encephalopathy. *Cochrane Database Syst Rev 4,* CD003311.
60. Khorshid, L., et al. (2005). Comparing mercury-in-glass, tympanic and disposable thermometers in measuring body temperature in healthy young people. *J Clin Nurs, 14,* 496.
61. Kim, S.M., et al. (2010). Improved care and growth outcomes by using hybrid humidified incubators in very preterm infants. *Pediatrics, 125,* e137.
62. Klaus, M.H., & Fanaroff, A.A. (2001). *Care of the high risk infant* (5th ed.). Philadelphia: Saunders.
63. Knobel, R., & Holditch-Davis, D. (2007). Thermoregulation and heat loss prevention after birth and during neonatal intensive-care unit stabilization of extremely low-birth weight infants. *J Obstet Gynecol Neonatal Nurs, 36,* 280.
64. Knobel, R., & Holditch-Davis, D. (2010). Thermoregulation and heat loss prevention after birth and during neonatal intensive-care unit stabilization of extremely low-birth-weight infants. *Adv Neonatal Care, 10,* S7.
65. Knobel, R.B., et al. (2009). Extremely low birth weight preterm infants lack vasomotor response in relationship to cold body temperatures at birth. *J Perinatol, 29,* 814.
66. Knobel, R.B., Holditch-Davis, D., & Schwartz, T.A. (2010). Optimal body temperature in transitional extremely low birth weight infants using heart rate and temperature as indicators. *J Obstet Gynecol Neonatal Nurs, 39,* 3.
67. Kornienko, I.A., & Gokhblit, I.I. (1980). Age differences of temperature regulation in children age 5-12 years. *Human Physiol, 6,* 443.
68. Kruse, J. (1988). Fever in children. *Am Fam Physician, 37,* 127.
69. Laptook, A.R., Salhab, W., & Bhaskar, B. (2007). Admission temperature of low birth weight infants: Predictors and associated morbidities. *Pediatrics, 119,* e643.
70. Laptook, A.R., & Watkinson, M. (2008). Temperature management in the delivery room. *Semin Fetal Neonatal Med, 13,* 383.
71. Laroia, N., Phelps, D.L., & Roy, J. (2007). Double wall versus single wall incubator for reducing heat loss in very low birth weight infants in incubator. *Cochrane Database Syst Rev 2,* CD004215.
72. Larsson, L., & Lindqvist, P.G. (2005). Low-impact exercise during pregnancy—a study of safety. *Acta Obstet Gynecol Scand, 84,* 34.
73. LeBlanc, M.H. (1987). The physics of thermal exchange between infants and their environment. *Med Instrum, 21,* 11.
74. Legault, M., & Goulet, C. (1995). Comparison of kangaroo and traditional methods of removing preterm infants from incubators. *J Obstet Gynecol Neonatal Nurs, 24,* 501.
75. Leick-Rude, M.K., & Bloom, L.F. (1998). A comparison of temperature taking methods in neonates. *Neonatal Netw, 17,* 21.
76. Lidell, M.E., & Enerbäck, S. (2010). Brown adipose tissue—a new role in humans? *Nat Rev Endocrinol, 6,* 319.
77. Lieberman, E., et al. (2000). Intrapartum maternal fever and neonatal outcome. *Pediatrics, 105,* 8.
78. Lynch, A.M., et al. (2007). Maternal physiological responses to swimming training during the second trimester of pregnancy. *Res Sports Med, 15,* 33.
79. Maastrup, R., & Greisen, G. (2010). Extremely preterm infants tolerate skin-to-skin contact during the first weeks of life. *Acta Paediatr, 99,* 1145.
80. Malaeb, S., & Dammann, O. (2009). Fetal inflammatory response and brain injury in the preterm newborn. *J Child Neurol, 24,* 1119.
81. Marshall, A. (1997). Humidifying the environment for the premature neonate: Maintenance of a thermoneutral environment. *J Neonatal Nurs, 3,* 32.
82. Mattson, M.P. (2010). Perspective: Does brown fat protect against diseases of aging? *Ageing Res Rev, 9,* 69.

83. McCall, E.M., et al. (2008). Interventions to prevent hypothermia at birth in preterm and/or low birthweight infants. *Cochrane Database Syst Rev 1,* CD004210.
84. McCarthy, P.L. (1998). Fever. *Pediatr Rev, 19,* 401.
85. McMurray, R.G., et al. (1993). Thermoregulation of pregnant women during aerobic exercise on land and in the water. *Am J Perinatol, 10,* 178.
86. Medves, J.M., & O'Brien, B. (2004). The effect of bather and location of first bath on maintaining thermal stability in newborns. *J Obstet Gynecol Neonatal Nurs, 33,* 175.
87. Miller, M.W., et al. (2007). Fetal thermal dose considerations during the obstetrician's watch: Implications for the pediatrician's observations. *Birth Defects Res C Embryo Today, 81,* 135.
88. Milunsky, A., et al. (1992). Maternal heat exposure and neural tube defects. *JAMA, 268,* 882.
89. Moretti, M.E., et al. (2005). Maternal hyperthermia and the risk for neural tube defects in offspring: Systematic review and meta-analysis. *Epidemiology, 16,* 216.
90. Nedergaard, J., & Cannon, B. (2012). Brown adipose tissue: Development and function. In R.A. Polin & W.W. Fox (Eds.), *Fetal and neonatal physiology* (4th ed.). Philadelphia: Saunders.
91. Panzer, O., et al. (1999). Shivering and shivering-like tremor during labor with and without epidural analgesia. *Anesthesiology, 90,* 1609.
92. Perlman, J.M., et al. (2010). International Consensus on Cardiopulmonary Resuscitation and Emergency Cardiovascular Care Science with Treatment Recommendations. Part 11. *Neonatal resuscitation, Circulation, 122* (Suppl 2), S516.
93. Pivarnik, J.M., Perkins, C.D., & Moyer-brailean, T. (2003). Athletics and pregnancy. *Clin Obstet Gynecol, 46,* 403.
94. Power, G.G. &, Blood, A.B.. (2012). Perinatal thermal physiology. In R.A. Polin, W.W. Fox, & S.H. Abman (Eds.), *Fetal and neonatal physiology* (4th ed.). Philadelphia: Saunders.
95. Previc, F.H. (2007). Prenatal influences on brain dopamine and their relevance to the rising incidence of autism. *Med Hypotheses, 68,* 46.
96. Ravussin, E., & Galgani, J.E. (2011). The implications of brown adipose tissue for humans. *Annu Rev Nutr, 21,* 33.
97. Riley, L.E., et al. (2011). Association of epidural-related fever and noninfectious inflammation in term labor. *Obstet Gynecol, 117,* 588.
98. Rowe, M.E., Weinberg, G., & Andrew, W. (1983). Reduction of neonatal heat loss by an insulated head cover. *J Pediatr Surg, 18,* 909.
99. Rutter, N. (1999). Thermal adaptation to extrauterine life. In C.H. Rodeck & M.J. Whittle (Eds.), *Fetal medicine: Basic science and clinical practice.* London: Churchill Livingstone.
100. Rutter, N. (2005). Temperature control and its disorders. In J.M. Rennie (Ed.), *Roberton's textbook of neonatology* (4th ed.). London: Churchill Livingstone.
101. Sahni, R., & Schulze, K. (2012). Temperature control in newborn infants. In R.A. Polin, W.W. Fox, & S.H. Abman (Eds.), *Fetal and neonatal physiology* (4th ed.). Philadelphia: Saunders.
102. Sedin, G. (2012). Physics and physiology of human neonatal incubation. In R.A. Polin, W.W. Fox, & S.H. Abman (Eds.), *Fetal and neonatal physiology* (4th ed.). Philadelphia: Saunders.
103. Sedin, G. (2011). Physical environment. In R.J. Martin, A.A. Fanaroff, & M.C. Walsh (Eds.), *Fanaroff & Martin's Neonatal-perinatal medicine: Diseases of the fetus and infant* (9th ed.). St. Louis: Mosby Elsevier.
104. Segal, S. (2010). Labor epidural analgesia and maternal fever. *Anesth Analg, 111,* 1467.
105. Selway, L.D. (2010). State of the science: Hypoxic ischemic encephalopathy and hypothermic intervention for neonates. *Adv Neonatal Care, 10,* 60.
106. Shah, P.S. (2010). Hypothermia: A systematic review and meta-analysis of clinical trials. *Semin Fetal Neonatal Med, 15,* 238.
107. Shankaran, S., et al. (2002). Whole-body hypothermia for neonatal encephalopathy: Animal observations as a basis for a randomized, controlled pilot study in term infants. *Pediatrics, 110,* 377.
108. Shankaran, S., et al. (2008). Outcomes of safety and effectiveness in a multicenter randomized controlled trial of whole-body hypothermia for neonatal hypoxic-ischemic encephalopathy. *Pediatrics, 122,* e791.
109. Shankaran, S. (2009). Neonatal encephalopathy: Treatment with hypothermia. *J Neurotrauma, 26,* 437.
110. Sheenan, M.S. (1996). Obtaining an accurate axillary temperature measurement. *J Neonatal Nurs, 2,* 6.
111. Short, M. (1998). A comparison of temperature in VLBW infants swaddled versus unswaddled in a double-walled incubator in skin control mode. *Neonatal Netw, 17,* 25.
112. Silva, J.E. (2006). Thermogenic mechanisms and their hormonal regulation. *Physiol Rev, 86,* 435.
113. Silva, J.E. (2011). Physiological importance and control of non-shivering facultative thermogenesis. *Front Biosci (Schol Ed), 3,* 352.
114. Simbruner, G., et al. (2005). Premature infants are less capable of maintaining thermal balance of head and body with increases of thermal environment than with decreases. *Am J Perinatol, 22,* 25.
115. Sinclair, J. (1992). Management of the thermal environment. In J.C. Sinclair & M.B. Brocker (Eds.), *Effective care of the newborn infant.* Oxford: Oxford University Press.
116. Sinclair, J. (2002). Servo-control for maintaining abdominal skin temperature at 36° C in low birth weight infants. *Cochrane Database Sys Rev 2,* CD001074.
117. Soll, R. (2008). Heat loss prevention in neonates. *J Perinatol, 28,* S57.
118. Soultanakis-Aligianni, H.N. (2003). Thermoregulation during exercise in pregnancy. *Clin Obstet Gynecol, 46,* 442.
119. Stern, L. (1979). Clinical aspects of thermoregulation in the newborn. *Contemp Obstet Gynecol, 13,* 109.
120. Suarez, L., Felkner, M., & Hendricks, K. (2004). The effect of fever, febrile illnesses, and heat exposure on the risk of neural-tube defects in a Texas-Mexico border population. *Birth Defects Res A Clin Mol Teratol, 70,* 815.
121. Swyer, P.R. (1987). Thermoregulation in the newborn. In L. Stern & P. Vert (Eds.), *Neonatal medicine.* New York: Masson.
122. te Pas, A.B., et al. (2010). Humidified and heated air during stabilization at birth improves temperature in preterm infants. *Pediatrics, 125,* e1427.
123. Templeman, M.C., & Bell, E.F. (1986). Head insulation for premature infants in servocontrolled incubators and radiant warmers. *Am J Dis Child, 140,* 940.
124. Thomas, K.A., & Burr, R. (1999). Preterm infant thermal care: Differing thermal environments produced by air versus skin servo-control incubators. *J Perinatol, 19,* 264.
125. Thomas, K.A. (2003). Preterm infant thermal responses to caregiving differ by incubator control mode. *J Perinatol, 23,* 640.
126. Thomas, K.A. (2003). Infant weight and gestational age effects on thermoneutrality in the home environment. *J Obstet Gynecol Neonatal Nurs, 32,* 745.
127. Trevisanuto, D., et al. (2010). Heat loss prevention in very preterm infants in delivery rooms: A prospective, randomized, controlled trial of polyethylene caps. *J Pediatr, 156,* 914.
128. Tsuzuki-Hayakawa, K., Tochihara, Y., & Ohnaka, T. (1995). Thermoregulation during heat exposure of young children compared to their mothers. *Eur J Appl Physiol Occup Physiol, 72,* 12.
129. Vaha-Eskeli, K., Erkkola, R., & Seppanen, A. (1991). Is the heat dissipating ability enhanced during pregnancy? *Eur J Obstet Gynecol Reprod Biol, 39,* 169.
130. Van Zanten, H.A., et al. (2007). The kangaroo method is safe for premature infants under 30 weeks of gestation during ventilator support. *J Neonatal Nurs, 12,* 186.
131. Varda, K.E., & Behnke, R.S. (2000). The effect of timing of initial bath on newborn's temperature. *J Obstet Gynecol Neonatal Nurs, 29,* 27.
132. Vento, M., et al. (2008). Using intensive care technology in the delivery room: A new concept for the resuscitation of extremely preterm neonates. *Pediatrics, 122,* 1113.

133. Virtanen, K.A., et al. (2009). Functional brown adipose tissue in healthy adults. *N Engl J Med, 360,* 1518.
134. Viscomi, C.M., & Manullang, T. (2000). Maternal fever, neonatal sepsis evaluation, and epidural labor analgesia. *Reg Anesth Pain Med, 25,* 549.
135. Vohra, S., et al. (2004). Heat Loss Prevention (HeLP) in the delivery room: A randomized controlled trial of polyethylene occlusive skin wrapping in very preterm infants. *J Pediatr, 145,* 750.
136. Wang, F., et al. (2009). Epidural analgesia in the latent phase of labor and the risk of cesarean delivery: A five-year randomized controlled trial. *Anesthesiology, 111,* 871.
137. Wrobel, L.C., et al. (2010). An overview of recent applications of computational modeling in neonatology. *Philos Transact A Math Phys Eng Sci, 368,* 2817.

Index

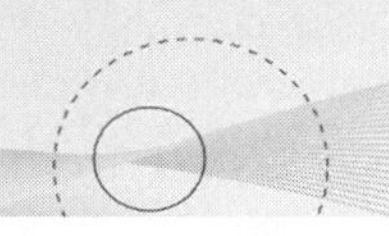

A

C

D

F

H

I

J

K

M

O

Q

R

S

T

U

X

Y

Z